WORKBOOK AND CASEBOOK

For Goodman and Gilman's
The Pharmacological Basis of Therapeutics

NOTICE

Medicine is an ever-changing science. As new research and clinical experience broaden our knowledge, changes in treatment and drug therapy are required. The authors and the publisher of this work have checked with sources believed to be reliable in their efforts to provide information that is complete and generally in accord with the standards accepted at the time of publication. However, in view of the possibility of human error or changes in medical sciences, neither the authors nor the publisher nor any other party who has been involved in the preparation or publication of this work warrants that the information contained herein is in every respect accurate or complete, and they disclaim all responsibility for any errors or omissions or for the results obtained from use of the information contained in this work. Readers are encouraged to confirm the information contained herein with other sources. For example and in particular, readers are advised to check the product information sheet included in the package of each drug they plan to administer to be certain that the information contained in this work is accurate and that changes have not been made in the recommended dose or in the contraindications for administration. This recommendation is of particular importance in connection with new or infrequently used drugs.

WORKBOOK AND CASEBOOK

For Goodman and Gilman's The Pharmacological Basis of Therapeutics

EDITORS

Douglas E. Rollins, MD, PhD
Professor Emeritus, Pharmacology & Toxicology
University of Utah
Salt Lake City, Utah

Donald K. Blumenthal, PhD
Associate Professor of Pharmacology & Toxicology
Associate Dean for Interprofessional Education & Assessment, College of Pharmacy
University of Utah
Salt Lake City, Utah

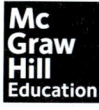

New York   Chicago   San Francisco   Lisbon   London   Madrid   Mexico City
Milan   New Delhi   San Juan   Seoul   Singapore   Sydney   Toronto

Workbook and Casebook for Goodman and Gilman's The Pharmacological Basis of Therapeutics

Copyright © 2016, by The McGraw-Hill Companies, Inc. All rights reserved. Printed in the United States of America. Except as permitted under the United States Copyright Act of 1976, no part of this publication may be reproduced or distributed in any form or by any means, or stored in a data base or retrieval system, without the prior written permission of the publisher.

1 2 3 4 5 6 7 8 9 0   RMN/RMN   19 18 17 16 15

ISBN 978-0-07-179336-0
MHID   0-07-179336-4

This book was set in Minion Pro by Cenveo® Publisher Services.
The editors were James Shanahan and Christie Naglieri.
The production supervisor was Richard Ruzycka.
Project management was provided by Sonam Arora, Cenveo Publisher Services.
The text designer was Alan Barnett.
The cover designer was Thomas DePierro.
The index was prepared by Kathrin Unger.
RR Donnelley was the printer and binder.

This book is printed on acid-free paper.

Library of Congress Cataloging-in-Publication Data

Workbook and casebook for Goodman and Gilman's the pharmacological basis of therapeutics / editors, Douglas E. Rollins, Donald K. Blumenthal.
   p. ; cm.
   Goodman and Gilman's the pharmacological basis of therapeutics
   Pharmacological basis of therapeutics
   Companion to Goodman & Gilman's the pharmacological basis of therapeutics / editor, Laurence L. Brunton; associate editors, Bruce A. Chabner, Bjorn C. Knollmann. 12th ed. 2011.
   Includes index.
   ISBN 978-0-07-179336-0 (pbk. : alk. paper) — ISBN 0-07-179336-4
   I. Rollins, Douglas E., editor.   II. Blumenthal, Donald Kamp, 1953- , editor.   III. Goodman & Gilman's the pharmacological basis of therapeutics. Companion to: IV. Title: Goodman and Gilman's pharmacological basis of therapeutics.   V. Title: Pharmacological basis of therapeutics.
   [DNLM: 1. Pharmacological Phenomena—Problems and Exercises.   2. Drug Therapy—Problems and Exercises. QV 18.2]
   RM105
   615.5076—dc23
                           2015028714

McGraw-Hill Education books are available at special quantity discounts to use as premiums and sales promotions, or for use in corporate training programs. To contact a representative please visit the Contact Us pages at www.mhprofessional.com.

CONTENTS

Preface..vi

SECTION I — 1
General Principles
1. Pharmacodynamics............................. 2
2. Pharmacokinetics.............................. 18
3. Clinical and Environmental Toxicity................ 40
4. Special Populations (Children and Elderly).......... 67

SECTION II — 79
Neuropharmacology
5. Neurotransmission............................ 80
6. Cholinergic Pharmacology...................... 95
7. Adrenergic, Dopaminergic, and Serotonergic Pharmacology...................... 118
8. Psychopharmacology.......................... 149
9. Hypnotics, Sedatives, and Ethanol................ 176
10. Opioid Pharmacology......................... 194
11. Anesthetic Agents and Therapeutic Gases.......... 210
12. Pharmacotherapy of the Epilepsies............... 225
13. Drug Therapy of Neurodegenerative Diseases....... 238
14. Drug Addiction.............................. 254

SECTION III — 267
Modulation of Cardiovascular Function
15. Drug Therapy of Hypertension, Edema, and Disorders of Sodium and Water Balance........... 268
16. Drug Therapy of Myocardial Ischemia............. 289
17. Pharmacotherapy of Heart Failure................ 301
18. Antiarrhythmic Drugs......................... 312
19. Drug Therapy of Thromboembolic Disorders....... 323
20. Drug Therapy of Dyslipidemias.................. 334

SECTION IV — 345
Inflammation, Immunomodulation, and Hematopoiesis
21. Histamine, Bradykinin, and Their Antagonists...... 346
22. Prostaglandins, NSAIDs, and Pharmacotherapy of Gout....................... 356
23. Immunotherapeutic Agents..................... 375
24. Pulmonary Pharmacology...................... 389
25. Hematopoietic Agents......................... 405

SECTION V — 421
Hormones and Hormone Antagonists
26. Introduction to Endocrinology: The Hypothalamic-Pituitary Axis................. 422
27. Thyroid and Antithyroid Drugs.................. 431
28. Estrogens, Progestins, Androgens, and Contraception............................ 441
29. ACTH, Adrenal Steroids, and Pharmacology of the Adrenal Cortex............. 459
30. Endocrine Pancreas and Pharmacotherapy of Diabetes Mellitus and Hypoglycemia........... 470
31. Drug Therapy of Mineral Ion Homeostasis and Bone Turnover Disorders.................. 480

SECTION VI — 489
Drugs Affecting Gastrointestinal Function
32. Pharmacotherapy of Gastric Acidity, Peptic Ulcers, and Gastroesophageal Reflux Disease....... 490
33. Drugs Used for the Treatment of Bowel Disorders... 497

SECTION VII — 511
Chemotherapy of Microbial Diseases
34. General Principles of Antimicrobial Therapy....... 512
35. Chemotherapy of Malaria....................... 520
36. Chemotherapy of Protozoal Infections: Amebiasis, Giardiasis, Trichomoniasis, Trypanosomiasis, Leishmaniasis, and Other Protozoal Infections...... 530
37. Chemotherapy of Helminth Infections............. 536
38. Sulfonamides, Trimethoprim-Sulfamethoxazole, Quinolones, and Agents for Urinary Tract Infections.............................. 542
39. Penicillins, Cephalosporins, and Other β-Lactam Antibiotics..................... 549
40. Aminoglycosides 559
41. Protein Synthesis Inhibitors and Miscellaneous Antibacterial Agents 568
42. Chemotherapy of Tuberculosis, *Mycobacterium Avium* Complex Disease, and Leprosy............. 578
43. Antifungal Agents 588
44. Antiviral Agents and Treatment of HIV Infection.............................. 600

SECTION VIII — 625
Chemotherapy of Neoplastic Diseases
45. Cancer Chemotherapy and Cytotoxic Agents....... 626
46. Targeted Anticancer Therapies................... 661

SECTION IX — 689
Special Systems Pharmacology
47. Ocular Pharmacology......................... 690
48. Dermatological Pharmacology................... 707

Index...728

PREFACE

This *Workbook and Casebook* derives from the 12th edition of *Goodman & Gilman's The Pharmacological Basis of Therapeutics*. The organization of the parent text has been retained and many of the tables and figures are the same. The editors have attempted to provide the most important concepts from the 12th edition of *G&G* in a user-friendly format without the elimination of salient pharmacological information. It is our intention that the *Workbook and Casebook* will complement the parent text and the second edition of *Goodman & Gilman's Manual of Pharmacology and Therapeutics* and be useful to students and educators who might need a companion text in an advanced pharmacology course.

The number of chapters in the *Workbook and Casebook* has been reduced from 67 to 48 by combining the substance of multiple chapters from the 12th edition into one *Workbook and Casebook* chapter. For example, Chapter 9 Muscarinic Receptor Agonists and Antagonists, Chapter 10 Anticholinesterase Agents, and Chapter 11 Agents Acting at the Neuromuscular Junction and Autonomic Ganglia in the 12th edition have been combined into one *Workbook* chapter entitled Cholinergic Pharmacology. An additional chapter, Chapter 4 Special Populations: Children and the Elderly, has been added to the *Workbook and Casebook* based in part on content that is published in Updates in the online version of *Goodman & Gilman* (Accessmedicine.com and Accesspharmacy.com).

Each *Workbook and Casebook* chapter begins with a statement of how it differs from the 12th edition so that the reader can refer to the parent text to obtain additional information if necessary. *Workbook and Casebook* chapters (except for chapters on general principles) are formatted as follows:

- Learning Objectives
- Drugs Included in the Chapter
- Mechanisms of Action (and, where appropriate, Mechanisms of Resistance) Table
- Clinical Cases
- Key Concepts
- Summary Quiz
- Summary Table of Drugs that includes Drug Class, Drug Name, Clinical Uses, and Common and Unique Clinically Important Toxicities

Additional Side Bars are included to highlight significant pharmacological information. Narrative pharmacological information is provided in the form of Clinical Cases to give a clinical context for the therapeutic use of drugs and their adverse events. We have omitted research data, chemical structures, references, and the pharmacokinetic data of Appendix II, all of which can be found on the *G&G* Web site on AccessMedicine.com and AccessPharmacy.com, along with pharmacotherapeutic updates and mechanistic animations.

We thank the contributors and editors of the 12th edition of *G&G*, Christie Naglieri and James Shanahan of McGraw Hill, and the long line of contributors and editors who have worked on *Goodman & Gilman* over 12 editions. It is an honor to follow in the path of Louis Goodman and Alfred Gilman, and it is a tribute to their writing and editing that their book is useful and relevant 74 years after the publication of the first edition.

Douglas E. Rollins
Donald K. Blumenthal

General Principles

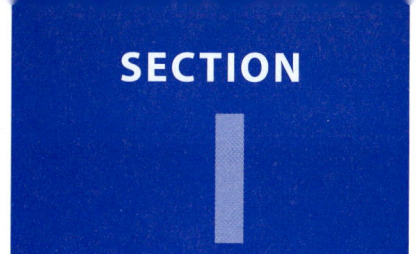

1. Pharmacodynamics 1
2. Pharmacokinetics 18
3. Clinical and Environmental Toxicity 40
4. Special Populations (Children and Elderly) 67

CHAPTER 1

Pharmacodynamics

PHARMACODYNAMIC CONCEPTS AND NOMENCLATURE (key terms are indicated in italics)

- *Pharmacodynamics* is the study of the biochemical and physiological effects of drugs and their mechanisms of action.
- Pharmacodynamics refers to the effects of a drug on the body; in contrast, the effects of the body on the actions of a drug are *pharmacokinetic* processes (see Chapter 2).
- The term drug *receptor* or drug *target* denotes the cellular macromolecule or macromolecular complex with which the drug interacts to elicit a cellular response.
- Drugs commonly alter the rate or magnitude of an intrinsic cellular response rather than create new responses.
- Drug receptors are often located on the surface of cells but may also be located in specific intracellular compartments.
- Many drugs also interact with *acceptors* within the body; acceptors are entities that do not directly cause any change in biochemical or physiological response.
- Proteins form the most important class of drug receptors. Examples include:
  - *Physiological receptors* for hormones, growth factors, transcription factors, and neurotransmitters (see Table 1-1)
  - Enzymes of crucial metabolic or regulatory pathways (eg, dihydrofolate reductase, acetylcholinesterase, and cyclic nucleotide phosphodiesterases)
  - Proteins involved in transport processes (eg, Na^+, K^+-ATPase); secreted glycoproteins (eg, Wnts)
  - Structural proteins (eg, tubulin)
- Specific binding of drugs to other cellular constituents such as DNA is also exploited for therapeutic purposes (eg, many cancer chemotherapeutic agents and antiviral drugs).
- Antibiotic and other anti-infectives often target enzymes and biochemical processes that are unique to the pathogen, resulting in cytotoxicity or inhibition of proliferation.

This chapter will be most useful after having a basic understanding of the material in Chapter 3, Pharmacodynamics: Molecular Mechanisms of Drug Action in *Goodman & Gilman's The Pharmacological Basis of Therapeutics*, 12th Edition. Additional information related to this chapter is provided in Chapter 1, Drug Invention and the Pharmaceutical Industry and Chapter 7, Pharmacogenetics. The drugs presented in this chapter are used to illustrate general pharmacodynamic principles. The mechanisms of action and therapeutic uses of drugs described in this chapter are discussed in more detail in subsequent chapters. Neither a Mechanisms of Action Table nor a Clinical Summary Table is included in this chapter because this information is provided in subsequent chapters.

In addition to the material presented here, *Goodman & Gilman's The Pharmacological Basis of Therapeutics*, 12th Edition contains:

- A description in Chapter 1 of the process of drug invention and FDA approval
- Table 1-1, Typical Characteristics of the Various Phases of the Clinical Trials Required for Marketing of New Drugs
- Figure 1-1, The Phases, Time Lines, and Attrition That Characterize the Invention of New Drugs
- A comprehensive description in Chapter 3 of the various mechanisms of drug action, including cellular pathways activated by physiological receptors, structural and functional families of physiological receptors, second messengers, ion channels, nuclear receptors, and transcription factors
- Chapter 3 also describes mechanisms of receptor desensitization and regulation, and an example of pharmacodynamic interactions in a multicellular context
- Chapter 7 includes a number of examples of genetic polymorphisms that affect drug pharmacodynamics, the impact of pharmacogenetics on drug development, and a discussion of pharmacogenetics in clinical practice

LEARNING OBJECTIVES

- ☑ Understand key concepts and terms related to pharmacodynamics, including drug receptor agonism and antagonism.
- ☑ Know concepts and terms that are used to quantify drug receptor interactions, including affinity, efficacy, potency, K_D and K_i.
- ☑ Understand how drug pharmacodynamic information is used to predict beneficial and toxic drug effects.
- ☑ Know the modern process of drug invention and FDA approval, and post-market surveillance.
- ☑ Know how genetic polymorphisms and other factors can affect the pharmacodynamic properties of drugs and lead to variability in individual patient responses to drugs.
- ☑ Know how pharmacodynamics is applied to populations of patients to estimate population therapeutic windows for drug dosing.

Pharmacodynamics

CHAPTER 1

TABLE 1-1 Physiological Receptors

STRUCTURAL FAMILY	FUNCTIONAL FAMILY	PHYSIOLOGICAL LIGANDS	EFFECTORS AND TRANSDUCERS	EXAMPLE DRUGS
G Protein-coupled receptors (GPCRs)	β Adrenergic receptors	NE, Epi, DA	G_s; AC	Dobutamine, propranolol
	Muscarinic cholinergic receptors	ACh	G_i and G_q; AC, ion channels, PLC	Atropine, carbachol
	Eicosanoid receptors	Prostaglandins, leukotrienes, thromboxanes	G_s, G_i, and G_q proteins	Misoprostol, montelukast
	Thrombin receptors (PAR)	Receptor peptide	$G_{12/13}$, GEFs	Vorapaxar
Ion channels	Ligand-gated	ACh (M_2), GABA, 5-HT	Na^+, Ca^{2+}, K^+, Cl^-	Nicotine, gabapentin
	Voltage-gated	None (activated by membrane depolarization)	Na^+, Ca^{2+}, K^+, other ions	Lidocaine, verapamil
Transmembrane enzymes	Receptor tyrosine kinases	Insulin, PDGF, EGF, VEGF, growth factors	SH2 domain and PTB-containing proteins	Herceptin, imatinib
	Membrane-bound GC Tyrosine phosphatases	Natriuretic peptides	Cyclic GMP	Neseritide
Transmembrane, non-enzymes	Cytokine receptors	Interleukins and other cytokines	Jak/STAT, soluble tyrosine kinases	Anakinra
	Toll-like receptors	LPS, bacterial products	MyD88, IARKs, NF-κB	(in development)
Nuclear receptors	Steroid receptors	Estrogen, testosterone	Co-activators	Estrogens, androgens, Cortisol
	Thyroid hormone receptors	Thyroid hormone		Thyroid hormone
	PPARγ, PPARα	Eiconsanoids, fatty acids	RXR	Thiazolidinediones
Intracellular enzymes	Soluble GC	NO, Ca^{2+}	Cyclic GMP	Nitrovasodilators

AC, adenylyl cyclase; DA, dopamine; GC, guanylyl cyclase; GEF, guanine nucleotide exchange factor; LPS, lipopolysaccharide; NE, norepinephrine; PAR, protease-activated receptor; PLC, phospholipase C; PPAR, peroxisome proliferator-activated receptor.

CASE 1-1

A man who suffers from hay fever is at his local pharmacy looking for a nonprescription drug that can provide relief of symptoms. One of the allergy medicines he finds on the shelf says the active ingredient is an antihistamine, diphenhydramine.

a. **What is an "active ingredient" in an allergy medication such as this?**

   Pharmaceuticals contain 1 or more pharmacologically active ingredients, which are termed active ingredients. The quantities of each active ingredient in each dose (eg, tablet, capsule, or volume of a liquid medication) are indicated on the packaging. In addition to active ingredients, most medications also contain other ingredients that are pharmacologically inactive, but may improve the pharmacokinetics, appearance, taste, shelf-life, or other properties that may enhance dosing and product effectiveness.

b. **What kind of drug is an "antihistamine" and why is it so named?**

   As the name indicates, an antihistamine is an agent that antagonizes the action of the endogenous mediator histamine. Histamine is released by mast cells and is involved in a variety of allergic and inflammatory responses (see Chapter 21). This man's hay fever is caused by mast cell release of histamine and other substances that result in his symptoms of sneezing, runny nose, itching of the nose and throat, and itchy, watery eyes. An antihistamine such as diphenhydramine will bind to histamine receptors on cells throughout the body and block the effects of histamine.

(Continued)

> **DRUG-RECEPTOR INTERACTIONS** (*key terms are indicated in italics*)
>
> - Many drugs act on physiological receptors and are particularly selective because physiological receptors have evolved to recognize and respond to individual signaling molecules with great selectivity.
> - Drugs that bind to physiological receptors and mimic the regulatory effects of the endogenous signaling compounds are termed *agonists*.
>   - A drug that binds to the same recognition site as the endogenous agonist (the *primary* or *orthosteric site* on the receptor) is said to be a *primary agonist*.
>
> *(continues)*

SECTION I

DRUG-RECEPTOR INTERACTIONS (key terms are indicated in italics) (Cont.)

- Drugs that can elicit the same maximal response as the endogenous ligand are termed *full agonists* (see Figure 1-1) and are said to possess full *efficacy*.
- Drugs that are only partly effective in activating a receptor regardless of the concentration employed are termed *partial agonists* (see Figure 1-1).
- A *syntopic interaction* is an interaction between ligands that bind to the same recognition site, or to recognition sites that overlap, on the receptor macromolecule (see Figure 1-2).
- *Allosteric (allotopic) agonists* bind to an *allosteric or allotopic site*, a region on the receptor that is different from the primary site (see Figure 1-2).
- Many receptors exhibit some constitutive activity in the absence of a regulatory ligand; drugs that stabilize such receptors in an inactive conformation are termed *inverse agonists* (see Figure 1-1).
- Drugs that block or reduce the action of an agonist are termed *antagonists* (see Figure 1-2).
  - Antagonism most commonly results from competition of a drug with an agonist for the primary site on the receptor (referred to as *competitive antagonists* because of a syntopic interaction; see Figure 1-2).
  - *Noncompetitive antagonism* results from an antagonist that covalently binds the receptor or dissociates extremely slowly from the receptor (*pseudo-irreversible*) such that the maximal response of the receptor is diminished with increasing concentration of antagonist (see Figure 1-2).
  - Noncompetitive antagonism can also occur with antagonists that interact with allosteric sites on the receptor (*allosteric antagonists*), reducing the affinity of the receptor for agonist.
  - Drugs that act by combining with the agonist are termed *chemical antagonists*.
  - *Functional antagonists* act by indirectly inhibiting the cellular or physiological effects of the agonist.

General Principles

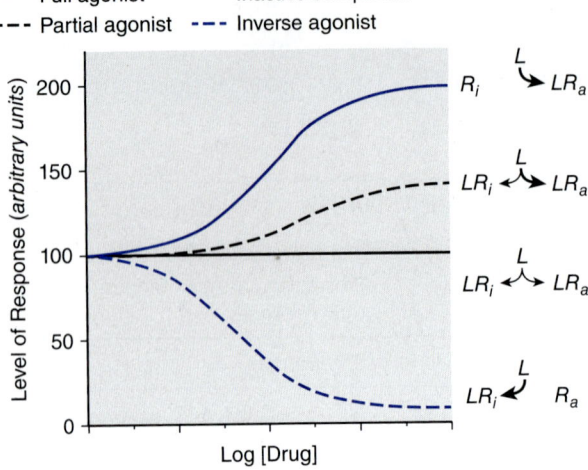

FIGURE 1-1 Regulation of the activity of a receptor with conformation-selective drugs. The ordinate is the activity of the receptor produced by R_a, the active receptor conformation (eg, stimulation of adenylyl cyclase by a β adrenergic receptor). If a drug L selectively binds to R_a, it will produce a maximal response. If L has equal affinity for R_i and R_a, it will not perturb the equilibrium between them and will have no effect on net activity; L would appear as an inactive compound. If the drug selectively binds to R_i, then the net amount of R_a will be diminished. If L can bind to receptor in an active conformation R_a but also bind to inactive receptor R_i with lower affinity, the drug will produce a partial response; L will be a partial agonist. If there is sufficient R_a to produce an elevated basal response in the absence of ligand (agonist-independent constitutive activity), then activity will be inhibited; L will then be an inverse agonist. Inverse agonists selectively bind to the inactive form of the receptor and shift the conformational equilibrium toward the inactive state. In systems that are not constitutively active, inverse agonists will behave like competitive antagonists, which helps explain why the properties of inverse agonists and the number of such agents previously described as competitive antagonists were only recently appreciated. Receptors that have constitutive activity and are sensitive to inverse agonists include benzodiazepine, histamine, opioid, cannabinoid, dopamine, bradykinin, and adenosine receptors.

c. What are histamine receptors and what kind of an antagonist is diphenhydramine?

Histamine receptors are G protein–coupled receptors (GPCRs; see Table 1-1). H_1 receptors couple to $G_{q/11}$ and activate the PLC–IP_3–Ca^{2+} pathway and its many possible sequelae, including activation of PKC, Ca^{2+}–calmodulin–dependent enzymes (eNOS and various protein kinases), and PLA_2. H_2 receptors link to G_s to activate the adenylyl cyclase–cyclic AMP–PKA pathway, whereas H_3 and H_4 receptors couple to $G_{i/o}$ to inhibit adenylyl cyclase and decrease cellular cyclic AMP. Activation of H_3 receptors also can activate mitogen-activated protein (MAP) kinase and inhibit the Na^+/H^+ exchanger, and activation of H_4 receptors mobilizes stored Ca^{2+} in some cells.

All the available H_1 receptor "antagonists" are actually inverse agonists (see Side Bar DRUG-RECEPTOR INTERACTIONS and Figure 1-1) that reduce constitutive activity of the receptor and compete with histamine. Whereas histamine binding to the receptor induces a fully active conformation, antihistamine binding yields an inactive conformation (see Figure 1-1). At the tissue level, the effect seen is proportional to receptor occupancy by the antihistamine.

d. The warning on the medication package says "marked drowsiness may occur." The package label also warns that "excitability may occur, especially in children." How are these side effects related to the "antihistamine" effects of the active ingredient?

Some antihistamines such as diphenhydramine can cross the blood-brain barrier (BBB) and have effects on histamine receptors in the central nervous system (CNS). There is substantial evidence that histamine functions as a neurotransmitter in

(Continued)

the CNS. Histamine, histidine decarboxylase, enzymes that metabolize histamine, and H_1, H_2, and H_3 receptors are distributed widely but nonuniformly in the CNS. Histamine-containing neurons control both homeostatic and higher brain functions, including regulation of the sleep-wake cycle, circadian and feeding rhythms, immunity, learning, memory, drinking, and body temperature.

(Continued)

DRUG-RECEPTOR INTERACTIONS (*key terms are indicated in italics*) (*Cont.*)

- Partial agonists and inverse agonists that compete with a full agonist at the same site on a receptor (ie, syntopic interaction) will behave as competitive antagonists.
- *Specificity* is a pharmacodynamic property of a drug that refers to a drug's ability to elicit a well-defined response in a specific tissue.
  ▸ The chemical structure of a drug contributes to its specificity for a given type of physiological receptor.
  ▸ A drug that interacts with a single type of receptor that is expressed on only a limited number of differentiated cells will exhibit *high (narrow) specificity*.
  ▸ Drugs acting on a type of receptor that is expressed ubiquitously on a variety of cells throughout the body will exhibit widespread effects, and could produce serious side effects or toxicities if the receptor serves important functions in multiple tissues.
  ▸ Many clinically important drugs exhibit a *low (broad) specificity* because the drug is able to interact with multiple receptors in different tissues; such broad specificity might enhance the clinical utility of a drug, but also contribute to a spectrum of adverse side effects due to *off-target interactions*.

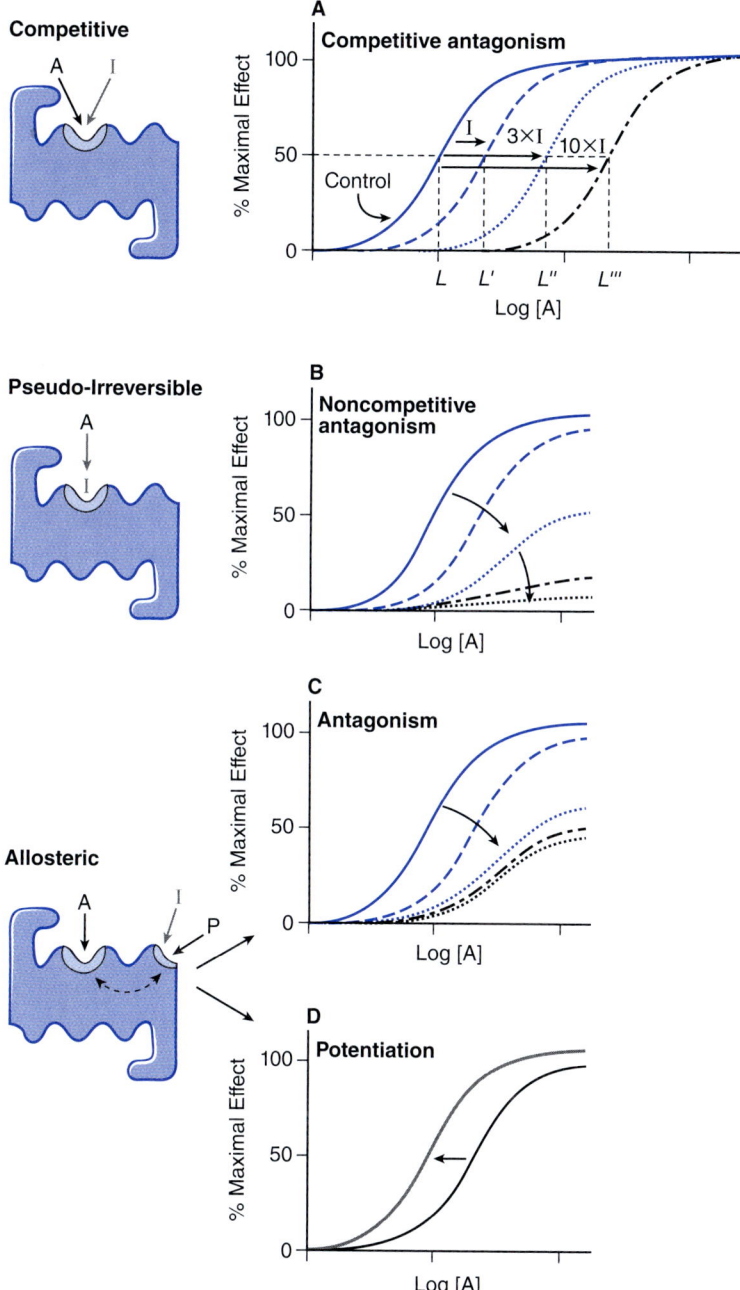

FIGURE 1-2 Mechanisms of receptor antagonism and potentiation. **A.** Competitive antagonism occurs when the agonist A and antagonist I compete for the same binding site on the receptor. Response curves for the agonist are shifted to the right in a concentration-related manner by the antagonist such that the EC_{50} for the agonist increases (eg, L versus L', L'', and L''') with the concentration of the antagonist. **B.** If the antagonist binds to the same site as the agonist but does so irreversibly or pseudo-irreversibly (slow dissociation but no covalent bond), it causes a shift of the dose-response curve to the right, with further depression of the maximal response. Allosteric effects occur when an allosteric ligand I or P binds to a different site on the receptor to either inhibit (I) the response (see panel C) or potentiate (P) the response (see panel D). This effect is saturable; inhibition or potentiation reaches a limiting value when the allosteric site is fully occupied.

SECTION 1

General Principles

QUANTITATIVE ASPECTS OF DRUG RECEPTOR INTERACTIONS

- Receptor occupancy theory assumes that response emanates from a receptor occupied by a drug, a concept that has its basis in the law of mass action.
- The *dose-response* (or *concentration-response*) curve is a depiction of the observed effect of a drug as a function of its concentration in the receptor compartment (see Figure 1-3).
  ‣ The maximal asymptotic response occurs when the drug occupies all the receptor sites.
  ‣ Some drug-receptor systems exhibit an inverted U-shaped dose-response relationship with low-dose stimulation and high-dose inhibition of response, an effect known as *hormesis*.
- The bimolecular drug-receptor interaction that results in receptor activation can be described as a series of 2 equilibrium reactions as shown in Equation 1-1.

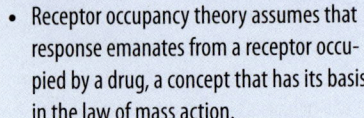

(Equation 1-1)

- The initial reaction is the reversible binding of drug (*L*) to a receptor (*R*) which leads to the formation of the drug-receptor complex (*LR*), and depends on both the forward or *association rate* (k_{+1}) and the reverse or *dissociation rate* (k_{-1}).
  ‣ The *equilibrium dissociation constant* (K_D) is defined as the ratio of the *off* and *on* rate constants (k_{-1}/k_{+1}; Equation 1-2); the *affinity* or *equilibrium association constant* (K_A) is the reciprocal of the equilibrium dissociation constant.

$$K_D = \frac{[L][R]}{[LR]} = \frac{k_{-1}}{k_{+1}}$$

(Equation 1-2)

  ‣ Thus a high-affinity drug has a low K_D and will bind a greater number of a particular receptor at a low concentration than a low-affinity drug.
  ‣ Depending on the characteristics of the drug (eg, full agonist, partial agonist, antagonist, inverse agonist; see Figure 1-1), the drug-receptor complex may undergo a conformational change that leads to the formation of the activated complex (*LR**).

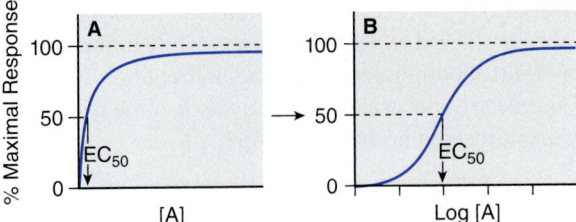

FIGURE 1-3 Graded responses (y axis as a percentage of maximal response) expressed as a function of the concentration of drug A present at the receptor. The hyperbolic shape of the curve in panel A becomes sigmoid when plotted semi-logarithmically, as in panel B. The concentration of drug that produces 50% of the maximal response quantifies drug activity and is referred to as the EC_{50} (effective concentration for 50% response). The range of concentrations needed to fully depict the dose-response relationship (~3 $\log_{10}$ units) is too wide to be useful in the linear format of Figure 1-3A; thus, most dose-response curves use log [Drug] on the x axis, as in Figure 1-3B. Dose-response curves presented in this way are sigmoidal in shape and have 3 properties: threshold, slope, and maximal asymptote. These 3 parameters quantitate the activity of the drug.

The first-generation H_1 antagonists can both stimulate and depress the CNS. Stimulation occasionally is encountered in patients given conventional doses; they become restless, nervous, and unable to sleep. Central excitation also is a striking feature of overdose, which commonly results in convulsions, particularly in infants. Central depression, on the other hand, usually accompanies therapeutic doses of the older H_1 antagonists. Diminished alertness, slowed reaction times, and somnolence are common manifestations. Patients vary in their susceptibility and responses to individual drugs. The ethanolamines (eg, diphenhydramine) are particularly prone to causing sedation. Thus, the development of second-generation "nonsedating" antihistamines was an important advance that allowed their general use. These newer H_1 antagonists do not cross the blood-brain barrier appreciably. Their sedative effects are similar to those of placebo.

e. Are there other pharmacological properties of H_1 antagonists that are clinically useful?

Many of the first-generation H_1 antagonists tend to inhibit responses to acetylcholine (ACh) that are mediated by muscarinic receptors and may be manifest during clinical use (see Chapter 6). Some H_1 antagonists also can be used to treat motion sickness; the anticholinergic properties of H_1 antagonists may be largely responsible for this effect. Indeed, promethazine (a first-generation H_1 antagonist) has perhaps the strongest muscarinic-blocking activity among these agents and is the most effective H_1 antagonist in combating motion sickness. The second-generation H_1 antagonists have no effect on muscarinic receptors.

CASE 1-2

A pharmaceutical company research and development team is working to develop new drugs that target a novel molecular entity that might play a role in diabetes. Preclinical data regarding the pharmacodynamics of a number of small molecules have been collected and are being analyzed to determine which lead compounds might be worth carrying forward into clinical trials in humans.

a. What are the steps that the team has taken to this point and what must be done before the drug is tested in humans?

Modern drug invention usually starts with a statement (or hypothesis) that a certain protein or pathway plays a critical role in the pathogenesis of a certain disease, and that altering the protein's activity would therefore be effective against that disease. The usual approach to invention of a small-molecule drug is to screen a collection of chemicals ("library") for compounds with the desired features.

(Continued)

Pharmacodynamics

An alternative is to synthesize and focus on close chemical relatives of a substance known to participate in a biological reaction of interest (eg, congeners of a specific enzyme substrate chosen to be possible inhibitors of the enzymatic reaction), a particularly important strategy in the discovery of anticancer drugs.

Several variables affect the frequency of hits obtained in a screen. Among the most important are the "drugability" of the target and the stringency of the screen in terms of the concentrations of compounds that are tested. The slang term "drugability" refers to the ease with which the function of a target can be altered in the desired fashion by a small organic molecule. If the protein target has a well-defined binding site for a small molecule (eg, a catalytic or allosteric site), chances are excellent that hits will be obtained. If the goal is to employ a small molecule to mimic or disrupt the interaction between 2 proteins, the challenge is much greater.

The validity of the target must also be confirmed. Modern techniques of molecular biology offer new and powerful tools for validation of potential drug targets, to the extent that the biology of model systems resembles human biology. Genes can be inserted, disrupted, and altered in mice. One can thereby create models of disease in animals or mimic the effects of long-term disruption or activation of a given biological process. If, for example, disruption of the gene encoding a specific enzyme or receptor has a beneficial effect in a valid murine model of a human disease, one may believe that the potential drug target has been validated. Mutations in humans can also provide extraordinarily valuable information.

Following the path just described can yield a potential drug molecule that interacts with a validated target and alters its function in the desired fashion (either enhancing or inhibiting the functions of the target). Now one must consider all aspects of the molecule in question—its affinity and selectivity for interaction with the target, its pharmacokinetic properties (absorption, distribution, excretion, metabolism), issues with regard to its large-scale synthesis or purification from a natural source, its pharmaceutical properties (stability, solubility, questions of formulation), and its safety.

(Continued)

CHAPTER 1

QUANTITATIVE ASPECTS OF DRUG RECEPTOR INTERACTIONS (Cont.)

- The *apparent dissociation constant*, K_{app}, is a macroscopic equilibrium constant that reflects both the ligand binding equilibrium and the subsequent equilibrium that results in the formation of the active receptor LR^*.

- The fractional occupancy of a receptor, f, is described by Equations 1-3 and 1-4; at a concentration of drug that results in 50% occupancy of the receptor ($f = 0.5$), the concentration of drug equals the K_D.

$$f = \frac{[\text{ligand-receptor complexes}]}{[\text{total receptors}]}$$

$$= \frac{[LR]}{[R] + [LR]} \quad \text{(Equation 1-3)}$$

$$f = \frac{K_A[L]}{1 + K_A[L]} = \frac{[L]}{[L] + K_D} \quad \text{(Equation 1-4)}$$

- The concentration of an agonist drug that produces 50% of the maximal response is termed the EC_{50} (the *half-maximally effective concentration*; see Figure 1-3).

- The ability of a drug to activate a receptor and generate a cellular response is a reflection of its efficacy; *relative efficacy* refers to a comparison of the maximal response of 2 agonists; the more *efficacious* drug exhibits a higher maximal response (see Figure 1-4).

  - A full agonist has full efficacy; a partial agonist has partial efficacy.

- Drug *potency* refers to a comparison of the concentrations of agonist drug required to elicit a given biological response and is a mixed function of both affinity and efficacy.

  - In comparing the EC_{50} of 2 drugs with the same efficacy, the drug with the lower EC_{50} is the more potent drug (see Figure 1-4).

- The affinity of a competitive antagonist (K_I) for its receptor can be determined in radioligand binding assays or by measuring the functional response of a system to a drug in the presence of the antagonist (see text and Equations 3-3 and 3-4 in Chapter 3 of *Goodman & Gilman's The Pharmacological Basis of Therapeutics*, 12th Edition).

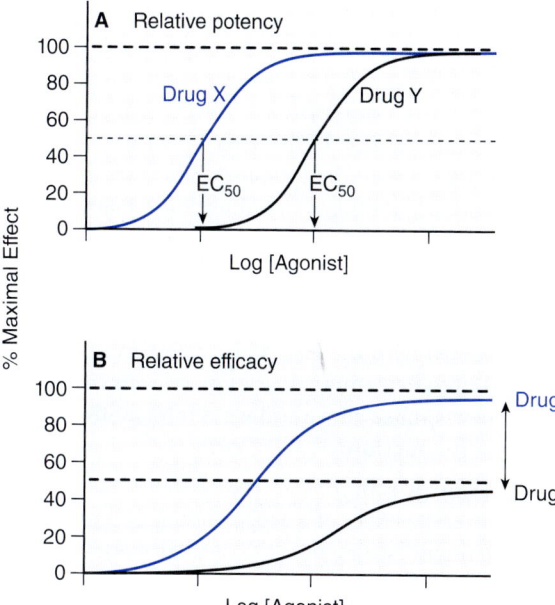

FIGURE 1-4 Two ways of quantifying agonism. **A.** The relative potency of 2 agonists (Drug X, blue line; Drug Y, black line) obtained in the same tissue is a function of their relative affinities and intrinsic efficacies. The EC_{50} of Drug X occurs at a concentration that is one-tenth the EC_{50} of Drug Y. Thus, Drug X is more potent than Drug Y. **B.** In systems where the 2 drugs do not both produce the same maximal response characteristic of the tissue, the observed maximal response is a non-linear function of their relative intrinsic efficacies. Drug X is more efficacious than Drug Y; their asymptotic fractional responses are 100% (Drug X) and 50% (Drug Y).

SECTION I General Principles

Before being administered to people, potential drugs are tested for general toxicity by monitoring the activity of various systems in 2 species of animals for extended periods of time. Compounds also are evaluated for carcinogenicity, genotoxicity, and reproductive toxicity. Animals are used for much of this testing, although the predictive value of results obtained in nonhuman species is certainly not perfect. Usually 1 rodent (usually mouse) and 1 nonrodent (often rabbit) species are used. In vitro and ex vivo assays are utilized when possible, both to spare animals and to minimize cost. If an unwanted effect is observed, an obvious question is whether it is mechanism-based (ie, caused by interaction of the drug with its intended target) or due to an off-target effect of the drug. If the latter, there is hope of minimizing the effect by further optimization of the molecule.

Before clinical trials of a potential new drug may proceed in the United States (ie, before the drug candidate can be administered to a human subject), the sponsor must file an IND (Investigational New Drug) application, which is a request to the United States. Food and Drug Administration (FDA) for permission to administer the drug to human test subjects. The IND describes the rationale and preliminary evidence for efficacy in experimental systems, as well as pharmacology, toxicology, chemistry, manufacturing, and so forth. It also describes the plan for investigating the drug in human subjects (see Chapter 3).

b. **In vitro binding studies show that K_D values of the drugs that are being considered for clinical studies range from 0.9 nM to 0.4 mM. What does a K_D measure and why is that value important to know?**

In general, the drug-receptor interaction is characterized by (1) binding of drug to receptor and (2) generation of a response in a biological system, as illustrated in Equation 1-1 where the drug or ligand is denoted as L and the inactive receptor as R. The equilibrium dissociation constant (K_D) is then described by ratio of the off and on rate constants (k_{-1}/k_{+1}) when L and R are at equilibrium with LR.

The affinity constant or equilibrium association constant (K_A) is the reciprocal of the equilibrium dissociation constant (ie, $K_A = 1/K_D$); thus a high-affinity drug has a low K_D and will bind a greater number of a particular receptor at a low concentration than a low-affinity drug. As a practical matter, the affinity of a drug is influenced most often by changes in its off-rate (k_{-1}) rather than its on-rate (k_{+1}).

Equation 1-3 shows the relationship of the fractional occupancy (f) of receptors by agonist L in terms of the concentration of L (ie, [L]), and either K_D (or K_A). This relationship illustrates that when the concentration of the drug equals the K_D (or $1/K_A$), $f = 0.5$, that is, the drug will occupy 50% of the receptors. Note that this relationship describes only receptor occupancy, not the eventual response that is often amplified by the cell. Many signaling systems reach a full biological response with only a fraction of receptors occupied (a phenomenon that might occur in a system with "spare receptors").

c. **Other preclinical studies were conducted with the target protein expressed in cultured cells. These studies were used to determine dose-response curves for each lead compound. What is a dose-response curve and what information can it provide regarding the drug-receptor interaction?**

The basic currency of receptor pharmacology is the dose-response (or concentration-response) curve, a depiction of the observed effect of a drug as a function of its concentration in the receptor compartment (see Figures 1-1 through 1-4). Drugs that bind to physiological receptors and mimic the regulatory effects of the endogenous signaling compounds are termed agonists. If the drug binds to the same recognition site as the endogenous agonist (the primary or orthosteric site on the receptor), the drug is said to be a primary agonist. Allosteric (allotopic) agonists bind to a different region on the receptor referred to as an allosteric or allotopic site. Drugs that block or reduce the action of an agonist are termed antagonists. Antagonism most commonly results from competition with an agonist for the same or overlapping site on the receptor (a syntopic interaction), but can also occur by

(*Continued*)

interacting with other sites on the receptor (allosteric antagonism), by combining with the agonist (chemical antagonism), or by functional antagonism by indirectly inhibiting the cellular or physiological effects of the agonist. Agents that are only partly as effective as agonists regardless of the concentration employed are termed partial agonists and are said to have lower efficacy than full agonists (see Figure 1-4, panel B). Many receptors exhibit some constitutive activity in the absence of a regulatory ligand; drugs that stabilize such receptors in an inactive conformation are termed inverse agonists (see bottom-most curve in Figure 1-1).

In addition to determining whether a ligand is an agonist or antagonist, dose-response curves as described here complement the in vitro binding studies described in part b previously and provide estimates of drug concentrations that might be appropriate for studies in animals and human subjects. In addition to estimating relative efficacy, the relative potency of agonist drugs can be estimated by comparison of EC_{50} values, the concentration of drug needed to obtain a half-maximal (ie, 50% of maximal) response. Dose response curves of antagonists generated in the presence of fixed concentrations of agonist can be used to estimate the affinity of a competitive antagonist for its receptor, the K_i (see text and Equations 3-3 and 3-4 in Chapter 3 of *Goodman & Gilman's The Pharmacological Basis of Therapeutics*, 12th Edition).

d. **Studies by this research group in rodent models showed that some of the lead compounds had unexpected side effects, including serious toxicities. What can cause such unexpected effects in a whole animal model?**

The chemical structure of a drug contributes to its affinity, intrinsic activity, as well as its specificity. A drug that interacts with a single type of receptor that is expressed on only a limited number of differentiated cells will exhibit high specificity. If however, a receptor is expressed ubiquitously on a variety of cells throughout the body, drugs acting on such a widely expressed receptor will exhibit widespread effects, and could produce serious side effects or toxicities if the receptor serves important functions in multiple tissues. Even if the primary action of a drug is localized, the subsequent physiological effects of the drug may be widespread. One example would be immunosuppressant drugs (see Chapter 23) that specifically inhibit cells of the immune system; their use is limited by the risk of opportunistic systemic infections.

Many clinically important drugs exhibit a broad (low) specificity because the drug is able to interact with multiple receptors in different tissues. Such broad specificity might enhance the clinical utility of a drug, but also contribute to a spectrum of adverse side effects due to off-target interactions. It should always be considered that a given drug has multiple mechanisms of action that depend on many factors, including receptor specificity, the tissue-specific expression of the receptor(s), drug access to target tissues, drug concentration in different tissues, pharmacogenetics (see Table 1-2), and interactions with other drugs (eg, see Chapters 2 to 7 in *Goodman & Gilman's The Pharmacological Basis of Therapeutics*, 12th Edition).

CASE 1-3

Following the FDA approval of a new short-acting hypnotic drug to enhance sleep following painful surgical procedures, postmarketing surveillance shows that toxic side effects are relatively common among elderly patients, but uncommon in younger adults.

a. **What is postmarketing surveillance?**

No drug is totally safe; all drugs produce unwanted effects in at least some people at some dose. Many unwanted and serious effects of drugs occur so infrequently, perhaps only once in several thousand patients, that they go undetected in the relatively small populations (a few thousand) in the standard Phase III clinical trial (see Table 1-1 in *Goodman & Gilman's The Pharmacological Basis of Therapeutics*, 12th Edition). To detect and verify that such events are in fact drug-related would require administration of the drug to tens or hundreds of thousands of people

(Continued)

SECTION I General Principles

TABLE 1-2 Examples of Genetic Polymorphisms Influencing Drug Response

GENE PRODUCT (*GENE*)	DRUGS[a]	RESPONSES AFFECTED
Targets and Receptors		
Angiotensin-converting enzyme (*ACE*)	ACE inhibitors (eg, enalapril)	Renoprotective effects, hypotension, left ventricular mass reduction, cough
Thymidylate synthase	5-Fluorouracil	Colorectal cancer response
Chemokine receptor 5 (*CCR5*)	Antiretrovirals, interferon	Antiviral response
β_2 Adrenergic receptor (*ADBR2*)	β_2 Antagonists (eg, albuterol, terbutaline)	Bronchodilation, susceptibility to agonist-induced desensitization, cardiovascular effects (eg, increased heart rate, cardiac index, peripheral vasodilation)
β_1 Adrenergic receptor (*ADBR1*)	β_1 Antagonists	Blood pressure and heart rate after β_1 antagonists
5-Lipoxygenase (*ALOX5*)	Leukotriene receptor antagonists	Asthma response
Dopamine receptors D_2, D_3, D_4	Antipsychotics (eg, haloperidol, clozapine, thioridazine, nemonapride)	Antipsychotic response (D_2, D_3, D_4), antipsychotic-induced tardive dyskinesia (D_3) and acute akathisia (D_3), hyperprolactinemia in females (D_2)
Estrogen receptor α	Estrogen hormone replacement therapy	High-density lipoprotein cholesterol
Serotonin transporter 5-HTT (*SLC6A4*)	Antidepressants (eg, clomipramine, fluoxetine, paroxetine, fluvoxamine)	Clozapine effects, 5-HT neurotransmission, antidepressant response
Serotonin receptor 5-HT$_{2A}$ (*HTR2A*)	Antipsychotics	Clozapine antipsychotic response, tardive dyskinesia, paroxetine antidepression response, drug discrimination
HMG-CoA reductase	Pravastatin	Reduction in serum cholesterol
Vitamin K oxidoreductase *VKORC1*	Warfarin[a]	Anticoagulant effect, bleeding risk
Corticotropin releasing hormone receptor (*CRHR1*)	Glucocorticoids	Bronchodilation, osteopenia
Ryanodine receptor (*RYR1*)	General anesthetics	Malignant hyperthermia
Modifiers		
Adducin	Diuretics	Myocardial infarction or strokes, blood pressure
Apolipoprotein E	Statins (eg, simvastatin), tacrine	Lipid-lowering; clinical improvement in Alzheimer disease
Human leukocyte antigen	Abacavir, carbamazepine, phenytoin	Hypersensitivity reactions
G6PD deficiency	Rasburicase[a], dapsone[a]	Methemoglobinemia
Cholesteryl ester transfer protein	Statins (eg, pravastatin)	Slowing atherosclerosis progression
Ion channels (*HERG, KvLQT1, Mink, MiRP1*)	Erythromycin, cisapride, clarithromycin, quinidine	Increased risk of drug-induced *torsade de pointes*, increased QT interval (Roden, 2003; Roden, 2004)
Methylguanine-methyltransferase	DNA methylating agents	Response of glioma to chemotherapy
Parkin	Levodopa	Parkinson disease response
MTHFR	Methotrexate	GI toxicity (Ulrich et al, 2001)
Prothrombin, factor V	Oral contraceptives	Venous thrombosis risk
Stromelysin-1	Statins (eg, pravastatin)	Reduction in cardiovascular events and in repeat angioplasty
Inosine triphosphatase (*ITPA*)	Azathioprine, mercaptopurine	Myelosuppression
Vitamin D receptor	Estrogen	Bone mineral density

[a]Information on genetics-based dosing, adverse events, or testing added to FDA-approved drug label (Grossman, 2007).

during clinical trials, adding enormous expense and time to drug development, and delaying access to potentially beneficial therapies. In general, the true spectrum and incidence of untoward effects becomes known only after a drug is released to the broader market and used by a large number of people (Phase IV, postmarketing surveillance; see Chapter 3, Case 3-2).

b. The preclinical trials of this drug showed a therapeutic index of 25. What is the therapeutic index and how is it calculated?

In preclinical studies of drugs, the median lethal dose (LD_{50}) is determined in experimental animals (see Figure 1-5, panel B). The LD_{50}/ED_{50} ratio is an indication of the therapeutic index, which is a quantitative statement of how selective the drug is in producing its desired effects versus its adverse effects. A therapeutic index of 25 indicates that the concentration of drug that is lethal in 50% of animals (LD_{50}) is 25-fold higher than the dose required to achieve a specific therapeutic effect in 50% of the population tested (the median effective dose, ED_{50}).

A similar term to therapeutic index, the therapeutic window, is the range of steady-state concentrations of drug that provides therapeutic efficacy with minimal toxicity (see Figure 1-6). In clinical studies, the dose, or preferably the concentration, of a drug required to produce toxic effects can be compared with the concentration required for therapeutic effects in the population to evaluate the clinical therapeutic index. Since pharmacodynamic variation in the population may be marked, the concentration or dose of drug required to produce a therapeutic effect in most of the population usually will overlap the concentration required to produce toxicity in some of the population, even though the drug's therapeutic index in an individual patient may be large. Also, the concentration-percent curves for efficacy and toxicity need not be parallel, adding yet another complexity to determination of the therapeutic index in patients. Finally, no drug produces a single effect, and the therapeutic index for a drug will vary depending on the effect being measured.

(Continued)

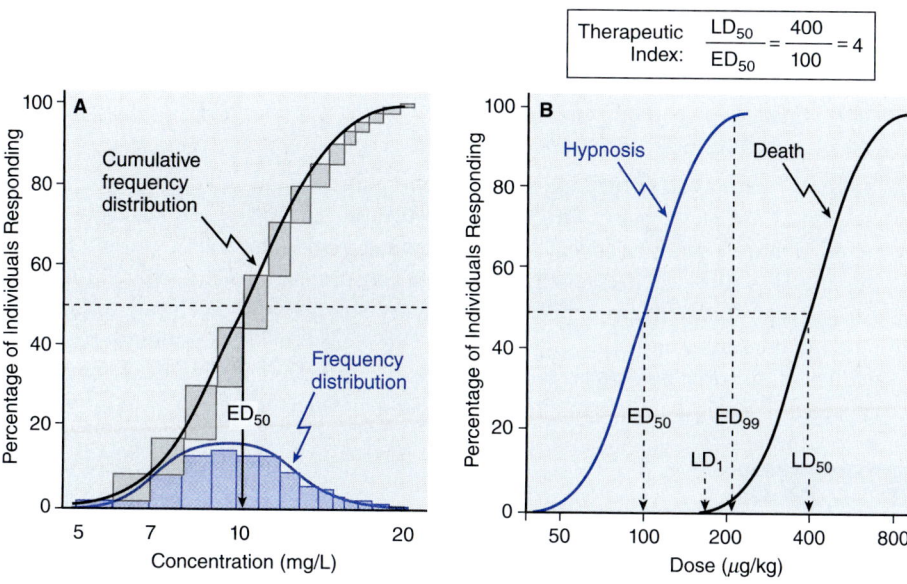

FIGURE 1-5 Frequency distribution curves and quantal concentration-effect and dose-effect curves. **A.** *Frequency distribution curves* An experiment was performed on 100 subjects, and the effective plasma concentration that produced a quantal response was determined for each individual. The number of subjects who required each dose is plotted, giving a log-normal frequency distribution (blue bars). The gray bars demonstrate that the normal frequency distribution, when summated, yields the cumulative frequency distribution—a sigmoidal curve that is a quantal concentration-effect curve. **B.** *Quantal dose-effect curves.* Animals were injected with varying doses of a drug and the responses were determined and plotted. The calculation of the therapeutic index, the ratio of the LD_{50} to the ED_{50}, is an indication of how selective a drug is in producing its desired effects relative to its toxicity. See Chapter 3 in *Goodman & Gilman's The Pharmacological Basis of Therapeutics*, 12th Edition for additional explanation.

SECTION I General Principles

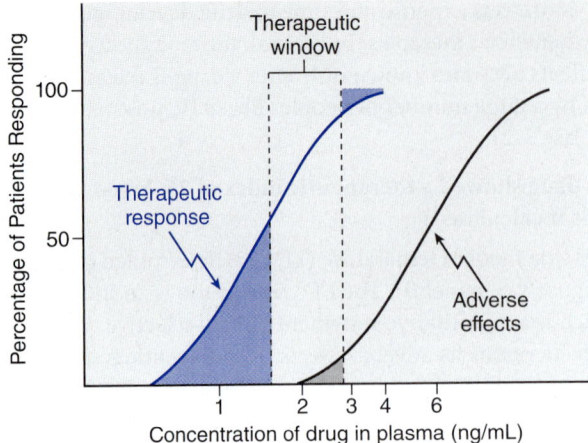

FIGURE 1-6 The relation of the therapeutic window of drug concentrations to the therapeutic and adverse effects in the population. The ordinate is linear; the abscissa is logarithmic.

c. Why might this toxicity primarily be seen in elderly patients in Phase IV trials?

Data on the correlation of drug levels with efficacy and toxicity must be interpreted in the context of the pharmacodynamic variability in the population (eg, genetics, age, disease, and the presence of coadministered drugs), as well as pharmacokinetic variables. Determinants of inter-individual variation in response to drugs that are due to pharmacokinetics include disease-related alterations such as impaired renal and liver clearance due to renal and hepatic disease, circulatory failure, altered drug binding to plasma proteins, impaired GI absorption, and pharmacokinetic drug interactions. The effects of these factors on variability of drug pharmacokinetics are described more thoroughly in Chapters 2 and 5 to 7 in *Goodman & Gilman's The Pharmacological Basis of Therapeutics*, 12th Edition.

If the Phase III clinical trials did not include large numbers of elderly patients, toxicities in this patient population might not be apparent until postmarketing surveillance has indicated an increased risk of toxicities in the elderly. Elderly patients may be more susceptible to toxicities for a variety of reasons, including age-related decreases in cardiac, renal and hepatic function, disease comorbidities, and poor nutritional status (see Chapter 3).

There is a quantal concentration-response curve for efficacy and adverse effects (see Figure 1-5B); for many drugs, the concentration that achieves efficacy in all the population may produce adverse effects in some individuals. Thus, a population therapeutic window expresses a range of concentrations at which the likelihood of efficacy is high and the probability of adverse effects is low (see Figure 1-6), but it does not guarantee either efficacy or safety. Therefore, use of the population therapeutic window to adjust dosage of a drug should be complemented by monitoring appropriate clinical and surrogate markers for drug effect(s).

CASE 1-4

A 64-year-old male patient diagnosed with atrial fibrillation is started on anticoagulant therapy with warfarin to lower his risk of stroke due to fibrin clots. Despite calculating initial warfarin dosing based on the patient's age, weight, and sex, laboratory monitoring of anticoagulant activity after the first week of therapy shows that the patient is receiving too much warfarin (his INR was too high indicating he is "over anti-coagulated"). After several weeks of dose adjustment, the patient's anticoagulant therapy is optimized at a warfarin concentration that is 10-fold lower than the initial dose.

a. What factors might have contributed to this patient's high sensitivity to warfarin?

Both pharmacokinetic and pharmacodynamic polymorphisms affect warfarin dosing (see Chapter 19). The anticoagulant warfarin is catabolized by CYP2C9, and warfarin's

(Continued)

action is partly dependent on the baseline level of reduced vitamin K (catalyzed by vitamin K epoxide reductase; Figure 1-7). Inactivating polymorphisms in *CYP2C9* are common, with 2 to 10% of most populations being homozygous for low-activity variants, and these polymorphisms are associated with lower warfarin clearance, a higher risk of bleeding complications, and lower dose requirements (see Table 30-2 in *Goodman & Gilman's The Pharmacological Basis of Therapeutics*, 12th Edition). Combined with genotyping for a common polymorphism in *VKORC1*, inherited variation in these 2 genes account for 20 to 60% of the variability in warfarin doses needed to achieve the desired INR (see Figure 1-7), and use of these tests in the clinic can result in fewer bleeding complications and a shorter time of trial-and-error dosing to achieve the desired steady-state level of anticoagulation.

The target of warfarin is *VKORC1*, an enzyme that reduces vitamin K epoxide to vitamin K hydroquinone (see Figure 1-7 and Table 1-2; Chapter 19). Warfarin inhibition of *VKORC1* blocks the reduction of vitamin K epoxide, which inhibits the synthesis of a number of vitamin K-dependent clotting factors. Several genetic variations in *VKORC1* are in strong linkage disequilibrium and have been designated haplotypes A and B (or non-A). *VKORC1* variants are more prevalent than those of *CYP2C9*. The prevalence of *VKORC1* genetic variants is higher in Asians, followed by European Americans and African Americans.

Polymorphism in *VKORC1* explains ~30% of the variability in warfarin dose requirements. Compared with *VKORC1* non-A/non-A homozygotes, the warfarin dose requirement is decreased by ~25% in heterozygotes and ~50% in A/A homozygotes.

The clinical relevance of these genetic polymorphisms remains uncertain. The goal of warfarin therapy is to maintain a patient within a target INR range, most often an INR value between 2 and 3. The risk of serious bleeding increases with INR values more than 4 and is highest during initiation of warfarin therapy. Variations in *VKORC1* have a greater effect than *CYP2C9* variants on warfarin responses early in therapy. Patients with *VKORC1* haplotype A have significantly higher INR values in the first week of warfarin therapy than non-A homozygotes; those with 1 or 2 *VKORC1* haplotype A alleles achieve a therapeutic INR more rapidly and are more likely to have an INR of 4 or greater than patients with 2 non-A alleles. Both the *VKORC1* haplotype and *CYP2C9* genotype have a significant effect on the warfarin dose after the first 2 weeks of therapy.

(Continued)

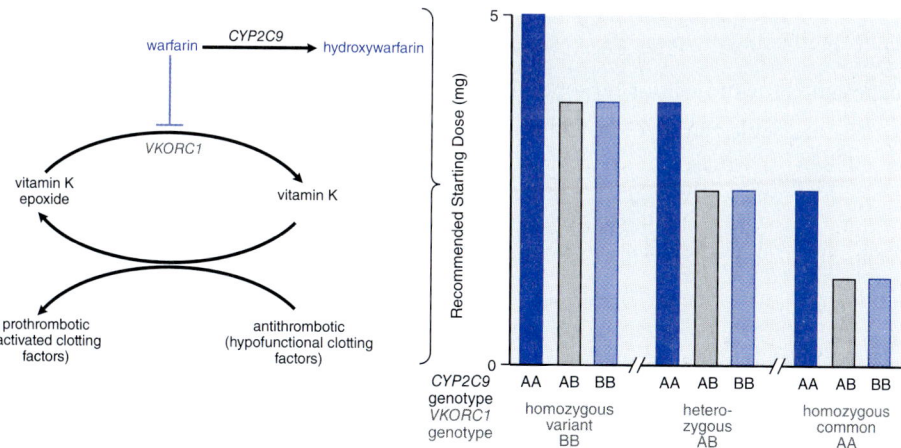

FIGURE 1-7 Pharmacogenetics of warfarin dosing. Warfarin is metabolized by *CYP2C9* to inactive metabolites, and exerts its anticoagulant effect partly via inhibition of *VKORC1* (vitamin K epoxide hydrolase), an enzyme necessary for reduction of inactive to active vitamin K. Common polymorphisms in both genes, *CYP2C9* and *VKORC1*, impact on warfarin pharmacokinetics and pharmacodynamics, respectively, to affect the population mean therapeutic doses of warfarin necessary to maintain the desired degree of anticoagulation (often measured by the international normalized ratio [INR] blood test) and minimize the risk of too little anticoagulation (thrombosis) or too much anticoagulation (bleeding).

SECTION I   General Principles

Based on evidence that genetic variations affect warfarin dose requirements and responses to therapy, the FDA amended the prescribing information for warfarin in 2007 to indicate that lower warfarin initiation doses be considered for patients with *CYP2C9* and *VKORC1* genetic variations. Efforts to facilitate the rational incorporation of genetic information into patient care have included the development of a warfarin dosing algorithm and point-of-care methods for *CYP2C9* and *VKORC1* genotyping. In a 2009 study of more than 4000 patients, the International Warfarin Pharmacogenetics Consortium compared the accuracy of a pharmacogenetic algorithm that included *VKORC1* and *CYP2C9* genotypes with 2 conventional clinical approaches: one based on clinical information to adjust the initial dose, and the other using a fixed-dose approach. The pharmacogenetic algorithm predicted the warfarin dose significantly better than the other 2 approaches. Moreover, the pharmacogenetic algorithm significantly improved the dose prediction for patients who required either high or low doses of warfarin (<21 mg/wk or >49 mg/wk).

Vitamin K is required for synthesis of functional clotting factors by serving as a cofactor (see Figure 1-7; Chapter 19). Relative deficiency of vitamin K may increase the sensitivity of patients to warfarin and may result from inadequate diet (eg, postoperative patients on parenteral fluids), especially when coupled with the elimination of intestinal flora by antimicrobial agents. Gut bacteria synthesize vitamin K and are an important source of this vitamin. Consequently, antibiotics can cause a high INR in patients who were previously adequately controlled on warfarin. In addition to an effect on reducing intestinal flora, cephalosporins containing heterocyclic side chains also inhibit steps in the vitamin K cycle. Low concentrations of coagulation factors may result from impaired hepatic function, congestive heart failure, or hypermetabolic states, such as hyperthyroidism; generally, these conditions increase the INR.

Frequently cited drug interactions that increase INR and enhance the risk of hemorrhage in patients taking warfarin include decreased metabolism due to CYP2C9 inhibition by amiodarone, azole antifungals, cimetidine, clopidogrel, cotrimoxazole, disulfiram, fluoxetine, isoniazid, metronidazole, sulfinpyrazone, tolcapone, or zafirlukast, and displacement from protein binding sites caused by loop diuretics or valproate.

CASE 1-5

A 42-year-old man is diagnosed with chronic myelogenous leukemia (CML). He is prescribed imatinib, a small molecule anticancer drug that targets a disease-causing enzyme in leukemic cells.

a. What is the molecular target of imatinib in CML?

The molecular target of imatinib in CML is the abnormal protein tyrosine kinase BCR-ABL, which is caused by a chromosomal translocation (see Chapter 46). BCR-ABL is constitutively active which causes the uncontrolled proliferation of leukemic cells. Imatinib binds at the active site of the kinase and blocks its activity, thus blocking cell proliferation.

Imatinib mesylate was the first molecularly targeted protein kinase inhibitor to receive FDA approval. Imatinib was identified through high-throughput screening against the BCR-ABL kinase. The lead compound of this series, a 2-phenylamino-pyrimidine, had low potency and poor specificity, inhibiting both serine/threonine and tyrosine kinases. The addition of a 3′-pyridyl group at the 3′ position of the pyrimidine enhanced its potency. Further modifications resulted in improved activity against PDGFR and c-KIT (2 other disease-causing tyrosine kinases) and loss of serine/threonine kinase inhibition. Introduction of *N*-methylpiperazine as a polar side chain greatly improved water solubility and oral bioavailability, yielding imatinib, an inhibitor of the closed, or inactive, configuration of the kinase.

(Continued)

Pharmacodynamics   CHAPTER 1

b. **The patient's cancer goes into remission for 24 months, but then comes back, despite daily doses of imatinib. What is the likely mechanism of resistance to imatinib that has developed in this patient?**

Resistance to imatinib and other small molecule tyrosine kinase inhibitors arises from point mutations in 3 separate segments of the kinase domain. The contact points between imatinib and the enzyme become sites of mutations in drug-resistant leukemic cells; these mutations prevent tight binding of the drug and lock the enzyme in its open configuration, in which it has access to substrate. Such mutations hold the enzyme in its open and enzymatically active confirmation. The most common resistance mutations affect amino acids 255 and 315, both of which serve as contact points for imatinib; these mutations confer high-level resistance to imatinib. Some mutations, such as at amino acids 351 and 355, confer low levels of resistance to imatinib.

c. **What is the therapeutic strategy to overcome resistance to imatinib in this patient?**

The strategy depends on the sites of mutation in BCR-ABL that lead to the resistance. Mutations at amino acids 351 and 355 might lead to a clinical response with dose escalation of imatinib. Mutations at other amino acids that confer high resistance to imatinib will require using a different tyrosine kinase inhibitor such as nilotinib or dasatinib. Dasatinib is unaffected by mutation at 255 but is ineffective in the presence of mutation at 315. Nilotinib retains inhibitory activity in the presence of most point mutations (except at 315) that confer resistance to imatinib.

KEY CONCEPTS

- Pharmacodynamics refers to the effects of a drug on the body.
- Most drugs act by binding to physiological receptors and alter the rate or magnitude of an intrinsic cellular response rather than create new responses.
- Important pharmacodynamic properties of a drug include its affinity, efficacy, and specificity.
- The effects of a drug depend on many pharmacodynamic factors, including receptor specificity, the tissue-specific expression of the receptor(s), drug concentration in the receptor compartment on target tissues, drug concentrations in different tissues expressing the receptor, pharmacogenetics, and interactions with other drugs at the receptor.
- No drug is totally safe; all drugs produce unwanted effects in at least some people at some dose.
- The concentration or dose of drug required to produce a therapeutic effect in most of the population usually will overlap the concentration required to produce toxicity in some of the population.

SUMMARY QUIZ

QUESTION 1-1 Pindolol and some other β adrenergic receptor antagonists have an additional property that is referred to as intrinsic sympathomimetic activity (ISA). This additional property indicates these agents are

a. full agonists.
b. inverse agonists.
c. partial agonists.
d. neutral antagonists.
e. noncompetitive antagonists.

SECTION I General Principles

QUESTION 1-2 A 28-year-old woman is brought to the emergency department after overdosing on oxycodone, an opiate analgesic. She is unconscious and barely breathing when she arrives at the hospital, but revives and is breathing normally within 2 minutes after receiving an injection of naloxone. After about an hour, she requires another dose of naloxone as the symptoms of opiate overdose begin to redevelop. Naloxone is likely acting as a

a. strong stimulant that counteracts the CNS-depressant effects of the opiate.
b. diuretic that increases renal excretion of the opiate.
c. drug that stimulates respiratory centers in the brain.
d. competitive antagonist of opioid receptors.
e. noncompetitive antagonist of opioid receptors.

QUESTION 1-3 The equilibrium dissociation constant (K_D) is a measure of a drug's

a. efficacy.
b. affinity for its receptor.
c. specificity.
d. safety.
e. solubility in water.

QUESTION 1-4 The therapeutic window is an indication of the

a. length of time a drug should be administered to achieve optimal effects.
b. time of day when a drug should be administered for optimal effects.
c. range of concentrations over which a drug is maximally effective for all patients.
d. range of concentrations over which a drug is safe and efficacious for most patients.
e. age range of patients that is optimal for a given drug.

QUESTION 1-5 Preclinical characterization of a new drug indicates that it is an inverse agonist for adenosine receptors. It interacts syntopically with adenosine. In the presence of adenosine, this drug will behave like a(n)

a. full agonist with additive effects to adenosine at high concentrations.
b. partial agonist with additive effects to adenosine at high concentrations.
c. partial agonist with inhibitory effects to adenosine at high concentrations.
d. inert compound with no additive or inhibitory effects to adenosine at high concentrations.
e. competitive antagonist with inhibitory effects on receptor activation.

SUMMARY QUIZ ANSWER KEY

QUESTION 1-1 Answer is **c.** Several β blockers (eg, pindolol, acebutolol, bucindolol) activate β receptors partially in the absence of catecholamines; however, the intrinsic activities of these drugs are less than that of a full agonist such as isoproterenol, epinephrine, or norepinephrine. Thus these are partial agonists and are said to have intrinsic sympathomimetic activity. Substantial sympathomimetic activity would be counterproductive to the response desired from a β antagonist; however, slight residual activity may, for example, prevent profound bradycardia or negative inotropy in a resting heart. The potential clinical advantage of this property, however, is unclear and may be disadvantageous in the context of secondary prevention of myocardial infarction.

Although only limited data are available, β blockers with slight partial agonist activity may produce smaller reductions in resting heart rate and blood pressure. Hence, such drugs may be preferred as antihypertensive agents in individuals with diminished cardiac reserve or a propensity for bradycardia.

Nonetheless, the clinical significance of partial agonism has not been substantially demonstrated in controlled trials but may be of importance in individual patients. Agents such as pindolol block exercise-induced increases in heart rate and cardiac output (see Chapters 15 and 16).

QUESTION 1-2 Answer is **d.** Naloxone is a competitive antagonist of various opioid receptors (see Chapter 10). Opioid antagonists, particularly naloxone, have an established use in the treatment of opioid-induced toxicity, especially respiratory depression. Its specificity is such that reversal by this agent is virtually diagnostic for the contribution of an opiate to the depression. Naloxone acts rapidly to reverse the respiratory depression associated with high doses of opioids.

It should be used cautiously because it also can precipitate withdrawal in dependent subjects and cause undesirable cardiovascular side effects. By carefully titrating the dose of naloxone, it usually is possible to rapidly antagonize the respiratory-depressant actions without eliciting a fully expressed withdrawal syndrome. The duration of action of naloxone is relatively short, and it often must be given repeatedly or by continuous infusion.

Under ordinary circumstances, opioid antagonists such as naloxone produce few effects in the absence of an exogenous agonist. However, under certain conditions (eg, shock), when the endogenous opioid systems are activated, the administration of an opioid antagonist alone may have visible consequences.

QUESTION 1-3 Answer is **b.** The equilibrium dissociation constant (K_D) is a measure of a drug's affinity for its receptor. It is the reciprocal of the affinity constant or equilibrium association constant (K_A; ie, $K_A = 1/K_D$). Thus a high-affinity drug has a low K_D and will bind a greater number of a particular receptor at a low concentration than a low-affinity drug.

QUESTION 1-4 Answer is **d.** A population therapeutic window expresses a range of concentrations at which the likelihood of efficacy is high and the probability of adverse effects is low (see Figure 1-6). It does not guarantee either efficacy or safety. Therefore, use of the population therapeutic window to adjust dosage of a drug should be complemented by monitoring appropriate clinical and surrogate markers for drug effect(s).

QUESTION 1-5 Answer is **e.** Many receptors exhibit some constitutive activity in the absence of a regulatory ligand. Inverse agonists selectively bind to the inactive form of such receptors and shift the conformational equilibrium toward the inactive state (see Figure 1-1). Inverse agonists typically bind such receptors at the same site as the endogenous agonist; ligands that interact syntopically with a full agonist will behave as competitive antagonists.

The characteristic pattern of competitive antagonism is the concentration-dependent production of a parallel shift to the right of the agonist dose-response curve with no change in the maximal response (see Figure 1-2A). The magnitude of the rightward shift of the curve depends on the concentration of the antagonist and its affinity for the receptor.

In systems that are not constitutively active, inverse agonists will behave like competitive antagonists, which helps explain why the properties of inverse agonists and the number of such agents previously described as competitive antagonists were only recently appreciated. Receptors that have constitutive activity and are sensitive to inverse agonists include benzodiazepine, histamine, opioid, cannabinoid, dopamine, bradykinin, and adenosine receptors.

CHAPTER 2

Pharmacokinetics

This chapter will be most useful after having a basic understanding of the material in Chapter 2, Pharmacokinetics in *Goodman & Gilman's The Pharmacological Basis of Therapeutics*, 12th Edition. This chapter also draws from content in Chapter 5, Membrane Transporters and Drug Response; Chapter 6, Drug Metabolism; and parts of Chapter 7, Pharmacogenetics. The drugs presented in this chapter are used to illustrate general pharmacokinetic principles. The pharmacokinetic, pharmacodynamic, and therapeutic uses of drugs described in Chapter 2 are discussed in more detail in subsequent chapters. Neither a Mechanisms of Action Table nor a Clinical Summary Table is included in this chapter because this information is provided in subsequent chapters.

In addition to the material presented here, the 12th Edition contains:

- A review in Chapter 2 of cell membranes and their physicochemical properties that affect the movement of drugs to their site of action
- A discussion in Chapter 2 of different routes of drug administration and their relative advantages and disadvantages
- A detailed discussion in Chapter 2 of renal drug excretion, biliary and fecal excretion, and excretion by other routes
- A comprehensive discussion of design and optimization of dosage regimens in Chapter 2, including examples of dosing calculations that take into consideration bioavailability, clearance, and distribution
- Appendix II Design Optimization of Dosage Regimens: Pharmacokinetic Data in *Goodman & Gilman's The Pharmacological Basis of Therapeutics*, 12th Edition provides a summary of basic pharmacokinetic data for a number of drugs that are in common clinical use, as well as information that is useful in individualizing dosing in a given patient
- Chapter 5 contains a detailed review of membrane transporters, including their role in absorption, distribution, and clearance of xenobiotics, and their role in adverse drug responses
- Table 5-1 Regulation of Transporter Expression by Nuclear Receptors provides detailed information about drug regulation of transporter expression mediated through specific nuclear receptors
- A description in Chapter 5 of the role of efflux transporters in the blood-brain barrier (BBB) and blood-cerebrospinal fluid (CSF) barrier
- Chapter 6 provides a comprehensive discussion of drug metabolism enzymes and illustrations that show many of the key chemical reactions catalyzed by these enzymes

CHARACTERISTICS OF A DRUG THAT PREDICT ITS MOVEMENT AND AVAILABILITY AT ITS SITES OF ACTION

- Molecular size and structural features
- Degree of ionization
- Relative lipid solubility of its ionized and nonionized forms
- Its binding to serum and tissue proteins

LEARNING OBJECTIVES

☑ Understand key concepts and terms that determine drug pharmacokinetics, including absorption, distribution, metabolism, and excretion.

☑ Understand the mechanisms by which drugs cross membranes and the physicochemical factors that influence this transfer.

☑ Be able to predict the ionization state of a drug that is a weak acid or base knowing the drug's pK_a and the pH of the fluid.

☑ Describe the role of membrane transporters in drug absorption, distribution, and clearance.

Pharmacokinetics

CHAPTER 2

- ☑ Know the major mechanisms by which drugs are metabolized and excreted from the body.
- ☑ Understand the major pharmacokinetic mechanisms that can result in drug interactions.
- ☑ Know the pharmacokinetic mechanisms that give rise to interpatient variability in drug response and toxicity.
- ☑ Understand the clinical pharmacokinetic principles used to calculate dosing required to achieve steady-state drug concentrations in plasma.
- ☑ Understand how route of administration can affect the bioavailability and clearance of drugs.

CASE 2-1

In Case 1-1, a gentleman is seeking an allergy medicine at his local pharmacy to relieve his hay fever symptoms. One of the nonprescription drugs he finds contains diphenhydramine, which can cause drowsiness or other CNS effects as discussed in part d of Case 1-1.

a. How is diphenhydramine able to cause CNS effects?

First-generation antihistamines such as diphenhydramine can cross the BBB and cause CNS depression such as somnolence. Diphenhydramine and the other first-generation antihistamines contain a tertiary amino group linked by a 2- or 3-atom chain to 2 aromatic substituents (see Figure 32-3 in *Goodman & Gilman's The Pharmacological Basis of Therapeutics*, 12th Edition). The only ionizable group in

(Continued)

PASSIVE TRANSPORT *VERSUS* ACTIVE TRANSPORT ACROSS CELLULAR BARRIERS

- *Passive transport* is the dominant transport mechanism in the disposition of most drugs (Figure 2-1).
  - In *passive diffusion*, the drug molecule usually penetrates cellular barriers by diffusion along a concentration gradient by virtue of its solubility in the lipid bilayer.
  - *Paracellular transport* through intercellular gaps occurs across capillary endothelium and is important in filtration across the glomerulus in the kidney but is limited in some tissues such as the CNS where capillaries have tight intercellular junctions.
  - *Facilitated diffusion* describes a carrier-mediated transport process in which there is no input of energy, and therefore enhanced movement of the involved substance is down a chemical gradient.
- *Active transport* is characterized by a direct requirement for energy, movement against an electrochemical gradient, saturability, selectivity, and competitive inhibition by cotransported compounds.

WEAK ELECTROLYTES AND THE INFLUENCE OF PH

- Many drugs are weak acids or bases that are present in solution as both the nonionized and ionized species.
  - Nonionized molecules are usually more lipid soluble and can diffuse readily across the cell membrane.
  - Ionized molecules usually are less able to penetrate the lipid membrane because of their low lipid solubility.
- The transmembrane distribution of a weak electrolyte is influenced by its pK_a and the pH gradient across the membrane.
- The ratio of nonionized to ionized drug at a given pH is readily calculated from the Henderson-Hasselbalch equation (Equation 2-1), where pK_a is the drug's acid dissociation constant.

$$\log \frac{[\text{protonated form}]}{[\text{unprotonated form}]} = pK_a - pH$$

(Equation 2-1)

(continues)

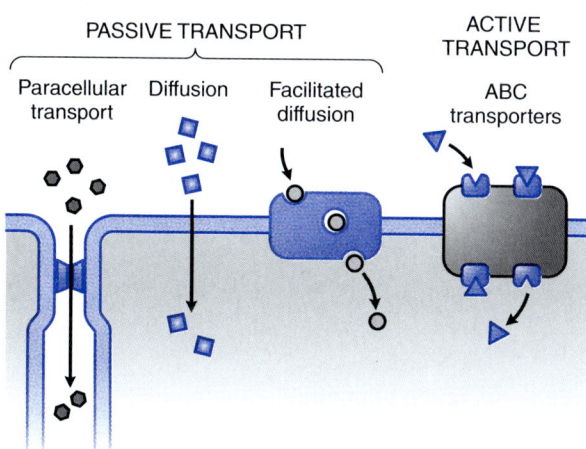

FIGURE 2-1 The variety of ways drugs move across cellular barriers in their passage throughout the body. Transmembrane movement of drug generally is limited to unbound drug; thus drug-protein complexes constitute an inactive reservoir of drug. Unbound drugs cross membranes either by passive processes or by mechanisms involving the active participation of components of the membrane. In passive transfer, the drug molecule usually penetrates by diffusion along a concentration gradient by virtue of its solubility in the lipid bilayer. Such transfer is directly proportional to the magnitude of the concentration gradient across the membrane, to the lipid-water partition coefficient of the drug, and to the membrane surface area exposed to the drug. The greater the partition coefficient, the higher is the concentration of drug in the membrane and the faster is its diffusion. After a steady-state is attained, the concentration of the unbound drug is the same on both sides of the membrane if the drug is a nonelectrolyte. For ionic compounds, the steady-state concentrations depend on the electrochemical gradient for the ion and on differences in pH across the membrane, which will influence the state of ionization of the molecule disparately on either side of the membrane and can effectively trap drug on 1 side of the membrane. Carrier-mediated active transport is characterized by a direct requirement for energy.

SECTION I

General Principles

WEAK ELECTROLYTES AND THE INFLUENCE OF PH (Cont.)

- Figure 2-2 illustrates the partitioning of a weak acid ($pK_a = 4.4$) between plasma (pH = 7.4) and gastric juice (pH = 1.4).
- At steady state, an acidic drug will accumulate on the more basic side of the membrane and a basic drug on the more acidic side, a phenomenon known as *ion trapping*.
- In the kidney tubules where a lipid soluble (uncharged) drug can be reabsorbed by passive diffusion, excretion of the drug can be promoted by altering the pH of the urine to favor the ionized state (A^- or BH^+).
  - Alkaline urine favors excretion of weak acids; for example, elevation of urine pH with sodium bicarbonate will increase the excretion of weak acids such as aspirin ($pK_a \sim 3.5$) and urate ($pK_a \sim 5.8$).
  - Acid urine favors excretion of weak bases.

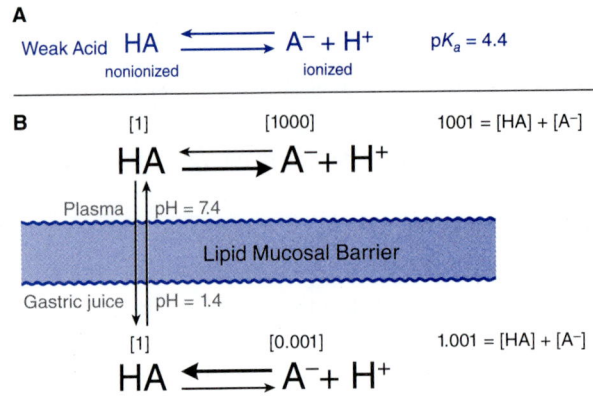

FIGURE 2-2 Influence of pH on the distribution of a weak acid between plasma and gastric juice separated by a lipid barrier. **A.** The dissociation of a weak acid, $pK_a = 4.4$. **B.** Dissociation of the weak acid in plasma (pH 7.4) and gastric acid (pH 1.4). The uncharged form, HA, equilibrates across the membrane. Blue numbers in brackets show relative concentrations of HA and A^-. In this example, the ratio of nonionized to ionized drug in plasma is 1:1000; in gastric juice, the ratio is 1:0.001, as given in brackets. The total concentration ratio between the plasma and the gastric juice therefore would be 1000:1 if such a system came to a steady-state. For a weak base with a pK_a of 4.4 (eg, chlordiazepoxide), the ratio would be reversed, as would the thick horizontal arrows, which indicate the predominant species at each pH. Accordingly, at steady state, an acidic drug will accumulate on the more basic side of the membrane and a basic drug on the more acidic side.

DRUG ABSORPTION, BIOAVAILABILITY, AND ROUTES OF ADMINISTRATION

- *Absorption* is the movement of a drug from its site of administration into the central compartment (Figure 2-3).
- *Bioavailability* is the fractional extent to which a dose of drug reaches its site of action or a biological fluid from which the drug has access to its site of action.
- A fraction of the administered and absorbed dose of drug will be inactivated or diverted in the intestine and liver before it can reach the general circulation and be distributed to its sites of action.
  - If the metabolic or excretory capacity of the liver and the intestine for the drug is large, bioavailability will be reduced substantially (*first-pass effect*).
- The *route of drug administration* can affect the time course of drug effects, extent of absorption, bioavailability, first-pass effect, variability of drug effects, and adverse effects (see Table 2-1).
- Knowledge of drugs that undergo significant metabolism or require active transport across the intestinal and hepatic membranes can be used to predict some pharmacokinetic interactions because drugs may compete for metabolism and transport.

diphenhydramine and these other agents is the tertiary amino group, which has a $pK_a \sim 9.0$. Thus, at physiological pH (pH 7.4), the drug is largely unionized (see Figure 2-2) and very lipophilic and can easily diffuse through lipid membranes, including the BBB.

b. Are there other antihistamines that this patient could take that do not cause drowsiness?

The second-generation antihistamines, such as loratadine (see Chapter 21), do not cause drowsiness. These second-generation histamine H_1 antagonists are ionized at physiological pH and as a consequence do not readily cross the BBB. For example, the pK_a of loratadine is ~4.3, and is thus largely ionized at pH 7.4 and not able to diffuse readily through lipid membranes.

(Continued)

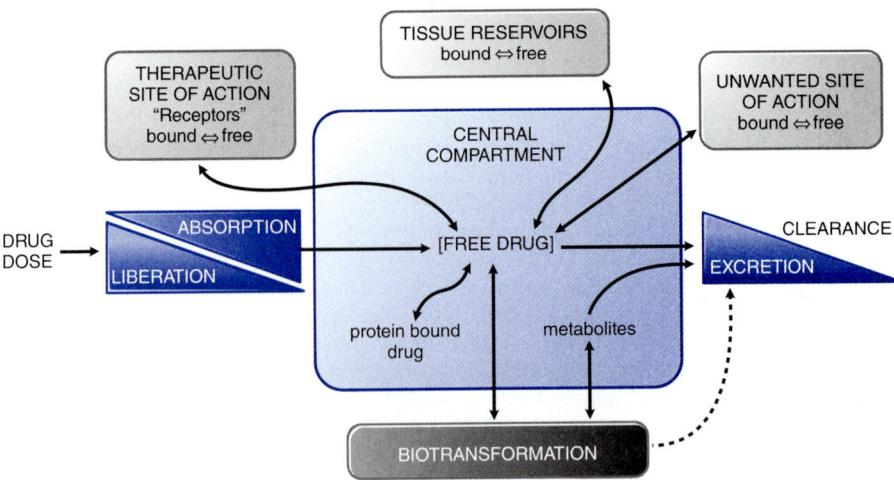

FIGURE 2-3 The interrelationship of the absorption, distribution, binding, metabolism, and excretion of a drug and its concentration at its sites of action. Possible distribution and binding of metabolites in relation to their potential actions at receptors are not depicted.

Pharmacokinetics CHAPTER 2

TABLE 2-1 Some Characteristics of Common Routes of Drug Administration

ROUTE	ABSORPTION PATTERN	SPECIAL UTILITY	LIMITATIONS AND PRECAUTIONS
Intravenous	Absorption circumvented Potentially immediate effects Suitable for large volumes and for irritating substances, or complex mixtures, when diluted	Valuable for emergency use Permits titration of dosage Usually required for high-molecular-weight protein and peptide drugs	Increased risk of adverse effects Must inject solutions *slowly* as a rule Not suitable for oily solutions or poorly soluble substances
Subcutaneous	Prompt from aqueous solution Slow and sustained from repository preparations	Suitable for some poorly soluble suspensions and for instillation of slow-release implants	Not suitable for large volumes Possible pain or necrosis from irritating substances
Intramuscular	Prompt from aqueous solution Slow and sustained from repository preparations	Suitable for moderate volumes, oily vehicles, and some irritating substances Appropriate for self-administration (eg, insulin)	Precluded during anticoagulant therapy May interfere with interpretation of certain diagnostic tests (eg, creatine kinase)
Oral ingestion	Variable, depends on many factors	Most convenient and economical; usually more safe	Requires patient compliance Bioavailability potentially erratic and incomplete

DISTRIBUTION OF DRUGS

- *Distribution* refers to the movement of drug into interstitial and intracellular fluids following absorption or systemic administration (see Figure 2-3).
- Distribution reflects a number of physiological factors and the particular physicochemical properties of the individual drug.
- Physiological factors that determine the rate of delivery and potential amount of drug distributed into tissue include:
  - Cardiac output
  - Regional blood flow
  - Capillary permeability
  - Tissue volume
- During the initial distribution phase, the liver, kidney, brain, and other well-perfused organs receive most of the drug.
- The second distribution phase to muscle, most viscera, skin, and fat is slower and may require minutes to several hours before the concentration of drug in tissue is in equilibrium with that in blood.
  - The second phase involves a far larger fraction of body mass (eg, muscle) than does the initial phase and generally accounts for most of the extravascularly distributed drug.
- With exceptions such as the brain, diffusion of drug into the interstitial fluid occurs rapidly because of the highly permeable nature of the capillary endothelial membrane.
- Tissue distribution is determined by the partitioning of drug between blood and the particular tissue.
  - Lipid solubility and transmembrane pH gradients are important determinants of tissue uptake for drugs that are either weak acids or bases; however, ion trapping associated with transmembrane pH gradients is generally not large because the pH difference between tissue and blood (~7.0 vs 7.4) is small.
  - The most important determinant of blood-tissue partitioning is the relative binding of drug to plasma proteins and tissue macromolecules that limits the concentration of free drug.

c. **Besides the CNS, where else in the body might the net charge of a drug be affected by pH?**

The partitioning of a weak acid (pK_a = 4.4) between plasma (pH = 7.4) and gastric juice (pH = 1.4) is depicted in Figure 2-2. Assume that the gastric mucosal membrane behaves as a simple lipid barrier with a high electrical resistance that is permeable only to the lipid-soluble, nonionized form of the acid. The ratio of nonionized to ionized drug at each pH is readily calculated from the Henderson-Hasselbalch equation (see Equation 2-1). In the example of Figure 2-2, the ratio of nonionized to ionized drug in plasma is 1:1000; in gastric juice, the ratio is 1:0.001, as given in brackets in Figure 2-2. The total concentration ratio between the plasma and the gastric juice therefore would be 1000:1 if such a system came to a steady-state. For a weak base with a pK_a of 4.4 (eg, chlordiazepoxide), the ratio would be reversed, as would the thick horizontal arrows in Figure 2-2, which indicate the predominant species at each pH. Accordingly, at steady state, an acidic drug will accumulate on the more basic side of the membrane and a basic drug on the more acidic side.

The effects of net charge are observable elsewhere in the body, such as in the kidney tubules. Urine pH can vary over a ride range, from 4.5 to 8. As urine pH drops (as [H^+] increases), weak acids (A^-) and weak bases (B) will exist to a greater extent in their protonated forms (HA and BH^+); the reverse is true as pH rises, where A^- and B will be favored. In the kidney tubules where a lipid-soluble (uncharged) drug can be reabsorbed by passive diffusion, excretion of the drug can be promoted by altering the pH of the urine to favor the ionized state (A^- or BH^+). Thus, alkaline urine

(Continued)

SECTION I

PLASMA PROTEIN BINDING OF DRUGS

- Many drugs circulate in the bloodstream bound to plasma proteins.
  - Albumin is a major carrier for acidic drugs.
  - α1-Acid glycoprotein binds basic drugs.
  - Certain drugs may bind to proteins that function as specific hormone carrier proteins, such as the binding of estrogen or testosterone to sex hormone–binding globulin or the binding of thyroid hormone to thyroxin-binding globulin.
- Plasma protein binding is a nonlinear, saturable process.
- Binding of a drug to plasma proteins limits its concentration in tissues and at its site of action because only unbound (free) drug is in equilibrium across membranes (see Figure 2-3).
- Appendix II in *Goodman & Gilman's The Pharmacological Basis of Therapeutics*, 12th Edition provides plasma protein binding percentages for a number of commonly used drugs.
- The extent of plasma protein binding also may be affected by disease-related factors.
  - Changes in protein binding due to disease states and drug–drug interactions are clinically relevant mainly for a small subset of the so-called high-clearance drugs of narrow therapeutic index that are administered intravenously.
- Drug excretion by the kidneys, transport, and metabolism can be limited by binding to plasma protein.

TISSUE BINDING OF DRUGS

- Many drugs accumulate in tissues at higher concentrations than those in the extracellular fluids and blood.
- Tissue accumulation may be a result of active transport or, more commonly, binding to cellular constituents such as proteins, phospholipids, or nuclear proteins.

(continues)

General Principles

favors excretion of weak acids; acid urine favors excretion of weak bases. Elevation of urine pH (by giving sodium bicarbonate) will promote urinary excretion of weak acids such as aspirin ($pK_a \sim 3.5$) and urate ($pK_a \sim 5.8$). This principle of ion trapping is an important process in drug distribution.

The establishment of concentration gradients of weak electrolytes across membranes with a pH gradient is a physical process and does not require an active electrolyte transport system. All that is necessary is a membrane preferentially permeable to one form of the weak electrolyte and a pH gradient across the membrane. The establishment of the pH gradient, however, is an active process.

CASE 2-2

A 68-year-old woman has symptoms of angina when she climbs stairs or engages in strenuous activity. She is prescribed nitroglycerin (glyceryl trinitrate, see Chapter 16) to take prophylactically before she engages in any activity that might cause angina symptoms.

a. The patient's pharmacist instructs her that she is to place the nitroglycerin tablet under her tongue a couple of minutes before strenuous activity to prevent angina. Why is this route of administration used for this drug?

Sublingual administration of nitroglycerin results in rapid onset of action (peak concentrations within 4 minutes of administration) and avoids the first-pass effect. Absorption from the oral mucosa has special significance for certain drugs despite the fact that the surface area available is small. Venous drainage from the mouth is to the superior vena cava, bypassing the portal circulation and thereby protecting the drug from rapid intestinal and hepatic first-pass metabolism. Nitroglycerin is effective when retained sublingually because it is nonionic and has very high lipid solubility. Thus, the drug is absorbed very rapidly. Nitroglycerin also is very potent; absorption of a relatively small amount produces the therapeutic effect ("unloading" of the heart; see Chapter 16). Nitroglycerin that is swallowed undergoes nearly complete first-pass metabolism as the result of enzymatic denitration in the liver. Thus, its bioavailability is only ~0.01 (ie, ~1%) when swallowed.

b. To prevent first-pass effects, what other routes of administration might be effective for this agent?

Because nitroglycerin has very high lipid solubility, it can be absorbed through the skin and administered via controlled-release transdermal patches. This route of administration is effective for patients requiring chronic administration of nitroglycerin to prevent symptoms of angina, but can result in the development of tolerance unless the patch is removed for 8-12 hours each day (see Case 16-1).

CASE 2-3

A 59-year-old man who was diagnosed with coronary artery disease undergoes angioplasty and receives a coronary stent. To prevent platelet thrombosis of the stent, he is prescribed a standard dosing regimen of clopidogrel, a drug that inhibits platelet aggregation (see Chapter 19). After several weeks of clopidogrel therapy, his platelet function is measured and it is determined that the dose of clopidogrel is too low to effectively inhibit platelet aggregation.

a. What kind of drug is clopidogrel and how might this explain the poor response to therapy with this agent?

Clopidogrel is a prodrug that requires bioactivation, primarily by CYP2C19. There is wide interindividual variability in the capacity of clopidogrel to inhibit platelet aggregation, and some patients are designated resistant to the antiplatelet effects

(Continued)

Pharmacokinetics

CHAPTER 2

TABLE 2-2 ABC Transporters Involved in Drug Absorption, Distribution, and Excretion Processes

TRANSPORTER NAME (GENE)	TISSUE DISTRIBUTION	PHYSIOLOGICAL FUNCTION	SUBSTRATES
MDR1 (*ABCB1*)	Liver, Kidney, Intestine, BBB, BTB, BPB	Natural detoxification system against xenobiotics	**Characteristics:** Neutral or cationic compounds with bulky structure **Anticancer drugs:** etoposide, doxorubicin, vincristine **Ca^{2+} channel blockers:** diltiazem, verapamil **HIV protease inhibitors:** indinavir, ritonavir **Antibiotics/Antifungals:** erythromycin, ketoconazole **Hormones:** testosterone, progesterone **Immunosuppressants:** cyclosporine, tacrolimus **Others:** digoxin, quinidine, fexofenadine, loperamide
MRP1 (*ABCC1*)	Ubiquitous (Kidney, BCSFB, BTB)	Leukotriene C_4 secretion from leukocyte	**Characteristics:** Amphiphilic with at least one negative net charge **Anticancer drugs:** vincristine (with GSH), methotrexate **Glutathione conjugates:** leukotriene C_4, glutathione conjugate of ethacrynic acid **Glucuronide conjugates:** estradiol-17-D-glucuronide, bilirubin mono(or bis)glucuronide **Sulfated conjugates:** estrone-3-sulfate (with GSH) **HIV protease inhibitors:** saquinavir **Antibiotics:** grepafloxacin **Others:** folate, GSH, oxidized glutathione
MRP2 (*ABCC2*)	Liver, Kidney, Intestine, BPB	Excretion of bilirubin glucuronide and GSH into bile	**Characteristics:** Amphiphilic with at least one negative net charge (similar to MRP1) **Anticancer drugs:** methotrexate, vincristine **Glutathione conjugates:** leukotriene C4, glutathione conjugate of ethacrynic acid **Glucuronide conjugates:** estradiol-17-D-glucuronide, bilirubin mono(or bis)glucuronide **Sulfate conjugate of bile salts:** taurolithocholate sulfate **Amphipathic organic anions:** statins, angiotensin II receptor antagonists, temocaprilat **HIV protease inhibitors:** indinavir, ritonavir **Others:** GSH, oxidized glutathione

TISSUE BINDING OF DRUGS (Cont.)

- Tissue binding is generally reversible and can serve as a reservoir that prolongs drug action in that same tissue or at a distant site reached through the circulation.
  ▸ Tissue binding and accumulation also can produce local toxicity.
- Many lipid-soluble drugs are stored by physical solution in the neutral fat; hence, fat may serve as a reservoir for lipid-soluble drugs.
- Some drugs, divalent metal ion chelating agents, and heavy metals may accumulate in bone by adsorption onto the bone crystal surface and eventual incorporation into the crystal lattice.

DRUG MEMBRANE TRANSPORTERS

- Transporters are membrane proteins that control the influx (uptake) of essential nutrients and ions, and the efflux of cellular waste, environmental toxins, drugs, and other xenobiotics.
- The functions of membrane transporters may be *facilitated* (*equilibrative*, not requiring energy) or *active* (requiring energy); see Figure 2-1.
- The transport of drugs is primarily mediated by 2 major superfamilies, ABC (ATP-binding cassette) and SLC (solute carrier) transporters.
  ▸ Most ABC proteins are primary active transporters, which rely on ATP hydrolysis to actively pump their substrates across membranes (Table 2-2).
    - There are 49 known genes for ABC protein which include *P*-glycoprotein (P-gp, encoded by *ABCB1*, also termed MDR1) and the cystic fibrosis transmembrane regulator (CFTR, encoded by *ABCC7*).
  ▸ The SLC superfamily includes genes that encode facilitated transporters and ion-coupled secondary active transporters (Table 2-3).
    - Approximately 315 SLC transporters have been identified in the human genome, many of which serve as drug targets or in drug absorption and disposition, including the serotonin (5-HT) and dopamine transporters (SERT, encoded by *SLC6A4*; DAT, encoded by *SLC6A3*).

(continues)

SECTION I — General Principles

DRUG MEMBRANE TRANSPORTERS (Cont.)

- Uptake and efflux transporters determine the plasma and tissue concentrations of endogenous compounds and xenobiotics, and thereby can influence the systemic or site-specific toxicity of drugs.
- Genetic mutations and polymorphisms in drug membrane transporters can lead to significant variability in individual patient drug disposition and response (for examples, see Table 2-4).

DISTRIBUTION OF DRUGS INTO THE CNS

- Distribution of drugs into the CNS from the blood is unique because:
  - Brain capillary endothelial cells have continuous tight junctions, thus drug penetration into the brain depends on transcellular rather than paracellular transport.
  - The BBB, which consists of brain capillary endothelial cells and pericapillary glial cells, have unique properties that limit drug transport.
  - At the choroid plexus, a blood-CSF barrier is present with epithelial cells that are joined by tight junctions, rather than endothelial cells.
- The more lipophilic a drug, the more likely it is to cross the BBB (see Case 2-1).
- Drugs may penetrate into the CNS by specific uptake transporters normally involved in the transport of nutrients and endogenous compounds from blood into the brain and CSF.
- The functional BBB and blood-CSF barrier involve efflux transporters that are capable of removing a large number of chemically diverse drugs from the CNS (see Figure 2-4, and Tables 2-2 and 2-3).
  - MDR1 (P-gp) and the organic anion–transporting polypeptide (OATP) are 2 of the more notable efflux transporters expressed in the BBB and blood-CSF barrier (BCSFB).
  - Efflux transporters are expressed in brain capillary endothelial cells and the choroid plexus.

TRANSPORTER NAME (GENE)	TISSUE DISTRIBUTION	PHYSIOLOGICAL FUNCTION	SUBSTRATES
MRP3 (*ABCC3*)	Liver Kidney Intestine	?	**Characteristics:** Amphiphilic with at least one negative net charge (Glucuronide conjugates are better substrates than glutathione conjugates.) **Anticancer drugs:** etoposide, methotrexate **Glutathione conjugates:** leukotriene C_4, glutathione conjugate of 15-deoxy-delta prostaglandin J2 **Glucuronide conjugates:** estradiol-17-D-glucuronide, etoposide glucuronide, morphine-3-glucuronide, morphine-6-glucuronide, acetaminophen glucuronide, hymecromone glucuronide, and harmol glucuronide **Sulfate conjugates of bile salts:** taurolithocholate sulfate **Bile salts:** glycocholate, taurocholate **Others:** folate, leucovorin
MRP4 (*ABCC4*)	Ubiquitous (Kidney, Prostate, Lung, Muscle, Pancreas, Testis, Ovary, Bladder, Gallbladder, BBB, BCSFB)	?	**Characteristics:** Nucleotide analogs **Anticancer drugs:** 6-mercaptopurine, methotrexate **Glucuronide conjugates:** estradiol-17-D-glucuronide **Sulfate conjugates:** dehydroepiandrosterone sulfate **Cyclic nucleotides:** cAMP, cGMP **Diuretics:** furosemide, trichlormethiazide **Antiviral drugs:** adefovir, tenofovir **Antibiotics:** cefazolin, ceftizoxime **Others:** folate, leucovorin, taurocholate (with GSH)
MRP5 (*ABCC5*)	Ubiquitous	?	**Characteristics:** Nucleotide analogs **Anticancer drugs:** 6-mercaptopurine **Cyclic nucleotides:** cAMP, cGMP **HIV protease inhibitors:** adefovir
MRP6 (*ABCC6*)	Liver Kidney	?	**Anticancer drugs:** doxorubicin*, etoposide* **Glutathione conjugates:** leukotriene C_4 **Other:** BQ-123 (cyclic peptide)
BCRP (MXR) (*ABCG2*)	Liver Intestine BBB	Normal heme metabolism/ transport during maturation of erythrocytes?	**Anticancer drugs:** methotrexate, mitoxantrone, camptothecins SN-38, topotecan, imatinib **Glucuronide conjugates:** 4-methylumbelliferone glucuronide, estradiol-17-D-glucuronide **Sulfate conjugates:** dehydroepiandrosterone sulfate, estrone-3-sulfate **Antibiotics:** nitrofurantoin, fluoroquinolones **Statins:** pitavastatin, rosuvastatin **Others:** cholesterol, estradiol, dantrolene, prazosin, sulfasalazine, phytoestrogens, PhIP, pheophorbide A

TRANSPORTER NAME (GENE)	TISSUE DISTRIBUTION	PHYSIOLOGICAL FUNCTION	SUBSTRATES
MDR3 (*ABCB4*)	Liver	Excretion of phospholipids into bile	**Characteristics:** Phospholipids
BSEP (*ABCB11*)	Liver	Excretion of bile salts into bile	**Characteristics:** Bile salts
ABCG5 and ABCG8	Liver Intestine	Excretion of plant sterols into bile and intestinal lumen	**Characteristics:** Plant sterols

Representative substrates and cytotoxic drugs with increased resistance (*) are included in this table (cytotoxicity with increased resistance is usually caused by the decreased accumulation of the drugs). Although MDR3 (*ABCB4*), BSEP (*ABCB11*), ABCG5, and ABCG8 are not directly involved in drug disposition, inhibition of these physiologically important ABC transporters will lead to unfavorable side effects.

BBB, blood-brain barrier; BTB, blood-testis barrier; BPB, blood-placental barrier; BCSFB, blood-cerebrospinal fluid barrier.

TABLE 2-3 Families in the Human Solute Carrier Superfamily

GENE NAME	FAMILY NAME	NUMBER OF FAMILY MEMBERS	SELECTED DRUG SUBSTRATES	EXAMPLES OF LINKED HUMAN DISEASES
SLC1	High-affinity glutamate and neutral amino acid transporter	7		Amyotrophic lateral sclerosis
SLC2	Facilitative GLUT transporter	14		
SLC3	Heavy subunits of the heteromeric amino acid transporters	2	Melphalan	Classic cystinuria type I
SLC4	Bicarbonate transporter	10		Hemolytic anemia, blindness-auditory impairment
SLC5	Na^+ glucose cotransporter	8	Dapagliflozin	Glucose-galactose malabsorption syndrome
SLC6	Na^+- and Cl^--dependent neurotransmitter transporter	16	Paraoxetine, fluoxetine	X-linked creatine deficiency syndrome
SLC7	Cationic amino acid transporter	14	Melphalan	Lysinuric protein intolerance
SLC8	Na^+/Ca^{2+} exchanger	3	N,N-Dimethylarginine	
SLC9	Na^+/H^+ exchanger	8	Thiazide diuretics	Congenital secretory diarrhea
SLC10	Na^+ bile salt cotransporter	6	Benzothiazepines	Primary bile salt malabsorption
SLC11	H^+ coupled metal ion transporter	2		Hereditary hemochromatosis
SLC12	Electroneutral cation-Cl^- cotransporter family	9		Gitelman's syndrome
SLC13	Na^+-sulfate/carboxylate cotransporter	5	Sulfate conjugates, cysteine conjugates	
SLC14	Urea transporter	2		Kidd antigen blood group
SLC15	H^+-oligopeptide cotransporter	4	Valacyclovir	

SECTION I General Principles

GENE NAME	FAMILY NAME	NUMBER OF FAMILY MEMBERS	SELECTED DRUG SUBSTRATES	EXAMPLES OF LINKED HUMAN DISEASES
SLC16	Monocarboxylate transporter	14	Salicylic acid, atorvastatin	Muscle weakness
SLC17	Vesicular glutamate transporter	8		Sialic acid storage disease
SLC18	Vesicular amine transporter	3	Reserpine	Myasthenic syndromes
SLC19	Folate/thiamine transporter	3	Methotrexate	Thiamine-responsive megaloblastic anemia
SLC20	Type III Na^+-phosphate cotransporter	2		
SLC21/SLC0	Organic anion transporter	11	Pravastatin	
SLC22	Organic cation/anion/zwitterion transporter	18	Pravastatin, metformin	Systemic carnitine deficiency syndrome
SLC23	Na^+-dependent ascorbate transporter	4	Vitamin C	
SLC24	$Na^+/(Ca^{2+}-K^+)$ exchanger	5		
SLC25	Mitochondrial carrier	27		Senger's syndrome
SLC26	Multifunctional anion exchanger	10	Salicylic acid, ciprofloxacin	Congenital Cl^--losing diarrhea
SLC27	Fatty acid transporter protein	6		
SLC28	Na^+-coupled nucleoside transport	3	Gemcitabine, cladribine	
SLC29	Facilitative nucleoside transporter	4	Dipyridamole, gemcitabine	
SLC30	Zinc efflux	9		
SLC31	Copper transporter	2	Cisplatin	
SLC32	Vesicular inhibitory amino acid transporter	1	Vigabatrin	
SLC33	Acetyl-CoA transporter	1		
SLC34	Type II Na^+-phosphate cotransporter	3		Autosomal-dominant hypophosphatemic rickets
SLC35	Nucleoside-sugar transporter	17		Leukocyte adhesion deficiency type II
SLC36	H^+-coupled amino acid transporter	4	D-Serine, cycloserine	
SLC37	Sugar-phosphate/phosphate exchanger	4		Glycogen storage disease (non-Ia)
SLC38	System A and N, Na^+-coupled neutral amino acid transporter	6		
SLC39	Metal ion transporter	14		Acrodermatitis enteropathica
SLC40	Basolateral iron transporter	1		Type IV hemochromatosis
SLC41	MgtE-like magnesium transporter	3		
SLC42	Rh ammonium transporter	3		Rh-null regulator
SLC43	Na^+-independent system-L-like amino acid transporter	2		

TABLE 2-4 Examples of Genetic Polymorphisms Influencing Drug Response

GENE PRODUCT (*GENE*)	DRUGS[a]	RESPONSES AFFECTED
Drug Metabolism and Transport		
CYP2C9	Tolbutamide, warfarin,[a] phenytoin, nonsteroidal anti-inflammatory	Anticoagulant effect of warfarin
CYP2C19	Mephenytoin, omeprazole, voriconazole,[a] hexobarbital, mephobarbital, propranolol, proguanil, phenytoin, clopidogrel	Peptic ulcer response to omeprazole; cardiovascular events after clopidogrel
CYP2D6	β blockers, antidepressants, anti-psychotics, codeine, debrisoquine, atomoxetine,[a] dextromethorphan, encainide, flecainide, fluoxetine, guanoxan, *N*-propylajmaline, perhexiline, phenacetin, phenformin, propafenone, sparteine, tamoxifen	Tardive dyskinesia from antipsychotics, narcotic side effects, codeine efficacy, imipramine dose requirement, β blocker effect; breast cancer recurrence after tamoxifen
CYP3A4/3A5/3A7	Macrolides, cyclosporine, tacrolimus, Ca^{2+} channel blockers, midazolam, terfenadine, lidocaine, dapsone, quinidine, triazolam, etoposide, teniposide, lovastatin, alfentanil, tamoxifen, steroids	Efficacy of immunosuppressive effects of tacrolimus
Dihydropyrimidine dehydrogenase	Fluorouracil, capecitabine[a]	5-Fluorouracil toxicity
N-acetyltransferase (*NAT2*)	Isoniazid, hydralazine, sulfonamides, amonafide, procainamide, dapsone, caffeine	Hypersensitivity to sulfonamides, amonafide toxicity, hydralazine-induced lupus, isoniazid neurotoxicity
Glutathione transferases (*GSTM1, GSTT1, GSTP1*)	Several anticancer agents	Decreased response in breast cancer, more toxicity and worse response in acute myelogenous leukemia
Thiopurine methyltransferase (*TPMT*)	Mercaptopurine,[a] thioguanine,[a] azathioprine[a]	Thiopurine toxicity and efficacy, risk of second cancers
UDP-glucuronosyl-transferase (*UGT1A1*)	Irinotecan,[a] bilirubin	Irinotecan toxicity
P-glycoprotein (*ABCB1*)	Natural product anticancer drugs, HIV protease inhibitors, digoxin	Decreased CD4 response in HIV-infected patients, decreased digoxin AUC, drug resistance in epilepsy
UGT2B7	Morphine	Morphine plasma levels
Organic anion transporter (*SLCO1B1*)	Statins, methotrexate, ACE inhibitors	Statin plasma levels, myopathy; methotrexate plasma levels, mucositis
COMT	Levodopa	Enhanced drug effect
Organic cation transporter (*SLC22A1, OCT1*)	Metformin	Pharmacologic effect and pharmacokinetics
Organic cation transporter (*SLC22A2, OCT2*)	Metformin	Renal clearance
Novel organic cation transporter (*SLC22A4, OCTN1*)	Gabapentin	Renal clearance
CYP2B6	Cyclophosphamide	Ovarian failure

[a] Information on genetics-based dosing, adverse events, or testing added to FDA-approved drug label.

| SECTION I | General Principles |

METABOLISM (BIOTRANSFORMATION) OF DRUGS

- The majority of therapeutic agents are lipophilic compounds filtered through the glomerulus and reabsorbed into the systemic circulation during passage through the renal tubules.
- The metabolism of drugs and other xenobiotics into more hydrophilic metabolites is essential for their elimination from the body, as well as for termination of their biological and pharmacological activity.
- In general, *biotransformation* reactions generate more polar, inactive metabolites that are readily excreted from the body through the urine or bile, but in some cases, metabolites with potent biological activity or toxic properties are generated.
- Drug metabolism or biotransformation reactions are classified as either phase I functionalization reactions or phase II biosynthetic (conjugation) reactions.
  ▸ *Phase 1 functionalization* reactions introduce or expose a functional group on the parent compound through oxidation, reduction, or hydrolytic reactions and generally result in the loss of pharmacological activity, although there are examples of retention or enhancement of activity.
    - Phase 1 enzymes lead to the introduction of functional groups such as –OH, –COOH, –SH, –O–, or NH_2.
    - *Prodrugs* are pharmacologically inactive compounds that are converted rapidly to biologically active metabolites, often by the hydrolysis of an ester or amide linkage.
  ▸ *Phase 2 conjugation* reactions lead to the formation of highly polar conjugates by covalent linkage of a functional group on the parent compound or phase I metabolite and endogenously derived glucuronic acid, sulfate, glutathione, amino acids, or acetate.
- Drugs that are poorly metabolized remain in the body for longer periods of time and their pharmacokinetic profiles show much longer elimination half-lives than drugs that are rapidly metabolized.

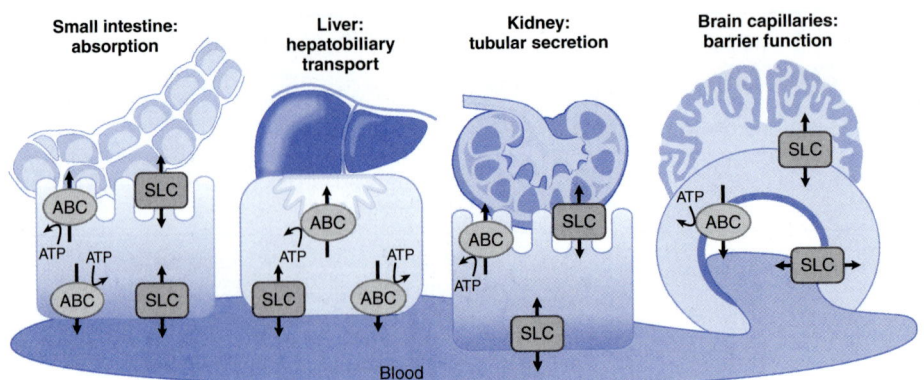

FIGURE 2-4 Transepithelial or transendothelial flux. Transepithelial or transendothelial flux of drugs requires distinct transporters at the 2 surfaces of the epithelial or endothelial barriers. These are depicted diagrammatically for transport across the small intestine (absorption), the kidney and liver (elimination), and the brain capillaries that comprise the BBB. Asymmetrical transport across a monolayer of polarized cells, such as the epithelial and endothelial cells of brain capillaries, is called vectorial transport. Vectorial transport is important in the efficient transfer of solutes across epithelial or endothelial barriers. From the viewpoint of drug absorption and disposition, vectorial transport plays a major role in hepatobiliary and urinary excretion of drugs from the blood to the lumen and in the intestinal absorption of drugs. In addition, efflux of drugs from the brain via brain endothelial cells and brain choroid plexus epithelial cells involves vectorial transport. The ABC transporters mediate only unidirectional efflux, whereas SLC transporters mediate either drug uptake or efflux.

of the drug. This variability reflects, at least in part, genetic polymorphisms in the CYPs involved in the metabolic activation of clopidogrel, most importantly CYP2C19. Clopidogrel-treated patients with the loss-of-function CYP2C19*2 allele exhibit reduced platelet inhibition compared with those with the wild-type CYP2C19*1 allele and experience a higher rate of cardiovascular events. Even patients with the reduced-function CYP2C19*3, *4, or *5 alleles may derive less benefit from clopidogrel than those with the full-function CYP2C19*1 allele. Although CYP3A4 also contributes to the metabolic activation of clopidogrel, polymorphisms in this enzyme do not appear to influence clopidogrel responsiveness.

b. What kinds of pharmacokinetic drug interactions might be expected with clopidogrel?

CYP2C19 is responsible for metabolizing a number of drugs (see Table 2-4) and there are potential drug interactions that can occur among these drugs. For example, omeprazole, a protein pump inhibitor, which is used to reduce gastric acidity (see Chapter 32), is also metabolized by CYP2C19 and can act as a CYP2C19 inhibitor. Concomitant administration of omeprazole and other proton pump inhibitors that are inhibitors of CYP2C19, with clopidogrel, produces a small reduction in the inhibitory effects of clopidogrel on platelet aggregation. This reduction in the antiplatelet effects of clopidogrel can increase the risk of cardiovascular events.

CASE 2-4

Acetaminophen is among the most widely used drugs and is an active ingredient in many over-the-counter analgesics and cold medications, as well as in many prescription products in combination with codeine and other analgesics.

a. How is acetaminophen normally metabolized?

Although many drugs require prior oxidative metabolism by phase 1 enzymes, acetaminophen and some other drugs can undergo phase 2 conjugation (glucuronidation and/or sulfation) without prior oxidative metabolism (see Table 2-6). One of

(Continued)

the important phase 2 enzymes that metabolizes acetaminophen are the sulfotransferase (SULT) SULT1 isoforms that are recognized as phenol SULTs, because they catalyze the sulfation of phenolic molecules such as acetaminophen, minoxidil, and 17α-ethinyl estradiol.

b. **Package labels on products containing acetaminophen warn of possible liver damage when daily dosing of acetaminophen exceeds 4000 mg. What is the mechanism of liver toxicity by acetaminophen?**

Acetaminophen, which is normally metabolized by glucuronidation and sulfation, is also a substrate for oxidative metabolism by CYP2E1 and CYP3A4, which generate the toxic metabolite N-acetyl-p-benzoquinone imine (NAPQI) that, under normal dosing, is readily neutralized through conjugation with glutathione (GSH). However, an overdose of acetaminophen can lead to depletion of cellular GSH levels, thereby increasing the potential for NAPQI to interact with other cellular components resulting in toxicity and cell death. Acetaminophen toxicity is associated with increased levels of NAPQI and hepatic necrosis (see Chapter 3).

CASE 2-5

A 26-year-old woman is filling a prescription for oral contraceptives and is asked by her pharmacist whether she is taking any other medications, including herbal remedies. The woman tells the pharmacist that she takes St John's wort, an over-the-counter herbal remedy used for depression.

a. **What are the possible drug interactions that might occur with St. John's wort?**

Hyperforin, a component of St. John's wort, activates a type 2 nuclear receptor, the pregnane X receptor (PXR). The type 2 nuclear receptors include the pregnane X receptor (PXR), constitutive androstane receptor (CAR), and the peroxisome

(Continued)

BIOTRANSFORMING ENZYMES (Xenobiotic-Metabolizing Enzymes; Table 2-5)

- Phase 1 oxidation reactions are carried out by cytochrome P-450s (CYPs), flavin-containing monooxygenases (FMO), and epoxide hydrolases (EH).
- Phase 2 enzymes include the glutathione-S-transferases (GST), UDP-glucuronosyltransferases (UGT), sulfotransferases (SULT), N-acetyltransferases (NAT), and methyltransferases (MT).
  - Conjugation reactions usually require the substrate to have oxygen (hydroxyl or epoxide groups), nitrogen, or sulfur atoms that serve as acceptor sites for a hydrophilic moiety, such as glutathione, glucuronic acid, sulfate, or an acetyl group.
- Xenobiotic metabolizing enzymes are found in most tissues in the body with the highest levels located in the GI tract (liver, small and large intestines).
  - The liver is considered the major "metabolic clearing house" for both endogenous chemicals (eg, cholesterol, steroid hormones, fatty acids, and proteins) and xenobiotics.
  - Drugs that are orally administered are absorbed by the gut and taken to the liver through the portal vein.
  - Xenobiotic-metabolizing enzymes located in the epithelial cells of the GI tract are responsible for the initial metabolic processing of most oral medications.
  - Following oral administration of a drug, a significant portion of the dose may be metabolically inactivated in either the intestinal epithelium or the liver before the drug reaches the systemic circulation; this so-called *first-pass metabolism* significantly limits the oral bioavailability of highly metabolized drugs.
  - Tissues of the nasal mucosa and lung play important roles in the metabolism of drugs that are administered through aerosol sprays and are also the first line of contact with hazardous chemicals that are airborne.
- Phase 1 oxidation enzymes are located primarily in the endoplasmic reticulum, whereas the phase 2 conjugation enzyme systems are mainly cytosolic.

TABLE 2-5 Xenobiotic Metabolizing Enzymes

ENZYMES	REACTIONS
Phase 1 "oxygenases"	
Cytochrome P450s (P450 or CYP)	C and O oxidation, dealkylation, others
Flavin-containing monooxygenases (FMO)	N, S, and P oxidation
Epoxide hydrolases (mEH, sEH)	Hydrolysis of epoxides
Phase 2 "transferases"	
Sulfotransferases (SULT)	Addition of sulfate
UDP-glucuronosyltransferases (UGT)	Addition of glucuronic acid
Glutathione-S-transferases (GST)	Addition of glutathione
N-acetyltransferases (NAT)	Addition of acetyl group
Methyltransferases (MT)	Addition of methyl group
Other enzymes	
Alcohol dehydrogenases	Reduction of alcohols
Aldehyde dehydrogenases	Reduction of aldehydes
NADPH-quinone oxidoreductase (NQO)	Reduction of quinones

mEH and sEH are microsomal and soluble epoxide hydrolase. UDP, uridine diphosphate; NADPH, reduced nicotinamide adenine dinucleotide phosphate.

SECTION I

CYTOCHROME P-450 SUPERFAMILY: THE CYPS

- The CYPs are a superfamily of enzymes, all of which contain a molecule of heme that is noncovalently bound to the polypeptide chain.
- CYPs use O_2, plus H^+ derived from the cofactor-reduced nicotinamide adenine dinucleotide phosphate (NADPH), to carry out the oxidation of substrates.
- CYPs catalyze diverse reactions, including N-dealkylation, O-dealkylation, aromatic hydroxylation, N-oxidation, S-oxidation, deamination, and dehalogenation (Table 2-6).
- The CYPs are promiscuous in their capacity to bind and metabolize multiple substrates; extensive overlapping substrate specificities by the CYPs is one of the underlying reasons for the predominance of drug–drug interactions involving drugs metabolized by CYPs.
  - When 2 coadministered drugs are both metabolized by a single CYP, they compete for binding to the enzyme's active site which can result in the inhibition of metabolism of 1 or both of the drugs, leading to elevated plasma levels.
- There are 57 putatively functional CYP genes in humans, which are named with the root CYP followed by a number designating the family, a letter denoting the subfamily, and another number designating the CYP form (eg, *CYP3A4* is family 3, subfamily A, and gene number 4).
- Most drugs are metabolized by only 12 CYPs (CYP1A1, 1A2, 1B1, 2A6, 2B6, 2C8, 2C9, 2C19, 2D6, 2E1, 3A4, and 3A5; see Figure 2-5).
  - The most active drug-metabolizing-CYPs are those in the CYP2C, CYP2D, and CYP3A subfamilies.
- CYP3A4, the most abundantly expressed CYP in liver, is involved in the metabolism of more than 50% of clinically used drugs (see Figure 2-5).
  - CYP1A, CYP1B, CYP2A, CYP2B, and CYP2E subfamilies are not significantly involved in the metabolism of therapeutic drugs, but they do catalyze the metabolic activation of many protoxins and procarcinogens to their ultimate reactive metabolites.

(continues)

General Principles

proliferator-activated receptors (PPARs). PXR, discovered because it is activated by the synthetic steroid pregnenolone-16α-carbonitrile, is also activated by a number of other drugs, including antibiotics (rifampicin and troleandomycin), Ca^{2+} channel blockers (nifedipine), statins (mevastatin), antidiabetic drugs (troglitazone), HIV protease inhibitors (ritonavir), and anticancer drugs (paclitaxel).

Activated PXR is an inducer of CYP3A4, which can metabolize steroids found in oral contraceptives. PXR also induces the expression of genes encoding certain drug transporters and phase 2 enzymes, including UDP-glucuronosyltransferases (UGTs) and sulfotransferases (SULTs). Thus, PXR facilitates the metabolism and elimination of many xenobiotics, including drugs, with notable consequences (see Figure 2-6).

b. How might concomitant administration of St. John's wort affect the efficacy of drugs this patient might be taking such as the oral contraceptives?

By activating PXR and inducing the expression CYP3A4, drugs that are metabolized by CYP3A4 will be cleared more quickly. CYP3A4 is the most abundantly expressed CYP in the liver and is responsible for metabolizing ~50% of all clinically useful drugs (see Figure 2-5 and Side Bar CYTOCHROME P-450 SUPERFAMILY: THE CYPS). Thus, the efficacy of the oral contraceptives this woman will be taking will be reduced, increasing the chance of an unplanned pregnancy.

CASE 2-6

A 63-year-old, 84-kg man with mild heart failure is started on a pharmacotherapy regimen with digoxin to improve cardiac output (see Chapter 17).

a. After administration of an intravenous dose of 500 μg of digoxin, the plasma concentration of drug is determined to be 0.75 ng/mL. What is the volume of distribution of digoxin in this patient?

Dividing the amount of drug in the body by the plasma concentration yields a volume of distribution for digoxin of ~667 L, or a value ~13 times greater than the total-body volume of an 84-kg man.

b. What might account for this surprisingly large volume of distribution?

Digoxin distributes preferentially to muscle and adipose tissue and to its specific receptors (Na^+, K^+-ATPase), leaving a very small amount of drug in the plasma to be measured. For drugs that are bound extensively to plasma proteins but that are not bound to tissue components, the volume of distribution will approach that of the plasma volume because drug bound to plasma protein is measurable in the assay of most drugs. In contrast, certain drugs have high volumes of distribution even though most of the drugs in the circulation are bound to albumin because these drugs are also sequestered elsewhere.

The volume of distribution may vary widely depending on the relative degrees of binding to high-affinity receptor sites, plasma and tissue proteins, the partition coefficient of the drug in fat, and accumulation in poorly perfused tissues. As might be expected, the volume of distribution for a given drug can differ according to patient's age, gender, body composition, and presence of disease.

c. How would the maintenance dose of oral digoxin be calculated in order to gradually bring this patient to therapeutic plasma concentrations?

A steady-state plasma concentration of 0.7 to 0.9 ng/mL is selected as an appropriate conservative target based on prior knowledge of the action of the drug in patients with heart failure to maintain levels at or below the 0.5 to 1.0 ng/mL range. Equation 2-11 (p. 38), the patient's creatinine clearance rate (CL_{CR} = 56 mL/min), and digoxin pharmacokinetic values (see Appendix II Design Optimization of Dosage Regimens: Pharmacokinetic Data in *Goodman and Gilman's*

(Continued)

Pharmacokinetics CHAPTER 2

The Pharmacological Basis of Therapeutics, 12th Edition) such as clearance ($CL = 0.88 \cdot CL_{CR} + 0.33$) and oral bioavailability ($F = 0.7 \pm 13$) are used to calculate the appropriate dosing rate, as described in the section on Maintenance Dose in Chapter 2 in *Goodman and Gilman's The Pharmacological Basis of Therapeutics*, 12th Edition. Digoxin clearance in this patient is estimated to be 77 mL/min (4.6 L/h). Using Equation 2-11, the maintenance dosing rate for this 84-kg man is calculated to be 0.12 mg/24 h (for details of the calculation, see Example in the Maintenance Dose section of Chapter 2 in *Goodman and Gilman's The Pharmacological Basis of Therapeutics*, 12th Edition).

In practice, the dosing rate would be rounded to the closest dosage size, 0.125 mg/24 h, which would result in a steady-state plasma concentration of 0.78 ng/mL (0.75 × 125/120). Digoxin is a well-characterized example of a drug that is difficult to dose and must be monitored regularly. While guidelines based on calculations of the sort suggested here are useful, it is clear that tablet sizes are limiting and tablet sizes intermediate to those available are often needed. Because the coefficient of variation for the clearance equation when used for digoxin treatment in this patient group is large (52%), it is common for patients who are not monitored regularly to require hospital admission to adjust medication. Monitoring the clinical status of patients (new or increased ankle edema, inability to sleep in a recumbent position, decreased exercise tolerance), whether accomplished by home health follow-up or regular visits to the clinician, is essential to avoid untoward results.

d. Digoxin has a narrow therapeutic index, and plasma levels ≤1.0 ng/mL usually are associated with efficacy and minimal toxicity. What are the maximum and minimum plasma concentrations associated with once-daily dosing with 0.125 mg of digoxin?

This calculation first requires estimation of digoxin's volume of distribution based on available pharmacokinetic data (Appendix II) and an estimate of digoxin's elimination $t_{1/2}$ as described in the Example in the section on Dosing Interval for Intermittent Dosage in Chapter 2 of *Goodman and Gilman's The Pharmacological Basis of Therapeutics*, 12th Edition. With once-daily dosing, the plasma concentrations would fluctuate minimally (0.7-0.88 ng/mL) about the steady-state concentration of 0.78 ng/mL, well within the recommended therapeutic range of 0.5-1.0 ng/mL. If twice the daily dose (2 × 0.125 mg) was given every other day, the average steady-state concentration would remain at 0.78 ng/mL, while the predicted maximum concentration would be 0.98 ng/mL and the minimum concentration would be 0.62 ng/mL. While this result would maintain a therapeutic concentration and avoid large excursions from the average steady-state concentration between doses, it does not favor patient compliance. Dosing must be compatible with the patient's routine and every other day dosing is problematic in this patient population.

e. After starting the patient on a maintenance dose of 0.125 mg of digoxin each day, how long will it take to reach a steady-state therapeutic level?

The rule of thumb for most drugs is that the time to reach 94% of steady-state concentrations after starting or changing dosing is four half-lives. Using Equation 2-10 (p. 38), the $t_{1/2}$ is 3.1 days (for details of the calculation, see Example in the Dosing Interval for Intermittent Dosage section of Chapter 2 in *Goodman and Gilman's The Pharmacological Basis of Therapeutics*, 12th Edition). Thus, it will take at least 12 days to reach steady-state concentrations of drug in this patient.

If target concentrations of drug need to be achieved more rapidly, it may be possible to use a loading dose. In the case of this patient, Equation 2-12 (p. 39) would be used to develop a loading dose strategy (for details of the calculation, see Example in the Loading Dose section of Chapter 2 in *Goodman and Gilman's The Pharmacological Basis of Therapeutics*, 12th Edition). Here a target C_p of 0.9 ng/mL is chosen as a target below the recommended maximum of 1.0 ng/mL. To avoid toxicity, this oral loading dose, would be given as an initial 0.25-mg dose followed by a 0.25-mg

(Continued)

CYTOCHROME P-450 SUPERFAMILY: THE CYPS *(Cont.)*

- There are large differences in levels of expression of each CYP among individuals due to the presence of genetic polymorphisms and differences in gene regulation.
- Human CYP genes that exhibit polymorphisms include *CYP2A6, CYP2C9, CYP2C19,* and *CYP2D6* (see Table 2-4).
- Some drugs are ligands for nuclear receptors and act as CYP inducers that can increase not only their own rates of metabolism, but also induce metabolism of other coadministered drugs (see Table 2-7 and Figure 2-6).
  - One potential consequence of CYP induction is a decrease in plasma drug concentration over the course of treatment, resulting in loss of drug efficacy.
  - In addition to inducing CYPs, drugs that are ligands for nuclear receptors can induce the transcription of a battery of target genes that affect pharmacokinetics, including drug transporters and phase 2 enzymes, which can lead to a variety of drug interactions.
  - CYP induction may also increase the rate of metabolic activation of protoxins and carcinogens, resulting in increased toxicity and carcinogenesis.
  - CYP3A4 is induced by nuclear receptors pregnane X receptor (PXR) and constitutive androstane receptor (CAR), thus its level is highly influenced by a number of drugs and other xenobiotics.

SECTION I — General Principles

TABLE 2-6 Major Reactions Involved in Drug Metabolism

REACTION		EXAMPLES
I. Oxidative reactions		
N-Dealkylation	$RNHCH_3 \rightarrow RNH_2 + CH_2O$	Imipramine, diazepam, codeine, erythromycin, morphine, tamoxifen, theophylline, caffeine
O-Dealkylation	$ROCH_3 \rightarrow ROH + CH_2O$	Codeine, indomethacin, dextromethorphan
Aliphatic hydroxylation	$RCH_2CH_3 \rightarrow RCHOHCH_3$	Tolbutamide, ibuprofen, phenobarbital, meprobamate, cyclosporine, midazolam
Aromatic hydroxylation	(arene → arene oxide → phenol)	Phenytoin, phenobarbital, propanolol, ethinyl estradiol, amphetamine, warfarin
N-Oxidation	$RNH_2 \rightarrow RNHOH$; $R_1R_2NH \rightarrow R_1R_2N{-}OH$	Chlorpheniramine, dapsone, meperidine
S-Oxidation	$R_1R_2S \rightarrow R_1R_2S{=}O$	Cimetidine, chlorpromazine, thioridazine, omeprazole
Deamination	$RCH(NH_2)CH_3 \rightarrow R{-}C(OH)(NH_2){-}CH_3 \rightarrow R{-}C({=}O){-}CH_3 + NH_3$	Diazepam, amphetamine
II. Hydrolysis reactions	(arene oxide → trans-dihydrodiol)	Carbamazepine (see Figure 6-4)
	$R_1COR_2 \rightarrow R_1COOH + R_2OH$	Procaine, aspirin, clofibrate, meperidine, enalapril, cocaine
	$R_1CNHR_2 \rightarrow R_1COOH + R_2NH_2$	Lidocaine, procainamide, indomethacin
III. Conjugation reactions		
Glucuronidation	$R + \text{UDP-glucuronic acid} \rightarrow R{-}O{-}\text{glucuronide} + UDP$	Acetaminophen, morphine, oxazepam, lorazepam
Sulfation	$PAPS + ROH \rightarrow R{-}O{-}SO_2{-}OH + PAP$	Acetaminophen, steroids, methyldopa
Acetylation	$CoAS{-}CO{-}CH_3 + RNH_2 \rightarrow RNH{-}CO{-}CH_3 + CoA{-}SH$	Sulfonamides, isoniazid, dapsone, clonazepam
Methylation	$RO{-}, RS{-}, RN{-} + AdoMet \rightarrow RO{-}CH_3 + AdoHomCys$	L-Dopa, methyldopa, mercaptopurine, captopril
Glutathionylation	$GSH + R \rightarrow R{-}GSH$	Adriamycin, fosfomycin, busulfan

PAPS, 3'-phosphoadenosine-5' phosphosulfate; PAP 3'-phosphoadenosine-5'-phosphate.

Pharmacokinetics

CHAPTER 2

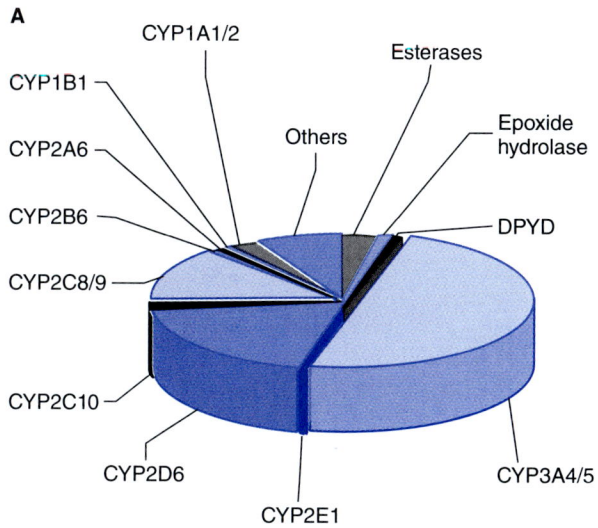

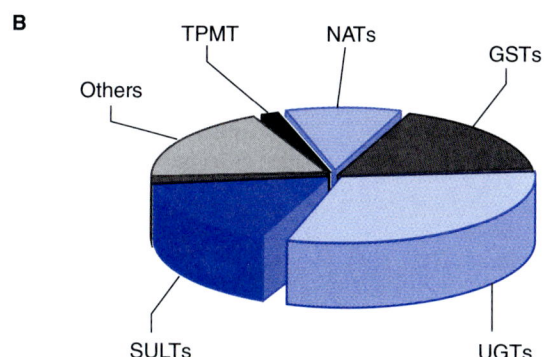

FIGURE 2-5 The fraction of clinically used drugs metabolized by the major phase 1 and phase 2 enzymes. The relative size of each pie section represents the estimated percentage of drugs metabolized by the major phase 1 (panel **A**) and phase 2 (panel **B**) enzymes, based on studies in the literature. In some cases, more than a single enzyme is responsible for metabolism of a single drug. CYP, cytochrome P-450; DPYD, dihydropyrimidine dehydrogenase; GST, glutathione-S-transferase; NAT, N-acetyltransferase; SULT, sulfotransferase; TPMT, thiopurine methyltransferase; UGT, UDP-glucuronosyltransferase

TABLE 2-7 Nuclear Receptors That Induce Drug Metabolism

RECEPTOR	LIGANDS
Aryl hydrocarbon receptor (AHR)	Omeprazole
Constitutive androstane receptor (CAR)	Phenobarbital
Pregnane X receptor (PXR)	Rifampin
Farnesoid X receptor (FXR)	Bile acids
Vitamin D receptor	Vitamin D
Peroxisome proliferator activated receptor (PPAR)	Fibrates
Retinoic acid receptor (RAR)	*all-trans*-Retinoic acid
Retinoid X receptor (RXR)	9-*cis*-Retinoic acid

EXCRETION OF DRUGS

- Drugs are eliminated from the body either unchanged by the process of excretion or converted to metabolites.
- Excretory organs, the lung excluded, eliminate polar compounds more efficiently than substances with high lipid solubility.
  ▸ Lipid-soluble drugs thus are not readily eliminated until they are metabolized to more polar compounds.
- The most important organ for excreting drugs and their metabolites is the kidney.
  ▸ Excretion of drugs and metabolites in the urine involves 3 distinct processes:
    - Glomerular filtration
    - Active tubular secretion
    - Passive tubular reabsorption
- Substances excreted in the feces are principally unabsorbed orally ingested drugs or drug metabolites excreted either in the bile or secreted directly into the intestinal tract and not reabsorbed.
- Excretion from the lung is important mainly for the elimination of anesthetic gases.
- Drugs excreted in breast milk are potential sources of unwanted pharmacological effects in the nursing infant.

CLINICAL PHARMACOKINETICS

- Clinical pharmacokinetics attempts to provide a quantitative relationship between dose and effect, and a framework within which to interpret measurements of concentrations of drugs in biological fluids and their adjustment through changes in dosing for the benefit of the patient.
- The 4 most important parameters governing drug disposition are:
  ▸ *Bioavailability*, the fraction of drug absorbed as such into the systemic circulation
  ▸ *Volume of distribution*, a measure of the apparent space in the body available to contain the drug based on how much is given versus what is found in the systemic circulation
  ▸ *Clearance*, a measure of the body's efficiency in eliminating drug from the systemic circulation

(*continues*)

33

SECTION I

General Principles

CLINICAL PHARMACOKINETICS (Cont.)

- *Elimination $t_{1/2}$,* the time it takes for the plasma concentration of a drug to be reduced by 50% and a measure of the rate of removal of drug from the systemic circulation

VOLUME OF DISTRIBUTION

- The volume of distribution (*V*) relates the amount of drug in the body to the concentration of drug (*C*) in the blood or plasma.
  - The volume of distribution defined in Equation 2-2 considers the body as a single homogeneous compartment (ie, a one-compartment model), in which all drug administration occurs directly into the central compartment, and distribution of drug is instantaneous throughout the volume (*V*).

  Amount of drug in body / *V* = *C* or
  V = amount of drug in the body / *C*
  (Equation 2-2)

- A drug's volume of distribution therefore reflects the extent to which it is present in extravascular tissues and not in the plasma.
- It is reasonable to view *V* as an imaginary volume, because for many drugs the volume of distribution exceeds the known volume of any and all body compartments.
- For drugs that are bound extensively to plasma proteins but that are not bound to tissue components, the volume of distribution will approach that of the plasma volume because drug bound to plasma protein is measurable in the assay of most drugs.
- Certain drugs have high volumes of distribution even though most of the drug in the circulation is bound to albumin because these drugs are also sequestered elsewhere.
- The volume of distribution may vary widely depending on:
  - The relative degrees of binding to high-affinity receptor sites, plasma, and tissue proteins
  - The partition coefficient of the drug in fat
  - Accumulation in poorly perfused tissues
- The volume of distribution for a given drug can differ according to a patient's:
  - Age
  - Gender
  - Body composition
  - Presence of disease

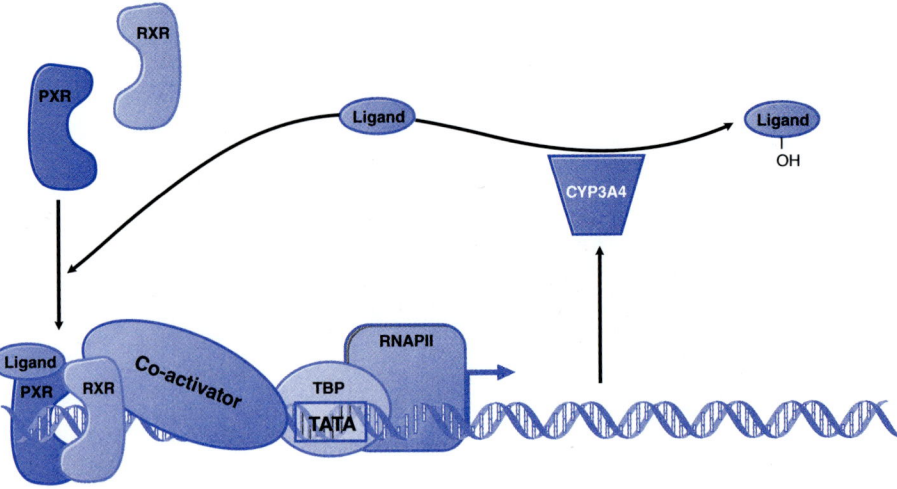

FIGURE 2-6 Induction of drug metabolism by nuclear receptor–mediated signal transduction. When a drug such as atorvastatin (Ligand) enters the cell, it can bind to a nuclear receptor such as the pregnane X receptor (PXR). PXR then forms a complex with the retinoid X receptor (RXR), binds to DNA upstream of target genes, recruits coactivator (which binds to the TATA box binding protein, TBP), and activates transcription by RNA polymerase II (RNAP II). Among PXR target genes are *CYP3A4*, which can metabolize the atorvastatin and decrease its cellular concentration. Thus, atorvastatin induces its own metabolism.

dose 6 to 8 hours later, with careful monitoring of the patient and the final 0.125-mg dose given 12 to 14 hours later.

f. If the patient's creatinine clearance was 20 mL/min, how would this affect the loading dose?

As shown in Equation 2-12 (p. 39), drug elimination rate is not a factor in determining the loading dose. Thus, the loading dose for a patient with renal insufficiency would be the same for a patient with normal renal function. However, the maintenance dose would have to be adjusted for the decreased clearance of the digoxin.

Additional information and examples regarding individualizing dosing for a given patient are provided in Appendix II of *Goodman and Gilman's The Pharmacological Basis of Therapeutics*, 12th Edition.

KEY CONCEPTS

➡ Understanding and employing pharmacokinetic principles can increase the probability of therapeutic success and reduce the occurrence of adverse drug effects.

➡ Absorption of drug from its site of administration into the central compartment is the first step in the drug reaching its site of action; bioavailability is the fractional extent to which an administered dose is absorbed and reaches its site of action.

➡ After absorption, a drug typically distributes most rapidly to well-perfused tissues (liver, kidney, brain), and more slowly to muscle, most viscera, skin, and fat.

➡ Tissue distribution is also determined by physicochemical properties of a drug, including lipid solubility, drug ionization, and the relative binding of drug to plasma proteins and tissue macromolecules.

➡ While many phase 1 reactions result in the biological inactivation of the drug, phase 2 reactions produce a metabolite with improved water solubility, a change that facilitates the elimination of the drug from the tissue, normally via efflux transporters.

Pharmacokinetics

CHAPTER 2

- Lipid-soluble drugs are not readily excreted until they are metabolized to more polar compounds.
- The kidney is the most important organ for excreting drugs and their metabolites.
- Pharmacokinetic drug–drug interactions are among the leading causes of adverse drug reactions (ADRs).
- When a constant drug dosage is given, steady state is not reached until at least four half-lives have passed.
- Genetic polymorphisms in membrane transporters and drug metabolizing enzymes can result in marked inter-patient responses to drugs, including serious drug toxicities.

SUMMARY QUIZ

QUESTION 2-1 The term "first-pass effect" refers to the
a. effect a new drug has on the body after its first administration.
b. time it takes for a drug to be detected in the urine or feces after oral administration.
c. ability of the intestines and liver to reduce the bioavailability of a drug.
d. time it takes for a drug to reach therapeutic concentrations in the target tissue.
e. initial effect a drug has on target tissues.

QUESTION 2-2 The term "blood-brain barrier" (BBB) refers to a
a. noncellular barrier that prevents drugs from entering the CNS unless transported by specific carriers.
b. cellular barrier that includes brain capillary endothelial cells that limits drug entry into the brain.
c. virtual or conceptual barrier that can explain the behavior of some drug effects on the CNS.
d. physical barrier that prevents blood from entering the brain.
e. device that is used to prevent blood-borne drugs from entering the brain.

QUESTION 2-3 Phase 1 drug metabolism differs from phase 2 metabolism in that
a. phase 1 metabolism always occurs prior to phase 2 metabolism.
b. phase 1 metabolism occurs in the intestine where orally administered drugs can first be metabolized, whereas phase 2 metabolism occurs in the blood.
c. phase 1 metabolism occurs in the liver soon after a drug is absorbed, whereas phase 2 metabolism occurs after a drug is excreted into the urine.
d. phase 1 metabolic enzymes activate prodrugs, whereas phase 2 metabolic enzymes inactivate drugs.
e. phase 1 metabolic reactions functionalize drugs, whereas phase 2 metabolic reactions conjugate drugs.

QUESTION 2-4 The most important pharmacokinetic concept to consider when designing a rational long-term pharmacotherapy is
a. bioavailability.
b. route of administration.
c. volume of distribution.
d. clearance.
e. elimination $t_{1/2}$.

DRUG CLEARANCE

- Clearance from the system circulation (CL) is the most important concept to consider when designing a long-term drug *dosing rate* that maintains *steady-state concentrations of a drug* (C_{ss}) within a *therapeutic window* (see Chapter 1 for definition of therapeutic window).
  - Assuming complete bioavailability, the steady-state concentration of drug in the body (C_{ss}) will be achieved when the rate of drug elimination (CL) equals the rate of drug administration (dosing rate) as described in Equation 2-3.

  $$\text{Dosing rate} = CL \cdot C_{ss}$$
  (Equation 2-3)

  - Systems for elimination of drugs such as metabolizing enzymes and transporters usually are not saturated, thus the absolute rate of elimination of the drug is essentially a linear function of its concentration in plasma (first-order kinetics), where a constant fraction of drug in the body is eliminated per unit of time.
  - If mechanisms for elimination of a given drug become saturated, the kinetics approach zero-order, in which a constant amount of drug is eliminated per unit of time, and the relationship of clearance (CL) to drug concentration (C) is described by Equation 2-4 which is analogous to the Michaelis-Menten equation where K_m represents the concentration at which half the maximal rate of elimination is reached (in units of mass/volume) and v_m is equal to the maximal rate of elimination (in units of mass/time).

  $$CL = v_m / (K_m + C) \quad \text{(Equation 2-4)}$$

  - Clearance of a drug (CL) is its rate of elimination by all routes normalized to the concentration of drug (C) in some biological fluid where measurement can be made as described in Equation 2-5.

  $$CL = \text{rate of elimination}/C$$
  (Equation 2-5)

  (continues)

SECTION I

General Principles

DRUG CLEARANCE (Cont.)

- For a single dose of a drug with complete bioavailability and first-order kinetics of elimination, systemic clearance may be determined from mass balance and the integration of Equation 2-5 over time as described in Equation 2-6 where AUC is the total area under the curve of drug concentration in the systemic circulation as a function of time from time zero to infinity as shown in Figure 2-7.

$$CL = Dose / AUC$$
(Equation 2-6)

RATE OF DISTRIBUTION AND EQUILIBRIUM OF DRUG INTO TISSUES

- The rate of distribution and equilibration of a drug into a tissue will depend on the ratio of the perfusion of the tissue to the partition of drug into the tissue.
- In many cases, groups of tissues with similar perfusion-partition ratios all equilibrate at essentially the same rate such that only one apparent phase of distribution is seen.
- If plasma and tissue reservoirs are in rapid equilibrium, drug distribution will appear as being in a single "central" compartment (see Figure 2-3).
- Clearance of drug from a single central compartment occurs in a first-order fashion, as defined in Equation 2-5.
- The decline of drug plasma concentration (C) with time for a drug introduced into this central compartment is depicted in Figure 2-8A and is described by Equation 2-7 where k is the elimination rate constant.

$$C = [dose / V][e^{-kt}]$$
(Equation 2-7)

- The multicompartment model of drug disposition can be viewed as though the blood and highly perfused lean organs such as heart, brain, liver, lung, and kidneys cluster as a single central compartment, whereas more slowly perfused tissues such as muscle, skin, fat, and bone behave as the final compartment (ie, the tissue compartment or reservoir; see Figure 2-3).

(continues)

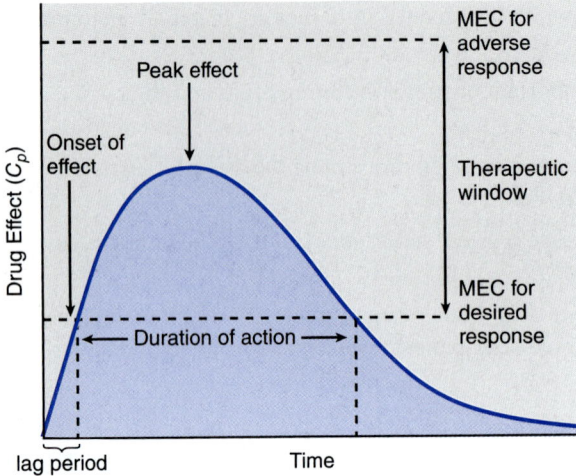

FIGURE 2-7 Temporal characteristics of drug effect and relationship to the therapeutic window (eg, single dose, oral administration). A lag period is present before the plasma drug concentration (C_p) exceeds the minimum effective concentration (MEC) for the desired effect. Following onset of the response, the intensity of the effect increases as the drug continues to be absorbed and distributed. This reaches a peak, after which drug elimination results in a decline in C_p and in the effect's intensity. Effect disappears when the drug concentration falls below the MEC. Accordingly, the duration of a drug's action is determined by the time period over which concentrations exceed the MEC. An MEC exists for each adverse response, and if drug concentration exceeds this, toxicity will result. The therapeutic goal is to obtain and maintain concentrations within the therapeutic window for the desired response with a minimum of toxicity. Drug response below the MEC for the desired effect will be sub-therapeutic; above the MEC for an adverse effect, the probability of toxicity will increase. Increasing or decreasing drug dosage shifts the response curve up or down the intensity scale and is used to modulate the drug's effect. Increasing the dose also prolongs a drug's duration of action but at the risk of increasing the likelihood of adverse effects. Unless the drug is nontoxic (eg, penicillins), increasing the dose is not a useful strategy for extending the duration of action. Instead, another dose of drug should be given, timed to maintain concentrations within the therapeutic window. The area under the blood concentration-time curve (area under the curve, or AUC, shaded region) can be used to calculate the clearance (see Equation 2-6) for first-order elimination. The AUC is also used as a measure of bioavailability (defined as 100% for an intravenously administered drug). Bioavailability will be less than 100% for orally administered drugs, due mainly to incomplete absorption and first-pass metabolism and elimination.

QUESTION 2-5 A drug that is a weak acid ($pK_a = 5$) is largely excreted unchanged by the kidneys. To increase its rate of excretion

a. the pH of the urine should be increased.
b. the pH of the urine should be decreased.
c. the pH of the urine should be left unchanged.
d. CYP liver enzymes should be induced to increase metabolism of the drug.
e. the patient should drink more water to increase urine output.

SUMMARY QUIZ ANSWER KEY

QUESTION 2-1 Answer is **c**. A drug given orally must be absorbed first from the GI tract, and the absorbed drug then passes through the liver, where metabolism and biliary excretion may occur before the drug enters the systemic circulation. Accordingly, a fraction of the administered and absorbed dose of drug will be inactivated or diverted in the intestine and liver before it can reach the general circulation and be distributed to its sites of action. If the metabolic or excretory capacity of the liver and the intestine for the drug is large, bioavailability will be reduced substantially (first-pass effect). This decrease in availability is a function of the anatomical site from which absorption

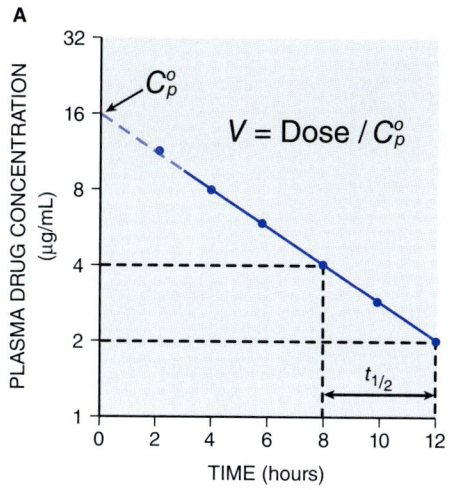 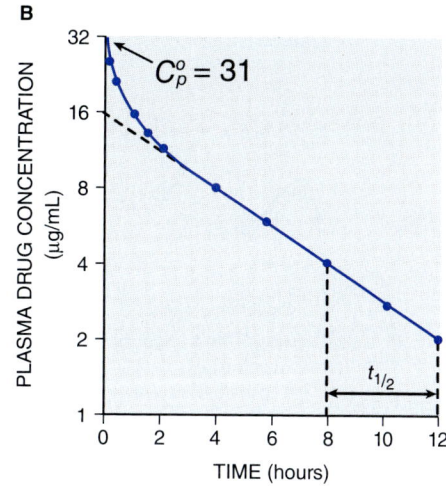

FIGURE 2-8 Plasma concentration-time curves following intravenous administration of a drug (500 mg) to a 70-kg patient. **A.** Drug concentrations are measured in plasma at 2-hour intervals following drug administration. The semilogarithmic plot of plasma concentration (C_p) versus time appears to indicate that the drug is eliminated from a single compartment by a first-order process (see Equation 2-7) with a $t_{1/2}$ of 4 hours ($k = 0.693/t_{1/2} = 0.173\ h^{-1}$). The volume of distribution (V) may be determined from the value of C_p obtained by extrapolation to $t = 0$ ($C_p^0 = 16\ \mu g/mL$). Volume of distribution (see Equation 2-2) for the 1-compartment model is 31.3 L, or 0.45 L/kg ($V = dose/C_p^0$). The clearance for this drug is 90 mL/min; for a 1-compartment model, $CL = kV$.
B. Sampling before 2 hours indicates that in fact the drug follows multiexponential kinetics. The terminal disposition $t_{1/2}$ is 4 hours, clearance is 84 mL/min (see Equation 2-6), V_{area} is 29 L (see Equation 2-7), and V_{ss} is 26.8 L. The initial or "central" distribution volume for the drug ($V_1 = dose/C_p^0$) is 16.1 L. The example chosen indicates that multicompartment kinetics may be overlooked when sampling at early times is neglected. In this particular case, there is only a 10% error in the estimate of clearance when the multicompartment characteristics are ignored. For many drugs, multicompartment kinetics may be observed for significant periods of time, and failure to consider the distribution phase can lead to significant errors in estimates of clearance and in predictions of the appropriate dosage. Also, the difference between the "central" distribution volume and other terms reflecting wider distribution is important in deciding a loading dose strategy. The idealized 1-compartment model discussed earlier does not describe the entire time course of the plasma concentration. That is, certain tissue reservoirs can be distinguished from the central compartment, and the drug concentration appears to decay in a manner that can be described by multiple exponential terms (Figure 2-8B).

RATE OF DISTRIBUTION AND EQUILIBRIUM OF DRUG INTO TISSUES (Cont.)

- The decline of drug plasma concentration with time for a multicompartment system is shown in Figure 2-8B.
- Two different terms have been used to describe the volume of distribution for drugs that follow multiple exponential decay.
  - V_{area} is the ratio of clearance to the rate of decline in concentration during the elimination (final) phase of the logarithmic concentration versus time curve (see Equation 2-8).

$$V_{area} = \frac{CL}{k} = \frac{dose}{k \cdot AUC}$$

(Equation 2-8)

  - The volume of distribution at steady-state (V_{ss}) represents the volume in which a drug would appear to be distributed during steady state if the drug existed throughout that volume at the same concentration as that in the measured plasma or blood (see Equation 2-9, where V_C is the volume of distribution in the central compartment and V_T is the volume term for drug in the tissue compartment).

$$V_{ss} = V_C + V_T$$

(Equation 2-9)

- Changes in the pattern or ratio of blood flow to various tissues changes will lead to changes in the rates of drug distribution to tissues.
  - Disease states that cause altered regional blood flow or reduced perfusion can lead to altered effects of drugs that vary depending on relative perfusion of specific tissues.

---

takes place; other anatomical, physiological, and pathological factors can influence bioavailability, and the choice of the route of drug administration must be based on an understanding of these conditions. Moreover, knowledge of drugs that undergo significant metabolism or require active transport across the intestinal and hepatic membranes instructs our understanding of adverse events in therapeutics, because some drugs are substrates for the same drug metabolizing enzymes or drug transporters and thus compete for metabolism and transport.

Diseases such as hepatic cirrhosis may affect "first-pass metabolism" by shunting of blood away from hepatic metabolizing enzymes.

QUESTION 2-2 Answer is **b.** The distribution of drugs into the CNS from the blood is unique. One reason for this is that the brain capillary endothelial cells have continuous tight junctions; therefore, drug penetration into the brain depends on transcellular rather than paracellular transport. The unique characteristics of brain capillary endothelial cells and pericapillary glial cells constitute the BBB. At the choroid plexus, a similar blood-CSF barrier is present, except that it is epithelial cells that are joined by tight junctions rather than endothelial cells. The lipid solubility of the nonionized and unbound species of a drug is therefore an important determinant of its uptake by the brain; the more lipophilic a drug, the more likely it is to cross the BBB. This situation

SECTION I

General Principles

DOSING REGIMENS TO ACHIEVE A STEADY-STATE DRUG CONCENTRATION

- Equation 2-3 indicates that a steady-state concentration eventually will be achieved when a drug is administered at a constant rate, that is, when the rate of drug elimination equals the rate of drug availability.
- With regular intermittent dosage the concentration of drug rises with absorption and falls by elimination during each dosing cycle, and at steady state, the entire cycle is repeated identically in each interdose interval (see Figure 2-9).
- Equation 2-10 provides an approximation of the time required to reach steady state after a dosage regimen is initiated or changed (ie, *four half-lives to reach ~94% of a new steady state*) and a means to estimate the appropriate dosing interval.

$$t_{1/2} \cong 0.693 \cdot V_{ss} / CL$$
(Equation 2-10)

- To maintain the chosen steady-state or target plasma drug concentration (C_p), the dosing rate is adjusted according to Equation 2-11 (where F is fractional bioavailability of the dose) such that the rate of input equals the rate of loss; Equation 2-11 is a similar relationship to what was previously described in Equation 2-3.

$$\text{Dosing rate} = \text{target } C_p \cdot CL/F$$
(Equation 2-11)

- The dosing interval for intermittent dosing depends on the total fluctuation in drug concentrations that can be tolerated.
  - If the dosing interval T were chosen to be equal to the $t_{1/2}$, then the total fluctuation would be 2-fold; this is often a tolerable variation.
  - If a drug is relatively nontoxic such that a concentration many times that necessary for therapy can be tolerated easily, the maximal-dose strategy can be used, and the dosing interval can be much longer than the elimination $t_{1/2}$ (for convenience).

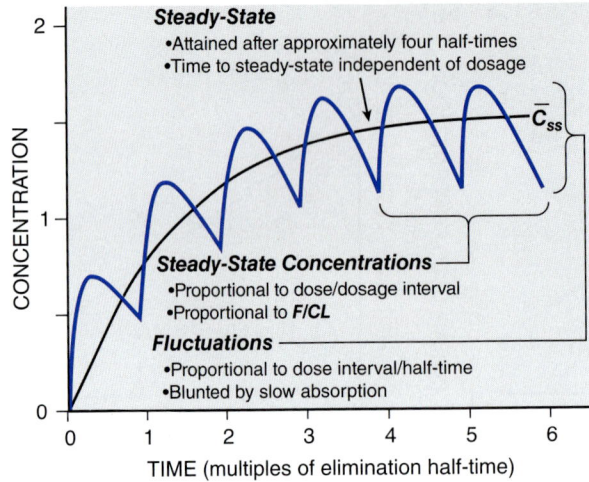

FIGURE 2-9 Fundamental pharmacokinetic relationships for repeated administration of drugs. The blue line is the pattern of drug accumulation during repeated administration of a drug at intervals equal to its elimination half-time when drug absorption is 10 times as rapid as elimination. As the rate of absorption increases, the concentration maxima approach 2 and the minima approach 1 during the steady state. The black line depicts the pattern during administration of equivalent dosage by continuous intravenous infusion. Curves are based on the 1-compartment model. Average concentration (C_{ss}) when the steady state is attained during intermittent drug administration:

$$F \cdot \text{dosing rate} = CL \cdot C_{ss}$$

where F is fractional bioavailability of the dose and T is dosage interval (time). By substitution of infusion rate for $F \cdot$ dosing rate, the formula is equivalent to Equation 2-3 and provides the concentration maintained at steady state during continuous intravenous infusion.

often is used in drug design to alter drug distribution to the brain; for example, the so-called second-generation antihistamines, such as loratadine, achieve far lower brain concentrations than do agents such as diphenhydramine and thus are nonsedating (see Case 2-1). Drugs may penetrate into the CNS by specific uptake transporters normally involved in the transport of nutrients and endogenous compounds from blood into the brain and CSF.

Another important factor in the functional BBB involves membrane transporters that are efflux carriers present in the brain capillary endothelial cell and capable of removing a large number of chemically diverse drugs from the cell. MDR1 (P-gp) and the organic anion–transporting polypeptide (OATP) are 2 of the more notable of these. The effects of these exporters are to dramatically limit access of the drug to the tissue expressing the efflux transporter.

QUESTION 2-3 Answer is **e**. Drug metabolism or biotransformation reactions are classified as either phase 1 functionalization reactions or phase 2 biosynthetic (conjugation) reactions.

Phase 1 reactions introduce or expose a functional group on the parent compound such as occurs in hydrolysis reactions. Phase 1 reactions generally result in the loss of pharmacological activity, although there are examples of retention or enhancement of activity. In rare instances, metabolism is associated with an altered pharmacological activity. Prodrugs are pharmacologically inactive compounds designed to maximize the amount of the active species that reaches its site of action. Inactive prodrugs are converted rapidly to biologically active metabolites often by the hydrolysis of an ester or amide linkage.

Phase 2 conjugation reactions lead to the formation of a covalent linkage between a functional group on the parent compound or phase 1 metabolite and endogenously derived glucuronic acid, sulfate, glutathione, amino acids, or acetate. These highly polar conjugates generally are inactive and are excreted rapidly in the urine and feces. An example of an active conjugate is the 6-glucuronide metabolite of morphine, which is a more potent analgesic than its parent (see Chapter 10).

QUESTION 2-4 Answer is **d**. Clearance is the most important concept to consider when designing a rational regimen for long-term drug administration. The clinician usually wants to maintain steady-state concentrations of a drug within a therapeutic window or range associated with therapeutic efficacy and a minimum of toxicity for a given agent. Assuming complete bioavailability, the steady-state concentration of drug in the body will be achieved when the rate of drug elimination equals the rate of drug administration (see Equation 2-3). Adjusting the dosing rate to achieve therapeutic steady-state concentration of drug thus requires an appreciation of the rate of clearance. When dosing rate is higher than clearance rate, drug will accumulate with possible toxic effects. When dosing rate is lower than clearance rate, subtherapeutic concentrations will result.

The concept of clearance is extremely useful in clinical pharmacokinetics because its value for a particular drug usually is constant over the range of concentrations encountered clinically. This is true because systems for elimination of drugs such as metabolizing enzymes and transporters usually are not saturated, and thus the absolute rate of elimination of the drug is essentially a linear function of its concentration in plasma. That is, the elimination of most drugs follows first-order kinetics, where a constant fraction of drug in the body is eliminated per unit of time.

QUESTION 2-5 Answer is **a**. To increase the rate of excretion of a drug that is a weak acid, the pH of the urine should be made more alkaline to increase the amount of drug in the urine that is ionized (see answer to Case 2-1c). In the proximal and distal tubules, the nonionized forms of weak acids and bases undergo net passive reabsorption. The concentration gradient for back-diffusion is created by the reabsorption of water with Na^+ and other inorganic ions. Because the tubular cells are less permeable to the ionized forms of weak electrolytes, passive reabsorption of these substances depends on the pH. When the tubular urine is made more alkaline, weak acids are largely ionized and thus are excreted more rapidly and to a greater extent. When the tubular urine is made more acidic, the fraction of drug ionized is reduced, and excretion is likewise reduced. Alkalinization and acidification of the urine have the opposite effects on the excretion of weak bases. In the treatment of drug poisoning, the excretion of some drugs can be hastened by appropriate alkalinization or acidification of the urine. Whether alteration of urine pH results in a significant change in drug elimination depends on the extent and persistence of the pH change and the contribution of pH-dependent passive reabsorption to total drug elimination. The effect is greatest for weak acids and bases with pK_a values in the range of urinary pH (5-8). However, alkalinization of urine can produce a 4- to 6-fold increase in excretion of a relatively strong acid such as salicylate when urinary pH is changed from 6.4 to 8.0 and the fraction of nonionized drug is reduced from 1% to 0.04%.

DOSING REGIMENS TO ACHIEVE A STEADY-STATE DRUG CONCENTRATION (*Cont.*)

- ▸ For drugs with a narrow therapeutic index, it may be important to estimate the maximal and minimal concentrations that will occur for a particular dosing interval (see the section Dosing Interval for Intermittent Dosage in Chapter 2 of *Goodman & Gilman's The Pharmacological Basis of Therapeutics*, 12th Edition for a detailed discussion and an example of the calculations).
- The *loading dose* is one or a series of doses that may be given at the onset of therapy with the aim of achieving the target concentration rapidly (ie, if the time required to attain steady state is long relative to the need to achieve therapeutic concentrations of drug).
  - ▸ Equation 2-12 provides an estimate for the magnitude of a loading dose.

  $$\text{Loading dose} = \text{target } C_p \cdot V_{ss}/F$$
  (Equation 2-12)

  - ▸ Note that the loading dose of a drug is not affected by drug elimination and thus is not routinely affected by hepatic or renal insufficiency.
  - ▸ Disadvantages of using a loading dose include abruptly exposing a patient to what may be a toxic concentration of drug and the long time required for drug concentration to fall if the concentration is excessive.
- Therapeutic drug monitoring to better estimate CL/F may be useful to refine dosing using Equation 2-11 to achieve desired target plasma concentrations.
  - ▸ When the goal of measurement is adjustment of dosage, the sample should be taken well after the previous dose, that is, just before the next planned dose, when the concentration is at its minimum, except for drugs that act only during the initial period of each dosing interval.
  - ▸ Although four half-lives are required to achieve steady-state concentrations with constant (nonloading) dosing, it may be important to monitor before steady-state has been achieved with drugs that are toxic to minimize damage.

CHAPTER 3

Clinical and Environmental Toxicity

SELECT ANTIDOTES, CARCINOGENS, AND METALS INCLUDED IN THIS CHAPTER[a,b,c]

- Acetylcysteine (MUCOMYST)
- Aflatoxin B_1
- Arsenic
- Atropine
- Benzo[a]pyrene
- Cadmium
- Chromium
- Deferasirox (EXJADE)
- Deferoxamine (DESFERAL)
- Dimercaprol
- Dimercaptosuccinic acid (DMSA), succimer (CHEMET)
- Diphenhydramine (BENEDRYL)
- EDTA $CaNa_2$
- Ethanol
- Flumazenil
- Fomepizole
- Lead
- Mercury
- Naloxone (NARCAN)
- Penicillamine
- Physostigmine
- Pralidoxime chloride (2-PAM)
- Sodium 2,3-dimercaptopropane sulfonate (DMPS)—not approved by FDA, but approved for use in Germany

[a] A complete list of antidotes is shown in Table 3-1; [b] examples of important carcinogens are shown in Table 3-2; [c] a list of toxic metals with frequent environmental or occupational exposure is shown in Table 3-3.

Chapter 3 Clinical and Environmental Toxicity is a compilation of Chapter 4, Drug Toxicity and Poisoning and Chapter 67 Environmental Toxicology: Carcinogens and Heavy Metals from *Goodman & Gilman's The Pharmacological Basis of Therapeutics*, 12th Edition. The specific pharmacology (including the mechanisms of action) of drugs mentioned in Chapter 3 is discussed in previous or subsequent chapters. The Mechanisms of Action and the Clinical Summary Tables are limited to the commonly used antidotes, toxic metals, and the metal chelators that are used therapeutically to treat heavy metal poisoning. In addition to the material presented here, the 12th Edition includes:

- A detailed description of drug toxicity testing in animals
- A detailed description of drug safety testing and clinical trials in humans
- A list of important resources for information related to drug toxicity and poisoning
- A description of various methods of decontaminating a poisoned patient
- A discussion of environmental risk assessment and risk management
- A detailed discussion of carcinogenesis and chemoprevention
- A discussion of the principles of the treatment of metal exposure

LEARNING OBJECTIVES

☑ Understand the dose-response relationship of drugs and how it is used to quantify efficacy and toxicity.

☑ Understand how drugs are tested for safety and efficacy in humans.

☑ Know the different types of therapeutic drug toxicity.

☑ Describe the different types of drug-drug interactions and know how they apply to drug therapy.

☑ Know the principles of managing a drug poisoning including the safe use of specific antidotes.

☑ Know the toxicity of acute and chronic heavy metal exposure.

☑ Understand the mechanisms of action and therapeutic uses of metal chelators for the treatment of acute metal exposure.

MECHANISMS OF ACTION OR TOXICITY OF SELECT ANTIDOTES, CARCINOGENS, AND HEAVY METALS

DRUG CLASS	DRUG	MECHANISM OF ACTION
Antidotes for Common Acute Poisons	Acetylcysteine	Binds with the toxic metabolite of acetaminophen
	Atropine	Muscarinic receptor antagonist (see Chapter 6)
	Diphenhydramine	H_1 histamine receptor antagonist (see Chapter 21)
	Deferoxamine	Chelates iron

Clinical and Environmental Toxicity — CHAPTER 3

DRUG CLASS	DRUG	MECHANISM OF ACTION
	Deferasirox	Chelates iron
	Ethanol	Competitive inhibitor of alcohol dehydrogenase (see Chapter 9)
	Fomepizole	Inhibitor of alcohol dehydrogenase (see Chapter 9)
	Flumazenil	Benzodiazepine receptor antagonist (see Chapter 9)
	Naloxone	Opiate receptor antagonist (see Chapter 10)
	Physostigmine	Cholinesterase inhibitor (see Chapter 6)
	Pralidoxime (2-PAM)	Cholinesterase reactivator (see Chapter 6)
Carcinogens	Aflatoxin B_1	8,9-epoxide metabolite reacts with amines in biological macromolecules Forms DNA adducts (see Figure 3-11)
	Benzo[a]pyrene	Genotoxic carcinogen that forms DNA adducts and reactive oxygen species
Toxic Heavy Metals	Arsenic	As^{3+} forms covalent bonds with sulfur and alters proteins containing cysteine
	Cadmium	Induces the formation of reactive oxygen species through an unknown mechanism
	Chromium	Cr^{VI} is taken into cells by anion transporters where it is reduced to Cr^{III}. Cr^{III} forms covalent adducts with DNA
	Lead	Inhibition of calcium transporters and channels that lead to alterations of almost all neurotransmitter pathways Inhibition of δ-aminolevulinate dehydratase Inhibition of ferrochelatase (see Figure 3-8)
	Mercury	Hg^{2+} and methylHg (MeHg) form covalent bonds with sulfur and alter proteins containing cysteine
Heavy Metal Chelators	Dimercaprol	Forms chelation complexes between its sulfhydryl groups and metals
	Sodium 2,3-dimercaptopropane sulfonate (DMPS)	Forms chelation complexes between its sulfhydryl groups and metals
	EDTA $CaNa_2$	Chelates divalent and trivalent metals
	Penicillamine	Chelator of copper, mercury, zinc, and lead
	Dimercaptosuccinic acid (DMSA), Succimer	Forms chelation complexes between its sulfhydryl groups and metals

SECTION I General Principles

TABLE 3-1 Some Common Antidotes and Their Indications

ANTIDOTE	POISONING INDICATION(S)
Acetylcysteine	Acetaminophen
Atropine sulfate	Organophosporus and carbamate pesticides
Benztropine	Drug-induced dystonia
Bicarbonate, sodium	Na^+ channel blocking drugs
Bromocriptine	Neuroleptic malignant syndrome
Calcium gluconate or chloride	Ca^{2+} channel blocking drugs, Fluoride
Carnitine	Valproate hyperammonemia
Crotalidae polyvalent immune Fab	North American crotaline snake envenomation
Dantrolene	Malignant hyperthermia
Deferoxamine	Iron
Digoxin immune Fab	Cardiac glycosides
Diphenhydramine	Drug-induced dystonia
Dimercaprol (BAL)	Lead, mercury, arsenic
EDTA, $CaNa_2$	Lead
Ethanol	Methanol, ethylene glycol
Fomepizole	Methanol, ethylene glycol
Flumazenil	Benzodiazepines
Glucagon hydrochloride	β adrenergic antagonists
Hydroxocobalamin hydrochloride	Cyanide
Insulin (high dose)	Ca^{2+} channel blockers
Leucovorin calcium	Methotrexate
Methylene blue	Methemoglobinemia
Naloxone hydrochloride	Opioids
Octreotide acetate	Sulfonylurea-induced hypoglycemia
Oxygen, hyperbaric	Carbon monoxide
Penicillamine	Lead, mercury, copper
Physostigmine salicylate	Anticholinergic syndrome
Pralidoxime chloride (2-PAM)	Organophosphorus pesticides
Pyridoxine hydrochloride	Isoniazid seizures
Succimer (DMSA)	Lead, mercury, arsenic
Thiosulfate, sodium	Cyanide
Vitamin K_1 (phytonadione)	Coumarin, indanedione

Clinical and Environmental Toxicity — CHAPTER 3

TABLE 3-2 Examples of Important Carcinogens[a]

CARCINOGEN CLASS	EXAMPLE	SOURCE	MECHANISM
Genotoxic			
Nitrosamines	Nicotine-derived nitrosaminoketone (NNK)	Tobacco products	Metabolic activation to form DNA adducts
Polycyclic aromatic hydrocarbons	Benzo[a]pyrene	Fossil fuel combustion, tobacco smoke, charbroiled food	Metabolic activation to form DNA adducts or ROS
Aromatic amines	2-Aminonaphthalene	Dyes	Metabolic activation to form DNA adducts
Fungal toxins	Aflatoxin B_1	Corn, peanuts, and other food	Metabolic activation to form DNA adducts
Non-genotoxic			
Liver toxicants	Ethanol	Beverages, environment	Toxicity and compensatory proliferation; depletion of GSH
Phorbol esters	Tetradecanoyl phorbol acetate	Horticulture; rubber and gasoline production	Activation of PKC isoforms
Estrogens	Diethylstilbestrol	Drugs, environment	Activation of estrogen-receptor signaling
Metals	Arsenic	Environment, occupation	Inhibition of DNA repair; activation of signal transduction pathways
Irritants	Asbestos	Environment, occupation	Stimulation of inflammation; formation of ROS
Dioxins	TCDD	Waste incineration, herbicides, paper-pulp bleaching	Activation of the aryl hydrocarbon receptor

[a]Compounds in this table are classified as group 1 carcinogens by the International Agency for Research on Cancer (IARC), with the exception of the phorbol esters, which have not been examined. TCDD, 2,3,7,8 tetrachlorodibenzo-p-dioxin; ROS, reactive oxygen species; GSH, glutathione; PKC, protein kinase C.

TABLE 3-3 Toxic Metals with Frequent Environmental or Occupational Exposure[a]

METAL	CERCLA PRIORITY	COMMON SOURCE OF EXPOSURE	ORGAN SYSTEMS MOST SENSITIVE TO TOXICITY	IARC CARCINOGEN CLASSIFICATION
As	1	Drinking water	CV, skin, multiple other	Group 1, carcinogenic to humans—liver, bladder, lung
Pb	2	Paint, soil	CNS, blood, CV, renal	Group 2A, probably carcinogenic
Hg	3	Air, food	CNS, renal	Group 2B, possibly carcinogenic ($MeHg^+$); group 3, not classifiable (Hg^0, Hg^{2+})
Cd	7	Occupational, food, smoking	Renal, respiratory	Group 1, carcinogenic to humans—lung
Cr^{6+}	18	Occupational	Respiratory	Group 1, carcinogenic to humans—lung
Be	42	Occupational, water	Respiratory	Group 1, carcinogenic to humans—lung
Co	49	Occupational, food, water	Respiratory, CV	Group 2B, possibly carcinogenic
Ni	53	Occupational	Respiratory, skin (allergy)	Group 1, carcinogenic (soluble Ni compounds); group 2B, possibly carcinogenic (metallic Ni)—lung

[a]The Agency for Toxic Substances and Disease Registry (ATSDR) has both detailed monographs and brief summaries for each of these compounds, available at http://www.atsdr.cdc.gov. The International Agency for Research on Cancer (IARC) also has monographs available at http://monographs.iarc.fr. CERCLA, Comprehensive Environmental Response, Compensation, and Liability Act. CNS, central nervous system; CV, cardiovascular.

SECTION I General Principles

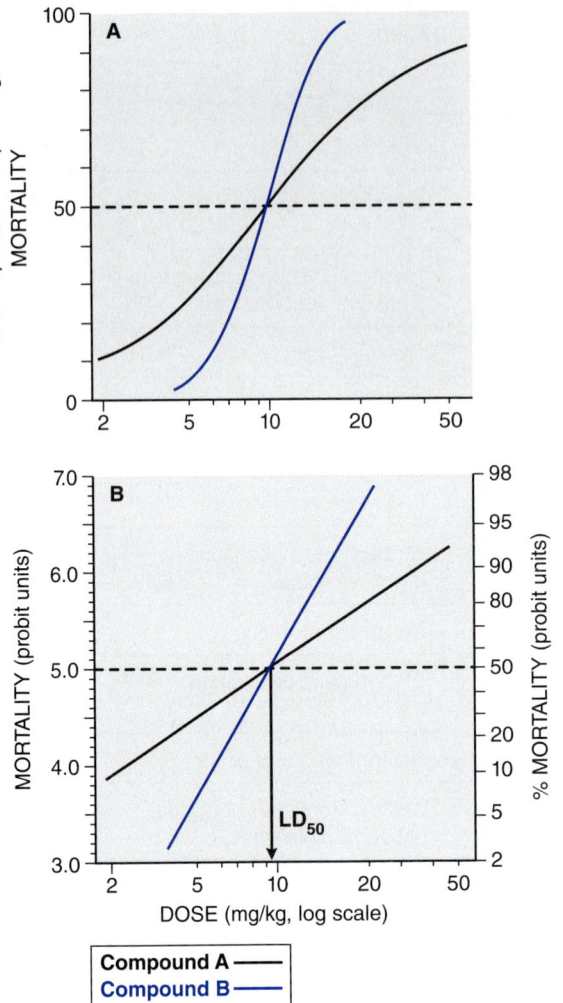

FIGURE 3-1 Dose-response relationships. **A.** The toxic response to a chemical is evaluated at several doses in the toxic or lethal range. The midpoint of the curve representing percent of population responding (response here is death) versus dose (log scale) represents the LD_{50}, or the concentration of drug that is lethal in 50% of the population. **B.** A linear transformation of the data in panel A is provided by plotting the log of the dose administered versus the percent of the population mortality, in probit units. For a discussion of probit units, see Chapter 4 in *Goodman and Gilman's The Pharmacological Basis of Therapeutics*, 12th Edition.

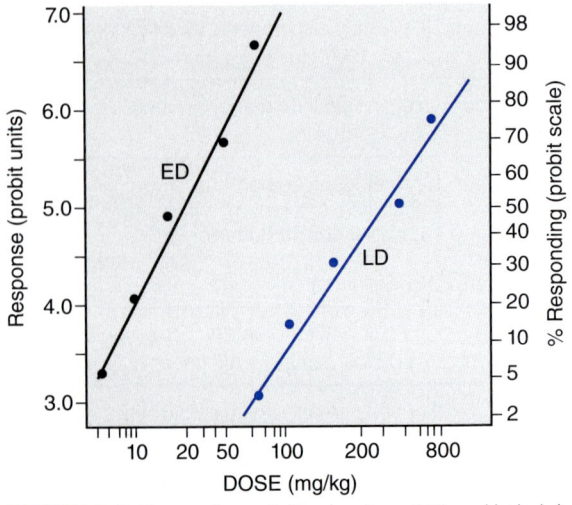

FIGURE 3-2 Comparison of effective dose (ED), and lethal dose (LD). For a discussion of probit units, see Chapter 4 in *Goodman and Gilman's The Pharmacological Basis of Therapeutics*, 12th Edition. Note that the abscissa is a logarithmic scale.

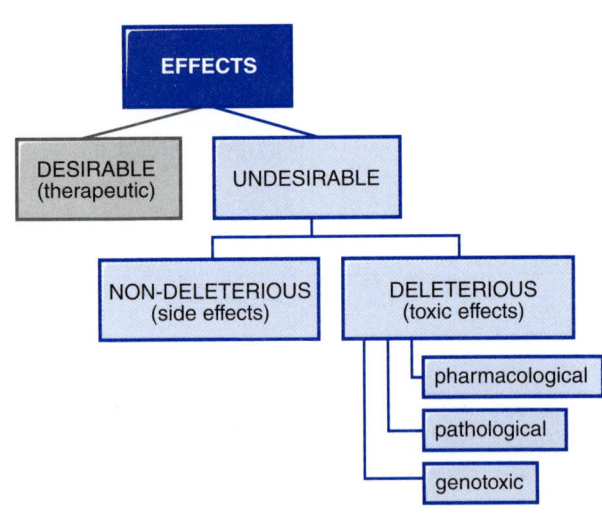

FIGURE 3-3 Spectrum of the effects of pharmaceuticals.

Clinical and Environmental Toxicity

CHAPTER 3

CASE 3-1

A new chemical is proposed for the treatment of hypertension.

a. Describe how the effects of the chemical are initially quantified?

Evaluation of the dose-response or the dose-effect relationship is crucially important to toxicologists. There is a graded dose-response relationship in an individual and a quantal dose-response relationship in the population (see Chapters 1 and 2). Graded doses of a drug given to an individual usually result in a greater magnitude of response as the dose is increased. In a quantal dose-response relationship, the percentage of the population affected increases as the dose is raised; the relationship is quantal in that the effect is specified to be either present or absent in a given individual (see Figure 3-1). This quantal dose-response phenomenon is extremely important in toxicology and is used to determine the median lethal dose (LD_{50}) of drugs and other chemicals. The LD_{50} of a compound is determined experimentally, usually by administration of the chemical to mice or rats (orally or intraperitoneally) at several doses in the lethal range.

b. Describe how the chemical's toxicity and "therapeutic index" are determined?

Figure 3-2 illustrates the relationship between a quantal dose-response curve for the therapeutic effect of a drug to generate a median effective dose (ED_{50}), the concentration of drug at which 50% of the population will have the desired response, and a quantal dose-response curve for lethality by the same agent. These 2 curves can be used to generate a therapeutic index (TI), which quantifies the relative safety of a drug.

$$TI = LD_{50}/ED_{50}$$

Drugs show a wide range of TI, from 1 to 2 to more than 100. Drugs with a low TI must be administered with caution. Agents that fall into this category include the cardiac glycoside digitalis (see Chapter 17) and cancer chemotherapeutic agents (see Chapters 45 and 46). Agents with very high TI are extremely safe and include some antibiotics (eg, penicillin) (see Chapter 39), unless there is a known allergic response.

GUIDELINES FOR THE STUDY OF NEW DRUGS IN HUMANS

PHASE OF STUDY	EXPLANATION
Notice of Claimed Investigational Exemption for a New Drug (IND)	Must be filed once a drug is judged ready to be studied in humans. Includes: • Information of composition and source • Chemical and manufacturing information • All data from animal studies • Proposed clinical plans and protocols • Names and credentials of physicians who will conduct clinical trials • Compilation of key data relevant to study the drug in humans made available to investigators in Institutional Review Boards
Phase I	Establish the effects of the drug as a function of dosage in 20-100 healthy volunteers: • Designed to prevent severe toxicity • Determine the probable limits of the safe clinical dosage range • Pharmacokinetic measurements are often conducted in this phase
Phase II	Performed in 100-200 patients with target disease: • Goal is to determine limited efficacy and the doses to be used in subsequent trials
Phase III	Performed in 1000 to 3000 patients: • To establish and confirm safety and efficacy • Double-blind and crossover study designs are often used • Drug formulated as intended for market
Phase IV	Post-marketing surveillance • FDA requires drug manufacturers to perform • FDA operates a voluntary reporting system available to physicians, pharmacists, and consumers • To identify additional drug toxicity not apparent during the drug development process

SECTION I General Principles

TYPES OF THERAPEUTIC DRUG TOXICITY[a]

TYPE OF TOXICITY	DESCRIPTION	EXAMPLE
Dose-dependent Reactions	Incidence and seriousness proportional to the concentration of the drug in the body and the duration of exposure	Drug overdose is a dramatic example
Pharmacological Toxicity	Progression of clinical effects to toxic effects dependent upon dose. May also occur at therapeutic doses	CNS depression produced by barbiturates from anxiolysis, to sedation, to somnolence, to coma. Phototoxicity associated with exposure to sunlight in patients treated with tetracycline
Pathological Toxicity	Drug in overdose produces a distinct pathological reaction	Acetaminophen overdose producing hepatic necrosis
Genotoxic Effects	Injury to DNA leading to mutagenic or carcinogenic toxicities	Aflatoxin exposure
Allergic Reactions	Result from previous sensitization to a particular chemical or to one that is structurally similar	Type I: Anaphylactic reactions mediated by IgE antibodies. Type II: Cytolytic reactions mediated by IgG and IgM antibodies. Type III: Arthrus reactions mediated predominantly by IgG. Type IV: Delayed hypersensitivity reactions mediated by sensitized T-lymphocyctes and macrophages
Idiosyncratic Reactions	An abnormal reaction to a chemical that is peculiar to a given individual. May take the form of extreme sensitivity to low doses or extreme insensitivity to high doses of drugs	Genetically determined resistance to the anticoagulant action of warfarin due to an alteration in vitamin K epoxide reductase (see Chapter 19)

[a] A complete discussion of the types of drug toxicity can be found in *Goodman and Gilman's The Pharmacological Basis of Therapeutics*, 12th Edition, Chapter 4.

CASE 3-2

A 35-year-old woman is being treated for esophageal reflux with a drug that has been recently approved by the Food and Drug Administration (FDA). After 2 months of therapy she is feeling better and nightly episodes of reflux are diminished, but her physician calls to tell her that the drug is being recalled because of a problem with cardiac arrhythmia, and a new drug will be prescribed.

a. **What is the process of drug approval by the FDA?**

   Fewer than one-third of the drugs tested in clinical trials reach the marketplace. Federal law in the United States and ethical considerations require that the study of new drugs in humans be conducted in accordance with stringent guidelines. See Side Bar GUIDELINES FOR THE STUDY OF NEW DRUGS IN HUMANS.

b. **What are the different types of therapeutic drug toxicity?**

   In therapeutics, a drug typically produces numerous effects, but usually only 1 is sought as the primary goal of treatment; most of the other effects are undesirable effects of that drug for that therapeutic indication (see Figure 3-3). Side effects of drugs usually are bothersome but not deleterious nor do they always necessitate the discontinuation of the drug; they include effects such as dry mouth occurring with tricyclic antidepressant therapy. Other undesirable effects may be characterized as toxic effects (see Side Bar TYPES OF THERAPEUTIC DRUG TOXICITY).

c. **Why can a drug approved by the FDA for use in humans and still cause serious toxicity?**

   Some toxicities of pharmaceuticals can be predicted based upon their known pharmacological mechanism; however, it is often not until the postmarketing period that the therapeutic toxicity profile of a drug becomes fully appreciated.

(Continued)

In the United States, the approval system for new drugs typically uses only 500 to 3000 exposed subjects. Such a system is likely to identify toxicities occurring in 1% or more of patients receiving a drug. The Adverse Event Reporting System of the FDA relies upon 2 signals to detect rare drug events. First, the FDA requires (Code of Federal Regulations, Title 21, Volume 5, Section 314.80) drug manufacturers to perform postmarketing surveillance of prescription drugs, and similar regulations exist for nonprescription products. Second, the FDA operates a voluntary reporting system MedWatch, available to both health professionals and consumers. Hospitals may also support adverse drug event committees to investigate potential adverse drug events, and these investigations may be made available to industry and the government. Unfortunately, any national dataset will significantly underestimate the morbidity and mortality attributable to adverse drug events because of underreporting and because it is difficult to estimate the denominator of total patient exposures for each event reported once a drug is available on the open market.

As an example, postmarketing surveillance identified the toxicity associated with the serotonin receptor-modulating drug cisapride. This drug was known to enhance GI motility and was marketed in the United States as a treatment for gastroesophageal reflux. Postmarketing surveillance revealed that cisapride was

(*Continued*)

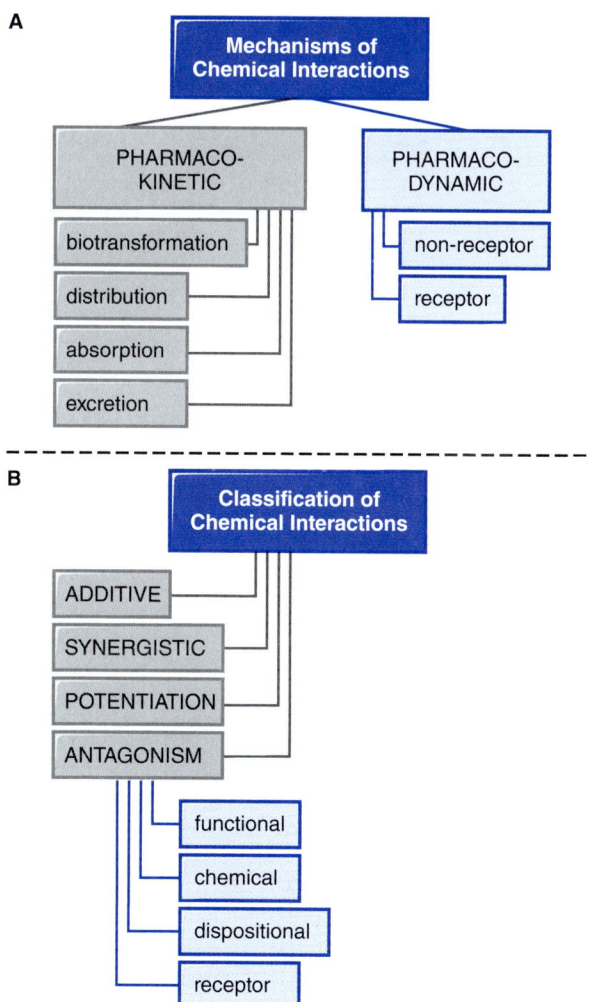

FIGURE 3-4 Mechanisms and classification of drug interactions.

SECTION I — General Principles

associated with prolongation of the QT interval and predisposition to ventricular arrhythmia. It was withdrawn from the market, and subsequent case-control studies demonstrated increased risk of arrhythmia. Cisapride is now limited in its distribution through an investigational access program managed by the manufacturer. Thus, the determination of drug toxicity extends beyond the stages of drug development and approval.

DRUG–DRUG INTERACTIONS

TYPE OF INTERACTION	DESCRIPTION	EXAMPLE
Absorption (Pharmacokinetic)	One drug causes an increase or decrease in the GI absorption of another drug	Ranitidine increases GI pH and may increase absorption of basic drugs such as triazolam
Protein Binding (Pharmacokinetic)	One drug displaces another from protein binding sites	The anticoagulant effects of warfarin may be enhanced by displacement from plasma proteins by valproic acid therapy
Metabolism (Pharmacokinetic)	A drug influences the metabolism of one or several other drugs by enhancing or inhibiting hepatic CYPs	Phenobarbital, phenytoin, and valproate increase the metabolism of carbamazepine. Metabolism of carbamazepine is inhibited by erythromycin (see Chapter 12)
Receptor Binding (Pharmacodynamic)	One drug binds to a receptor and prevents the pharmacological action of another drug at that receptor	Buprenorphine binds opioid receptors with high affinity, and can prevent euphoria from concomitant use of abused opioid drugs
Therapeutic Action (Pharmacodynamic)	The therapeutic effect of 1 drug impacts the therapeutic effect of another drug	When aspirin, an inhibitor of platelet aggregation, is given concomitantly with heparin, an anticoagulant, there may be an increased risk of bleeding

CLASSIFICATION OF DRUG–DRUG INTERACTIONS

- Additive—the combined effect of 2 drugs equals the sum of the effect of each agent given alone
- Synergistic—the combined effect of 2 drugs exceeds the sum of the effects of each drug given alone
- Potentiation—the creation of a toxic effect of 1 drug due to the presence of another drug
- Antagonism—the interference of 1 drug with the action of another drug
  - Chemical antagonism—reaction between 2 chemicals to neutralize their effects
  - Dispositional antagonism—alteration of the disposition of a substance so that less of the agent reaches the target organ
  - Receptor antagonism—blockade of the effect of 1 drug with another drug that competes at the receptor site

CASE 3-3

A 38-year-old man is being treated for a seizure disorder with carbamazepine. Although his seizure frequency is decreased, valproic acid is added to further reduce the seizure frequency.

a. Is a drug–drug interaction of concern in this patient?

Patients are commonly treated with more than 1 drug, have individual dietary choices, and may also be using over-the-counter (OTC) medications, vitamins, and other "natural" supplements. This polypharmaceutical nature of health care requires consideration of potential drug interactions (see Figure 3-4).

A drug can frequently influence the metabolism of 1 or several other drugs (see Chapter 2), and this is especially notable with hepatic CYPs. Acetaminophen is partially transformed by CYP2E1 to the toxic metabolite NAPQI (see Figure 3-6). Intake of ethanol, a potent inducer of the 2E1 isoenzyme, may lead to increased susceptibility to acetaminophen poisoning after overdose. Similarly, a number of second-generation piperidine antihistamines (terfenadine, astemizole) were removed from the market when they were noted to lead to QT interval prolongation and tachydysrhythmias when coadministered with macrolide antibiotics.

b. What are the different types of drug–drug interactions?

Drug interactions generally involve drug absorption, protein binding, metabolism, receptor binding, or therapeutic action (see Side Bar DRUG–DRUG INTERACTIONS). Further drug–drug interactions can be classified as additive, synergistic, potentiation, or antagonism (see Side Bar CLASSIFICATION OF DRUG–DRUG INTERACTIONS).

Clinical and Environmental Toxicity — CHAPTER 3

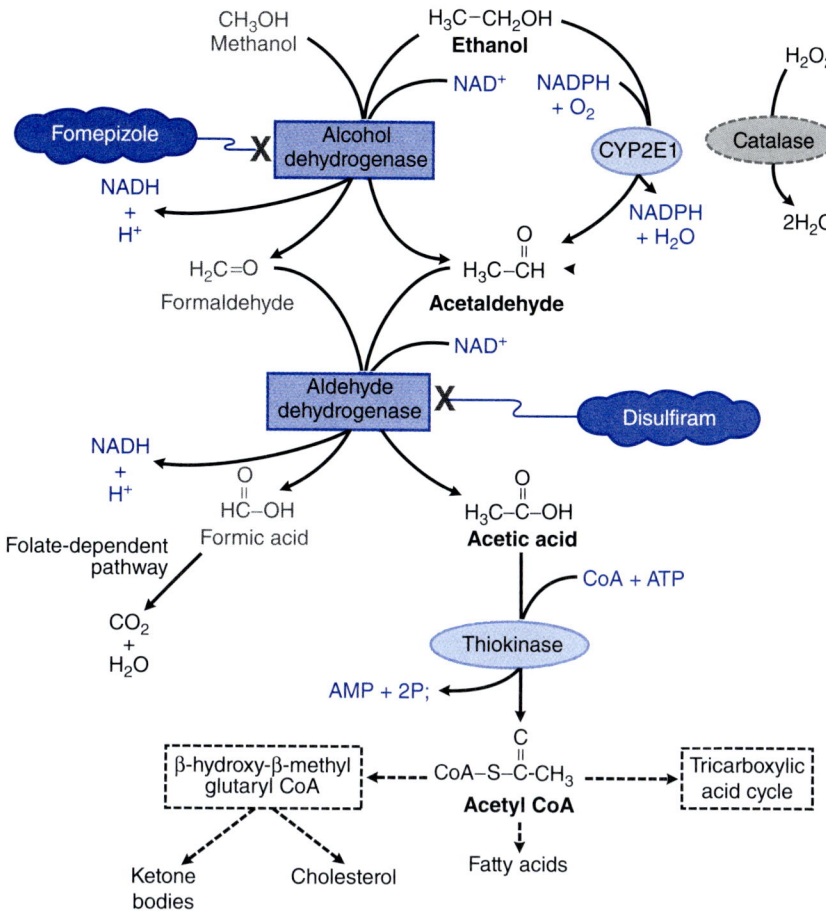

FIGURE 3-5 Metabolism of ethanol and methanol.

CASE 3-4

A 20-year-old man goes to a college party. A person at the party offers to spike his punch from an unlabeled flask. An hour later the man is experiencing an intense headache and blurred vision. He is taken to the emergency room where it is determined that he has been poisoned with methanol.

a. How does methanol produce toxicity?

One carbon alcohol, methanol (CH_3OH), is also known as methyl and wood alcohol. It is an important industrial reagent and solvent found in products such as paint removers, shellac, and antifreeze; methanol is added to industrial-use ethanol to make it unsafe for human consumption.

Severe metabolic acidosis can develop due to the accumulation of formic acid (see Figure 3-5), and the respiratory depression can be severe, especially in the context of coma. The visual disturbances associated with methanol intoxication are a prominent part of the clinical picture and occur as a consequence of injury to ganglion cells of the retina caused by the metabolite, formic acid, with subsequent inflammation, atrophy, and potential bilateral blindness.

b. What are the signs and symptoms of methanol poisoning?

Methanol poisoning consists of headache, GI distress, and pain (partially related to pancreatic injury), difficulty breathing, restlessness, and blurred vision associated with hyperemic optic disks. The clinical picture can also include necrosis of the pancreas.

(Continued)

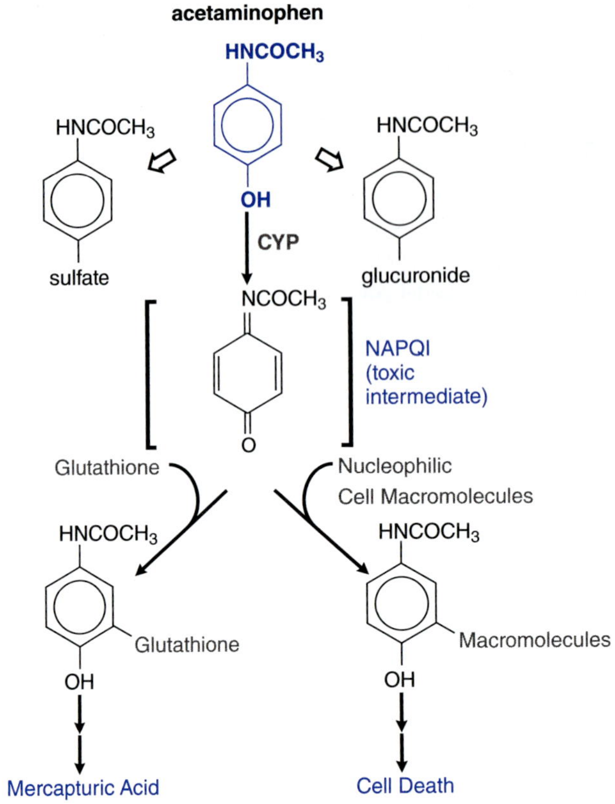

SECTION I — General Principles

FIGURE 3-6 Pathways of acetaminophen metabolism and toxicity. The toxic intermediate NAPQI is *N*-acetyl-*p*-benzoquinoneimine.

c. **What are the treatment options for this patient?**

Table 3-1 lists common antidotes and their indications. Methanol is rapidly absorbed via the oral route, inhalation, and through the skin, with the latter 2 routes being most relevant to industrial settings. Methanol also is metabolized (see Figure 3-5) by ADH and ALDH, with damaging consequences. Competition between methanol and ethanol for ADH forms the basis of the use of ethanol as an antidote in methanol poisoning. Fomepizole (4-methylpyrazole), an ADH inhibitor, is useful in methanol and ethylene glycol poisoning.

Following the inhibition of metabolism of methanol with either ethanol or fomepizole, hemodialysis is used to effectively remove the remaining methanol.

CASE 3-5

A 16-year-old woman is brought to the emergency room because she took an overdose of acetaminophen. Her vital signs are normal and she appears stable except for being distraught at having attempted suicide.

a. **What are the general principles of the management of a poisoned patient?**

The majority of poisoning exposures reported to US poison control centers are judged to be nontoxic or only minimally toxic. When toxicity is expected, or does occur, the priority of poisoning treatment is to support vital functions until the drug or chemical is eliminated from the body. Because of the acute onset of action and finite duration of action of most drugs, the treatment of poisoning must be prompt and goal directed. The first goal is to protect vital physiological functions from impairment. The second goal is to keep the concentration of poison in tissues as low as possible by preventing absorption and enhancing elimination. The third goal is to combat the toxicological effects of the poison at the effector sites.

(Continued)

CHAPTER 3
Clinical and Environmental Toxicity

TABLE 3-4 Top Five Agents Involved in Drug-Related Deaths

Cocaine
Opioids
Benzodiazepines
Alcohol
Antidepressants

U.S. DHHS.

Knowledge of the relative toxicity of drugs is the beginning to the proper management of a poisoned patient. The following tables put human poisonings in perspective: Table 3-4 lists the top 5 agents involved in drug-related deaths; Table 3-5 lists the substances most frequently involved in human poisoning exposures; Table 3-6 lists the poisons associated with the largest number of human fatalities.

The "ABC" mnemonic of emergency care (airway, breathing, circulation) is popularly taught and applies to the treatment of acute poisoning, but with the addition of elements D (disability) and E (exposure) (see Table 3-7). In severe cases, endotracheal intubation, mechanical ventilation, pharmacological blood pressure support, and/or extracorporeal circulatory support may be necessary and appropriate.

A carefully obtained medical history may create a list of available medications or chemicals that might be implicated in a poisoning event. Often, an observation of physical symptoms and signs may be the only additional clues to a poisoning diagnosis. Groups of physical signs and symptoms associated with specific poisoning syndromes are known as toxidromes. Table 3-8 describes commonly encountered toxidromes.

The most typically available urine drug toxicology test is an immunoassay designed to detect common drugs of abuse such as amphetamines, barbiturates, benzodiazepines, cannabis, cocaine, and opiates. Acute poisoning with these substances can usually be determined on clinical grounds, and the results of these assays are infrequently available fast enough to guide stabilization. Additionally, detection of drugs or their metabolites on a urine immunoassay does not mean that the detected drug is responsible for the currently observed poisoning illness. When ingestion

(Continued)

TABLE 3-5 Substances Most Frequently Involved in Human Poisoning Exposures

SUBSTANCE	%
Analgesics	12.5
Personal care products	9.1
Cleaning substances	8.7
Sedatives/hypnotics/antipsychotics	6.2
Foreign bodies	5.1
Topical preparations	4.5
Cold and cough medications	4.5
Antidepressants	4.0

Data from Bronstein AC, Spyker DA, Cantilena LR, et al. 2007. Annual Report of the American Association of Poison Control Centers' National Poison Data System (NPDS): 25th annual report. *Clin Toxicol*, 2008, 46:927–1057.

SECTION I General Principles

TABLE 3-6 Poisons Associated with the Largest Number of Human Fatalities

Sedatives/hypnotics/antipsychotics
Acetaminophen
Opioids
Antidepressants
Cardiovascular drugs
Stimulants and street drugs
Alcohols

Bronstein AC, Spyker DA, Cantilena LR, et al. 2007. Annual Report of the American Association of Poison Control Centers' National Poison Data System (NPDS): 25th annual report. *Clin Toxicol*, 2008, 46:927–1057.

of acetaminophen or aspirin cannot clearly be excluded via the exposure history, serum quantification of these drugs is recommended. An electrocardiogram (ECG) may be useful at detecting heart blocks, Na^+ channel blockade, or K^+ channel blockade associated with specific medication classes. Further laboratory analysis, such as use of blood gas determinations, serum chemistries, complete blood counts, and other testing, should be tailored to the individual poisoning circumstance.

b. How are the principles of absorption, distribution, metabolism, and elimination different for a drug after excessive exposure than after a therapeutic dose?

The principles of pharmacokinetics (absorption, distribution, metabolism, and elimination) are described in Chapter 2. Toxicokinetics (the pharmacokinetics of a drug under circumstances that produce toxicity or excessive exposure) may differ significantly after poisoning, and these differences may profoundly alter treatment decisions and prognosis. Ingesting larger than therapeutic doses of a pharmaceutical may prolong its absorption, alter its protein binding and apparent volume of distribution, and change its metabolic fate.

When confronted with a potential poisoning, 2 toxicokinetic questions should be foremost in the clinician's mind:

- How long does an asymptomatic patient need to be monitored (drug absorption and dynamics)?
- How long will it take an intoxicated patient to get better (drug elimination and dynamics)?

(Continued)

TABLE 3-7 ABCDE: Initial Treatment Approach for Acute Poisoning

Airway	Maintain patency
Breathing	Maintain adequate oxygenation and ventilation
Circulation	Maintain perfusion of vital organs
Disability	Assess for central nervous system dysfunction *If neurological disability is noted, consider:* • *Oxygen administration (check pulse oximetry)* • *Dextrose administration (check blood glucose concentration)* • *Naloxone administration (consider empiric trial)* • *Thiamine (for adult patients receiving dextrose)*
Exposure	Assess "toxidrome" (see Table 3-8)

TABLE 3-8 Common Toxidromes

DRUG CLASS	EXAMPLE(S)	MENTAL STATUS	HR	BP	RR	T	PUPIL SIZE	OTHER
Sympathomimetic	Cocaine, Amphetamine	Agitation	↑	↑		↑	↑	Tremor, diaphoresis
Anticholinergic	Diphenhydramine, *Belladonna atropa*	Delirium	↑	↑		↑	↑	Ileus, flushing
Cholinergic	Organophosphates	Somnolence/coma			↑		↓	SLUDGE,[a] fasciculation
Opioid	Heroin, Oxycodone	Somnolence/coma	↓		↓		↓	
Sedative-hypnotic	Benzodiazepines, Barbiturates	Somnolence/coma		↓	↓			
Salicylate	Aspirin	Confusion	↑		↑	↑		Diaphoresis, vomiting
Ca^{2+} channel blocker	Verapamil		↓	↓				

HR, heart rate; BP, blood pressure; RR, respiratory rate; T, temperature. [a]SLUDGE, muscarinic effects of Salivation, Lacrimation, Urination, Defecation, Gastric cramping, and Emesis.

c. How does acetaminophen produce toxicity?

Acetaminophen is metabolized to nontoxic glucuronide and sulfate conjugates, and to a highly reactive metabolite *N*-acetyl-*p*-benzoquinoneimine (NAPQI) via CYP isoforms. NAPQI is referred to as a biologically reactive intermediate, and such intermediates often arise due to drug metabolism. At therapeutic dosing, NAPQI binds to nucleophilic glutathione; but, in overdose, glutathione depletion may lead to the pathological finding of hepatic necrosis (see Figure 3-6). The highly reactive NAPQI metabolite binds covalently to cell macromolecules, leading to dysfunction of enzymatic systems and structural and metabolic disarray. Furthermore, depletion of intracellular GSH renders the hepatocytes highly susceptible to oxidative stress and apoptosis.

Acute overdose can cause severe hepatic damage, and the number of accidental or deliberate poisonings with acetaminophen continues to grow. Chronic use of less than 2 g/day is not typically associated with hepatic dysfunction, but overuse of acetaminophen-containing narcotic and over-the-counter combination products marketed in the United States has led to heightened awareness of the possibility of toxicity.

Acute ingestion of more than 7.5 g of acetaminophen, or repeat use of supratherapeutic doses, can result in toxicity. The most serious acute adverse effect of an overdose of acetaminophen is a potentially fatal hepatic necrosis. Renal tubular necrosis and hypoglycemic coma also may occur.

In adults, hepatotoxicity may occur after ingestion of a single dose of 10 to 15 g (150-250 mg/kg) of acetaminophen; doses of 20 to 25 g or more are potentially fatal. Conditions of CYP induction (eg, heavy alcohol consumption) or GSH depletion (eg, fasting or malnutrition) increase the susceptibility to hepatic injury, which has been documented, albeit uncommonly, with doses in the therapeutic range.

Symptoms that occur during the first 2 days of acute poisoning by acetaminophen reflect gastric distress (eg, nausea, abdominal pain, anorexia) and belie the potential seriousness of the intoxication. Plasma hepatic transaminases become elevated, sometimes markedly so, beginning ~12 to 36 hours after ingestion. Clinical indications of hepatic damage manifest within 2 to 4 days of ingestion of toxic doses, with right subcostal pain, tender hepatomegaly, jaundice, and coagulopathy. Renal impairment or frank renal failure may occur. Liver enzyme abnormalities typically peak 72 to 96 hours after ingestion. The onset of hepatic encephalopathy or worsening coagulopathy beyond this time indicates a poor prognosis. Biopsy of the liver reveals centrilobular necrosis with sparing of the periportal area. In nonfatal cases, the hepatic lesions are reversible over a period of weeks or months.

(Continued)

SECTION I   General Principles

d. How is the diagnosis of acetaminophen toxicity established?

Acetaminophen overdose constitutes a medical emergency. Severe liver damage occurs in 90% of patients with plasma concentrations of acetaminophen more than 300 μg/mL at 4 hours after ingestion or 45 μg/mL at 15 hours after the ingestion of the drug. Minimal hepatic damage can be anticipated when the drug concentration is less than 120 μg/mL at 4 hours or 30 μg/mL at 12 hours after ingestion.

e. How should acetaminophen poisoning be treated?

Early diagnosis and treatment of acetaminophen overdose is essential to optimize outcome. Perhaps 10% of poisoned patients who do not receive specific treatment develop severe liver damage; 10 to 20% of these eventually die of hepatic failure despite intensive supportive care. Activated charcoal, if given within 4 hours of ingestion, decreases acetaminophen absorption by 50 to 90% and is the preferred method of gastric decontamination. Gastric lavage generally is not recommended.

N-acetylcysteine (NAC)(see Table 3-1) is indicated for those at risk of hepatic injury. NAC therapy should be instituted in suspected cases of acetaminophen poisoning before blood concentrations become available, with treatment terminated if assay results subsequently indicate that the risk of hepatotoxicity is low. NAC functions by detoxifying NAPQI. It both repletes GSH stores and may conjugate directly with NAPQI by serving as a GSH substitute. There is some evidence that in cases of established acetaminophen toxicity, NAC may protect against extrahepatic injury by its antioxidant and anti-inflammatory properties. Even in the presence of activated charcoal, there is ample absorption of NAC, and neither should activated charcoal be avoided nor NAC administration be delayed because of concerns of a charcoal-NAC interaction.

Adverse reactions to NAC include rash (including urticaria, which does not require drug discontinuation), nausea, vomiting, diarrhea, and rare anaphylactic reactions. An oral loading dose of 140 mg/kg is given, followed by the administration of 70 mg/kg every 4 hours for 17 doses. Where available, the intravenous loading dose is 150 mg/kg by intravenous infusion in 200 mL of 5% dextrose over 60 minutes, followed by 50 mg/kg by intravenous infusion in 500 mL of 5% dextrose over 4 hours, then 100 mg/kg by intravenous infusion in 1000 mL of 5% dextrose over 16 hours.

In addition to NAC therapy, aggressive supportive care is warranted. This includes management of hepatic and renal failure if they occur and intubation if the patient becomes obtunded. Hypoglycemia can result from liver failure, and plasma glucose should be monitored closely. Fulminant hepatic failure is an indication for liver transplantation, and a liver transplant center should be contacted early in the course of treatment of patients who develop severe liver injury despite NAC therapy.

CASE 3-6

A 2-year-old-girl is brought to the emergency room after ingesting some of her pregnant mother's iron tablets.

a. How should iron poisoning be established in this patient?

A history of ingestion by a parent is frequently sufficient to initiate therapy. A confirmation of the diagnosis is made with the measurement of a plasma iron.

In the evaluation of a child thought to have ingested iron, a color test for iron in the gastric contents and an emergency determination of the concentration of iron in plasma can be performed. If the latter is less than 63 μmol (3.5 mg/L), the child is not in immediate danger. However, vomiting should be induced when there is iron in the stomach, and an x-ray should be taken to evaluate the number of pills remaining in the small bowel (iron tablets are radiopaque).

Large amounts of ferrous salts are toxic, but fatalities are rare in adults. Most deaths occur in children, particularly between the ages of 12 and 24 months. As little as 1 to 2 g of iron may cause death, but 2 to 10 g usually is ingested in fatal cases. The frequency of iron poisoning relates to its availability in the household, particularly

(Continued)

Clinical and Environmental Toxicity — CHAPTER 3

the supply that remains after a pregnancy. The colored sugar coating of many of the commercially available tablets gives them the appearance of candy. All iron preparations should be kept in childproof bottles.

b. What are the signs and symptoms of iron poisoning and how does iron produce toxicity?

Signs and symptoms of severe poisoning may occur within 30 minutes after ingestion or may be delayed for several hours. They include abdominal pain, diarrhea, or vomiting of brown or bloody stomach contents containing pills. Of particular concern are pallor or cyanosis, lassitude, drowsiness, hyperventilation due to acidosis, and cardiovascular collapse. If death does not occur within 6 hours, there may be a transient period of apparent recovery, followed by death in 12 to 24 hours. The corrosive injury to the stomach may result in pyloric stenosis or gastric scarring. Hemorrhagic gastroenteritis and hepatic damage are prominent findings at autopsy.

c. How should this patient be treated?

Iron in the upper GI tract can be precipitated by lavage with sodium bicarbonate or phosphate solution, although the clinical benefit is questionable. When the plasma concentration of iron is greater than the total iron-binding capacity (63 µmol; 3.5 mg/L), deferoxamine should be administered. Shock, dehydration, and acid-base abnormalities should be treated in the conventional manner. Most important is the speed of diagnosis and therapy. With early effective treatment, the mortality from iron poisoning can be reduced from as high as 45% to as low as 1%.

Deferoxamine is isolated as the iron chelate from *Streptomyces pilosus* and is treated chemically to obtain the metal-free ligand. Deferoxamine has the desirable properties of a remarkably high affinity for ferric iron ($K_a = 10^{31}$) coupled with a very low affinity for calcium ($K_a = 10^2$). In vitro, it removes iron from hemosiderin and ferritin and, to a lesser extent, from transferrin. Iron in hemoglobin or cytochromes is not removed by deferoxamine.

Deferoxamine is poorly absorbed after oral administration, and parenteral administration is required. For severe iron toxicity (serum iron levels greater than 500 µg/dL), the intravenous route is preferred. The drug is administered at 10 to 15 mg/kg/hour by constant infusion. Faster rates of infusion (45 mg/kg/h) have been used in a few cases; rapid boluses usually are associated with hypotension. Deferoxamine may be given intramuscularly in moderately toxic cases (serum iron 350-500 µg/dL) at a dose of 50 mg/kg with a maximum dose of 1 g. Hypotension also can occur with the intramuscular route.

d. What are the toxic effects of deferoxamine therapy?

Deferoxamine causes a number of allergic reactions, including pruritus, wheals, rash, and anaphylaxis. Other adverse effects include dysuria, abdominal discomfort, diarrhea, fever, leg cramps, and tachycardia. Occasional cases of cataract formation have been reported. Deferoxamine may cause neurotoxicity during long-term, high-dose therapy for transfusion-dependent thalassemia major; both visual and auditory changes have been described. A "pulmonary syndrome" has been associated with high-dose (10-25 mg/kg/h) deferoxamine therapy; tachypnea, hypoxemia, fever, and eosinophilia are prominent symptoms. Contraindications to the use of deferoxamine include renal insufficiency and anuria; during pregnancy, the drug should be used only if clearly indicated.

CASE 3-7

A 48-year-old man has a community-acquired pneumonia. He is prescribed an oral penicillin product. Within 15 minutes of taking the first dose, he develops tightness in his chest, and numbness and swelling of his lips. His wife calls emergency services; he is treated in his home and transported to the hospital.

a. What are the different types of adverse reactions to medications?

The different types of toxicity to drugs include dose-dependent reactions that may be an extension of a drug's therapeutic effect, pathological toxicity, genotoxicity,

(Continued)

allergic reactions, and idiosyncratic reactions (see Side Bar TYPES OF THERAPEUTIC DRUG TOXICITY).

b. He does not remember ever-receiving penicillin before so what type of reaction is this?

He may have received penicillin as a child and not known what the medication was. An allergy is an adverse reaction that results from previous sensitization to a particular chemical or to one that is structurally similar. Such reactions are mediated by the immune system. For a low-molecular-weight chemical to cause an allergic reaction, it or its metabolic product usually acts as a hapten, combining with an endogenous protein to form an antigenic complex. Such antigens induce the synthesis of antibodies, usually after a latent period of at least 1 to 2 weeks. Subsequent exposure to the chemical results in an antigen-antibody interaction that provokes the typical manifestations of allergy. Dose-response relationships usually are not apparent for the provocation of allergic reactions. Allergic responses have been divided into 4 general categories based on the mechanism of immunological involvement (see Side Bar TYPES OF THERAPEUTIC DRUG TOXICITY).

Anaphylaxis is mediated by IgE antibodies. The Fc portion of IgE can bind to receptors on mast cells and basophils. If the Fab portion of the antibody molecule then binds antigen, various mediators (eg, histamine, leukotrienes, and prostaglandins) are released and cause vasodilation, edema, and an inflammatory response. The main targets of this type of reaction are the gastrointestinal (GI) tract (food allergies), the skin (urticaria and atopic dermatitis), the respiratory system (rhinitis and asthma), and the vasculature (anaphylactic shock). These responses tend to occur quickly after challenge with an antigen to which the individual has been sensitized and are termed immediate hypersensitivity reactions.

c. What would be the treatment for this type of reaction?

The use of epinephrine to immediately treat drug-induced anaphylaxis is introduced in Chapter 7 of *Goodman and Gilman's The Pharmacological Basis of Therapeutics*, 12th Edition.

CASE 3-8

A 56-year-old woman previously developed a severe thrombocytopenia after receiving sulfamethoxazole-trimethoprim fixed-dose product (SEPTRA) for a urinary tract infection. She is now in the hospital for hip replacement surgery. Her hospital chart has a sticker "Allergic to SEPTRA" on the front cover. Following her surgery she develops a urinary tract infection and is given BACTRIM.

a. What is the issue with the administration of BACTRIM to this patient?

BACTRIM is another trade name for a fixed-dose combination of sulfamethoxazole-trimethoprim (see Chapter 38). So there should be concern that BACTRIM will cause the same type of adverse reaction as SEPTRA. This type of medication error is obviously preventable and stems from the lack of knowledge by hospital staff about the medications being administered. In this case, apparently the pharmacy staff either did not know that the patient had a history of a prior reaction to SEPTRA, or that BACTRIM was a similar product.

b. How can medication errors be avoided?

Over the past decade considerable attention has been given to the reduction of medication errors and adverse drug events (ADEs). Medication errors can occur in any part of the medication prescribing or use process, while ADEs are injuries related to the use or nonuse of medications. It is believed that medication errors are 50 to 100 times more common than ADEs. Some ADEs, such as previously unknown allergies, are unpreventable, but most medication errors can be prevented. Traditionally, the "5 Rights" of safe medication administration have been taught on hospital wards:

Right drug, right patient, right dose, right route, right time. *(Continued)*

Clinical and Environmental Toxicity

CHAPTER 3

However, accomplishing a reduction in medication errors involves scrutiny of the systems involved in prescribing, documenting, transcribing, dispensing, administering, and monitoring a therapy.

c. **How can medication errors be prevented?**

Good medication use practices have mandatory and redundant checkpoints, such as having a pharmacist, a doctor, and a nurse all review and confirm that an ordered dose of a medication is appropriate for a patient prior to the drug's administration. In such a system, medication errors occur only when several "holes" in the medication administration safeguards exist and are simultaneously aligned. Several practical strategies have been suggested to reduce medication errors within hospitals and other health care settings (see Table 3-9), and these strategies are being constantly revised.

CASE 3-9

A 3-year-old boy is brought to a medical clinic because of the recent onset of lethargy and behavior changes. The diagnosis of lead intoxication is made.

a. **How could this child have been exposed to lead?**

In the United States, paint containing lead for use in and around households was banned in 1978, while the use of tetraethyl lead in gasoline was phased out and eventually eliminated between 1976 and 1996. The economic benefit of the reduction in lead exposure due to these 2 measures is estimated at hundreds of billions of dollars per year. Despite these bans, past use of lead carbonate and lead oxide in paint and tetraethyl lead in gasoline remain the primary sources of lead exposure. Lead is not degradable and remains throughout the environment in dust, soil, and the paint of older homes. Young children often are exposed to lead by nibbling sweet-tasting paint chips or eating dust and soil in and around older homes. Renovation or demolition of older buildings may cause substantial lead exposure. Tetraethyl lead was used as an antiknock agent in gasoline, which resulted in high levels of lead in air pollution. Removal of lead from gasoline caused lead levels in air pollution to drop by more than 90% between 1982 and 2002. Lead was commonly used in plumbing and can leach into drinking water. Acidic foods and beverages dissolve lead when stored in containers with lead in their glaze or lead-soldered cans, which was a significant problem through the middle of the 20th century and remains a problem in developing countries. Lead exposure also has been traced to other sources such as lead toys,

(Continued)

HEALTH EFFECTS OF LEAD TOXICITY

- Neurotoxicity
  - Cognitive delays and behavior changes in children
  - Neuromuscular defects—lead palsy
  - Encephalopathy
- Cardiovascular effects
  - Increased blood pressure
- Renal effects
  - Depressed glomerular filtration
- Hematological effects
  - Hypochromic microcytic anemia
  - Immunosupression
- Gastrointestinal effects
  - Severe intestinal pain—lead colic
- Carcinogenesis
  - Probably carcinogenic to humans—cancers of lung, brain, kidney, and stomach

TABLE 3-9 Best Practice Recommendations to Reduce Medication Administration Errors[a]

Short Term
- Maintain unit-dose distribution systems for nonemergency medications
- Have pharmacies prepare intravenous solutions
- Remove inherently dangerous medications (eg, concentrated KCl) from patient care areas
- Develop special procedures for high-risk drugs
- Improve drug-related clinical information resources
- Improve medication administration education for clinicians
- Educate patients about the safe and accurate use of medications
- Improve access of bedside clinicians to pharmacists

Long Term
Implement technology-based safeguards:
- Computerized order entry
- Computerized dose and allergy checking
- Computerized medication tracking
- Use of bar codes or electronic readers for medication preparation and administration

[a]See Massachusetts Hospital Association.
http://macoalition.org/documents/Best_Practice_Medication_Errors.pdf

SECTION I   General Principles

Succinyl CoA + Glycine
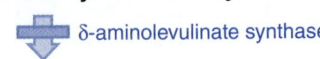
δ-Aminolevulinate (δ-ALA)
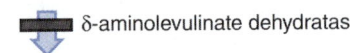
Porphobilinogen
 porphobilinogen deaminase
uroporphyrinogen III cosynthase
Uroporphyrinogen III
 uroporphyrinogen decarboxylase
Coproporphyrinogen III
 coproporphyrinogen oxidase
Protoporphyrin IX
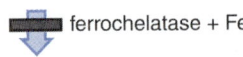
Heme

Action produced by lead:
■ Inhibition
■ Postulated inhibition

FIGURE 3-7 Heme biosynthesis and actions of lead. Lead interferes with the biosynthesis of heme at several enzymatic steps. Steps that definitely are inhibited by lead are indicated by black blocks. Steps at which lead is thought to act but where evidence for this is inconclusive are indicated by blue blocks.

non-Western folk medicines, cosmetics, retained bullets, artists' paint pigments, ashes and fumes from painted wood, jewelers' wastes, home battery manufacture, and lead-type. Blood lead levels in the general population have steadily decreased since the 1970s. Between 1976 and 2002, mean blood levels in children 1 to 5 years of age dropped from 15 to 1.9 μg/dL. The Centers for Disease Control and Prevention (CDC) recommends screening of children at 6 months of age and the use of aggressive lead abatement for children with blood lead levels greater than 10 μg/dL.

Lead exposure occurs through ingestion or inhalation. GI absorption of lead varies considerably with age and diet. Children absorb a much higher percentage of ingested lead (~40% on average) than adults (<20%).

b. What is the mechanism of lead toxicity?

Lead toxicity results from molecular mimicry of other divalent metals. Lead takes the place of zinc or calcium in a number of important proteins. Because of its size and electron affinity, lead alters protein structure and can inappropriately activate or inhibit protein function. Specific organ systems that are targets for lead are CNS, cardiovascular, renal, hematopoietic, and gastrointestinal.

c. What are the health effects of lead poisoning?

Figure 3-7 shows the sites of action of the actions of lead on heme biosynthesis. Lead causes a hypochromic microcytic anemia. Figure 3-8 shows the health effects of lead poisoning in relation to the blood lead concentration.

d. What are the treatment options for this patient?

The most important response to lead poisoning is removal of the source of lead exposure. Supportive measures should be undertaken to relieve symptoms.

Chelation therapy is warranted for children and adults with high blood lead levels (>45 μg/dL and >70 μg/dL, respectively) and/or acute symptoms of lead poisoning. Although chelation therapy is effective at lowering blood lead levels and relieving immediate symptoms, it does not reduce the chronic effects of lead beyond the benefit of lead abatement alone. In rats, chelators enhance mobilization of lead from the soft tissues to the brain and may increase the adverse neurodevelopmental effects of lead.

Chelators effective in treating acute lead poisoning are listed in the Summary Table at the end of the chapter.

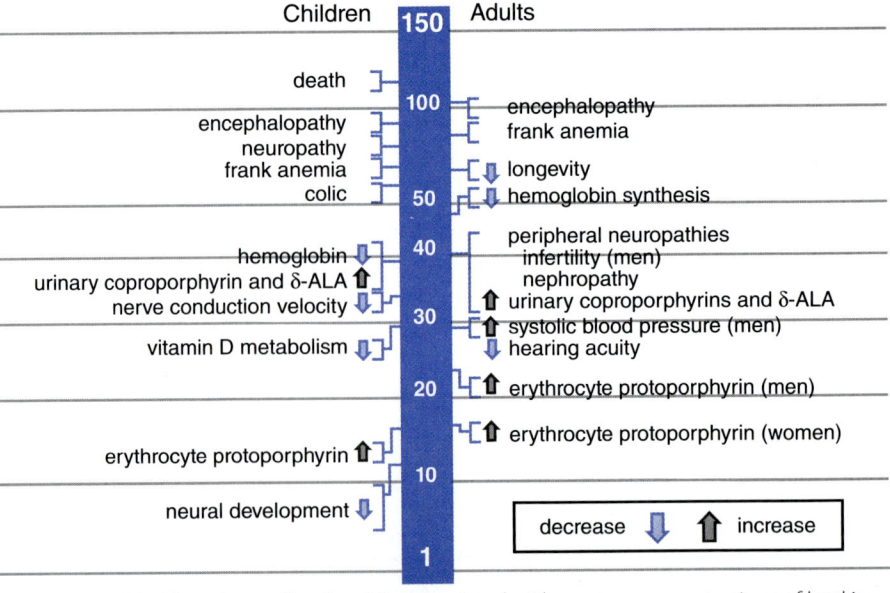

FIGURE 3-8 Manifestations of lead toxicity associated with varying concentrations of lead in the blood of children and adults. δ-ALA, δ-aminolevulinate

Clinical and Environmental Toxicity — CHAPTER 3

CASE 3-10

A 12-month-old boy is brought to the hospital because of weakness, nausea, vomiting, diarrhea, and dyspnea for the past week. His father admitted to bringing home elemental mercury so that his older children could shine silver coins. The older children admitted to pushing the liquid mercury around the table some of which fell onto the carpet. So that it would not be detected the older children spread it around with their feet. Neither the parents nor the 3 older children were ill. A 24-hour urine collected from the toddler showed an elevated mercury concentration.

a. Why was the youngest child intoxicated when the older children or the adults were not?

Most likely it is because he was crawling or close to the floor which would have the highest concentration of mercury vapor.

Figure 3-9 shows the health effects of mercury in relation to the concentration in air and the corresponding urinary concentrations.

Metallic mercury (Hg^0) vapor is readily absorbed through the lungs (~70-80%), but GI absorption of metallic mercury is negligible. Once absorbed, Hg^0 distributes throughout the body and crosses membranes such as the blood-brain barrier (BBB) and the placenta via diffusion. Hg^0 is oxidized by catalase in the erythrocytes and other cells to form Hg^{2+}. Shortly after exposure, some Hg^0 is eliminated in exhaled air. After a few hours, distribution and elimination of Hg^0 resemble the properties of Hg^{2+}. After exposure to Hg^0 vapor, it is oxidized to Hg^{2+} and retained in the brain.

Inhalation of high levels of mercury vapor over a short duration is acutely toxic to the lung. Respiratory symptoms of mercury exposure start with cough and tightness in the chest and can progress to interstitial pneumonitis and severely compromised respiratory function. Other initial symptoms include weakness, chills, metallic taste, nausea, vomiting, diarrhea, and dyspnea. Acute exposure to high doses of mercury is toxic to the CNS with symptoms, including tremor, emotional lability, insomnia, muscular atrophy, parathesia, and cognitive deficits.

b. How can this exposure be limited?

It is unlikely that the metallic mercury can be removed by cleaning the carpet in place. The carpet will need to be removed from the house and discarded properly.

(Continued)

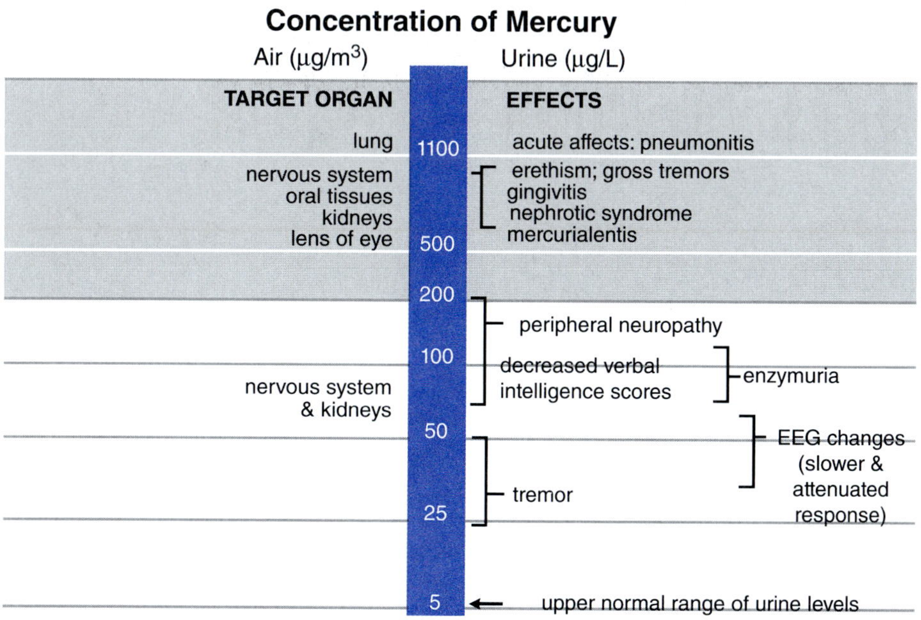

Concentration of Mercury

Target Organ	Air (µg/m³) / Urine (µg/L)	Effects
lung	1100	acute affects: pneumonitis
nervous system, oral tissues, kidneys, lens of eye	500	erethism; gross tremors; gingivitis; nephrotic syndrome; mercurialentis
	200	
	100	peripheral neuropathy; decreased verbal intelligence scores; enzymuria
nervous system & kidneys	50	
	25	tremor; EEG changes (slower & attenuated response)
	5	upper normal range of urine levels

FIGURE 3-9 The concentration of mercury vapor in the air and related concentrations of mercury in urine are associated with a variety of toxic effects.

c. What are the treatment options for this patient?

With exposure to metallic mercury, termination of exposure is critical and respiratory support may be required. Emesis may be used within 30 to 60 minutes of oral exposure to inorganic mercury, provided the patient is awake and alert and there is no corrosive injury. This would not be necessary in this patient who was poisoned with mercury vapor. Maintenance of electrolyte balance and fluids is important for patients exposed to inorganic mercury. Chelation therapy is beneficial in patients with acute inorganic or metallic mercury exposure. For specific mercury chelators, see the Summary Table at the end of this chapter.

CASE 3-11

A 33-year-old man, recently arrived from Kenya, is suspected of having liver cancer due to aflatoxin B_1 exposure.

a. What are some common carcinogens? How do environmental contaminants cause cancer?

Figure 3-10 shows the steps that lead from an environmental carcinogen exposure to carcinogenesis. Table 3-2 lists some important carcinogens.

b. How do humans become exposed to excessive amounts of aflatoxin B_1?

Aflatoxins are produced by *Aspergillus flavus*, a fungus that is a common contaminant of foods, especially corn, peanuts, cottonseed, and tree nuts. *A. flavus* is abundant in regions with hot and wet climates, and as a result, hepatocellular carcinoma is a serious problem in subtropical and tropical regions of Latin America, Africa, and Southeast Asia. Human exposure to aflatoxin in the United States is very rare and not thought to have a significant impact on health.

c. What is the mechanism by which aflatoxin B_1 is thought to be carcinogenic?

The mechanism of aflatoxin carcinogenesis has been extensively studied (see Figure 3-11). The 8,9-epoxide of aflatoxin B_1 readily reacts with amines in biological macromolecules. Aflatoxin B_1 8,9-epoxide forms adducts with deoxyguanosine and albumin that can be detected in the blood or urine of humans and laboratory animals exposed to aflatoxin, providing evidence for the activity of this pathway in vivo. Aflatoxin primarily forms DNA adducts at deoxyguanosine residues, reacting at either the N1 or N7 position. The N7-guanine adduct mispairs with adenine, leading to G → T transversions. Human aflatoxin exposure is associated with hepatocellular carcinomas bearing an AGG to AGT mutation in codon 249 of the p53

(Continued)

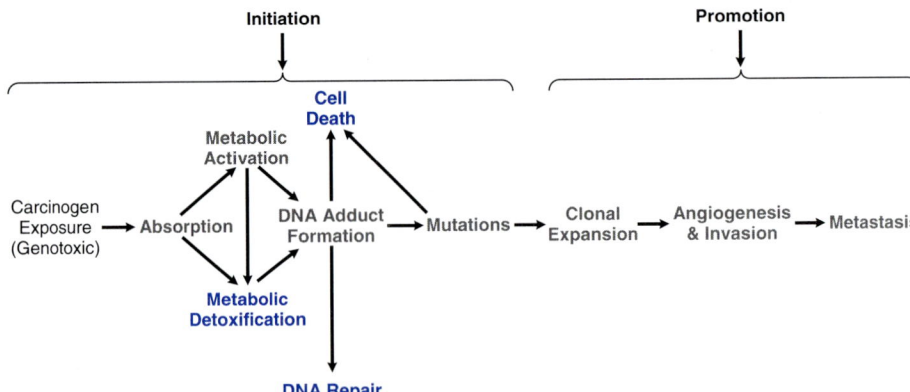

FIGURE 3-10 Carcinogenesis: initiation and promotion. There are many steps that occur between the exposure to a genotoxic carcinogen and the development of cancer. Processes in gray lead to the development of cancer, while those in blue reduce the risk. Nongenotoxic carcinogens act by enhancing steps leading to cancer and/or inhibiting protective processes. A chemopreventive agent acts by inhibiting steps leading to cancer or by increasing protective processes.

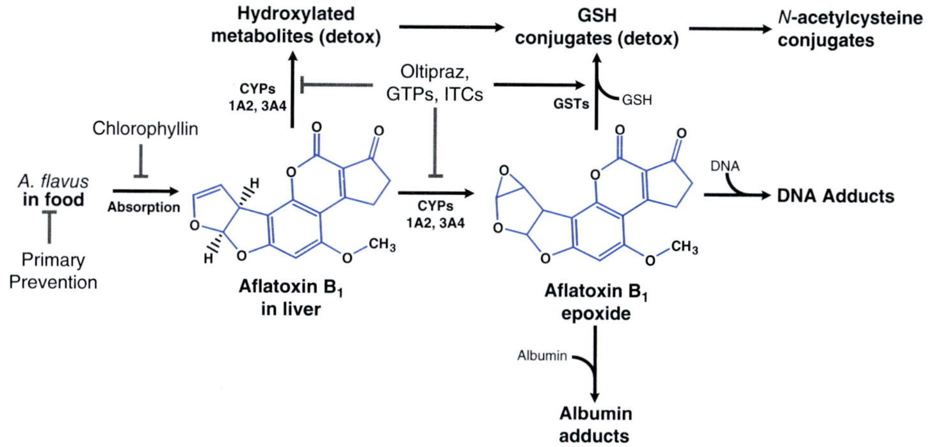

FIGURE 3-11 Metabolism and actions of aflatoxin B_1. Following absorption, aflatoxin B_1 undergoes activation by CYPs to its 8,9-epoxide, which can be detoxified by glutathione S-transferases (GSTs) or by spontaneous hydration. Alternatively, it can react with cellular macromolecules such as DNA and protein, leading to toxicity and cancer. Oltipraz, green tea polyphenols (GTPs), and isothiocyanates (ITCs) decrease aflatoxin carcinogenesis by inhibiting the CYPs involved in activating aflatoxin and increasing the synthesis of the cofactor GSH for GSTs involved in detoxification.

tumor suppressor gene, resulting in the replacement of an arginine with cysteine. This mutation is almost never observed in geographical regions with limited aflatoxin exposure.

Aflatoxin exposure and hepatitis B virus work synergistically to cause hepatocellular carcinoma. Many of the regions with elevated aflatoxin exposure also have a high level of endemic hepatitis B infection. Separately, aflatoxin or hepatitis B exposure increases the risk of hepatocellular carcinoma 3.4- or 7.3-fold, respectively; those exposed to both have a 59-fold increased risk of cancer compared to unexposed individuals.

The interaction between aflatoxin and hepatitis B that is responsible for the increased incidence of hepatocellular carcinoma is not well understood. Hepatitis B influences the metabolism of aflatoxin B_1 by upregulating CYPs, including 3A4, and decreasing glutathione S-transferase activity. In addition, hepatocellular proliferation to repair damage done by hepatitis B infection increases the likelihood that aflatoxin-induced DNA adducts will cause mutations. The hepatotoxic and tumor-promoting effects of hepatitis B also could provide a more favorable environment for the proliferation and invasion of initiated cells.

d. What treatment options are available for a person likely to be exposed to aflatoxin?

The clear relationship between aflatoxin metabolism (see Figure 3-11) and its carcinogenicity makes it an appealing target for chemopreventive strategies that modify its metabolism. Inhibiting CYP activity or increasing glutathione conjugation will reduce the intracellular concentration of the 8,9-epoxide and thus prevent DNA adduct formation. Oltipraz, green tea polyphenols (GTPs), and isothiocyanates (ITCs) decrease aflatoxin carcinogenesis by inhibiting the CYPs involved in activating aflatoxin and increasing the synthesis of the cofactor GSH for GSTs involved in detoxification (see Figure 3-11).

Chemoprevention of hepatocellular carcinoma in people exposed to aflatoxin also can be achieved by limiting infections with hepatitis B. Because of the strong interaction between hepatitis B and aflatoxin in carcinogenesis, the hepatitis B vaccine will reduce the sensitivity of people to the induction of cancer by aflatoxin. Primary prevention of aflatoxin exposure through hand or fluorescent sorting of crops to remove those with fungal contamination can also reduce human exposure. A more cost-effective primary prevention approach is to improve food storage to limit the spread of *A. flavus*, which requires a warm and humid environment.

(Continued)

SECTION I General Principles

Yet another approach used for the chemoprevention of aflatoxin hepatocarcinogenesis is the use of "interceptor molecules." Chlorophyllin, an over-the-counter mixture of water-soluble chlorophyll salts, binds tightly to aflatoxin in the GI tract, forming a complex that is not absorbed (see Figure 3-11).

KEY CONCEPTS

- Pharmacology intersects with toxicology when the physiological response to a drug is an adverse effect.
- The therapeutic index (TI) quantifies the relative safety of a drug.
- Toxicokinetics (the pharmacokinetics of a drug under circumstances that produce toxicity or excessive exposure) may differ significantly after poisoning.
- The effects of chemicals observed in laboratory animals, when properly qualified, apply to human toxicity.
- Exposure of experimental animals to toxic agents in high doses is a necessary and valid method to discover possible hazards to humans exposed to much lower doses.
- Federal law in the United States and ethical considerations require that the study of new drugs in humans be conducted in accordance with stringent guidelines (see Side Bar GUIDELINES FOR THE STUDY OF NEW DRUGS IN HUMANS).
- Medication errors are believed to be 50 to 100 times more common than adverse drug events.
- The priority of poisoning treatment is to support vital functions until the drug or chemical is eliminated from the body; specific antidotes are uncommonly needed.
- With environmental exposures, one has to consider population exposures to low-dose toxicants over long periods of time.
- The transformation of a normal cell to a malignancy is a multistage process, and exogenous chemicals can act at 1 or more of these stages.
- Metals are an important class of environmental toxicants; they are ubiquitous environmental contaminants that come from both natural and anthropogenic sources.
- The most important response to exposure to metals is to eliminate the source of the exposure.
- Treatment for acute metal intoxication often involves the use of chelators.
- Following chronic exposure to toxic metals, chelation therapy does not show clinical benefits beyond those of cessation of exposure alone, and in some cases may do more harm than good.

SUMMARY QUIZ

QUESTION 3-1 Five drugs each have one of the therapeutic indexes shown below. Which drug will require the closest monitoring to avoid toxicity?

a. TI = 2
b. TI = 5
c. TI = 50
d. TI = 10
e. TI = 100

QUESTION 3-2 A mother with 3 children less than the age of 5 years is concerned about strategies to prevent poisoning in her children. One effective strategy is to

a. tell the children not to take medicine unless it is given to them by an adult.
b. keep all medicine in a high cabinet.

c. make certain that all medicine is in a child-resistant package.
d. keep all cleaning products under the kitchen sink and tell the children not to open the door.
e. keep pesticides in the garage.

QUESTION 3-3 A 28-year-old man is brought to the emergency room. Physical examination reveals that he has salivation, lacrimation, urination, diarrhea, stomach pain, vomiting, increased heart rate, and constricted pupils. It is likely that he has been poisoned with

a. heroin.
b. aspirin.
c. methanol.
d. organophosphate pesticide.
e. diazepam.

QUESTION 3-4 A 23-year-old woman with a suspected drug overdose is brought to the emergency room. On physical examination, she is unresponsive and her respirations are shallow. Her initial therapy should be to

a. cause emesis.
b. make certain that she is well oxygenated.
c. get a toxicology test to determine what poison she has ingested.
d. get a chest x-ray.
e. get an electrocardiogram.

QUESTION 3-5 A 35-year-old man is being treated with $CaNa_2EDTA$ for acute exposure to

a. mercury.
b. arsenic.
c. iron.
d. copper.
e. lead.

QUESTION 3-6 After a chronic exposure to lead, a 43-year-old man should be treated with

a. EDTA $CaNa_2$.
b. dimercaprol.
c. deferoxamine.
d. succimer.
e. none of the above.

QUESTION 3-7 A 27-year-old woman is diagnosed with arsenic poisoning. A likely source of her exposure is

a. drinking water.
b. hair spray.
c. her husband.
d. syphilis treatment.
e. dental fillings.

QUESTION 3-8 Benzo[a]pyrene, a key carcinogen in tobacco smoke, is a carcinogen because it forms adducts with

a. epinephrine.
b. DNA.

SECTION I — General Principles

   c. cysteine.

   d. leucine.

   e. dopamine.

SUMMARY QUIZ ANWSER KEY

QUESTION 3-1 Answer **a.** The therapeutic index (TI), quantifies the relative safety of a drug. Clearly, the higher the ratio, the safer the drug. TI = LD_{50}/ED_{50} (see Figure 3-2). Drugs show a wide range of TI, from 1 to more than 100. Drugs with a low TI must be administered with caution. Agents that fall into this category include the cardiac glycoside digitalis and cancer chemotherapeutic agents. Agents with very high TI are extremely safe and include some antibiotics (eg, penicillin), unless there is a known allergic response.

QUESTION 3-2 Answer **c.** Poisoning prevention strategies may be categorized as being passive, requiring no behavior change on the part of the individual, or active, requiring sustained adaptation to be successful. Passive prevention strategies are the most effective, and several types of passive poisoning prevention are described in Table 4-7 in Chapter 4 of *Goodman and Gilman's The Pharmacological Basis of Therapeutics*, 12th Edition. One effective strategy is to make certain that all medications are in child-resistant containers.

QUESTION 3-3 Answer **d.** Often, an observation of physical symptoms and signs may be the only additional clues to a poisoning diagnosis. Groups of physical signs and symptoms associated with specific poisoning syndromes are known as toxidromes. Table 3-8 describes commonly encountered toxidromes. This patient has the characteristic signs and symptoms of organophosphate poisoning.

QUESTION 3-4 Answer **b.** The "ABC" mnemonic of emergency care is popularly taught and applies to the treatment of acute poisoning (see Table 3-7). In severe cases, endotracheal intubation, mechanical ventilation, pharmacological blood pressure support, and/or extracorporeal circulatory support may be necessary and appropriate.

QUESTION 3-5 Answer **e.** EDTA $CaNa_2$ is effective for the treatment of acute lead poisoning, particularly in combination with dimercaprol, but is not an effective chelator of mercury or arsenic in vivo.

QUESTION 3-6 Answer **e.** A chelator is a compound that forms stable complexes with metals, typically as 5- or 6-membered rings. Formation of complexes between chelators and metals should prevent or reverse metal binding to biological ligands. In cases of acute exposure to high doses of most metals, chelation therapy reduces toxicity. However, following chronic exposure, chelation therapy does not show clinical benefits beyond those of cessation of exposure alone and, in some cases, does more harm than good. Chelation therapy may increase the neurotoxic effects of heavy metals and is only recommended for acute poisonings.

QUESTION 3-7 Answer **a.** The primary source of exposure to arsenic is through drinking water. Arsenic naturally leaches out of soil and rocks into well and spring water. Levels of arsenic in drinking water average 2 µg/L (ppb) in the United States but can be more than 50 µg/L (5 times the EPA standard) in private well water, particularly in California, Nevada, and Arizona. Drinking water from other parts of the world where well water has been promoted to prevent waterborne illness, particularly Taiwan, China, Argentina, Chile, Bangladesh, and eastern India, sometimes is contaminated with much higher levels of arsenic (sometimes several hundred micrograms per liter), and widespread poisonings have resulted.

Clinical and Environmental Toxicity — CHAPTER 3

QUESTION 3-8 Answer **b.** Benzo[a]pyrene, a key carcinogen in tobacco smoke, is an example of a genotoxic carcinogen that forms both direct DNA adducts and reactive oxygen species (ROS).

SUMMARY TABLE OF SELECT ANTIDOTES, HEAVY METALS, AND HEAVY METAL CHELATORS[a]

CLASS AND SUBCLASSES	NAMES	CLINICAL USES	TOXICITIES COMMON	TOXICITIES UNIQUE: CLINICALLY IMPORTANT
Antidotes for Common Acute Poisons	Acetylcysteine	Treatment of acute acetaminophen poisoning	Nausea Rash	Rare anaphylaxis
	Atropine	Treatment of poisoning with organophosphate and carbamate pesticides	Anticholinergic symptoms (see Chapter 6)	See Chapter 6
	Diphenhydramine	Treatment of drug-induced dystonia	Sedation, dry mouth, dry eyes (see Chapter 21)	See Chapter 21
	Deferoxamine	Parenteral treatment of acute and chronic iron poisoning	Pruritus, wheals, rash, dysuria, abdominal pain, diarrhea, and fever	Anaphylaxis Cataract formation has been reported
	Deferasirox	Oral treatment of chronic iron overload		
	Ethanol	Used to treat acute methanol and ethylene glycol poisoning	See Chapter 9	See Chapter 9
	Fomepizole	Used to treat acute methanol and ethylene glycol poisoning		
	Flumazenil	Treatment of the CNS depression produced by benzodiazepines	See Chapter 9	See Chapter 9
	Naloxone	Treatment of opiate-induced CNS depression	See Chapter 10	See Chapter 10
	Physostigmine	Treatment of anticholinergic syndrome	See Chapter 6	See Chapter 6
	Pralidoxime (2-PAM)	Cholinesterase reactivator used in the treatment of organophosphate poisoning	See Chapter 6	See Chapter 6
Toxic Heavy Metals	Lead			See Figure 3-7 Cognitive delays and behavior changes, encephalopathy, neuromuscular deficits (lead palsy), elevated blood pressure, hypochromic microcytic anemia (see Figure 3-8), abdominal pain (lead colic), anorexia, and constipation
	Mercury			See Figure 3-9 Tremors, emotional lability, muscular atrophy, parathesia, and cognitive deficits
	Cadmium			Local irritation along absorption route Inhaled cadmium results in lung irritation and pneumonitis Nausea, vomiting, and diarrhea

SECTION I — General Principles

CLASS AND SUBCLASSES	NAMES	CLINICAL USES	TOXICITIES — COMMON	TOXICITIES — UNIQUE: CLINICALLY IMPORTANT
	Chromium			Tubular and glomerular renal injury Inhaled chromium results in lung and upper respiratory tract irritation and decreased lung function GI pain, vomiting, and diarrhea
	Arsenic			Myocardial ischemia, cardiac arrhythmia, peripheral vascular disease (blackfoot disease) Hyperkeratinization of the palms of hands and soles of feet GI cramping, vomiting, GI hemorrhaging Headache, lethargy, seizures, coma Anemia and leukopenia
Heavy Metal Chelators	Dimercaprol	Used to treat acute exposures to arsenic, gold, mercury, and in combination with EDTA $CaNa_2$ to treat lead exposure	Increased blood pressure Nausea, vomiting, headache, burning sensation in mouth and throat, and abdominal pain	Painful sterile abscess at injection site Contraindicated for treatment of chronic exposure to heavy metals because it does not prevent neurotoxic effects
	Sodium 2,3-dimercaptopropane sulfonate (DMPS)	Treatment of acute exposure to lead, arsenic, and mercury		
	EDTA $CaNa_2$	Treatment of acute lead poisoning	Malaise, fatigue, excessive thirst	Rapid IV administration causes hypocalcemic tetany Renal toxicity due to chelation of essential metals, particularly zinc, in proximal renal tubular cells Used in pregnancy only under conditions where benefits outweigh risks
	Penicillamine	Used for treatment of exposure to copper, mercury, zinc, and lead	Dryness and scaling of skin	Long-term treatment results in cutaneous reactions such as urticaria, maculopapular reactions, pemphigoid lesions, lupus erythematosus, and dermatomyositis
	Dimercaptosuccinic acid (DMSA), Succimer	Approved for the treatment of children with acute lead poisoning Used off label for treatment of adults with lead, arsenic, and mercury poisoning	Nausea, vomiting, diarrhea, and loss of appetite	Transient elevations in hepatic transaminases

[a]carcinogens are not appropriate for this summary table. Only the toxicities of select heavy metals are shown.

Special Populations (Children and Elderly)

CHAPTER 4

There is no specific chapter on the topic of pharmacotherapy of special populations (children and elderly) in *Goodman & Gilman's The Pharmacological Basis of Therapeutics*, 12th Edition. However, this is an important area of clinical pharmacology because the pharmacotherapy of children and the elderly requires consideration of the differences in pharmacokinetics and pharmacodynamics that can significantly affect the safety and efficacy of drugs used in these special populations. Moreover, most randomized controlled clinical trials exclude young children and the aged, which makes it difficult for the clinician to make evidence-based decisions regarding appropriate drugs and dosing regimens to use in these patients.

The content of this chapter is drawn from a variety of sources, including a number of chapters in *Goodman & Gilman's The Pharmacological Basis of Therapeutics*, 12th Edition including Chapters 1 to 3 in Section I: General Principles, and later chapters in which the pharmacotherapy of children or the elderly is discussed in the context of specific agents. Content regarding general principles of pharmacotherapy in these special populations is drawn from online Updates published as part of the online version of *Goodman & Gilman's The Pharmacological Basis of Therapeutics*, 12th Edition related to pediatric pharmacology (specifically, *The History of Pediatric Drug Therapy: Learning from Errors Not Trials* and *Pediatric Pharmacokinetics: Why Kids Are Not Small Adults*), and from *Hazzard's Geriatric Medicine and Gerontology*, 6th Edition (specifically, Chapter 8 General Principles of Pharmacology and Chapter 24 Appropriate Approach to Prescribing). Neither a Mechanisms of Action Table nor a Clinical Summary Table is included in this chapter because this information is provided for specific agents in subsequent chapters. In addition to the material provided here, *Goodman & Gilman's The Pharmacological Basis of Therapeutics*, 12th Edition contains:

- Appendix II with pharmacokinetic data for a number of drugs with differences in pharmacokinetic parameters that occur in children, the aged, and individuals with specific disease states

Hazzard's Geriatric Medicine and Gerontology, 6th Edition contains:

- Table 8-5 Changes in Pharmacokinetics and Pharmacodynamics with Aging and Suggested Dose Adjustments for Older Patients

LEARNING OBJECTIVES

- ☑ Describe the important pharmacokinetic and pharmacodynamic differences between adults and children that can affect safety and efficacy of drugs used in infants and children.
- ☑ Know the FDA's role in providing information to clinicians to improve safe and effective use of drugs in young children, including breast-feeding infants.
- ☑ Describe the important changes in the pharmacokinetics and pharmacodynamics of drugs that occur in older adults.
- ☑ Know the classes of medications that should be avoided in older adults because of central nervous system (CNS) effects.
- ☑ Know the steps that should be taken to optimize drug regimens in older adults.

PEDIATRIC PHARMACOKINETICS—ABSORPTION

- Absorption of drugs from the gastrointestinal (GI) tract is reduced in neonates and changes with maturation making prediction of medication bioavailability of orally administered drugs very difficult.
  - ▸ Young children have higher gastric pH than adults; adult levels of gastric acidity are not reached until 3 to 7 years of age.
  - ▸ Acid-labile drugs (eg, penicillin, ampicillin, and nafcillin) have greater bioavailability.
  - ▸ Weak acids (eg, phenobarbital, phenytoin) are ionized in the GI tract of the neonate and young child and thus are more slowly absorbed than in adults.
  - ▸ Weak bases (eg, penicillin, ampicillin, and erythromycin) will be more quickly absorbed than in the adult GI tract.
  - ▸ Neonates and infants have prolonged rates of gastric emptying compared to adults, with adult rates of gastric emptying not developing until 6 to 8 months of age.
  - ▸ Biliary function develops over the first month of life; the reduced levels of bile acid salts and pancreatic enzymes in the neonate may reduce the absorption of lipophilic drugs.
  - ▸ β-Glucuronidase and UDP-glucuronyl transferase have higher activities in the neonate GI tract than in adults which may reduce drug absorption.
  - ▸ The development of intestinal flora in the neonate, which depends primarily on diet, can contribute to differences in drug metabolism compared with adults.
- Dermal absorption is higher in neonates and infants due to underdeveloped stratum corneum and increased skin hydration.
- Intramuscular injections are generally avoided in neonates, infants, and children because intramuscular absorption is unpredictable due to decreased muscle tone and contraction, and variable blood flow and oxygenation.

SECTION I

PEDIATRIC PHARMACOKINETICS—DISTRIBUTION

- Volume of distribution (V) is important in children due to age-related changes in body composition.
  - Premature infants have a higher percentage of body weight that is water (85% total body water) than term infants (75% total body water).
  - Adult total body water (55%) is reached by 12 years of age.
  - The V of drugs that distribute in total body water and extracellular fluid are higher for infants than adults.
- Body fat increases with age and development.
  - Premature infants do not have appreciable body fat compared to term infants (16% body fat).
  - Drugs that are fat soluble have lower V in infants and children than adults.
  - Premature infants have increased membrane permeability allowing easier access of drugs into compartments such as the CNS.
  - Infants have an immature blood-brain barrier (BBB), which allows toxic substances to more readily cross into and damage the brain.
- Protein binding, both α1-acid glycoprotein and albumin, are decreased in the neonate.
  - Serum albumin concentrations do not reach adult levels until 1 year of age.
  - Neonatal serum albumin is 80% of that in adults and has decreased binding affinity for many drugs.
  - Bilirubin and free fatty acids are present in higher concentrations in neonates and compete with some drugs that bind to albumin (see Case 4-1).
  - The reduced plasma protein binding of drugs results in a larger fraction of free drug in neonatal serum and thus greater drug effect.

General Principles

CASE 4-1

In 1956, newborns receiving the antibiotic sulfisoxazole were found to have a high incidence of kernicterus, which leads to yellow discoloration of the brain, seizures, and death.

a. **What is kernicterus and what causes it?**

Kernicterus refers to the yellow discoloration of the brain that is caused by high concentrations of bilirubin in the brain. It is a condition only seen in young children and can lead to brain damage and death if not treated.

Bilirubin is a yellow pigment that is the breakdown product of heme, 80% of which originates from circulating hemoglobin and 20% from other heme-containing proteins such as the CYPs. Bilirubin is hydrophobic, associates with serum albumin, and must be metabolized further by glucuronidation to assure its elimination. The failure to efficiently metabolize bilirubin by glucuronidation leads to elevated serum levels and a clinical symptom called hyperbilirubinemia or jaundice. High levels of free bilirubin in the plasma can enter the brain causing kernicterus.

b. **How did sulfisoxazole lead to kernicterus in these newborns?**

Bilirubin is metabolized by glucuronosyl transferase (UGT1A1) and the glucuronidated bilirubin is excreted in the urine. Infants have limited expression of glucuronosyl transferase and thus cannot efficiently metabolize bilirubin. Sulfisoxazole displaces bilirubin from plasma proteins, thus increasing the free fraction of bilirubin in the plasma and enhancing the movement of bilirubin into the brain. Moreover, infants also have an immature BBB, which allows more of the free bilirubin to cross into and damage the brain.

c. **What other infant drug toxicities have resulted from low glucuronosyl transferase expression in newborns?**

In 1959, gray baby syndrome was described in premature infants receiving the antibiotic chloramphenicol. This syndrome was caused by chloramphenicol accumulation and resulted in hypothermia, vomiting, acidosis, hypotension, cyanosis, a characteristic gray color, and death in some infants. Because of immature glucuronosyl transferase, infants cannot metabolize chloramphenicol to the inactive chloramphenicol glucuronate. Infants also have reduced renal capacity and diminished renal excretion of chloramphenicol and its metabolites also contributed to the accumulation of the drug in these children.

d. **What other drugs have altered metabolism in children because of immature phase 2 metabolic enzymes?**

Morphine is metabolized by glucuronosyl transferase to the 20-fold more active metabolite, 6-glucuronide morphine. Thus, higher serum concentrations of morphine are required for infants to obtain effective analgesia.

CASE 4-2

An 83-year-old man has occasional pain from mild osteoarthritis. He also has hypertension and is overweight.

a. **What are the considerations in using a nonsteroidal anti-inflammatory drug (NSAID; Chapter 22) to treat this patient's arthritis symptoms?**

Epidemiologic and clinical studies have demonstrated an association between NSAID use and GI bleeds and renal impairment in older persons. The effects of NSAIDs on renal function increase salt and water retention, which will contribute to this patient's hypertension. Age generally is correlated with an increased probability of developing serious adverse reactions to NSAIDs (see Chapter 22), and caution is warranted such as choosing a lower starting dose for elderly patients.

(Continued)

Special Populations (Children and Elderly) — CHAPTER 4

NSAIDs are labeled with a black box warning related to cardiovascular risks and are specifically contraindicated following coronary artery bypass graft (CABG) surgery. Patients at increased risk of cardiovascular disease or thrombosis are likely to be particularly prone to cardiovascular adverse events while on NSAIDs. This includes patients with rheumatoid arthritis as the relative risk of myocardial infarction is increased in these patients compared to patients with osteoarthritis or no arthritis. The risk appears to be related to factors influencing drug exposure, such as dose, $t_{1/2}$, degree of COX-2 selectivity, potency, and treatment duration. Thus, the lowest possible dose should be prescribed for the shortest possible period.

b. What are the alternatives to NSAIDs in this patient?

Alternative approaches should be considered before NSAIDs are prescribed for indications such as osteoarthritis in elderly patients. Possible non-pharmacologic approaches, such as gentle exercise and weight reduction, may be beneficial alternatives to treatment with NSAIDs.

When pharmacologic therapy is required, a drug therapy with a less-adverse event profile, such as acetaminophen, should be used.

CASE 4-3

A 90-year-old woman develops symptoms of a cold and buys an over-the-counter cold medication at the grocery store. The medication contains diphenhydramine, acetaminophen, and phenylephrine. She takes the recommended adult dose but soon after taking the medication she becomes very confused and disoriented.

a. What is likely causing the signs of confusion?

Diphenhydramine is a first-generation antihistamine that is a common ingredient in over-the-counter cold and allergy medications (see Chapter 21). This agent is able to cross the BBB where it has significant anticholinergic effects, including confusion and somnolence. The elderly have reduced BBB function and are also at a higher risk of adverse drug effects when taking drugs that have anticholinergic properties.

b. What symptoms are associated with strong anticholinergic drugs in older patients?

In the elderly, drugs with strong anticholinergic properties are associated with adverse effects such as confusion, dry mouth, dry eyes, urinary retention, constipation, and postural hypotension.

c. What other drugs have strong anticholinergic properties that should be avoided in elderly patients?

The 2012 Beers Criteria (see Side Bar POTENTIALLY INAPPROPRIATE MEDICATIONS FOR THE ELDERLY) lists the following medications with strong anticholinergic properties that should be avoided in older adults.

First-generation antihistamines, as a single agent or as part of a combination product (see Chapter 21):

- Brompheniramine
- Carbinoxamine
- Chlorpheniramine
- Clemastine
- Cyproheptadine

(Continued)

PEDIATRIC PHARMACOKINETICS—EXCRETION

- Infants and small children have reduced renal function (20-40% of adult function).
- Adult filtration rates are not reached until approximately 3 years of age.
- Reduced renal function in children is due to:
  - Reduced glomerular filtration rate (GFR)
  - Tubular cell immaturity
  - Reduced nephron length
  - Reduced solute gradient
  - Decreased responsiveness to antidiuretic hormone
- Even when normalized for body surface area, renal plasma flow, glomerular filtration, tubular secretion, tubular reabsorption, and the concentrating and acidifying functions of the kidney are low compared with adults.
- Renal clearance of drugs excreted almost entirely by glomerular filtration (eg, aminoglycosides and vancomycin) will change in a manner that corresponds to maturation of renal function.
- Premature infants have lower filtration rates and are slow to develop the renal capacity that term neonates will have developed by 1 week of age.
  - Premature infants require lower doses, longer dosing intervals, or both to maintain the same steady-state plasma concentrations as the full-term infant.
- Excretion of drugs that depend on tubular secretion (eg, penicillins, sulfonamides, furosemide, and chloramphenicol) has reduced rates of clearance in the neonate.

SECTION I

General Principles

PEDIATRIC PHARMACKINETICS—METABOLISM

- Infants have reduced hepatic drug metabolism enzymes.
- Neonatal phase 1 activity (functionalization reactions catalyzed by CYPs, see Chapter 2) are intact but not at full capacity until 6 months to 1 year of age.
  - As a result, oxidation of many drugs is impaired in the neonate.
  - Lack of one CYP enzyme may be compensated for by another.
- Neonatal phase 2 activity (conjugation reactions, see Chapter 2) is 50 to 70% of the adult rate.
  - Glucuronidation is significantly reduced in the neonate and drug glucuronidation is much less than in the adult (eg, acetaminophen glucuronidation).
  - The glucuronidation pathway may take up to 3 to 4 years to fully develop which can slow metabolism of endogenous substrates such as bilirubin and drugs such as morphine and chloramphenicol.
    - Higher serum concentrations of morphine are required for infants because infants cannot metabolize morphine to the active 6-glucuronide metabolite.
  - The sulfation pathway is well developed in neonates and partly compensates for the low rates of glucuronidation (eg, acetaminophen is excreted in the urine primarily as sulfate conjugates in the neonate, whereas adults excrete acetaminophen in the urine primarily as the glucuronide conjugate).

Dexbrompheniramine
Dexchlorpheniramine
Diphenhydramine (oral)
Doxylamine
Hydroxyzine
Promethazine
Triprolidine

Antispasmodics (see Chapter 6)
  Belladonna alkaloids
  Clidinium-chlordiazepoxide
  Dicyclomine
  Hyoscyamine
  Propantheline
  Scopolamine

Antiarrhythmics (see Chapter 18)
  Disopyramide

Tertiary tricyclic antidepressants (TCAs), alone or in combination (see Chapter 8)
  Amitriptyline
  Chlordiazepoxide-amitriptyline
  Clomipramine
  Doxepin more than 6 mg/d
  Imipramine
  Perphenazine-amitriptyline
  Trimipramine

Antipsychotics (see Chapter 8)
  Thioridazine
  Mesoridazine

Skeletal muscle relaxants (see Chapter 9)
  Carisoprodol
  Chlorzoxazone
  Cyclobenzaprine
  Metaxalone
  Methocarbamol
  Orphenadrine

Special Populations (Children and Elderly)

CHAPTER 4

CASE 4-4

A 72-year-old woman occasionally takes diazepam when she feels anxious and has trouble sleeping. Her physician has prescribed diazepam for her since she was 50. Recently the patient has had trouble maintaining her balance after taking diazepam.

a. **What might be causing this patient's difficulty in maintaining her balance.**

Older adults have increased sensitivity to benzodiazepines (see Chapter 9), which increases the risk of falls, fractures, motor vehicle accidents, cognitive impairment, and delirium in older adults. Benzodiazepines and other hypnotic drugs increase postural sway, which may contribute to this patient's difficulty in maintaining balance.

b. **What are the factors that increase benzodiazepine sensitivity in older adults?**

The increased sensitivity of older adults to benzodiazepines is due to 3 factors: (1) drug clearance is reduced; (2) there is increased distribution of benzodiazepines to the brain due to changes in lean body mass; (3) based on studies in animal models, there is increased pharmacodynamic sensitivity of the brain to any given concentration of benzodiazepine.

c. **Are there benzodiazepines that are safer in older adults?**

Longer-acting benzodiazepines like diazepam are more likely to produce CNS adverse events such as daytime somnolence, confusion, and impaired motor coordination. Although short-acting benzodiazepines might reduce the risk of falls, all benzodiazepines increase risk of cognitive impairment, delirium, falls, fractures, and motor vehicle accidents in older adults.

Benzodiazepines may be appropriate in some older adults to treat seizure disorders, rapid eye movement sleep disorders, benzodiazepine withdrawal, ethanol withdrawal, severe generalized anxiety disorder, periprocedural anesthesia, and in end-of-life care. If a benzodiazepine is determined to be appropriate in treating an older adult, a prudent approach would be to avoid using agents with long elimination half-life and high doses of benzodiazepine therapy.

Nonbenzodiazepine hypnotics (ie, eszopiclone, zolpidem, zaleplon) are benzodiazepine receptor agonists that have adverse effects in older adults similar to those of benzodiazepines and have minimal improvement in sleep latency and duration. Chronic use (longer than 90 days) should be avoided with these agents.

d. **What other medications have greater CNS effects in the elderly?**

Older adults are more sensitive to the effects of opiates, anesthetic agents, and psychotropic agents including antipsychotics (see Side Bar CHANGES IN RESPONSE TO DRUGS WITH AGING).

In the case of opiate analgesics, pharmacokinetics do not change with aging, but studies in animal models indicate increased sensitivity may be due to altered expression of opiate receptors. In contrast, sensitivity to anesthetic induction doses of thiopentone is increased in older adults due to drug distribution, not an age-related change in receptor sensitivity. Reduced clearance of thiopentone from the central drug compartment produces higher drug concentrations in the CNS.

KEY CONCEPTS

- Neonates and young children have very different pharmacokinetics (drug absorption, distribution, metabolism, and excretion) and pharmacodynamics compared to adults, which can significantly reduce medication safety and efficacy.

- Older adults constitute a very heterogeneous group ranging from healthy, fit, community-dwelling individuals taking no regular medication to frail institutionalized individuals with multiple comorbidities and polypharmacy.

- The most consistent and marked change in pharmacokinetics in older adults is the increase in interindividual variability.

PEDIATRIC MEDICATION SAFETY AND THE FDA

- Once a drug is approved for either adults or older children, it is frequently used off-label for other ages and indications.

- Pediatric product development studies, other than for vaccines or some childhood illnesses such as otitis media, tend to be small due to the limited number of children available for clinical trial participation.

- Postmarket pediatric experience is crucial to understand safe use in the pediatric population.

- Federal legislation in the past several years has expanded the FDA'a authority to expand clinical studies of drugs in the pediatric population (see FDA Pediatric Product Development http://www.fda.gov/Drugs/DevelopmentApprovalProcess/DevelopmentResources/ucm049867.htm).

- In 2012, as part of the Food and Drug Administration Safety and Innovation Act, or FDASIA, Congress permanently reauthorized the Best Pharmaceuticals for Children Act of 2002 (BPCA) and the Pediatric Research Equity Act of 2003 (PREA), and gave FDA new authorities to encourage more research into, and more development of, treatments for children.

  ▸ BPCA provides an incentive for drug companies to conduct FDA-requested pediatric studies by granting an additional 6 months of marketing exclusivity.

  ▸ PREA requires drug companies to study their products in children under certain circumstances; when required, pediatric studies must be conducted with the same drug and for the same use for which they were approved in adults.

  ▸ FDA can waive studies in children if the studies are not necessary and can grant extensions for deferred pediatric studies at a sponsor's request if there is good cause for a delay in completing the studies.

- Before BPCA and PREA became law, more than 80% of the drugs approved for adult use were being used in children, even though the safety and effectiveness had not been established in children; today that number has been reduced to about 50%.

(Continued)

SECTION I

PEDIATRIC MEDICATION SAFETY AND THE FDA (CONT.)

- The FDA Safety and Innovation Act of 2012 has had a dramatic impact on pediatric labeling of drugs, and labeling of drugs for breast-feeding women.
- FDA's Office of Pediatric Therapeutics (OPT) was created by a mandate of Congress to assure access for children to innovative, safe and effective medical products, and in collaboration with another branch of the agency (Center for Drug Evaluation and Research [CDER]) developed the New Pediatric Labeling Information Database which contains pediatric labeling changes based on key pediatric information from the studies submitted in response to PREA and BPCA (http://www.accessdata.fda.gov/scripts/sda/sdNavigation.cfm?sd=labelingdatabase).
- In 2014, FDA published a final rule setting standards for how information about medicines used during pregnancy and breast-feeding is presented in the labeling of prescription drugs and biological products.
  - This labeling replaces the previous product letter categories—A, B, C, D, and X—used to classify the risks of using prescription drugs during pregnancy.
  - The final rule requires the use of 3 subsections in the labeling titled "Pregnancy," "Lactation," and "Females and Males of Reproductive Potential" that provide details about use of the drug or biological product.
  - The "Pregnancy" and "Lactation" subsections also includes 3 subheadings: "risk summary," "clinical considerations," and "data."

General Principles

➡ Reduced hepatic and renal clearance are generally the most significant pharmacokinetic changes in aging, which can affect maintenance dose and dosing interval.

➡ Available methods to estimate renal function in older adults are not reliable, particularly in frail or acutely ill older adults.

➡ There is an increased risk of adverse drug effects in older adults.

➡ When prescribing drug therapies in older adults, it is important to use the minimal dose required to obtain benefit.

➡ Optimal drug therapy in the older patient should include:
  ➡ An assessment of the aims of therapy in the individual
  ➡ Risks of drug therapy
  ➡ Possible drug–drug interactions
  ➡ The effect of disease on drug effects
  ➡ Monitoring of drug efficacy and adverse drug effects once drug therapy is initiated

SUMMARY QUIZ

QUESTION 4-1 The dosing of morphine in an infant to control pain typically requires using higher doses than an adult. The major reason for the higher dosing is

a. increased binding of drug to plasma proteins.
b. reduced entry of drug into the CNS.
c. reduced opiate sensitivity in young children.
d. reduced metabolism of drug.
e. increased clearance of drug.

QUESTION 4-2 The bioavailability of orally administered drugs is difficult to predict in infants because

a. the rate of transit of drugs through the infant GI tract is very rapid.
b. infants have very high first-pass metabolism.
c. absorption of drugs from the GI tract is reduced in neonates and changes with maturation.
d. the clearance of drugs by the kidney is very rapid in infants.
e. all of the above.

QUESTION 4-3 Nonsteroidal anti-inflammatory drugs (NSAIDs) such as ibuprofen should be avoided in the elderly because NSAIDs

a. have little efficacy in treating pain in older adults.
b. are more readily converted to toxic metabolites in older adults.
c. impair renal function in older adults.
d. impair hepatic function in older adults.
e. impair uptake of many nutrients from the GI tract in older adults.

QUESTION 4-4 Certain tricyclic antidepressants such as amitriptyline should be avoided in elderly patients because they

a. have anticholinergic effects.
b. have effects on the heart that increase the risk of arrhythmias.
c. cannot be adequately monitored for adherence.
d. can cause serious GI bleeding.
e. are ineffective in most elderly patients.

Special Populations (Children and Elderly)

CHAPTER 4

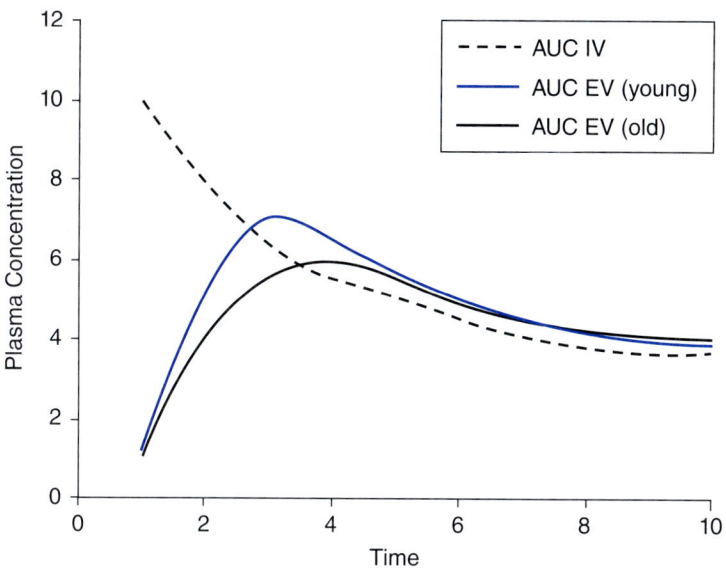

FIGURE 4-1 Theoretical plasma concentration–time curves for the same drug given intravascularly (IV) and extravascularly (EV) in a young adult versus an elderly adult. The bioavailability is the ratio of the area under the curve (AUC) for the EV route to the AUC for the IV route. The intravascular AUC is not affected by age. With aging, the extravascular curve shows delayed and lower maximal plasma concentration and AUC may be increased for drugs that undergo first-pass hepatic metabolism. *(Reproduced with permission from Halter JB, Ouslander JG, Tinetti ME, Studenski S, High KP, & Asthana S (Eds). Hazzard's Geriatric Medicine and Gerontology, 6th ed. McGraw-Hill, Inc., 2009. Fig 8-1.)*

PHARMACOKINETICS IN THE ELDERLY— ABSORPTION AND BIOAVAILABILITY

- Absorption of drugs is often slower in the aged (see Figure 4-1) so the maximal plasma concentration is reached later (longer T_{max}) and is lower (lower C_{max}).
- The extent of absorption is usually complete in older adults so the area under the curve (bioavailability) is not affected.
- Oral bioavailability may be decreased for drugs that require an acidic environment in older adults with age-related hypochlorhydria secondary to atrophic gastritis (5-10% of older adults) and in those taking medications that raise gastric pH such as H_2-antagonists and proton pump inhibitors.
- Factors associated with age-related changes in absorption and bioavailability are shown in Table 4-1.

TABLE 4-1 Factors Associated with Bioavailability of Drugs Administered Through Common Extravascular Routes and Description of Age-Related Changes

ROUTE	PROPERTIES OF DRUG	ABSORPTION		FIRST-PASS CLEARANCE	
		DESCRIPTION	AGE-RELATED CHANGES	DESCRIPTION	AGE-RELATED CHANGES
Oral	Particle size formulation Lipid solubility Ionization	Gut lumen decomposition	Gastric pH may be less acidic, altering ionisation	Gut wall CYP450 metabolism	Not known
		Passive absorption	Complete but slower – Increased by longer gastrointestinal transit time and possible increase in permeability of epithelium – Decreased by reduced perfusion	Hepatic metabolism	Reduced 30–50%
		Active transport (e.g., iron, vitamin B-12)	Probably decreased		
		Gut wall P-glycoprotein transports drugs back into lumen	Not known		
Sublingual	Particle size Lipid solubility Potency	Rapid into blood vessels at base of tongue	Not known ?Reduced perfusion	Nil	
Rectal (local and systemic action)	Lipid solubility Ionisation	Varies with rectal contents	Not known ?Reduced perfusion	Nil	

(Continued)

SECTION I — General Principles

ROUTE	PROPERTIES OF DRUG	ABSORPTION DESCRIPTION	ABSORPTION AGE-RELATED CHANGES	FIRST-PASS CLEARANCE DESCRIPTION	FIRST-PASS CLEARANCE AGE-RELATED CHANGES
Subcutaneous Injection	Particle size (small particles absorbed by capillaries, large particles absorbed by lymphatics) Protein complex pH Use of vasoconstrictors	Slow	Not known ?Reduced perfusion ?Changes to lymphatics	Nil ?Proteolysis of protein drugs in lymph nodes	
Intramuscular Injection	Lipid solubility Particle size (small particles absorbed by capillaries, large particles absorbed by lymphatics)	Slow (faster than subcutaneous due to better perfusion)	Not known ?Reduced perfusion ?Changes to lymphatics	Nil ?Proteolysis of protein drugs in lymph nodes	
Percutaneous	Lipid solubility	Slow Heat dependent	Not known ?Reduced perfusion	Nil	
Intranasal (local and systemic)	Lipid solubility	Variable	Not known ?Reduced perfusion	Nil	
Inhaled (local and systemic)	Particle size – Powders – Aerosol solutions inhaler (type and how used) Gases: gas partition coefficient (blood)	Minimal systemic absorption	Not known ?Effects of reduced alveolar area, low-grade inflammation, ventilation/perfusion mismatch, decreased diffusion and transport across alveolar capillary membrane	Lung metabolism and clearance	Not known
Ophthalmic (topical)	Formulation: drops, suspensions, ointments	Minimal (drainage through nasolacrimal canal)	Not known	Nil	

Reproduced with permission from Halter JB, Ouslander JG, Tinetti ME, Studenski S, High KP, & Asthana S (Eds). *Hazzard's Geriatric Medicine and Gerontology*, 6th ed. McGraw-Hill, Inc., 2009. Table 8-1.

PHARMACOKINETICS IN THE ELDERLY—DISTRIBUTION

- Age-related changes in plasma protein binding, tissue binding properties, and body fat/body water ratios can alter the V (Table 4-2).
- The BBB may become less effective with aging.
- Tissue perfusion may decrease with aging, which may slow distribution, particularly to less highly perfused tissues such as muscle and fat.
- It may be necessary to change loading dose of drugs in older adults because of changes in V.

SUMMARY QUIZ ANSWER KEY

QUESTION 4-1 Answer is **d**. Morphine is metabolized by glucuronosyl transferase to the 20-fold more active metabolite, 6-glucuronide morphine. The phase 2 glucuronidation pathway is significantly reduced in the neonate and as a result, drug glucuronidation is much less than in the adult. The glucuronidation pathway may take up to 3 to 4 years to fully develop. Thus, higher serum concentrations of morphine are required for infants to obtain effective analgesia.

QUESTION 4-2 Answer is **c**. Absorption of drugs from the GI tract is reduced in neonates and changes with maturation making prediction of bioavailability of orally administered drugs very difficult (see Side Bar PEDIATRIC PHARMACOKINETICS—ABSORPTION). Some of the factors that alter absorption of drugs in the GI tract that change with age during the first several years of life include gastric pH, gastric emptying time, biliary function, metabolic enzymes in the GI tract, and development of intestinal flora.

Special Populations (Children and Elderly)

CHAPTER 4

QUESTION 4-3 Answer is **c**. Epidemiologic and clinical studies have demonstrated an association between NSAID use and GI bleeds and renal impairment in older persons (see Case 4-2). Age generally is correlated with an increased probability of developing serious adverse reactions to NSAIDs, and caution is warranted such as choosing a lower starting dose for elderly patients and limiting use to the shortest time possible. NSAIDs are labeled with a black box warning related to cardiovascular risks and are specifically contraindicated following coronary artery bypass graft (CABG) surgery.

QUESTION 4-4 Answer is **a**. Tertiary tricyclic antidepressants should be avoided in older adults because they have strong anticholinergic effects (see Case 4-3). In the elderly, drugs with strong anticholinergic properties are associated with adverse effects such as confusion, dry mouth, dry eyes, urinary retention, constipation, and postural hypotension.

PHARMACOKINETICS IN THE ELDERLY—METABOLISM AND CLEARANCE

- A number of age-related changes in hepatic blood flow and function alter metabolism of drugs in the elderly (Table 4-3).
- Hepatic blood flow is reduced by ~50% with normal aging, which reduces clearance of flow-limited drugs by ~50% but has no effect on capacity-limited drugs (see Figure 4-2).
- Hepatic blood flow may also be reduced in diseases prevalent in the elderly such as heart failure.
- Phase 1 metabolism is reduced by 30 to 50% in normal aging.
- Phase 2 metabolism appears to be maintained in normal aging, but reduced in frail aging.
- In older adults with reduced hepatic metabolism there may be a higher dose requirement for prodrugs to obtain the same AUC for the active drug (ie, the metabolite) as in a young person.
- Decreased drug clearance associated with aging results in an increase in drug half-life, and is prolonged even more for lipid-soluble drugs due to an increase in V (see Figure 4-3).

TABLE 4-2 Factors That Determine Volume of Distribution: Effects of Aging

FACTOR	EFFECT ON V	AGE-RELATED CHANGES	CLINICAL APPLICATION
Plasma protein binding	Highly protein bound drugs are generally less able to cross membranes and have smaller V	Decreased albumin which binds acidic drugs, eg, warfarin, NSAIDs, phenytoin. Increased α 1-acid glycoprotein which binds basic drugs, eg, verapamil, propranolol.	Not usually clinically significant.
Tissue binding properties	Drugs which are tightly bound to tissues have large V	Changes in body composition (sarcopenia, increased adiposity) may affect V.	Drugs bound to muscle, eg, digoxin, have decreased V with aging. Therefore decreased loading dose required.
Lipid: water coefficient	Lipid soluble drugs can pass through lipid membranes of cells more easily and have higher V than water soluble drugs	Relative increase in proportion of body fat and decrease in body water (muscle mass). Therefore, higher V for lipid soluble drugs and lower V for water soluble drugs with aging.	Loading dose of water soluble drugs, eg, gentamicin, digoxin, decreased with aging to avoid toxicity from high initial Cp.
Transporters	Passive facilitated diffusion (move drug in same direction as concentration gradient). Active transport (use ATP to move drug against concentration gradient).	Unknown.	Drug interactions may occur at level of transporters. Passive transporters include the Organic Anion Transport Proteins (OAT-P) for benzyl penicillin, digoxin, and pravastatin. Active transporters include MDR1 (P-gp) for many cationic or neutral drugs, eg, digoxin, macrolide antibiotics, verapamil.

Reproduced with permission from Halter JB, Ouslander JG, Tinetti ME, Studenski S, High KP, & Asthana S (Eds). *Hazzard's Geriatric Medicine and Gerontology*, 6th ed. McGraw-Hill, Inc., 2009. Table 8-2.

SECTION I

General Principles

PHARMACOKINETICS IN THE ELDERLY—EXCRETION

- Renal drug clearance is reduced with aging (Table 4-4).
- GFR is reduced by 10 to 40% with aging.
  - Much of the age-related decline in renal function may be related to disease, particularly hypertension, atherosclerosis, and heart failure, rather than normal aging.
- Available methods to estimate renal function in older adults are not reliable, particularly in frail or acutely ill older adults.
  - The Cockcroft–Gault equation (see below) can give an estimate of renal function for dose adjustment of renally excreted drugs; however, the maintenance dose of drugs with narrow therapeutic indices should be guided by therapeutic drug monitoring and clinical response.
- Tubular secretion is reduced with aging, to a similar or greater extent than GFR.
- Tubular secretion may be further reduced by polypharmacy that increases competition of drugs for transporters.
- Overall tubular function is decreased in the elderly, with impaired ability to concentrate or dilute urine maximally.

Cockcroft–Gault Equation

$$\text{Creatinine clearance (mL/min)} = \frac{(140 - \text{age}) \times \text{weight (kg)}}{72 \times \text{serum creatinine (mg/dL)}} \times 0.85 \text{ for females}$$

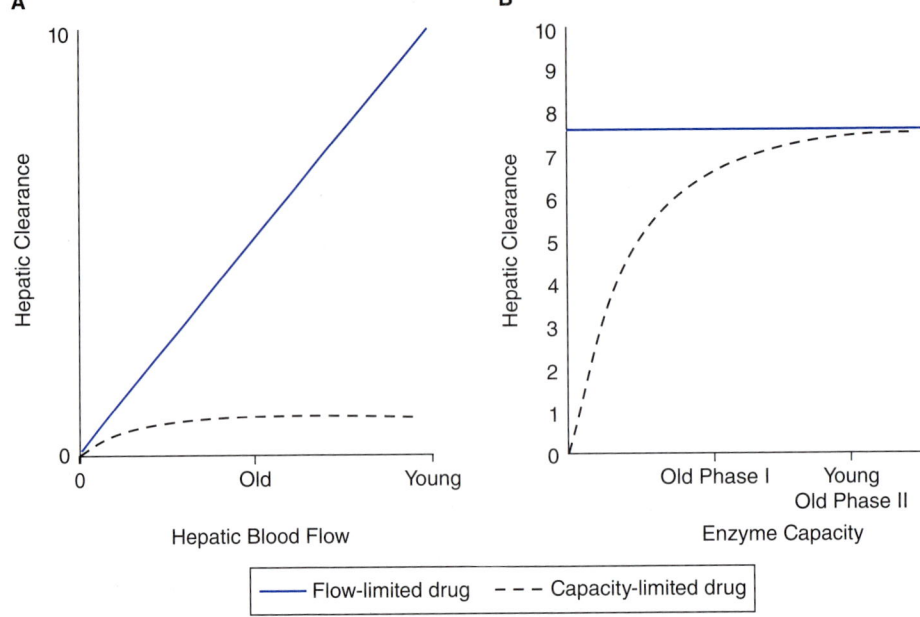

FIGURE 4-2 The effects of normal aging on hepatic drug clearance. With aging, hepatic blood flow is reduced by approximately 50%, which is associated with a 50% reduction in clearance of flow-limited drugs, but has little effect on clearance of capacity-limited drugs **(A)**. In normal aging, phase 1 metabolism is reduced, which reduces hepatic clearance of capacity-limited drugs metabolized by these enzymes, while phase 2 metabolism is probably preserved, although it may be reduced in frailty. Changes in enzyme capacity do not affect the clearance of flow-limited drugs **(B)**. *(Reproduced with permission from Halter JB, Ouslander JG, Tinetti ME, Studenski S, High KP, & Asthana S [Eds]. Hazzard's Geriatric Medicine and Gerontology, 6th ed. McGraw-Hill, Inc., 2009. Figs 8-3A&B.)*

TABLE 4-3 Changes in Hepatic Clearance with Aging

PROCESS OF HEPATIC CLEARANCE	DESCRIPTION	AGE-RELATED CHANGES	CLINICAL APPLICATION
Hepatic blood flow	Portal venous flow (~80%) and hepatic arterial flow (~20%)	Decreases by 30-50%	Reduced clearance by 30-50% of high extraction ratio drugs, eg, morphine and verapamil. Less impact on low extraction ratio drugs, eg, carbamazepine, warfarin, diazepam.
Protein binding	Only free drug is cleared. Protein binding affected by disease and competition from other drugs.	Decreased albumin: acidic drugs have higher fraction unbound and increased hepatic clearance. Increased α1-acid glycoprotein: basic drugs have lower fraction unbound and decreased hepatic clearance.	Only significant for drugs that are highly protein bound (>90%) with low hepatic extraction ratios, eg, warfarin, phenytoin, diazepam.
Scavenger cells	Kupffer cells scavenge large protein drugs. Liver sinusoidal endothelial cells (LSECs) may scavenge smaller particles.	Possible reduction in scavenger function (in animal studies).	Not known. May reduce hepatic clearance.

(Continued)

Special Populations (Children and Elderly)

CHAPTER 4

PROCESS OF HEPATIC CLEARANCE	DESCRIPTION	AGE-RELATED CHANGES	CLINICAL APPLICATION
Transfer into hepatocyte	Transfer across the LSECs and the hepatocyte apical membrane by passive or active transport.	Structural changes in LSECs and the space of Disse may reduce transfer. Changes in hepatocyte membrane transport not known.	Not known. May reduce hepatic clearance.
Metabolism	Biotransformation to more hydrophilic metabolites that may be equally, less or more active than parent drug	Reduced phase I metabolism in vivo in normal aging by 30–50%. Phase II metabolism appears to be maintained in healthy aging, reduced in frail aged.	Probably preserved clearance of drugs that undergo capacity-limited phase II metabolism in healthy aging, eg, temazepam, salicylic acid.
Transfer into bile ductule	Active transport into bile canaliculi. Bile enters small intestine and drug or metabolite reabsorbed (enterohepatic cycle) or excreted in faeces.	Unknown. In aged rodents, increased biliary P-glycoprotein expression and function.	Unknown.

Reproduced with permission from Halter JB, Ouslander JG, Tinetti ME, Studenski S, High KP, & Asthana S (Eds). *Hazzard's Geriatric Medicine and Gerontology*, 6th ed. McGraw-Hill, Inc., 2009. Table 8-3.

CHANGES IN RESPONSE TO DRUGS WITH AGING

- Decreased sensitivity of the baroreceptor reflex occurs with aging which changes the cardiovascular response to many drugs.
  - β-Adrenergic receptor antagonists (see Chapter 7) may be less effective in controlling hypertension (see Chapter 15) in the elderly.
  - The acute blood pressure response to calcium channel blockers (see Chapter 15) may be greater in the aged.
- Aging increases the sensitivity to many CNS drugs.
  - Older adults are more sensitive to the sedative and respiratory depressant effects of benzodiazepines (see Chapter 9), and experience more cognitive impairment.
  - Older adults are more sensitive to opiates (see Chapter 10) and general anesthetics (see Chapter 11).
  - Exposure to any psychotropic medication (see Chapter 8), regardless of class, is associated with an almost twofold increased risk of falls in older adults.
  - Psychotropic (see Chapter 8) and anticholinergic (see Chapter 6) medications are strongly associated with cognitive impairment and delirium in the aged, as well as anticholinergic adverse effects such as urinary retention and postural hypotension (see Chapter 6), and may reduce the effectiveness of cholinesterase inhibitor therapy in managing Alzheimer disease and related dementias.
  - Antipsychotic drugs increase the risk of drug-induced parkinsonism in the elderly which might be misdiagnosed as a new medical condition (ie, Parkinson disease).

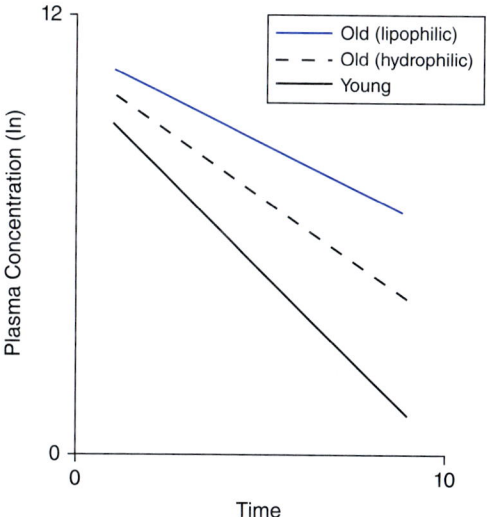

FIGURE 4-3 The theoretical effects of aging on half-life. The decrease in clearance with aging prolongs half-life. For lipid-soluble drugs, the increase in volume of distribution (V) prolongs half-life further. For water-soluble drugs, the decrease in V reduces half-life, but in most cases, the size of the effect of aging on V is smaller than the effect on clearance, resulting in an overall increase in half-life compared to young subjects. The half-life determines the time course of drug accumulation and elimination, and the choice of dose interval. The increase in half-life that is observed for many drugs with aging means that it will take longer for drugs to reach steady-state, longer to be eliminated after they are ceased, and dosing intervals may need to be increased. *(Reproduced with permission from Halter JB, Ouslander JG, Tinetti ME, Studenski S, High KP, & Asthana S [Eds]. Hazzard's Geriatric Medicine and Gerontology, 6th ed. McGraw-Hill, Inc., 2009. Fig 8-4.)*

STEPS IN OPTIMIZING DRUG REGIMENS IN OLDER ADULTS

- Review current drug therapy.
- Discontinue unnecessary drug therapy.
- Consider any new symptom to be caused by adverse drug events.
- Consider nonpharmacologic therapies.
- Substitute with safer alternatives (see Side Bar POTENTIALLY INAPPROPRIATE MEDICATIONS FOR THE ELDERLY).
- Reduce the dose.

SECTION I

POTENTIALLY INAPPROPRIATE MEDICATIONS FOR THE ELDERLY

- The American Geriatric Society (AGS) has developed and regularly updates the Beers Criteria (medication list of Potentially Inappropriate Medications for the Elderly) based on evidence-based recommendations:
  - https://www.dcri.org/trial-participation/the-beers-list
- The list is updated based on a comprehensive, systematic review and grading of the evidence on drug-related problems and adverse drug events in older adult.
- The 2012 AGS Beers Criteria for Potentially Inappropriate Medication Use in Older Adults is available online at:
  - http://www.americangeriatrics.org/files/documents/beers/2012AGSBeersCriteriaCitations.pdf

General Principles

TABLE 4-4 Changes in Renal Drug Clearance with Aging

PROCESS OF RENAL CLEARANCE	EFFECTS OF AGE	CLINICAL APPLICATION	EXAMPLE
Glomerular filtration	Decreased GFR, extent unclear, ~10-40%	Estimates used to adjust maintenance doses of drugs for renal impairment	Gentamicin clearance correlates with Cockcroft-Gault estimates of creatinine clearance.
Tubular secretion (active)	Decreased	Reduction in renal clearance may be greater than reduction in GFR. With polypharmacy, increased risk of drug-drug interactions through competition for transporters.	Ratio of procainamide clearance to creatinine clearance decreases with aging. Digoxin excreted by passive glomerular filtration and active tubular secretion. Serum digoxin levels increase with number of concurrent P-gp inhibitors, e.g., verapamil, erythromycin, amiodarone, spironolactone, atorvastatin.
Tubular reabsorption (passive)	Unknown	If impaired, would reduce the effect of reduced glomerular filtration on clearance.	Changes in clearance of lithium, which, like sodium, is freely filtered at glomerulus and 80% reabsorbed in the proximal tubule, consistent with changes in GFR with aging.

Reproduced with permission from Halter JB, Ouslander JG, Tinetti ME, Studenski S, High KP, & Asthana S (Eds). *Hazzard's Geriatric Medicine and Gerontology*, 6th ed. McGraw-Hill, Inc., 2009. Table 8-4.

Neuropharmacology

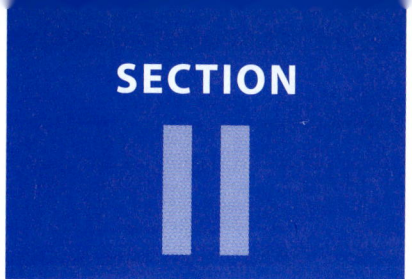

5. Neurotransmission 80
6. Cholinergic Pharmacology 95
7. Adrenergic, Dopaminergic, and Serotonergic Pharmacology 118
8. Pyschopharmacology 149
9. Hypnotics, Sedatives, and Ethanol 176
10. Opioid Pharmacology 194
11. Anesthetic Agents and Therapeutic Gases 210
12. Pharmacotherapy of the Epilepsies 225
13. Drug Therapy of Neurodegenerative Diseases 238
14. Drug Addiction 254

CHAPTER 5

Neurotransmission

DRUGS INCLUDED IN THIS CHAPTER

The pharmacology of specific drugs is not included in this chapter. The drugs presented in the cases are used as examples to illustrate various aspects of neurotransmission; the specific pharmacology of these drugs is presented in the subsequent chapters of this section.

Chapter 5, Neurotransmission is a compilation of Chapter 8 Neurotransmission: The Autonomic and Somatic Motor Nervous Systems, and Chapter 14 Neurotransmission and the Central Nervous System in *Goodman & Gilman's The Pharmacological Basis of Therapeutics*, 12th Edition. An understanding of the material in these chapters will be helpful in following the material presented in this chapter. In addition to the material presented here, the 12th Edition includes:

- A detailed discussion of the peripheral and central nervous systems (CNS)
- An intricate discussion of the neurotransmitters in the peripheral and CNS, their synthesis, storage, mechanisms of release and termination of effect
- Details of the cholinergic, adrenergic, and somatic nervous systems that are also addressed in Chapters 6 and 7 of this book
- A detailed discussion of chemical transmission of impulses in the CNS

LEARNING OBJECTIVES

- ☑ Understand the characteristics of the parasympathetic, sympathetic, and enteric nervous systems.
- ☑ Understand the difference between the autonomic and somatic nervous systems.
- ☑ Know the predominant transmitters at ganglionic sites in the parasympathetic and sympathetic nerves.
- ☑ Know the transmitters and their target receptors in parasympathetic and sympathetic nervous system.
- ☑ Know the effect that agonist and antagonists have at each target receptor.
- ☑ Understand the blood-brain barrier (BBB).
- ☑ Understand the intricacies of chemical transmission within the CNS and how the interaction of central neurons control the pharmacological effects of drugs acting in the brain.

CASE 5-1

A 47-year-old woman is given a drug to treat her overactive bladder. She is told that the drug is similar to atropine and that it will decrease her frequency of urination. She is cautioned to be aware of the possibility of dry eyes, dry mouth, blurred vision, constipation, drowsiness, dizziness, and confusion.

a. **What are the divisions of the peripheral autonomic nervous system that describe the diverse actions of this drug?**

The efferent nerves of the involuntary (autonomic) nervous system supply all innervated structures of the body except skeletal muscle, which is served by the somatic nerves (see Figures 5-1 and 5-2). The peripheral autonomic nervous system is composed of the sympathetic, parasympathetic, and enteric divisions (see Side Bar DIVISIONS OF THE PERIPHERAL AUTONOMIC NERVOUS SYSTEM).

b. **Why does this drug have such a broad constellation of side effects involving so many different organs?**

Atropine is a drug that blocks cholinergic muscarinic receptors located on the membranes of many effector organs (see Figure 5-1 and Table 5-1), and it blocks all the peripheral actions of acetylcholine, the parasympathetic neurotransmitter

(Continued)

Neurotransmission   CHAPTER 5

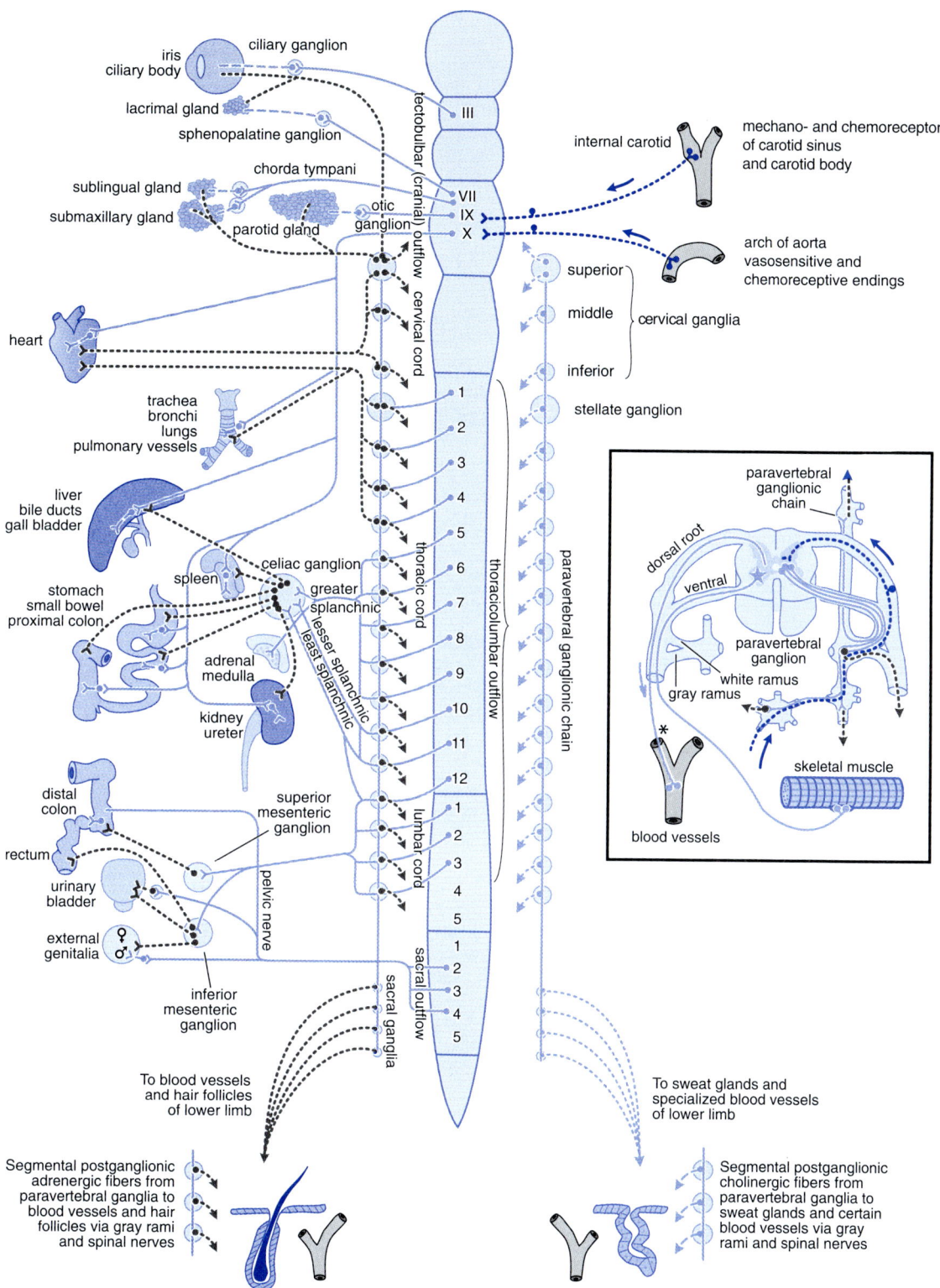

FIGURE 5-1 The autonomic nervous system. Schematic representation of the autonomic nerves and effector organs based on chemical mediation of nerve impulses. Blue, cholinergic; grey, adrenergic; dotted blue, visceral afferent; solid lines, preganglionic; broken lines, postganglionic. In the rectangle at the right are shown the finer details of the ramifications of adrenergic fibers at any 1 segment of the spinal cord, the path of the visceral afferent nerves, the cholinergic nature of somatic motor nerves to skeletal muscle, and the presumed cholinergic nature of the vasodilator fibers in the dorsal roots of the spinal nerves. The asterisk (*) indicates that it is not known whether these vasodilator fibers are motor or sensory or where their cell bodies are situated.

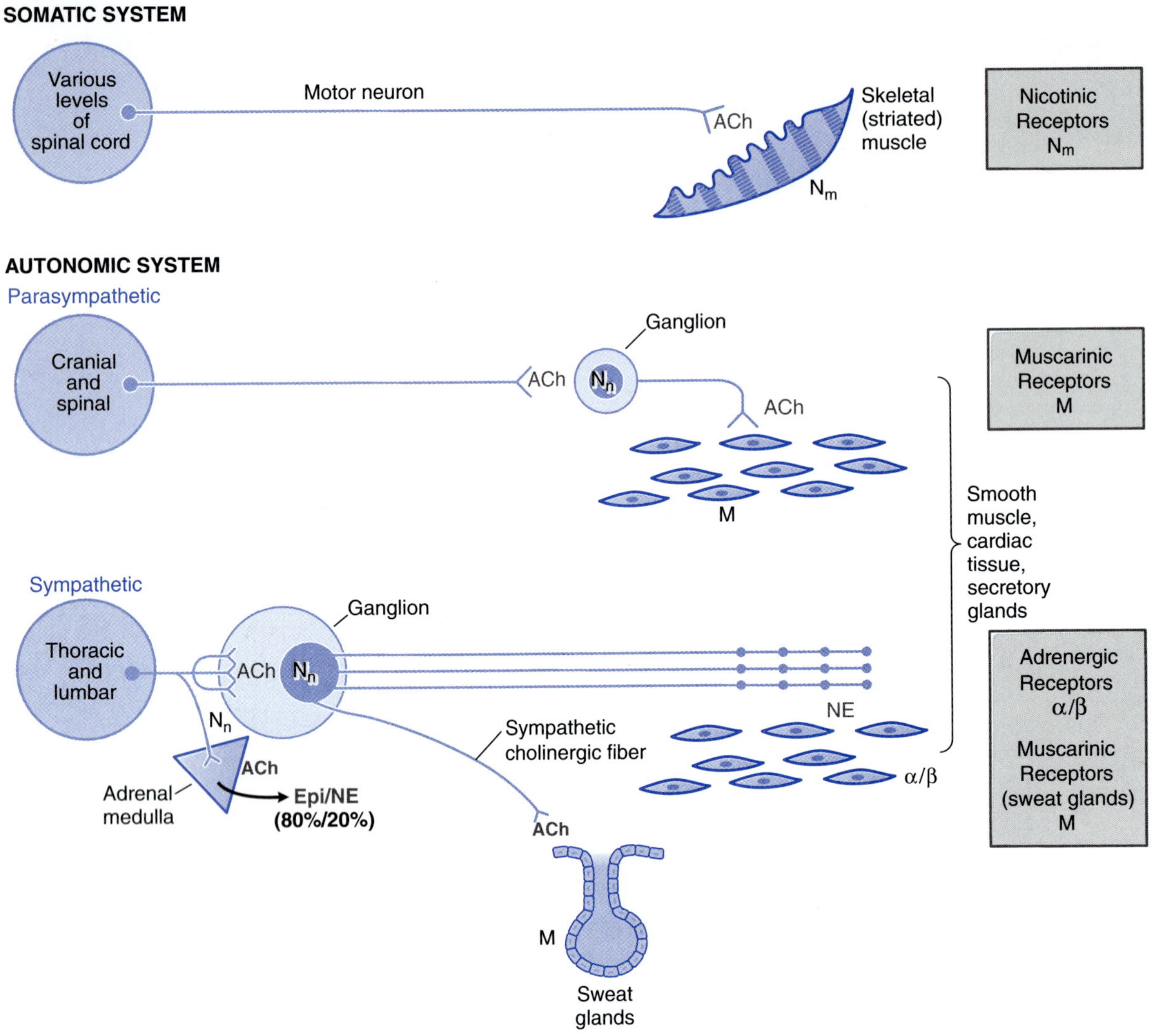

SECTION II Neuropharmacology

SOMATIC SYSTEM

AUTONOMIC SYSTEM
Parasympathetic

Sympathetic

FIGURE 5-2 Schematic representation of the somatic motor nerves and the efferent nerves of the autonomic nervous system. The principal neurotransmitters, acetylcholine (ACh) and norepinephrine (NE), are shown in grey. The receptors for these transmitters, nicotinic (N) and muscarinic (M) cholinergic receptors, α and β adrenergic receptors are shown in grey rectangles to the right. The somatic nerves innervate skeletal muscle directly without a ganglionic relay. The autonomic nerves innervate smooth muscles, cardiac tissue, and glands. Both parasympathetic and sympathetic systems have ganglia where ACh is the transmitter of the preganglionic fibers; ACh acts on nicotinic receptors on the postganglionic nerves. ACh is also the neurotransmitter at cells of the adrenal medulla, where it acts on nicotinic ACh receptors to cause release of the catecholamines epinephrine (Epi) and NE into the circulation. Epi represents ~80% of the released catecholamines. ACh is the predominant neurotransmitter of postganglionic parasympathetic nerves and acts on muscarinic receptors. NE is the principal neurotransmitter of postganglionic sympathetic nerves, acting on α or β adrenergic receptors. Note that somatic nerves form a specialized synaptic junction, termed the motor end plate. Autonomic nerves form a more diffuse pattern with multiple synaptic sites. The ganglia in the parasympathetic system are near or within the organ being innervated with generally a one-to-one relationship between pre- and postganglionic fibers. In the sympathetic system, the ganglia are generally far from the effector cells (eg, within the sympathetic chain ganglia). Preganglionic sympathetic fibers may make contact with a large number of postganglionic fibers.

(see Chapter 6). Thus, it is easy to see why its side effects involve so many organs. Although atropine has minimal effects on the CNS, there are definitely muscarinic receptors in the brain and their antagonism may lead to drowsiness and confusion.

c. **What is the enteric nervous system?**

The processes of mixing, propulsion, and absorption of nutrients in the GI tract are controlled locally through a restricted part of the peripheral nervous system called the enteric nervous system (ENS; see Chapter 33). The ENS actually comprises components of the sympathetic and parasympathetic nervous systems and has sensory nerve connections through the spinal and nodose ganglia.

(Continued)

Neurotransmission — CHAPTER 5

TABLE 5-1 Responses of Effector Organs to Autonomic Nerve Impulses

ORGAN SYSTEM	SYMPATHETIC EFFECT[a]	ADRENERGIC RECEPTOR SUBTYPE[b]	PARASYMPATHETIC EFFECT[a]	CHOLINERGIC RECEPTOR SUBTYPE[b]
Eye				
Radial muscle, iris	Contraction (mydriasis)++	α_1		
Sphincter muscle, iris			Contraction (miosis)+++	M_3, M_2
Ciliary muscle	Relaxation for far vision+	β_2	Contraction for near vision+++	M_3, M_2
Lacrimal glands	Secretion+	α	Secretion+++	M_3, M_2
Heart[c]				
Sinoatrial node	↑ in heart rate++	$\beta_1 > \beta_2$	↓ in heart rate+++	$M_2 \gg M_3$
Atria	↑ in contractility and conduction velocity++	$\beta_1 > \beta_2$	↓ in contractility++ and shortened AP duration	$M_2 \gg M_3$
Atrioventricular node	↑ in automaticity and conduction velocity++	$\beta_1 > \beta_2$	↓ in conduction velocity; AV block+++	$M_2 \gg M_3$
His-Purkinje system	↑ in automaticity and conduction velocity	$\beta_1 > \beta_2$	Little effect	$M_2 \gg M_3$
Ventricle	↑ in contractility, conduction velocity, automaticity and rate of idioventricular pacemakers+++	$\beta_1 > \beta_2$	Slight ↓ in contractility	$M_2 \gg M_3$
Blood Vessels (Arteries and arterioles)[d]				
Coronary	Constriction+; dilation[e]++	$\alpha_1, \alpha_2; \beta_2$	No innervation[h]	—
Skin and mucosa	Constriction+++	α_1, α_2	No innervation[h]	—
Skeletal muscle	Constriction; dilation[e,f]++	$\alpha_1; \beta_2$	Dilation[h] (?)	—
Cerebral	Constriction (slight)	α_1	No innervation[h]	—
Pulmonary	Constriction+; dilation	$\alpha_1; \beta_2$	No innervation[h]	—
Abdominal viscera	Constriction +++; dilation +	$\alpha_1; \beta_2$	No innervation[h]	—
Salivary glands	Constriction+++	α_1, α_2	Dilation[h]++	M_3
Renal	Constriction++; dilation++	$\alpha_1, \alpha_2; \beta_1, \beta_2$	No innervation[h]	
(Veins)[d]	Constriction; dilation	$\alpha_1, \alpha_2; \beta_2$		
Endothelium	—	—	↑NO synthase[h]	M_3
Lung				
Tracheal and bronchial smooth muscle	Relaxation	β_2	Contraction	$M_2 = M_3$
Bronchial glands	↓ secretion, ↑ secretion	α_1 β_2	Stimulation	M_2, M_3
Stomach				
Motility and tone	↓ (usually)[i]+	$\alpha_1, \alpha_2; \beta_1, \beta_2$	↑[i]+++	$M_2 = M_3$
Sphincters	Contraction (usually)+	α_1	Relaxation (usually)+	M_3, M_2
Secretion	Inhibition	α_2	Stimulation++	M_3, M_2
Intestine				
Motility and tone	Decrease[h]+	$\alpha_1, \alpha_2; \beta_1, \beta_2$	↑[i]+++	M_3, M_2
Sphincters	Contraction+	α_1	Relaxation (usually)+	M_3, M_2
Secretion	↓	α_2	↑++	M_3, M_2
Gallbladder and Ducts	Relaxation+	β_2	Contraction+	M
Kidney				
Renin secretion	↓+; ↑++	$\alpha_1; \beta_1$	No innervation	—
Urinary Bladder				
Detrusor	Relaxation+	β_2	Contraction+++	$M_3 > M_2$
Trigone and sphincter	Contraction++	α_1	Relaxation++	$M_3 > M_2$
Ureter				
Motility and tone	↑	α_1	↑ (?)	M
Uterus	Pregnant contraction	α_1		
	Relaxation	β_2	Variable[j]	M
	Nonpregnant relaxation	β_2		

(Continued)

SECTION II Neuropharmacology

ORGAN SYSTEM	SYMPATHETIC EFFECT[a]	ADRENERGIC RECEPTOR SUBTYPE[b]	PARASYMPATHETIC EFFECT[a]	CHOLINERGIC RECEPTOR SUBTYPE[b]
Sex Organs, male	Ejaculation+++	α_1	Erection+++	M_3
Pilomotor muscles	Contraction++	α_1	—	
Sweat glands	Localized secretion[k]++	α_1	—	
	—		Generalized secretion+++	M_3, M_2
Spleen Capsule	Contraction+++	α_1	—	—
	Relaxation+	β_2	—	
Adrenal Medulla	—		Secretion of epinephrine and norepinephrine	$N(\alpha_3)_2(\beta_4)_3$; M (secondarily)
Skeletal Muscle	Increased contractility; glycogenolysis; K+ uptake	β_2	—	—
Liver	Glycogenolysis and gluconeogenesis+++	α_1 β_2	—	—
Pancreas				
Acini	↓ secretion+	α	Secretion++	M_3, M_2
Islets (β cells)	↓ secretion+++	α_2	—	
	↑ secretion+	β_2		
Fat Cells[l]	Lipolysis+++; thermogenesis	$\alpha_1; \beta_1, \beta_2, \beta_3$	—	—
	Inhibition of lipolysis	α_2		
Salivary Glands	K+ and water secretion+	α_1	K+ and water secretion+++	M_3, M_2
Nasopharyngeal Glands	—		Secretion++	M_3, M_2
Pineal Glands	Melatonin synthesis	β	—	
Posterior Pituitary	ADH secretion	β_1	—	
Autonomic Nerve Endings				
Sympathetic terminal				
Autoreceptor	Inhibition of NE release	$\alpha_{2A} > \alpha_{2C}(\alpha_{2B})$		
Heteroreceptor	—		Inhibition of NE release	M_2, M_4
Parasympathetic terminal				
Autoreceptor	—		Inhibition of ACh release	M_2, M_4
Heteroreceptor	Inhibition ACh release	$\alpha_{2A} > \alpha_{2C}$	—	—

[a]Responses are designated + to +++ to provide an approximate indication of the importance of sympathetic and parasympathetic nerve activity in the control of the various organs and functions listed.

[b]Adrenergic receptors: α_1, α_2 and subtypes thereof; β_1, β_2, β_3. Cholinergic receptors: nicotinic (N); muscarinic (M), with subtypes 1-4. When a designation of subtype is not provided, the nature of the subtype has not been determined, unequivocally. Only the principal receptor subtypes are shown. Transmitters other than ACh and NE contribute to many of the responses.

[c]In the human heart, the ration of β_1 to β_2 is about 3:2 in atria and 4:1 in ventricles. While M_2 receptors predominate, M_3 receptors are also present.

[d]The predominant α_1 receptor subtype in most blood vessels (both arteries and veins) is α_{1A}, although other α_1 subtypes are present in specific blood vessels. The α_{1D} is the predominant subtype in the aorta.

[e]Dilation predominates *in situ* owing to metabolic autoregulatory mechanisms.

[f]Over the usual concentration range of physiologically released circulating epinephrine, the β receptor response (vasodilation) predominates in blood vessels of skeletal muscle and liver; β receptor response (vasoconstriction) in blood vessels of other abdominal viscera. The renal and mesenteric vessels also contain specific dopaminergic receptors whose activation causes dilation.

[g]Sympathetic cholinergic neurons cause vasodilation in skeletal muscle beds, but this is not involved in most physiological responses.

[h]The endothelium of most blood vessels releases NO, which causes vasodilation in response to muscarinic stimuli. However, unlike the receptors innervated by sympathetic cholinergic fibers in skeletal muscle blood vessels, these muscarinic receptors are not innervated and respond only to exogenously added muscarinic agonists in the circulation.

[i]While adrenergic fibers terminate at inhibitory β receptors on smooth muscle fibers and at inhibitory β receptors on parasympathetic (cholinergic) excitatory ganglion cells of the myenteric plexus, the primary inhibitory response is mediated *via* enteric neurons through NO, P2Y receptors, and peptide receptors.

[j]Uterine responses depend on stages of menstrual cycle, amount of circulating estrogen and progesterone, and other factors.

[k]Palms of hands and some other sites ("adrenergic sweating").

[l]There is significant variation among species in the receptor types that mediate certain metabolic responses. All three β adrenergic receptors have been found in human fat cells. Activation of β_3 receptors produces a vigorous thermogenic response as well as lipolysis. The significance is unclear. Activation of β receptors also inhibits leptin release from adipose tissue.

ADH, antidiuretic hormone; AP, action potential; AV, atrioventricular

Neurotransmission

CHAPTER 5

DIVISIONS OF THE PERIPHERAL AUTONOMIC NERVOUS SYSTEM

- Sympathetic nervous system
- Parasympathetic nervous system
- Enteric nervous system

d. What are the differences between the parasympathetic and sympathetic nervous systems?

The sympathetic system is distributed to effectors throughout the body, whereas parasympathetic distribution is much more limited (see Figure 5-1). The ganglia in the parasympathetic system are near or within the organ being innervated with generally a one-to-one relationship between pre- and postganglionic fibers (see Figure 5-2). In the sympathetic system the ganglia are generally far from the effector cells. Preganglionic sympathetic fibers may make contact with a large number of postganglionic fibers.

In contrast to the parasympathetic and sympathetic nervous systems, somatic nerves innervate skeletal muscle directly without a ganglionic relay (see Case 5-2).

Acetylcholine (ACh) is the predominant neurotransmitter of postganglionic parasympathetic nerves and acts on muscarinic receptors. Norepinephrine (NE) is the principal neurotransmitter of postganglionic sympathetic nerves acting on α or β adrenergic receptors.

Both parasympathetic and sympathetic systems have ganglia where ACh is the transmitter of the preganglionic fibers; ACh acts on nicotinic receptors on the postganglionic nerves. ACh is also the transmitter at cells of the adrenal medulla, where it acts on nicotinic receptors to cause release of epinephrine and norepinephrine into the circulation.

STEPS INVOLVED IN JUNCTIONAL TRANSMISSION

- Transmitter synthesis
- Transmitter storage
- Transmitter release
- Transmitter recognition and binding by target receptor
- Termination of action

CASE 5-2

A 35-year-old man is undergoing abdominal surgery. The anesthesiologist explains in a presurgery meeting with the patient that a neuromuscular blocking drug will be administered to cause complete muscle relaxation prior to the initiation of surgery.

a. What is the difference between the autonomic nervous system that innervates many visceral organs and the somatic nervous system that innervates skeletal muscle?

The somatic nerves innervate skeletal muscle directly without a ganglion relay (see Figure 5-2). At each neuromuscular junction, the axon terminal loses its myelin sheath and forms a terminal aborization that lies in apposition to a specialized surface of the muscle membrane termed the motor end plate (see Chapter 6).

b. What are the steps involved in the transmission of a nerve impulse?

The steps involved in excitatory and inhibitory neurotransmission are depicted schematically in Figure 5-3. The steps involved in the junctional transmission of the nerve impulse are outlined in the Side Bar STEPS INVOLVED IN JUNCTIONAL TRANSMISSION, the details of which are characteristic of a specific nerve transmission system, that is, parasympathetic, sympathetic, somatic, and in the CNS.

Transmitter synthesis: Small molecules like ACh and NE (see Side Bar NEUROTRANSMITTERS for a list of neurotransmitters) are synthesized in nerve terminals; peptides are synthesized in cell bodies and transported to nerve terminals.

Transmitter storage: Synaptic vesicles store transmitters, often in association with various proteins and frequently with ATP.

Transmitter release: Release of transmitter occurs by exocytosis. Depolarization results in an influx of Ca^{++}, which in turn appears to bind proteins called synaptotagmins. The storage vesicles dock and then fuse with scaffolding proteins on the presynaptic membrane, which is followed by exocytotic release of their contents into the synaptic cleft (see Figure 5-3).

Transmitter recognition: Receptors exist on postsynaptic cells, which recognize the transmitter (see Side Bar NEUROTRANSMITTERS). Binding of a neurotransmitter to its receptor initiates a signal transduction event (see Figures 5-4 and 5-6).

(Continued)

SECTION II

Neuropharmacology

NEUROTRANSMITTERS

PERIPHERAL	CENTRAL
Acetylcholine	Acetylcholine
Norepinephrine	Norepinephrine
Epinephrine	Epinephrine
Dopamine	Dopamine
Serotonin	Serotonin
	Amino acids
	γ-amino-butyric acid (GABA)
	Glycine
	Aspartic acid
	Glutamic acid
	Peptide neurotransmitters or neuromodulators (see Table 14-7 *Goodman and Gilman's The Pharmacological Basis of Therapeutics,* 12th Edition)

Termination of action: A variety of mechanisms terminate the action of synaptically released transmitter, including hydrolysis and reuptake into neurons by specific transporters (see Chapters 6 and 7 for specific examples).

c. What is the role of ion channels in the promulgation of the nerve impulse and controlling neuronal excitability?

Voltage-dependent ion channels provide for rapid changes in ion permeability along axons and within dendrites and for excitation-secretion coupling that releases neurotransmitters from presynaptic sites.

The electrical excitability of neurons is achieved through modification of ion channels in neuronal plasma membranes (see Figures 5-3 through 5-6). The relatively high extracellular concentration of Na^+ ($\approx$140 mM) compared to its concentration intracellularly ($\approx$14 mM) means that increases in permeability to Na^+ causes depolarization, ultimately leading to the generation of action potentials.

Increases in the concentration of intracellular Ca^{++} affects multiple processes in the cell and are critical to the release of neurotransmitters. Table 5-2 lists the various subtypes of Ca^{++} channels.

The Cl^- gradient across the plasma membrane explains the fact that activation of Cl^- channels causes an inhibitory postsynaptic potential (IPSP) that dampens neuronal excitability and inactivation of these channels can lead to hyperexcitability. Figure 14-3 in *Goodman and Gilman's The Pharmacological Basis of Therapeutics,* 12th Edition shows the structures of 3 families of Cl^- channels.

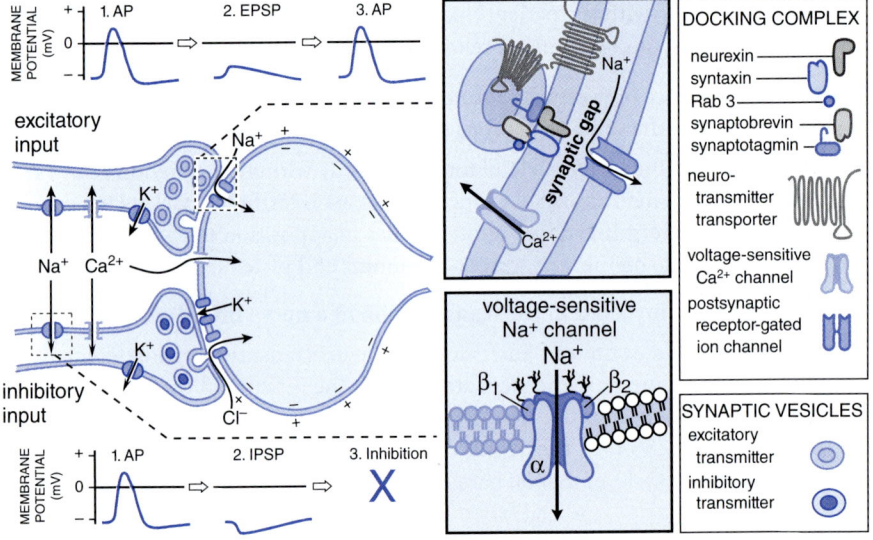

FIGURE 5-3 Steps involved in excitatory and inhibitory neurotransmission. **1.** The nerve action potential (AP) consists of a transient self-propagated reversal of charge on the axonal membrane. (The internal potential E_i goes from a negative value, through zero potential, to a slightly positive value primarily through increases in Na^+ permeability and then returns to resting values by an increase in K^+ permeability.) When the AP arrives at the presynaptic terminal, it initiates release of the excitatory or inhibitory transmitter. Depolarization at the nerve ending and entry of Ca^{2+} initiate docking and then fusion of the synaptic vesicle with the membrane of the nerve ending. Docked and fused vesicles are shown. **2.** Combination of the excitatory transmitter with postsynaptic receptors produces a localized depolarization, the excitatory postsynaptic potential (EPSP), through an increase in permeability to cations, most notably Na^+. The inhibitory transmitter causes a selective increase in permeability to K^+ or Cl^-, resulting in a localized hyperpolarization, the inhibitory postsynaptic potential (IPSP). **3.** The EPSP initiates a conducted AP in the postsynaptic neuron; this can be prevented, however, by the hyperpolarization induced by a concurrent IPSP. The transmitter is dissipated by enzymatic destruction, by reuptake into the presynaptic terminal or adjacent glial cells, or by diffusion. Depolarization of the postsynaptic membrane can permit Ca^{2+} entry if voltage-gated Ca^{2+} channels are present. (Reproduced with permission from Brunton L, Parker K, Blumenthal D, Buxton I (eds). *Goodman & Gilman's Manual of Pharmacology and Therapeutics.* New York: McGraw-Hill, 2008, p 94. Copyright © 2008 by The McGraw-Hill Companies, Inc. All rights reserved.)

Neurotransmission   CHAPTER 5

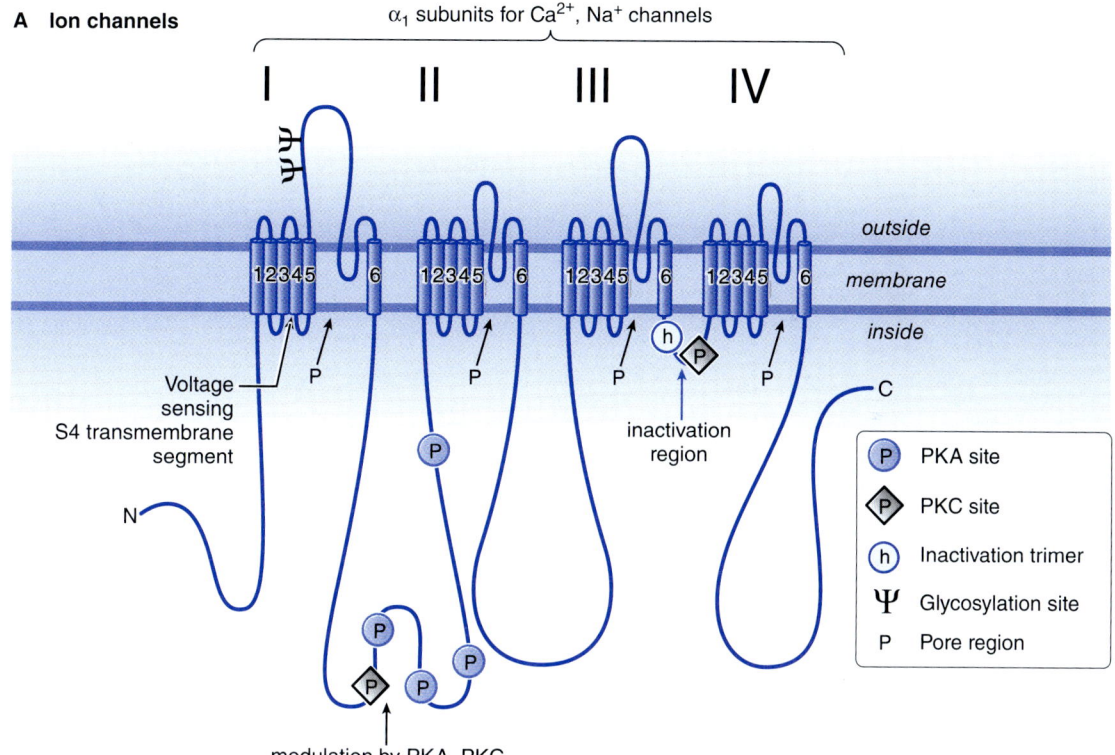

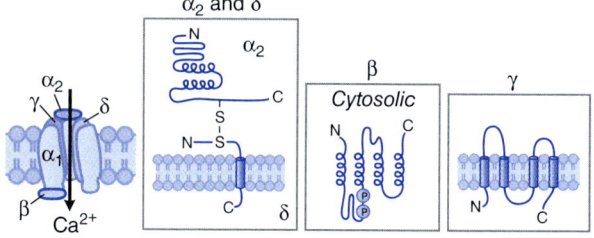

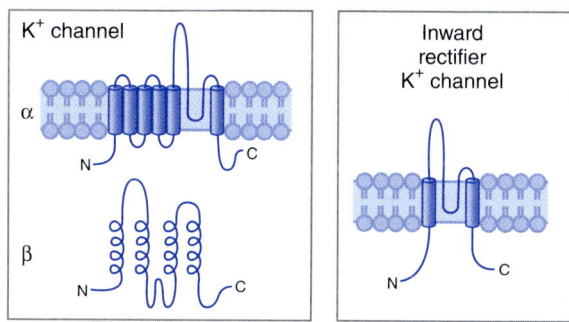

FIGURE 5-4 Structural similarities of voltage-dependent Na^+, Ca^{2+}, and K^+ channels. **A.** The α subunit in both Ca^{2+} and Na^+ channels contains 4 subunits, each with 6 transmembrane hydrophobic domains. The hydrophobic regions that connect segments 5 and 6 in each domain form the pore of the channel. Segment 4 in each domain includes the voltage-sensor. (Adapted with permission from Catterall W. From ionic currents to molecular mechanisms: The structure and function of voltage-gated sodium channels. *Neuron, 2000, 26:13–25. Copyright © Elsevier.*) **B.** The Ca^{2+} channel also requires several auxiliary small proteins ($α_2$, β, γ, and δ). The $α_2$ and δ subunits are linked by a disulfide bond. Regulatory subunits also exist for Na^+ channels. **C.** Voltage-sensitive K^+ channels (K_V) and the rapidly activating K^+ channel (K_A) share a similar putative hexaspanning structure similar in overall configuration to 1 repeat unit within the Na^+ and Ca^{2+} channel structure, while the inwardly rectifying K^+ channel protein (K_{ir}) retains the general configuration of just loops 5 and 6. Regulatory β subunits (cystosolic) can alter K_V channel functions. Channels of these 2 overall motifs can form heteromultimers.

SECTION II Neuropharmacology

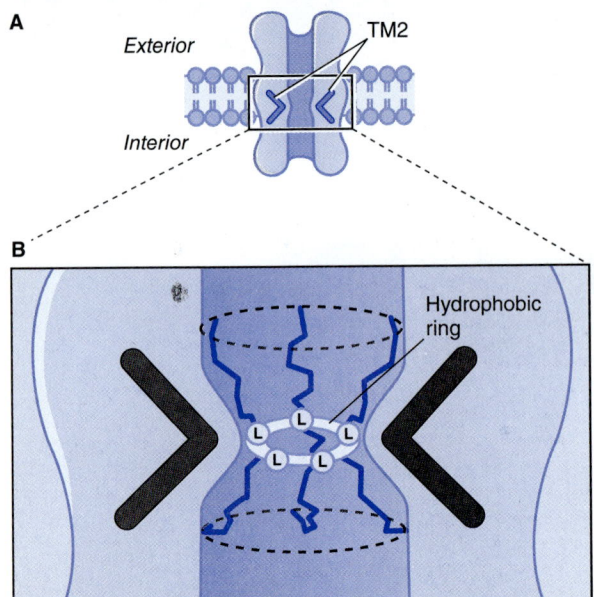

FIGURE 5-5 Predicted 3-D structure of a ligand-gated ion channel receptor in a postsynaptic membrane. **A.** These channels consist of a cylindrical membrane-embedded structure with a central pore. The second transmembrane domain (TM2) of each subunit lines the pore and bends inward to block ion flow through the channel. **B.** A highly conserved leucine residue (L) in the TM2 bend of each subunit is believed to protrude into the pore to form a tight hydrophobic ring, which may act as a barrier to the flow of hydrated ions across the channel. (Redrawn with permission from Nestler EJ, Hyman SE, Malenka RC (eds). *Molecular Neuropharmacology*, 2nd ed. New York: McGraw-Hill, 2009, p 174. Copyright © 2009 by The McGraw-Hill Companies, Inc. All rights reserved.)

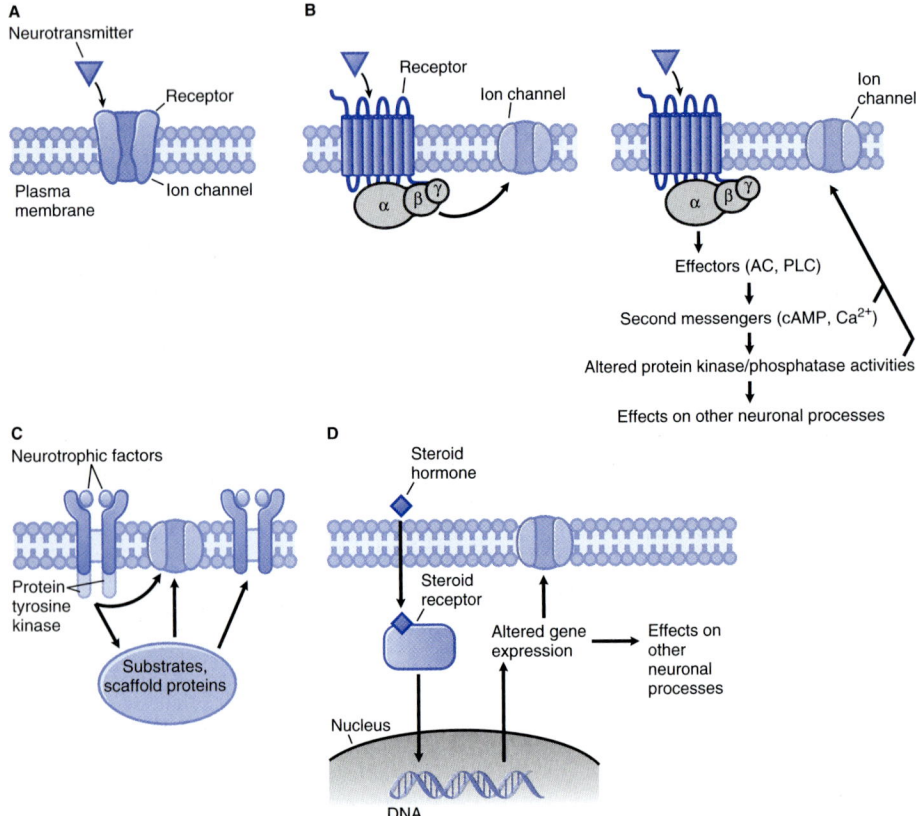

FIGURE 5-6 General patterns of signal transduction in the brain. **A.** Neurotransmitter activation of a receptor that contains an integral ion channel. **B.** Neurotransmitter activation of G protein–coupled receptor. After activation, the βγ subunits of the G protein can directly regulate an ion channel (*left*), and the α subunit can activate second messenger-dependent signaling involving protein kinases and protein phosphatases, which can, in turn, affect ion channels and other neuronal processes (*right*). **C.** Neurotrophic factors promote receptor dimerization, which leads to activation of receptor protein tyrosine kinase activity and its sequelae. **D.** Steroid hormone activation of a cytoplasmic receptor. After the receptor-hormone complex forms, it enters the nucleus and regulates gene expression. (Redrawn with permission from Nestler EJ, Hyman SE, Malenka RC (eds). *Molecular Neuropharmacology*, 2nd ed. New York: McGraw-Hill, 2009, p 76. Copyright © 2009 by The McGraw-Hill Companies, Inc. All rights reserved.)

Neurotransmission — CHAPTER 5

TABLE 5-2 Subtypes of Ca^{2+} Channel[a]

Ca^{2+} CHANNEL	UNOFFICIAL NAME	Ca^{2+} CURRENT TYPE	PRIMARY LOCATIONS	ANTAGONISTS	FUNCTION
Ca_v 1.1	BK channel	L	Skeletal muscle	DHP, PAA, BZP	EC coupling
Ca_v 1.2		L	Cardiac muscle Endocrine cells Neurons	DHP, PAA, BZP	EC coupling Ca^{2+} homeostasis Regulation of transcription
Ca_v 1.3		L	Endocrine cells Neurons	DHP, PAA, BZP	Hormone secretion Regulation of transcription
Ca_v 1.4		L	Retina	DHP, PAA, BZP	Tonic neurotransmitter release
Ca_v 2.1	SK1	P/Q	Nerve terminals Dendrites	ω-Agatoxin IVA	Neurotransmitter release Dendrite Ca^{2+} transients
Ca_v 2.2	SK2	N	Nerve terminals Dendrites	ω-CTX-GVIA Riluzole	Neurotransmitter release Dendrite Ca^{2+} transients
Ca_v 2.3	SK3	R	Cell bodies Dendrites Nerve Terminals	SNX-482	Ca^{2+}-dependent action potentials Dendritic Ca^{2+} transients
Ca_v 3.1	Gardos channel	T	Cardiac muscle Skeletal muscle Neurons	Mibefradil	Repetitive firing of pacemaker cells
Ca_v 3.2		T	Cardiac muscle Neurons	Mibefradil	Repetitive firing of pacemaker cells
Ca_v 3.3		T	Neurons	Mibefradil	Repetitive firing of pacemaker cells

DHP = dihydropyridines (nifedipine). PAA = Phenylalkylamines (verapamil). BZP = benzothiazepines (diltiazem). ω-CTX = ω-conotoxin
[a]Five classes of Ca^{2+} channel identified as L, P/Q, N, R, and T channels exist.

CASE 5-3

A 6-year-old boy is accidentally exposed to a large oral dose of the pesticide malathione, a cholinesterase inhibitor.

a. Why are the symptoms that this boy might experience predictable?

Acetylcholinesterase catalyzes the hydrolysis of the neurotransmitter acetylcholine (ACh) (see Chapter 6). When the enzyme is inhibited, there is an abundance of ACh at the ganglion in parasympathetic and sympathetic fibers, at the parasympathetic effector organs, and at the somatic neuromuscular junctions (see Figure 5-2). Although poisoning by anticholinesterase agents is complex (see Chapter 6), knowing the organs innervated by parasympathetic, sympathetic, and somatic fibers can allow for the prediction of symptoms to be experienced by this boy (see Figure 5-1 and Table 5-1).

b. How are the actions of neurotransmitters terminated?

Figure 5-7 shows the various mechanisms by which neurotransmitters are terminated. Released neurotransmitter is inactivated by reuptake into the nerve terminal (dopamine, NE, GABA), by degradation (ACh, peptides), or by uptake and metabolism by glial cells in the CNS (glutamate).

CASE 5-4

A 23-year-old woman develops seasonal allergies, involving severe itching eyes, lacrimation, and rhinorrhea. She commonly takes an over-the-counter product that contains diphenhydramine (a first-generation antihistamine), but it makes her drowsy

(Continued)

RECEPTORS IN THE PERIPHERAL AND CENTRAL NERVOUS SYSTEMS

- Muscarinic acetylcholine
- Nicotinic acetylcholine
- α Adrenergic
- β Adrenergic
- Serotinergic
- Dopamine
- Amino acid receptors (GABA, Glutamate, Aspartate, Glycine)
- Opioid receptors (δ, κ, μ) (see Chapter 10)
- Somatostatin
- Neurotensin
- Cholecystokinin
- Purinergic receptors (see Table 14-10)

Goodman and Gilman's The Pharmacological Basis of Therapeutics, 12th Edition)

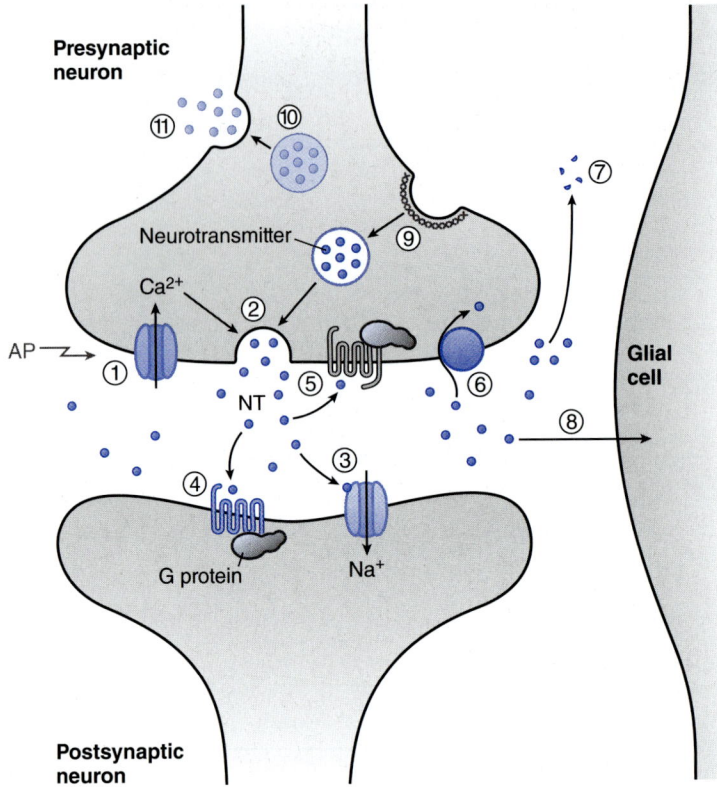

FIGURE 5-7 Transmitter release, action, and inactivation. Depolarization opens voltage-dependent Ca²⁺ channels in the presynaptic nerve terminal. (1) The influx of Ca²⁺ during an action potential (AP) triggers (2) the exocytosis of small synaptic vesicles that store neurotransmitter (NT) involved in fast neurotransmission. Released neurotransmitter interacts with receptors in the postsynaptic membranes that either couple directly with ion channels (3) or act through second messengers, such as (4) GPCRs. Neurotransmitter receptors in the presynaptic nerve terminal membrane (5) can inhibit or enhance subsequent exocytosis. Released neurotransmitter is inactivated by reuptake into the nerve terminal by (6) a transport protein coupled to the Na⁺ gradient, for example, DA, NE, and GABA; by (7) degradation (ACh, peptides); or by (8) uptake and metabolism by glial cells (Glu). The synaptic vesicle membrane is recycled by (9) clathrin-mediated endocytosis. Neuropeptides and proteins are stored in (10) larger, dense core granules within the nerve terminal. These dense core granules are released from (11) sites distinct from active zones after repetitive stimulation.

and she is unable to work productively (see Chapter 21). Her doctor recommends that she switch to loratadine, which should make her less sleepy.

a. What is the difference between diphenhydramine and loratadine?

The antihistamines are discussed in detail in Chapter 21 (see specifically Case 21-1). Both diphenhydramine and loratadine are antagonists of histamine H_1 receptors. Diphenhydramine is an ethanolamine and readily penetrates the CNS causing the drowsiness experienced by this patient. Loratadine is a tricyclic piperidine that does not penetrate the CNS and does not cause drowsiness.

b. What process in the brain keeps loratadine from producing sleepiness?

Drugs acting in the CNS have to cross the blood-brain barrier (BBB) or the blood-CSF barrier (see Chapter 2). These 2 barriers are formed by brain capillary endothelial cells and epithelial cells of the choroid plexus, respectively. Lipophilic molecules such as diphenhydramine diffuse freely across the BBB and accumulate in the brain. Loratadine is less lipophilic and does not cross the BBB. In addition, diphenhydramine is an anticholinergic and interacts with muscarinic receptors, whereas loratadine does not inhibit muscarinic receptors.

Chapter 5: Neurotransmission

CASE 5-5

A 62-year-old man with a diagnosis of Alzheimer's disease has mild cognitive loss. He is given a drug that may improve his cognition, but his doctor explains to the family that the patient's loss of cognitive ability will likely progress (see Chapter 13).

a. How is the pharmacological treatment of a disorder of the CNS different from treating a disorder in the peripheral nervous system?

The identification of targets for drugs that affect the CNS and behavior is a difficult scientific challenge. Complicating this effort is the fact that a CNS-active drug (such as this patient is receiving to improve cognition) may act at multiple sites with disparate and even opposing effects. In addition, many CNS disorders involve multiple brain regions and pathways, which can frustrate efforts to use a single therapeutic agent.

b. What are the neurotransmitters in the CNS?

The neurotransmitters in the CNS are generally the same as in the peripheral nervous system (see Side Bar NEUROTRANSMITTERS). In addition, there are many other neurotransmitters in the CNS such as amino acids and peptides (see Table 5-3).

c. How does this difference make it difficult to treat disorders of the CNS?

In the peripheral nervous system, there are limited transmitters and receptors which recognize them; thus, agonists or antagonists have specific predictable effects. In the CNS there are more transmitters and receptors that function to regulate brain activity and behavior. Figure 5-6 shows the multiple patterns of signal transduction in the brain. Specific therapeutic approaches to neurological and psychiatric disorders are discussed in Chapters 8, 9, 12, 13, and 14.

TABLE 5-3 Examples of Neuropeptides

Calcitonin Family
Calcitonin
Calcitonin gene-related peptide (CGRP)
Hypothalamic Hormones
Oxytocin
Vasopressin
Hypothalamic Releasing and Inhibitory Hormones
Corticotropin-releasing factor (CRF or CRH)
Gonadotropin-releasing hormone (GnRH)
Growth hormone releasing hormone (GHRH)
Somatostatin (SST)
Thyrotropin releasing hormone (TRH)
Neuropeptide Y Family
Neuropeptide Y (NPY)
Neuropeptide YY (PYY)
Pancreatic polypeptide (PP)
Opioid Peptides
β-endorphin (also pituitary hormone)
Dynorphin peptides
Leu-enkephalin
Met-enkephalin
Pituitary Hormones
Adrenocorticotropic hormone (ACTH)
α-Melanocyte-stimulating hormone (α-MSH)
Growth hormone (GH)
Follicle-stimulating hormone (FSH)
β-lipotropin (β-LPH)
Luteinizing hormone (LH)

Tachykinins
Neurokinin A (substance A)
Neurokinin B
Neuropeptide K
Substance P
VIP-Glucagon Family
Glucagon
Glucagon-like peptide (GLP-1)
Pituitary adenylyl cyclase—activating peptide (PACAP)
Vasoactive intestinal polypeptide (VIP)
Some Other Peptides
Agouti-related peptide (ARP)
Bombesin
Bradykinin (BK)
Cholecystokinin (CCK; multiple forms)
Cocaine- and amphetamine-regulated transcript (CART)
Galanin
Ghrelin
Melanin-concentrating hormone (MCH)
Neurotensin
Nerve growth factor (NGF)
Orexins (or Hypocretins)
Orphanin GQ (or Nociceptin) (also grouped with opioids)

Modified with permission from Nestler EJ, Hyman SE, Malenka RC (eds). *Molecular Neuropharmacology, 2nd ed.* New York: McGraw-Hill, 2009, p 184, Table 7-1. Copyright © 2009 by The McGraw-Hill Companies, Inc. All rights reserved.

SECTION II Neuropharmacology

CASE 5-6

A 56-year-old woman with advanced breast cancer is prescribed morphine for pain. Although the morphine effectively diffuses the pain, the patient develops severe constipation.

a. What is meant by drug specificity and nonspecificity in the CNS?

The effect of a drug in the CNS is considered to be specific when it affects an identifiable molecular mechanism unique to target cells that bear receptors for that drug. Conversely, a drug is regarded as being nonspecific when it produces effects at a variety of different target cells, thus affecting a diverse set of neurobiological systems.

Although relief of pain is the goal when administering an opiate, one must also contend with potential off-target effects, including respiratory depression and constipation (see Chapter 10).

CASE 5-7

A 75-year-old woman has been taking alprazolam for anxiety and sleep for the past 10 years. Lately she has developed mild dementia and has forgotten to refill her prescription. After 3 days without taking her alprazolam, she becomes extremely anxious and shaky and has a tonic-clonic seizure.

a. What property of CNS drugs has led to this state of hyperexcitability in this patient?

Alprazolam is a CNS depressant used commonly to treat anxiety and insomnia (see Chapter 9).

Acute, excessive stimulation of the cerebrospinal axis (not the case with this patient) normally is followed by depression, which is in part a consequence of neuronal fatigue and exhaustion of stores of transmitters. Acute, drug-induced depression (also not the case with this patient) is not followed by stimulation. However, chronic drug-induced sedation or depression (such as with this patient) may be followed by prolonged hyperexcitability upon abrupt cessation of the medication. This effect is also common in alcohol withdrawal (see Chapter 9).

KEY CONCEPTS

- The autonomic nervous system, also called the vegetative, visceral, or involuntary nervous system, regulates body functions that occur without control (see Table 5-1).
- The autonomic nervous system consists of nerves, ganglia, and plexuses that innervate the heart, blood vessels, glands, other visceral organs, and smooth muscle in various tissues (see Figure 5-1).
- The autonomic nervous system comprises the parasympathetic, sympathetic, and enteric nervous systems.
- The somatic nervous system innervates skeletal muscle.
- The CNS is made up of various anatomic regions—cerebral cortex, limbic system, diencephalon, midbrain and brainstem, cerebellum, and spinal cord with a complex assembly of interacting neurons and nuclei that regulate their own and each other's activities generally through chemical neurotransmission.
- The parasympathetic and sympathetic systems have ganglia where ACh is the transmitter of the preganglionic fibers (see Figure 5-2). In these ganglia, ACh acts on nicotinic receptors on the postganglionic nerves.
- ACh is also the neurotransmitter at cells of the adrenal medulla where it acts on nicotinic ACh receptors.

Neurotransmission CHAPTER 5

- ACh is the predominant neurotransmitter of postganglionic parasympathetic nerves and acts on muscarinic receptors in the target tissues.
- NE is the principal neurotransmitter of postganglionic sympathetic nerves acting on α and β adrenergic receptors.
- In the CNS there are several other transmitters beside ACh and NE, including neuropeptides (see Side Bar NEUROTRANSMITTERS and Table 5-3).
- In the peripheral nervous system, the actions of agonists and antagonist are predictable based on their interactions with specific receptors (see Table 5-1).
- In the CNS, the actions of agonist and antagonists are not as predictable as in the peripheral nervous system due to interacting neurons and nuclei.

SUMMARY QUIZ

QUESTION 5-1 A 42-year-old man has just been prescribed a new drug. After several doses he notices dry mouth, dry eyes, and a rapid heart rate. This is most likely due to an inhibition of which of the following neurotransmitter:

a. Norepinephrine
b. Serotonin
c. Glutamate
d. Acetylcholine
e. Epinephrine

QUESTION 5-2 A 23-year-old man is accosted by 3 men late at night. Immediately his heart rate increases due to an increase in epinephrine in his circulation. This release of epinephrine from the adrenal medulla is the result of the action of acetylcholine on

a. muscarinic receptors.
b. α adrenergic receptors.
c. nicotinic receptors.
d. β adrenergic receptors.
e. glutamate receptors.

QUESTION 5-3 A 56-year-old woman goes to an ophthalmologist for an eye examination. The ophthalmologist administers an eye drop to dilate her pupils prior to the eye examination. The medication in the eye drop is most likely acting on

a. serotonin receptors.
b. $α_1$ adrenergic receptors.
c. $β_2$ adrenergic receptors.
d. nicotinic receptors.
e. acetylcholinesterase.

QUESTION 5-4 The neurotransmitter at the neuromuscular junction is

a. acetylcholine.
b. norepinephrine.
c. serotonin.
d. aspartate.
e. epinephrine.

SECTION II — Neuropharmacology

QUESTION 5-5 A 33-year-old woman with a brain infection (meningitis) is administered her antibiotic directly into the cerebrospinal fluid because the

a. bacteria causing the brain infection are not sensitive to the antibiotic.
b. blood brain barrier excludes the antibiotic if it is administered systemically.
c. antibiotic binds to brain cells and is not available to the bacteria.
d. antibiotic is activated by the cerebrospinal fluid.
e. bacteria are mostly located in the cerebrospinal fluid.

QUESTION 5-6 An 80-year-old woman is administered a CNS depressant drug for anxiety. When she abruptly stops the drug, after taking it for many years, she is likely to experience

a. increased sedation.
b. hyperexcitability.
c. a depressed mood.
d. nausea.
e. blurred vision.

SUMMARY QUIZ ANSWER KEY

QUESTION 5-1 Answer **d**. ACh is the predominant neurotransmitter of postganglionic parasympathetic nerves. A cholinergic antagonist acts on muscarinic receptors to produce the side effects noted in this patient (see Figures 5-1 and 5-2, and Table 5-1).

QUESTION 5-2 Answer **c**. ACh is the neurotransmitter at cells of the adrenal medulla, where it acts on nicotinic ACh receptors to cause the release of the catecholamines, epinephrine (80%) and norepinephrine (20%), into the circulation.

QUESTION 5-3 Answer **b**. The eye drop used is most likely an α_1 adrenergic agonist that is acting on receptors to cause contraction (mydriasis) of the radial muscle in the iris (see Table 5-1).

QUESTION 5-4 Answer **a**. ACh is the transmitter at the neuromuscular junction of somatic nerves (see Figure 5-2).

QUESTION 5-5 Answer **b**. Drugs acting in the CNS have to cross the BBB or the blood-CSF barrier (see Chapter 2). These 2 barriers are formed by brain capillary endothelial cells and epithelial cells of the choroid plexus, respectively. Lipophilic molecules diffuse freely across the BBB and accumulate in the brain, whereas less lipophilic drugs (such as most antibiotics) do not easily penetrate the brain and are often administered directly into the cerebrospinal fluid thus bypassing the BBB (see Case 5-4.)

QUESTION 5-6 Answer **b**. Chronic drug-induced sedation or depression (such as with this patient) may be followed by prolonged hyperexcitability upon abrupt cessation of the medication (see Case 5-7.)

Chapter 6

Cholinergic Pharmacology

Chapter 6 Cholinergic Pharmacology is a combination of Chapter 9 Muscarinic Receptor Agonists and Antagonists Chapter 10 Anticholinesterase Agents, and Chapter 11 Agents Acting at the Neuromuscular Junction and Autonomic Ganglia in *Goodman and Gilman's The Pharmacological Basis of Therapeutics*, 12th Edition. An understanding of the material in these chapters will be helpful in following the material presented in this chapter. In addition to the material presented here the above chapters in the 12th Edition include:

- A complete discussion of the properties and subtypes of muscarinic receptors
- The pharmacological effects of acetylcholine (ACh)
- A detailed discussion of the pharmacological effects of atropine, a muscarinic receptor antagonist
- A discussion of the toxicology of drugs with antimuscarinic properties
- A review of the structure of acetylcholinesterase (AChE)
- A discussion of the mechanism of AChE
- A description of the nicotinic acetylcholine receptor
- A description of the actions of neuromuscular blocking agents on various organ systems
- A discussion of the pathophysiology and treatment of malignant hyperthermia
- A discussion of ganglionic transmission
- A description of the pharmacological actions of nicotine

LEARNING OBJECTIVES

- ☑ Understand cholinergic pharmacology, including the different types and subtypes of cholinergic receptors expressed in the central nervous system (CNS), autonomic nervous system (ANS), and neuromuscular junction.
- ☑ Know the mechanisms of synthesis, storage, release, and destruction of ACh in the CNS, parasympathetic and sympathetic ganglia, parasympathetic nerve fibers, and the neuromuscular junction.
- ☑ Know the uses and toxicities of muscarinic receptor agonists and antagonists.
- ☑ Know the uses and toxicities of drugs and agents that inhibit AChE.
- ☑ Describe the uses and toxicities of drugs that block neuromuscular transmission.

DRUGS (OR AGENTS) INCLUDED IN THIS CHAPTER

Acetylcholine (MIOCHOL-E)
Aldicarb (TEMIK)—Insecticide
Ambenonium chloride (MYTELASE)
Atracurium (TACRIUM, others)
Atropine
Benztropine mesylate (COGENTIN, others); see Chapter 13
Bethanechol (URECHOLINE)
Carbachol (MIOSTAT, ISOPTOCARBACHOL)
Carbaryl (SEVIN)—Insecticide
Cevimeline (EVOXAC)
Chlorpyrifos (DURSBAN, LORSBAN)—Insecticide
Cisatracurium (NIMBEX)
Cyclopentolate hydrochloride (CYCLOGYL, others)
Dantrolene (DANTRIUM, others)
Darifenacin (ENABLEX)
Diazinon (SPECTRICIDE, others)—Insecticide
Dicyclomine hydrochloride (BENTYL, others)
Donepezil (ARICEPT)
Doxacurium
Edrophonium
Fesoterodine (TOVIAZ)
Flavoxate (Urispas)
Galantamine (REMINYL)
Glycopyrrolate (ROBINUL, others)
Homatropine hydrobromide (ISOPTO HOMATROPRINE)
Ipratropium (ATROVENT, others)
Malathion (CHEMATHION, MALA-SPRAY)—Insecticide
Mecamylamine (INVERSINE)
Methacholine (PROVOCHOLINE)
Methscopolamine bromide (PAMINE)
Mivacurium (Not available in the United States)
Neostigmine bromide (PROSTIGMIN-oral)

(continues)

MECHANISM OF ACTION MUSCARINIC AGONISTS AND ANTAGONISTS

DRUG CLASS	DRUG	MECHANISM OF ACTION
Muscarinic Receptor Agonists	Acetylcholine	Neurotransmitter at nicotinic and muscarinic receptors (see Figures 5-2, 6-1, and Table 6-1 for details)
	Pilocarpine	Muscarinic receptor agonist
	Methacholine	Muscarinic receptor agonist
	Carbachol	Muscarinic receptor agonist
	Bethanechol	Muscarinic receptor agonist
	Cevimeline	Muscarinic receptor agonist

SECTION II

Neuropharmacology

DRUGS (OR AGENTS) INCLUDED IN THIS CHAPTER (Cont.)

- Neostigmine methylsulfate (PROSTIGMIN-parenteral)
- Nicotine gum or lozenge (NICOTINE POLACRILEX, NICORETTE, COMMIT, THRIVE, others)
- Nicotine nasal spray or vapor inhaler (NICOTROL)
- Nicotine transdermal patch (HABITROL, others)
- Onabotulinum toxin A (BOTOX)
- Oxybutynin (DITROPAN, others; OXYTROL-transdermal; GELNIQUE-gel)
- Pancuronium
- Physostigmine salicylate (ANTILIRIUM)
- Pilocarpine (ISOPTO CARPINE)
- Pilocarpine hydrochloride (SALAGEN, others)
- Pipecuronium
- Pralidoxime (2-PAM; PROTOPAM CHLORIDE)
- Propoxur (BAYGON)—Insecticide
- Pyridostigmine bromide (MESTINON-oral; REGINOL, MESTINON-parenteral)
- Rimabotulinum toxin B (MYOBLOC)
- Rivastigmine (EXELON)
- Rocuronium (ZEMURON, others)
- Sarin—Nerve gas
- Scopolamine (TRANSDERM SCOP)
- Solifenacin (VESICARE)
- Soman—Nerve gas
- Succinylcholine (ANECTINE, QUELICIN)
- Tabun—Nerve gas
- Tacrine (COGNEX)
- Tiotropium (SPIRIVA)
- Tolterodine (DETROL)
- Trihexyphenidyl hydrochloride (ARTANE, others); see Chapter 13
- Trimethaphan
- Tropicamide (MYDRIACYL, others)
- Trospium chloride (SANCTURA)
- Varenicline (CHANTIX)
- Vecuronium (NORCURON, others)

DRUG CLASS	DRUG	MECHANISM OF ACTION
Muscarinic Receptor Antagonists	Atropine	Muscarinic receptor antagonist
	Scopolamine	Muscarinic receptor antagonist
	Ipratropium	Muscarinic receptor antagonist
	Tiotropium	Muscarinic receptor antagonist
	Oxybutynin	Muscarinic receptor antagonist
	Tolterodine	Muscarinic receptor antagonist
	Trospium chloride	Muscarinic receptor antagonist
	Darifenacin	Muscarinic receptor antagonist
	Solifenacin	Muscarinic receptor antagonist
	Fesoterodine	Muscarinic receptor antagonist
	Flavoxate	Muscarinic receptor antagonist
	Glycopyrrolate	Muscarinic receptor antagonist
	Dicyclomine hydrochloride	Muscarinic receptor antagonist
	Homatropine hydrobromide	Muscarinic receptor antagonist
	Cyclopentolate hydrochloride	Muscarinic receptor antagonist
	Tropicamide	Muscarinic receptor antagonist
	Benztropine mesylate	Muscarinic receptor antagonist
	Trihexyphenidyl hydrochloride	Muscarinic receptor antagonist
	Methscopolamine bromide	Muscarinic receptor antagonist

CASE 6-1

A 65-year-old man with urinary retention and inadequate emptying of the bladder is being treated with bethanechol.

a. Why is he treated with this drug?

Bethanechol is a muscarinic receptor agonist. Parasympathetic stimulation causes detrusor muscle contraction, increased voiding pressure, and ureteral peristalsis (see Tables 5-1, 6-2, and 6-3). Bethanechol has utility in treating urinary retention and inadequate emptying of the bladder when organic obstruction is absent, as in postoperative retention, diabetic autonomic neuropathy, and certain types of neurogenic bladder.

b. What side effects should he be aware of while taking bethanechol?

The side effects this patient might experience are a predictable consequence of muscarinic receptor stimulation (see Table 5-1), for example, diaphoresis, diarrhea, abdominal cramps, lacrimation, salivation, bradycardia, and bronchial secretion.

c. What are the contraindications to the use of bethanechol?

The important contraindications to using bethanechol are asthma, chronic obstructive pulmonary disease (COPD), urinary or GI tract obstruction, acid-peptic disease, cardiovascular disease accompanied by bradycardia, hypotension, and hyperthyroidism (muscarinic agonists may precipitate atrial fibrillation in hyperthyroid patients).

Cholinergic Pharmacology   CHAPTER 6

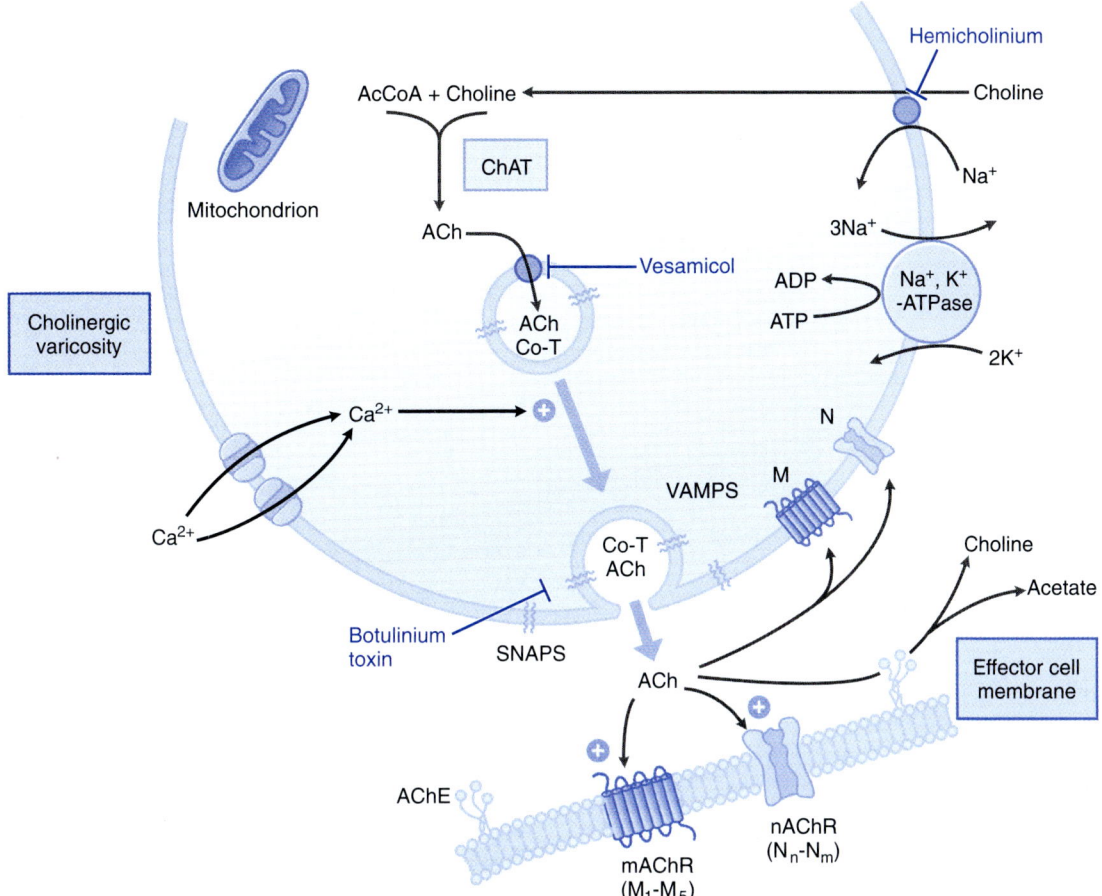

FIGURE 6-1 A cholinergic neuroeffector junction showing features of the synthesis, storage, and release of acetylcholine (ACh) and receptors on which ACh acts. The synthesis of ACh in the varicosity depends on the uptake of choline via a sodium-dependent carrier. This uptake can be blocked by hemicholinium. Choline and the acetyl moiety of acetyl coenzyme A, derived from mitochondria, form ACh, a process catalyzed by the enzyme choline acetyl transferase (ChAT). ACh is transported into the storage vesicle by another carrier that can be inhibited by vesamicol. ACh is stored in vesicles along with other potential cotransmitters (Co-T) such as ATP and VIP at certain neuroeffector junctions. Release of ACh and the Co-T occurs on depolarization of the varicosity, which allows the entry of Ca^{2+} through voltage-dependent Ca^{2+} channels. Elevated $[Ca^{2+}]_{in}$ promotes fusion of the vesicular membrane with the cell membrane, and exocytosis of the transmitters occurs. This fusion process involves the interaction of specialized proteins associated with the vesicular membrane (VAMPs, vesicle-associated membrane proteins) and the membrane of the varicosity (SNAPs, synaptosome-associated proteins). The exocytotic release of ACh can be blocked by botulinum toxin. Once released, ACh can interact with the muscarinic receptors (M), which are GPCRs, or nicotinic receptors (N), which are ligand-gated ion channels, to produce the characteristic response of the effector. ACh also can act on presynaptic mAChRs or nAChRs to modify its own release. The action of ACh is terminated by metabolism to choline and acetate by acetylcholinesterase (AChE), which is associated with synaptic membranes.

CASE 6-2

A 56-year-old man reports to the emergency room after eating mushrooms that he has foraged. He has brought some of the whole, uncooked mushrooms with him.

a. Although his symptoms now, one hour after ingesting the mushrooms, only include mild abdominal pain and diarrhea, what symptoms should one look for?

It is important to identify the specific mushroom, if possible, to be able to be aware of the possible toxicities. *Amanita muscaria* mushrooms contain muscarine, a potent muscarinic receptor agonist, and symptoms will be related to stimulation of muscarinic receptors (see Table 5-1). Mushrooms of the *Psilocybe* or *Panaeolus* species contain psilocybin which will cause short-lasting hallucinations. Mushrooms of the *Amanita phalloides* or related species contain amatoxins which can cause hepatic and renal failure, and ultimately death.

(Continued)

TABLE 6-1 Characteristics of Subtypes of Nicotinic Acetylcholine Receptors (nAChRs)

RECEPTOR (Primary Receptor Subtype)[a]	MAIN SYNAPTIC LOCATION	MEMBRANE RESPONSE	MOLECULAR MECHANISM	AGONISTS	ANTAGONISTS
Skeletal Muscle (N_m) $(\alpha_1)_2\beta_1\epsilon\delta$ adult $(\alpha_1)_2\beta_1\gamma\delta$ fetal	Skeletal neuromuscular junction (postjunctional)	Excitatory; end-plate depolarization; skeletal muscle contraction	Increased cation permeability (Na^+; K^+)	ACh Nicotine Succinylcholine	Atracurium Vecuronium d-Tubocurarine Pancuronium α-Conotoxin α-Bungarotoxin
Peripheral Neuronal (N_n) $(\alpha_3)_2(\beta_4)_3$	Autonomic ganglia; adrenal medulla	Excitatory; depolarization; firing of postganglion neuron; depolarization and secretion of catecholamines	Increased cation permeability (Na^+; K^+)	ACh Nicotine Epibatidine Dimethylphenyl-piperazinium	Trimethaphan Mecamylamine
Central Neuronal (CNS) $(\alpha_4)_2(\beta_4)_3$ (α-btox-insensitive)	CNS; pre- and postjunctional	Pre- and postsynaptic excitation Prejunctional control of transmitter release	Increased cation permeability (Na^+; K^+)	Cytosine, epibatidine Anatoxin A	Mecamylamine Dihydro-β-erythrodine Erysodine Lophotoxin
$(\alpha_7)_5$ (α-btox-sensitive)	CNS; pre- and postsynaptic	Pre- and postsynaptic excitation Prejunctional control of transmitter release	Increased permeability (Ca^{2+})	Anatoxin A	Methyllycaconitine α-Bungarotoxin α-Conotoxin Iml

[a]Nine α (α_2–α_{10}) and three β (β_2–β_4) subunits have been identified and cloned in human brain, which combine in various conformations to form individual receptor subtypes. The structure of individual receptors and the subtype composition are incompletely understood. Only a finite number of naturally occurring functional nAChR constructs have been identified. α-btox, β-bungarotoxin.

TABLE 6-2 Characteristics of Muscarinic Acetylcholine Receptor Subtypes (mAChRs)

RECEPTOR	SIZE; CHROMOSOME	CELLULAR AND TISSUE LOCATION[a]	CELLULAR RESPONSE[b]	FUNCTIONAL RESPONSE[c]	DISEASE RELEVANCE
M_1	460 aa 11q 12–13	CNS; Most abundant in cerebral cortex, hippocampus, striatum and thalamus Autonomic ganglia Glands (gastric and salivary) Enteric nerves	Couples by $G_{q/11}$ Activation of PLC; ↑ IP_3 and ↑ DAG → ↑ Ca^{2+} and PKC Depolarization and excitation (↑ sEPSP) Activation of PLD_2, PLA_2; ↑ AA	Increased cognitive function (learning and memory) Increased seizure activity Decrease in dopamine release and locomotion Increase in depolarization of autonomic ganglia Increase in secretions	Alzheimer's disease Cognitive dysfunction Schizophrenia
M_2	466 aa 7q 35–36	Widely expressed in CNS, hind brain, thalamus, cerebral cortex, hippocampus, striatum, heart, smooth muscle, autonomic nerve terminals	Couples by G_i/G_o (PTX-sensitive) Inhibition of AC, ↓ cAMP Activation of inwardly rectifying K^+ channels Inhibition of voltage-gated Ca^{2+} channels Hyperpolarization and inhibition	**Heart:** SA node: slowed spontaneous depolarization; hyperpolarization, ↓ HR AV node: decrease in conduction velocity Atrium: ↓ refractory period, ↓ contraction Ventricle: slight ↓ contraction **Smooth muscle:** ↑ Contraction **Peripheral nerves:** Neural inhibition via autoreceptors and heteroreceptor ↓ Ganglionic transmission **CNS:** Neural inhibition ↑ Tremors; hypothermia; analgesia	Alzheimer's disease Cognitive dysfunction Pain

Cholinergic Pharmacology — CHAPTER 6

RECEPTOR	SIZE; CHROMOSOME	CELLULAR AND TISSUE LOCATION[a]	CELLULAR RESPONSE[b]	FUNCTIONAL RESPONSE[c]	DISEASE RELEVANCE
M_3	590 aa 1q 43–44	Widely expressed in CNS (< than other mAChRs), cerebral cortex, hippocampus Abundant in smooth muscle and glands Heart	Couples by $G_{q/11}$ Activation of PLC; ↑ IP_3 and ↑ DAG → ↑ Ca^{2+} and PKC Depolarization and excitation (↑ sEPSP) Activation of PLD_2, PLA_2; ↑ AA	**Smooth muscle:** ↑ contraction (predominant in some, eg, bladder) **Glands:** ↑ secretion (predominant in salivary gland) Increases food intake, body weight fat deposits Inhibition of DA release Synthesis of NO	Chronic obstructive pulmonary disease (COPD) Urinary incontinence Irritable bowel disease
M_4	479 aa 11p 12–11.2	Preferentially expressed in CNS, particularly forebrain, also striatum, cerebral cortex, hippocampus	Couples by G_i/G_o (PTX-sensitive) Inhibition of AC, ↓ cAMP Activation of inwardly rectifying K^+ channels Inhibition of voltage-gated Ca^{2+} channels Hyperpolarization and inhibition	Autoreceptor- and heteroreceptor-mediated inhibition of transmitter release in CNS and periphery. Analgesia; cataleptic activity Facilitation of DA release	Parkinson disease Schizophrenia Neuropathic pain
M_5	532 aa 15q 26	Substantia nigra Expressed in low levels in CNS and periphery Predominant mAChR in neurons in VTA and substantia nigra	Couples by $G_{q/11}$ Activation of PLC; ↑ IP_3 and ↑ DAG → ↑ Ca^{2+} and PKC Depolarization and excitation (↑ sEPSP) Activation of PLD_2, PLA_2; ↑ AA	Mediator of dilation in cerebral arteries and arterioles (?) Facilitates DA release Augmentation of drug-seeking behavior and reward (eg, opiates, cocaine)	Drug dependence Parkinson disease Schizophrenia

[a]Most organs, tissues, and cells express multiple mAChRs.
[b]M_1, M_3, and M_5 mAChRs appear to couple to the same G proteins and signal through similar pathways. Likewise, M_2 and M_4 mAChRs couple through similar G proteins and signal through similar pathways.
[c]Despite the fact that in many tissues, organs, and cells multiple subtypes of mAChRs coexist, one subtype may predominate in producing a particular function; in others, there may be equal predominance.
PLC, phospholipase C; IP_3, inositol-1,4,5-triphosphate; DAG, diacylglycerol; PLD_2, phospholipase D; AA, arachidonic acid; PLA, phospholipase A; AC, adenylyl cyclase; DA, dopamine; cAMP, cyclic AMP; SA node, sinoatrial node; AV node, atrioventricular node; HR, heart rate; PTX, pertussis toxin; VTA, ventral tegmentum area.

TABLE 6-3 Some Pharmacological Properties of Choline Esters and Natural Alkaloids

| MUSCARINIC AGONIST | SUSCEPTIBILITY TO CHOLINESTERASES | MUSCARINIC ACTIVITY ||||| NICOTINIC ACTIVITY |
		CARDIOVASCULAR	GASTROINTESTINAL	URINARY BLADDER	EYE (TOPICAL)	ANTAGONISM BY ATROPINE	
Acetylcholine	+++	++	++	++	+	+++	++
Methacholine	+	+++	++	++	+	+++	+
Carbachol	−	+	+++	+++	++	+	+++
Bethanechol	−	±	+++	+++	++	+++	−
Muscarine[a]	−	++	+++	+++	++	+++	−
Pilocarpine	−	+	+++	+++	++	+++	−

[a]Not used therapeutically

b. The mushrooms he has with him have been identified as *Amanita muscaria*. What is the treatment for this type of mushroom poisoning?

Treatment with atropine effectively blocks the effects of muscarinic receptor stimulation. Large doses may be required. If the patient is showing signs of CNS excitation and hallucinations, these symptoms should be treated with a benzodiazepine (see Chapter 9). Atropine often exacerbates the delirium.

CASE 6-3

A 48-year-old woman is being treated with oxybutynin for low bladder capacity and urinary frequency.

a. What kind of drug is oxybutynin and why is it effective in this patient?

Oxybutynin is a muscarinic receptor antagonist that is indicated for the treatment of overactive bladder (see Table 6-4). This drug lowers intravesicular pressure, increases bladder capacity, and reduces the frequency of contractions by antagonizing parasympathetic control of the bladder (see Tables 5-1 and 6-3).

b. What side effects should she be cautioned about?

The side effects of oxybutynin are a predictable consequence of muscarinic receptor antagonism (see Table 5-1). These effects include xerostomia, blurred vision, constipation, and dyspepsia. CNS-related antimuscarinic effects, including drowsiness, dizziness, and confusion can occur and are particularly problematic in elderly patients. Dry mouth and dry eyes are the most common reasons for discontinuation.

MECHANISMS OF ACTION OF ACETYLCHOLINESTERASE (AChE) INHIBITORS

DRUG CLASS	DRUG	MECHANISM OF ACTION
"Reversible" AChE Inhibitors	Edrophonium	AChE inhibition
	Physostigmine salicylate	AChE inhibition
	Neostigmine bromide	AChE inhibition
	Neostigmine methylsulfate	AChE inhibition
	Ambenonium chloride	AChE inhibition
	Pyridostigmine bromide	AChE inhibition
	Tacrine	AChE inhibition
	Donepezil	AChE inhibition
	Rivastigmine	AChE inhibition
	Galantamine	AChE inhibition
Carbamate Insecticides	Carbaryl (SEVIN) Insecticide	AChE inhibition
	Propoxur	AChE inhibition
	Aldicarb	AChE inhibition
Organophosphate Insecticides	Diazinon	AChE inhibition
	Chlorpyrifos	AChE inhibition
	Malathion	AChE inhibition
Organophosphate Nerve Gases	Tabun	AChE inhibition
	Sarin	AChE inhibition
	Soman	AChE inhibition
Cholinesterase Reactivators	Pralidoxime (2-PAM)	AChE reactivator

Cholinergic Pharmacology

CHAPTER 6

TABLE 6-4 Muscarinic Receptor Antagonists Used in the Treatment of Overactive Urinary Bladder

NONPROPRIETARY NAME	TRADE NAME	$t_{1/2}$ (hours)	PREPARATIONS[a]	DAILY DOSE (ADULT)
Oxybutynin	DITROPAN, others	2-5	IR	10-20 mg[b]
			ER	5-30 mg[b]
	OXYTROL		Transdermal patch	3.9 mg
	GELNIQUE		Topical gel	100 mg
Tolterodine	DETROL	2-9.6[c]	IR	2-4 mg[b,d]
		6.9-18[c]	ER	4 mg[b,d]
Trospium chloride	SANCTURA	20	IR	20-40 mg[e]
		35	ER	60 mg[e]
Solifenacin	VESICARE	55	IR	5-10 mg[b]
Darifenacin	ENABLEX	13-19	ER	7.5-15 mg[f]
Fesoterodine	TOVIAZ	7	ER	4-8 mg

[a]Preparations are designated as follows: IR, immediate-release tablet; ER, extended-release tablet or capsule.
[b]Doses may need to be reduced in patients taking drugs that inhibit CYP3A4.
[c]Longer times in indicated ranges are seen in poor metabolizers.
[d]Doses should be reduced in patients with significant renal or hepatic impairment.
[e]Doses should be reduced in patients with significant renal impairment; dosage adjustments also may be needed in patients with hepatic impairment.
[f]Doses may need to be reduced in patients taking drugs that inhibit CYPs 3A4 or 2D6.

CASE 6-4

A 14-year-old boy is brought to the emergency room after drinking a tea made with jimson weed seeds.

a. What is jimson weed and what are the likely symptoms this boy may experience?

Jimson weed is a common plant that contains atropine and other belladonna alkaloids. The seeds contain high concentrations of these alkaloids and poisoning results from their ingestion. The symptoms of various doses of atropine are shown in Table 6-5 and are predictable as a consequence of muscarinic receptor antagonism.

(Continued)

POTENTIAL EFFECTS OF AGENTS THAT INHIBIT AChE

- Stimulation of muscarinic receptor responses at autonomic effector organs
- Stimulation, followed by depression or paralysis, of all autonomic ganglion and skeletal muscle (nicotinic actions)
- Stimulation, with occasional subsequent depression, of cholinergic receptor sites in the CNS

TABLE 6-5 Effects of Atropine in Relation to Dose

DOSE (mg)	EFFECTS
0.5	Slight cardiac slowing; some dryness of mouth; inhibition of sweating
1	Definite dryness of mouth; thirst; acceleration of heart, sometimes preceded by slowing; mild dilation of pupils
2	Rapid heart rate; palpitation; marked dryness of mouth; dilated pupils; some blurring of near vision
5	Above symptoms marked; difficulty in speaking and swallowing; restlessness and fatigue; headache; dry, hot skin; difficulty in micturition; reduced intestinal peristalsis
≥10	Above symptoms more marked; pulse rapid and weak; iris practically obliterated; vision very blurred; skin flushed, hot, dry, and scarlet; ataxia, restlessness, and excitement; hallucinations and delirium; coma

The clinical picture of a high (toxic) dose of atropine may be remembered by an old mnemonic device that summarizes the symptoms: *Red as a beet, Dry as a bone, Blind as a bat, Hot as firestone, and Mad as a hatter.*

SECTION II — Neuropharmacology

SYMPTOMS OF ACUTE ORGANOPHOSPHATE POISONING

Muscarinic—Mild
- Miosis
- Ocular pain
- Conjunctival congestion
- Diminished vision
- Salivation
- Lacrimation
- Rhinorrhea
- Bronchoconstriction
- Increased bronchial secretions
- Anorexia
- Nausea and vomiting
- Diarrhea
- Abdominal cramps

Muscarinic—Severe
- Extreme salivation, lacrimation, and sweating
- Involuntary defecation and urination
- Penile erection
- Bradycardia
- Hypotension

Nicotinic—Mild
- Generalized muscle weakness
- Fatigability
- Involuntary twitching and scattered fasciculations

Nicotinic—Severe
- Severe muscle weakness
- Paralysis

Central Nervous System
- Confusion
- Ataxia
- Slurred speech
- Loss of reflexes
- Generalized seizures
- Coma
- Central respiratory paralysis

b. If his symptoms are serious and life threatening, what is the appropriate treatment?

Measures to limit absorption of the atropine should be initiated without delay if the poison has been taken orally, as in this case. For symptomatic treatment, slow intravenous injection of physostigmine (an AChE inhibitor) will increase ACh at muscarinic receptors. Physostigmine will rapidly abolish the delirium and coma caused by high doses of atropine, but carries some risk in mild atropine intoxication. Because physostigmine is metabolized rapidly, the patient may again lapse into a coma within 1 to 2 hours and repeated doses may be needed. If marked excitement is present, and more specific treatment is not available, a benzodiazepine (see Chapter 9) is the most appropriate treatment to induce sedation and prevent seizures. Support of respiration and control of hyperthermia may be necessary.

CASE 6-5

A 23-year-old woman is brought to the emergency room after deliberately ingesting a bottle of organophosphate insecticide.

a. Why is it important to identify the specific product this woman ingested?

There are two types of insecticides in this class: carbamate insecticides and organophosphate insecticides (see Table 6-6). The carbamate insecticides are "reversible" and inhibit AChE in a fashion identical to other carbamoylating agents (physostigmine and neostigmine), while the organophosphate insecticides inhibit AChE in an irreversible manner by alkylphosphorylation. The organophosphate inhibition of AChE is initially reversible, but "ages" into an enzyme inhibition that is resistant to hydrolysis and reactivation (see Figure 6-2). The symptoms of poisoning from both insecticides resemble each other, but poisoning from an organophosphate insecticide will benefit from the early administration of an AChE reactivator (see below).

b. What symptoms is she likely to experience and what is the timeframe that these symptoms may appear?

The effects of acute intoxication by anticholinesterase (anti-ChE) insecticides are manifested by stimulation of muscarinic and nicotinic receptors (see Table 5-1). In addition, there may be CNS effects except with those agents that have low lipid solubility that cannot cross the blood-brain barrier. The symptoms of poisoning with AChE inhibitors are highlighted in the Side Bar SYMPTOMS OF ACUTE ORGANOPHOSPHATE POISONING.

After the inhalation of vapors or aerosols, systemic effects may occur within minutes, whereas the systemic effects are delayed after GI or percutaneous absorption. The duration of toxic symptoms is determined largely by the properties of the compound: its lipid solubility, whether it must be activated to form the oxon, the stability of the organophosphate-AChE bond, and whether "aging" of the phosphorylated enzyme has occurred. Delayed symptoms appearing after 1 to 4 days and marked by persistent low blood ChE and severe muscle weakness are termed the "intermediate syndrome."

c. What is the appropriate treatment for this ingestion?

Atropine in sufficient dosage (large doses may be required) effectively antagonizes the effects at muscarinic receptor sites. Atropine is virtually without effect against the peripheral neuromuscular junction (nicotinic) effects.

The nicotinic effects of acute organophosphate poisoning can be reversed by pralidoxime (2-PAM), a cholinesterase reactivator. The mechanism of action of pralidoxime is shown in Figure 6-2. The reactivation of AChE is most pronounced at the skeletal neuromuscular junction. Because pralidoxime has weak anti-ChE activity, it is not recommended for the treatment of overdosage with physostigmine or neostigmine or poisoning with the carbamoylating insecticides such as carbaryl.

Cholinergic Pharmacology — CHAPTER 6

TABLE 6-6 Chemical Classification of Representative Organophosphorus Compounds of Particular Pharmacological or Toxicological Interest

General formula: $\begin{array}{c} R_1 \\ R_2 \end{array}\!\!\!>\!\!P\!\!\!\begin{array}{c} \nearrow O\ (S) \\ \searrow X \end{array}$

Group **A**, X = halogen, cyanide, or thiocyanate leaving group; group **B**, X = alkylthio, arylthio, alkoxy, or aryloxy leaving group; group **C**, thionophosphorus or thio-thionophosphorus compounds; group **D**, quaternary ammonium leaving group. R_1 can be an alkyl (phosphonates), alkoxy (phosphorates) or an alkylamino (phosphoramidates) group.

GROUP	STRUCTURAL FORMULA	COMMON, CHEMICAL, AND OTHER NAMES	COMMENTS
A	(structure: diisopropyl fluorophosphate)	DFP; Isoflurophate; diisopropyl fluorophosphate	Potent, irreversible inactivator
	(structure: Tabun)	Tabun; Ethyl N-dimethylphosphoramidocyanidate	Extremely toxic "nerve gas"
	(structure: Sarin)	Sarin (GB); Isopropyl methylphosphonofluoridate	Extremely toxic "nerve gas"
	(structure: Soman)	Soman (GD); Pinacolyl methylphosphonofluoridate	Extremely toxic "nerve gas"; greatest potential for irreversible action/rapid aging
B	(structure: Paraoxon)	Paraoxon (MINTACOL), E 600; O,O-Diethyl O-(4-nitrophenyl)-phosphate	Active metabolite of parathion
	(structure: Malaoxon)	Malaoxon; O,O-Dimethyl S-(1,2-dicarboxyethyl)-phosphorothioate	Active metabolite of malathion
C	(structure: Parathion)	Parathion; O,O-Diethyl O-(4-nitrophenyl)-phosphorothioate	Agricultural insecticide, resulting in numerous cases of accidental poisoning; phased out in 2003
	(structure: Diazinon)	Diazinon, Dimpylate; O,O-Diethyl O-(2-isopropyl-6-methyl-4-pyrimidinyl) phosphorothioate	Insecticide; use limited to non-residential agricultural settings
	(structure: Chlorpyrifos)	Chlorpyrifos; O,O-Diethyl O-(3,5,6-trichloro-2-pyridyl) phosphorothioate	Insecticide; use limited to non-residential agricultural settings
	(structure: Malathion)	Malathion; O,O-Dimethyl S-(1,2-dicarbethoxyethyl) phosphorodithioate	Widely employed insecticide of greater safety than parathion or other agents because of rapid detoxification by higher organisms
D	(structure: Echothiophate)	Echothiophate (PHOSPHOLINE IODIDE), MI-217; Diethoxyphosphinylthiocholine iodide	Extremely potent choline derivative; administered locally in treatment of glaucoma; relatively stable in aqueous solution

SECTION II   Neuropharmacology

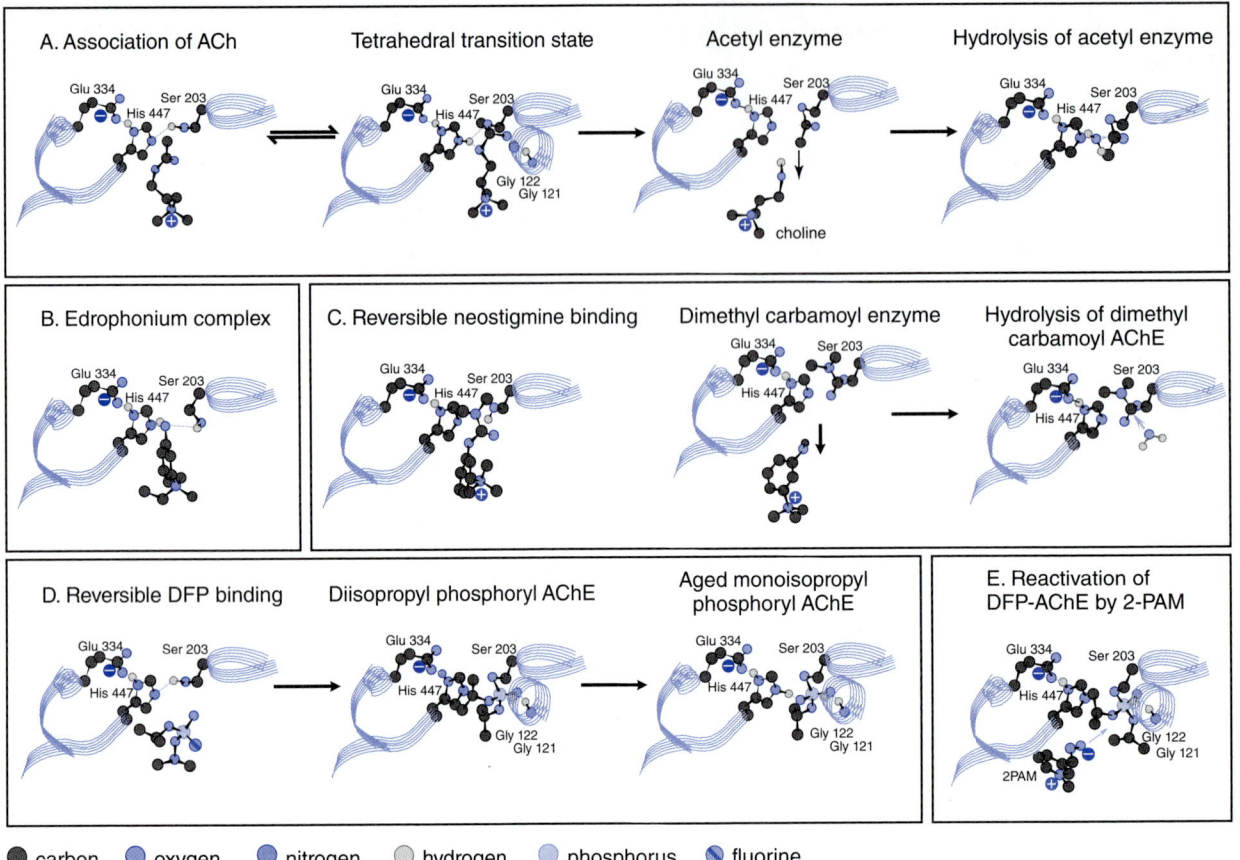

FIGURE 6-2 Steps involved in the hydrolysis of acetylcholine by acetylcholinesterase and in the inhibition and reactivation of the enzyme. Only the 3 residues of the catalytic triad are depicted. The associations and reactions shown are: **A.** Acetylcholine (ACh) catalysis: binding of ACh, formation of a tetrahedral transition state, formation of the acetyl enzyme with liberation of choline, rapid hydrolysis of the acetyl enzyme with return to the original state. **B.** Reversible binding and inhibition by edrophonium. **C.** Neostigmine reaction with and inhibition of AChE: reversible binding of neostigmine, formation of the dimethyl carbamoyl enzyme, slow hydrolysis of the dimethyl carbamoyl enzyme. **D.** Diisopropyl fluorophosphate (DFP) reaction and inhibition of AChE: reversible binding of DFP, formation of the diisopropyl phosphoryl enzyme, formation of the aged monoisopropyl phosphoryl enzyme. Hydrolysis of the diisopropyl enzyme is very slow and is not shown. The aged monoisopropyl phosphoryl enzyme is virtually resistant to hydrolysis and reactivation. The tetrahedral transition state of ACh hydrolysis resembles the conjugates formed by the tetrahedral phosphate inhibitors and accounts for their potency. Amide bond hydrogens from Gly121 and Gly122 stabilize the carbonyl and phosphoryl oxygens. **E.** Reactivation of the diisopropyl phosphoryl enzyme by pralidoxime (2-PAM). 2-PAM attack of the phosphorus on the phosphorylated enzyme will form a phospho-oxime with regeneration of active enzyme. The individual steps of phosphorylation reaction and oxime reaction have been characterized by mass spectrometry.

CASE 6-6

A 35-year-old woman with myasthenia gravis is being treated with ambenonium chloride.

a. What is myasthenia gravis?

Myasthenia gravis is a neuromuscular disease characterized by weakness and marked fatigability of skeletal muscle; exacerbations and partial remissions occur frequently. The defect in myasthenia gravis is in synaptic transmission at the neuromuscular junction (see Figure 6-3). Myasthenia gravis is caused by an autoimmune response primarily to the ACh receptor at the postjunctional end plate. A related disease is Lambert-Eaton syndrome, in which antibodies are directed against Ca^{++} channels that are necessary for presynaptic release of ACh.

b. How is edrophonium used in the diagnosis of myasthenia gravis?

Although the diagnosis of myasthenia gravis usually can be made from the history, signs, and symptoms, the use of the anti-ChE medication, edrophonium, is often useful in confirming the diagnosis. The edrophonium test is performed

(Continued)

Cholinergic Pharmacology

CHAPTER 6

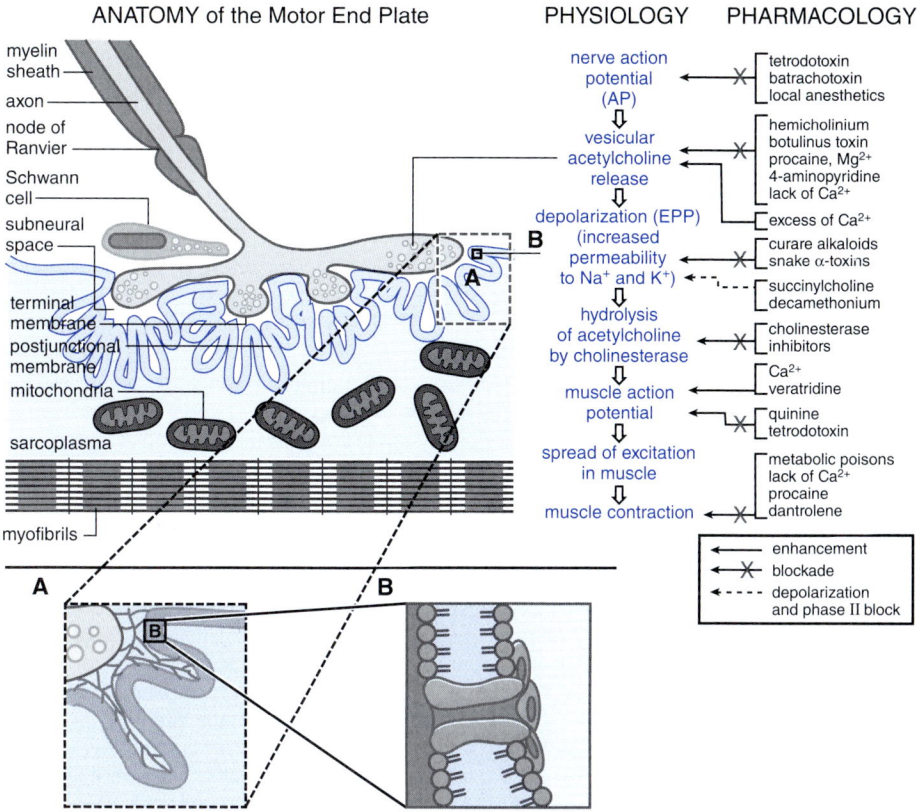

FIGURE 6-3 Sites of action of agents at the neuromuscular junction and adjacent structures. The anatomy of the motor end plate, shown at the left, and the sequence of events from liberation of acetylcholine (ACh) by the nerve action potential (AP) to contraction of the muscle fiber, indicated by the middle column, are described in Chapter 8 of *Goodman and Gilman's The Pharmacological Basis of Therapeutics*, 12th Edition. The modification of these processes by various agents is shown on the right; an arrow marked with an X indicates inhibition or block; an unmarked arrow indicates enhancement or activation. The insets are enlargements of the indicated structures. The highest magnification depicts the receptor in the bilayer of the postsynaptic membrane.

by rapid intravenous injection of 2 mg of edrophonium chloride, followed 45 seconds later by an additional 8 mg if the first dose is without effect; a positive response consists of improvement in strength, unaccompanied by lingual fasciculations.

c. **Why is ambenonium chloride used to treat this patient?**

Ambenonium chloride along with pyridostigmine and neostigmine is the standard anti-ChE drug used in the symptomatic treatment of myasthenia gravis. Following AChE inhibition, receptors at the end plate presumably are exposed to concentrations of ACh that are sufficient for channel opening and production of a postsynaptic endplate potential (see Figures 6-1, 6-3, and 6-4).

d. **What are the expected side effects of this treatment?**

An excessive dose of an anti-ChE drug results in a cholinergic crisis. This condition is characterized by weakness resulting from generalized depolarization of the motor endplate and other features resulting from stimulation of muscarinic receptors. The weakness may resemble myasthenia weakness. Cholinergic crisis and myasthenia gravis can be distinguished by cautiously performing the edrophonium test, limiting the dose to 2 mg and with facilities for respiratory resuscitation available. A further decrease in strength indicates cholinergic crisis, while improvement signifies myasthenia weakness.

SECTION II Neuropharmacology

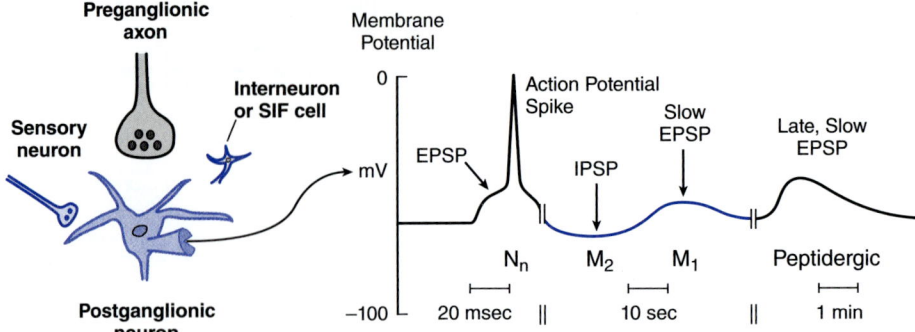

FIGURE 6-4 Postsynaptic potentials recorded from an autonomic postganglionic nerve cell body after stimulation of the preganglionic nerve fiber. The preganglionic nerve releases ACh onto postganglionic cells. The initial excitatory postsynaptic potential (EPSP) results from the inward Na$^+$ current (and perhaps Ca^{2+} current) through the nicotinic receptor channel. If the EPSP is of sufficient magnitude, it triggers an action potential spike, which is followed by a slow inhibitory postsynaptic potential (IPSP), a slow EPSP, and a late, slow EPSP. The slow IPSP and slow EPSP are not seen in all ganglia. The electrical events subsequent to the initial EPSP are thought to modulate the probability that a subsequent EPSP will reach the threshold for triggering a spike. Other interneurons, such as catecholamine-containing, small, intensely fluorescent (SIF) cells, and axon terminals from sensory, afferent neurons also release transmitters and that may influence the slow potentials of the postganglionic neuron. A number of cholinergic, peptidergic, adrenergic, and amino acid receptors are found on the dendrites and soma of the postganglionic neuron and the interneurons. The preganglionic fiber releases ACh and peptides; the interneurons store and release catecholamines, amino acids, and peptides; the sensory afferent nerve terminals release peptides. The initial EPSP is mediated through nicotinic (N_n) receptors, the slow IPSP and EPSP through M_2 and M_1 muscarinic receptors, and the late, slow EPSP through several types of peptidergic receptors.

MECHANISMS OF ACTION OF DRUGS ACTING AT THE NEUROMUSCULAR JUNCTION (NMJ) AND AUTONOMIC GANGLIA

DRUG CLASS	DRUG	MECHANISM OF ACTION
Depolarizing Neuromuscular Blocking Agents	Succinylcholine (see Table 6-7)	Block ACh at nicotinic receptors
Competitive Neuromuscular Blocking Agents	Pancuronium (see Table 6-7)	Block ACh at nicotinic receptors
	Atracurium (see Table 6-7)	Block ACh at nicotinic receptors
	Vecuronium (see Table 6-7)	Block ACh at nicotinic receptors
	Pipecuronium (see Table 6-7)	Block ACh at nicotinic receptors
	Doxacurium (see Table 6-7)	Block ACh at nicotinic receptors
	Mivacurium (see Table 6-7)	Block ACh at nicotinic receptors
	Rocuronium (see Table 6-7)	Block ACh at nicotinic receptors
	Cisatracurium (see Table 6-7)	Block ACh at nicotinic receptors
Botulinum Toxins	Onabotulinum toxin A	Block presynaptic release of Ach
	Rimabotulinum toxin B	Block presynaptic release of Ach
Antispasticity and Antirigidity Agents	Dantrolene	Inhibits Ca^{++} release of sarcoplasmic reticulum of skeletal muscle
Ganglionic Stimulating Agents	Nicotine	Stimulation of cholinergic receptors on autonomic ganglia; eventually blocks these receptors by persistent depolarization
Nicotinic ACh Receptor Agonists	Varenicline	Partial to full agonist at nicotinic ACh receptors
Ganglionic Blocking Drugs	Mecamylamine (see Table 6-8)	Block ACh at ganglionic nicotinic receptors
	Trimethaphan (see Table 6-8)	Block ACh at ganglionic nicotinic receptors

Cholinergic Pharmacology — CHAPTER 6

TABLE 6-7 Classification of Neuromuscular Blocking Agents

AGENT	CHEMICAL CLASS	PHARMACOLOGICAL PROPERTIES	TIME OF ONSET (MIN)[a]	CLINICAL DURATION (MIN)[a]	MODE OF ELIMINATION
Succinyl choline (ANECTINE, others)	Dicholine ester	Ultrashort duration; depolarizing	0.8-1.4	6-11	Hydrolysis by plasma cholinesterases
D-Tubocurarine[b]	Natural alkaloid (cyclic benzyl-isoquinoline)	Long duration; competitive	6	80	Renal and hepatic elimination
Metocurine[b]	Benzylisoquinoline	Long duration; competitive	4	110	Renal elimination
Atracurium (TRACRIUM, others)	Benzylisoquinoline	Intermediate duration; competitive	3	45	Hofmann elimination; hydrolysis by plasma esterases
Cisatracurium (NIMBEX)	Benzylisoquinoline	Intermediate duration; competitive	2-8	45-90	Hofmann and renal elimination
Doxacurium[b]	Benzylisoquinoline	Long duration; competitive	4-8	120	Renal elimination
Mivacurium	Benzylisoquinoline	Short duration; competitive	2-3	15-21	Hydrolysis by plasma cholinesterases
Pancuronium (generic)	Ammonio steroid	Long duration; competitive	3-4	85-100	Renal and hepatic elimination
Pipecuronium[b]	Ammonio steroid	Long duration; competitive	3-6	30-90	Renal elimination; hepatic metabolism and clearance
Rocuronium (ZEMURON, others)	Ammonio steroid	Intermediate duration; competitive	0.9-1.7	36-73	Hepatic elimination
Vecuronium (NORCURON, others)	Ammonio steroid	Intermediate duration; competitive	2-3	40-45	Hepatic and renal elimination
Gantacurium[c]	Asymmetric mixed-onium chlorofumarate	Ultra-short duration, competitive	1-2	5-10	Cysteine adduction and ester hydrolysis

[a]Time of onset and clinical duration achieved from therapeutic doses.
[b]D-Tubocurarine, doxacurium, metocurine, and pipecuronium are no longer available in the United States.
[c]Gantacurium is in investigational status.

TABLE 6-8 Usual Predominance of Sympathetic or Parasympathetic Tone at Various Effector Sites, and Consequences of Autonomic Ganglionic Blockade

SITE	PREDOMINANT TONE	EFFECT OF GANGLIONIC BLOCKADE
Arterioles	Sympathetic (adrenergic)	Vasodilation; increased peripheral blood flow; hypotension
Veins	Sympathetic (adrenergic)	Dilation: peripheral pooling of blood; decreased venous return; decreased cardiac output
Heart	Parasympathetic (cholinergic)	Tachycardia
Iris	Parasympathetic (cholinergic)	Mydriasis
Ciliary muscle	Parasympathetic (cholinergic)	Cycloplegia—focus to far vision
Gastrointestinal tract	Parasympathetic (cholinergic)	Reduced tone and motility; constipation; decreased gastric and pancreatic secretions
Urinary bladder	Parasympathetic (cholinergic)	Urinary retention
Salivary glands	Parasympathetic (cholinergic)	Xerostomia
Sweat glands	Sympathetic (cholinergic)	Anhidrosis
Genital tract	Sympathetic and parasympathetic	Decreased stimulation

SECTION II — Neuropharmacology

CASE 6-7

A 48-year-old man is undergoing abdominal surgery. Succinylcholine is used as a muscle relaxant during the surgery.

a. What is succinylcholine and how does it act?

Succinylcholine is a depolarizing neuromuscular blocking agent. Its initial action is to open channels in the same manner as ACh (see Figures 6-1 and 6-3). However, it persists longer than ACh primarily because of its resistance to AChE. The long-lasting depolarization results in a brief period of repetitive excitation (resulting in muscle fasciculations) followed by block of neuromuscular transmission and flaccid paralysis.

b. What are the contraindications for the use of succinylcholine?

Succinylcholine and other depolarizing agents can release K^+ from intracellular sites. This may be a factor in the production of the prolonged apnea in patients receiving these drugs. This is a life-threatening complication and precludes the use of succinylcholine in patients with soft-tissue trauma, burns, or patients with congestive heart failure who are receiving digoxin or diuretics. Succinylcholine is also contraindicated or should be given with great caution to patients with nontraumatic rhabdomyolysis, ocular lacerations, spinal cord injuries with paraplegia or quadriplegia, or muscular dystrophies.

Hepatic disease that results in a deficiency of butyrylcholinesterase (which is responsible for the rapid hydrolysis of succinylcholine) may also be responsible for a prolonged apnea.

CASE 6-8

A 49-year-old man is undergoing abdominal surgery. Vecuronium is used as a muscle relaxant during the surgery.

a. What is vecuronium, how does it act, and how does it differ from succinylcholine?

Vecuronium is a competitive blocker at the neuromuscular junction (see Figure 6-3). It combines with the nicotinic ACh receptor at the end plate and thereby competitively blocks the binding of ACh. Table 6-7 shows the classification and differences between the neuromuscular blocking agents.

b. What are the contraindications for the use of vecuronium?

Vecuronium is eliminated by hepatic metabolism and caution should be exercised when using this drug in patients with hepatic dysfunction.

CASE 6-9

A 2-year-old girl is brought to the emergency room after having ingested 3 of her mother's nicotine patches.

a. What is the danger from this ingestion?

Nicotine is a ganglionic stimulating agent and is readily absorbed from the intestine. The major action of nicotine consists initially of transient stimulation and subsequently of a more persistent depression of all autonomic ganglia and neuromuscular blockade by receptor desensitization. Nicotine markedly stimulates the CNS presumably due to the release of excitatory amino acids.

b. What are the symptoms of nicotine poisoning?

The toxic effects of acute nicotine poisoning are shown in the Side Bar EFFECTS OF ACUTE NICOTINE POISONING.

c. What is the appropriate treatment for this patient?

Treatment options are limited. Attempts to limit absorption should be instituted (see Chapter 3). Treatment of seizures with a benzodiazepine (see Chapter 9) may be appropriate. Respiratory assistance and treatment of shock may be necessary.

EFFECTS OF ACUTE NICOTINE POISONING

- Nausea
- Salivation
- Abdominal pain
- Vomiting
- Headache
- Cold sweat
- Dizziness
- Disturbed hearing and vision
- Mental confusion
- Muscle weakness
- Hypotension
- Seizures
- Death from respiratory failure

Cholinergic Pharmacology

CHAPTER 6

KEY CONCEPTS

- Muscarinic acetylcholine receptors in the peripheral nervous system are located primarily on effector organs that are innervated by postganglionic parasympathetic nerves (see Figure 5-2).
- Muscarinic acetylcholine receptors are also located in the CNS.
- The effects of drugs that are muscarinic receptor agonists and antagonist can be predicted from knowledge of parasympathetic nerve innervation (see Tables 5-1 and 6-3).
- Acetylcholine (ACh) is the neurotransmitter that interacts with muscarinic receptors at the postganglionic parasympathetic nerve endings (see Figure 6-1).
- ACh is also the neurotransmitter at nicotinic acetylcholine receptors of the parasympathetic and sympathetic autonomic ganglia (see Figure 5-2).
- ACh is also the neurotransmitter at nicotinic acetylcholine receptor at the motor end plate of skeletal muscle (see Figures 5-2 and 6-3).
- ACh at these synaptic sites is destroyed by acetylcholine esterase (AChE) (see Figure 6-2).
- Drugs and other agents that are inhibitors of AChE have effects that are predicted from knowledge of an excess of ACh at the above synaptic sites (see Table 5-1).
- Drugs that block the nicotinic acetylcholine receptor at the motor endplate of skeletal muscle are used as adjuvants during surgery to relax muscles.

SUMMARY QUIZ

QUESTION 6-1 A 35-year-old man has ingested *Amanita muscaria* mushrooms. He is experiencing a heart rate of 40 beats per minute. This bradycardia is most likely due to an interaction of the chemical(s) in the mushrooms with which receptors at the sinoatrial node?

a. α_1 Adrenergic
b. β_1 Adrenergic
c. β_2 Adrenergic
d. M_2 muscarinic
e. Nicotinic

QUESTION 6-2 A 49-year-old woman is treated with pilocarpine hydrochloride for xerostomia (dry mouth) following head and neck radiation treatments. As a result of taking this drug she may experience which of the following side effects?

a. Sweating
b. Dry eyes
c. Dry skin
d. Confusion
e. Tachycardia

QUESTION 6-3 A 54-year-old woman is receiving Botox injections to remove facial wrinkles. Botox (*botulinum* toxin) acts by

a. stimulating the release of ACh.
b. stimulating the release of norepinephrine.
c. blocking the release of ACh.
d. blocking the release of norepinephrine.
e. blocking muscarinic receptors.

SECTION II

Neuropharmacology

QUESTION 6-4 A 23-year-old man has deliberately ingested an organophosphate insecticide. His initial symptoms of salivation, lacrimation, and diarrhea are a consequence of inhibition of

a. butyrylcholinesterase.
b. acetylcholinesterase.
c. Na^+, K^+-ATPase.
d. tyrosine hydroxylase.
e. monoamine oxidase.

QUESTION 6-5 The patient in Question 6-4 should be treated with atropine and which additional drug in the following list?

a. Physostigmine
b. Bethanechol
c. Pralidoxime
d. Morphine
e. Gentamicin

QUESTION 6-6 A 65-year-old man with the diagnosis of Alzheimer's disease is being treated with donepezil. This drug acts by

a. stimulating the release of ACh.
b. blocking the reuptake of norepinephrine.
c. inhibiting monamine oxidase.
d. blocking the release of ACh.
e. inhibiting AChE.

QUESTION 6-7 A 53-year-old man is scheduled to receive vecuronium as an adjuvant muscle relaxant during abdominal surgery. The dose of vecuronium may have to be adjusted if this patient is also receiving

a. gentamicin.
b. penicillin.
c. ibuprofen.
d. acetaminophen.
e. prednisone.

QUESTION 6-8 A 72-year-old woman receives succinylcholine as an adjuvant muscle relaxant during knee surgery. This drug acts by

a. blocking ACh at nicotinic receptors of neuromuscular endplate.
b. blocking ACh at nicotinic receptors in the adrenal medulla.
c. increasing Na^+ and K^+ permeability of the postsynaptic neuromuscular membrane.
d. blocking the transmission of the action potential along the nerve axon.
e. blocking the release of ACh from neuromuscular presynaptic vesicles.

QUESTION 6-9 A 3-year-old boy is brought to the emergency room because he has ingested a large amount of a nicotine-containing product. Serious nicotine toxicity in this child is the result of

a. blockade of transmission at autonomic ganglia and neuromuscular junctions.
b. blockade of muscarinic receptors.
c. stimulation of adrenergic receptors.
d. blockade of adrenergic receptors.
e. stimulation of muscarinic receptors.

Cholinergic Pharmacology

CHAPTER 6

SUMMARY QUIZ ANSWER KEY

QUESTION 6-1 Answer is **d.** Although the concentration of muscarine is low in these mushrooms, the symptom of bradycardia observed in this patient is most likely attributable to muscarine. Other chemicals that may be involved in the neurotoxicity of mushrooms of the *Amanita* species are muscimol, ibotenic acid, and other isoxazole derivatives. The receptors in the sinoatrial node innervated by parasympathetic nerves are M_2 muscarinic receptors (see Table 5-1).

QUESTION 6-2 Answer is **a.** Side effects with pilocarpine treatment typify cholinergic stimulation, with sweating being the most common complaint. The other answers would be side effects seen after treatment with a muscarinic receptor antagonist.

QUESTION 6-3 Answer is **c.** Botulinum toxins act peripherally to reduce muscle contraction. The anaerobic bacterium *Clostridium botulinum* produces a family of toxins targeted to presynaptic proteins that block the release of ACh (see Figure 6-1). By blocking ACh release, BOTOX produces flaccid paralysis of skeletal muscle and diminished activity of parasympathetic and sympathetic cholinergic synapses. The FDA has issued a safety alert for BOTOX, warning of respiratory paralysis from unexpected spread of the toxin from the site of injection.

QUESTION 6-4 Answer is **b.** The effects of acute intoxication by anti-ChE agents such as an organophosphate insecticide are manifested by muscarinic and nicotinic signs and symptoms, and, except for compounds of extremely low lipid solubility, by signs referable to the CNS (see Side Bar SYMPTOMS OF ACUTE ORGANOPHOSPHATE POISONING).

QUESTION 6-5 Answer is **c.** The AChE reactivator pralidoxime can be of great benefit in the therapy of anti-ChE intoxication, but its use is supplemental to the administration of atropine. Although the phosphorylated esteratic site of AChE undergoes hydrolytic regeneration at a slow or negligible rate, nucleophilic agents such as the oxime, pralidoxime, reactivate the enzyme more rapidly than does spontaneous hydrolysis (see Figure 6-2). The reactivating action of oximes is most marked at the skeletal neuromuscular junction.

QUESTION 6-6 Answer is **e.** A deficiency of intact cholinergic neurons, particularly those extending from subcortical areas such as the nucleus basalis of Meynert, has been observed in patients with progressive dementia of the Alzheimer type (see Chapter 13). Donepezil along with tacrine and rivastigmine are AChE inhibitors, which have the requisite affinity and hydrophobicity to cross the blood-brain barrier and exhibit a prolonged duration of action. They tend to slow the decline in cognitive function and behavioral manifestations for limited intervals of time.

QUESTION 6-7 Answer is **a.** Vecuronium is a competitive-type neuromuscular blocking drug. Gentamicin is an aminoglycoside antibiotic (see Chapter 40) that also produces neuromuscular blockade by inhibiting ACh release from the preganglionic terminal (through competition with Ca^{++}) and to a lesser extent by noncompetitively blocking the ACh receptor (see Figure 6-1).

QUESTION 6-8 Answer is **c.** Succinylcholine is a depolarizing neuromuscular blocking drug that acts to depolarize the membrane in the same manner as ACh by opening ligand-gated ion channels (ie, N_m acetylcholine receptors; see Figures 6-1 and 6-3). However, succinylcholine persists for a longer duration at the neuromuscular junction because of its resistance to AChE. The initial depolarization is followed by block of neuromuscular transmission and flaccid paralysis.

QUESTION 6-9 Answer is **a.** The major action of nicotine consists initially of transient stimulation and subsequently of a more persistent depression of all autonomic ganglia. The effects of high doses of nicotine on the neuromuscular junction are similar to those on ganglia.

SECTION II — Neuropharmacology

SUMMARY TABLE CHOLINERGIC PHARMACOLOGY

CLASS AND SUBCLASSES	NAMES	CLINICAL USES	TOXICITIES COMMON	TOXICITIES UNIQUE; CLINICALLY IMPORTANT
Muscarinic Receptor Agonists	Acetylcholine	Neurotransmitter at nicotinic and muscarinic receptor sites; used topically to induce miosis during ophthalmologic surgery		
	Pilocarpine	Used topically for treatment of glaucoma and to induce miosis; treatment of xerostomia following head and neck radiation or Sjögren syndrome	Parasympathomimetic effects if absorbed systemically	Of limited concern if used topically; but caution should be taken in patients with asthma, COPD, urinary or GI obstruction, or cardiovascular disease accompanied by hypotension or bradycardia
	Methacholine	Administered cautiously by inhalation for the diagnosis of bronchial airway hyper-reactivity	Parasympathomimetic effects if absorbed systemically	Emergency resuscitation equipment and medications to treat severe bronchospasm should be available during testing
	Carbachol	Used topically for treatment of glaucoma and to induce miosis	Parasympathomimetic effects if absorbed systemically	Of limited concern if used topically; but caution should be taken in patients with asthma, COPD, urinary or GI obstruction, or cardiovascular disease accompanied by hypotension or bradycardia
	Bethanechol	Treatment of urinary retention and inadequate emptying of the bladder when obstruction is absent Treatment of decreased GI motility and decreased lower esophageal sphincter pressure	Parasympathomimetic effects if absorbed systemically	Caution should be taken in patients with asthma, COPD, urinary or GI obstruction, or cardiovascular disease accompanied by hypotension or bradycardia
	Cevimeline	Long-lasting sialogogic effect and enhances lacrimal secretions in Sjögren syndrome	May have fewer side effects than pilocarpine	Caution should be taken in patients with asthma, COPD, urinary or GI obstruction, or cardiovascular disease accompanied by hypotension or bradycardia
Muscarinic Receptor Antagonists	Atropine	Treatment of patients with acute MI in whom excessive vagal tone causes bradycardia; treatment of *Amanita muscaria* poisoning; treatment of AChE poisoning	Predictable effects of muscarinic blockade (see Tables 5-1 and 6-2): xerostomia, constipation, blurred vision, dyspepsia, and cognitive impairment	Urinary or GI obstruction, angle-closure glaucoma Use with extreme caution in patients with benign prostatic hyperplasia
	Scopolamine	Treatment of motion sickness	Xerostomia, drowsiness, and blurred vision in some individuals	Mydriasis and cycloplegia can occur by inadvertent transfer of drug to the eye; rare but severe psychotic episodes are possible
	Ipratropium	Treatment of chronic obstructive pulmonary disease (COPD; see Chapter 24)	Predictable consequences of muscarinic receptor blockade (see Tables 5-1 and 6-2)	Urinary or GI obstruction, angle-closure glaucoma Use with extreme caution in patients with benign prostatic hyperplasia

Cholinergic Pharmacology — CHAPTER 6

CLASS AND SUBCLASSES	NAMES	CLINICAL USES	TOXICITIES COMMON	UNIQUE; CLINICALLY IMPORTANT
	Tiotropium	Treatment of chronic obstructive pulmonary disease (see Chapter 24)	Predictable consequences of muscarinic receptor blockade (see Tables 5-1 and 6-2)	Urinary or GI obstruction, angle-closure glaucoma Use with extreme caution in patients with benign prostatic hyperplasia
	Oxybutynin	Treatment of overactive bladder by increasing capacity and reducing frequency	Predictable consequences of muscarinic receptor blockade (see Tables 5-1 and 6-2)	Reduce dose in patients taking drugs that inhibit CYP3A4 Urinary or GI obstruction, angle-closure glaucoma Use with extreme caution in patients with benign prostatic hyperplasia
	Tolterodine	Treatment of overactive bladder by increasing capacity and reducing frequency	Predictable consequences of muscarinic receptor blockade (see Tables 5-1 and 6-2)	Reduce dose in patients taking drugs that inhibit CYP3A4 Urinary or GI obstruction, angle-closure glaucoma Use with extreme caution in patients with benign prostatic hyperplasia
	Trospium chloride	Treatment of overactive bladder by increasing capacity and reducing frequency	Predictable consequences of muscarinic receptor blockade (see Tables 5-1 and 6-2)	Dosage adjustment is necessary for patients with impaired renal function Urinary or GI obstruction, angle-closure glaucoma Use with extreme caution in patients with benign prostatic hyperplasia
	Darifenacin	Treatment of overactive bladder by increasing capacity and reducing frequency	Predictable consequences of muscarinic receptor blockade (see Tables 5-1 and 6-2)	Reduce dose in patients taking drugs that inhibit CYP3A4 or CYP2D6 Urinary or GI obstruction, angle-closure glaucoma Use with extreme caution in patients with benign prostatic hyperplasia
	Solifenacin	Treatment of overactive bladder by increasing capacity and reducing frequency	Predictable consequences of muscarinic receptor blockade (see Tables 5-1 and 6-2)	Reduce dose in patients taking drugs that inhibit CYP3A4
	Fesoterodine	Treatment of overactive bladder by increasing capacity and reducing frequency	Predictable consequences of muscarinic receptor blockade (see Tables 5-1 and 6-2)	Urinary or GI obstruction, angle-closure glaucoma Use with extreme caution in patients with benign prostatic hyperplasia
	Flavoxate	Treatment of overactive bladder by increasing capacity and reducing frequency	Predictable consequences of muscarinic receptor blockade (see Tables 5-1 and 6-2)	Urinary or GI obstruction, angle-closure glaucoma Use with extreme caution in patients with benign prostatic hyperplasia
	Glycopyrrolate	Used to reduce GI tone and motility (see Chapter 33)		
	Dicyclomine hydrochloride	Used for the treatment of diarrhea-predominant irritable bowel syndrome (see Chapter 33)	Predictable consequences of muscarinic receptor blockade (see Tables 5-1 and 6-2)	Urinary or GI obstruction, angle-closure glaucoma Use with extreme caution in patients with benign prostatic hyperplasia

SECTION II Neuropharmacology

CLASS AND SUBCLASSES	NAMES	CLINICAL USES	TOXICITIES	
			COMMON	UNIQUE; CLINICALLY IMPORTANT
	Homatropine hydrobromide	Topical administration to produce mydriasis and cycloplegia	Predictable consequences of muscarinic receptor blockade (see Tables 5-1 and 6-2)	Urinary or GI obstruction, angle-closure glaucoma. Use with extreme caution in patients with benign prostatic hyperplasia
	Cyclopentolate hydrochloride	Topical administration to produce mydriasis and cycloplegia	Predictable consequences of muscarinic receptor blockade (see Tables 5-1 and 6-2)	Urinary or GI obstruction, angle-closure glaucoma. Use with extreme caution in patients with benign prostatic hyperplasia
	Tropicamide	Topical administration to produce mydriasis and cycloplegia	Predictable consequences of muscarinic receptor blockade (see Tables 5-1 and 6-2)	Urinary or GI obstruction, angle-closure glaucoma. Use with extreme caution in patients with benign prostatic hyperplasia
	Benztropine mesylate	Used to treat Parkinson's disease and drug-induced extrapyramidal symptoms (see Chapters 8 and 13)	Predictable consequences of muscarinic receptor blockade (see Tables 5-1 and 6-2)	Urinary or GI obstruction, angle-closure glaucoma. Use with extreme caution in patients with benign prostatic hyperplasia
	Trihexyphenidyl hydrochloride	Used to treat Parkinson's disease and drug-induced extrapyramidal symptoms (see Chapters 8 and 13)	Predictable consequences of muscarinic receptor blockade (see Tables 5-1 and 6-2)	Urinary or GI obstruction, angle-closure glaucoma. Use with extreme caution in patients with benign prostatic hyperplasia
	Methscopolamine bromide	Used in certain combination products for the temporary relief of symptoms of allergic rhinitis, sinusitis, and the common cold	Predictable consequences of muscarinic receptor blockade (see Tables 5-1 and 6-2)	Urinary or GI obstruction, angle-closure glaucoma. Use with extreme caution in patients with benign prostatic hyperplasia
"Reversible" AChE Inhibitors	Edrophonium	Used for the diagnosis of myasthenia gravis	Predictable consequences of muscarinic receptor stimulation (see Tables 5-1 and 6-2)	See Side Bar POTENTIAL EFFECTS OF ANTI-CHE AGENTS
	Physostigmine salicylate	Used to treat intoxication by anticholinergic drugs or substances	Predictable consequences of muscarinic receptor stimulation (see Tables 5-1 and 6-2)	See Side Bar POTENTIAL EFFECTS OF ANTI-CHE AGENTS; cardiac arrhythmias if administered rapidly
	Neostigmine bromide (oral)	Used for the treatment of myasthenia gravis	Predictable consequences of muscarinic receptor stimulation (see Tables 5-1 and 6-2)	See Side Bar POTENTIAL EFFECTS OF ANTI-CHE AGENTS
	Neostigmine methylsulfate (parenteral)	Used for the treatment of myasthenia gravis	Predictable consequences of muscarinic receptor stimulation (see Tables 5-1 and 6-2)	See Side Bar POTENTIAL EFFECTS OF ANTI-CHE AGENTS
	Ambenonium chloride	Used for the treatment of myasthenia gravis	Predictable consequences of muscarinic receptor stimulation (see Tables 5-1 and 6-2)	See Side Bar POTENTIAL EFFECTS OF ANTI-CHE AGENTS
	Pyridostigmine bromide	Used for the treatment of myasthenia gravis	Predictable consequences of muscarinic receptor stimulation (see Tables 5-1 and 6-2)	See Side Bar POTENTIAL EFFECTS OF ANTI-CHE AGENTS

Cholinergic Pharmacology — CHAPTER 6

CLASS AND SUBCLASSES	NAMES	CLINICAL USES	TOXICITIES COMMON	TOXICITIES UNIQUE; CLINICALLY IMPORTANT
	Tacrine	Approved for the treatment of Alzheimer's disease	Predictable consequences of muscarinic receptor stimulation (see Tables 5-1 and 6-2)	See Side Bar POTENTIAL EFFECTS OF ANTI-CHE AGENTS
	Donepezil	Approved for the treatment of Alzheimer's disease	Predictable consequences of muscarinic receptor stimulation (see Tables 5-1 and 6-2)	See Side Bar POTENTIAL EFFECTS OF ANTI-CHE AGENTS
	Rivastigmine	Approved for the treatment of Alzheimer's disease	Predictable consequences of muscarinic receptor stimulation (see Tables 5-1 and 6-2)	See Side Bar POTENTIAL EFFECTS OF ANTI-CHE AGENTS
	Galantamine	Approved for the treatment of Alzheimer's disease	Predictable consequences of muscarinic receptor stimulation (see Tables 5-1 and 6-2)	See Side Bar POTENTIAL EFFECTS OF ANTI-CHE AGENTS
Carbamate Insecticides	Carbaryl	Insecticide	Excessive muscarinic receptor stimulation (see Tables 5-1 and 6-2); low toxicity from dermal absorption	Acute toxicity results from excessive stimulation of muscarinic and nicotinic receptors
	Propoxur	Insecticide	Excessive muscarinic receptor stimulation (see Tables 5-1 and 6-2)	Acute toxicity results from excessive stimulation of muscarinic and nicotinic receptors
	Aldicarb	Insecticide	Excessive muscarinic receptor stimulation (see Tables 5-1 and 6-2)	Acute toxicity results from excessive stimulation of muscarinic and nicotinic receptors
Organophosphate Insecticides	Diazinon	Insecticide	Excessive muscarinic receptor stimulation (see Tables 5-1 and 6-2)	Acute toxicity results from excessive stimulation of muscarinic and nicotinic receptors. Stability of phosphorylated cholinesterase is enhanced through "aging"
	Chlorpyrifos	Insecticide	Excessive muscarinic receptor stimulation (see Tables 5-1 and 6-2)	Acute toxicity results from excessive stimulation of muscarinic and nicotinic receptors. Stability of phosphorylated cholinesterase is enhanced through "aging"
	Malathion	Insecticide	Excessive muscarinic receptor stimulation (see Tables 5-1 and 6-2)	Acute toxicity results from excessive stimulation of muscarinic and nicotinic receptors. Acute toxicity arises only from deliberate poisoning because mammals detoxify malathion by a plasma carboxyl-esterase which dictates species resistance. Stability of phosphorylated cholinesterase is enhanced through "aging"

SECTION II Neuropharmacology

CLASS AND SUBCLASSES	NAMES	CLINICAL USES	TOXICITIES COMMON	UNIQUE; CLINICALLY IMPORTANT
Organophosphate Nerve Gases	Tabun	Nerve gas agent		Potent toxin; toxicity is due to stimulation of muscarinic and nicotinic receptors Stability of phosphorylated cholinesterase is enhanced through "aging"
	Sarin	Nerve gas agent		Potent toxin; toxicity is due to stimulation of muscarinic and nicotinic receptors Stability of phosphorylated cholinesterase is enhanced through "aging"
	Soman	Nerve gas agent		Potent toxin; toxicity is due to stimulation of muscarinic and nicotinic receptors Stability of phosphorylated cholinesterase is enhanced through "aging"
Cholinesterase Reactivators	Pralidoxime (2-PAM)	Used to reactivate cholinesterase after an organo-phosphate intoxication		Reverses peripheral neuromuscular blockade of organo-phosphate poisoning; does not enter the CNS
Depolarizing Neuromuscular Blocking Agents	Succinylcholine	Depolarizing neuromuscular blocking agent used as an adjuvant during surgical anesthesia to obtain relaxation of skeletal muscle	Should be administered only by an anesthesiologist in a setting where facilities for respiratory and cardiovascular resuscitation are available (see Chapter 11)	Life-threatening hyperkalemia; rarely may cause ganglionic blockade Histamine release which may result in bronchospasm, hypotension, and excessive bronchial and salivary secretion
Competitive Neuromuscular Blocking Agents	Pancuronium	Competitive neuromuscular blocking agent used as an adjuvant during surgical anesthesia to obtain relaxation of skeletal muscle; long duration of action	Should be administered only by an anesthesiologist in a setting where facilities for respiratory and cardiovascular resuscitation are available (see Chapter 11)	Persistent blockade with difficulty in complete reversal of blockade
	Atracuium	Competitive neuromuscular blocking agent used as an adjuvant during surgical anesthesia to obtain relaxation of skeletal muscle; intermediate duration of action	Should be administered only by an anesthesiologist in a setting where facilities for respiratory and cardiovascular resuscitation are available (see Chapter 11)	Histamine release which may result in bronchospasm, hypotension, and excessive bronchial and salivary secretion
	Vecuronium	Competitive neuromuscular blocking agent used as an adjuvant during surgical anesthesia to obtain relaxation of skeletal muscle Intermediate duration of action	Should be administered only by an anesthesiologist in a setting where facilities for respiratory and cardiovascular resuscitation are available (see Chapter 11)	
	Pipecuronium	Competitive neuromuscular blocking agent used as an adjuvant during surgical anesthesia to obtain relaxation of skeletal muscle; long duration of action	Should be administered only by an anesthesiologist in a setting where facilities for respiratory and cardiovascular resuscitation are available (see Chapter 11)	Persistent blockade with difficulty in complete reversal of blockade

Cholinergic Pharmacology — CHAPTER 6

CLASS AND SUBCLASSES	NAMES	CLINICAL USES	TOXICITIES COMMON	TOXICITIES UNIQUE; CLINICALLY IMPORTANT
	Doxacurium	Competitive neuromuscular blocking agent used as an adjuvant during surgical anesthesia to obtain relaxation of skeletal muscle; long duration of action	Should be administered only by an anesthesiologist in a setting where facilities for respiratory and cardiovascular resuscitation are available (see Chapter 11)	Persistent blockade with difficulty in complete reversal of blockade
	Mivacurium	Competitive neuromuscular blocking agent used as an adjuvant during surgical anesthesia to obtain relaxation of skeletal muscle; short duration of action (Not available in the United States)		Histamine release which may result in bronchospasm, hypotension, and excessive bronchial and salivary secretion
	Rocuronium	Competitive neuromuscular blocking agent used as an adjuvant during surgical anesthesia to obtain relaxation of skeletal muscle; intermediate duration of action but with rapid onset	Should be administered only by an anesthesiologist in a setting where facilities for respiratory and cardiovascular resuscitation are available (see Chapter 11)	
	Cisatracurium	Competitive neuromuscular blocking agent used as an adjuvant during surgical anesthesia to obtain relaxation of skeletal muscle; intermediate duration of action	Should be administered only by an anesthesiologist in a setting where facilities for respiratory and cardiovascular resuscitation are available (see Chapter 11)	
Botulinum Toxins	Onabotulinum toxin A	Treatment of strabismus and blepharospasm and as a cosmetic procedure to reduce facial wrinkles (see Chapter 48)		Diplopia, eyelid drop, and distant spread of toxin with paralysis of respiratory muscles
	Rimabotulinum toxin B	Treatment of strabismus and blepharospasm and as a cosmetic procedure to reduce facial wrinkles (see Chapter 48)		Diplopia, eyelid drop, and distant spread of toxin with paralysis of respiratory muscles
Antispasticity and Antirigidity Agents	Dantrolene	Treatment of malignant hyperthermia; treatment of spasticity and rigidity in nonambulatory patients		Hepatotoxicity has been reported and continued use requires monitoring of liver function
Ganglionic Stimulating Agents	Nicotine	Presence in tobacco products conferring dependence on its users (see Chapter 14)		Nicotine poisoning from the accidental ingestion of nicotine-containing insecticides, or, in children, from ingestion of tobacco products; death from respiratory failure may occur rapidly
Nicotinic ACh Receptor Agonists	Varenicline	Used as an aid to smoking cessation		FDA has issued a warning about mood and behavioral changes
Ganglionic Blocking Drugs	Mecamylamine	Initially used to treat hypertension, but now surpassed by safer agents (see Table 6-8)	Visual disturbances, dry mouth, urinary hesitancy, decreased sexual potency, diarrhea, abdominal pain	Marked hypotension, constipation, syncope, urinary retention, paralytic ileus, and cycloplegia
	Trimethaphan	Initially used to treat hypertension, but now surpassed by safer agents (see Table 6-8)	Visual disturbances, dry mouth, urinary hesitancy, decreased sexual potency, diarrhea, abdominal pain	Marked hypotension, constipation, syncope, urinary retention, paralytic ileus, and cycloplegia

CHAPTER 7

Adrenergic, Dopaminergic, and Serotonergic Pharmacology

DRUGS INCLUDED IN THIS CHAPTER

- Acebutolol (SECTRAL, others)
- Albuterol (VENTOLIN-HFA, PROVENTIL-HFA, others)
- Alfuzosin (UROXATRAL)
- Almotriptan (AXERT)
- Alosetron (LOTRONEX)
- Apomorphine (APOKYN)
- Apraclonidine (IOPIDINE)
- Arformeterol (BROVENA)
- Aripiprazole (ABILIFY)
- Atenolol (TENORMIN, others)
- Betaxolog (BETAOPTIC, others)
- Betaxolol (LOKREN, KERCONE, others)
- Bitolterol (TORNALATE)—discontinued in the United States
- Brimonidine (ALPHAGAN, others)
- Bromocriptine (PARLODEL)
- Bucindolol (SANDORMIN)
- Bunazosin—not available in the United States
- Buspirone (BUSPAR, others)
- Cabergoline (DOSTINEX)
- Carteolol (OCCUPRES, others)
- Carvedilol (COREG)
- Celiprolol (SELECTOL)
- Citralopam (CELEXA)
- Clonidine (CATAPRES, others; Transdermal, CATAPRES-TTS)
- Clozapine (FAZACLO)
- Desvenlafaxine (PRISTIQ)
- Dexmedetomide (PRECEDEX)
- Dexmethylphenidate (FOCALIN, FOCALIN XR)
- Dextroamphetamine (DEXIDRINE, ADDERAL XR, others)
- Dobutamine (DOBUTREX)
- Dolasetron (ANZEMET)
- Dopamine
- Dopexamine (DOPACARD)—not currently available in the United States

(continues)

This chapter is a combination of Chapter 12 Adrenergic Agonists and Antagonists and Chapter 13 5-Hydroxytryptamine (Serotonin) from *Goodman and Gilman's The Pharmacological Basis of Therapeutics*, 12th Edition. An understanding of the material in those chapters will be helpful in following the material presented in this chapter. Further details of the therapeutic use of the drugs mentioned in this chapter can be found in subsequent chapters. In addition to the material presented here the above chapters in the 12th Edition include:

- Table 12-1 Chemical Structures and Main Clinical Uses of Important Sympathomimetic Drugs
- A detailed discussion of the pharmacology of the endogenous catecholamines epinephrine (E), norepinephrine (NE), and dopamine (DA)
- The pharmacology of miscellaneous sympathomimetic amines, including amphetamine, methamphetamine, methylphenidate, and ephedrine
- A discussion of the therapeutic uses of sympathomimetic drugs in shock, hypotension, cardiac arrhythmias, nasal decongestion, allergic reactions, narcolepsy, weight reduction, and attention deficit/hyperactivity disorder (ADHD)
- Details of the physiological functions of serotonin, including the multiple receptor subtypes of 5-HT
- A discussion of the pharmacology of ergot and the ergot alkaloids, including lysergic acid diethylamide (LSD)
- The physiological functions of dopamine, including a detailed discussion of dopamine receptor subtypes

LEARNING OBJECTIVES

☑ Understand the pharmacology of the major adrenergic and serotonergic agonists and antagonists.

☑ Know the mechanisms of action of the adrenergic and serotonergic agonists and antagonists.

☑ Know the therapeutic uses, adverse effects, toxicities, and contraindications of the adrenergic and serotonergic agonists and antagonists.

MECHANISM OF ACTION OF ENDOGENOUS CATECHOLAMINES

DRUG CLASS	DRUG	MECHANISM OF ACTION
Endogenous Catecholamines (see Figure 7-1)	Epinephrine (E)	Stimulates both α and β adrenergic receptors Responses are shown in Table 5-1
	Norepinephrine (NE)	Neurotransmitter at postganglionic sympathetic nerves Potent α and $β_1$ adrenergic receptor agonist (see Table 5-1)
	Dopamine (DA)	Immediate metabolic precursor of NE and E; central neurotransmitter important for the regulation of movement and behavior (see Figure 7-2)
Dopamine Derivatives	Fenoldopam	Agonist for peripheral D_1 receptors and binds with moderate affinity to $α_2$ receptors
	Dopexamine	Intrinsic activity at D_1 and D_2 receptors as well as $β_2$ receptors

Adrenergic, Dopaminergic, and Serotonergic Pharmacology

CHAPTER 7

MECHANISM OF ACTION OF α-ADRENERGIC RECEPTOR AGONISTS AND ANTAGONISTS

DRUG CLASS	DRUG	MECHANISM OF ACTION
α_1-Selective Adrenergic Receptor Agonists (see Figure 7-3)	Phenylephrine	Agonist at α_1 adrenergic receptors (see Table 5-1)
	Mephentermine	Agonist at α_1 adrenergic receptors (see Table 5-1)
	Meteraminol	Agonist at α_1 adrenergic receptors (see Table 5-1)
	Midodrine	Agonist at α_1 adrenergic receptors (see Table 5-1)
α_2-Selective Adrenergic Receptor Agonists (see Figure 7-3)	Clonidine	Agonist at α_2 adrenergic receptors (see Table 5-1) Suppresses the outflow of the sympathetic nervous system activity from the brain See Chapter 15
	Dexmedetomidine	Agonist at α_2 adrenergic receptors (see Table 5-1) Suppresses the outflow of the sympathetic nervous system activity from the brain See Chapter 15
	Apraclonidine	Agonist at α_2 adrenergic receptors (see Table 5-1) α_2 Receptor–mediated reduction in the formation of aqueous humor (see Chapter 47) Does not cross the blood-brain barrier (BBB)
	Brimonidine	Agonist at α_2 adrenergic receptors (see Table 5-1) α_2 Receptor–mediated reduction in the formation of aqueous humor (see Chapter 47) Can cross the BBB
	Guanfacine	Agonist at α_2 adrenergic receptors (see Table 5-1) Suppresses the outflow of the sympathetic nervous system activity from the brain See Chapter 15
	Guanabenz	Agonist at α_2 adrenergic receptors (see Table 5-1) Suppresses the outflow of the sympathetic nervous system activity from the brain See Chapter 15
	Methyldopa	Metabolized to α-methylnorepinephrine in the brain where it activates α_2 receptors and suppresses the outflow of the sympathetic nervous system activity from the brain See Chapter 15
	Tizanidine	Agonist at α_2 adrenergic receptors (see Table 5-1) See Chapter 15
α_1 Adrenergic Receptor Antagonists (see Figure 7-4)	Prazosin	Antagonist at α_1 adrenergic receptors (see Table 5-1) to inhibit vasoconstriction induced by endogenous catecholamines See Chapter 15
	Terazosin	Antagonist at α_1 adrenergic receptors (see Table 5-1) to inhibit vasoconstriction induced by endogenous catecholamines See Chapter 15
	Doxazosin	Antagonist at α_1 adrenergic receptors (see Table 5-1) to inhibit vasoconstriction induced by endogenous catecholamines See Chapter 15
	Alfuzosin	Antagonist at α_1 adrenergic receptors (see Table 5-1) with affinity for all α_1 receptor subtypes
	Tamsulosin	Antagonist at α_1 adrenergic receptors (see Table 5-1); some selectivity for α_{1A} in prostate
	Silodosin	Antagonist at α_1 adrenergic receptors (see Table 5-1) some selectivity for α_{1A} in prostate

DRUGS INCLUDED IN THIS CHAPTER (Cont.)

- Doxazosin (CARDURA, others)
- Duloxetine (CYMBALTA)
- Eletriptan (RELPAX)
- Ephedrine
- Epinephrine (solution for injection, EPIPEN)
- Escitralopam (LEXAPRO)
- Esmolol (BREVIBLOC, others)
- Fenoldopam (CORLOPAM)
- Fenoterol (BEROTEC)—withdrawn from market
- Fluoxetine (PROZAC, others)
- Fluvoxamine (LUVOX, others)
- Formoterol (FORADIL, others)
- Frovatriptan (FROVAL)
- Granisetron (KYTRIL, others)
- Guanabenx (WYTENSIN)
- Guanfacine (TENEX, others; INTUNIV, sustained release)
- Indoramin—not available in the United States
- Isocarboxazid (MARPLAN)
- Isoetharine (BRONKOSOL)—no longer marketed in the United States
- Isoproterenol (ISUPREL)
- Ketanserin (SUFREXAL)—not available in the United States
- Levalbuterol (XOPENEX)
- Levobetaxolol (BETAXON, others)
- Levobunolol (BETAGAN, others)
- Lisdexamfetamine (VYVANASE)
- Mephentermine—discontinued in the United States
- Metaproterenol (ALUPENT, orciprenaline in Europe)
- Metaraminol
- Methamphetamine (DESOXYN)
- Methyldopa (ALDOMET, others)
- Methylphenidate (RITALIN, RITALIN SR, CONCERTA, META-DATE, others; DAYTRANA, transdermal)
- Methylsergide (SANSERT)
- Metipranolol (OPTIPRANOLOL, others)
- Metoprolol (LOPRESSOR, others)
- Midodrine (PROAMATINE, others)

(continues)

SECTION II

DRUGS INCLUDED IN THIS CHAPTER (Cont.)

- Milnacipran (SAVELLA)
- Modafinil (PROVIGIL)
- Naphazoline (PRIVINE, NAPHCON, others)
- Naratriptan (AMERGE)
- Nebivolol (NEBILET, BYSTOLIC)
- Norepinephrine (LEVOPHED)
- Olanzapine (ZYPREXA)
- Ondansetron (ZOFRAN, others)
- Oxymetazoline (AFRIN, OCU-CLEAR, others)
- Palonosetron (ALOXI)
- Paroxetine (PAXIL)
- Pemoline (CYLERT, others)—discontinued in the United States
- Pergolide (PERMAX)
- Phenelzine (NARDIL)
- Phenoxybenzamine (DIBENZYLINE)
- Phentolamine (ORAVERSE)
- Phenylephrine (NEO-SYNEPHRINE, others)
- Pindolol (VISKEN, others)
- Pirbuterol (MAXAIR)
- Pramipexole (MIRAPEX)
- Prazosin (MINIPRES, others)
- Procaterol (MASCACIN)—not available in the United States
- Propranolol (INDERAL, INDERAL LA, others)
- Propylhexedrine (BENZEDREX, others)
- Pseudoephedrine (SUDAPHED, others)
- Quetiapine (SEROQUEL)
- Respiridone (RISPERDAL, others)
- Ritodrine—not available in the United States
- Rizatriptan (MAXALT, others)
- Ropinirole (REQUIP)
- Rotigotine (NEUPRO)
- Salmeterol (SEREVENT)
- Sertraline (ZOLOFT)
- Sibutramine (MERIDIA)
- Silodosin (RAPAFLO)
- Sumatriptan (IMITREX, others)
- Tamsulosin (FLOMAX)
- Terazosin (HYTRIN, others)
- Terbutaline (BRETHINE)
- Timolol (TIMOPTIC, others, for ophthalmic use; BLOCADREN, others, for systemic use)
- Tizanidine (ZANAFLEX, others)

(continues)

Neuropharmacology

DRUG CLASS	DRUG	MECHANISM OF ACTION
α_2 Adrenergic Receptor Antagonists (see Figure 7-4)	Yohimbine	Competitive antagonist that is selective for α_2-adrenergic receptors
	Phenoxybenzamine	Nonselective antagonist at α_2 adrenergic receptors
	Phentolamine	Nonselective antagonist at α_2 adrenergic receptors
Additional α Adrenergic Receptor Antagonists (see Figure 7-4)	Ergot Alkaloids	Partial agonists and antagonists at α receptors, DA receptors, and serotonin receptors
	Indoramin	Selective α_1 receptor antagonist
	Ketanserin	Antagonist at α_1 receptors and 5-HT receptors
	Urapidil	Antagonist at α_1 adrenergic receptors
	Bunazosin	An α_1 selective antagonist

MECHANISM OF ACTION OF MISCELLANEOUS SYMPATHOMIMETIC AGONISTS

DRUG CLASS	DRUG	MECHANISM OF ACTION
Miscellaneous Sympathomimetic Agonists (see Figure 7-3)	Amphetamine	Amphetamine exerts most of its effects in the CNS through the release of biogenic amines from their storage sites by targeting the neuronal dopamine transporter (DAT) and the vesicular monoamine transporter 2 (VMAT2) (see Table 7-1 and Figure 7-2)
	Methamphetamine	In the brain, methamphetamine releases DA and other biogenic amines, and inhibits neuronal and vesicular monoamine transporters as well as MAO
	Methylphenidate	In the brain, methylphenidate is predominantly a dopamine and norepinephrine uptake inhibitor
	Dexmethylphenidate	Mechanism of action is similar to methylphenidate
	Lisdexamphetamine	Mechanism of action is similar to methylphenidate
	Pemoline	Dopaminergic but precise mechanism of action has not been determined
	Ephedrine	Agonist at both α and β adrenergic receptors; also enhances the release of NE from sympathetic neurons
	Propylhexedrine	Sympathomimetic drug that acts as a vasoconstrictor for local application to the nasal mucosa or the eye
	Naphazoline	Sympathomimetic drug that acts as a vasoconstrictor for local application to the nasal mucosa or the eye
	Oxymetazoline	Sympathomimetic drug that acts as a vasoconstrictor for local application to the nasal mucosa or the eye
	Xylometazoline	Sympathomimetic drug that acts as a vasoconstrictor for local application to the nasal mucosa or the eye
	Pseudoephedrine	Stereoisomer of ephedrine with vasoconstrictor activity
	Modafinil	CNS stimulant with actions on NE, DA, and 5-HT neurons, but precise mechanism of action has not been determined

Adrenergic, Dopaminergic, and Serotonergic Pharmacology

CHAPTER 7

DRUGS INCLUDED IN THIS CHAPTER (Cont.)

- Tranylcypromine (PARNATE, others)
- Urapidil—not available in the United States
- Venlafaxine (EFFEXOR)
- Xylometazoline (OTRIVIN, others)
- Yohimbine (YOCON, APHRODYNE)
- Zolmitriptan (ZOMIG)

CASE 7-1

A 56-year-old woman is being treated with prazosin for her elevated blood pressure.

a. What class of drug is prazosin and how is it used to treat hypertension?

The major effects of prazosin result from its blockade of α_1 receptors in arterioles and veins (see Figure 7-4). This leads to a fall in peripheral vascular resistance and in venous return to the heart. Unlike other vasodilating drugs, administration of prazosin usually does not increase heart rate (see answer to b below). In addition, prazosin decreases cardiac preload and thus has little tendency to increase cardiac

(Continued)

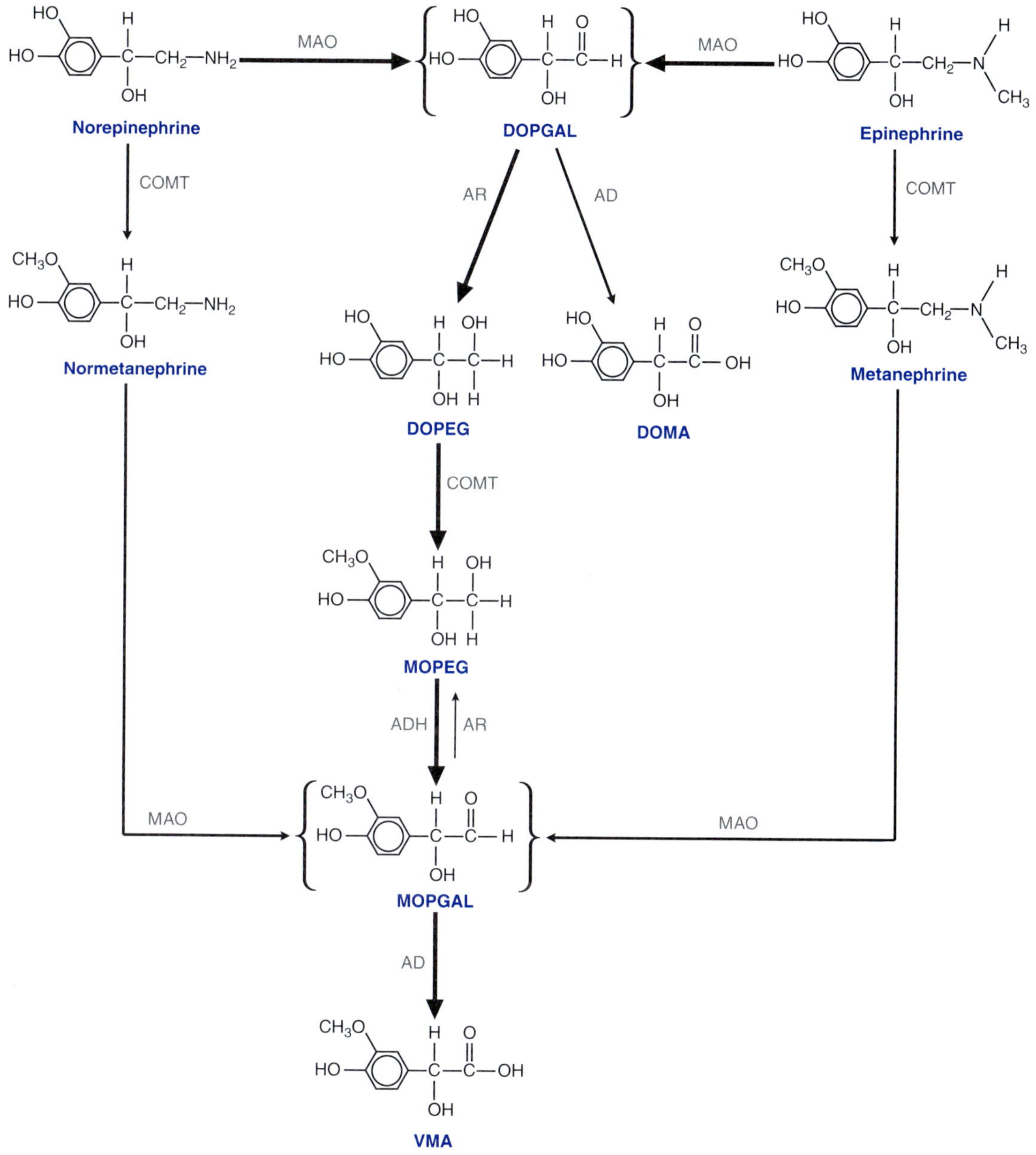

FIGURE 7-1 Steps in the metabolic disposition of catecholamines. Norepinephrine and epinephrine are first oxidatively deaminated to a short-lived intermediate (DOPGAL) by monoamine oxidase (MAO). DOPGAL then undergoes further metabolism to more stable alcohol or acid deaminated metabolites. Aldehyde dehydrogenase (AD) metabolizes DOPGAL to 3,4-dihydroxymandelic acid (DOMA) while aldehyde reductase (AR) metabolizes DOPGAL to 3,4-dihydroxyphenyl glycol (DOPEG). Under normal circumstances DOMA is a minor metabolite with DOPEG being the major metabolite produced from norepinephrine and epinephrine. Once DOPEG leaves the major sites of its formation (sympathetic nerves; adrenal medulla), it is converted to 3-methoxy, 4-hydroxyphenylglycol (MOPEG) by catechol-O-methyl transferase (COMT). MOPEG is then converted to the unstable aldehyde (MOPGAL) by alcohol dehydrogenase (ADH) and finally to vanillyl mandelic acid (VMA) by aldehyde dehydrogenase. VMA is the major end product of norepinephrine and epinephrine metabolism. Another route for the formation of VMA is conversion of norepinephrine or epinephrine into normetanephrine or metanephrine by COMT either in the adreneal medulla or extraneuronal sites, with subsequent metabolism to MOPGAL and thence to VMA.

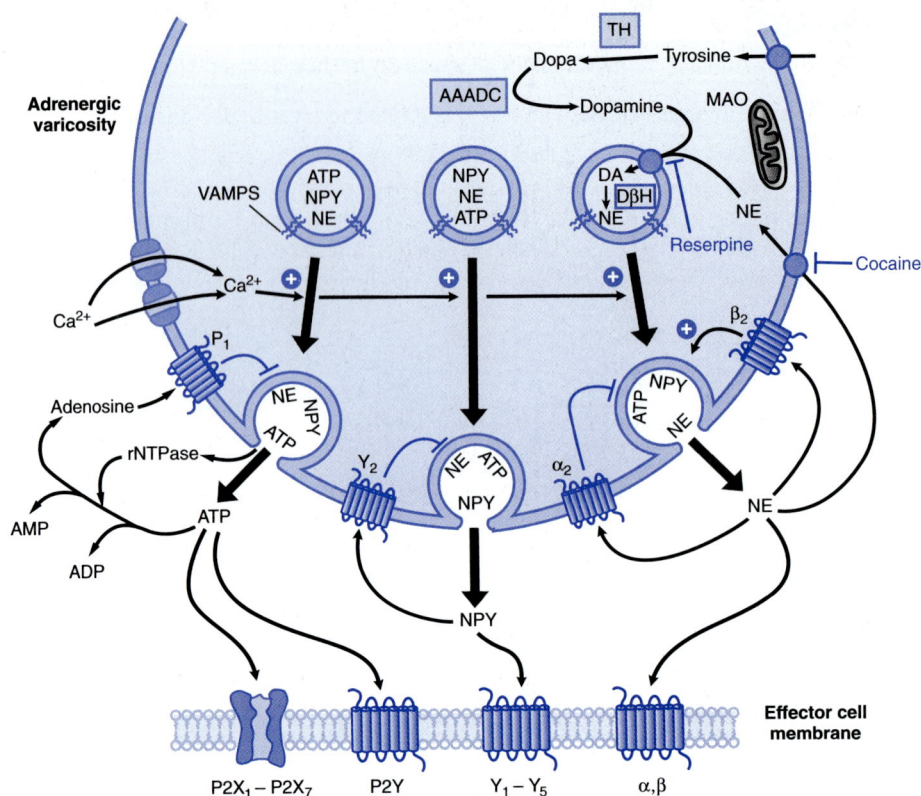

FIGURE 7-2 An adrenergic neuroeffector junction showing features of the synthesis, storage, release, and receptors for norepinephrine (NE), the cotransmitters neuropeptide Y (NPY), and ATP. Tyrosine is transported into the varicosity and is converted to DOPA by tyrosine hydroxylase (TH) and DOPA to dopamine (DA) by the action of aromatic L-amino acid decarboxylase (AAADC). Dopamine is taken up into the vesicles of the varicosity by a transporter, VMAT2, that can be blocked by reserpine. Cytoplasmic NE also can be taken up by this transporter. Dopamine is converted to NE within the vesicle via the action of dopamine-β-hydroxylase (DβH). NE is stored in vesicles along with other cotransmitters, NPY and ATP, depending on the particular neuroeffector junction. Release of the transmitters occurs upon depolarization of the varicosity, which allows entry of Ca^{2+} through voltage-dependent Ca^{2+} channels. Elevated levels of Ca^{2+} promote the fusion of the vesicular membrane with the membrane of the varicosity, with subsequent exocytosis of transmitters. This fusion process involves the interaction of specialized proteins associated with the vesicular membrane (VAMPs, vesicle-associated membrane proteins) and the membrane of the varicosity (SNAPs, synaptosome-associated proteins). In this schematic representation, NE, NPY, and ATP are stored in the same vesicles. Different populations of vesicles, however, may preferentially store different proportions of the cotransmitters. Once in the synapse, NE can interact with α and β adrenergic receptors to produce the characteristic response of the effector. The adrenergic receptors are GPCRs. α and β Receptors also can be located presynaptically where NE can either diminish ($α_2$), or facilitate (β) its own release and that of the cotransmitters. The principal mechanism by which NE is cleared from the synapse is via a cocaine-sensitive neuronal uptake transporter, NET. Once transported into the cytosol, NE can be restored in the vesicle or metabolized by monoamine oxidase (MAO). NPY produces its effects by activating NPY receptors, of which there are at least five types (Y_1 through Y_5). NPY receptors are GPCRs. NPY can modify its own release and that of the other transmitters via presynaptic receptors of the Y_2 type. NPY is removed from the synapse by metabolic breakdown by peptidases. ATP produces its effects by activating P2X receptors or P2Y receptors. P2X receptors are ligand-gated ion channels; P2Y receptors are GPCRs. There are multiple subtypes of both P2X and P2Y receptors. As with the other cotransmitters, ATP can act prejunctionally to modify its own release via receptors for ATP or via its metabolic breakdown to adenosine that acts on P1 (adenosine) receptors. ATP is cleared from the synapse primarily by releasable nucleotidases (rNTPase) and by cell-fixed ectonucleotidases.

Adrenergic, Dopaminergic, and Serotonergic Pharmacology

CHAPTER 7

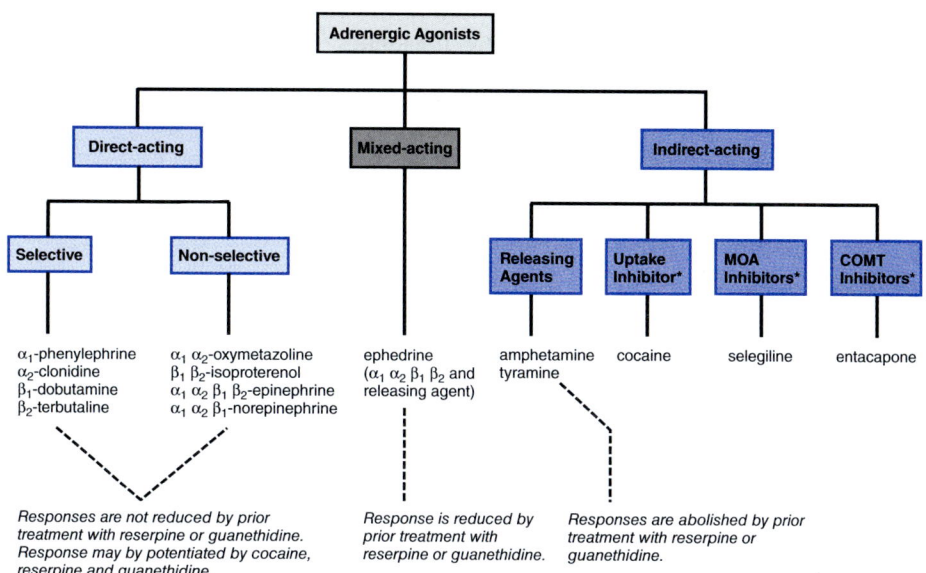

MECHANISMS BY WHICH INDIRECT-ACTING SYMPATHOMIMETIC DRUGS INCREASE NE AND E TO STIMULATE ADRENERGIC RECEPTORS

- Release or displace NE from sympathetic nerve varicosities
- Block the transport of NE into sympathetic nerve terminals
- Block the catecholamine metabolizing enzymes MAO and COMT

FIGURE 7-3 Classification of adrenergic receptor agonists (sympathomimetic amines) or drugs that produce sympathomimetic-like effects. For each category, a prototypical drug is shown. (*Not actually sympathetic drugs but produce sympathomimetic-like effects.)

output and rate, in contrast to vasodilators such as hydralazine that have minimal dilatory effects on veins (see Chapter 15).

b. What is prazosin's mechanism of action?

Blockade of α_1 adrenergic receptors inhibits vasoconstriction induced by endogenous catecholamines; vasodilation may occur in both arteriolar resistance vessels and in veins. The result is a fall in blood pressure due to decreased peripheral resistance. The magnitude of such effects depends on the activity of the sympathetic nervous system at the time the antagonist is administered, and thus is less in supine than in upright subjects and is particularly marked if there is hypovolemia. For most α receptor antagonists, the fall in blood pressure is opposed by baroreceptor reflexes that cause increases in heart rate as well as fluid retention. Prazosin appears to depress baroreflex function in hypertensive patients.

(Continued)

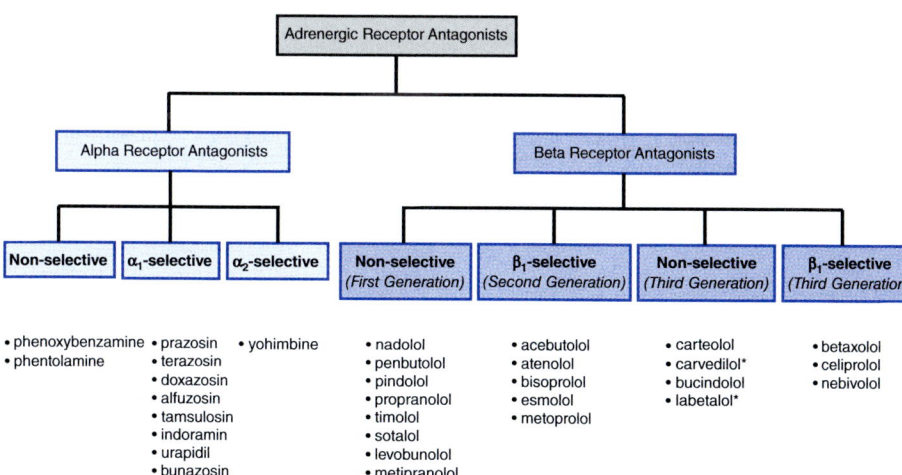

FIGURE 7-4 Classification of adrenergic receptor antagonists. Drugs marked by an asterisk (*) also block α_1 receptors.

SECTION II — Neuropharmacology

TABLE 7-1 Characteristics of Plasma Membrane Transporters for Endogenous Catecholamines

TYPE OF TRANSPORTER	SUBSTRATE SPECIFICITY	TISSUE	REGION/CELL TYPE	INHIBITORS
Neuronal				
NET	DA > NE > Epi	All sympathetically innervated tissue Adrenal medulla Liver Placenta	Sympathetic nerves Chromaffin cells Capillary endothelial cells Syncytiotrophoblast	Desipramine Cocaine Nisoxetine
DAT	DA > NE > Epi	Kidney Stomach Pancreas	Endothelium Parietal and endothelial cells Pancreatic duct	Cocaine Imazindol
Non-neuronal				
OCT1	DA > Epi >> NE	Liver Intestine Kidney (not human)	Hepatocytes Epithelial cells Distal tubule	Isocyanines Corticosterone
OCT2	DA >> NE > Epi	Kidney Brain	Medullary proximal and distal tubules Glial cells of DA-rich regions, some nonadrenergic neurons	Isocyanines Corticosterone
ENT (OCT 3)	Epi >> NE > DA	Liver Brain Heart Blood vessels Kidney Placenta Retina	Hepatocytes Glial cells, others Myocytes Endothelial cells Cortex, proximal and distal tubules Syncytiotrophoblasts (basal membrane) Photoreceptors, ganglion amacrine cells	Isocyanines Corticosterone O-methyl-isoproterenol

NET, norepinephrine transporter, originally known as uptake 1; DAT, dopamine transporter; ENT (OCT3), extraneuronal transporter, originally known as uptake 2; OCT 1, OCT 2, organic cation transporters; Epi, epinephrine; NE, norepinephrine; DA, dopamine.

c. **What are the major side effects of prazosin that this patient should be aware of?**

A major potential adverse effect of prazosin and its congeners is the first-dose effect; marked postural hypotension and syncope sometimes are seen 30 to 90 minutes after an initial dose of prazosin. Syncopal episodes also have occurred with a rapid increase in dosage or with the addition of a second antihypertensive drug to the regimen of a patient who already is taking a large dose of prazosin. It is recommended that patients take their first dose immediately prior to bedtime.

CASE 7-2

A 48-year-old man with the diagnoses of essential hypertension is being treated with clonidine.

a. **What type of drug is clonidine?**

Clonidine, an α_2-selective adrenergic agonist (see Figure 7-3), is used primarily for the treatment of systemic hypertension (see Chapter 15). Clonidine's efficacy as an antihypertensive agent is somewhat surprising, because many blood vessels contain postsynaptic α_2 adrenergic receptors that promote vasoconstriction. Indeed, clonidine, the prototypic α_2 agonist, was initially developed as a vasoconstricting nasal decongestant.

b. **What is clonidine's mechanism of action?**

Clonidine's capacity to lower blood pressure results from activation of α_2 receptors in the cardiovascular control centers of the CNS; such activation suppresses the outflow of sympathetic nervous system activity from the brain. Although the exact mechanism by which clonidine lowers blood pressure is not completely understood, the effect appears to result, at least in part, from activation of α_2 receptors in the lower brainstem region.

(Continued)

Adrenergic, Dopaminergic, and Serotonergic Pharmacology

CHAPTER 7

c. What side effects of clonidine should this patient be warned about?

The major adverse effects of clonidine are dry mouth and sedation. These responses occur in at least 50% of patients and may require drug discontinuation. However, they may diminish in intensity after several weeks of therapy. Sexual dysfunction also may occur. Marked bradycardia is observed in some patients.

Withdrawal reactions follow abrupt discontinuation of long-term therapy with clonidine in some hypertensive patients.

MECHANISM OF ACTION OF β ADRENERGIC RECEPTOR AGONISTS AND ANTAGONISTS

DRUG CLASS	DRUG	MECHANISM OF ACTION
β Adrenergic Receptor Agonists (see Figure 7-3)	Isoproterenol	Potent β adrenergic receptor agonist with very low affinity for α receptors; powerful effect on all β receptors and almost no action on α receptors (see Table 5-1)
	Dobutamine	Direct agonist interactions with α- and β-adrenergic receptors
β_2 Selective Adrenergic Receptor Agonists (see Figure 7-3)	Metaproterenol	Agonist at β_2 adrenergic receptors (see Table 5-1) See Chapter 24
	Albuterol	Agonist at β_2 adrenergic receptors (see Table 5-1) See Chapter 24
	Levalbuterol	Agonist at β_2 adrenergic receptors (see Table 5-1) See Chapter 24
	Pirbuterol	Agonist at β_2 adrenergic receptors (see Table 5-1) See Chapter 24
	Terbutaline	Agonist at β_2 adrenergic receptors (see Table 5-1) See Chapter 24
	Isoetharine	Agonist at β_2 adrenergic receptors (see Table 5-1)
	Bitolterol	Agonist at β_2 adrenergic receptors (see Table 5-1)
	Fenoterol	Agonist at β_2 adrenergic receptors (see Table 5-1)
	Procaterol	Agonist at β_2 adrenergic receptors (see Table 5-1)
	Salmeterol	Agonist at β_2 adrenergic receptors (see Table 5-1) See Chapter 24
	Formoterol	Agonist at β_2 adrenergic receptors (see Table 5-1) See Chapter 24
	Arformoterol	Agonist at β_2 adrenergic receptors (see Table 5-1) See Chapter 24
	Ritodrine	Agonist at β_2 adrenergic receptors (see Table 5-1)
Nonselective β Adrenergic Receptor Antagonists (see Figure 7-4)	Carteolol	Antagonist at β_1 and β_2 adrenergic receptors (see Table 5-1) See Chapter 47
	Propranolol	Antagonist at β_1 and β_2 adrenergic receptors (see Table 5-1) See Chapters 15, 16, 17, and 18
	Nadolol	Antagonist at β_1 and β_2 adrenergic receptors (see Table 5-1) See Chapters 15, 16, 17, and 18
	Levobunolol	Antagonist at β_1 and β_2 adrenergic receptors (see Table 5-1) See Chapter 47
	Metipranolol	Antagonist at β_1 and β_2 adrenergic receptors (see Table 5-1) See Chapter 47

(Continued)

SECTION II — Neuropharmacology

DRUG CLASS	DRUG	MECHANISM OF ACTION
	Timolol	Antagonist at β_1 and β_2 adrenergic receptors (see Table 5-1) See Chapters 15, 16, 17, 18, and 47
	Pindolol	Antagonist at β_1 and β_2 adrenergic receptors (see Table 5-1) See Chapters 15, 16, 17, and 18
β_1 Selective Adrenergic Receptor Antagonists (see Figure 7-4)	Metoprolol	Antagonist at β_1 adrenergic receptors See Chapters 15, 16, 17, and 18
	Betaxolol	Antagonist at β_1 adrenergic receptors See Chapter 47
	Levobetaxolol	Antagonist at β_1 adrenergic receptors See Chapter 47
	Bisoprolol	Antagonist at β_1 adrenergic receptors See Chapters 15, 16, 17, and 18
	Acebutolol	Antagonist at β_1 adrenergic receptors See Chapters 15, 16, 17, and 18
	Atenolol	Antagonist at β_1 adrenergic receptors See Chapters 15, 16, 17, and 18
	Esmolol	Antagonist at β_1 adrenergic receptors that has a very short duration of action
β Adrenergic Receptor Antagonists with Additional Cardiovascular Effects ("Third Generation" β Blockers) (see Figure 7-4)	Labetalol	Competitive antagonist at α_1 and β adrenergic receptors See Chapter 15
	Carvedilol	Competitive antagonist at α_1 and β adrenergic receptors, but also has antioxidant and anti-inflammatory effects (see Figure 7-5) See Chapters 15 and 17
	Bucindolol	Antagonist at β adrenergic receptors with weak α_1 adrenergic receptor blocking properties
	Celiprolol	Third-generation β_1 adrenergic receptor antagonist
	Nebivolol	Third-generation β_1 adrenergic receptor antagonist with endothelial NO-mediated vasodilator activity (see Figure 7-5)

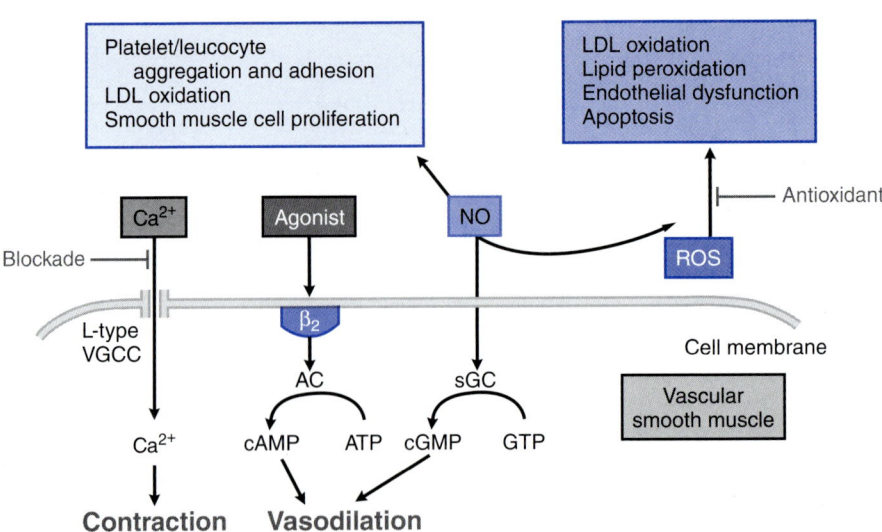

FIGURE 7-5 Mechanisms underlying actions of vasodilating β blockers in blood vessels. ROS, reactive oxygen species; sGC, soluble guanylyl cyclase; AC adenylyl cyclase; L-type VGCC, L-type voltage gated Ca²⁺ channel. *(Modified with permission from Toda N. Vasodilating β-adrenoceptor blockers as cardiovascular therapeutics. Pharmacol Ther, 2003;100:215-234. Copyright © Elsevier.)*

Adrenergic, Dopaminergic, and Serotonergic Pharmacology

CHAPTER 7

CASE 7-3

A 62-year-old woman with chronic obstructive airway disease is being treated with albuterol.

a. What kind of drug is albuterol?

Albuterolol, a selective β_2 receptor agonist (see Figure 7-3), is administered either by inhalation or orally for the symptomatic relief of bronchospasm. Some of the major adverse effects of β receptor agonists in the treatment of asthma or obstructive pulmonary disease (COPD) are caused by stimulation of β_1 receptors in the heart. Accordingly, drugs with preferential affinity for β_2 receptors compared with β_1 receptors have been developed. However, this selectivity is relative, not absolute, and is lost at high concentrations of these drugs.

b. How does albuterol affect airways so that this patient might expect improvement?

In the treatment of asthma and COPD, β receptor agonists are used to activate pulmonary receptors that relax bronchial smooth muscle and decrease airway resistance. Although this action appears to be a major therapeutic effect of these drugs in patients with asthma, evidence suggests that β receptor agonists also may suppress the release of leukotrienes and histamine from mast cells in lung tissue, enhance mucociliary function, decrease microvascular permeability, and possibly inhibit phospholipase A_2. See Chapter 24 for a detailed discussion of the treatment of pulmonary disease with β_2 receptor agonists.

c. What adverse effects should this patient be alerted to?

The major adverse effects of β receptor agonists occur as a result of excessive activation of β receptors. Tachycardia is a common adverse effect of systemically administered β receptor agonists. Stimulation of heart rate occurs primarily by means of β_1 receptors. Patients with underlying cardiovascular disease are particularly at risk for significant reactions. However, the likelihood of adverse effects can be greatly decreased in patients with lung disease by administering the drug by inhalation rather than orally or parenterally.

The risk of adverse cardiovascular effects also is increased in patients who are receiving MAO inhibitors. In general, at least 2 weeks should elapse between the use of MAO inhibitors and administration of β_2 agonists or other sympathomimetics.

Tremor is a relatively common adverse effect of the β_2-selective receptor agonists. Tolerance generally develops to this effect. Feelings of restlessness, apprehension, and anxiety may limit therapy with these drugs, particularly oral or parenteral administration.

CASE 7-4

A 51-year-old man has suffered a myocardial infarction. In the intensive care unit, he is started on the β blocker, metoprolol.

a. Why is this patient started on a β blocker soon after the onset of his myocardial infarction?

A great deal of interest has focused on the use of β receptor antagonists in the treatment of acute myocardial infarction and in the prevention of recurrences for those who have survived an initial attack. Numerous trials have shown that β receptor antagonists administered during the early phases of acute myocardial infarction and continued long-term may decrease mortality by ~25%.

b. What is the mechanism of action of metoprolol?

The pharmacodynamics and pharmacokinetic parameters of β receptor antagonists are shown in Table 7-2. The precise mechanism by which β receptor antagonists

(Continued)

TABLE 7-2 Pharmacological/Pharmacokinetic Properties of β Adrenergic Receptor Blocking Agents

DRUG	MEMBRANE STABILIZING ACTIVITY	INTRINSIC AGONIST ACTIVITY	LIPID SOLUBILITY	EXTENT OF ABSORPTION (%)	ORAL AVAILABILITY (%)	PLASMA $t_{1/2}$ (HOURS)	PROTEIN BINDING (%)
Classical non-selective β blockers: First generation							
Nadolol	0	0	Low	30	30-50	20-24	30
Penbutolol	0	+	High	~100	~100	~5	80-98
Pindolol	+	+++	Low	>95	~100	3-4	40
Propranolol	++	0	High	<90	30	3-5	90
Timolol	0	0	Low to moderate	90	75	4	<10
$β_1$-Selective β blockers: Second generation							
Acebutolol	+	+	Low	90	20-60	3-4	26
Atenolol	0	0	Low	90	50-60	6-7	6-16
Bisoprolol	0	0	Low	≤90	80	9-12	~30
Esmolol	0	0	Low	NA	NA	0.15	55
Metoprolol	+*	0	Moderate	~100	40-50	3-7	12
Non-selective β blockers with additional actions: Third generation							
Carteolol	0	++	Low	85	85	6	23-30
Carvedilol	++	0	Moderate	>90	~30	7-10	98
Labetalol	+	+	Low	>90	~33	3-4	~50
$β_1$-selective β blockers with additional actions: Third generation							
Betaxolol	+	0	Moderate	>90	~80	15	50
Celiprolol	0	+	Low	~74	30-70	5	4-5
Nebivolol	0	0	Low	NA	NA	11-30	

*Detectable only at doses much greater than required for β blockade.

decrease mortality and morbidity after a myocardial infarction is not known, but the favorable effects may stem from decreased myocardial oxygen demand, redistribution of myocardial blood flow, and antiarrhythmic actions. There is likely much less benefit if β adrenergic receptor antagonists are administered for only a short time. In studies of secondary prevention, the most extensive, favorable clinical trial data are available for propranolol, metoprolol, and timolol. In spite of these proven benefits, many patients with myocardial infarction do not receive a β adrenergic receptor antagonist.

c. **What are the adverse effects of β blockers?**

The most common adverse effects of β receptor antagonists arise as pharmacological consequences of blockade of β receptors (see Table 5-1); serious adverse effects unrelated to β receptor blockade are rare. β Receptor blockade may cause or exacerbate heart failure in patients with decompensated heart failure, acute myocardial infarction, or cardiomegaly. Abrupt discontinuation of β receptor antagonists after long-term treatment can exacerbate angina and may increase the risk of sudden death.

(Continued)

Adrenergic, Dopaminergic, and Serotonergic Pharmacology

CHAPTER 7

A major adverse effect of β receptor antagonists is caused by blockade of β_2 receptors in bronchial smooth muscle. Drugs with selectivity for β_1 receptors or those with intrinsic sympathomimetic activity at β_2 receptors seem less likely to induce bronchospasm. Since the selectivity of current β blockers for β_1 receptors is modest, these drugs should be avoided if at all possible in patients with asthma.

The adverse effects of β receptor antagonists that are referable to the CNS may include fatigue, sleep disturbances (including insomnia and nightmares), and depression.

β Adrenergic blockade may blunt recognition of hypoglycemia by diabetic patients; it also may delay recovery from insulin-induced hypoglycemia. β Receptor antagonists should be used with great caution in patients with diabetes who are prone to hypoglycemic reactions; β_1-selective agents may be preferable for these patients.

CASE 7-5

A 58-year-old woman has suffered from mild heart failure for 5 years. She has been treated with carvedilol. She recently changed to a different physician who questions the use of a β blocker to treat heart failure.

a. **Why would her new physician question the use of a β blocker to treat heart failure?**

It is a common clinical observation that administration of β receptor antagonists can worsen markedly or even precipitate congestive heart failure in compensated patients with multiple forms of heart disease, such as ischemic or congestive cardiomyopathy. Consequently, the hypothesis that β receptor antagonists might be efficacious in the long-term treatment of heart failure originally seemed counterintuitive to many physicians.

Carvedilol, metoprolol, and bisoprolol all have been shown to reduce the mortality rate in large cohorts of patients with stable chronic heart failure regardless of severity. Treatment of patients with congestive heart failure with β receptor antagonists should only be undertaken by physicians with experience in using these drugs for this purpose.

b. **What is the mechanism of action of carvedilol for this indication?**

A number of mechanisms have been proposed to play a role in the beneficial effects of β receptor antagonists in heart failure. Since chronic excess catecholamines may be toxic to the heart, especially through activation of β_1 receptors, inhibition of the pathway may help preserve myocardial function. Also, antagonism of β receptors in the heart may attenuate cardiac remodeling, which ordinarily might have deleterious effects on cardiac function. Interestingly, activation of β receptors and elevation of cellular cyclic AMP may promote myocardial cell death by apoptosis. In addition, properties of certain β receptor antagonists that are due to other, unrelated properties of these drugs may be potentially important. For example, afterload reduction by drugs such as carvedilol may be clinically relevant (see Table 7-3 and Figure 7-5).

TABLE 7-3 Third Generation β Receptor Antagonists with Putative Additional Mechanisms of Vasodilation

NITRIC OXIDE PRODUCTION	β_2 RECEPTOR AGONISM	α_1 RECEPTOR ANTAGONISM	Ca^{2+} ENTRY BLOCKADE	K^+ CHANNEL OPENING	ANTIOXIDANT ACTIVITY
Celiprolol[a]	Celiprolol[a]	Carvedilol	Carvedilol	Tilisolol[a]	Carvedilol
Nebivolol	Carteolol	Bucindolol[a]	Betaxolol		
Carteolol	Bopindolol[a]	Bevantolol[a]	Bevantolol[a]		
Bopindolol[a]		Nipradilol[a]			
Nipradilol[a]		Labetalol			

[a]Not currently available in the United States, where most are under investigation for use.

SECTION II — Neuropharmacology

MECHANISM OF ACTION OF DRUGS ACTING AT SEROTINERGIC AND DOPAMINERGIC RECEPTORS

DRUG CLASS	DRUG	MECHANISM OF ACTION
Selective Serotonin (5-HT) Reuptake Inhibitors (SSRIs)	Fluoxetine Citalopram Escitalopram Fluvoxamine Paroxetine Sertraline	Inhibition of presynaptic reaccumulation of neuronally released 5-HT
Serotonin (5-HT)/Norepinephrine (NE) Reuptake Inhibitors (SNRIs)	Duloxetine Venlafaxine Desvenlafaxine Minacipran Sibutramine	Selective reuptake inhibitor of 5-HT and NE
MAO Inhibitors That Alter 5-HT Concentrations	Phenelzine Tranylcypromine Isocarboxazid	MAO inhibition that results in alteration of 5-HT (see Figure 7-6)
5-HT Receptor Agonists	Buspirone	$5\text{-}HT_{1A}$ receptor-selective partial agonist
	Almotripan Eletriptan Frovatriptan Naratriptan Rizatriptan Sumatriptan Zolmitriptan	$5\text{-}HT_{1B/1D}$ receptor-selective agonist (see Table 7-4)
Ergot Alkaloid Derivative	Methylsergide	$5\text{-}HT_{2A/2C}$ receptor antagonist with some partial agonist activity (see Table 7-4)
5-HT Receptor Antagonists	Ondansetron Dolasetron Granisetrol Palonosetron Alosetron	$5\text{-}HT_{3}$ receptor antagonist (see Table 7-4)
	Clozapine	$5\text{-}HT_{2A/2C}$ receptor antagonist (see Table 7-4 and Chapter 8)
	Respiradone	$5\text{-}HT_{2A}$ and D_2 receptor antagonist (see Table 7-4 and Chapter 8)
	Quetiapine	5-HT and DA receptor antagonist (see Table 7-4 and Chapter 8)
	Olanzepine	5-HT and DA receptor antagonist (see Table 7-4 and Chapter 8)
Dopamine (DA) Receptor Agonists	Bromocriptine	Ergot derivative that is a D_1/D_2 receptor agonist
	Pergolide	Ergot derivative that is a D_1/D_2 receptor agonist
	Cabergoline	Ergot derivative that is a strong D_2 receptor agonist
	Apomorphine	Non-ergot alkaloid with agonist properties at dopamine receptors with an order of potency $D_4>D_2>D_3>D_5$
	Rotigotine	Dopamine receptor agonist with preferential binding to D_2 and D_3 receptors
	Pramipexole	Selective D_2 receptor agonist (see Chapter 13)
	Ropinirole	Selective D_2 receptor agonist (see Chapter 13)
Dopamine (DA) Receptor Antagonists	Aripiprazole	Partial agonist at D_2 receptors (see Chapter 8)

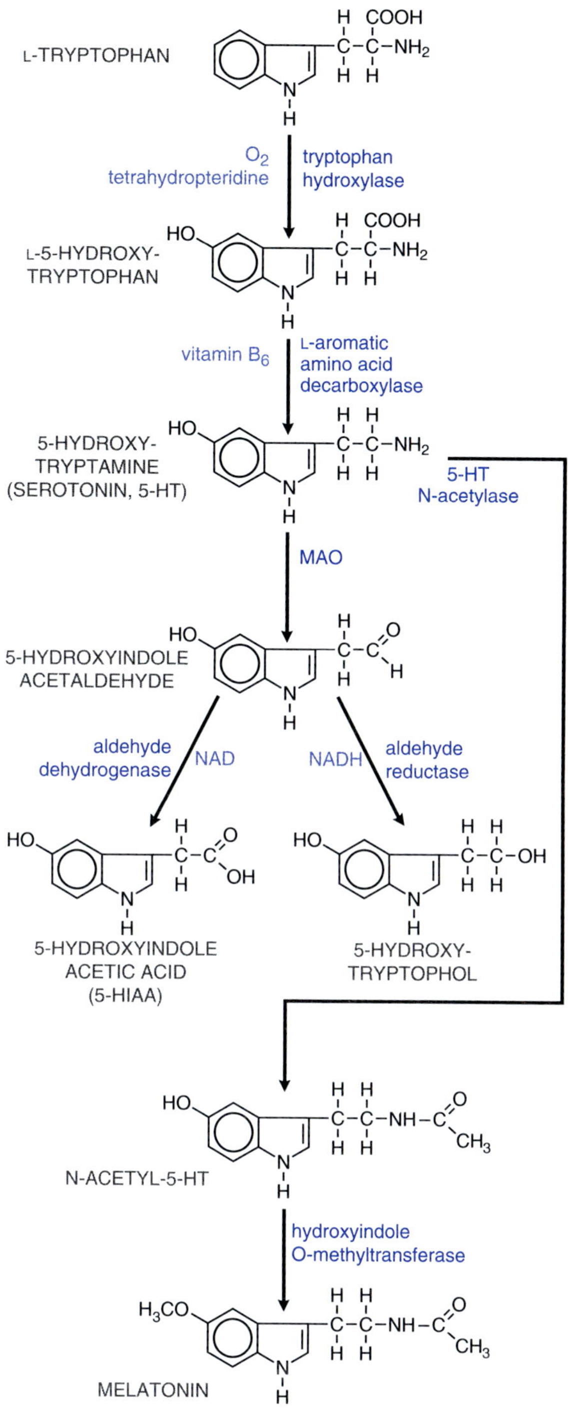

Adrenergic, Dopaminergic, and Serotonergic Pharmacology

CHAPTER 7

FIGURE 7-6 Synthesis and inactivation of serotonin. Enzymes and co-factors are shown in blue.

CASE 7-6

A 36-year-old woman has been going through a difficult divorce for the past year. Two weeks ago her father died. She now presents to her physician with moderate situational depression and is started on the selective serotonin reuptake inhibitor (SSRI) fluoxetine.

a. Why is a drug that modulates serotonin (5-HT) at nerve endings effective in treating depression?

The synthesis and inactivation of serotonin is shown in Figure 7-6 and the actions and clinical indications of serotonergic drugs are presented in Table 7-5. A multitude

(Continued)

TABLE 7-4 Serotonin Receptor Subtypes

STRUCTURAL FAMILIES

5-HT$_1$, 5-HT$_2$, 5-HT$_{4-7}$: G protein–coupled receptor

5-HT$_3$: 5-HT–gated ion channel

SUBTYPE	GENE STRUCTURE	SIGNAL TRANSDUCTION	LOCALIZATION	FUNCTION	SELECTIVE AGONIST	SELECTIVE ANTAGONIST
5-HT$_{1A}$	Intronless	↓ AC	Raphe nuclei Cortex Hippocampus	Autoreceptor	8-OH-DPAT	WAY 100135
5-HT$_{1B}$[a]	Intronless	↓ AC	Subiculum Globus pallidus Substantia nigra	Autoreceptor	—	—
5-HT$_{1D}$	Intronless	↓ AC	Cranial blood vessels Globus pallidus Substantia nigra	Vasoconstriction	Sumatriptan	—
5-HT$_{1E}$	Intronless	↓ AC	Cortex Striatum	—	—	—
5-HT$_{1F}$[b]	Intronless	↓ AC	Brain and periphery	—	—	—
5-HT$_{2A}$ (D receptor)	Introns	↑ PLC and ↑ PLA$_2$	Platelets Smooth muscle Cerebral cortex	Aggregation Contraction Neuronal excitation	α-Methyl-5-HT, DOI, MCPP	Ketanserin LY53857 MDL 100, 907
5-HT$_{2B}$	Introns	↑ PLC	Stomach fundus	Contraction	α-Methyl-5-HT, DOI	LY53857 SB206553
5-HT$_{2C}$	Introns	↑ PLC ↑ PLA$_2$	Choroid plexus Hypothalamus	CSF production Neuronal excitation	α-Methyl-5-HT, DOI, MK 2.2	LY53857 SB 2022084 Mesulergine
5-HT$_3$ (M receptor)	Introns	Ligand-operated ion channel	Parasympathetic nerves Solitary tract Area postrema	Neuronal excitation	2-Methyl-5-HT	Ondansetron Tropisetron
5-HT$_4$	Introns	↑ AC	Hippocampus GI tract	Neuronal excitation	Renzapride	GR 113808
5-HT$_{5A}$	Introns	↓ AC	Hippocampus	Unknown	—	—
5-HT$_{5B}$	Introns	Unknown	—	Pseudogene	—	—
5-HT$_6$	Introns	↑ AC	Hippocampus Striatum Nucleus accumbens	Neuronal excitation	—	SB 271046
5-HT$_7$	Introns	↑ AC	Hypothalamus Hippocampus GI tract	Unknown	5-carboxamino-tryptamine	

[a]Also referred to as 5-HT$_{1DB}$.
[b]Also referred to as 5-HT$_{1EB}$.
AC, adenylyl cyclase; PLC, phospholipase C; PLA$_2$, phospholipase A$_2$; 8-OH-DPAT, 8-hydroxy-(2-N,N-dipropylamino)-tetraline; DOI, 1-(2,5-dimethoxy-4-iodophenyl) isopropylamine;
MCPP, metachlorphenylpiperazine; MK212.

of brain functions are influenced by 5-HT, including sleep, cognition, sensory perception, motor activity, temperature regulation, nociception, mood, appetite, sexual behavior, and hormone secretion. All of the cloned 5-HT receptors are expressed in the brain, often in overlapping domains (see Table 7-4). Although patterns of 5-HT receptor expression in individual neurons have not been extensively defined, it is likely that multiple 5-HT receptor subtypes with similar or opposing actions are expressed in individual neurons, leading to a tremendous diversity of actions.

(Continued)

Adrenergic, Dopaminergic, and Serotonergic Pharmacology

CHAPTER 7

TABLE 7-5 Serotonergic Drugs: Primary Actions and Clinical Indications

RECEPTOR	ACTION	DRUG EXAMPLES	CLINICAL DISORDER
5-HT$_{1A}$	Partial agonist	Buspirone, ipsaperone	Anxiety, depression
5-HT$_{1D}$	Agonist	Sumatriptan	Migraine
5-HT$_{2A/2C}$	Antagonist	Methysergide, risperidone, ketanserin	Migraine, depression, schizophrenia
5-HT$_3$	Antagonist	Ondansetron	Chemotherapy-induced emesis
5-HT$_4$	Agonist	Cisapride	GI disorders
SERT (5-HT transporter)	Inhibitor	Fluoxetine, sertraline	Depression, obsessive-compulsive disorder, panic disorder, social phobia, post-traumatic stress disorder

The effects of 5-HT–active drugs in anxiety and depressive disorders, like the effects of selective serotonin reuptake inhibitors (SSRIs), strongly suggest a role for 5-HT in the neurochemical mediation of these disorders.

b. What are the adverse effects of fluoxetine?

Excessive stimulation of brain 5-HT$_2$ receptors may result in insomnia, increased anxiety, irritability, and decreased libido, effectively worsening prominent depressive symptoms. Excess activity at spinal 5-HT$_2$ receptors causes sexual side effects, including erectile dysfunction, anorgasmia, and ejaculatory delay.

Stimulation of 5-HT$_3$ receptors in the CNS and periphery contributes to GI effects, which are usually limited to nausea but may include diarrhea and emesis. Some patients experience an increase in anxiety, especially with the initial dosing of SSRIs. With continued treatment, some patients also report a dullness of intellectual abilities and concentration. In addition, a phenomenon of a residual "flat affect" can occur in an otherwise successful treatment with SSRIs.

c. Although this patient is otherwise healthy and is taking no other drugs, of what drug interactions should she be warned?

Most antidepressants, including the SSRIs, exhibit drug–drug interactions based on their routes of metabolism CYPs (see Chapter 8). Paroxetine and, to a lesser degree, fluoxetine are potent inhibitors of CYP2D6. The other SSRIs, outside of fluvoxamine, are at least moderate inhibitors of CYP2D6. This inhibition can result in disproportionate increases in plasma concentrations of drugs metabolized by CYP2D6.

Another important drug–drug interaction with SSRIs occurs via a pharmacodynamic mechanism. MAOIs enhance the effects of SSRIs due to inhibition of serotonin metabolism (see Figure 7-6 and Chapters 5 and 8). Administration of these drugs together can produce synergistic increases in extracellular brain serotonin, leading to the serotonin syndrome. Symptoms of the serotonin syndrome include hyperthermia, muscle rigidity, myoclonus, tremors, autonomic instability, confusion, irritability, and agitation; this can progress toward coma and death.

> **EVIDENCE SUGGESTING THAT 5-HT IS A KEY MEDIATOR IN THE PATHOGENESIS OF MIGRAINE**
>
> - Plasma and platelet concentrations of 5-HT vary with the different phases of the migraine attack.
> - Urinary concentrations of 5-HT and its metabolites are elevated during most migraine attacks.
> - Migraine may be precipitated by agents (eg, reserpine and fenfluramine) that release 5-HT from intracellular storage sites.

CASE 7-7

A 23-year-old woman suffers from migraine headaches. She is given a prescription for the 5-HT receptor agonist sumitriptan and told to take it as soon as a migraine starts.

a. Why is she given a drug that is a 5-HT receptor agonist?

The evidence that 5-HT is important in the pathogenesis of migraine headaches is shown in the Side Bar EVIDENCE SUGGESTING THAT 5-HT IS A KEY MEDIATOR IN THE PATHOGENESIS OF MIGRAINE. Consistent with this 5-HT hypothesis, 5-HT receptor agonists have become a mainstay for acute treatment of migraine headaches. The triptans are effective, acute antimigraine agents. Their

(Continued)

SECTION II Neuropharmacology

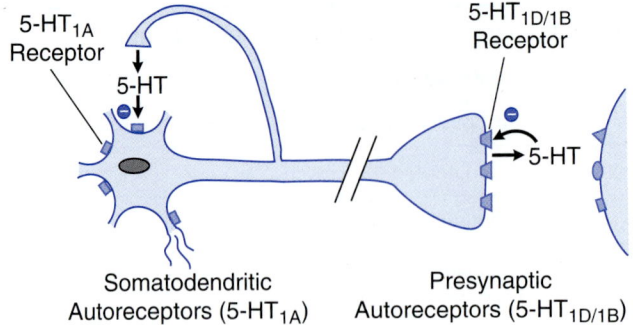

FIGURE 7-7 Two classes of 5-HT autoreceptors with differential localizations. Somatodendritic 5-HT$_{1A}$ autoreceptors decrease raphe cell firing when activated by 5-HT released from axon collaterals of the same or adjacent neurons. The receptor subtype of the presynaptic autoreceptor on axon terminals in the forebrain has different pharmacological properties and has been classified as 5-HT$_{1D}$ (in humans) or 5-HT$_{1B}$ (in rodents). This receptor modulates the release of 5-HT. Postsynaptic 5-HT$_1$ receptors are also indicated.

ability to decrease, rather than exacerbate, the nausea and vomiting of migraine is an important advance in the treatment of the condition.

b. What is the mechanism of action of sumitriptan?

There remains a controversy about the relative importance of vascular versus neurological dysfunction in migraine; thus the mechanism of the efficacy of 5-HT$_{1B/1D}$ agonists in migraine is not resolved.

According to a prominent pathophysiological model of migraine, unknown events lead to the abnormal dilation of carotid arteriovenous anastomoses in the head and shunting of carotid arterial blood flow, producing cerebral ischemia and hypoxia. Based on this model, an effective antimigraine agent would close the shunts and restore blood flow to the brain. Indeed, sumatriptan has the capacity to produce this vascular effect with a pharmacological specificity that mirrors the effects of these agents on 5-HT$_{1B}$ and 5-HT$_{1D}$ receptor subtypes.

An alternative hypothesis concerning the significance of one or more 5-HT$_1$ receptors in migraine pathophysiology relates to the observation that both 5-HT$_{1B}$ and 5-HT$_{1D}$ receptors serve as presynaptic autoreceptors, modulating neurotransmitter release from neuronal terminals (see Figure 7-7). 5-HT$_1$ agonists may block the release of proinflammatory neuropeptides at the level of the nerve terminal in the perivascular space, which could account for their efficacy in the acute treatment of migraine.

c. What are the adverse effects of sumitriptan?

Rare but serious cardiac events have been associated with the administration of 5-HT$_1$ agonists, including coronary artery vasospasm, transient myocardial ischemia, atrial and ventricular arrhythmias, and myocardial infarction, predominantly in patients with risk factors for coronary artery disease. Orally administered triptans can cause paresthesias; asthenia and fatigue; flushing; feelings of pressure, tightness, or pain in the chest, neck, and jaw; drowsiness; dizziness; nausea; and sweating.

The triptans are contraindicated in patients who have a history of ischemic or vasospastic coronary artery disease (including history of stroke or transient ischemic attacks), cerebrovascular or peripheral vascular disease, hemiplegic or basilar migraines, other significant cardiovascular diseases, or ischemic bowel diseases.

KEY CONCEPTS

- Catecholamines and sympathomimetic drugs are classified as direct-acting, indirect-acting, or mixed-acting (see Figures 7-3 and 7-4).
- The pharmacological effects of adrenergic agonists and antagonists can be predicted from the distribution of α and β adrenergic receptors (see Table 5-1).

(Continued)

Adrenergic, Dopaminergic, and Serotonergic Pharmacology
CHAPTER 7

➡ Drugs that are selective for a particular adrenergic receptor subtype may have therapeutic benefits, but the selectivity is relative, not absolute, and is often lost at higher concentrations.

➡ Adverse effects and toxicity of adrenergic agonists and antagonist can mostly be predicted from the distribution of α and β adrenergic receptors (see Table 5-1).

➡ Adrenergic agonists and antagonists have broad and varied therapeutic uses, including the treatment of shock, hypotension, hypertension, cardiac arrhythmias, congestive heart failure, nasal decongestion, asthma and chronic pulmonary disease (COPD), allergic reactions, glaucoma, narcolepsy, weight reduction, and attention-deficit/hyperactivity disorder (ADHD).

➡ Serotonin (5-HT) and dopamine (DA) are neurotransmitters in the CNS and also have prominent peripheral actions.

➡ The multiple actions of 5-HT and DA involve interaction with distinct 5-HT and DA receptor subtypes, respectively.

➡ Many of the therapeutic effects of 5-HT and DA agonists and antagonists in the CNS are discussed in detail in Chapter 8 Psychopharmacology and Chapter 13 Drug Therapy of Neurodegenerative Diseases.

SUMMARY QUIZ

QUESTION 7-1 Despite its ability to stimulate receptors in the sympathetic nervous system, norepinephrine has relatively little capacity to increase bronchial airflow because the receptors in bronchial smooth muscle are largely of the

a. $β_2$ subtype.
b. $α_1$ subtype.
c. D_2 subtype.
d. $5-HT_4$ subtype.
e. M_3 subtype.

QUESTION 7-2 A 38-year-old man is taking tranylcypromine, an MAO inhibitor, for depression. After a celebratory dinner, he develops a severe headache and chest pain. At hospital his blood pressure is 190/135 mm Hg. His hypertensive crisis is likely due to the ingestion of

a. green salad.
b. chocolate cake.
c. red wine.
d. broiled salmon.
e. wheat bread.

QUESTION 7-3 A 53-year-old woman with COPD is using an albuterol inhaler for symptomatic relief of bronchospasm. She does not like using her inhaler because it causes

a. her lips to turn black.
b. her heart to beat faster.
c. numbness in her fingers and toes.
d. transient blindness.
e. transient diminished hearing.

QUESTION 7-4 A 23-year-old male college student is taking amphetamine on a regular basis to stay alert while studying. The mechanism of action of amphetamine that causes this effect is

a. due to the release of epinephrine (E) from the adrenal medulla.
b. due to the release of histamine from mast cells.

SECTION II Neuropharmacology

   c. due to the stimulation of β receptors in the frontal cortex of the brain.

   d. due to the release of norepinephrine (NE) from central adrenergic neurons.

   e. the result of inhibition of monoamine oxidase (MAO).

QUESTION 7-5 A 34-year-old woman has been frequently using a nasal spray containing the α adrenergic receptor agonist oxymetazoline for nasal decongestion. She has recently noticed that it is less effective and her symptoms are worse. This loss of efficacy is most likely due to

   a. the fact that her spray container is empty.

   b. degradation of the oxymetazoline.

   c. a manufacturing defect in the nasal spray container.

   d. a loss of innervation to her nasal mucosa.

   e. rebound hyperemia of her nasal mucosa.

QUESTION 7-6 A 32-year-old woman with the diagnosis of a pheochromocytoma is scheduled for surgery to remove her adrenal tumor. The best drug to control her episodes of severe hypertension prior to surgery would be

   a. a nonselective α adrenergic antagonist such as phenoxybenzamine.

   b. a selective $α_2$ adrenergic receptor agonist such as clonidine.

   c. a selective $β_2$ adrenergic receptor agonist such as terbutaline.

   d. a nonselective β adrenergic receptor antagonist such as propranolol.

   e. a selective $α_1$ adrenergic receptor antagonist such as terazosin.

QUESTION 7-7 The typical dose of oral propranolol for the treatment of hypertension is 320 mg/day. The typical dose of IV propranolol to treat a life-threatening arrhythmia is 1 to 3 mg administered slowly. The reason for the discrepancy in these doses is

   a. β adrenergic receptors are more sensitive to IV than oral propranolol.

   b. the IV dose avoids the "first pass" metabolism of oral propranolol.

   c. treatment of hypertension requires a higher dose of propranolol than does treatment of a cardiac arrhythmia.

   d. the density of $β_2$ receptors in the heart is greater than the density of $β_2$ receptors on blood vessels.

   e. oral propranolol is excreted by the kidney at a faster rate than IV propranolol.

QUESTION 7-8 A 32-year-old woman is taking sertraline for mild depression. This drug increases the availability of serotonin (5-HT) at the postsynaptic membrane because it

   a. stimulates $5-HT_4$ receptors.

   b. enhances the release of 5-HT from presynaptic nerve endings.

   c. inhibits the presynaptic uptake of 5-HT.

   d. blocks MAO which degrades 5-HT.

   e. enhances the synthesis of 5-HT.

QUESTION 7-9 A 35-year-old man is taking buspirone for anxiety. This drug acts as a(n)

   a. partial agonist at $5-HT_{1A}$ receptors.

   b. inhibitor of 5-HT reuptake into presynaptic nerve terminals.

   c. agonist at dopamine receptors.

   d. agonist at $α_2$ adrenergic receptors.

   e. antagonist at M_3 receptors.

QUESTION 7-10 A major mechanism for the termination of dopamine's (DA) postsynaptic effect is

   a. downregulation of DA postsynaptic receptors.

   b. degradation of DA in postsynaptic nerve terminals.

Adrenergic, Dopaminergic, and Serotonergic Pharmacology

c. decreased synthesis of DA.
d. blockage of postsynaptic β adrenergic receptors.
e. reuptake of DA into presynaptic nerve terminals.

SUMMARY QUIZ ANSWER KEY

QUESTION 7-1 Answer is **a.** An important factor in the response of any cell or organ to sympathomimetic amines is the density and proportion of α- and β adrenergic receptors (see Table 5-1). For example, NE has relatively little capacity to increase bronchial airflow, since the receptors in bronchial smooth muscle are largely of the β_2 subtype.

QUESTION 7-2 Answer is **c.** MAO is an enzyme involved in the inactivation of catecholamines (see Figure 7-1). Patients who have received MAO inhibitors may experience severe hypertensive crises if they ingest cheese, beer, or red wine. These and related foods, which are produced by fermentation, contain a large quantity of tyramine, and to a lesser degree, other phenylethylamines. When GI and hepatic MAOs are inhibited, the large quantity of tyramine that is ingested is absorbed rapidly and reaches the systemic circulation in high concentration. A massive and precipitous release of NE can result with consequent hypertension that can be severe enough to cause myocardial infarction or a stroke (see Figures 7-1 and 7-2).

QUESTION 7-3 Answer is **b.** Some of the major adverse effects of β receptor agonists in the treatment of asthma or chronic obstructive pulmonary disease (COPD) are caused by stimulation of β_1 receptors in the heart. Accordingly, drugs with preferential affinity for β_2 receptors compared with β_1 receptors have been developed. However, this selectivity is relative, not absolute, and is lost at high concentrations of these drugs. Moreover up to 40% of the β receptors in the human heart are β_2 receptors, activation of which can cause cardiac stimulation.

QUESTION 7-4 Answer is **d.** The alerting effect of amphetamine, its anorectic effect, and at least a component of its locomotor-stimulating action presumably are mediated by release of NE from central noradrenergic neurons. Amphetamine appears to exert most or all of its effects in the CNS by releasing biogenic amines from their storage sites in nerve terminals; the neuronal dopamine transporter (DAT) and the vesicular monoamine transporter 2 (VMAT2) appear to be two of the principal targets of amphetamine's action (see Figure 7-2).

QUESTION 7-5 Answer is **e.** α-Adrenergic receptor agonists are used extensively as nasal decongestants in patients with allergic or vasomotor rhinitis and in acute rhinitis in patients with upper respiratory infections. These drugs probably decrease resistance to airflow by decreasing the volume of the nasal mucosa; this may occur by activation of α adrenergic receptors in venous capacitance vessels in nasal tissues that have erectile characteristics.

Intense constriction of these vessels may cause structural damage to the mucosa. A major limitation of therapy with nasal decongestants is loss of efficacy, "rebound" hyperemia, and worsening of symptoms with chronic use or when the drug is stopped. Although the mechanisms are uncertain, possibilities include receptor desensitization and damage to the mucosa.

QUESTION 7-6 Answer is **a.** One use of phenoxybenzamine is in the treatment of pheochromocytoma. Pheochromocytomas are tumors of the adrenal medulla and sympathetic neurons that secrete enormous quantities of catecholamines into the circulation. The usual result is hypertension, which may be episodic and severe. The vast majority of pheochromocytomas are treated surgically; however, phenoxybenzamine is often used in preparing the patient for surgery. The drug controls episodes of severe hypertension and minimizes other adverse effects of catecholamines, such as contraction of plasma volume and injury of the myocardium. β-Receptor antagonists also are used to treat pheochromocytoma, but only after the administration of a nonselective α-receptor antagonist.

Neuropharmacology

QUESTION 7-7 Answer is **b**. Propranolol is highly lipophilic and is almost completely absorbed after oral administration. However, much of the drug is metabolized by the liver during its first passage through the portal circulation; on average, only ~25% reaches the systemic circulation.

QUESTION 7-8 Answer is **c**. A highly specific mechanism for altering synaptic availability of 5-HT is inhibition of presynaptic reaccumulation of neuronally released 5-HT. Through this mechanism serotonin reuptake inhibitors (SSRIs), such as sertraline, potentiate and prolong the action of 5-HT released by neuronal activity.

Newly formed 5-HT is rapidly accumulated in synaptic vesicles (through VMAT2), where it is protected from MAO. 5-HT released by nerve-impulse flow is reaccumulated into the presynaptic terminal by the 5-HT transporter, SERT (SLC6A4) (see Chapter 2). Presynaptic reuptake is a highly efficient mechanism for terminating the action of 5-HT released by nerve-impulse flow. MAO localized in postsynaptic elements and surrounding cells rapidly inactivates 5-HT that escapes neuronal reuptake and storage.

QUESTION 7-9 Answer is **a**. Long-chain arylpiperazines such as buspirone are selective partial agonists at 5-HT$_{1A}$ receptors. Other closely related arylpiperazines act as 5-HT$_{1A}$-receptor antagonists. Buspirone, the first clinically available drug in this series, has been effective in the treatment of anxiety (see Chapter 8).

QUESTION 7-10 Answer is **e**. Synaptically released DA is subject to both transporter clearance and metabolism (see Figure 7-8). The DA transporter (DAT) is not selective

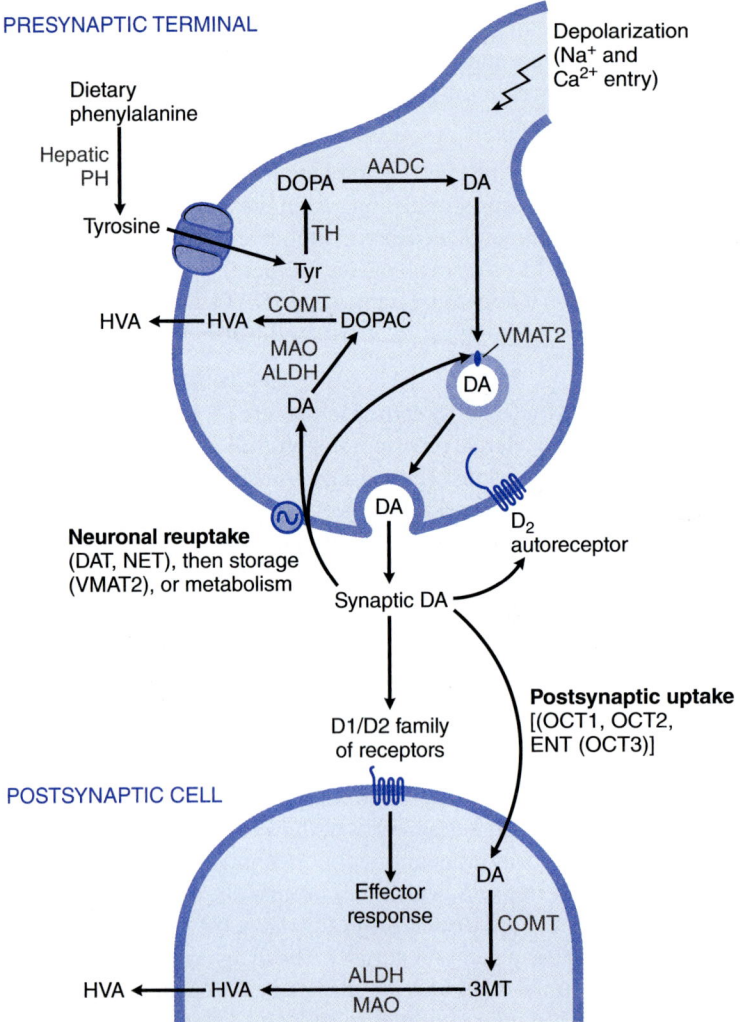

FIGURE 7-8 Dopaminergic terminal. Illustrated are the sequence of events (synthesis, release, postsynaptic receptors, reuptake, and metabolism) that take place at synaptic terminals.

Adrenergic, Dopaminergic, and Serotonergic Pharmacology

CHAPTER 7

for DA; moreover, DA can also be cleared from the synapse by the NE transporter, NET. Reuptake of DA by the DA transporter is the primary mechanism for termination of DA action and allows for either vesicular repackaging of transmitter or metabolism.

SUMMARY TABLE ADRENERGIC, DOPAMINERGIC, AND SEROTONERGIC PHARMACOLOGY

CLASS AND SUBCLASSES	NAMES	CLINICAL USES	TOXICITIES COMMON	TOXICITIES UNIQUE; CLINICALLY IMPORTANT
Endogenous Catecholamines	Epinephrine (E)	Used to provide rapid, emergency relief of anaphylactic reactions. Used in combination with local anesthetics to prolong their action (see Chapter 11). Used to restore cardiac rhythm in patients in cardiac arrest	Restlessness, throbbing headaches, tremor, and palpitations	Contraindicated in patients who are receiving a nonselective β adrenergic receptor antagonist, since unopposed actions on vascular α_1 receptors may lead to severe hypertension. Cerebral hemorrhage and cardiac arrhythmia
	Norepinephrine (NE)	Used as a vasoconstrictor to raise or support blood pressure under certain intensive care conditions	Similar to epinephrine	Excessive dose may result in severe hypertension; extravasation at the site of IV injection may result in tissue necrosis
	Dopamine (DA)	Used in treatment of severe congestive heart failure. Also used to treat cardiogenic and septic shock	Nausea, vomiting, tachycardia, anginal pain, arrhythmia, headache, hypertension	Extravasation may cause tissue necrosis. Should be avoided or used with reduced dose in patients receiving a MAO inhibitor
Dopamine Derivatives	Fenoldopam	Dopamine derivative used for control of severe hypertension	Headache, flushing, dizziness	Tachycardia or bradycardia
	Dopexamine	Used to treat congestive heart failure, sepsis, and shock		Tachycardia and hypotension at high infusion rates
α_1-Selective Adrenergic Receptor Agonists (see Figure 7-3)	Phenylephrine	Used as a nasal decongestant and a mydriatic		
	Mephentermine	Used to prevent hypotension which accompanies spinal anesthesia (Discontinued in the United States)	CNS stimulation	Excessive rise in blood pressure and arrhythmias
	Meteraminol	Used in the treatment of hypotensive states		
	Midodrine	Used to treat autonomic insufficiency and postural hypotension	Supine hypertension	
α_2-Selective Adrenergic Receptor Agonists (see Figure 7-3)	Clonidine	Used to treat hypertension (see Chapter 15). Used off-label to treat diarrhea in patients with autonomic neuropathy and useful in treating withdrawal in patients addicted to narcotic, alcohol, and tobacco. Used preoperatively for sedation and anxiolysis. Transdermal administration may be useful to treat menopausal hot flashes	Dry mouth and sedation. Sexual dysfunction may occur	Marked bradycardia. Contact dermatitis with transdermal patch. Withdrawal reaction upon abrupt discontinuation of long-term therapy. Use with caution in patients with cardiovascular disease
	Dexmedetomidine	Used to treat hypertension (see Chapter 15). Used off-label to treat diarrhea in patients with autonomic neuropathy and useful in treating withdrawal in patients addicted to narcotic, alcohol, and tobacco. Used preoperatively for sedation and anxiolysis	Dry mouth and sedation. Sexual dysfunction may occur	Marked bradycardia. Withdrawal reaction upon abrupt discontinuation of long-term therapy. Use with caution in patients with cardiovascular disease

SECTION II Neuropharmacology

CLASS AND SUBCLASSES	NAMES	CLINICAL USES	TOXICITIES	
			COMMON	UNIQUE; CLINICALLY IMPORTANT
	Apraclonidine	Used topically to reduce intraocular pressure	Minimal effects on systemic cardiovascular parameters	Use with caution in patients with cardiovascular disease
	Brimonidine	Used topically to reduce intraocular pressure	Hypotension and sedation	Use with caution in patients with cardiovascular disease
	Guanfacine	Used to treat hypertension (see Chapter 15) Used off-label to treat diarrhea in patients with autonomic neuropathy and useful in treating withdrawal in patients addicted to narcotic, alcohol, and tobacco A sustained-release form is approved for treatment of attention deficit/hyperactivity disorder (ADHD) in children aged 6-17 years	Dry mouth and sedation Sexual dysfunction may occur	Marked bradycardia Withdrawal reaction upon abrupt discontinuation of long-term therapy Use with caution in patients with cardiovascular disease
	Guanabenz	Used to treat hypertension (see Chapter 15)	Dry mouth and sedation	Use with caution in patients with cardiovascular disease
	Methyldopa	Used to treat hypertension (see Chapter 15)		Use with caution in patients with cardiovascular disease
	Tizanidine	Muscle relaxant used for the treatment of spasticity	Dry mouth and sedation	Use with caution in patients with cardiovascular disease
α_1 Adrenergic Receptor Antagonists (see Figure 7-4)	Prazosin	Used to treat hypertension	Syncopal reaction after first dose Headache and dizziness rarely limit treatment	Orthostatic hypotension
	Terazosin	Used to treat hypertension Also used to manage benign prostatic hypertrophy (BPH)	Syncopal reaction after first dose Headache and dizziness rarely limit treatment	Orthostatic hypotension
	Doxazosin	Used to treat hypertension Also used to manage BPH	Syncopal reaction after first dose Headache and dizziness rarely limit treatment	Orthostatic hypotension
	Alfuzosin	Used to treat BPH	Syncopal reaction after first dose Headache and dizziness rarely limit treatment	Orthostatic hypotension
	Tamsulosin	Used to treat BPH	Syncopal reaction after first dose Headache and dizziness rarely limit treatment	Orthostatic hypotension Impaired ejaculation has been reported
	Silodosin	Used to treat BPH	Syncopal reaction after first dose Headache and dizziness rarely limit treatment	Orthostatic hypotension

(Continued)

Adrenergic, Dopaminergic, and Serotonergic Pharmacology — CHAPTER 7

CLASS AND SUBCLASSES	NAMES	CLINICAL USES	TOXICITIES COMMON	TOXICITIES UNIQUE; CLINICALLY IMPORTANT
α_2 Adrenergic Receptor Antagonists (see Figure 7-4)	Yohimbine	Although not approved, it is used off-label to treat male sexual dysfunction	Enhanced motor activity and tremors	
	Phenoxybenzamine	Used in the treatment of pheochromocytoma		Hypotension and reflex cardiac stimulation may cause alarming tachycardia, arrhythmias, or ischemic cardiac events
	Phentolamine	Used in the treatment of pheochromocytoma; used to prevent dermal necrosis after the inadvertent extravasation of an α receptor agonist; Use to reverse the duration of soft-tissue anesthesia		Hypotension and reflex cardiac stimulation may cause alarming tachycardia, arrhythmias, or ischemic cardiac events; Should be used with caution in patients with peptic ulcer disease because of enhanced gastric acid secretion
Additional α Adrenergic Receptor Antagonists (see Figure 7-4)	Ergot Alkaloids	Used in the treatment of migraine (see narrative in Chapter 13 of *Goodman and Gilman's* 12th Edition)	Nausea and vomiting; Leg weakness, numbness and tingling of fingers and toes	Contraindicated in women who are, or who may become pregnant due to increased motor activity of the uterus; Contraindicated in patients with coronary artery disease, hypertension, impaired hepatic or renal function
	Indoramin	Used for the treatment of hypertension, BPH, and the prophylaxis of migraine		
	Ketanserin	Used to treat hypertension		
	Urapidil	Used to treat hypertension		
	Bunazosin	Used to treat hypertension		
Miscellaneous Sympathomimetic Agonists (see Figure 7-3)	Amphetamine	Used for the treatment of narcolepsy and ADHD	Excessive CNS stimulation, with dizziness, tremor, and hyperactive reflexes	Aggressiveness, changes in libido, paranoid hallucinations, panic states, and suicidal tendencies; Cardiovascular effects include hypertension and arrhythmias; Potential for abuse (see Chapter 14)
	Methamphetamine	Schedule II drug with a high potential for abuse; Used off-label for weight reduction	Excessive CNS stimulation, with dizziness, tremor, and hyperactive reflexes	Aggressiveness, changes in libido, paranoid hallucinations, panic states, and suicidal tendencies; Cardiovascular effects include hypertension and arrhythmias; Potential for abuse (see Chapter 14)
	Methylphenidate Dex-methylphenidate Lisdexamphetamine	Used to treat narcolepsy and ADHD	Insomnia, abdominal pain, anorexia, weight loss	Large doses may lead to convulsions; Contraindicated in patients with glaucoma
	Pemoline	Used to treat ADHD; discontinued for use in the United States	Insomnia, abdominal pain, anorexia, weight loss	Large doses may lead to convulsions

(Continued)

CLASS AND SUBCLASSES	NAMES	CLINICAL USES	TOXICITIES	
			COMMON	UNIQUE; CLINICALLY IMPORTANT
	Propylhexedrine	Used to treat allergic or vasomotor rhinitis	Tachycardia and restlessness	Loss of efficacy and rebound hyperemia Use with caution in patients with cardiovascular disease and men with prostatic enlargement Contraindicated in patients taking MAO inhibitors
	Naphazoline	Used to treat conjunctival hyperemia and irritation (see Chapter 47)		Loss of efficacy and rebound hyperemia Use with caution in patients with cardiovascular disease and men with prostatic enlargement Contraindicated in patients taking MAO inhibitors
	Oxymetazoline	Used to treat conjunctival hyperemia and irritation (see Chapter 47) Also used as a nasal decongestant		Loss of efficacy and rebound hyperemia Use with caution in patients with cardiovascular disease and men with prostatic enlargement Contraindicated in patients taking MAO inhibitors
	Xylometazoline	Used to treat conjunctival hyperemia and irritation (see Chapter 47)		Loss of efficacy and rebound hyperemia Use with caution in patients with cardiovascular disease and men with prostatic enlargement Contraindicated in patients taking MAO inhibitors
	Pseudoephedrine	Used to treat allergic or vasomotor rhinitis	Tachycardia and restlessness	Use with caution in patients with cardiovascular disease and men with prostatic enlargement Contraindicated in patients taking MAO inhibitors
	Modafinil	Used to treat narcolepsy	Tachycardia and restlessness	Use with caution in patients with cardiovascular disease and men with prostatic enlargement Contraindicated in patients taking MAO inhibitors
β Adrenergic Receptor Agonists (see Figure 7-3)	Isoproterenol	Used in emergencies to stimulate heart rate in patients with bradycardia, heart block, or torsades de pointes	Palpitations, tachycardia, headache, and flushing	Cardiac ischemia and arrhythmias may occur in patients with coronary artery disease
	Dobutamine	Indicated for the short-term treatment of cardiac decompensation that may occur after cardiac surgery or in patients with congestive heart failure or myocardial infarction	Increased blood pressure and heart rate	Patients with atrial fibrillation are at risk of marked increases in ventricular rate because dobutamine facilitates AV conduction May increase size of a myocardial infarct by increasing myocardial O_2 demand

(Continued)

Adrenergic, Dopaminergic, and Serotonergic Pharmacology — CHAPTER 7

CLASS AND SUBCLASSES	NAMES	CLINICAL USES	TOXICITIES COMMON	TOXICITIES UNIQUE; CLINICALLY IMPORTANT
β_2-Selective Adrenergic Receptor Agonists (see Figure 7-3)	Metaproterenol	Used for the long-term treatment of obstructive airway diseases, asthma, and acute bronchospasm (see Chapter 24)	Muscle tremor, anxiety, restlessness, tachycardia Selectivity is relative and is lost at high concentrations	Dysrhythmias and cardiac effects
	Albuterol	Used for the long-term treatment of obstructive airway diseases and for treatment of acute bronchospasm (see Chapter 24)	Muscle tremor, anxiety, restlessness, tachycardia Selectivity is relative and is lost at high concentrations	Dysrhythmias and cardiac effects
	Levalbuterol	Used for the long-term treatment of obstructive airway diseases and for treatment of acute bronchospasm (see Chapter 24)	Muscle tremor, anxiety, restlessness, tachycardia Selectivity is relative and is lost at high concentrations	Dysrhythmias and cardiac effects
	Pirbuterol	Used for the long-term treatment of obstructive airway diseases and for treatment of acute bronchospasm (see Chapter 24)	Muscle tremor, anxiety, restlessness, tachycardia Selectivity is relative and is lost at high concentrations	Dysrhythmias and cardiac effects
	Terbutaline	Used for the long-term treatment of obstructive airway diseases and for treatment of acute bronchospasm (see Chapter 24)	Muscle tremor, anxiety, restlessness, tachycardia Selectivity is relative and is lost at high concentrations	Dysrhythmias and cardiac effects
	Isoetharine	Used for the long-term treatment of obstructive airway diseases and for treatment of acute bronchospasm (see Chapter 24)	Muscle tremor, anxiety, restlessness, tachycardia Selectivity is relative and is lost at high concentrations	Dysrhythmias and cardiac effects
	Bitolterol	Used for the long-term treatment of obstructive airway diseases and for treatment of acute bronchospasm (see Chapter 24)	Muscle tremor, anxiety, restlessness, tachycardia Selectivity is relative and is lost at high concentrations	Dysrhythmias and cardiac effects
	Fenoterol	Used for the long-term treatment of obstructive airway diseases and for treatment of acute bronchospasm (see Chapter 24)	Muscle tremor, anxiety, restlessness, tachycardia Selectivity is relative and is lost at high concentrations	Dysrhythmias and cardiac effects
	Procaterol	Used for the long-term treatment of obstructive airway diseases and for treatment of acute bronchospasm (see Chapter 24)	Muscle tremor, anxiety, restlessness, tachycardia Selectivity is relative and is lost at high concentrations	Dysrhythmias and cardiac effects
	Salmeterol	Prolonged duration of action (>12 hours) Used for the long-term treatment of obstructive airway diseases Agent of choice for nocturnal asthma (see Chapter 24)	Muscle tremor, anxiety, restlessness, tachycardia Selectivity is relative and is lost at high concentrations	Dysrhythmias and cardiac effects Increased risk of fatal or near fatal asthma attacks

(Continued)

SECTION II Neuropharmacology

CLASS AND SUBCLASSES	NAMES	CLINICAL USES	TOXICITIES	
			COMMON	UNIQUE; CLINICALLY IMPORTANT
	Formoterol	Prolonged duration of action (>12 hours) Used for the long-term treatment of obstructive airway diseases Agent of choice for nocturnal asthma Approved for prophylaxis of exercise-induced bronchospasm (see Chapter 24)	Muscle tremor, anxiety, restlessness, tachycardia Selectivity is relative and is lost at high concentrations	Dysrhythmias and cardiac effects Increased risk of fatal or near fatal asthma attacks
	Arformoterol	Prolonged duration of action (>12 hours) Used for the long-term treatment of obstructive airway diseases, including chronic bronchitis (see Chapter 24)	Selectivity is relative and is lost at high concentrations Skeletal muscle tremor, insomnia, and increases in blood glucose	Dysrhythmias and cardiac effects Increased risk of fatal or near fatal asthma attacks
	Ritodrine	Used as a uterine muscle relaxant to arrest preterm labor	Muscle tremor, anxiety, restlessness, tachycardia Selectivity is relative and is lost at high concentrations	May actually increase maternal morbidity
Nonselective β Adrenergic Receptor Antagonists (see Figure 7-4)	Carteolol	Used in the treatment of chronic open-angle glaucoma (see Chapter 47)		Use with caution in patients with pulmonary disease or congestive heart failure
	Propranolol	Used in the treatment of hypertension, angina, acute coronary syndromes and congestive heart failure The later use should only be undertaken by physicians experienced in the use of β blockers to treat CHF (see Chapters 15, 16, 17, and 18)	Use of β blockers may increase fatigue, sleep disturbances, and depression May blunt recognition of hypoglycemia	Use with caution in patients with congestive heart failure May exacerbate asthma or COPD Abrupt discontinuation after long-term use may exacerbate angina and increase the risk of sudden death
	Levobunolol	Used in the treatment of chronic open-angle glaucoma (see Chapter 47)		Use with caution in patients with pulmonary disease or congestive heart failure
	Metipranolol	Used in the treatment of chronic open-angle glaucoma (see Chapter 47)		Use with caution in patients with pulmonary disease or congestive heart failure
	Nadolol	Used in the treatment of hypertension, angina, acute coronary syndromes and congestive heart failure The later use should only be undertaken by physicians experienced in the use of β blockers to treat CHF (see Chapters 15, 16, 17, and 18)	Use of β blockers may increase fatigue, sleep disturbances, and depression May blunt recognition of hypoglycemia	Used with caution in patients with congestive heart failure May exacerbate asthma or COPD Abrupt discontinuation after long-term use may exacerbate angina and increase the risk of sudden death

(Continued)

Adrenergic, Dopaminergic, and Serotonergic Pharmacology — CHAPTER 7

CLASS AND SUBCLASSES	NAMES	CLINICAL USES	TOXICITIES COMMON	TOXICITIES UNIQUE; CLINICALLY IMPORTANT
	Timolol	Ophthalmic preparations used in the treatment of chronic open-angle glaucoma (see Chapter 47) Also used for the treatment of hypertension, angina, acute coronary syndromes and congestive heart failure The later use should only be undertaken by physicians experienced in the use of β blockers to treat CHF (see Chapters 15, 16, 17, and 18)	Use of β blockers may increase fatigue, sleep disturbances, and depression May blunt recognition of hypoglycemia	Use with caution in patients with congestive heart failure May exacerbate asthma or COPD Abrupt discontinuation after long-term use may exacerbate angina and increase the risk of sudden death
	Pindolol	Used in the treatment of chronic open-angle glaucoma Also used for the treatment of hypertension, angina, acute coronary syndromes and congestive heart failure The later use should only be undertaken by physicians experienced in the use of β blockers to treat CHF (see Chapters 15, 16, 17, and 18)	Use of β blockers may increase fatigue, sleep disturbances, and depression May blunt recognition of hypoglycemia	Used with caution in patients with congestive heart failure May exacerbate asthma or COPD Abrupt discontinuation after long-term use may exacerbate angina and increase the risk of sudden death
β_1 Selective Adrenergic Receptor Antagonists (see Figure 7-4)	Metoprolol	Used to treat hypertension, angina, tachycardia, heart failure, vasovagal syncope, and as secondary prevention of myocardial infarction Also used for migraine prophylaxis (see Chapters 15, 16, and 17)	Use of β blockers may increase fatigue, sleep disturbances, and depression May blunt recognition of hypoglycemia	Selectivity is relative and dependent on dose Should be avoided if possible in patients with asthma or COPD Contraindicated for the treatment of acute myocardial infarction in patients with heart rates <45 bpm, heart block greater than first degree, systolic blood pressure <100 mm Hg, or moderate to severe chronic heart failure
	Betaxolol	Used to treat hypertension, angina pectoris, and glaucoma	Use of β blockers may increase fatigue, sleep disturbances, and depression May blunt recognition of hypoglycemia	Selectivity is relative and dependent on dose Should be avoided if possible in patients with asthma or COPD
	Levobetaxolol	Used to treat hypertension, angina pectoris, and glaucoma	Use of β blockers may increase fatigue, sleep disturbances, and depression May blunt recognition of hypoglycemia	Selectivity is relative and dependent on dose Should be avoided if possible in patients with asthma or COPD
	Bisoprolol	Used to treat hypertension and moderate to severe chronic heart failure, cardiac arrhythmias, and ischemic heart disease (see Chapters 15, 16, 17, and 18)	Use of β blockers may increase fatigue, sleep disturbances, and depression May blunt recognition of hypoglycemia	Selectivity is relative and dependent on dose Should be avoided if possible in patients with asthma or COPD

(Continued)

SECTION II Neuropharmacology

CLASS AND SUBCLASSES	NAMES	CLINICAL USES	TOXICITIES	
			COMMON	UNIQUE; CLINICALLY IMPORTANT
	Acebutolol	Used to treat hypertension, ventricular and atrial cardiac arrhythmias, and acute myocardial infarction (see Chapters 15, 16, and 18)	Use of β blockers may increase fatigue, sleep disturbances, and depression May blunt recognition of hypoglycemia	Selectivity is relative and dependent on dose Should be avoided if possible in patients with asthma or COPD
	Atenolol	Used to treat hypertension, angina, tachycardia, and as secondary prevention of myocardial infarction (see Chapters 15, 16, and 17) Also used to treat Graves' disease until anti-thyroid medications can take effect (see Chapter 27)	Use of β blockers may increase fatigue, sleep disturbances, and depression May blunt recognition of hypoglycemia	Selectivity is relative and dependent on dose Should be avoided if possible in patients with asthma or COPD
	Esmolol	Used when short duration of β blockade is needed such as during surgery to control heart rate or in the treatment of supraventricular tachycardia (see Chapter 18)		
β Adrenergic Receptor Antagonists with Additional Cardiovascular Effects ("Third Generation" β Blockers) (see Figure 7-4)	Labetalol	Used to treat hypertension (see Chapter 15)	Use of β blockers may increase fatigue, sleep disturbances, and depression May blunt recognition of hypoglycemia	Should be avoided in patients with asthma or COPD
	Carvedilol	Used to treat hypertension, mild to severe congestive heart failure, and acute myocardial infarction (see Chapters 15, 16, and 17)	Use of β blockers may increase fatigue, sleep disturbances, and depression May blunt recognition of hypoglycemia	Should be avoided in patients with asthma or COPD
	Bucindolol	Used to treat hypertension, mild to severe congestive heart failure, and acute myocardial infarction (see Chapters 15, 16, and 17)	Use of β blockers may increase fatigue, sleep disturbances, and depression May blunt recognition of hypoglycemia	Should be avoided in patients with asthma or COPD
	Celiprolol	Used to treat hypertension and angina	Use of β blockers may increase fatigue, sleep disturbances, and depression May blunt recognition of hypoglycemia	Should be avoided in patients with asthma or COPD
	Nebivolol	Used to treat hypertension	Use of β blockers may increase fatigue, sleep disturbances, and depression May blunt recognition of hypoglycemia	Should be avoided in patients with asthma or COPD
Selective Serotonin (5-HT) Reuptake Inhibitors (SSRIs)	Fluoxetine Citalopram Escitalopram Fluvoxamine Paroxetine Sertraline	Used to treat depression and anxiety (see Chapter 8)	Sedation (see Chapter 8)	Significant drug interactions due to inhibition of CYPs (see Chapter 8)

(Continued)

Adrenergic, Dopaminergic, and Serotonergic Pharmacology — CHAPTER 7

CLASS AND SUBCLASSES	NAMES	CLINICAL USES	TOXICITIES COMMON	UNIQUE; CLINICALLY IMPORTANT
Serotonin(5-HT)/ Norepinephrine (NE) Reuptake Inhibitors (SNRIs)	Duloxetine	Used to treat depression, anxiety, peripheral neuropathy, and fibromyalgia (see Chapter 8)	See Chapter 8	See Chapter 8
	Venlafaxine	Used to treat depression, anxiety, and panic disorders (see Chapter 8)	See Chapter 8	See Chapter 8
	Desvenlafaxine	Used to treat depression, anxiety, and panic disorders (see Chapter 8)	See Chapter 8	See Chapter 8
	Minacipran	Approved for fibromyalgia		
Inhibitor of the Reuptake of 5-HT, NE, and DA (dopamine)	Sibutramine	Used as an appetite suppressant		
MAO Inhibitors That Alter 5-HT Concentrations	Phenelzine Tranylcypromine Isocarboxazid	Used to treat depression (see Chapter 8)	See Chapter 8	See Chapter 8
5-HT Receptor Agonists	Buspirone	Used to treat anxiety (see Chapter 8)	See Chapter 8	See Chapter 8
	Almotripan Eletriptan Frovatriptan Naratriptan Rizatriptan Sumatriptan Zolmitriptan	Used to treat an acute attack of migraine, but not intended for use in the prophylaxis of migraine	Paresthesias, asthenia and fatigue, flushing, tightness in the chest, dizziness, nausea, and sweating	Contraindicated in patients who have a history of ischemic or vasospastic coronary artery disease, cerebrovascular or peripheral vascular disease, hemiplegic or basilar migraines, or other significant cardiovascular diseases, or ischemic bowel disease. Naratriptan is also contraindicated in patients with severe renal or hepatic impairment. Eletriptan is contraindicated in hepatic disease. Almotriptan, rizatriptan, sumatriptan, and zolmitriptan are contraindicated in patients who have taken an MAO inhibitor within the preceding 2 weeks (see Chapter 8)
	Methylsergide	Used for the prophylactic treatment of migraine (not available in the United States)		A complication of prolonged treatment is inflammatory pulmonary, coronary, and endocardial fibrosis
5-HT Receptor Antagonists	Ondansetron Dolasetron Granisetrol Palonosetron	Used to treat chemotherapy-induced nausea (see Chapter 33)	See Chapter 33	See Chapter 33
	Alosetron	Used in the treatment of irritable bowel syndrome (see Chapter 33)	See Chapter 33	See Chapter 33
	Ketanserin	Used to treat hypertension (not available in the United States)		
	Clozapine Respiradone Quetiapine Olanzepine	Atypical antipsychotics	See Chapter 8	See Chapter 8

(Continued)

SECTION II — Neuropharmacology

CLASS AND SUBCLASSES	NAMES	CLINICAL USES	TOXICITIES COMMON	TOXICITIES UNIQUE; CLINICALLY IMPORTANT
Dopamine (DA) Receptor Agonists	Bromocriptine	Used for the treatment of Parkinson's disease (see Chapter 13) Also used to treat acromegaly (see Chapter 26)	Nausea, dizziness, and headache	Hallucination and other CNS effects such as psychosis
	Pergolide	Used for the treatment of Parkinson's disease (see Chapter 13) Used off-label to treat hyper-prolactinemia (see Chapter 26)		Has been linked to valvular heart disease
	Cabergoline	Used to treat hyper-prolactinemia (see Chapter 26)	Hypotension, nausea, dizziness	Has been linked to valvular heart disease
	Apomorphine	Used to treat Parkinson's disease (see Chapter 13)	See Chapter 13	See Chapter 13
	Rotigotine	Used to treat Parkinson's disease (see Chapter 13; not available in the United States due to problems with patch release of drug)	See Chapter 13	See Chapter 13
	Pramipexole	Used to treat Parkinson's disease (see Chapter 13)	Sedation	
	Ropinirole	Used to treat Parkinson's disease (see Chapter 13) Also used to treat restless leg syndrome	Sedation	
Dopamine (DA) Receptor Antagonists	Aripiprazole	An atypical antipsychotic (see Chapter 8)	See Chapter 8	See Chapter 8

CHAPTER 8

Psychopharmacology

Chapter 8 Psychopharmacology is a combination of Chapter 15, Drug Therapy of Depression and Anxiety Disorders and Chapter 16, Pharmacology of Psychosis and Mania from *Goodman and Gilman's The Pharmacological Basis of Therapeutics*, 12th Edition. An understanding of the material in those chapters will be helpful in following the material presented in this chapter. In addition to the material presented here, the above chapters in the 12th Edition include:

- A characterization of depressive and anxiety disorders
- Table 15-2, The Potencies of Antidepressants at the Human Transporters for Norepinephrine (NET), Serotonin (SERT), and Dopamine (DAT)
- Table 15-4, Potencies of Selected Antidepressants at Muscarinic, Histamine H_1, and alpha$_1$-Adrenergic Receptors
- A discussion of the long-term adaptive effects of antidepressants that enhance the effectiveness of therapy
- A discussion of the pathophysiology of psychosis
- A discussion of the chemistry of antipsychotic agents
- The role of dopamine and serotonin receptors in antipsychotic therapy
- A detailed discussion of the use antipsychotic agents for nonpsychotic disorders
- A discussion of the adverse effects of antipsychotic agents that are not predicted by monoamine receptor affinities
- Novel treatments for psychosis and mania

LEARNING OBJECTIVES

- ☑ Understand the mechanisms of action, therapeutic uses, and adverse effects of antidepressant drugs.
- ☑ Know how antidepressant drugs are used to manage depression.
- ☑ Know the mechanisms of action, therapeutic uses, and adverse effects of antipsychotic drugs and drugs used to treat mania.
- ☑ Understand the pharmacotherapy of acute and chronic psychoses and bipolar disorder.

DRUGS INCLUDED IN THIS CHAPTER

- Amitriptyline (ELAVIL, others)
- Amoxapine (ASENDIN)
- Aripiprazole (ABILIFY)
- Asenapine (SAPHRIS, others)
- Atomoxetine (STRATTERA)
- Bupropion (WELLBUTRIN, ZYBAN, others)
- Buspirone (BUSPAR)
- Carbamazepine (TEGRETOL, others)
- Chlorpromazine (THORAZINE, others)
- Citalopram (CELEXA)
- Clomipramine (ANAFRANIL)
- Clozapine (CLOZARIL, others)
- Desipramine (NORPRAMIN)
- Desvenlafaxine (PRISTIQ)
- Doxepin (ADAPIN, SINEQUAN)
- Droperidol (INAPSIN, others)
- Duloxetine (CYMBALTA)
- Escitalopram (LEXAPRO)
- Fluoxetine (PROSAC, SYMBYAX, others)
- Fluphenazine (PROLIXIN, others)
- Fluvoxamine (LUVOX)
- Haloperidol (HALDOL, others)
- Iloperidone (FANAPT)
- Imipramine (TOFRANIL, others)
- Isocarboxazid (MARPLAN)
- Lamotrigine (LAMICTAL)
- Lithium
- Loxapine (LOXITANE)
- Maprotiline (LUDIOMIL)
- Mianserin (DEPNON, others)—not approved in the United States
- Milnacipran (IXEL, others)—not approved in the United States
- Mirtazapine (REMERON, others)
- Molindone (MOBAN)—use discontinued
- Nefazodone (DUTONIN, others)

(*continues*)

SECTION II

DRUGS INCLUDED IN THIS CHAPTER (Cont.)

- Nortriptyline (PAMELOR)
- Olanzapine (ZYPREXA)
- Paliperidone (INVEGA)
- Paroxetine (PAXIL)
- Perphenazine (TRILAFON, others)
- Phenelzine (NARDIL)
- Protriptyline (VIVACTIL)
- Quetiapine (SEROQUEL)
- Reboxetine (EDRONAX)—not available in the United States
- Risperidone (RESPERDAL)
- Selegiline (EMSAM)
- Sertindole (SERDOLECT, others)—not approved in the United States
- Sertraline (ZOLOFT)
- Tranylcypromine (PARNATE)
- Trazodone (DESYREL)
- Trifluoperazine (STELAZINE, others)
- Trimipramine (SURMONTIL)
- Valproic acid, divalproex sodium (DEPAKENE, DEPAKOTE, others)
- Venlafaxine (EFFEXOR)
- Ziprasidone (GEODON)

Neuropharmacology

MECHANISMS OF ACTION OF PSYCHOPHARMACOLOGICAL AGENTS

DRUG CLASS	DRUG	MECHANISM OF ACTION
Monamine Oxidase Inhibitors (MAOIs)	Tranylcypromine Phenelzine Isocarboxazid Selegiline	Irreversible inhibitors of MAO-A and MAO-B that increase noradrenergic and serotonergic neurotransmission by inhibiting the catabolism of norepinephrine (NE) and serotonin (5-HT) (see Figure 8-1) Selegiline is a selective MAO-B inhibitor that is also used to treat Parkinson's disease (see Chapter 13)
Serotonin, Norepinephrine Reuptake Inhibitors (SNRIs) Tertiary Amine Tricyclics (Tricyclic Antidepressants, TCAs)	Amitriptyline Doxepin Imipramine Clomipramine Trimipramine	Increase noradrenergic and serotonergic neurotransmission by blocking the norepinephrine (NET) and serotonin (SERT) transporters at presynaptic terminals (see Figure 8-1) Clomipramine is somewhat selective for inhibition of serotonin uptake
Serotonin, Norepinephrine Reuptake Inhibitors (SNRIs) Secondary Amine Tricyclics, Tricyclic Antidepressants (TCAs)	Amoxapine Desipramine Maprotiline Nortriptyline Protriptyline	Increase noradrenergic and serotonergic neurotransmission by blocking the norepinephrine (NET) and serotonin (SERT) transporters at presynaptic terminals (see Figure 8-1)
Selective Serotonin Reuptake Inhibitors (SSRIs)	Fluoxetine Fluvoxamine Paroxetine Sertraline Citalopram Escitalopram	Blockade of serotonin reuptake results in enhanced and prolonged serotonergic neurotransmission
Atypical Antidepressants and SNRIs	Duloxetine Venlafaxine Desvenlafaxine Milnacipran	Inhibit the reuptake of both NE and 5-HT, but do not have a tricyclic structure and thus avoid some of the side effects of TCAs
	Atomoxetine	Inhibits the reuptake of NE
	Trazodone Nefazodone Mirtazapine Mianserin	Antagonist of the 5-HT$_2$ family of receptors
	Bupropion	Enhances both noradrenergic and dopaminergic neurotransmission via reuptake inhibition of NE and dopamine (DA) and may involve the presynaptic release of NE and DA
	Reboxetine	NE reuptake inhibitor
Anxiolytic Drugs (Benzodiazepines)	See Chapter 9	See Chapter 9
Anxiolytic Drugs (not benzodiazepines)	Buspirone	Partial agonist at 5-HT$_{1A}$ receptors and antagonist at D$_2$ receptors
Typical Antipsychotic Drugs (Phenothiazines)	Chlorpromazine Perphenazine Trifluoperazine Fluphenazine	Dopamine antagonists, but also antiadrenergic, anticholinergic, antiserotonergic, and antihistaminergic (see Figure 8-2)

Psychopharmacology — CHAPTER 8

DRUG CLASS	DRUG	MECHANISM OF ACTION
Typical Antipsychotic Drugs (Other)	Molindone Loxapine Haloperidol Droperidol	Dopamine antagonists, but also antiadrenergic, anticholinergic, antiserotonergic, and antihistaminergic (see Figure 8-2)
Atypical Antipsychotic Drugs	Aripiprazole Olanzapine Quetiapine Risperidone Asenapine Clozapine Ziprasidone Paliperidone Iloperidone Sertindole	Reduced dopaminergic neurotransmission through 2 mechanisms: (1) D_2 antagonism (olanzapine) and (2) partial D_2 agonism (aripiprazole) Many of the atypical antipsychotic drugs also are antagonists at serotonin receptors (eg, olanzapine, iloperidone, clozapine, asenapine, paliperidone, risperidone, quetiapine, sertindole, and ziprasidone) Some atypical antipsychotics are antagonists at adrenergic, cholinergic, and histaminergic receptors as well (see Figure 8-2)
Anticonvulsants Used to Treat Mania	Valproic acid Carbamazepine Lamotrigine	Valproate exhibits non-specific binding to voltage-gated Na^+ channels (see Chapter 12) Carbamazepine and lamotrigine have specific high affinity for the open-channel configuration of the alpha subunit of the Na^+ channel (see Chapter 12)
Lithium	Lithium carbonate Lithium citrate	Plausible mechanisms of action of Li^+ a. Li^+ is not a substrate for the Na^+ pump and therefore cannot maintain membrane potential b. Li^+ can interfere with the activity of both stimulatory and inhibitory G proteins (G_s and G_i) by keeping them in their inactive state c. Inhibition of inositol monophosphatase and interference with phosphatidylinositol pathway (see Figure 8-2) leading to decreased cerebral inositol concentrations d. Li^+ treatment also leads to consistent decreases in the functioning of protein kinases in brain tissue, including PKC e. Li^+ and valproate treatment also inhibits the activity of glycogen synthase kinase-3β (GSK-3β) f. Li^+ and valproate both reduce arachidonic acid turnover in brain membrane phospholipids g. Li^+ and valproate both interact with nuclear regulatory factors that affect gene expression, including increased expression of Bcl-2, which is associated with protection against neuronal degeneration/apoptosis

SECTION II
Neuropharmacology

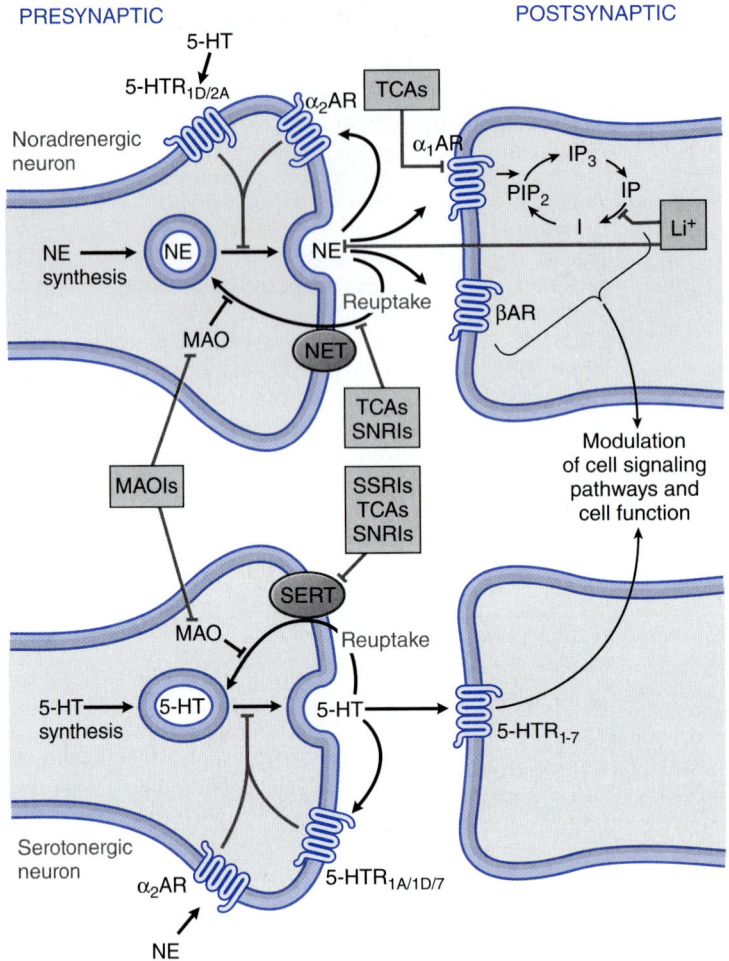

FIGURE 8-1 Sites of action of antidepressants. Schematics representing noradrenergic (top) and serotonergic (bottom) nerve terminals. SSRIs, SNRIs, and TCAs increase noradrenergic or serotonergic neurotransmission by blocking the norepinephrine or serotonergic transporter at presynaptic terminals (NET, SERT). MAOIs inhibit the catabolism of norepinephrine and serotonin. Some antidepressants such as trazodone and related drugs have direct effects on serotonergic receptors that contribute to their clinical effects. Chronic treatment with a number of antidepressants desensitizes presynaptic autoreceptors and heteroreceptors, producing long-lasting changes in monoaminergic neurotransmission. Post-receptor effects of antidepressant treatment, including modulation of GPCR signaling and activation of protein kinases and ion channels, are involved in the mediation of the long-term effects of antidepressant drugs. Note that NE and 5-HT also affect each other's neurons.

CASE 8-1

A 39-year-old woman is taking amitriptyline for major depression.

a. How do antidepressants act to elevate the mood of patients?

Many different antidepressants have established track records of efficacy for treating major depression. However, they all suffer some limitations in efficacy, since at least 20% of all depressed patients are refractory to multiple different antidepressants at adequate doses. In monoamine systems, reuptake of the transmitter is the main mechanism by which neurotransmission is terminated; thus, inhibition of reuptake can enhance neurotransmission, presumably by slowing clearance of the transmitter from the synapse and prolonging the dwell-time of the transmitter in the synapse. Enhancing neurotransmission may subsequently lead to adaptive changes (see Figure 8-1).

(Continued)

Psychopharmacology CHAPTER 8

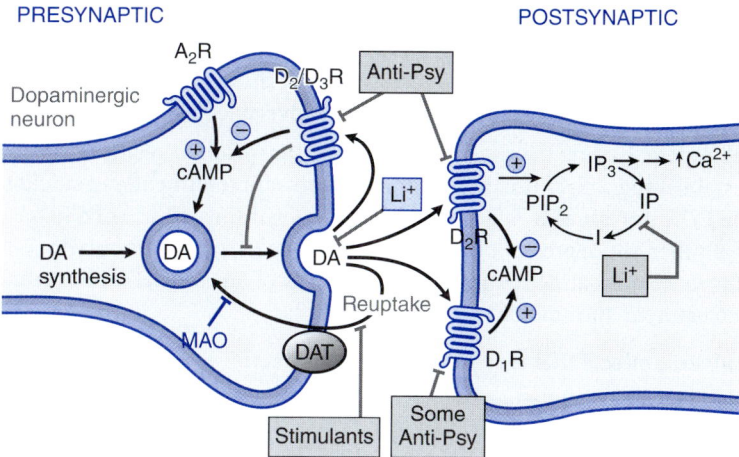

FIGURE 8-2 Sites of action of antipsychotic agents and Li+. In varicosities ("terminals") along terminal arborizations of dopaminergic neurons projecting from midbrain to forebrain, DA is synthesized and stored in vesicles. Following exocytotic release, DA interacts with postsynaptic receptors (R) of D_1 and D_2 types, and presynaptic D_2 and D_3 autoreceptors. Termination of DA action occurs primarily by active transport of DA into presynaptic terminals via the DA transporter DAT, with secondary deamination by mitochondrial monoamine oxidase (MAO). Stimulation of postsynaptic D_1 receptors activates the G_s-adenylyl cyclase-cAMP pathway. D_2 receptors couple through G_i to inhibit adenylyl cyclase and through G_q to activate the PLC-IP_3-Ca^{2+} pathway. Activation of the G_i pathway can also activate K+ channels, leading to hyperpolarization. Lithium inhibits the phosphatase that liberates inositol (I) from inositol phosphate (IP). Li+ can also inhibit depolarization-evoked release of DA and NE, but not 5-HT. D_2-like autoreceptors suppress synthesis of DA by diminishing phosphorylation of rate-limiting TH, and by limiting DA release. In contrast, presynaptic A_2 adenosine receptors (A_2R) activate AC and, through cyclic AMP production, TH activity. All antipsychotic agents act at D_2 receptors and autoreceptors; some also block D_1 receptors. Stimulant agents inhibit DA reuptake by DAT, thereby prolonging the dwell time of synaptic DA. Initially in antipsychotic treatment, DA neurons release more DA, but following repeated treatment, they enter a state of physiological depolarization inactivation, with diminished production and release of DA, in addition to continued receptor blockade. ("T-line"), inhibition or blockade; +, elevation of activity; –, reduction of activity.

Long-term effects of antidepressant drugs evoke adaptive or regulatory mechanisms that enhance the effectiveness of therapy. These responses include increased adrenergic or serotonergic receptor density or sensitivity, increased receptor-G protein coupling and cyclic nucleotide signaling, induction of neurotrophic factors, and increased neurogenesis in the hippocampus. Persistent antidepressant effects depend on the continued inhibition of 5-HT or NE transporters, or enhanced serotonergic or noradrenergic neurotransmission achieved by an alternative pharmacological mechanism. For example, chronic treatment with some antidepressants that interact directly with monoamine transporters (eg, SSRIs, SNRIs, or NE reuptake inhibitors) reduces the expression and activity of 5-HT or NE transporters in the brain, which results in enhanced serotonergic or noradrenergic neurotransmission.

b. What are the major considerations when starting an antidepressant medication?

Following initiation of antidepressant drug treatment, there is generally a "therapeutic lag" lasting 3 to 4 weeks before a measurable therapeutic response becomes evident. This is the reason that electroconvulsive therapy may be the treatment of choice for agitated, depressed patients with a high risk of suicide. Some patients may respond to antidepressant treatment sooner than 3 to 4 weeks; others may require more than 8 weeks for an adequate response. In general, if a patient does not respond to a given antidepressant after an 8-week trial on an adequate dose, then switching to another antidepressant with a different mechanism of action is a reasonable next step (eg, SSRI to SNRI). If a partial response has been observed, other drugs may be added to the primary SSRI or SNRI medications; these additive medications include the antidepressant drug bupropion, thyroid hormone (triiodothyronine), or an atypical antipsychotic (aripiprazole or olanzapine).

(Continued)

SECTION II   Neuropharmacology

After the successful initial treatment phase, a 6- to 12-month maintenance treatment phase is typical, after which the drug is gradually withdrawn. If a patient has experienced 2 separate episodes of major depression or is chronically depressed (ie, >2 years), lifelong treatment with an antidepressant is advisable.

A controversial issue regarding the use of all antidepressants is their relationship to suicide. Data establishing a clear link between antidepressant treatment and suicide are lacking. The FDA has issued a "black box" warning regarding the use of SSRIs and a number of other antidepressants in children and adolescents, particularly during the early phase of treatment, due to the possibility of an association between antidepressant treatment and suicide.

c. **What are the adverse effects that this patient might expect?**

Amitriptyline is a tricyclic antidepressant. TCAs are potent anticholinergics and antagonists at histamine H_1 receptors; H_1 receptor antagonism contributes to the sedative effects of TCAs (Table 8-1). Antagonism of muscarinic acetylcholine receptors contributes to cognitive dulling as well as a range of adverse effects mediated by the parasympathetic nervous system (blurred vision, dry mouth, tachycardia, constipation, difficulty urinating). Some tolerance does occur for these anticholinergic effects, which are mitigated by titration strategies to reach therapeutic doses over a reasonable period of time. Antagonism of α_1-adrenergic receptors contributes to orthostatic hypotension and sedation. Weight gain is another side effect of this class of antidepressants.

TCAs also have quinidine-like effects on cardiac conduction that can be life-threatening with overdose and limit the use of TCAs in patients with coronary heart disease. This is the primary reason that no more than a 1-week supply should be provided to a new patient; even during maintenance treatment, only a very limited supply should be available to the patient at any given time. Like other antidepressant drugs, TCAs also lower the seizure threshold.

d. **What are this patient's options if the side effects of amitriptyline become intolerable?**

The SSRIs are also effective in treating major depression. All of the SSRIs show a clear improvement in safety margin compared to the TCAs and are much safer in overdose, and in clinical practice have affected a broad range of psychiatric, behavioral, and medical conditions, for which they are used, on- and off-label.

In addition to use as antidepressants, SSRIs also are anxiolytics with demonstrated efficacy in the treatment of generalized anxiety, panic, social anxiety, and obsessive-compulsive disorders.

CASE 8-2

A 48-year-old man has developed depression after the death of his wife. He is prescribed venlafaxine.

a. **How does venlafaxine differ from other antidepressants?**

Many older TCAs block both SERT and NET, but with a high side effect burden. Four medications with a nontricyclic structure that inhibit the reuptake of both 5-HT and norepinephrine have been approved for use in the United States for treatment of depression, anxiety disorders, and pain: venlafaxine and its demethylated metabolite, desvenlafaxine; duloxetine; and milnacipran (approved only for fibromyalgia pain in the United States). The rationale behind the development of these newer agents was that targeting both SERT and NET, analogous to the effects of some TCAs, might improve overall treatment response.

(Continued)

TABLE 8-1 Antidepressants: Chemical Structures, Dose and Dosage Forms, and Side Effects

NONPROPRIETARY NAME (TRADE NAME)	Usual[a] Dose (mg/day)	Dosage Form	AMINE EFFECTS	Agitation	Seizures	Sedation	Hypotension	Anticholinergic Effects	GI Effects	Weight Gain	Sexual Effects	Cardiac Effects
Norepinephrine Reuptake Inhibitors: Tertiary Amine Tricyclics												
Amitriptyline (ELAVIL and others)	100-200	O, I	NE, 5-HT	0	2+	3+	3+	3+	0/+	2+	2+	3+
Clomipramine (ANAFRANIL)	100-200	O	NE, 5-HT	0	3+	2+	2+	3+	+	2+	3+	3+
Doxepin (ADAPIN, SINEQUAN)	100-200	O	NE, 5-HT	0	2+	3+	2+	2+	0/+	2+	2+	3+
Imipramine (TOFRANIL and others)	100-200	O, I	NE, 5-HT	0/+	2+	2+	2+	2+	0/+	2+	2+	3+
(±)-Trimipramine (SURMONTIL)	75-200	O	NE, 5-HT	0	2+	3+	2+	3+	0/+	2+	2+	3+
Norepinephrine Reuptake Inhibitors: Secondary Amine Tricyclics												
Amoxapine (ASENDIN)	200-300	O	NE, DA	0	2+	+	2+	+	0/+	+	2+	2+
Desipramine (NORPRAMIN)	100-200	O	NE	+	+	0/+	+	+	0/+	+	2+	2+
Maprotiline (LUDIOMIL)	100-150	O	NE	0/+	3+	2+	2+	2+	0/+	+	2+	2+
Nortriptyline (PAMELOR)	75-150	O	NE	0	+	+	+	+	0/+	+	2+	2+
Protriptyline (VIVACTIL)	15-40	O	NE	2+	2+	0/+	+	2+	0/+	+	2+	3+
Selective Serotonin Reuptake Inhibitors												
(±)-Citalopram (CELEXA)	20-40	O	5-HT	0/+	0	0/+	0	0	3+	0	3+	0
(+)-Escitalopram (LEXAPRO)	10-20	O	5-HT	0/+	0	0/+	0	0	3+	0	3+	0
(±)-Fluoxetine (PROZAC)	20-40	O	5-HT	+	0/+	0/+	0	0	3+	0/+	3+	0/+
Fluvoxamine (LUVOX)	100-200	O	5-HT	0	0	0/+	0	0	3+	0	3+	0
(−)-Paroxetine (PAXIL)	20-40	O	5-HT	+	0	0/+	0	0/+	3+	0	3+	0

SECTION II Neuropharmacology

NONPROPRIETARY NAME (TRADE NAME)	DOSE AND DOSAGE FORMS	AMINE EFFECTS	SIDE EFFECTS							
(+)-Sertraline (ZOLOFT)	100-150 O	5-HT	+	0	0/+	0	0	3+	0	3+	0
(±)-Venlafaxine (EFFEXOR)	75-225 O	5-HT, NE	0/+	0	0	0	0	3+	0	3+	0/+
Atypical Antidepressants											
(−)-Atomoxetine (STRATTERA)	40-80 (children: mg/kg) O	NE	0	0	0	0	0	0/+	0	0	0
Bupropion (WELLBUTRIN)	200-300 O	DA, ?NE	3+	4+	0	0	0	2+	0	0	0
(+)-Duloxetine (CYMBALTA)	80-100 O	NE, 5-HT	+	0	0/+	0/+	0	0/+	0/+	0/+	0/+
(±)-Mirtazapine (REMERON)	15-45 O	5-HT, NE	0	0	4+	0/+	0	0/+	0/+	0	0/+
Nefazodone (SERZONE)	200-400 O	5-HT	0	0	3+	0	0	2+	0/+	0/+	0/+
Trazodone (DESYREL)	150-200 O	5-HT	0	0	3+	0	0	2+	+	+	0/+
Monoamine Oxidase Inhibitors											
Phenelzine (NARDIL)	30-60 O	NE, 5-HT, DA	0/+	0	+	+	0	0/+	+	3+	0
Tranylcypromine (PARNATE)	20-30 O	NE, 5-HT, DA	2+	0	0	0	0	0/+	+	2+	0
(−)-Selegiline (ELDEPRYL)	10 O	DA, ?NE, ?5-HT	0	0	0	0	0	0	0	+	0

Note: Most of the drugs are hydrochloride salts, but SURMONTIL and LUVOX are maleates; CELEXA is a hydrobromide, and REMERON is a free-base. Selegiline is approved for early Parkinson disease, but may have antidepressant effects, especially at daily doses 20 mg, and is under investigation for administration by transdermal patch.

[a]Both higher and lower doses are sometimes used, depending on an individual patient's needs and response to the drug; see the literature and FDA-approved dosage recommendations.

O, oral tablet or capsule; I, injectable; NE, norepinephrine; 5-HT, serotonin, DA, dopamine; 0, negligible; 0/+, minimal; +, mild; 2+, moderate; 3+, moderately severe; 4+, severe. Other significant side effects for individual drugs are described in the Summary Table.

b. **Why is there a delay in the onset of antidepressant effect with SSRI antidepressants and SNRIs such as venlafaxine?**

SNRIs inhibit both SERT and NET. Depending on the drug, the dose, and the potency at each site, SNRIs cause enhanced serotonergic and/or noradrenergic neurotransmission. Similar to the action of SSRIs, the initial inhibition of SERT induces activation of $5\text{-}HT_{1A}$ and $5\text{-}HT_{1D}$ autoreceptors. This action decreases serotonergic neurotransmission by a negative feedback mechanism until these serotonergic autoreceptors are desensitized. Then, the enhanced serotonin concentration in the synapse can interact with postsynaptic 5-HT receptors.

c. **What side effects might this patient expect with venlafaxine?**

The side effects of venlafaxine are shown in Table 8-1. Venlafaxine dose reductions are suggested for patients with renal or hepatic impairment (see Table 8-2). The SNRIs have desirable safety advantages over the TCAs. SNRIs have a side effect profile similar to that of the SSRIs, including nausea, constipation, insomnia, headaches, and sexual dysfunction. The immediate release formulation of venlafaxine can induce sustained diastolic hypertension (systolic blood pressure > 90 mm Hg at consecutive weekly visits) in 10 to 15% of patients at higher doses; this risk is reduced with the extended-release form.

CASE 8-3

A 53-year-old man with mild depression has been treated with a monoamine oxidase inhibitor. His physician is now switching his antidepressant therapy to fluoxetine.

a. **What drug interactions should he be cautioned about while taking the SSRI?**

Most antidepressants, including the SSRIs, exhibit drug–drug interactions based on their routes of metabolism (see Table 8-2). Paroxetine and, to a lesser degree, fluoxetine are potent inhibitors of CYP2D6. The other SSRIs, outside of fluvoxamine, are at least moderate inhibitors of CYP2D6. This inhibition can result in disproportionate increases in plasma concentrations of drugs metabolized by CYP2D6 when doses of these drugs are increased. Fluvoxamine directly inhibits CYP1A2 and CYP2C19; fluoxetine and fluvoxamine also inhibit CYP3A4. See Chapter 2 for a list of drugs metabolized by these CYPs.

b. **He had previously been taking tranylcypromine, an MAO inhibitor. What concerns are there for switching his medication to an SSRI?**

Another important drug–drug interaction with SSRIs occurs via a pharmacodynamic mechanism. MAOIs enhance the effects of SSRIs due to inhibition of serotonin metabolism. Administration of these drugs together can produce synergistic increases in extracellular brain serotonin, leading to the serotonin syndrome. Symptoms of the serotonin syndrome include hyperthermia, muscle rigidity, myoclonus, tremors, autonomic instability, confusion, irritability, and agitation; this can progress toward coma and death. Other drugs that may induce the serotonin syndrome include substituted amphetamines such as methylenedioxymethamphetamine (Ecstasy), which directly releases serotonin from nerve terminals. The primary treatment is stopping all serotonergic drugs, administering nonselective serotonin antagonists, and supportive measures.

Since currently available MAOIs bind irreversibly to MAO and block the enzymatic metabolism of monoaminergic neurotransmitters, SSRIs should not be started until at least 14 days following discontinuation of treatment with an MAOI; this allows for synthesis of new MAO. For all SSRIs but fluoxetine, at least 14 days should pass prior to beginning treatment with an MAOI following the end of treatment with an SSRI. Since the active metabolite of fluoxetine, norfluoxetine, has a $t_{1/2}$ of 1 to 2 weeks, at least 5 weeks should pass between stopping fluoxetine and beginning an MAOI.

(Continued)

TABLE 8-2 Disposition of Antidepressants

DRUG	ELIMINATION $t_{1/2}$ (h) PARENT DRUG (Active Metabolite)	TYPICAL C_p (ng/mL)	PREDOMINANT CYP INVOLVED IN METABOLISM
Tricyclic Antidepressants			
Amitriptyline	16 (30)	100-250	2D6, 2C19, 3A3/4, 1A2
Amoxapine	8 (30)	200-500	
Clomipramine	32 (70)	150-500	
Desipramine	30	125-300	
Doxepin	18 (30)	150-250	
Imipramine	12 (30)	175-300	
Maprotiline	48	200–400	
Nortriptyline	31	60-150	
Protriptyline	80	100-250	
Trimipramine	16 (30)	100-300	
Selective Serotonin Reuptake Inhibitors			
R,S-Citalopram	36	75-150	3A4, 2C19
S-Citalopram	30	40-80	3A4, 2C19
Fluoxetine	53 (240)	100-500	2D6, 2C9
Fluvoxamine	18	100-200	2D6, 1A2, 3A4, 2C9
Paroxetine	17	30-100	2D6
Sertraline	23 (66)	25-50	2D6
Serotonin-Norepinephrine Reuptake Inhibitors			
Duloxetine	11	—	2D6
Venlafaxine	5 (11)	—	2D6, 3A4
Other Antidepressants			
Atomoxetine	5-20 (child: 3)	—	2D6, 3A3/4
Bupropion	11	75-100	2B6
Mirtazapine	16	—	2D6
Nefazodone	2–4	—	3A3/4
Reboxetine	12	—	—
Trazodone	6	800-1600	2D6

Values shown are elimination $t_{1/2}$ values for a number of clinically used antidepressant drugs; numbers in parentheses are $t_{1/2}$ values of active metabolites. Fluoxetine (2D6), fluvoxamine (1A2, 2C8, 3A3/4), paroxetine (2D6), and nefazodone (3A3/4) are potent inhibitors of CYPs; sertraline (2D6), citalopram (2C19), and venlafaxine are less potent inhibitors. Plasma concentrations are those observed at typical clinical doses. Information was obtained from manufacturers' summaries and Appendix II in *Goodman and Gilman's The Pharmacological Basis of Therapeutics*, 12th Edition, which the reader should consult for important details.

Psychopharmacology — CHAPTER 8

CASE 8-4

A 49-year-old man is in hospital for surgery on a herniated vertebral disc. On the second day following surgery, he becomes agitated, belligerent, paranoid, and aggressive. He is given haloperidol to control his behavior.

a. **What kind of drug is haloperidol and how does it act?**

Like most antipsychotic drugs haloperidol is an antagonist at D_2 receptors (see Figure 8-2; Tables 8-3 and 8-4).

b. **What are the advantages of using a drug such as haloperidol in this setting?**

Delirium following surgery generally requires only short-term therapy. Because anticholinergic drug effects may worsen delirium and dementia, high-potency typical antipsychotic drugs (eg, haloperidol) or atypical antipsychotic agents with limited antimuscarinic properties (eg, risperidone) are often the drugs of choice.

c. **While not a consideration in this setting, what are the side effects of the chronic use of haloperidol?**

Excessive D_2 blockade, as is often the case with the use of high-potency typical agents (eg, haloperidol), not only increases risk for motor neurological effects (eg, muscular rigidity, bradykinesia, tremor, akathisia) (see Figure 8-3), but also slows mentation (bradyphrenia), and interferes with central reward pathways, resulting in patient complaints of anhedonia. Rarely used are low-potency typical agents (eg, chlorpromazine), which also have high affinities for H_1, M, and α_1 receptors that cause many undesirable effects (sedation, anticholinergic properties, orthostasis). Concerns regarding QT_c prolongation (eg, thioridazine) further limit their clinical usefulness.

d. **What are other options in treating this patient?**

Intramuscular (IM) administration of ziprasidone, aripiprazole, or olanzapine represents an option for treating agitated and minimally cooperative patients, and presents less risk of drug-induced parkinsonism than haloperidol. QT_c prolongation associated with intramuscular droperidol and intravenous administration of haloperidol have curtailed the use of those particular formulations. Treatment continues until agitated or hallucinatory behaviors are controlled and the underlying etiologies are addressed.

CASE 8-5

A 32-year-old woman with a long history of drug abuse has been diagnosed with schizophrenia.

a. **What are the goals of short-term therapy with this patient?**

The immediate goals of acute antipsychotic treatment are the reduction of agitated, disorganized, or hostile behavior, decreasing the impact of hallucinations, the improvement of organization of thought processes, and the reduction of social withdrawal. Doses used are often higher than those required for maintenance treatment of stable patients.

b. **What are the goals of long-term therapy with this patient?**

The need for long-term treatment poses issues almost exclusively to the chronic psychotic illnesses, schizophrenia and schizoaffective disorder, although long-term antipsychotic treatment is sometimes used for manic patients, for ongoing psychosis in dementia patients, for L-dopa psychosis, and for adjunctive use in SSRI-unresponsive major depression.

The choice of antipsychotic agents for long-term schizophrenia treatment is based primarily on avoidance of adverse effects and, when available, prior history of patient response. Since schizophrenia spectrum disorders are lifelong diseases, treatment acceptability is paramount to effective illness management. Whether atypical antipsychotic agents are superior to typical antipsychotic agents has been the subject of significant and contentious debate.

(Continued)

SECTION II Neuropharmacology

TABLE 8-3 Chemical Structures, Dosages for Acute Psychosis and Schizophrenia Maintenance, and Metabolic Risk Profile[a]

NONPROPRIETARY NAME (TRADE NAME)	ORAL DOSAGE (MG/DAY)				METABOLIC SIDE EFFECTS		
	ACUTE PSYCHOSIS		MAINTENANCE				
DOSAGE FORMS	1ST EPISODE	CHRONIC	1ST EPISODE	CHRONIC	WEIGHT GAIN	LIPIDS	GLUCOSE
Typical Antipsychotic Agents							
Phenothiazines							
Chlorpromazine (THORAZINE) **O, S, IM**	200-600	400-800	150-600	250-750	+++	+++	++
Perphenazine (TRILAFON) **O, S, IM**	12-50	24-48	12-48	24-60	+/−	−	−
Trifluoperazine (STELAZINE) **O, S, IM**	5-30	10-40	2.5-20	10-30	+/−	−	−
Fluphenazine (PROLIXIN) **O, S, IM**	2.5-15	5-20	2.5-10	5-15	+/−	−	−
Fluphenazine decanoate **Depot IM**	Not for acute use		5-75 mg/2 wks		+/−	−	−
Other Typical Agents							
Molindone (MOBAN) **O, S**	15-50	30-60	15-50	30-60	−	−	−
Loxapine (LOXITANE) **O, S, IM**	15-50	30-60	15-50	30-60	+	−	−
Haloperidol (HALDOL) **O, S, IM**	2.5-10	5-20	2.5-10	5-15	+/−	−	−
Haloperidol decanoate **Depot IM**	Not for acute use		100-300 mg/month		+/−	−	−
Atypical Antipsychotic Agents							
Aripiprazole (ABILIFY) **O, S, ODT, IM**	10-20	15-30	10-20	15-30	+/−	−	−
Asenapine (SAPHRIS, SYCREST) **ODT**	10	10-20	10	10-20	+/−	−	−
Clozapine (CLOZARIL, FAZCLO) **O, ODT**	200-600	400-900	200-600	300-900	++++	+++	+++

(Continued)

Psychopharmacology

NONPROPRIETARY NAME (TRADE NAME)	ORAL DOSAGE (MG/DAY)					METABOLIC SIDE EFFECTS		
	ACUTE PSYCHOSIS		MAINTENANCE					
DOSAGE FORMS	1ST EPISODE	CHRONIC	1ST EPISODE	CHRONIC	WEIGHT GAIN	LIPIDS	GLUCOSE	
Iloperidone (FANAPT) **O**		12-24[b]		8-16	+	+/-	+/-	
Olanzapine (ZYPREXA) **O, ODT, IM**	7.5-20	10-30	7.5-15	15-30	++++	+++	+++	
Paliperidone (INVEGA) **O**	6-9	6-12	3-9	6-15	+	+/-	+/-	
Paliperidone palmitate (SUSTENNA)[c] **Depot IM**	See note[c] on dosing				+	+/-	+/-	
Quetiapine (SEROQUEL, SEROQUEL XR) **O**	200-600	400-900	200-600	300-900	+	+	+/-	
Risperidone (RISPERDAL) **O, S, ODT**	2-4	3-6	2-6	3-8	+	+/-	+/-	
RISPERDAL CONSTA **Depot IM**	Not for acute use		25-50 mg/2 wks					
Sertindole (SERDOLECT, SERLECT)[d] **O**	4-16	12-20	12-20	12-32	+/-	–	–	
Ziprasidone (GEODON, ZELDOX)[e] **O, IM**	120-160	120-200	80-160	120-200	+/-	–	–	

Dosage Forms: O, tablet; S, solution; IM, acute intramuscular; ODT, orally dissolving tablet.

[a] For further information on antipsychotic dosing in psychotic disorders, see Expert Consensus Panel for Optimizing Pharmacologic Treatment of Psychotic Disorders. The expert consensus guideline series. Optimizing pharmacologic treatment of psychotic disorders. *J Clin Psychiatry,* 2003, 64(Suppl 12):2–97.

Note that doses in first-episode, younger, or antipsychotic-naïve patients are lower than for chronic schizophrenia patients. Dose in elderly schizophrenia patients is approximately 50% of that used in younger adults with schizophrenia; dosing for dementia-related psychosis is approximately 25%.

[b] Due to orthostasis risk, dose titration of iloperidone is 1 mg bid on day 1, increasing to 2, 4, 6, 8, 10, and 12 mg bid on days 2, 3, 4, 5, 6, and 7 (as needed). Safety data exist for daily doses up to 16 mg bid.

[c] Paliperidone palmitate dosing: in acute schizophrenia, deltoid IM loading doses of 234 mg at day 1 and 156 mg at day 8 provide paliperidone levels equivalent to 6 mg oral paliperidone during the first week, and peaking on day 15 at a level comparable to 12 mg oral paliperidone. No oral antipsychotic needed in first week. Maintenance IM doses can be given in deltoid or gluteus every 4 weeks after day 8. Maintenance dose options: 39, 78, 117, 156, or 234 mg every 4 weeks. Failure to give initiation doses (except for those switching from depot) will result in subtherapeutic levels for months.

[d] Not available in the United States.

[e] Oral dose must be given with food (500 kcal) to facilitate absorption. Food increases the absorption of single doses of 20-, 40-, and 80-mg capsules by 48%, 87%, and 101%, respectively.

Neuropharmacology

TABLE 8-4 Potencies of Antipsychotic Agents at Neurotransmitter Receptors[a]

	DOPAMINE D_2	SEROTONIN 5-HT_{1A}	5-HT_{2A}	5-HT_{2C}	$5HT_{2A}/D_2$ RATIO	DOPAMINE D_1	D_4	MUSCARINIC M_1	ADRENERGIC α_{1A}	α_{2A}	HISTAMINE H_1
Typical Agents											
Haloperidol	1.2	2100	57	4500	47	120	5.5	>10,000	12	1130	1700
Fluphenazine	0.8	1000	3.2	990	3.9	17	29	1100	6.5	310	14
Thiothixene	0.7	410	50	1360	72	51	410	>10,000	12	80	8
Perphenazine	0.8	420	5.6	130	7.4	37	40	1500	10	810	8.0
Loxapine	11	2550	4.4	13	0.4	54	8.1	120	42	150	4.9
Molindone	20	3800	>5000	10,000	>250	>10,000	>2000	>10,000	2600	1100	2130
Thioridazine	8.0	140	28	53	3.5	94	6.4	13	3.2	130	16
Chlorpromazine	3.6	2120	3.6	16	1	76	12	32	0.3	250	3.1
Atypical Agents											
Asenapine[b]	1.4	2.7	0.1	0.03	0.05	1.4	1.1	>10,000	1.2	1.2	1.0
Ziprasidone	6.8	12	0.6	13	0.1	30	39	>10,000	18	160	63
Sertindole[b]	2.7	280	0.4	0.90	0.2	12	13	>5000	1.8	640	130
Zotepine[b]	8.0	470	2.7	3.2	0.3	71	39	330	6.0	210	3.2
Risperidone	3.2	420	0.2	50	0.05	240	7.3	>10,000	5.0	16	20
Paliperidone	4.2	20	0.7	48	0.2	41	54	>10,000	2.5	4.7	19
Iloperidone	6.3	90	5.6	43	0.9	130	25	4900	0.3	160	12
Aripiprazole	1.6	6.0	8.7	22	5.0	1200	510	6800	26	74	28
Sulpiride[b]	6.4	>10,000	>10,000	>10,000	>1000	>10,000	54	>10,000	>10000	>5000	>10,000
Olanzapine	31	2300	3.7	10	0.1	70	18	2.5	110	310	2.2
Quetiapine	380	390	640	1840	2.0	990	2020	37	22	2900	6.9
Clozapine	160	10	5.4	9.4	0.03	270	24	6.2	1.6	90	1.1

[a]Data are averaged K_i values (nM) from published sources determined by competition with radioligands for binding to the indicated cloned human receptors. Data derived from receptor binding to human or rat brain tissue is used when cloned human receptor data is lacking.
[b]Not available in the United States.
NIMH Psychoactive Drug Screening Program (PDSP) K_i Database: http://pdsp.med.unc.edu/pdsp.php (Accessed June 30, 2009).

c. She is prescribed the atypical antipsychotic drug aripiprazole. What is the mechanism of action of aripiprazole?

Presently, antipsychotic agents include many different chemical structures with a range of activities at different neurotransmitter receptors (eg, 5-HT_{2A} antagonism, 5-HT_{1A} partial agonism). As a result, structure-function relationships that were relied upon in the past have become less important. Instead, receptor-function relationships and functional assays are more clinically relevant. Aripiprazole represents a good example of how an examination of the structure provides little insight into its mechanism, which is based on dopamine receptor partial agonism. Detailed knowledge of receptor affinities (see Table 8-4) and the functional effect at specific

(Continued)

Psychopharmacology

CHAPTER 8

USE OF ANTIPSYCHOTIC AGENTS IN NONPSYCHOTIC DISORDERS

- Anxiety disorders
- Tourette disorder
- Huntington's disease
- Autism
- Antiemetic use

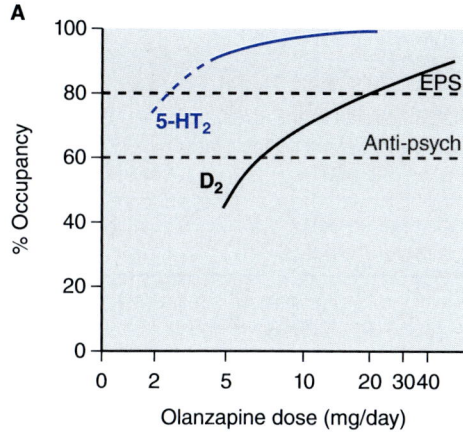

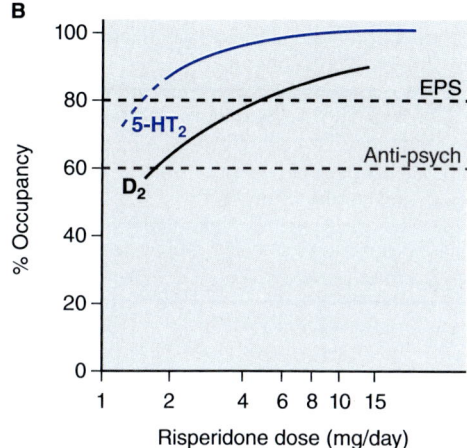

FIGURE 8-3 Receptor occupancy and clinical response for antipsychotic agents. Typically, in D_2 receptor occupancy by the drug more than 60% provides antipsychotic effects, receptor occupancy more than 80% causes extrapyramidal symptoms (EPS). Atypical agents combine weak D_2 receptor blockade with more potent 5-HT$_{2A}$ antagonism/inverse agonism. Inverse agonism at 5-HT$_2$ receptor subtypes may contribute to the reduced EPS risk of olanzapine (Panel A) and risperidone (Panel B) and efficacy at lower D_2 receptor occupancy (olanzapine, Panel A). Aripiprazole is a partial D_2 agonist that can achieve only 75% functional blockade.

receptors (eg, full, partial, or inverse agonism or antagonism) can provide important insight into the therapeutic and adverse effects of antipsychotic agents.

The reduction in dopaminergic neurotransmission is presently achieved through 1 of 2 mechanisms: D_2 antagonism or partial D_2 agonism, of which aripiprazole is the only current example.

d. What are expected side effects of aripiprazole?

While concerns over extrapyramidal symptoms (EPS) and tardive dyskinesia have abated with the introduction of the atypical antipsychotic agents into clinical practice, there has been increased concern over metabolic effects of antipsychotic treatment (see Table 8-3): weight gain, dyslipidemia (particularly hypertriglyceridemia), and an adverse impact on glucose-insulin homeostasis, including new-onset type 2 DM, and diabetic ketoacidosis (DKA), with reported fatalities from the latter. Clozapine and olanzapine have the highest metabolic risk and are only used as last resort. Olanzapine has been relegated in most treatment algorithms to third-tier status and is considered only after failure of more metabolically benign agents such as aripiprazole, ziprasidone, asenapine, iloperidone, risperidone, and paliperidone.

SECTION II Neuropharmacology

ADVERSE EFFECTS OF LITHIUM

ORGAN SYSTEM	ADVERSE EFFECT
CNS	Fine postural hand tremor, incoordination, ataxia, slurred speech, seizures reported at therapeutic plasma concentrations, central appetite stimulation with weight gain
Renal	Decreased ability to concentrate urine, polydipsia, polyuria, and a picture of nephrogenic diabetes insipidus
Endocrine	Benign, diffuse, nontender thyroid enlargement in patients with normal thyroid function; 7-10% of patients develop overt hypothyroidism
Cardiovascular	Benign and reversible T wave and the appearance of U waves on ECG; rare reports of effects on cardiac conduction
Skin	Allergic reactions such as dermatitis, folliculitis, and vasculitis; worsening of other dermatological conditions is common
Reproductive	Pregnancy category risk D; risk of cardiovascular abnormalities in newborn if used early in pregnancy; Li^+ freely crosses the placenta and may cause fetal or neonatal Li^+ toxicity such as neonatal goiter, CNS depression, hypotonia, and cardiac murmur
Other	Benign increase in circulating polymorphonuclear leukocytes; metallic taste; worsening of myasthenia gravis

CASE 8-6

A 38-year-old woman is being treated with lithium for bipolar disorder.

a. What is bipolar disorder and how effective is Li^+ in treating the mania and depression associated with bipolar disorder?

Patients who experience periods of hypomania and major depression have bipolar II disorder, those with mania at any time have bipolar I, and those with hypomania, but less severe forms of depression have cyclothymia.

Treatment with Li^+ ideally is conducted in patients with normal cardiac and renal function. Occasionally, patients with severe systemic illnesses are treated with Li^+, provided that the indications are compelling, but the need for diuretics, nonsteroidal anti-inflammatory agents, or other medications that pose potential pharmacokinetic problems often precludes lithium use in those with multiple medical problems. Treatment of acute mania and the prevention of recurrences of bipolar illness in adults or adolescents are uses of Li^+ approved by the FDA.

While Li^+, valproate, and carbamazepine have efficacy in acute mania, in clinical practice these are usually combined with atypical antipsychotic drugs, even in manic patients without psychotic features, due to their delayed onset of action. Li^+, carbamazepine, and valproic acid preparations are only effective with daily dosing that maintains adequate serum levels, and require serum level monitoring.

b. What are the options for this patient?

Li^+ is effective in acute mania but is rarely employed as a sole treatment for reasons noted above, and because 5 to 7 days are required for clinical effect. The anticonvulsant sodium valproate provides more rapid antimanic effects than Li^+, with therapeutic benefit seen within 3 to 5 days. The most common form of valproate in use is divalproex sodium, which is preferred over valproic acid due to lower incidence of GI and other adverse effects.

Carbamazepine is effective for acute mania. Immediate release forms of carbamazepine cannot be loaded or rapidly titrated over 24 hours as with valproate due to the

(Continued)

development of neurological adverse effects such as dizziness or ataxia, even within the therapeutic range (6-12 µg/mL); the extended-release form of carbamazepine is FDA-approved for acute mania.

c. **What therapeutic options are there for prophylaxis for future depressive episodes?**

The choice of ongoing prophylaxis is determined by the need for continued antipsychotic drug use and for use of a mood-stabilizing agent. Both aripiprazole and olanzapine are effective as monotherapy for mania prophylaxis, but olanzapine use is eschewed out of concern for metabolic effects, and aripiprazole shows no benefit for prevention of depressive relapse.

The overriding concern guiding bipolar treatment is the high recurrence rate. Individuals who experience mania have an 80 to 90% lifetime risk of subsequent manic episodes. As with schizophrenia, lack of insight, poor psychosocial support, and substance abuse all interfere with treatment adherence. The anticonvulsants lamotrigine, carbamazepine, and divalproex have data supporting their use in bipolar prophylaxis.

Lamotrigine was effective in 2 large, 18-month-long maintenance trials for bipolar patients whose most recent mood episode was manic or depressed, with greater effect on depressive relapse. The ability to provide prophylaxis for future depressive episodes combined with data in acute bipolar depression has made lamotrigine a useful choice for bipolar treatment, given that bipolar I and II patients spend large amounts of time in depressive phases (32 and 50%, respectively).

Bipolar disorder is a lifetime illness with high recurrence rates. Individuals who experience an episode of mania should be educated about the probable need for ongoing treatment. Stopping mood stabilizer therapy can be considered in patients who have experienced only 1 lifetime manic episode, particularly when there may have been a pharmacological precipitant (eg, substance or antidepressant use), and who have been euthymic for extended periods. For bipolar II patients, the impact of hypomania is relatively limited, so the decision to recommend prolonged maintenance treatment with a mood stabilizer is based on clinical response and risk:benefit ratio. Discontinuation of maintenance Li^+ treatment in bipolar I patients carries a high risk of early recurrence and of suicidal behavior over a period of several months, even if the treatment had been successful for several years.

CASE 8-7

A 71-year-old man with bipolar disorder has been treated successfully with Li^+ since age 40. He now has developed hypertension, mild congestive heart failure, and osteoarthritis.

a. **What are issues that might arise from the coadministration of drugs for these conditions?**

The majority of older patients on Li^+ therapy are those maintained for years on the medication. Less than 10% of individuals with bipolar disorder experience their first manic episode at age 50 or above. Elderly patients frequently take numerous medications for other illnesses and the potential for contraindications or drug–drug interactions is substantial. For patients naïve to Li^+, these issues can be addressed relatively easily prior to commencement of Li^+ treatment. The more difficult clinical decision revolves around switching treatment in stable patients who have taken Li^+ for years or decades with excellent clinical response. In addition, age-related reductions in total body water and creatinine clearance reduce the safety margin for Li^+ treatment in older patients. Targeting lower maintenance serum levels (0.6-0.8 mEq/L) may reduce the risk of toxicity. As GFR drops below 60 mL/min, strong consideration must be given to a search for alternative agents, despite lithium's therapeutic advantages. Li^+ toxicity occurs more frequently in elderly patients, in part as the result of concurrent use of loop diuretics and angiotensin-converting enzyme inhibitors. Anticonvulsants, especially extended-release divalproex, are a reasonable alternative to Li^+.

(Continued)

SECTION II

Neuropharmacology

Li⁺ is completely filtered, and 80% is reabsorbed in the proximal tubules. Li⁺ competes with Na⁺ for reabsorption, and Li⁺ retention can be increased by Na⁺ loss related to diuretic use, or febrile, diarrheal, or other GI illness. Heavy sweating leads to a preferential secretion of Li⁺ over Na⁺; however, the repletion of excessive sweating using free water without electrolytes can cause hyponatremia, and promote Li⁺ retention. Thiazide diuretics deplete Na⁺ and can cause significant reductions in Li⁺ clearance that result in toxic levels. The K⁺-sparing diuretics triamterene, spironolactone, and amiloride have modest effects on the excretion of Li⁺, with concomitantly smaller increases in serum levels. Loop diuretics such as furosemide seem to have limited impact on Li⁺ levels. Renal excretion can be increased by administration of osmotic diuretics or acetazolamide, but not sufficiently for the management of acute Li⁺ intoxication.

Through alteration of renal perfusion, some nonsteroidal anti-inflammatory agents can facilitate renal proximal tubular resorption of Li⁺ and thereby increase serum concentrations. This interaction appears to be particularly prominent with indomethacin, but also may occur with ibuprofen, naproxen, and COX-2 inhibitors, and possibly less so with sulindac and aspirin. Angiotensin-converting enzyme inhibitors, particularly the renally cleared lisinopril, also cause Li⁺ retention, with isolated reports of toxicity among stable lithium-treated patients switched from fosinopril to lisinopril.

b. How should his bipolar disorder be managed in light of his age and coexisting medical conditions?

Because of the low therapeutic index for Li⁺, periodic determination of serum concentrations is crucial. Li⁺ cannot be used with adequate safety in patients who cannot be tested regularly. Concentrations considered to be effective and acceptably safe are between 0.6 and 1.5 mEq/L. The range of 1.0 to 1.5 mEq/L is favored for treatment of acutely manic or hypomanic patients. Somewhat lower values (0.6-1.0 mEq/L) are considered adequate and are safer for long-term prophylaxis. Serum concentrations of Li⁺ have been found to follow a clear dose-effect relationship between 0.4 and 1.0 mEq/L, but with a corresponding dose-dependent rise in polyuria and tremor as indices of adverse effects. Nonetheless, patients who maintain trough levels of 0.8 to 1.0 mEq/L experience decreased relapse risk compared to those maintained at lower serum concentrations. There are patients who may do well with serum levels of 0.5 to 0.8 mEq/L, but there are no current clinical or biological predictors to permit a priori identification of these individuals. Individualization of serum levels is often necessary to obtain a favorable risk-benefit relationship.

The concentration of Li⁺ in blood usually is measured at a trough of the daily oscillations that result from repetitive administration (ie, from samples obtained 10-12 hours after the last oral dose of the day). Peaks can be 2 or 3 times higher than trough levels at steady state. When the peaks are reached, intoxication may result, even when concentrations in morning samples of plasma at the daily nadir are in the acceptable range of 0.6 to 1 mEq/L. Single daily doses generate relatively large oscillations of plasma Li⁺ concentration but lower mean trough levels than with multiple daily dosing and are associated with a reduction in the extent and risk for polyuria; moreover, single nightly dosing means that peak serum levels occur during sleep, so complaints regarding CNS adverse effects are minimized. While relatively uncommon, GI complaints are a compelling reason for multiple daily dosing or using delayed release Li⁺ preparations, bearing in mind the increased polyuria risk from these strategies.

CASE 8-8

A 28-year-old woman is taking lithium for management of the mania phase of bipolar disorder. She has entered the depressive phase of the disorder and takes an overdose of her lithium.

a. What are the acute toxic effects of lithium overdose?

The occurrence of toxicity is related to the serum concentration of Li⁺ and its rate of rise following administration. Acute intoxication is characterized by vomiting,

(Continued)

profuse diarrhea, coarse tremor, ataxia, coma, and convulsions. Symptoms of milder toxicity are most likely to occur at the absorptive peak of Li⁺ and include nausea, vomiting, abdominal pain, diarrhea, sedation, and fine tremor. The more serious effects involve the nervous system and include mental confusion, hyperreflexia, gross tremor, dysarthria, seizures, and cranial nerve and focal neurological signs, progressing to coma and death. Sometimes both cognitive and motor neurological damage may be irreversible, with persistent cerebellar tremor being the most common. Other toxic effects are cardiac arrhythmias, hypotension, and albuminuria.

b. What is the treatment for acute overdose of lithium?

There is no specific antidote for Li⁺ intoxication, and treatment is supportive (see Chapter 3), including intubation if indicated, and continuous cardiac monitoring. Levels greater than 1.5 mEq/L are considered toxic, but inpatient medical admission is usually not indicated (in the absence of symptoms) until levels exceed 2 mEq/L. Care must be taken to assure that the patient is not Na⁺- and water-depleted. Dialysis is the most effective means of removing Li⁺ and is necessary in severe poisonings, that is, in patients exhibiting symptoms of toxicity or patients with serum Li⁺ concentrations more than or equal to 3 mEq/L in acute overdoses. A review of 213 case reports of acute Li⁺ toxicity between 1948 and 1984 found that complete recovery occurred with an average maximal level of 2.5 mEq/L, permanent neurological symptoms with mean levels of 3.2 mEq/L, and death with mean maximal levels of 4.2 mEq/L. The most common neurological sequelae are due to cerebellar damage, and manifest clinically as ataxia, tremor, dysarthria, and dysmetria.

KEY CONCEPTS

- Inhibition of monoamine reuptake is a major mechanism by which antidepressant drugs enhance neurotransmission (see Figure 8-1).
- Monoamine oxidase inhibitor (MAOI) antidepressants inhibit monoamine metabolism (see Figure 8-1).
- With antidepressant drugs there is a "therapeutic lag" lasting 3 to 4 weeks before a measurable response becomes evident.
- Sudden withdrawal of antidepressants can precipitate a withdrawal syndrome.
- TCAs are potent antagonists at histamine H_1 and muscarinic receptors that account for many of their side effects (see Chapters 6 and 21).
- MAOIs have many serious food and drug interactions.
- All antipsychotic drugs reduce dopaminergic neurotransmission by D_2 blockade (or in the case of aripiprazole modulation of DA activity by virtue of being a partial D_2 agonist).
- A Parkinson-like syndrome, a risk of long-term therapy with antipsychotic drugs that is dose- and drug-dependent, can be predicted based on receptor occupancy (see Figure 8-3).
- Alteration of a patient's metabolic profile (see Table 8-3) is also a serious side effect of some antipsychotic medications.
- Bipolar disorder is generally treated with Li⁺; the anticonvulsants valproic acid and carbamazepine, and antipsychotic drugs are useful to manage the acute manic phase.
- The narrow therapeutic indices for Li⁺, valproic acid, and carbamazepine requires careful monitoring of their plasma concentrations.

SUMMARY QUIZ

QUESTION 8-1 A 56-year-old man who has a 30-year history of smoking cigarettes is being treated for schizophrenia with clozapine. He is hospitalized for an acute exacerbation of his psychoses; his clozapine therapy is continued. During the third week of his hospital stay, he has a seizure that is thought to be due to clozapine toxicity. The clozapine toxicity in this patient is likely due to

a. increased GI absorption of clozapine.
b. decreased renal excretion of clozapine.
c. a decrease in his blood-brain barrier function.
d. decreased metabolism of clozapine.
e. a pharmacy mistake.

QUESTION 8-2 A 54-year-old woman is taking Li$^+$ for bipolar disorder. Her Li$^+$ plasma concentrations have consistently been 0.8 mEq/L (therapeutic range 0.6-1.5 mEq/L). She has developed osteoarthritis for which she is prescribed ibuprofen. One week later during a routine visit it is noted that her Li$^+$ plasma concentration is 1.5 mEq/L. The cause of the rise in this patient's plasma Li$^+$ concentration is due to the effect of ibuprofen to

a. increase Li$^+$ GI absorption.
b. facilitate Li$^+$ reabsorption in the renal proximal tubule.
c. decrease Li$^+$ metabolism in the liver.
d. displace Li$^+$ from serum albumin.
e. facilitate Li$^+$ reabsorption from the distal colon.

QUESTION 8-3 A 22-year-old woman is being treated with amitriptyline for depression. She, and her family, should be cautioned about not seeing a therapeutic effect for

a. 24 hours.
b. 12 hours.
c. 3 days.
d. 1 week.
e. 3 to 4 weeks.

QUESTION 8-4 A 75-year-old man with obsessive compulsive disorder is treated with risperidone. After 3 weeks of therapy, he develops bradykinesia, masked facies, and reduced arm movements when walking. These symptoms are due to

a. α_1-adrenergic receptor antagonism.
b. β-adrenergic receptor antagonism.
c. 5-HT receptor stimulation.
d. D$_2$ receptor antagonism.
e. blockade of norepinephrine uptake into presynaptic terminals.

QUESTION 8-5 An 86-year-old man with severe dementia has become very aggressive and poses a danger to himself and his family. His geriatrician is reluctant to prescribe an antipsychotic medication to control his behavior because of the risk of

a. increased mortality.
b. increased dementia.
c. decreased peripheral blood perfusion.
d. skin cancer.
e. glaucoma.

QUESTION 8-6 A 43-year-old woman is being treated with olanzapine for schizophrenia. Although olanzapine appeared to be improving her behavioral symptoms, she stopped using the drug likely due to

a. an unusual taste.
b. increased libido.
c. weight gain.
d. her urine turned green.
e. hirsutism.

Psychopharmacology

CHAPTER 8

QUESTION 8-7 A 32-year-old woman is treated for schizophrenia with clozapine. Her physician insists on regular monitoring of

a. serum aminotransferases.

b. serum Na$^+$.

c. serum K$^+$.

d. serum Ca^{++}.

e. complete blood count (CBC).

QUESTION 8-8 A 43-year-old man with the diagnosis of bipolar disorder has developed a particularly severe form of mania with psychotic symptoms. The patient's physician should begin treatment with which of the following anticonvulsants?

a. Phenytoin

b. Gabapentin

c. Valproic acid

d. Lamotrigine

e. Topiramate

SUMMARY QUIZ ANSWER KEY

QUESTION 8-1 Answer is **d.** Changes in smoking status can be especially problematic for clozapine-treated patients and will alter serum levels by 50% or more. Within 2 weeks of smoking discontinuation (eg, hospitalization in nonsmoking environment), the absence of aryl hydrocarbons will cause upregulated CYP1A2 activity to return to baseline levels, with a concomitant rise in serum clozapine concentrations (see Table 8-5).

QUESTION 8-2 Answer is **b.** Through alteration of renal perfusion, some nonsteroidal anti-inflammatory agents can facilitate renal proximal tubular resorption of Li$^+$ and thereby increase serum concentrations.

QUESTION 8-3 Answer is **e.** Following initiation of antidepressant drug treatment, there is generally a "therapeutic lag" lasting 3 to 4 weeks before a measurable therapeutic response becomes evident (see Case 8-1).

QUESTION 8-4 Answer is **d.** With the exception of the D$_2$ partial agonist aripiprazole, all other antipsychotic agents possess D$_2$ antagonist properties, the strength of which determines the likelihood for extrapyramidal syndrome (EPS), akathisia, long-term tardive dyskinesia risk, and hyperprolactinemia. The manifestations of EPS are described in Table 8-6, along with the usual treatment approach (also see Figure 8-3).

Parkinsonism resembling its idiopathic form occurs when striatal D$_2$ occupancy exceeds 78%, and often responds to dose reduction or switching to an antipsychotic with weaker D$_2$ antagonism. In situations where this is neither possible nor desirable, anti-parkinsonian medication may be employed. Clinically, there is a generalized slowing and impoverishment of volitional movement (bradykinesia) with masked facies and reduced arm movements during walking. The syndrome characteristically evolves gradually over days to weeks as the risk of acute dystonia diminishes. The most noticeable signs are slowing of movements, and sometimes rigidity and variable tremor at rest, especially involving the upper extremities. Bradykinesia and masked facies may be mistaken for clinical depression. Elderly patients are at greatest risk.

QUESTION 8-5 Answer is **a.** Perhaps the least understood adverse effect is the increased risk for cerebrovascular events and all-cause mortality among elderly dementia patients exposed to antipsychotic medications. All antipsychotic agents carry a mortality warning in the drug label regarding their use in dementia patients. The cerebrovascular adverse event rates in 10-week dementia trials range from 0.4 to 0.6% for placebo to 1.3 to 1.5% for risperidone, olanzapine, and aripiprazole. The mortality

(Continued)

TABLE 8-5 Metabolism of Common Antipsychotic Drugs

AGENT	METABOLIC PATHWAYS	EFFECT OF CYP INHIBITION	EFFECT OF CYP INDUCTION
Atypical Antipsychotic Agents			
Aripiprazole	2D6 and 3A4 convert aripiprazole to active metabolite dehydro-aripiprazole. Metabolite has longer $t_{1/2}$ (75 vs. 94 hours) and represents 40% of AUC at steady state.	2D6 PMs experience 80% ↑ in aripiprazole AUC, and 30% ↓ in metabolite AUC (net effect is 60% ↑ in AUC for active moiety). Aripiprazole $t_{1/2}$ ≈ 146 hrs in PM. 2D6 inhibitors ↑ aripiprazole AUC by 112% and ↓ metabolite AUC by 35%. Ketoconazole (a potent 3A4 inhibitor) with a 15-mg single dose of aripiprazole ↑ the AUC of aripiprazole and its active metabolite by 63% and 77%, respectively.	3A4 induction ↓ maximum concentration and AUC of aripiprazole and metabolite by 70%.
Asenapine	Primarily glucuronidation (UGT 1A4), and limited oxidation via CYP 1A2, and to a lesser extent 2D6 and 3A4. No active metabolites.	Fluvoxamine, 25 mg twice daily for 8 days, ↑ C_{max} by 13% and AUC 29%. Paroxetine ↓ both C_{max} and AUC by 13%. Valproate, a UGT 1A4 inhibitor, ↑ C_{max} 2%, and ↓ AUC 1%.	Smoking had no effect on clearance or other kinetic parameters. Carbamazepine ↓ both C_{max} and AUC by 16%.
Clozapine	Multiple enzymes convert clozapine to active metabolite N-desmethylclozapine. The mean contributions of CYPs 1A2, 2C19, 3A4, 2C9, and 2D6 are 30%, 24%, 22%, 12%, and 6%, respectively. CYP1A2 is the most important form at low concentrations, which is in agreement with clinical findings.	Fluvoxamine ↑ C_p 5-10 fold. 2D6 inhibition may ↑ levels as much as 100%.	Loss of smoking-related 1A2 induction ↑ serum levels by 50%. Carbamazepine ↓ clozapine levels on average by 50%.
Iloperidone	2D6 and 3A4 convert iloperidone to active metabolites P88 and P95. In 2D6 EM, the $t_{1/2}$ of P88 and P95 are 26 and 23 hours, respectively; in PM, 37 and 31 hours, respectively. Only P88 has affinity for D_2. P88 accounts for 19.5% and 34.0% of total exposure in EM and PM, respectively. P95 has K_i of 3.91 nM for $5HT_{2A}$ and 4.7 nM for α_{1A}, and accounts for 48% and 25% of total exposure in EM and PM, respectively.	Ketoconazole ↑ AUC of a single 3-mg iloperidone dose and its metabolites P88 and P95 by 57%, 55%, and 35%, respectively. Fluoxetine ↑ 3-mg single dose AUC of iloperidone and P88 metabolite 2-3 fold, and P95 AUC by 50%. Paroxetine ↑ AUC of iloperidone and P88 metabolite 1.6-fold, and reduces P95 AUC by 50%. Paroxetine (8-12 mg twice daily) ↑ steady state C_{max} of iloperidone and P88 by 1.6-fold, and ↓ steady state C_{max} of P95 by 50%. Combined use ↑ steady state C_{max} of iloperidone and P88 by 1.4-fold, and ↓ steady state C_{max} of P95 1.4-fold.	Impact of 3A4 inducers not documented.
Olanzapine	Direct glucuronidation or 1A2 mediated oxidation to N-desmethylolanzapine (inactive).	Increase in olanzapine C_{max} following fluvoxamine is 54% in female nonsmokers and 77% in male smokers. The mean increase in olanzapine AUC is 52% and 108%, respectively.	Carbamazepine use ↑ clearance by 50%. Olanzapine C_p lower in smokers (with equal dosing).
Paliperidone	59% excreted unchanged in urine, 32% excreted as metabolites. Phase 2 metabolism accounts for no more than 10%.	Unlikely to have much of an effect.	Carbamazepine use ↓ steady state C_{max} and AUC by 37%.

Psychopharmacology   CHAPTER 8

AGENT	METABOLIC PATHWAYS	EFFECT OF CYP INHIBITION	EFFECT OF CYP INDUCTION
Quetiapine	3A4 mediated sulfoxidation to active metabolite norquetiapine, $t_{1/2} \approx$ 12 hours. Steady state mean C_{max} and AUC of norquetiapine are ~25% and ~50% of that for quetiapine.	Ketoconazole (200 mg once daily for 4 days), ↓ oral clearance of quetiapine by 84%, resulting in a 335% ↑ in maximum C_p.	Phenytoin increases clearance 5-fold.
Risperidone	2D6 converts risperidone to active metabolite 9-OH risperidone. In 2D6 PMs, half-lives are: risperidone, 20 hours; 9-OH risperidone, 30 hours	Fluoxetine and paroxetine ↑ risperidone concentration ~ 2.5 fold and 3-9 fold, respectively. Fluoxetine did not affect 9-OH risperidone conc., but paroxetine lowered 9-OH risperidone (13%). Net effect: 2D6 inhibition ↑ levels of active moiety up to 75%.	In a drug interaction study of risperidone 6 mg/day × 3 weeks, followed by 3 weeks of carbamazepine, concentration of active moieties (risperidone + 9-OH risperidone) was decreased 50%.
Ziprasidone	3A4 (~1/3) Aldehyde Oxidase (~2/3)	Concomitant ketoconazole ↑ AUC by 35%	Carbamazepine ↓ AUC by 35%.
Haloperidol	Multiple CYP pathways, particularly 2D6, 3A4, and minor pathway 1A2. Only active metabolite, reduced haloperidol (formed by ketone reductase). Reduced haloperidol inhibits CYP2D6 and may be re-oxidized to the parent drug. Therapeutic serum levels not well defined; 5-20 ng/mL used as a target for dosing.	Half-life prolonged in CYP 2D6 PMs Individuals with only one functional 2D6 allele experience 2-fold greater trough serum levels, those with no functioning alleles 3-4 fold higher.	Carbamazepine and phenytoin ↑ haloperidol clearance ~32%, with ↓ C_p (mean, 47%). Discontinuation of carbamazepine ↑ C_p 2-3 fold.
Chlorpromazine	CYP2D6. Over 10 identified human metabolites, most inactive. Chlorpromazine is a moderate 2D6 inhibitor, and also induces its own metabolism. Levels drop 25-33% during weeks 1-3 of treatment.	Case report of fluoxetine-chlorpromazine interaction, but no serum level data on extent of effect.	3A4/PGP inducers (eg, phenobarbital, carbamazepine) decrease chlorpromazine levels by ~35%. Carbamazepine discontinuation ↑ C_p (30-80%).

AUC, area under the curve; PM, poor metabolizer; EM, extensive metabolizer; $t_{1/2}$, half life; C_p, plasma concentration; C_{max}, maximum plasma concentration.

[a]May have multiphasic elimination with much longer terminal $t_{1/2}$.

warning indicates a 1.6 to 1.7-fold increased mortality risk for drug versus placebo. Mortality is due to heart failure, sudden death, or pneumonia. The underlying etiology for antipsychotic-related cerebrovascular and mortality risk is unknown, but the finding of virtually equivalent mortality risk for typical agents compared to atypical antipsychotic drugs (including aripiprazole) suggests an impact of reduced D_2 signaling regardless of individual antipsychotic mechanisms.

QUESTION 8-6 Answer is **c**. Weight gain is a significant problem during long-term use of antipsychotic drugs and represents a major barrier to medication adherence, as well as a significant threat to the physical and emotional health of the patient (see Table 8-3). Weight gain has effectively replaced concerns over EPS as the adverse effect causing the most consternation among patients and clinicians alike. Appetite stimulation is the primary mechanism involved, with little evidence to suggest that decreased activity (due to sedation) is a main contributor to antipsychotic-related weight gain. Recent animal studies indicate that medications with significant H_1 antagonism induce appetite stimulation through effects at hypothalamic sites. The low-potency phenothiazine chlorpromazine and the atypical antipsychotic drugs olanzapine and clozapine are the agents of highest risk, but weight gain of some extent is seen with nearly all antipsychotic drugs, partly related to the fact that acutely psychotic patients may lose weight; in placebo-controlled acute schizophrenia trials, the placebo cohort inevitably loses weight. For clozapine and olanzapine, massive weight gains of 50 kg or more are not uncommon,

(Continued)

TABLE 8-6 Neurological Side Effects of Antipsychotic Drugs

REACTION	FEATURES	TIME OF ONSET AND RISK INFO	PROPOSED MECHANISM	TREATMENT
Acute dystonia	Spasm of muscles of tongue, face, neck, back	Time: 1-5 days. Young, antipsychotic naïve patients at highest risk	Acute DA antagonism	Anti-parkinsonian agents are diagnostic and curative[a]
Akathisia	Subjective and objective restlessness; *not* anxiety or "agitation"	Time: 5-60 days	Unknown	Reduce dose or change drug; clonazepam, propranolol more effective than anti-parkinsonian agents[b]
Parkinsonism	Bradykinesia, rigidity, variable tremor, mask facies, shuffling gait	Time: 5-30 days. Elderly at greatest risk	DA antagonism	Dose reduction; change medication; anti-parkinsonian agents[c]
Neuroleptic malignant syndrome	Extreme rigidity, fever, unstable BP, myoglobinemia; can be fatal	Time: weeks-months. Can persist for days after stopping antipsychotic	DA antagonism	Stop antipsychotic immediately; supportive care; dantrolene and bromocriptine[d]
Perioral tremor ("rabbit syndrome")	Perioral tremor (may be a late variant of parkinsonism)	Time: months or years of treatment	Unknown	Anti-parkinsonian agents often help[c]
Tardive dyskinesia	Orofacial dyskinesia; rarely widespread choreoathetosis or dystonia	Time: months, years of treatment. Elderly at 5-fold greater risk. Risk ∝ potency of D_2 blockade	Postsynaptic DA receptor supersensitivity, up-regulation	Prevention crucial; treatment unsatisfactory. May be reversible with early recognition and drug discontinuation

[a]Treatment: diphenhydramine 25-50 mg IM, or benztropine 1-2 mg IM. Due to long antipsychotic $t_{1/2}$, may need to repeat, or follow with oral medication.
[b]Propranolol often effective in relatively low doses (20-80 mg/day in divided doses). β_1-Selective adrenergic receptor antagonists are less effective.
Non-lipophilic β adrenergic antagonists have limited CNS penetration and are of no benefit (eg, atenolol).
[c]Use of amantadine avoids anticholinergic effects of benztropine or diphenhydramine.
[d]Despite the response to dantrolene, there is no evidence of abnormal Ca^{2+} transport in skeletal muscle; with persistent antipsychotic effects (eg, long-acting injectable agents), bromocriptine may be tolerated in large doses (10-40 mg/day). Anti-parkinsonian agents are not effective.

and mean annual weight gains of 13 kg are reported in schizophrenia clinical trials, with 20% of subjects gaining more than or equal to 20% of baseline weight.

QUESTION 8-7 Answer is **e**. Clozapine possesses a host of unusual adverse effects aside from seizure induction, the most concerning of which is agranulocytosis. Clozapine's introduction in the United States was based on its efficacy in refractory schizophrenia, but came with FDA-mandated CBC monitoring that is overseen by industry-created registries. Now that several generic forms of clozapine are available in addition to proprietary CLOZARIL, clinicians must verify with each manufacturer the history of prior exposure. The overall agranulocytosis incidence is slightly under 1%, with highest risk during the initial 6 months of treatment, peaking at months 2 to 3 and diminishing rapidly thereafter. The mechanism is immune-mediated, and patients who have verifiable clozapine-related agranulocytosis should not be rechallenged. Increased risk is associated with certain HLA types and advanced age. An extensive algorithm guiding clinical response to agranulocytosis, and lesser forms of neutropenia, is available from manufacturer Web sites, and must be followed, along with the current recommended CBC monitoring frequency.

Psychopharmacology

CHAPTER 8

QUESTION 8-8 Answer is **c**. The pharmacology and chemistry of the anticonvulsants with significant data for acute mania (valproic acid compounds, carbamazepine) and for bipolar maintenance (lamotrigine) are covered extensively in Chapter 12. These compounds are of diverse chemical classes, but share the common property of functional blockade of voltage-gated Na^+ channels, albeit with differing binding sites. Valproate exhibits non-specific binding to voltage-gated Na^+ channels, while carbamazepine (and its congeners) and lamotrigine have specific high affinity for the open-channel configuration of the alpha subunit of voltage-gated Na^+ channels. These anticonvulsants have varying affinities for voltage-dependent Ca^{2+} channels, and differ in their ability to facilitate GABA-ergic (valproate) or inhibit glutamatergic neurotransmission (lamotrigine). The extent to which any of these actions is necessary for antimanic or other mood stabilizing activity is unknown, but the failure of phenytoin, gabapentin, and topiramate to be effective antimanic and mood-stabilizing medications suggests that potent blockade of voltage-gated Na^+ channels (which gabapentin and topiramate lack) is necessary but not sufficient, since phenytoin is very active at these channels.

While Li^+, valproate, and carbamazepine have efficacy in acute mania, in clinical practice these are usually combined with atypical antipsychotic drugs, even in manic patients without psychotic features, due to their delayed onset of action.

Li^+ is effective in acute mania, but is rarely employed as a sole treatment for reasons noted above, and because 5 to 7 days are required for clinical effect. The anticonvulsant sodium valproate provides more rapid antimanic effects than Li^+, with therapeutic benefit seen within 3 to 5 days.

Lamotrigine has no role in acute mania due to the slow, extended titration necessary to minimize risk of Stevens-Johnson syndrome.

SUMMARY TABLE PSYCHOPHARMACOLOGICAL DRUGS

CLASS AND SUBCLASSES	NAMES	CLINICAL USES	TOXICITIES COMMON	TOXICITIES UNIQUE: CLINICALLY IMPORTANT
Monoamine Oxidase Inhibitors (MAOIs)	Tranylcypromine Phenelzine Isocarboxazid Selegiline	Used to treat depression Selegiline is also used to treat Parkinson's disease (see Chapter 13)	See Table 8-1	Hypertensive crisis resulting from foods containing tyramine Drug interactions—opioid agonist and SSRIs and SNRIs may cause serotonin syndrome and other antidepressants such as TCAs and buprorion should be avoided
Serotonin, Norepinephrine Reuptake Inhibitors (SNRIs)—Tertiary Amine Tricyclics (TCAs)	Amitriptyline Doxepin Imipramine Clomipramine Trimipramine	Used to treat depression	Blurred vision, dry mouth, tachycardia, difficulty urinating, constipation, and sedation Weight gain (see Table 8-1)	Quinidine-like effects on cardiac conduction Lowering of seizure threshold Orthostatic hypotension from antagonism of $α_1$-adrenergic receptors
Serotonin, Norepinephrine Reuptake Inhibitors (SNRIs)—Secondary Amine Tricyclics (TCAs)	Amoxapine Desipramine Maprotiline Nortriptyline Protriptyline	Used to treat depression	Blurred vision, dry mouth, tachycardia, difficulty urinating, constipation, and sedation Weight gain (see Table 8-1)	Quinidine-like effects on cardiac conduction Lowering of seizure threshold Orthostatic hypotension from antagonism of $α_1$-adrenergic receptors

SECTION II Neuropharmacology

CLASS AND SUBCLASSES	NAMES	CLINICAL USES	TOXICITIES COMMON	UNIQUE: CLINICALLY IMPORTANT
Selective Serotonin Reuptake Inhibitors (SSRIs)	Fluoxetine Fluvoxamine Paroxetine Sertraline Citalopram Escitalopram	Effective in treating depression, generalized anxiety, panic social anxiety, and obsessive compulsive disorder (OCD) Fluvoxamine is approved for OCD but not for depression Citalopram is approved for use in premenstrual dysphoric disorder	Insomnia, increased anxiety, irritability, and decreased libido (see Table 8-1)	Abrupt withdrawal may precipitate dizziness, headache, nervousness, nausea, and insomnia This withdrawal may be more intense for paroxetine Paroxetine is associated with an increase risk of congenital cardiac malformations
Serotonin-Norepinephrine Reuptake Inhibitors (SNRIs)	Venlafaxine Desvenlafaxine Duloxetine Milnacipran	Treatment of depression, anxiety disorders, and fibromyalgia and neuropathic pain (duloxetine) Milnacipran is approved only for fibromyalgia pain	Nausea, constipation, insomnia, headache, and sexual dysfunction (see Table 8-1)	The immediate release form of venlafaxine can induce sustained diastolic hypertension Abrupt withdrawal of venlafaxine may precipitate a withdrawal syndrome
Atypical Antidepressants	Atomoxetine	Approved for attention deficit hyperactivity disorder in children, adolescents, and adults	Insomnia, nausea, constipation, headache, erectile dysfunction (see Table 8-1)	Suicide-related events, emotional lability Contraindicated in patients with symptomatic cardiovascular disease
	Trazodone Nefazodone Mirtazapine Mianserin	Effective antidepressants	Somnolence, weight gain, increased appetite Mirtazapine and mianserin are quite sedating (see Table 8-1)	Trazodone is associated with priapism Mirtazapine is associated with agranulocytosis Nefazodone withdrawn from market after rare cases of liver failure; generic nefazodone still available (see Table 8-1)
	Bupropion	Used to treat depression, prevention of seasonal depressive disorder, and as a smoking cessation treatment	See Table 8-1	Seizures at high doses (see Table 8-1)
	Reboxetine	Used for the treatment of depression	Insomnia, dry mouth, constipation	Glaucoma Suicidal ideation Aggressive behavior
Anxiolytic Drugs (Benzodiazepines)	See Chapter 9	See Chapter 9	See Chapter 9	See Chapter 9
Anxiolytic Drugs (Not benzodiazepines)	Buspirone	Used to treat general anxiety disorder	Dizziness Somnolence	Contraindicated in patients with severe renal or liver impairment and in patients with symptomatic cardiovascular disease
Typical Antipsychotic Drugs—Phenothiazines	Chlorpromazine Perphenazine Trifluoperazine Fluphenazine	Low-potency drugs used for the treatment of acute and chronic psychoses, including schizophrenia	Anticholinergic symptoms of dry mouth, blurred vision, constipation, and urinary retention	Lowers seizure threshold (see Tables 8-3 and 8-6)

Psychopharmacology — CHAPTER 8

CLASS AND SUBCLASSES	NAMES	CLINICAL USES	TOXICITIES COMMON	TOXICITIES UNIQUE: CLINICALLY IMPORTANT
Other Typical Antipsychotic Drugs	Molindone Loxapine Haloperidol Droperidol	High-potency drugs used for the treatment of acute and chronic psychoses, including schizophrenia	Anticholinergic symptoms of dry mouth, blurred vision, constipation, and urinary retention	Extrapyramidal symptoms at doses that exceed 80% receptor occupancy (see Figure 8-3) Haloperidol is associated with prolonged QT interval Metabolic side effects (see Table 8-3) Neuroleptic malignant syndrome (NMS)
Atypical Antipsychotic Drugs	Aripiprazole Olanzapine Quetiapine Risperidone Asenapine Clozapine Ziprasidone Paliperidone Iloperidone Sertindole	Used for the treatment of acute and chronic psychoses Most antipsychotics (except quetiapine) are ineffective as monotherapy for bipolar depression	Weight gain, anxiety, insomnia	Extrapyramidal symptoms at doses that exceed 80% receptor occupancy (see Figure 8-3) Metabolic side effects (see Table 8-3)
Anticonvulsants Used to Treat Mania	Valproic acid Carbamazepine Lamotrigine	Used to treat acute mania (valproic acid, carbamazepine) and for bipolar maintenance (lamotrigine) (see Chapter 12)	See Chapter 12	See Chapter 12
Lithium	Lithium carbonate Lithium citrate	Treatment of bipolar disorder Also used for augmentation of unipolar depression in patients who are inadequate responders to antidepressant therapy	See Side Bar ADVERSE EFFECTS OF LITHIUM Fine postural hand tremor Ataxia, slurred speech, and incoordination Weight gain	See Side Bar ADVERSE EFFECTS OF LITHIUM Low therapeutic index and requires periodic measurement of serum concentrations Seizures reported at therapeutic concentrations Nephrogenic diabetes insipidus

CHAPTER 9

Hypnotics, Sedatives, and Ethanol

DRUGS INCLUDED IN THIS CHAPTER

- Acamprosate (CAMPRAL)
- Alprazolam (XANAX)
- Amobarbital (AMYTAL)
- Butabarbital (BUTISOL, others)
- Carisoprodol (SOMA)
- Clomethiazole—not approved in the United States
- Chloral Hydrate (NOCTEC)
- Chlorazepate (TRANXENE, others)
- Chlordiazepoxide (LIBRIUM, others)
- Clonazepam (KLONIPIN)
- Diazepam (VALIUM, others)
- Disulfiram (ANTABUSE)
- Estazolam (PROSOM, others)
- Eszopiclone (LUNESTA)
- Etomidate (AMIDATE)
- Flumazenil (ROMAZICON)
- Flurazepam (DALMANE, others)
- Lorazepam (ATIVAN)
- Mephobarbital (MEBERAL)
- Meprobamate
- Methohexital (BREVITAL)
- Midazolam (VERSED)
- Nalmefene (REVEX)
- Naltrexone (REVIA, VIVITROL)
- Oxazepam (SERAX)
- Paraldehyde—no longer used in the United States
- Pentobarbital (NEMBUTAL)
- Phenobarbital (LUMINAL, others)
- Propofol (DIPRIVAN)
- Quazepam (DORAL)
- Ramelteon (ROZEREM)
- Secobarbital (SECONAL)
- Temazepam (RESTORIL)
- Thiopental (PENTOTHAL)
- Triazolam (HALCION)
- Zaleplon (SONATA)
- Zolpidem (AMBIEN)

Chapter 9 Hypnotics, Sedatives, and Ethanol is a combination of Chapter 17, Hypnotics and Sedatives and Chapter 23, Ethanol and Methanol from *Goodman and Gilman's The Pharmacological Basis of Therapeutics*, 12th Edition. An understanding of the material in those chapters will be helpful in following the material presented in this chapter. In addition to the material presented here, the above chapters in the 12th Edition include:

- A detailed discussion of the pharmacological properties of benzodiazepines, including animal models of anxiety, the effects of benzodiazepines on the electroencephalogram (EEG) and sleep stages, the molecular targets of benzodiazepines, and $GABA_A$ receptor–mediated electrical events
- Table 17-1 Benzodiazepines: Names and Structures
- A discussion of miscellaneous sedative hypnotic drugs used less commonly today
- A detailed discussion of the management of insomnia
- The history of ethanol consumption details of the pharmacological effects of ethanol

In addition, the mechanisms of action of methanol and acute methanol poisoning, including treatment with ethanol and fomepizole are covered in this book Chapter 3 Clinical and Environmental Toxicity.

LEARNING OBJECTIVES

- ☑ Know the pharmacological effects, mechanisms of action, untoward effects, and therapeutic uses of benzodiazepines.
- ☑ Know the pharmacological effects, mechanisms of action, untoward effects, and therapeutic uses of barbiturates.
- ☑ Understand the management of insomnia.
- ☑ Know the effects of ethanol on physiological systems.
- ☑ Describe the issues of physical dependence and tolerance of chronic ethanol use.
- ☑ Understand the genetics of ethanol disposition.
- ☑ Know the drugs used to treat alcoholism.

MECHANISMS OF ACTION OF SEDATIVES, HYPNOTICS, AND DRUGS USED TO TREAT ALCOHOLISM

DRUG CLASS	DRUG	MECHANISM OF ACTION
Benzodiazepines	Alprazolam Chlordiazepoxide Clonazepam Chlorazepate Diazepam Estazolam Flurazepam Lorazepam Midazolam Oxazepam Quazepam Temazepam Triazolam	Figure 9-1 shows the benzodiazepine binding site on the $GABA_A$ receptor • Unlike barbiturates, benzodiazepines do not activate $GABA_A$ receptors directly; rather benzodiazepines act allosterically by modifying the effects of GABA • Benzodiazepines and related compounds can act as agonists, antagonists, or inverse agonists • Agonists at the binding site increase, and inverse agonists decrease, the amount of chloride current generated by $GABA_A$ receptor activation

Hypnotics, Sedatives, and Ethanol

DRUG CLASS	DRUG	MECHANISM OF ACTION
Novel Benzodiazepine Receptor Agonists	Zolpidem	Zolpidem is a nonbenzodiazepine that acts as an agonist on $GABA_A$ receptors
	Zaleplon	Zaleplon is a nonbenzodiazepine that preferentially binds to the benzodiazepine-binding site on $GABA_A$ receptors containing the α1 receptor subunit
	Eszopiclone	Eszopiclone is believed to act by enhancing $GABA_A$ receptor function
Benzodiazepine Receptor Antagonist	Flumazenil	Flumazenil binds with high affinity to specific sites on the $GABA_A$ receptor, where it competitively antagonizes the binding and allosteric effects of benzodiazepines and other ligands
Melatonin Congeners	Ramelteon	Agonist at melatonin MT_1 and MT_2 receptors to promote sleep
Barbiturates	Amobarbital Butabarbital Mephobarbital Methohexital Pentobarbital Phenobarbital Secobarbital Thiopental	Mechanism of action of barbiturates on $GABA_A$ receptors (see Figure 9-1): • Barbiturates enhance the binding of GABA to $GABA_A$ receptors in a Cl^- dependent fashion; however, barbiturates also promote the binding of benzodiazepines • Barbiturates potentiate GABA-induced Cl^- currents by prolonging periods during which bursts of channel opening occur • Only α and β (not γ) subunits of $GABA_A$ receptors are required • Barbiturate-induced increases in Cl^- conductance are not affected by the deletion of the tyrosine and threonine residues in the β subunit that govern the sensitivity of $GABA_A$ receptors to activation by agonists
Miscellaneous Sedative-Hypnotic Drugs	Paraldehyde	General central nervous system (CNS) depressant no longer used in the United States
	Chloral Hydrate	Rapidly metabolized to trichloroethanol which exerts barbiturate-like effects on the $GABA_A$ receptor
	Meprobamate	Mechanism of action is not clear
	Carisoprodol	Metabolized to meprobamate
	Etomidate	Intravenous anesthetic (see Chapter 11)
	Clomethiazole	Probably acts as an allosteric modulator at the barbiturate site on the $GABA_A$ receptor
	Propofol	Mechanism is not entirely known but thought to act through enhancement of $GABA_A$ receptor function
Drugs Used to Treat Alcoholism	Naltrexone	Opioid antagonist (see Chapter 10)
	Disulfiram	Inhibits aldehyde dehydrogenase (ALDH) causing accumulation of acetaldehyde (see Figure 9-2)
	Nalmefene	Opioid antagonist (see Chapter 10)
	Acamprosate	An analog of GABA, it is an agonist at $GABA_A$ receptors and is probably an allosteric modulator

SECTION II

CATEGORIES OF BENZODIAZEPINES BASED ON THEIR ELIMINATION $t_{1/2}$

- Ultra-short acting—midazolam
- Short-acting agents ($t_{1/2}$ <6 hours)—triazolam, the nonbenzodiazepine zolpidem ($t_{1/2}$ ~2 hours), and eszopiclone ($t_{1/2}$ 5-6 hours)
- Intermediate-acting agents ($t_{1/2}$ 6-24 hours), including estazolam and temazepam
- Long-acting agents ($t_{1/2}$ >24 hours), including flurazepam, diazepam, and quazepam

CATEGORIES OF INSOMNIA

- Transient insomnia lasts less than 3 days and usually is caused by a brief environmental or situational stressor
- Short-term insomnia lasts from 3 days to 3 weeks and is usually caused by a personal stressor such as illness, grief, or job problems
- Long-term insomnia is insomnia that has lasted for more than 3 weeks; no specific stressor may be identifiable

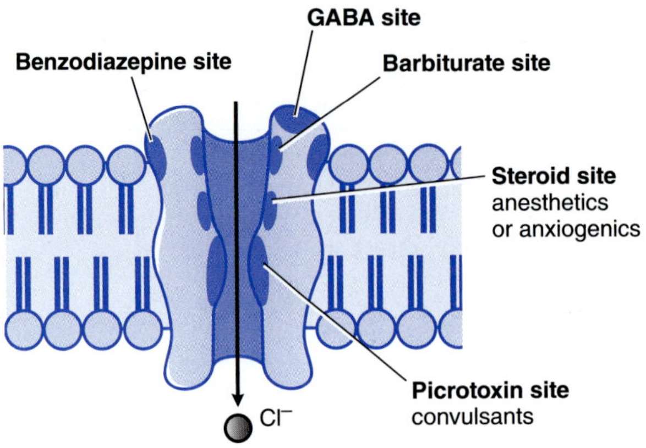

Neuropharmacology

FIGURE 9-1 Pharmacologic binding sites on the $GABA_A$ receptor. *(Reproduced with permission from Nestler EJ, Hyman SE, Malenka RC (eds). Molecular Neuropharmacology, 2nd ed. New York: McGraw-Hill, 2009, p 135. Copyright © 2009 by The McGraw-Hill Companies, Inc. All rights reserved.)*

CASE 9-1

A 35-year-old woman comes to her physician complaining of not being able to sleep for the past week. She is prescribed zolpidem to be taken at bedtime.

a. What type of drug is zolpidem and what is its mechanism of action?

Zolpidem is a nonbenzodiazepine sedative-hypnotic drug approved for the short-term treatment of insomnia. Although the actions of zolpidem are due to agonist effects on

(Continued)

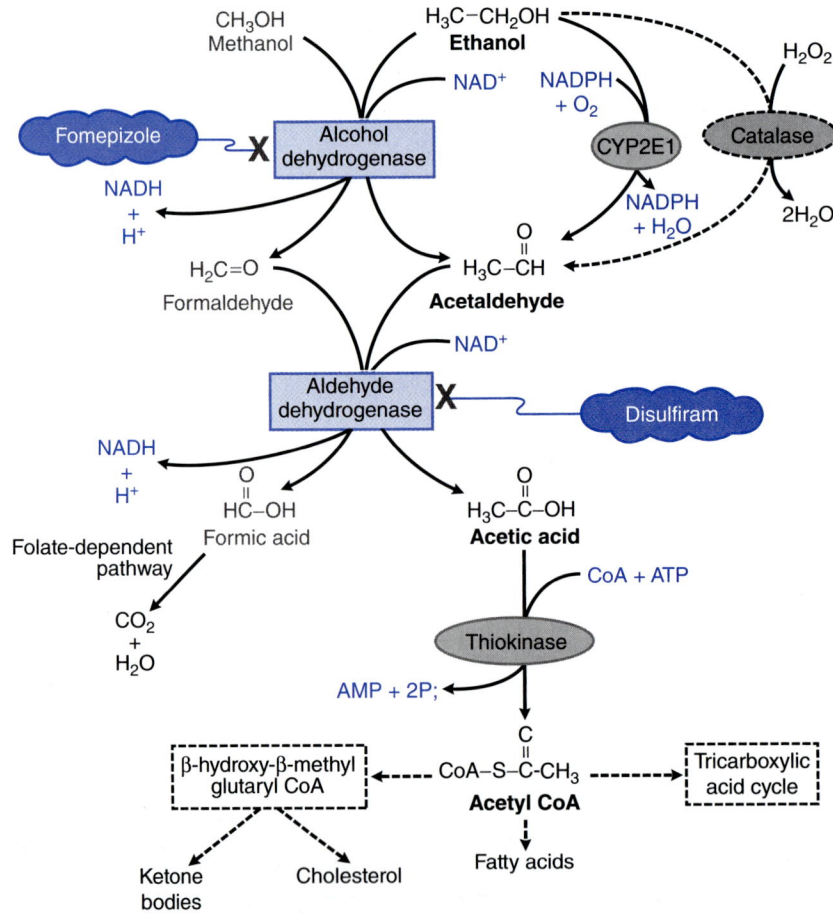

FIGURE 9-2 Metabolism of ethanol and methanol.

GABA$_A$ receptors and generally resemble those of benzodiazepines, it produces only weak anticonvulsant effects in experimental animals, and its relatively strong sedative actions appear to mask anxiolytic effects in various animal models of anxiety.

b. What side effects should this woman be warned of?

After discontinuation of zolpidem, the beneficial effects on sleep reportedly persist for up to 1 week, but mild rebound insomnia on the first night also has occurred. Tolerance and physical dependence develop only rarely and under unusual circumstances. At therapeutic doses (5-10 mg), zolpidem infrequently produces residual daytime sedation or amnesia, and the incidence of other adverse effects (eg, GI complaints or dizziness) also is low. As with the benzodiazepines, large overdoses of zolpidem do not produce severe respiratory depression unless other agents (eg, ethanol) also are ingested. Hypnotic doses increase the hypoxia and hypercarbia of patients with obstructive sleep apnea.

c. What considerations should her physician be aware of when treating insomnia in this patient?

The categories of insomnia are shown in the Side Bar CATEGORIES OF INSOMNIA. This patient's insomnia would be classified as short-term and hypnotics such as zolpidem should be used intermittently, perhaps even skipping a dose after 1 to 2 nights of good sleep. However, if her insomnia persists and becomes a long-term problem, it raises a new set of issues. Side effects of hypnotic agents may limit their usefulness for insomnia management (see Summary Table at the end of the chapter). The use of hypnotics for long-term insomnia is problematic for many reasons. Long-term hypnotic use leads to a decrease in effectiveness and may produce rebound insomnia on discontinuance. If a sedative-hypnotic has been used regularly for more than 2 weeks, it should be tapered rather than discontinued abruptly. In some patients on hypnotics with a short $t_{1/2}$, it is easier to switch first to a hypnotic with a long $t_{1/2}$ and then to taper. The onset of withdrawal symptoms from medications with a long $t_{1/2}$ may be delayed. Consequently, the patient should be warned about the symptoms associated with withdrawal effects.

Hypnotics that act at GABA$_A$ receptors, including the benzodiazepine hypnotics and the newer agents zolpidem, zopiclone, and zaleplon, are preferred to barbiturates because they have a greater therapeutic index, are less toxic in overdose, have smaller effects on sleep architecture, and have less abuse potential. Compounds with a shorter $t_{1/2}$ are favored in patients with sleep-onset insomnia but without significant daytime anxiety who need to function at full effectiveness during the day. These compounds also are appropriate for the elderly because of a decreased risk of falls and respiratory depression. However, the patient and physician should be aware that early-morning awakening, rebound daytime anxiety, and amnestic episodes could also occur. These undesirable side effects are more common at higher doses of the benzodiazepines.

CASE 9-2

A 23-year-old male college student is brought to the ER because he cannot be aroused. The patient has a history of depression and he has been acting depressed over his classes lately. The patient has a prescription for lorazepam for anxiety and insomnia. In the ER he is given flumazenil intravenously.

a. What type of drug is flumazenil and what is its role in treating a benzodiazepine overdose?

Flumazenil, the only member of this class, is an imidazobenzodiazepine that behaves as a specific benzodiazepine receptor antagonist. Flumazenil binds with high affinity to specific sites on the GABA$_A$ receptor, where it competitively antagonizes the binding and allosteric effects of benzodiazepines and other ligands. Flumazenil antagonizes both the electrophysiological and behavioral effects of agonist and inverse-agonist benzodiazepines. The drug is given intravenously.

(Continued)

The primary indications for the use of flumazenil are the management of suspected benzodiazepine overdose and the reversal of sedative effects produced by benzodiazepines administered during either general anesthesia or diagnostic and/or therapeutic procedures.

b. What cautions should be taken with this patient?

The administration of a series of small injections of flumazenil is preferred to a single bolus injection. A total of 1 mg flumazenil given over 1 to 3 minutes usually is sufficient to abolish the effects of therapeutic doses of benzodiazepines; patients with suspected benzodiazepine overdose should respond adequately to a cumulative dose of 1 to 5 mg given over 2 to 10 minutes; a lack of response to 5 mg flumazenil strongly suggests that a benzodiazepine is not the major cause of sedation. Additional courses of treatment with flumazenil may be needed within 20 to 30 minutes should sedation reappear. Flumazenil is not effective in single-drug overdoses with either barbiturates or tricyclic antidepressants. To the contrary, the administration of flumazenil in these settings may be associated with the onset of seizures, especially in patients poisoned with tricyclic antidepressants. Seizures or other withdrawal symptoms also may be precipitated in patients who had been taking benzodiazepines for protracted periods and in whom tolerance and/or dependence may have developed.

CASE 9-3

A 66-year-old man is brought to the ER with extreme anxiety, agitation, irritation, and confusion. It is learned that, because of early dementia, he recently did not renew his prescription for alprazolam, which he had been taking for the past 3 years for anxiety.

a. What is the likely cause of this patient's change in mental status?

Chronic benzodiazepine use poses a risk for development of dependence and abuse. Mild dependence may develop in many patients who have taken therapeutic doses of benzodiazepines on a regular basis for prolonged periods. Withdrawal symptoms may include temporary intensification of the problems that originally prompted their use (eg, insomnia or anxiety). Dysphoria, irritability, sweating, unpleasant dreams, tremors, anorexia, and faintness or dizziness also may occur, especially when withdrawal of the benzodiazepine occurs abruptly. Hence, it is prudent to taper the dosage gradually when therapy is to be discontinued.

b. What are the options for treating this patient?

One option would be to reinstitute the alprazolam and once it has its calming effects, begin a slow tapering of the dose. Another option would be to begin a benzodiazepine with a longer $t_{1/2}$ such as flurazepam and once it has its calming effects, discontinue its use and let the long half-life taper the effects and avoid withdrawal. Each of these options would depend on the ability of the patient or a caregiver to administer the drug.

CASE 9-4

A 43-year-old woman has been treated with secobarbital for insomnia for the past 10 years.

a. What distinguishes secobarbital from other barbiturates?

Table 9-1 shows the distinguishing features of selected barbiturates, including secobarbital. Secobarbital has a relatively short $t_{1/2}$ compared to other barbiturates such as phenobarbital.

b. What is the mechanism of action of barbiturates?

See the Mechanisms of Action Table above. The barbiturates reversibly depress the activity of all excitable tissues. The barbiturates exert several distinct effects on excitatory and inhibitory synaptic transmission. For example, (−)-pentobarbital

(Continued)

TABLE 9-1 Structures, Trade Names, and Major Pharmacological Properties of Selected Barbiturates

$$(\text{or } S=)^a \; O=C_2 \begin{array}{c} R_3 \\ N-C \\ | \quad \; \; \; 5 \\ N-C \\ H \end{array} \begin{array}{c} O \\ \diagdown \\ R_{5a} \\ \diagup \\ R_{5b} \\ O \end{array}$$

COMPOUND (TRADE NAMES)	R_3	R_{5a}	R_{5b}	DOSAGE FORMS[b]	$t_{1/2}$ (hours)	THERAPEUTIC USES	COMMENTS
Amobarbital (AMYTAL)	—H	—C_2H_5	—$CH_2CH_2CH(CH_3)_2$	IM, IV	10-40	Insomnia, pre-op sedation, emergency management of seizures	Only Na^+ salt administered parenterally
Butabarbital (BUTISOL, others)	—H	—C_2H_5	—$CH(CH_3)CH_2CH_3$	Oral	35-50	Insomnia, pre-op sedation	Redistribution shortens duration of action of single dose to 8 hours
Mephobarbital (MEBARAL)	—CH_3	—C_2H_5	—phenyl	Oral	10-70	Seizure disorders, daytime sedation	Second-line anticonvulsant
Methohexital (BREVITAL)	—CH_3	—$CH_2CH=CH_2$	—$CH(CH_3)C\equiv CCH_2CH_3$	IV	3-5[c]	Induction and maintenance of anesthesia	Only Na^+ salt available; single dose provides 5-7 min of Anesthesia[c]
Pentobarbital (NEMBUTAL)	—H	—C_2H_5	—$CH(CH_3)CH_2CH_2CH_3$	Oral, IM, IV, rectal	15-50	Insomnia, pre-op sedation, emergency management of seizures	Only Na^+ salt administered parenterally
Phenobarbital (LUMINAL, others)	—H	—C_2H_5	—phenyl	Oral, IM, IV	80-120	Seizure disorders, status epilepticus, daytime sedation	First-line anticonvulsant; only Na^+ salt administered parenterally
Secobarbital (SECONAL)	—H	—$CH_2CH=CH_2$	—$CH(CH_3)CH_2CH_2CH_3$	Oral	15-40	Insomnia, preoperative Sedation	Only Na^+ salt available
Thiopental (PENTOTHAL)	—H	—C_2H_5	—$CH(CH_3)CH_2CH_2CH_3$	IV	8-10[c]	Induction and maintenance of anesthesia, pre-op sedation, emergency management of seizures	Only Na^+ salt available; single dose provides brief of anesthesia[c]

[a] O except in thiopental, where it is replaced by S. [b] IM, intramuscular injection; IV, intravenous administration. [c] Value represents terminal $t_{1/2}$ due to metabolism by the liver; redistribution following parenteral administration produces effects lasting only a few minutes

potentiates GABA-induced increases in chloride conductance and depresses voltage-activated Ca^{2+} currents at similar concentrations (<10 µM) in isolated hippocampal neurons. Barbiturates can produce all degrees of depression of the CNS, ranging from mild sedation to general anesthesia.

c. **Why are barbiturates now not commonly used as sedatives?**

The barbiturates were once used extensively as sedative-hypnotic drugs, but are associated with physical dependence. Except for a few specialized uses, they have been largely replaced by the much safer benzodiazepines.

d. **Describe the tolerance and physical dependence that occurs with barbiturates.**

Pharmacodynamic (functional) and pharmacokinetic tolerance to barbiturates can occur. The former contributes more to the decreased effect than does the latter.

(Continued)

SECTION II

Neuropharmacology

Tolerance to the effects on mood, sedation, and hypnosis occurs more readily and is greater than that to the anticonvulsant and lethal effects; thus, as tolerance increases, the therapeutic index decreases. Pharmacodynamic tolerance to barbiturates confers cross-tolerance to all general CNS-depressant drugs, including ethanol.

Chronic administration of barbiturates markedly increases the protein and lipid content of the hepatic smooth endoplasmic reticulum, as well as the activities of glucuronyl transferase and CYPs 1A2, 2C9, 2C19, and 3A4. The induction of these enzymes increases the metabolism of a number of drugs and endogenous substances, including steroid hormones, cholesterol, bile salts, and vitamins K and D. This also results in an increased rate of barbiturate metabolism, which partly accounts for the tolerance to barbiturates. Repeated administration, especially of phenobarbital, shortens the $t_{1/2}$ of barbiturates that are metabolized as a result of the induction of microsomal enzymes.

Like other CNS depressant drugs, barbiturates are abused, and some individuals develop a dependence on them (see Chapter 14). Moreover, the barbiturates may have euphoriant effects.

Withdrawal from barbiturates can be serious, resulting in seizures and death.

e. What are the adverse effects that can be seen with the chronic use of barbiturates?

Drowsiness may last for only a few hours after a hypnotic dose of barbiturate, but residual CNS depression sometimes is evident the following day, and subtle distortions of mood and impairment of judgment and fine motor skills may be demonstrable. Residual effects also may take the form of vertigo, nausea, vomiting, or diarrhea, or sometimes may be manifested as overt excitement. The user may awaken slightly intoxicated and feel euphoric and energetic; later, as the demands of daytime activities challenge possibly impaired faculties, the user may display irritability and temper.

Rarely, exfoliative dermatitis may be caused by phenobarbital and can prove fatal; the skin eruption may be associated with fever, delirium, and marked degenerative changes in the liver and other parenchymatous organs.

Barbiturates combine with other CNS depressants to cause severe depression; ethanol is the most frequent offender, and interactions with first-generation antihistamines also are common.

Barbiturates competitively inhibit the metabolism of certain other drugs; however, the greatest number of drug interactions results from induction of hepatic CYPs and the accelerated disappearance of many drugs and endogenous substances (see answer to Case 9-4d above).

Because barbiturates enhance porphyrin synthesis, they are absolutely contraindicated in patients with acute intermittent porphyria or porphyria variegata.

DISTINGUISHING FEATURES OF FETAL ALCOHOL SYNDROME

- A cluster of craniofacial abnormalities
- CNS dysfunction
- Pre- and/or postnatal stunting of growth

CASE 9-5

A 35-year-old woman has been an abstainer from alcohol all of her adult life. Recently she has read on the Internet that the French population have a relatively low mortality from coronary heart disease and that this "protection" is due to their widespread wine consumption. She talks to her physician about this issue.

a. Should this patient be advised to consume alcohol in moderate amounts?

In most countries, the risk of mortality due to coronary heart disease (CHD) is correlated with a high dietary intake of saturated fat and elevated serum cholesterol levels. France is an exception to this rule, with relatively low mortality from CHD despite the consumption of high quantities of saturated fats (the "French paradox"). Epidemiological studies suggest that widespread wine consumption

(Continued)

(20-30 g ethanol per day) is 1 of the factors conferring a cardioprotective effect, with 1 to 3 drinks per day resulting in a 10 to 40% decreased risk of coronary heart disease compared with abstainers. One possible mechanism by which alcohol could reduce the risk of CHD is through its effects on blood lipids. Changes in plasma lipoprotein levels, particularly increases in high-density lipoprotein (HDL; see Chapter 20), have been associated with the protective effects of ethanol.

b. Should abstainers from alcohol be advised to consume ethanol in moderate amounts?

The answer is no. There have been no randomized clinical trials to test the efficacy of daily alcohol use in reducing rates of coronary heart disease and mortality, and it is inappropriate for physicians to advocate alcohol ingestion solely to prevent heart disease.

c. What are the effects of ethanol on various physiological systems?

Table 9-2 lists the effects of ethanol on various physiological systems. Most notable are the CNS where ethanol is a general CNS depressant and perturbs the balance between excitatory and inhibitory influences in the brain, resulting in anxiolysis, ataxia, and sedation; the cardiovascular system where ethanol can result in cardiomyopathy; skeletal muscle where ethanol results in decreased strength, and the gastrointestinal system where ethanol can produce significant pathology in the pancreas and liver.

TABLE 9-2 Effects of Ethanol on Physiological Systems

PHYSIOLOGICAL SYSTEM	EFFECT
Central Nervous System	Ethanol is a general CNS depressant. Chronic abuse leads to dependence, tolerance, and craving for ethanol (see Chapter 14). Alcoholism is a progressive illness, and brain damage from chronic alcohol abuse contributes to the deficits in cognitive functioning and judgment seen in alcoholics. Alcoholism is a leading cause of dementia in the United States. Chronic alcohol abuse results in shrinkage of the brain owing to loss of both white and gray matter. It is important to note that ethanol itself is neurotoxic, and although malnutrition or vitamin deficiencies probably play roles in complications of alcoholism such as Wernicke encephalopathy and Korsakoff's psychosis, most of the alcohol-induced brain damage in Western countries is due to alcohol itself. Additional severe neurological syndromes associated with chronic heavy use of alcohol include cerebellar degeneration with associated atrophy of the cerebellar vermis, and a peripheral neuropathy. Heavy doses of ethanol over multiple days or weeks are also associated with several temporary but disturbing "alcohol-induced" psychiatric syndromes.
Neurochemical Pathways	Alcohol perturbs the balance between excitatory and inhibitory influences in the brain, resulting in anxiolysis, ataxia, and sedation. This is accomplished by either enhancing inhibitory or antagonizing excitatory neurotransmission. Ethanol likely produces its effects by simultaneously altering the functioning of a number of proteins that can affect neuronal excitability (see Table 9-3). Many of the prominent effects are on ligand-gated and voltage-gated ion channels and GPCR systems. While no definitive data on the mechanisms for alcohol-induced psychiatric conditions are available, it is logical to assume that alcohol-related changes in CNS pathways (NE and 5-HT levels, the balance between $GABA_A$ and NMDA receptor activity, dopaminergic activity) may operate in a manner similar to those seen in depression, anxiety, and schizophrenic disorders.
Ion Channels	Substantial data implicate the $GABA_A$ receptor as an important target for the in vivo actions of ethanol. Stimulation of this multisubunit, ligand-gated Cl^- channel system contributes to feelings of sleepiness, muscle relaxation, and the acute anticonvulsant properties associated with all GABA-boosting drugs. The nicotinic ACh receptor is also sensitive to the effects of ethanol. Drinking acutely increases ACh in the ventral tegmental area, with a subsequent increase in DA in the nucleus accumbens. Ethanol inhibits the function of the NMDA and kainate receptor subtypes; AMPA receptors are largely resistant to alcohol. Ethanol enhances the activity of large-conductance, Ca^{2+}-activated K^+ channels in neurohypophyseal terminals, perhaps contributing to the reduced release of oxytocin and vasopressin after ethanol consumption.

(Continued)

PHYSIOLOGICAL SYSTEM	EFFECT
Other Neurotransmitter Systems	Dopamine-related systems have central importance regarding the feelings of reward and craving associated with all intoxicating substances. Of special importance are alterations in DA activity in the ventral tegmental and related areas, especially the nucleus accumbens, which are likely to play a major role in feelings of euphoria and reward. Acute alcohol intoxication results in an increase in synaptic DA; repeated alcohol administration is associated with changes in both D_2 and D_4 receptors that may be important in the perpetuation of alcohol use as well as in relapse. The acute administration of ethanol is associated with a significant increase in 5-HT in the synaptic space; continued use of ethanol produces an upregulation of 5-HT receptors. Cannabinoid receptors, especially CB_1 encoded by the gene CNR1, are also affected by ethanol. Activation of CB_1 occurs with acute ethanol administration and affects the release of DA, GABA, and glutamate, and reward circuits of the brain. Antagonists of CB_1 receptors, such as rimonabant, may block the effect of ethanol on dopaminergic systems.
Protein Kinases and Intracellular Signaling Enzymes	Intracellular signal-transduction cascades, such as MAPK, tyrosine kinases, and neurotrophic factor receptors, also are thought to be affected by ethanol. Ethanol enhances the activities of several isoforms of adenylyl cyclase, with AC7 being the most sensitive. This promotes increased production of cyclic AMP and thus increased activity of PKA. Ethanol's actions appear to be mediated by activation of G_s and promotion of the interaction between G_s and adenylyl cyclase.

Cardiovascular System	Ethanol intake greater than 3 standard drinks per day elevates the risk for heart attacks and bleeding-related strokes. Indeed, vascular-related diseases are among the leading causes of early death in alcohol-dependent individuals. The risk includes a sixfold increased risk for coronary artery disease, a heightened risk for cardiac arrhythmias, and an elevated risk of congestive heart failure.
	Serum Lipoproteins and Cardiovascular Effects
	  In France, there is relatively low mortality from coronary heart disease (CHD) despite the consumption of high quantities of saturated fats (the "French paradox"). Epidemiological studies suggest that widespread wine consumption (20-30 g ethanol per day) is one of the factors conferring a cardioprotective effect, with 1-3 drinks per day resulting in a 10-40% decreased risk of coronary heart disease compared with abstainers. In contrast, daily consumption of greater amounts of alcohol leads to an increased incidence of noncoronary causes of cardiovascular failure, such as arrhythmias, cardiomyopathy, and hemorrhagic stroke, offsetting the beneficial effects of alcohol on coronary arteries; that is, alcohol has a J-shaped dose-mortality curve. One possible mechanism by which alcohol could reduce the risk of CHD is through its effects on blood lipids. Changes in plasma lipoprotein levels, particularly increases in high-density lipoprotein (HLD) (see Chapter 20), have been associated with the protective effects of ethanol.
	Hypertension
	  Heavy alcohol use can raise diastolic and systolic blood pressure. The prevalence of hypertension attributable to excess alcohol consumption is not known, but studies suggest a range of 5-11%.
	Cardiac Arrhythmias
	  Alcohol has a number of pharmacological effects on cardiac conduction, including prolongation of the QT interval, prolongation of ventricular repolarization, and sympathetic stimulation. Atrial arrhythmias associated with chronic alcohol use include supraventricular tachycardia, atrial fibrillation, and atrial flutter.
	Cardiomyopathy
	  Ethanol is known to have dose-related toxic effects on both skeletal and cardiac muscle. Numerous studies have shown that alcohol can depress cardiac contractility and lead to cardiomyopathy.
	Stroke
	  Clinical studies indicate an increased incidence of hemorrhagic and ischemic stroke in persons who drink more than 40-60 g alcohol per day.

Skeletal Muscle	Chronic, heavy, daily alcohol consumption is associated with decreased muscle strength, even when adjusted for other factors such as age, nicotine use, and chronic illness. Heavy doses of alcohol also can cause irreversible damage to muscle, reflected by a marked increase in the activity of creatine kinase in plasma.
Body Temperature	Ingestion of ethanol causes a feeling of warmth because alcohol enhances cutaneous and gastric blood flow. Increased sweating also may occur. Heat, therefore, is lost more rapidly, and the internal body temperature falls. After consumption of large amounts of ethanol, the central temperature-regulating mechanism becomes depressed, and the fall in body temperature may become pronounced.
Diuresis	Alcohol inhibits the release of vasopressin (antidiuretic hormone) from the posterior pituitary gland, resulting in enhanced diuresis. The volume loading that accompanies imbibing complements the diuresis that occurs as a result of reduced vasopressin secretion.

(Continued)

PHYSIOLOGICAL SYSTEM	EFFECT
Gastrointestinal System	**Esophagus** Alcohol frequently is either the primary etiologic factor or one of multiple causal factors associated with esophageal dysfunction. **Stomach** Heavy alcohol use can disrupt the gastric mucosal barrier and cause acute and chronic gastritis. Alcohol is not thought to play a role in the pathogenesis of peptic ulcer disease. Unlike acute and chronic gastritis, peptic ulcer disease is not more common in alcoholics. Nevertheless, alcohol exacerbates the clinical course and severity of ulcer symptoms. It appears to act synergistically with *Helicobacter pylori* to delay healing (see Chapter 32). **Intestines** Many alcoholics have chronic diarrhea as a result of malabsorption in the small intestine. The major symptom is frequent loose stools. The rectal fissures and *pruritus ani* that frequently are associated with heavy drinking probably are related to chronic diarrhea. **Pancreas** Heavy alcohol use is the most common cause of both acute and chronic pancreatitis in the United States. While pancreatitis has been known to occur after a single episode of heavy alcohol use, prolonged heavy drinking is common in most cases. Acute alcoholic pancreatitis is characterized by the abrupt onset of abdominal pain, nausea, vomiting, and increased levels of serum or urine pancreatic enzymes. **Liver** Ethanol produces a constellation of dose-related deleterious effects in the liver. The primary effects are fatty infiltration of the liver, hepatitis, and cirrhosis. Because of its intrinsic toxicity, alcohol can injure the liver in the absence of dietary deficiencies. The accumulation of fat in the liver is an early event and can occur in normal individuals after the ingestion of relatively small amounts of ethanol. This accumulation results from inhibition of both the tricarboxylic acid cycle and the oxidation of fat, in part owing to the generation of excess NADH produced by the actions of ADH and ALDH (see Figure 9-2). Fibrosis, resulting from tissue necrosis and chronic inflammation, is the underlying cause of alcoholic cirrhosis. **Vitamins and Minerals** The almost complete lack of protein, vitamins, and most other nutrients in alcoholic beverages predisposes those who consume large quantities of alcohol to nutritional deficiencies. Alcoholics often present with these deficiencies owing to decreased intake, decreased absorption, or impaired utilization of nutrients. The peripheral neuropathy, Korsakoff's psychosis, and Wernicke's encephalopathy seen in alcoholics probably are caused by deficiencies of the B complex of vitamins (particularly thiamine), although direct toxicity produced by alcohol itself has not been ruled out.
Sexual Function	Despite the widespread belief that alcohol can enhance sexual activities, the opposite effect is generally noted. Both acute and chronic alcohol use can lead to impotence in men. Increased blood alcohol concentrations lead to decreased sexual arousal, increased ejaculatory latency, and decreased orgasmic pleasure. Many female alcoholics complain of decreased libido, decreased vaginal lubrication, and menstrual cycle abnormalities.
Hematological and Immunological Effects	Chronic alcohol use is associated with anemia. Microcytic anemia can occur because of chronic blood loss and iron deficiency. Macrocytic anemia and increases in mean corpuscular volume are common and may occur in the absence of vitamin deficiencies. Normochromic anemia also can occur owing to effects of chronic illness on hematopoiesis. Alcohol also affects granulocytes and lymphocytes. Effects include leukopenia, alteration of lymphocyte subsets, decreased T-cell mitogenesis, and changes in immunoglobulin production.

TABLE 9-3 Impact of Ethanol on Key Neurochemical Systems

NEUROTRANSMITTER SYSTEM	EFFECTS
$GABA_A$	GABA release, ↑ receptor density
NMDA	Inhibition of postsynaptic NMDA receptors; with chronic use, up-regulation
DA	↑ Synaptic DA, ↑ effects on ventral tegmentum/nucleus accumbens reward
ACTH	↑ CNS and blood levels of ACTH
Opioid	Release of β endorphins, activation of μ receptors
5-HT	↑ in 5-HT synaptic space
Cannabinoid	↑ CB1 activity → changes in DA, GABA, glutamate activity

SECTION II — Neuropharmacology

CASE 9-6

A 43-year-old man has been chronically abusing alcohol (up to one-fifth of whisky per day) over the past 10 years. He is recently incarcerated and has had no access to alcohol for the past 3 days.

a. What is this man at risk of?

Physical dependence to ethanol is demonstrated by the elicitation of a withdrawal syndrome when alcohol consumption is terminated. The symptoms and severity are determined by the amount and duration of alcohol consumption and include sleep disruption, autonomic nervous system (sympathetic) activation, tremors, and in severe cases, seizures. In addition, 2 or more days after withdrawal, some individuals experience delirium tremens, characterized by hallucinations, delirium, fever, and tachycardia. Delirium tremens can be fatal.

b. How should alcohol withdrawal be treated?

Alcohol withdrawal syndrome should be treated with sedatives such as a long-acting benzodiazepine, and general supportive care such as intravenous fluids and seizure precautions.

CASE 9-7

A 40-year-old man has been consuming 4 to 5 alcoholic drinks each night after work and an additional 2 to 3 drinks each night at home. Recently, he has been consuming alcohol prior to leaving for work in the morning. He is seeking help for his drinking behavior.

a. What are the goals of any alcohol treatment program?

The core of care is a process of interventions and sessions that help enhance changes in how the person views their problem, along with efforts to help them alter the problematic behaviors. With cognitive-behavioral approaches serving as the core of treatment, and a 20% or greater rate of spontaneous remission in alcohol use disorders, the role of medications can be difficult to evaluate. Thus, only those pharmacological approaches that have been shown to be superior to placebo through double-blind control trials are worth considering in clinical practice.

b. What is the role of pharmacotherapy of alcoholism?

Currently, 3 drugs are approved in the United States for treatment of alcoholism: disulfiram, naltrexone, and acamprosate (see Table 9-4). Disulfiram has a long history of use but has fallen into disfavor because of its side effects and problems with patient adherence to therapy. Naltrexone and acamprosate were introduced more recently. The goal of these medications is to assist the patient in maintaining abstinence.

(Continued)

TABLE 9-4 Oral Medications for Treating Alcohol Abuse

MEDICATION	USUAL DOSE	MECHANISM/EFFECT
Disulfiram	250 mg/day (range 125-500 mg/day)	Inhibits ALDH with resulting ↑ acetaldehyde after drinking. Abstinence is reinforced to avoid the resulting adverse reaction.
Naltrexone	50 mg/day	μ Opioid receptor antagonist; felt to ↓ drinking through ↓ feelings of reward with alcohol and/or ↓ craving.
Acamprosate	666 mg three times daily	Weak antagonist of NMDA receptors, activator of $GABA_A$ receptors; may ↓ mild protracted abstinence syndromes with ↓ feelings of a "need" for alcohol.

c. **What are the drugs available to treat alcoholism?**

Naltrexone helps to maintain abstinence by reducing the urge to drink and increasing control when a "slip" occurs. It is not a "cure" for alcoholism and does not prevent relapse in all patients. Naltrexone works best when used in conjunction with some form of psychosocial therapy, such as cognitive behavioral therapy. There is evidence that naltrexone blocks activation by alcohol of dopaminergic pathways in the brain that are thought to be critical to reward.

Acamprosate is an analogue of GABA. A number of double-blind, placebo-controlled studies have demonstrated that acamprosate (1.3-2 g/d) decreases drinking frequency and reduces relapse drinking in abstinent alcoholics and appears to have efficacy similar to that of naltrexone.

Disulfiram, given alone, is a relatively nontoxic substance, but it inhibits aldehyde dehydrogenase (ALDH) activity (see Figure 9-2) and causes the blood acetaldehyde concentration to rise to 5 to 10 times above the level achieved when ethanol is given to an individual not pretreated with disulfiram. Acetaldehyde, produced as a result of the oxidation of ethanol by alcohol dehydrogenase (ADH), ordinarily does not accumulate in the body because it is further oxidized almost as soon as it is formed. Following the administration of disulfiram, both cytosolic and mitochondrial forms of ALDH are irreversibly inactivated to varying degrees, and the concentration of acetaldehyde rises.

The ingestion of alcohol by individuals previously treated with disulfiram gives rise to marked signs and symptoms of acetaldehyde poisoning. Within 5 to 10 minutes, the face feels hot and soon afterward becomes flushed and scarlet in appearance. As the vasodilation spreads over the whole body, intense throbbing is felt in the head and neck, and a pulsating headache may develop. Respiratory difficulties, nausea, copious vomiting, sweating, thirst, chest pain, considerable hypotension, orthostatic syncope, marked uneasiness, weakness, vertigo, blurred vision, and confusion are observed. The facial flush is replaced by pallor, and the blood pressure may fall to shock levels.

CASE 9-8

A 22-year-old pregnant woman continues to drink 4 to 5 beers and 2 to 3 glasses of wine each day despite being cautioned against the use of alcohol while she is pregnant

a. **What are possible teratogenic effects of ethanol?**

Children born to alcoholic mothers display a common pattern of distinct dysmorphology known as fetal alcohol syndrome (FAS). The diagnosis of FAS typically is based on the observance of a triad of abnormalities shown in the Side Bar DISTINGUISHING FEATURES OF FETAL ALCOHOL SYNDROME.

b. **What is the likelihood that the child of this woman will have FAS?**

The incidence of FAS is believed to be in the range of 0.5 to 1 per 1000 live births in the general US population, with rates as high as 2 to 3 per 1000 in African American and Native American populations. A lower socioeconomic status of the mother rather than racial background per se appears to be primarily responsible for the higher incidence of FAS observed in those groups. Children who do not meet all the criteria for a diagnosis of FAS still may show physical and mental deficits consistent with a partial phenotype, termed fetal alcohol effects (FAEs) or alcohol-related neurodevelopmental disorders.

The incidence of FAEs is likely higher than that of FAS, making alcohol consumption during pregnancy a major public health problem.

SECTION II — Neuropharmacology

KEY CONCEPTS

- Benzodiazepine can be categorized based on their elimination $t_{1/2}$ (see Side Bar CATEGORIES OF BENZODIAZEPINES BASED ON THEIR ELIMINATION $t_{1/2}$).
- Benzodiazepines are pharmacologically interchangeable.
- Benzodiazepines act by modulating the effects of GABA at the $GABA_A$ receptor.
- Most benzodiazepines are metabolized extensively by hepatic CYPs; oxazepam and lorazepam are conjugated directly (see Table 9-5).
- Flumazenil is a benzodiazepine antagonist used to reverse effects of benzodiazepines.
- The novel benzodiazepine agonists zolpidem, zaleplon, and zopiclone have largely replaced benzodiazepines in the treatment of insomnia.
- Ethanol is metabolized by sequential hepatic oxidation first to acetaldehyde by ADH, and then to acetic acid by ALDH (see Figure 9-2).
- Ethanol has serious and long-lasting effects on many physiological systems (see Table 9-2).

TABLE 9-5 Major Metabolic Relationships among Some of the Benzodiazepines[a]

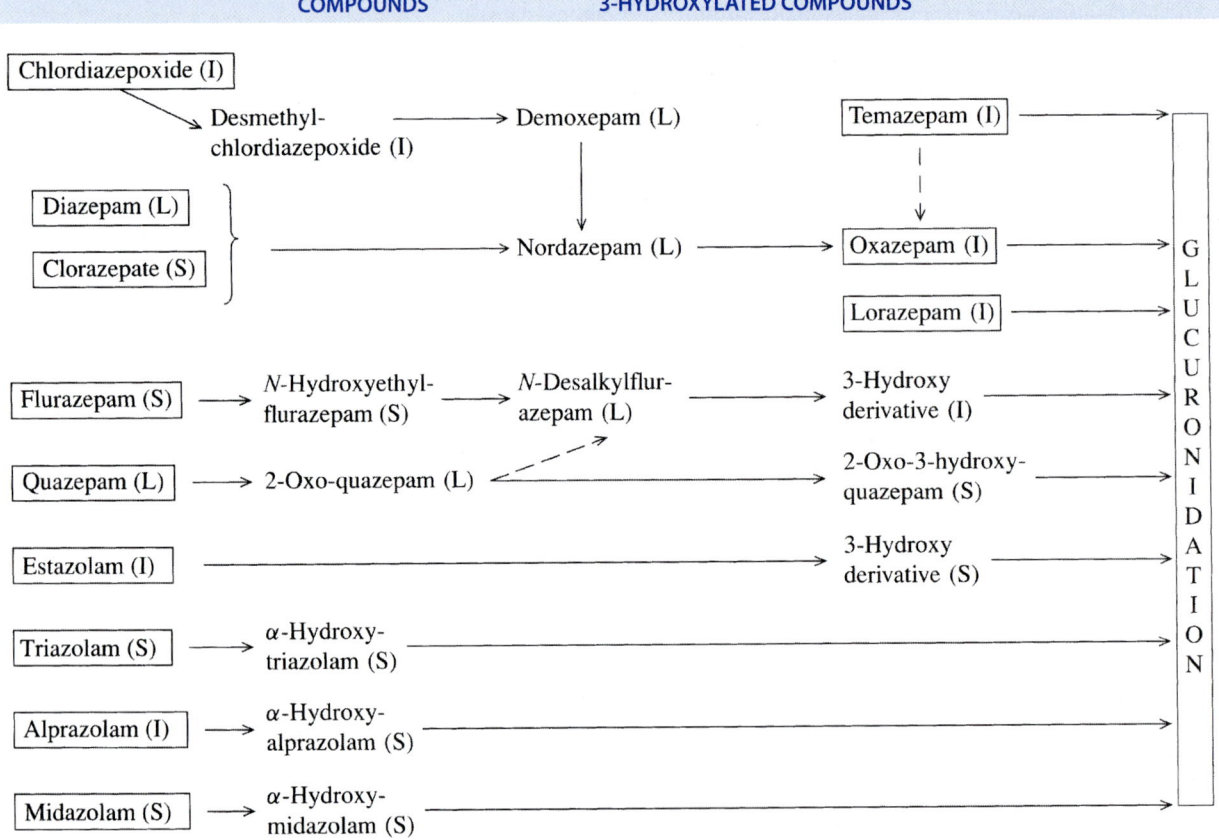

[a]Compounds enclosed in boxes are marketed in the United States. The approximate half-lives of the various compounds are denoted in parentheses; S (short-acting), $t_{1/2}$ <6 hours; I (intermediate-acting), $t_{1/2}$ = 6-24 hours; L (long-acting), $t_{1/2}$ = >24 hours. All compounds except clorazepate are biologically active; the activity of 3-hydroxydesalkylflurazepam has not been determined. Clonazepam (not shown) is an N-desalkyl compound, and it is metabolized primarily by reduction of the 7-NO_2 group to the corresponding amine (inactive), followed by acetylation; its $t_{1/2}$ is 20-40 hours.

Hypnotics, Sedatives, and Ethanol — CHAPTER 9

SUMMARY QUIZ ANSWER KEY

QUESTION 9-1 A 43-year-old man with severe hepatic cirrhosis requires a sedative for insomnia. Which of the following sedatives would be the best choice for this patient?

a. Phenobarbital
b. Diazepam
c. Lorazepam
d. Secobarbital
e. Flurazepam

QUESTION 9-2 A 19-year-old college student has overdosed on phenobarbital. After standard supportive care, the physician in the ER should do which of the following to hasten the elimination of phenobarbital?

a. Acidify the urine
b. Acidify the blood
c. Alkalinize the blood
d. Alkalinize the urine
e. Use a drug to stimulate hepatic CYP 2C19

QUESTION 9-3 A 32-year-old woman is taking ramelteon for chronic insomnia. Ramelteon binds to

a. melatonin receptors M_1 and M_2.
b. muscarinic receptors M_3.
c. nicotinic receptors.
d. α_1-adrenergic receptors.
e. D_2 dopaminergic receptors.

QUESTION 9-4 A 43-year-old woman is prescribed a benzodiazepine for anxiety. The choice of which benzodiazepine to prescribe should be based on

a. volume of distribution.
b. plasma half-life.
c. protein binding.
d. the indications approved by the FDA.
e. creatinine clearance.

QUESTION 9-5 A 53-year-old man with 15 years of alcohol abuse has developed weakness in his legs and the onset of heart failure. The primary treatment is

a. digoxin.
b. metoprolol.
c. creatine.
d. abstinence from alcohol.
e. thiamine.

QUESTION 9-6 A 33-year-old Japanese man becomes flushed and light-headed after one glass of wine. This reaction is likely due to

a. the rate he drank the glass of wine.
b. increased absorption of the alcohol.
c. inhibition of monoamine oxidase.
d. decreased renal excretion of alcohol.
e. a variant in aldehyde dehydrogenase.

SECTION II   Neuropharmacology

SUMMARY QUIZ ANSWER KEY

QUESTION 9-1 Answer is **c**. The benzodiazepines are metabolized extensively by hepatic CYPs, particularly CYPs 3A4 and 2C19. Some benzodiazepines, such as oxazepam and lorazepam, are conjugated directly and are not metabolized by these enzymes. Thus, the benzodiazepine of choice in a patient who might have diminished hepatic metabolism by CYPs would be either oxazepam or lorazepam.

QUESTION 9-2 Answer is **d**. The treatment of acute barbiturate intoxication is based on general supportive measures, which are applicable in most respects to poisoning by any CNS depressant. Hemodialysis or hemoperfusion is necessary only rarely, and the use of CNS stimulants is contraindicated because they increase the mortality rate. If renal and cardiac functions are satisfactory, and the patient is hydrated, forced diuresis and alkalinization of the urine will hasten the excretion of phenobarbital. Measures to prevent or treat atelectasis should be taken, and mechanical ventilation should be initiated when indicated. See Chapter 3 Clinical and Environmental Toxicity.

QUESTION 9-3 Answer is **a**. Ramelteon is a synthetic tricyclic analog of melatonin. Binding of agonists, such as melatonin, to MT_1 receptors promotes the onset of sleep while melatonin binding to MT_2 receptors shifts the timing of the circadian system. Ramelteon binds to both MT_1 and MT_2 receptors with high affinity but, unlike melatonin, it does not bind appreciably to quinone reductase 2, the structurally unrelated MT_3 receptor. Ramelteon is not known to bind to any other classes of receptors, such as nicotinic, acetylcholine, neuropeptide, dopamine, or opiate receptors, or the benzodiazepine-binding site on $GABA_A$ receptors.

QUESTION 9-4 Answer is **b**. The therapeutic uses and routes of administration of individual benzodiazepines that are marketed in the United States are summarized in Table 9-6. Most benzodiazepines can be used interchangeably. For example, diazepam can be used for alcohol withdrawal, and most benzodiazepines work as hypnotics. In general, the therapeutic choice of a given benzodiazepine depends on its $t_{1/2}$ (see Side Bar CATEGORIZATION OF BENZODIAZEPINES BASED ON THEIR ELIMINATION $t_{1/2}$) and may not match the FDA-approved indications. Benzodiazepines that are useful as anticonvulsants have a long $t_{1/2}$, and rapid entry into the brain is required for efficacy in treatment of status epilepticus. A short elimination $t_{1/2}$ is desirable for hypnotics, although this carries the drawback of increased abuse liability and severity of withdrawal after drug discontinuation. Antianxiety agents, in contrast, should have a long $t_{1/2}$ despite the drawback of the risk of neuropsychological deficits caused by drug accumulation.

QUESTION 9-5 Answer is **d**. Ethanol is known to have dose-related toxic effects on both skeletal and cardiac muscle. Numerous studies have shown that alcohol can depress cardiac contractility and lead to cardiomyopathy. Echocardiography demonstrates global hypokinesis. Approximately half of all patients with idiopathic cardiomyopathy are alcohol-dependent. Although the clinical signs and symptoms of idiopathic and alcohol-induced cardiomyopathy are similar, alcohol-induced cardiomyopathy has a better prognosis if patients are able to stop drinking. Since 40 to 50% of persons with alcohol-induced cardiomyopathy who continue to drink die within 3-5 years, abstinence remains the primary treatment.

QUESTION 9-6 Answer is **e**. Homozygotes with a nonfunctional aldehyde dehydrogenase 2*2 (ALDH2*2) occur in 5 to 10% of Japanese, Chinese, and Korean individuals, for whom severe adverse reactions occur after consumption of one drink or less. Consequently, their risk for severe repetitive heavy drinking is close to zero. This reaction operates through the same mechanism that occurs with drinking after taking the ALDH2 inhibitor, disulfiram (see Figure 9-2). Heterozygotes for this polymorphism (ALDH2*2, 2*1) make up 30 to 40% of Asian individuals who, after consuming ethanol, experience a facial flush and an enhanced sensitivity to beverage alcohol, but who do not necessarily report an overall adverse response to ethanol.

TABLE 9-6 Trade Names, Routes of Administration, and Therapeutic Uses of Benzodiazepines

COMPOUND (TRADE NAME)	ROUTES OF ADMINISTRATION[a]	EXAMPLES OF THERAPEUTIC USES[b]	COMMENTS	$t_{1/2}$, Hours[c]	USUAL SEDATIVE-HYPNOTIC DOSAGE, mg[d]
Alprazolam (XANAX)	Oral	Anxiety disorders, agoraphobia	Withdrawal symptoms may be especially severe	12±2	—
Chlordiazepoxide (LIBRIUM, others)	Oral, IM, IV	Anxiety disorders, management of alcohol withdrawal, anesthetic premedication	Long-acting and self-tapering because of active metabolites	10±3.4	50-100, qd–qid[e]
Clonazepam (KLONOPIN)	Oral	Seizure disorders, adjunctive treatment in acute mania and certain movement disorders	Tolerance develops to anticonvulsant effects	23±5	—
Clorazepate (TRANXENE, others)	Oral	Anxiety disorders, seizure disorders	Prodrug; activity due to formation of nordazepam during absorption	2.0±0.9	3.75-20, bid–qid[e]
Diazepam (VALIUM, others)	Oral, IM, IV, rectal	Anxiety disorders, status epilepticus, skeletal muscle relaxation, anesthetic premedication	Prototypical benzodiazepine	43±13	5-10, tid–qid[e]
Estazolam (PROSOM)	Oral	Insomnia	Contains triazolo ring; adverse effects may be similar to those of triazolam	10–24	1-2
Flurazepam (DALMANE)	Oral	Insomnia	Active metabolites accumulate with chronic use	74±24	15-30
Lorazepam (ATIVAN)	Oral, IM, IV	Anxiety disorders, preanesthetic medication	Metabolized solely by Conjugation	14±5	2-4
Midazolam (VERSED)	IV, IM	Preanesthetic and intraoperative medication	Rapidly inactivated	1.9±0.6	—[f]
Oxazepam (SERAX)	Oral	Anxiety disorders	Metabolized solely by Conjugation	8.0±2.4	15-30, tid–qid[e]
Quazepam (DORAL)	Oral	Insomnia	Active metabolites accumulate with chronic use	39	7.5-15
Temazepam (RESTORIL)	Oral	Insomnia	Metabolized mainly by Conjugation	11±6	7.5-30
Triazolam (HALCION)	Oral	Insomnia	Rapidly inactivated; may cause disturbing daytime side effects	2.9±1.0	0.125-0.25

[a]IM, intramuscular injection; IV, intravenous administration; qd, once a day; bid, twice a day; tid, three times a day; qid, four times a day. [b]The therapeutic uses are identified as examples to emphasize that most benzodiazepines can be used interchangeably. In general, the therapeutic uses of a given benzodiazepine are related to its $t_{1/2}$ and may not match the marketed indications.
[c]Half-life of active metabolite may differ. [d]For additional dosage information, see Chapter 11 (anesthesia), and Chapter 12 (seizure disorders).
[e]Approved as a sedative-hypnotic only for management of alcohol withdrawal; doses in a nontolerant individual would be smaller.
[f]Recommended doses vary considerably depending on specific use, condition of patient, and concomitant administration of other drugs.

SUMMARY TABLE: SEDATIVE HYPNOTIC DRUGS AND DRUGS USED TO TREAT ALCOHOLISM

CLASS AND SUBCLASSES	NAMES	CLINICAL USES	TOXICITIES COMMON	UNIQUE: CLINICALLY IMPORTANT
Benzodiazepines	Alprazolam, Chlordiazepoxide, Clonazepam, Chlorazepate, Diazepam, Estazolam, Flurazepam, Lorazepam, Midazolam, Oxazepam, Quazepam, Temazepam, Triazolam	The therapeutic uses and routes of administration of benzodiazepines are summarized in Table 9-6. In general, the therapeutic uses of a given benzodiazepine depend on its elimination $t_{1/2}$ (see Side Bar CATEGORIZATION OF BENZODIAZEPINES BASED ON THEIR ELIMINATION HALF-LIFE) and may not match FDA-approved indications	At peak concentrations hypnotic doses can be expected to cause varying degrees of lightheadedness, lassitude, increased reaction time, impaired mental and motor functions, confusion, and amnesia; these effects can impair driving skills, particularly when combined with ethanol	The paradoxical effect of nightmares has been reported with flurazepam. Amnesia, restlessness, sleepwalking, and hypomania have been reported with various benzodiazepines. Disinhibition reactions are also reported. Chronic benzodiazepine use is associated with dependence, abuse, and withdrawal
Novel Benzodiazepine Receptor Agonists	Zolpidem	Approved for the short-term treatment of insomnia	May produce daytime sedation or amnesia	Hypnotic doses increase the hypoxia and hypercarbia of patients with obstructive sleep apnea
	Zaleplon	Used to treat chronic or transient insomnia		Dependence and a withdrawal syndrome may be less than for other sedatives
	Eszopiclone	Used for long-term treatment of insomnia	Bitter taste	Minor withdrawal syndrome of abnormal dreams, anxiety, and nausea
Benzodiazepine Receptor Antagonist	Flumazenil	Available only for IV use to treat benzodiazepine overdose (see Chapter 3) and to reverse the sedative effects of benzodiazepines administered during surgery or diagnostic procedures	Duration of clinical effect usually only 30 to 60 minutes. A series of small injections is preferred to a single large injection; additional courses of treatment may be required should sedation reappear	Flumazenil will precipitate withdrawal in patients who have been using benzodiazepines chronically
Melatonin Congeners	Ramelteon	Approved for the treatment of insomnia. Not a controlled substance	Dizziness, nausea, fatigue	No tolerance to its reduction in sleep onset
Barbiturates	Amobarbital, Butabarbital, Mephobarbital, Methohexital, Pentobarbital, Phenobarbital, Secobarbital, Thiopental	All are used as sedatives, mephobarbital and phenobarbital are also used to treat seizures. See Table 9-1 for details of differences in plasma $t_{1/2}$ and uses	Residual CNS depression the day after administration. Residual effects may also include vertigo, nausea, vomiting, or diarrhea. Barbiturates may produce excitement rather than depression in some patients and may worsen a patient's perception of pain	Pharmacodynamic and pharmacokinetic tolerance to barbiturates can occur. Depression of respiratory drive. Induction of liver microsomal drug-metabolizing enzymes. Exfoliative dermatitis caused by phenobarbital. Severe CNS depression especially when combined with other CNS depressants such as ethanol. Because barbiturates cause enhanced porphyrin synthesis they are contraindicated in patients with acute intermittent porphyria or porphyria variegata

Hypnotics, Sedatives, and Ethanol — CHAPTER 9

CLASS AND SUBCLASSES	NAMES	CLINICAL USES	TOXICITIES COMMON	TOXICITIES UNIQUE: CLINICALLY IMPORTANT
Miscellaneous Sedative-Hypnotic Drugs	Paraldehyde	General CNS depressant no longer used in the United States	Irritating to throat and stomach after oral use	Intravenous use is associated with injuries to tissues
	Chloral hydrate	May be used to treat patients with paradoxical reactions to benzodiazepines		
	Meprobamate	Used as a sedative anti-anxiety agent	Drowsiness and ataxia	Abuse potential is high. Impairment of motor coordination and prolongation of reaction time. Withdrawal syndrome on abruptly stopping
	Carisoprodol	Muscle relaxant. Major metabolite is meprobamate	Drowsiness and ataxia	Has abuse potential as a popular street drug. Impairment of motor coordination and prolongation of reaction time. Withdrawal syndrome on abruptly stopping
	Etomidate	Used as an IV anesthetic (see Chapter 11)	See Chapter 11	See Chapter 11
	Clomethiazole	Used for hypnosis in elderly and institutionalized patients especially for withdrawal from ethanol		Physical dependence and tolerance can occur and are associated with a withdrawal syndrome upon abruptly stopping the drug
	Propofol	Used in the induction and maintenance of general anesthesia (see Chapter 11)	See Chapter 11	See Chapter 11
Drugs Used to Treat Alcoholism	Naltrexone	Approved for the treatment of ethanol dependence	Nausea, abdominal cramps	Excessive doses can cause liver damage. Contraindicated in patients with liver failure or acute hepatitis
	Disulfiram	Used to promote abstinence from ethanol	By itself disulfiram may cause lassitude, urticarial rash, restlessness, tremor, headache, dizziness, and mild GI disturbances	Severe reaction when ethanol, even in small quantities, is co-ingested. Reactions may include nausea, vomiting, flushing, sweating, chest pain, hypotension, blurred vision, and confusion
	Nalmefene	Approved for use in treatment of opiate overdose (see Chapter 10). Oral dosage forms used to treat ethanol dependence are not approved in the United States	Dizziness, nausea, vomiting	Agitation, hypotension, hallucinations
	Acamprosate	Promotes abstinence from ethanol	Insomnia, sexual impotence, headaches	Diarrhea, low or high blood pressure, irregular heart rhythm

CHAPTER 10

Opioid Pharmacology

DRUGS INCLUDED IN THIS CHAPTER

- Alfentanil (ALFENTA)
- Benzonatate (TESSALON, others)
- Buprenorphine; injection (BUPRENEX); oral (SUBUTEX); in combination with naloxone (SUBOXONE)
- Butorphanol (STADOL, others)
- Codeine
- Dextromethorphan marketed for over-the-counter sales
- Difenoxin (MOTOFEN) available only in combination with atropine
- Diphenoxylate (LOMOTIL, others) available only in combination with atropine
- Fentanyl citrate (SUBLIMAZE, others); transdermal patch (DURAGESIC, others); fentanyl buccal tablets, buccal film, lollipop-like lozenges (FENTORA, ONSOLIS, ACTIQ, others)
- Hydrocodone (LORTAB, VICODIN, others)
- Hydromorphone (DILAUDID, others)
- Levorphanol (LEVO-DROMORAN)
- Loperamide (IMODIUM, others)
- Meperidine (pethidine, DEMEROL, others)
- Methadone (DOLOPHINE, others)
- Methylnaltrexone (RELISTOR)
- Morphine sulfate; liposomal formulation (DEPODUR); preservative-free for spinal delivery (DURAMORPH, DEPODUR, others)
- Nalbuphine (NUBAIN, others)
- Nalmefene—no longer marketed in the United States
- Nalorphine (NALLINE, others)
- Naloxone (NARCAN, others)
- Naltrexone (REVIA, VIVITROL, others)
- Naltrindole (δ receptor antagonist used only for biomedical research)
- Oxycodone (PERCODAN); in combination with acetaminophen (PERCOCET); extended release (OXYCONTIN)
- Oxymorphone (NUMORPHAN, others)

(continues)

This chapter will be most useful after having a basic understanding of the material in Chapter 18, Opioids, Analgesia, and Pain Management in *Goodman & Gilman's The Pharmacological Basis of Therapeutics*, 12th Edition. In addition to the material presented here, the 12th Edition includes:

- A history of analgesic use
- A detailed description of the endogenous opioid systems: ligands and receptors
- A discussion of opioid receptor classes, distribution, binding/coupling requirements for opiate ligands, and the functional consequences of acute and chronic opiate receptor activation
- Figure 18-8 Structures of morphine-related opiate agonists and antagonists
- Figure 18-9 Chemical structures of piperidine and phenylpiperidine analgesics
- Details of the cellular and molecular mechanisms of opioid tolerance, dependence, and withdrawal
- Nonanalgesic therapeutic uses of opioids
- Table 18-4 Resources for Pain Management
- Table 18-5 World Health Organization Analgesic Ladder

LEARNING OBJECTIVES

- ☑ Understand the mechanisms of action, adverse effects, and therapeutic uses of opiate receptor agonists.
- ☑ Know the mechanisms of action and therapeutic uses of opiate receptor antagonists.
- ☑ Know the role of opiate receptor agonists in the management of acute and chronic pain.
- ☑ Know the different methods of administration of opiate receptor agonists that improve analgesic efficacy while reducing side effects.

ACTIONS AND SELECTIVITIES OF SOME OPIOIDS AT μ, δ, κ RECEPTORS

OPIATE LIGANDS	RECEPTOR TYPES		
	μ	δ	κ
Agonists			
Fentanyl	+++		
Hydromorphone	+++		
Levorphanol	+++		
Methadone	+++		
Morphine[a]	+++		
Sufentanil	+++	+	+
Buprenorphine	P		--
Butorphanol	P		+++

(Continued)

Opioid Pharmacology

CHAPTER 10

DRUGS INCLUDED IN THIS CHAPTER (Cont.)

- Pentazocine (TALWIN); in combination with acetaminophen (TALCEN); in combination with naloxone (TALWIN NX)
- Propoxyphene (DARVON, others)
- Propoxyphene napsylate (DARVON-N)
- Remifentanil (ULTIVA)
- Sufentanil (SUFENTA, others)
- Tapentadol (NUCYNTA)
- Tramadol (ULTRAM)

OPIATE LIGANDS	RECEPTOR TYPES		
	μ	δ	κ
Nalbuphine	–		++
Antagonists			
Naloxone[b]	– – –	–	– –
Naltrexone[b]	– – –	–	– – –
Naltrindole[b]	–	– – –	–

[a] Prototypical μ-preferring.
[b] antagonist; P partial agonist. The number of + or – symbols is an indication of potency.
Adapted with permission from Raynor K, Kong H, Chen Y, Yasuda K, Yu L, Bell GI, Reisine T, Pharmacological characterization of the cloned kappa-, delta-, and mu-opioid receptors. *Mol Pharmacol*, 1994;45:330-334.

MECHANISMS OF ACTION OF OPIOID AGONISTS AND ANTAGONISTS

DRUG CLASS	DRUG	MECHANISM OF ACTION
Opioid Receptor Agonist	Morphine Codeine Hydromorphone Hydrocodone Oxycodone Oxymorphone Meperidine Methadone Propoxyphene Fentanyl Alfentanil Sufentanil Remifentanil Levorphanol Tramadol Tapentadol	Morphine and its congeners act through activation (Side Bar ACTIONS AND SELECTIVITIES OF SOME OPIOIDS AT μ, δ, AND κ RECEPTORS) of the GPCR receptors: μ (mu opioid receptor, MOR); δ (delta opioid receptor, DOR); or κ (kappa opioid receptor, KOR) (see also Figure 10-1) Agonist binding results in conformational changes in the GPCR, initiating G protein activation (see Chapter 1); the G_i/G_o coupling results in a large number of intracellular events, including: • Inhibition of adenyl cyclase activity • Reduced opening of voltage-gated Ca^{2+} channels • Stimulation of K^+ current through several channels • Activation of PKC and PLC_β Tramadol and tapentadol also inhibit uptake of norepinephrine and serotonin
Opioid Receptor Agonists/Antagonists and Partial Agonists	Nalbuphine	MOR antagonist and KOR agonist
	Butorphanol	MOR antagonist and KOR agonist
	Pentazocine	Weak MOR antagonist or partial MOR agonist and KOR agonist
	Buprenorphine	Partial MOR agonist
Antidiarrheal Agents	Diphenoxylate	Congener of meperidine that activates MOR to produce constipation (see Chapter 33); only available in combination with atropine to reduce abuse liability
	Difenoxin	Metabolite of diphenoxylate that acts similar to parent compound
	Loperamide	Congener of meperidine that activates MOR to produce constipation (see Chapter 33)
Opioid Receptor Antagonist	Naloxone	Opioid receptor antagonist
	Naltrexone	Opioid receptor antagonist
	Methylnaltrexone	Opioid receptor antagonist at peripheral sites

(Continued)

SECTION II Neuropharmacology

FACTORS EXACERBATING OPIATE-INDUCED RESPIRATORY DEPRESSION

- **Other medications**
  Other depressant medications such as alcohol, tranquilizers, sedative-hypnotics
- **Sleep**
  Natural sleep produces a decrease in the sensitivity to CO_2
  Obstructive sleep apnea increases the likelihood of fatal respiratory depression
- **Age**
  Newborns and elderly patients are at greater risk
- **Disease**
  Patients with chronic cardiopulmonary or renal diseases can manifest a desensitization to increased CO_2
- **COPD**
  Enhanced respiratory depression is seen in patients with chronic obstructive pulmonary disease (COPD)
- **Relief of pain**
  Removal of a painful condition (which can stimulate respiration) will reduce the ventilatory drive and lead to apparent respiratory depression

DRUG CLASS	DRUG	MECHANISM OF ACTION
Antitussives	Dextromethorphan	Congener of the codeine analog methorphan NMDA-receptor antagonist Antitussive MOA is not clear (see Chapter 24)
	Benzonatate	Antitussive action is believed to be mediated through stretch or cough receptors in the lung, as well as by a central mechanism (see Chapter 24)

CASE 10-1

A 22-year-old man is brought to the emergency room following a skiing injury to his knee. Although he is in considerable pain, it is relieved by a small dose of morphine. He reports that his pain is still present, but it is less bothersome. He says the morphine "feels good."

a. What are the mechanisms for the different causes of pain?

All pain is not the same and a number of variables contribute to the patient's pain report and therefore to the effect of the analgesic. Many clinical pain syndromes, such as found in cancer, typically represent a combination of inflammatory and neuropathic mechanisms. The Side Bar PAIN STATES differentiates the various types of

(Continued)

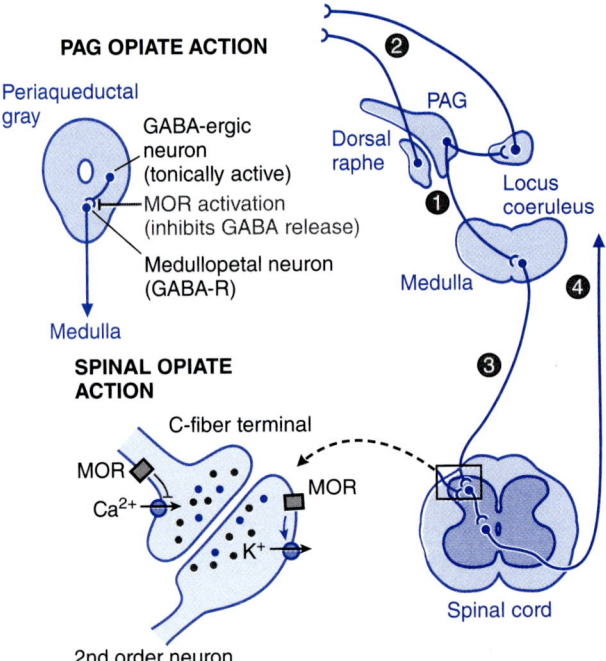

FIGURE 10-1 Mechanisms of opiate action in producing analgesia. Top left: Schematic of organization of opiate action in the periaqueductal gray (PAG). Top right: Opiate-sensitive pathways in PAG μ opiate actions block the release of GABA from tonically active systems that otherwise regulate the projections to the medulla (1) leading to an activation of PAG outflow resulting in activation of forebrain (2) and spinal (3) monoamine receptors that regulate spinal cord projections (4) which provide sensory input to higher centers and mood.
Bottom left: Schematic of primary afferent synapse with second order dorsal horn spinal neuron, showing pre- and postsynaptic opiate receptors coupled to Ca^{2+} and K^+ channels, respectively. Opiate receptor binding is highly expressed in the superficial spinal dorsal horn (substantia gelatinosa). These receptors are located presynaptically on the terminals of small primary afferents (C-fibers) and postsynaptically on second-order neurons. Presynaptically, activation of MOR blocks the opening of the voltage-sensitve Ca^{2+} channel, which otherwise initiates transmitter release. Postsynaptically, MOR activation enhances opening of K^+ channels, leading to hyperpolarization. Thus, an opiate agonist acting at these sites jointly serves to attenuate the afferent-evoked excitation of the second-order neuron.

Opioid Pharmacology

CHAPTER 10

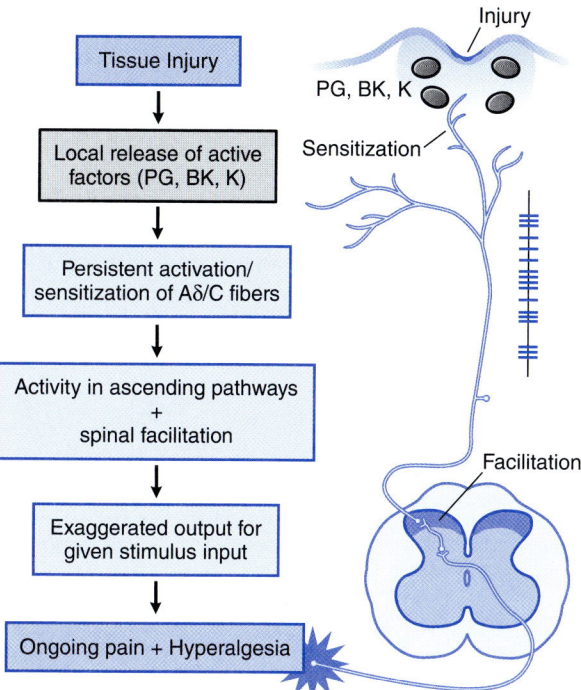

FIGURE 10-2 Mechanistic flow diagram of tissue injury–evoked nociception. BK, bradykinin; K, cytokines; PG, prostagladins.

pain and Figures 10-2 and 10-3 show mechanistic diagrams of these types of pain. Although nociceptive pain (as in this patient) usually is responsive to opioid analgesics, neuropathic pain is typically considered to respond less well to opioid analgesics.

b. What are the mechanisms of action for morphine and other opiate ligands to produce analgesia?

The analgesic actions of opiates after systemic delivery are believed to represent actions in the brain (supraspinal), spinal cord, and in some instances in the periphery. The supraspinal and spinal actions of opiates are shown schematically in Figure 10-1.

c. What are the mechanisms of action by which morphine and other opiate ligands alter mood and have rewarding properties that may be important in addiction?

The mechanisms by which opioids produce euphoria, tranquility, and other alterations of mood (including rewarding properties) are complex and not entirely clear.

(Continued)

PAIN STATES

- **Acute nociception**

  Acute activation of small high-threshold sensory afferents (Aδ and C fibers) generates transient input into the spinal cord, which in turn leads to activation of neurons that project contralateral to the thalamus and thence to the somatosensory cortex; examples include a hot coffee cup, a needle stick, or an incision

- **Tissue injury (Figure 10-2)**

  Following tissue injury or local inflammation (eg, local skin burn, toothache, rheumatoid joint), an ongoing pain state arises that is characterized by burning, throbbing, or aching, and an abnormal pain response (hyperalgesia); such tissue injury-evoked pain is often referred to as "nociceptive" pain

- **Nerve injury (Figure 10-3)**

  Injury to a peripheral nerve yields complex anatomical and biochemical changes in the nerve and spinal cord that induce spontaneous dysesthesias (shooting, burning pain) and allodynia (light touch hurts); this pain state is said to be neuropathic

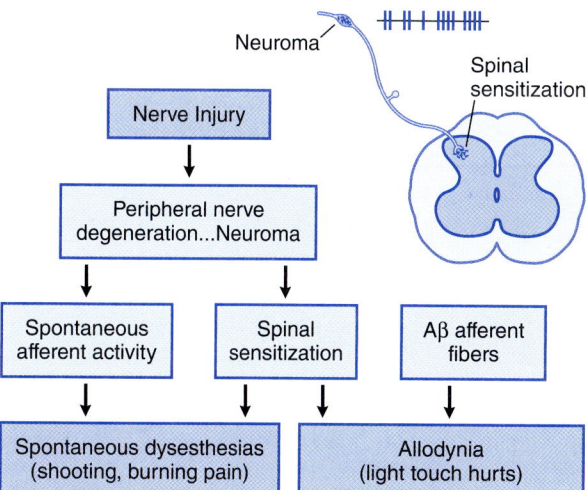

FIGURE 10-3 Mechanistic flow diagram of nerve injury–evoked nociception.

SECTION II Neuropharmacology

Neural systems thought to mediate opioid reinforcement overlap with, but are distinct from, those involved in physical dependence and analgesia. Behavioral and pharmacological data point to a pivotal role of the mesocorticolimbic (MCL) dopamine system, a basal forebrain circuit long implicated in reward and motivation (see Figure 10-4).

CASE 10-2

Following surgery for a hip replacement, a 64-year-old woman is treated with a parenteral opiate for pain. Upon release from hospital, she is given a prescription for oral oxycodone for pain. Three days after discharge she is complaining of constipation.

a. What is the cause of her constipation?

Opiates have important effects upon all aspects of GI function (see Chapter 33). It is estimated that 40 to 95% of patients treated with opioids develop constipation and that changes in bowel function can be demonstrated even with acute dosing. Opiate agonists suppress local neurogenic networks that provide a rhythmic

(Continued)

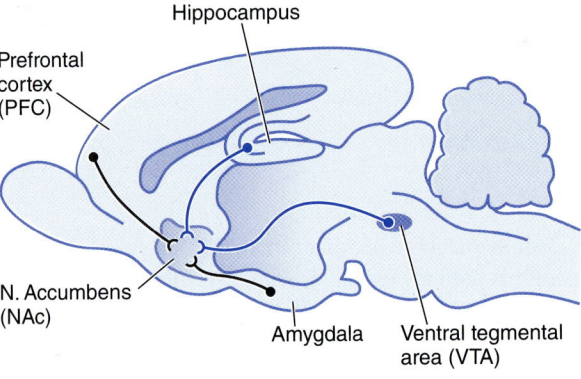

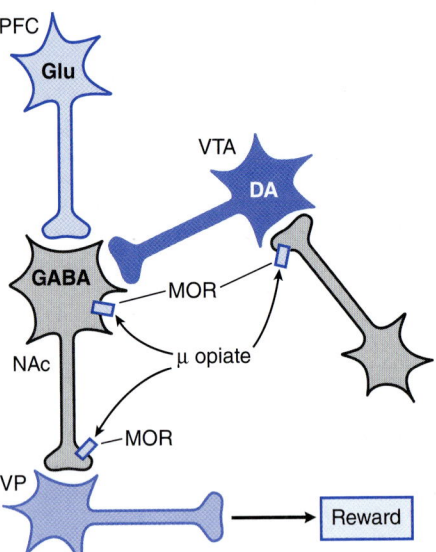

FIGURE 10-4 Schematic pathways underlying rewarding properties of opiates.
Upper panel: This sagittal section of rat brain displays simplified DA and GABA inputs from the ventral tegmental area (VTA) and prefrontal cortex (PFC), respectively, into the nucleus accumbens (NAc).
Lower panel: Neurons are labeled with their primary neurotransmitters. At a cellular level, MOR agonists reduce excitability and transmitter release at the sites indicated by inhibiting Ca^{2+} influx and enhancing K^+ current (see Figure 10-1). Thus, opiate-induced inhibition in the VTA on GABA-ergic interneurons or in the NAc reduce GABA-mediated inhibition and increase outflow from the ventral pallidum (VP), which appears to correlate with a positive reinforcing state (enhanced reward).

inhibition of muscle tone leading to concurrent increases in basal tone in the circular muscle of the small and large intestine. This results in enhanced high-amplitude phasic contractions, which are nonpropulsatile. The upper part of the small intestine, particularly the duodenum, is affected more than the ileum. A period of relative atony may follow the hypertonicity. The reduced rate of passage of the intestinal contents, along with reduced intestinal secretion, leads to increased water absorption, increasing viscosity of the bowel contents, and constipation.

b. What are the options for treatment of this patient?

The peripherally limited antagonists such as methylnaltrexone have a very important role in the management of the constipation and the reduced GI motility present in the patient undergoing chronic opioid therapy (as for chronic pain or methadone maintenance) and have been approved by the FDA for that use. With distribution restricted to the periphery, these agents do not alter central opioid agonist actions. Worrisome reports of GI perforation in this setting are under review by FDA. Other strategies for the management of opioid-induced constipation are described in Chapter 33.

CASE 10-3

A 43-year-old markedly obese man with the history of sleep apnea is being treated with hydrocodone for chronic back pain.

a. What considerations should be taken into account when treating chronic pain with opiates?

Management of pain is an important element in any therapeutic intervention. Failure to adequately manage pain can have important negative consequences on physiological function such as autonomic hyper-reactivity (increased blood pressure, heart rate, suppression of gastrointestinal motility, reduced secretions), reduced mobility leading to deconditioning, muscle wasting, joint stiffening, and decalcification, and can contribute to deleterious changes in the psychological state (depression, helplessness syndromes, anxiety). By many hospital-accrediting organizations, and by law in many states, appropriate pain assessment and adequate pain management are considered to be standard of care, with pain being considered the "fifth vital sign."

Table 10-1 shows dosing data for clinically employed opioid analgesics. These are only guidelines, but they can give a place to start a patient's treatment.

Numerous societies and agencies have published guidelines for the use of strong opioids in treating pain, including the American Academy of Pain Medicine, the American Pain Society, the Federation of State Medical Boards (FSMB), and the Drug Enforcement Agency. While slightly different in particulars, all guidelines to date share the criteria established by the FSMB (see Table 10-2).

b. Why is this patient at risk of respiratory depression while taking the hydrocodone?

This patient's history of sleep apnea puts him at increased risk of respiratory depression with opiate therapy (see Side Bar FACTORS EXACERBATING OPIATE-INDUCED RESPIRATORY DEPRESSION). Although effects on respiration are readily demonstrated, clinically significant respiratory depression rarely occurs with standard analgesic doses in the absence of other contributing variables. It should be stressed, however, that respiratory depression represents the primary cause of morbidity secondary to opiate therapy.

c. What is a possible mechanism for respiratory depression in this patient?

Morphine-like opioids depress respiration through MOR and DOR receptors in part by a direct depressant effect on rhythm generation, with changes in respiratory pattern and rate observed at lower doses than changes in tidal volume. A key property

(Continued)

SECTION II — Neuropharmacology

TABLE 10-1 Dosing Data for Clinically Employed Opioid Analgesics

DRUG	APPROXIMATE EQUI-ANALGESIC ORAL DOSE	APPROXIMATE EQUI-ANALGESIC PARENTERAL DOSE	RECOMMENDED STARTING DOSE (ADULTS >50 KG) ORAL	RECOMMENDED STARTING DOSE (ADULTS >50 KG) PARENTERAL	RECOMMENDED STARTING DOSE (CHILDREN AND ADULTS <50 KG)[a] ORAL	RECOMMENDED STARTING DOSE (CHILDREN AND ADULTS <50 KG)[a] PARENTERAL
Opioid Agonists						
Morphine[b]	30 mg q3–4h (around-the-clock dosing) 60 mg q3–4h (single dose or intermittent dosing)	10 mg q3–4h	15 mg q3–4h	5 mg q3–4h	0.3 mg/kg q3–4h	0.1 mg/kg q3–4h
Codeine[c]	130 mg q3–4h	75 mg q3–4h	30 mg q3–4h	30 mg q2h (IM/SC)	1 mg/kg q3–4h[d]	Not recommended
Hydromorphone (DILAUDID)[b]	7.5 mg q3–4h	1.5 mg q3–4h	4 mg q3–4h	1 mg q3–4h	0.06 mg/kg q3–4h	0.015 mg/kg q3–4h
Hydrocodone (in LORCET, LORTAB, VICODIN, others, typically with acetominophen)	30 mg q3–4h	Not available	5 mg q3–4h	Not available	0.2 mg/kg q3–4h[d]	Not available
Levorphanol	4 mg q6–8h	2 mg q6–8h	2 mg q6–8h	1 mg q6–8h	0.04 mg/kg q6–8h	0.02 mg/kg q6–8h
Meperidine (DEMEROL)	300 mg q2–3h	100 mg q3h	Not recommended	50 mg q3h	Not recommended	0.75 mg/kg q2–3h
Methadone (DOLOPHINE, others)	20 mg q6–8h	10 mg q6–8h	2.5 mg q12h	2.5 mg q12h	0.2 mg/kg q12h	0.1 mg/kg q6–8h
Oxycodone (REXICODONE, OXYCONTIN, also in PERCOCET, PERCODAN, TYLOX, others)[g]	30 mg q3–4h	Not available	5 mg q3–4h	Not available	0.2 mg/kg q3–4h[d]	Not available
Oxymorphone[b] (NUMORPHAN)	Not available	1 mg q3–4h	Not available	1 mg q3–4h	Not recommended	Not recommended
Propoxyphene (DARVON)	130 mg[e]	Not available	65 mg q4–6h[e]	Not available	Not recommended	Not recommended
Tramadol[f] (ULTRAM)	100 mg[e]	100 mg	50–100 mg q6h[e]	50–100 mg q6h[e]	Not recommended	Not recommended
Opioid Agonist-Antagonists or Partial Agonists						
Buprenorphine (BUPRENEX)	Not available	0.3–0.4 mg q6–8h	Not available	0.4 mg q6–8h	Not available	0.004 mg/kg q6–8h
Butorphanol (STADOL)	Not available	2 mg q3–4h	Not available	2 mg q3–4h	Not available	Not recommended
Nalbuphine (NUBAIN)	Not available	10 mg q3–4h	Not available	10 mg q3–4h	Not available	0.1 mg/kg q3–4h

Published tables vary in the suggested doses that are equi-analgesic to morphine. Clinical response is the criterion that must be applied for each patient; titration to clinical response is necessary. Because there is not complete cross-tolerance among these drugs, it is usually necessary to use a lower than equi-analgesic dose when changing drugs and to retitrate to response. *Caution:* Recommended doses do not apply to patients with renal or hepatic insufficiency or other conditions affecting drug metabolism and kinetics.

[a]*Caution:* Doses listed for patients with body weight less than 50 kg cannot be used as initial starting doses in babies less than 6 months of age. Consult the *Clinical Practice Guideline for Acute Pain Management: Operative or Medical Procedures and Trauma* section on management of pain in neonates for recommendations. [b]For morphine, hydromorphone, and oxymorphone, rectal administration is an alternate route for patients unable to take oral medications, but equi-analgesic doses may differ from oral and parenteral doses because of pharmacokinetic differences.
[c]*Caution:* Codeine doses above 65 mg often are not appropiate due to diminishing incremental analgesia with increasing doses but continually increasing constipation and other side effects.
[d]*Caution:* Doses of aspirin and acetaminophen in combination opi-oid/NSAID preparations must also be adjusted to the patient's body weight. Maximum acetaminophen dose: 4 g/day in adults, 90 mg/kg/day in children.
[e]Doses for moderate pain not necessarily equivalent to 30 mg oral or 10 mg parenteral morphine.
[f]Risk of seizures: parenteral formulation not available in the United States.
[g]Oxycontin is an extended-release preparation containing up to 160 mg of oxycodone per tablet and recommended for use every 12 hours. It has been subject to substantial abuse. Modified from Agency for Healthcare Policy and Research, 1992.

TABLE 10-2 Guidelines for the Use of Opioids to Treat Chronic Pain

- *Evaluation of the patient*: A complete medical history and physical must be conducted and documented in the medical record.
- *Treatment plan*: The treatment plan should state objectives that are used to determine treatment success.
- *Informed consent and agreement*: The physician should discuss the risks, benefits, and alternatives to chronic opioid therapy with the patient. Many practitioners have developed an "opioid contract" that outlines the responsibilities of the physician and the patient for continued prescription of controlled substances.
- *Periodic review*: At reasonable intervals, the patient should be seen by the physician to review the course of treatment and document results of consultation, diagnostic, testing, laboratory results, and the success of treatment.
- *Consultation*: The physician should refer the patient for consultation when appropriate.
- *Documentation/medical records*: The physician should keep actual and complete medical records that include: (a) medical history and physical examination; (b) diagnostic, therapeutic, and laboratory results; (c) evaluations and consultations; (d) treatment objectives; (e) discussion of risks and benefits; (f) treatment; (g) medications including date, type, dosage, and quantity prescribed; (h) instructions and agreements; and (i) periodic reviews.
- *Compliance with controlled substances law and regulations*: To prescribe, dispense or administer controlled substances, the physician must be licensed in the state and comply with applicable state and federal regulations.

of opiate effects on respiration is the depression of the ventilatory response to increased PCO_2. The ventilatory response to increased PCO_2 is important in patients with sleep apnea. This effect is mediated by opiate depression of the excitability of brainstem chemosensory neurons. In addition to the effects on the CO_2 response, opiates will depress ventilation otherwise driven by hypoxia through an effect upon carotid and aortic body chemosensors. Importantly, with opiates, hypoxic stimulation of chemoreceptors still may be effective when opioids have decreased the responsiveness to CO_2, and inhalation of O_2 may remove the residual drive resulting from the elevated PCO_2 and produce apnea.

CASE 10-4

A 56-year-old woman with advanced breast cancer is being treated with methadone for her pain.

a. Why is methadone a good choice for this patient?

The outstanding properties of methadone are its analgesic activity, its efficacy by the oral route, its extended duration of action in suppressing withdrawal symptoms in physically dependent individuals, and its tendency to show persistent effects with repeated administration.

b. What are the major considerations in using methadone to treat this patient's pain?

Side effects, toxicity, and conditions that alter sensitivity, as well as the treatment of acute intoxication, are similar to those described for morphine. During long-term administration, there may be excessive sweating, lymphocytosis, and increased concentrations of prolactin, albumin, and globulins in the plasma. Rifampin and phenytoin accelerate the metabolism of methadone and can precipitate withdrawal symptoms. Unlike other opioids, methadone is associated with long QT syndrome and is additive with agents known to prolong the QT interval. Serious cardiac arrhythmias, including torsades de pointes, have been observed during treatment with methadone.

Care must be taken when escalating the dosage because of the prolonged $t_{1/2}$ of the drug and its tendency to accumulate over a period of several days with repeated dosing. Iatrogenic overdoses have occurred during initiation of therapy and dosing titration with methadone because of too-rapid titration or the concomitant use of depressant drugs. The peak respiratory depressant effects of methadone typically occur later and persist longer than the peak analgesic effects so it is necessary to exercise vigilance and strongly caution patients against self-medicating with CNS depressants, particularly during treatment initiation and dose titration.

(Continued)

TABLE 10-3 Oral Morphine to Methadone Conversion Guidelines

DAILY MORPHINE DOSE (mg/24 h, ORALLY)	CONVERSION RATIOS		
	MORPHINE (oral)	:	METHADONE (oral)
<100	3	:	1
101-300	5	:	1
301-600	10	:	1
601-800	12	:	1
801-1000	15	:	1
>1000	20	:	1

While not necessarily relevant to this patient, Table 10-3 shows the oral morphine to methadone guidelines.

The pain state (see Side Bar PAIN STATES) in any given clinical condition is not typically constant and will vary over time. In chronic pain states, the daily course of the pain may fluctuate, for example, being greater in the morning hours or upon awakening. Arthritic states display flares that are associated with an exacerbated pain condition. Changes in the magnitude of pain occur during the daily routine resulting in "breakthrough pain" during episodic events such as dressing changes (incident pain). These examples emphasize the need for individualized management of increased or decreased pain levels with baseline analgesic dosing supplemented with the use of short-acting "rescue" medications as required. In the face of ongoing severe pain, analgesics should be dosed in continuous or "around-the-clock" fashion rather than on an as-needed basis. This provides more consistent analgesic levels and avoids unnecessary suffering.

c. **What are other options for the treatment of this patient's pain?**

There are a variety of routes of administration of opiates for the treatment of chronic pain.

Patient-controlled analgesia (PCA)

With this modality, the patient has limited control of the dosing of opioid from an infusion pump programmed within tightly mandated parameters. PCA can be used for intravenous, epidural, or intrathecal administration of opioids. This technique avoids delays inherent in administration by a caregiver and generally permits better alignment between pain control and individual differences in pain perception and responsiveness to opioids.

Spinal delivery

Administration of opioids into the epidural or intrathecal space provides more direct access to the first pain-processing synapse in the dorsal horn of the spinal cord. This permits the use of doses substantially lower than those required for oral or parenteral administration

Local drug action

Opioid receptors on peripheral sensory nerves respond to locally applied opioids during inflammation. Peripheral analgesia permits the use of lower doses, applied locally, than those necessary to achieve a systemic effect.

Rectal administration

This route is an alternative for patients with difficulty swallowing or other oral pathology and who prefer a less invasive route than parenteral administration.

(Continued)

Inhalation

Opioids can be delivered by nebulizer. However, this delivery method is rarely used due to erratic absorption from the lung and highly variable therapeutic effect.

Oral transmucosal administration

Opioids can be absorbed through the oral mucosa more rapidly than through the stomach. Bioavailability is greater owing to avoidance of first-pass metabolism, and lipophilic opioids are absorbed better by this route than are hydrophilic compounds such as morphine. A transmucosal delivery system that suspends fentanyl in a dissolvable sugar-based lollipop or rapidly dissolving buccal tablet have been approved for the treatment of cancer pain; in this setting, transmucosal fentanyl relieves pain within 15 minutes, and patients easily can titrate the appropriate dose.

Transnasal administration

Butorphanol, a(n) KOR agonist/MOR antagonist, has been employed intranasally. A transnasal pectin-based fentanyl spray is currently in clinical trials for the treatment of cancer-related pain.

Transdermal and iontophoretic administration

Transdermal fentanyl patches are approved for use in sustained pain. The opioid permeates the skin, and a "depot" is established in the stratum corneum layer.

Iontophoresis is the transport of soluble ions through the skin by using a mild electric current. This technique has been employed with morphine. Unlike transdermal opioids, a drug reservoir does not build up in the skin, thus limiting the duration of both desired and undesired effects. Patient-controlled iontophoretic transdermal fentanyl systems have been developed, but none is currently marketed.

CASE 10-5

A 19-year-old man is brought to the emergency room with a suspected heroin overdose. He is unresponsive and his respirations are depressed. He was discharged from 30 days in a detoxification program earlier in the day. Naloxone is administered intravenously.

a. **What is naloxone and why is it effective in this patient?**

   A variety of agents bind competitively to 1 or more of the opioid receptors, display little or no intrinsic activity, and robustly antagonize the effects of opiate receptor agonists. Opioid antagonists, particularly naloxone, have an established use in the treatment of opioid-induced toxicity, especially respiratory depression. Its specificity is such that reversal by this agent is virtually diagnostic for the contribution of an opiate to the respiratory depression. Naloxone acts rapidly to reverse the respiratory depression associated with high doses of opioids.

b. **What precautions must be taken with the administration of naloxone?**

   It should be used cautiously because it also can precipitate withdrawal in dependent subjects and cause undesirable cardiovascular side effects. By carefully titrating the dose of naloxone, it usually is possible to rapidly antagonize the respiratory-depressant actions without eliciting a fully expressed withdrawal syndrome. The duration of action of naloxone is relatively short, and it often must be given repeatedly or by continuous infusion.

c. **What are other therapeutic uses of opiate antagonists?**

   There is considerable interest in the use of opiate antagonists such as naltrexone as an adjuvant in treating a variety of nonopioid dependency syndromes such as alcoholism (see Chapters 9 and 14), where an opiate antagonist decreases the chance of relapse.

   Buprenorphine in a fixed-dose combination with naloxone is approved for the treatment of opioid dependence.

(Continued)

The potential utility of opiate antagonists in the treatment of shock, stroke, spinal cord and brain trauma, and other disorders that may involve mobilization of endogenous opioid peptides has been reported; but opioid antagonists have failed to demonstrate neuroprotective benefits and their study in trauma has been largely abandoned.

CASE 10-6

A 17-year-old boy is brought to the emergency room following an injury to his arm while playing soccer. He is administered meperidine by intramuscular injection for pain.

a. What is meperidine and how does it act as an analgesic?

Meperidine is predominantly an MOR agonist that produces a pattern of effects similar but not identical to those already described for morphine. The major use of meperidine is for analgesia. Unlike morphine and its congeners, meperidine is not used for the treatment of cough or diarrhea. The analgesic effects of meperidine are detectable ~15 minutes after oral administration, peak in 1 to 2 hours, and subside gradually.

b. What cautions should be taken with the use of meperidine?

The pattern and overall incidence of untoward effects that follow the use of meperidine are similar to those observed after equi-analgesic doses of morphine, except that constipation and urinary retention may be less common.

Meperidine and its congeners are contraindicated in patients taking MAO inhibitors or within 14 days after discontinuation of an MAO inhibitor. Severe reactions may follow the administration of meperidine to patients being treated with MAO inhibitors. Two basic types of interactions can be observed. The most prominent is an excitatory reaction ("serotonin syndrome") with delirium, hyperthermia, headache, hyper- or hypotension, rigidity, convulsions, coma, and death. This reaction may be due to the ability of meperidine to block neuronal reuptake of 5-HT, resulting in serotonergic overactivity. Conversely, the MAO inhibitor interaction with meperidine may resemble acute narcotic overdose owing to the inhibition of hepatic CYPs.

Meperidine is *N*-demethylated to normeperidine, which then may be hydrolyzed to normeperidinic acid and subsequently conjugated. In patients or addicts who are tolerant to the depressant effects of meperidine, large doses repeated at short intervals may produce an excitatory syndrome including hallucinations, tremors, muscle twitches, dilated pupils, hyperactive reflexes, and convulsions. These excitatory symptoms are due to the accumulation of normeperidine, which has a $t_{1/2}$ of 15 to 20 hours, compared to 3 hours for meperidine. Since normeperidine is eliminated by the kidney and the liver, decreased renal or hepatic function increases the likelihood of toxicity. As a result of these properties, meperidine is not recommended for the treatment of chronic pain because of concerns over metabolite toxicity. It should not be used for longer than 48 hours or in doses more than 600 mg/d.

KEY CONCEPTS

- Opioids are a mainstay of pain treatment, but rational therapy may involve, depending on the pain state, 1 or more drug classes, such as NSAIDs, anticonvulsants, and antidepressants (see Table 10-4).
- Opioid analgesics provide symptomatic relief of pain, but the underlying disease remains.
- Opioids activate μ, δ, and κ opiate receptors to produce their pharmacological effects.
- Sustained administration of an opiate agonist leads to tolerance, physical dependence, and a withdrawal syndrome upon abrupt discontinuation.

(Continued)

TABLE 10-4 Summary of Drug Target and Site of Action of Common Drug Classes and Relative Efficacy by Pain State

DRUG CLASS (REPRESENTATIVE AGENTS IN PARENTHESES)	DRUG ACTION	SITE OF ACTION[a]	RELATIVE EFFICACY IN PAIN STATES[b]
NSAIDs (ibuprofen, aspirin acetominophen)	Nonspecific COX inhibitors	Peripheral and spinal	Tissue injury >> acute stimuli = nerve injury = 0
COX 2 inhibitor (celecoxib)	COX2-selective inhibitor	Peripheral and spinal	Tissue injury >> acute stimuli = nerve injury = 0
Opioids (morphine)	μ receptor agonist	Supraspinal and spinal	Tissue injury = acute stimuli ≥ nerve injury > 0 (see this chapter)
Anticonvulsants (gabapentin)	Na$^+$ channel block, α$_2$δ subunit of Ca^{2+} channel	Supraspinal and spinal	Nerve injury > tissue injury = acute stimuli = 0
Tricyclic antidepressants (amitryptiline)	Inhibit uptake of 5-HT/NE	Supraspinal and spinal	Nerve injury ≥ tissue injury >> acute stimuli = 0

[a]Studies based on local delivery in preclinical models, eg, intracranial microinjection or intraventricular injections, lumbar intrathecal delivery or topical/subcutaneous application at injury site.
[b]Pain states are defined by preclinical models: acute: hot plate/tail flick/acute mechanical compression; tissue injury: intraplantar injections of irritants, focal thermal injury; nerve injury: compression/ligation of sciatic nerve or its branches or of nerve roots; systemic delivery of chemotherapeutics.

- Respiratory depression represents the primary cause of morbidity secondary to opiate therapy.
- The majority of patients treated with opioids develop constipation.
- Naloxone and naltrexone are centrally acting opioid antagonists; methylnaltrexone is a peripherally acting opioid antagonist.
- In addition to the traditional oral and parenteral formulations for opioids, many other methods of administration have been developed in an effort to improve therapeutic efficacy and reduce side effects (see Case 10-4c).
- Morphine and meperidine should be avoided in patients with impaired renal function due to metabolite toxicity.

SUMMARY QUIZ

QUESTION 10-1 A 55-year-old woman is having a colonoscopy. Aside from other medications for sedation, it is likely she will receive which of the following analgesics?

a. Methadone
b. Meperidine
c. Buprenorphine
d. Fentanyl
e. Pentazocine

QUESTION 10-2 A 42-year-old man with chronic pain is brought to the emergency room because of over-sedation and respiratory depression while using fentanyl patches. He is given intravenous naloxone. He is not given oral naloxone because naloxone

a. is not absorbed from the GI tract.
b. undergoes first-pass metabolism in the liver.
c. is metabolized to an inactive metabolite in the GI lining.
d. is excreted unchanged in the urine.
e. is destroyed by stomach acid.

SECTION II Neuropharmacology

QUESTION 10-3 A 48-year-old man is being treated with a long-acting opiate for pain associated with terminal cancer. He is also prescribed a transmucosal fentanyl formulation (lollipop) for "breakthrough" pain. The transmucosal formulation is an effective analgesic because it

a. avoids first pass metabolism of fentanyl.
b. avoids nausea and vomiting that is associated with the systemic use of fentanyl.
c. delivers fentanyl directly to opiate receptors in the mouth.
d. avoids constipation.
e. avoids respiratory depression.

QUESTION 10-4 A 50-year-old woman with back pain is administered an opiate agonist. After 2 weeks of therapy, she notices that she needs to increase the dose to get the same analgesic effect. She is experiencing

a. physical dependence.
b. addiction.
c. tolerance.
d. withdrawal.
e. drug-seeking behavior.

QUESTION 10-5 A 43-year-old man with postsurgical pain is placed on an intravenous patient-controlled analgesia pump with morphine as the analgesic. This form of analgesic administration is preferred to oral administration because morphine

a. is not absorbed orally.
b. administered orally is rapidly eliminated in the urine.
c. administered orally does not penetrate the brain.
d. administered orally causes more severe constipation.
e. administered parenterally bypasses first-pass metabolism.

QUESTION 10-6 The morphine metabolite that may be responsible for most of morphine's analgesic activity is

a. desmethylmorphine.
b. morphine-6-glucuronide.
c. morphine sulfate.
d. *N*-acetylmorphine.
e. hydroxymorphine.

QUESTION 10-7 A 20-year-old man is given codeine to relieve the pain of a sprained ankle. After two days the man returns to his doctor saying that the codeine is not effective. A likely cause is due to

a. poor absorption.
b. rapid urinary excretion.
c. poor metabolism.
d. high protein binding.
e. poor brain penetration.

QUESTION 10-8 A 53-year-old man is requesting meperidine for his chronic back pain. His physician is reluctant to use meperidine for the treatment of chronic pain because of

a. metabolite toxicity.
b. poor oral absorption.
c. increased addiction potential.
d. patient noncompliance.
e. likelihood that meperidine will be diverted for sale on the street.

QUESTION 10-9 A 32-year-old woman has been taking an oxycodone-acetaminophen product for chronic arthritic pain. On a follow-up appointment her serum aminotransferases are elevated and she is slightly jaundiced. She admits to increasing the dose of the oxycodone combination product over the past several weeks. The most likely cause of her liver injury is

a. oxycodone.

b. hepatitis A.

c. hepatitis C.

d. arthritis.

e. acetaminophen.

SUMMARY QUIZ ANSWER KEY

QUESTION 10-1 Answer is **d.** Fentanyl citrate and sufentanil citrate have widespread popularity as anesthetic adjuvants (see Chapter 11). They are used commonly either intravenously, epidurally, or intrathecally. The analgesic effects of fentanyl and sufentanil are similar to those of morphine and other opioids. Fentanyl is ~100 times more potent than morphine, and sufentanil is ~1000 times more potent than morphine. The time to peak analgesic effect after intravenous administration of fentanyl and sufentanil (~5 minutes) is notably less than that for morphine and meperidine (~15 minutes). Recovery from analgesic effects also occurs more quickly.

QUESTION 10-2 Answer is **b.** Although absorbed readily from the GI tract, naloxone is almost completely metabolized by the liver before reaching the systemic circulation and thus must be administered parenterally. The drug is absorbed rapidly from parenteral sites of injection and is metabolized in the liver primarily by conjugation with glucuronic acid; other metabolites are produced in small amounts. The $t_{1/2}$ of naloxone is ~1 hour, but its clinically effective duration of action can be even less.

QUESTION 10-3 Answer is **a.** Opioids can be absorbed through the oral mucosa more rapidly than through the stomach. Bioavailability is greater owing to avoidance of first-pass metabolism, and lipophilic opioids are better absorbed by this route than are hydrophilic compounds such as morphine. A transmucosal delivery system that suspends fentanyl in a dissolvable sugar-based lollipop or rapidly dissolving buccal tablet have been approved for the treatment of cancer pain; in this setting, transmucosal fentanyl relieves pain within 15 minutes, and patients easily can titrate the appropriate dose.

QUESTION 10-4 Answer is **c.** Sustained administration of an opiate agonist (days to weeks) leads to progressive loss of drug effect. Here tolerance refers to a decrease in the apparent effectiveness of a drug with continuous or repeated agonist administration, and with the removal of the agonist tolerance disappears over several weeks. This tolerance is reflected by a reduction in the maximum achievable effect or a right-shift in the dose-effect curve.

QUESTION 10-5 Answer is **e.** With most opioids, including morphine, the effect of a given dose is less after oral than after parenteral administration because of variable but significant first-pass metabolism in the liver. For example, the bioavailability of oral preparations of morphine is only ~25%. The shape of the time-effect curve also varies with the route of administration, so the duration of action often is somewhat longer with the oral route. If adjustment is made for variability of first-pass metabolism and clearance, adequate relief of pain can be achieved with oral administration of morphine.

QUESTION 10-6 Answer is **b.** Morphine-6-glucuronide has pharmacological actions indistinguishable from those of morphine. Morphine-6-glucuronide given systemically is approximately twice as potent as morphine in animal models and in humans. With chronic administration, the 6-glucuronide accounts for a significant portion

(Continued)

of morphine's analgesic actions. Indeed, with chronic oral dosing, the blood levels of morphine-6-glucuronide typically exceed those of morphine. Given its greater MOR potency and its higher concentration, morphine-6-glucuronide may be responsible for most of morphine's analgesic activity in patients receiving chronic oral morphine.

QUESTION 10-7 Answer is **c.** Codeine has an exceptionally low affinity for opioid receptors, and the analgesic effect of codeine is due to its conversion to morphine. CYP2D6 catalyzes the conversion of codeine to morphine. Well-characterized genetic polymorphisms in CYP2D6 lead to the inability to convert codeine to morphine thus making codeine ineffective as an analgesic for ~10% of the Caucasian population.

QUESTION 10-8 Answer is **a.** Meperidine is N-demethylated to normeperidine, which then may be hydrolyzed to normeperidinic acid and subsequently conjugated. In patients or addicts who are tolerant to the depressant effects of meperidine large doses repeated at short intervals may produce an excitatory syndrome, including hallucinations, tremors, muscle twitches, dilated pupils, hyperactive reflexes, and convulsions. These excitatory symptoms are due to the accumulation of normeperidine, which has a $t_{1/2}$ of 15 to 20 hours, compared to 3 hours for meperidine. As a result of these properties, meperidine is not recommended for the treatment of chronic pain because of concerns over metabolite toxicity. It should not be used for longer than 48 hours or in doses more than 600 mg/d.

QUESTION 10-9 Answer is **e.** Doses of acetaminophen greater than 4 g/day may result in hepatotoxicity (see Chapters 2 and 22). This amount of acetaminophen is easily reached in patients who are taking an acetaminophen-opiate combination product, and who escalate their dose of the opiate-acetaminophen analgesic when tolerance occurs. Recently the FDA has lowered the amount of acetaminophen that can be formulated in combination with opiate analgesics. Patients will still have access to over-the-counter products that contain acetaminophen, which they may use to supplement their pain therapy.

SUMMARY TABLE OF OPIOID PHARMACOLOGY

CLASS AND SUBCLASSES	NAMES	CLINICAL USES	TOXICITIES COMMON	TOXICITIES UNIQUE; CLINICALLY IMPORTANT
Opioid Receptor Agonist	Morphine Codeine Hydromorphone Hydrocodone Oxycodone Oxymorphone Meperidine	Treatment of acute and chronic pain	Nausea, vomiting, dizziness, constipation, pruritus, tolerance, and physical dependence	Respiratory depression (see Side Bar FACTORS EXACERBATING OPIOID-INDUCED RESPIRATORY DEPRESSION) Mental clouding, urinary retention, hypotension Propoxyphene has been associated with cardiac toxicity
	Methadone	Long-acting MOR agonist used for treatment of chronic pain and opioid abstinence syndrome Treatment of heroin users		
	Propoxyphene	Used to treat mild to moderate pain		
	Fentanyl Alfentanil Sufentanil Remifentanil	Potent MOR agonist with short duration of action used for acute pain and as an adjunct to general anesthesia Fentanyl topical patch and other forms of oral mucosal delivery are used for chronic pain Remifentanil is used for short painful procedures requiring rapid onset and offset		

Opioid Pharmacology — CHAPTER 10

CLASS AND SUBCLASSES	NAMES	CLINICAL USES	TOXICITIES COMMON	TOXICITIES UNIQUE; CLINICALLY IMPORTANT
	Levorphanol	Available for IV, IM, and PO administration as an analgesic		
	Tramadol Tapentadol	Synthetic codeine analogues that are weak MOR agonists Used to treat mild to moderate pain Possess monoamine reuptake inhibitor activity	Nausea, vomiting, dizziness, dry mouth, sedation and headache Less constipating than equivalent doses of morphine	Less respiratory depression than equi-analgesic doses of morphine Abrupt discontinuation may precipitate withdrawal syndrome
Opioid Receptor Agonist/ Antagonists and Partial Agonists	Nalbuphine	Generally considered to be a KOR agonist and MOR antagonist that is used as an analgesic		Should not be used in combination with MOR agonists
	Butorphanol	Generally considered to be a KOR agonist and MOR antagonist that is used to treat acute pain		
	Pentazocine	Used to treat mild to moderate pain		
	Buprenorphine	MOR partial agonist used as an analgesic Fixed-dose combination with naloxone is used to treat opioid dependence		May produce an abstinence syndrome in patients taking MOR agonist for several weeks
Antidiarrheal Agents	Diphenoxylate	Used to treat diarrhea (see Chapter 33)		Available only in combination with atropine because of abuse liability
	Difenoxin			
	Loperamide			Low abuse liability because of poor solubility and CNS penetration
Opioid Receptor Antagonists	Naloxone Naltrexone	Used to treat opioid-induced toxicity		Will precipitate a withdrawal syndrome in long-term opiate users
	Methylnaltrexone	Used in the management of opioid-induced constipation		Does not alter central opiate actions Reports of GI perforation
Antitussives	Dextromethorphan	Over-the-counter treatment for cough often in combination with antihistamines, decongestants, expectorants, and bronchodilators	Produces fewer subjective or GI side effects than codeine	Should not be used to suppress a productive cough
	Codeine	Also used as a cough suppressant (see Chapter 24)		
	Benzonatate	Used in the treatment of cough	Drowsiness, dizziness, and dysphagia	Should not be used to suppress a productive cough

CHAPTER 11

Anesthetic Agents and Therapeutic Gases

DRUGS INCLUDED IN THIS CHAPTER

- Articaine (SEPTOCAINE)
- Benzocaine (large number of preparations for topical application)
- Bupivicane (MARCAINE, SENSORCAINE, others)
- Carbon dioxide
- Chloroprocaine (NESACAINE)
- Cocaine
- Desflurane (SUPRANE)
- Dexmedetomidine (PRECEDEX)
- Dibucaine (NUPERCAINAL, others)
- Dyclonine (over-the-counter products such as SUCRETS, ORAJEL and OVERNIGHT COLD SORE PATCH, and SKIN SHIELD LIQUID BANDAGE)
- Enflurane (ETHRANE)
- Etomidate (AMIDATE)
- Fospropofol (LUSEDRA)
- Halothane (FLUOTHANE)
- Helium
- Isoflurane (FORANE, others)
- Ketamine (KETALAR)
- Lidocaine (XYLOCAINE, others); transdermal patch (LIDODERM); oral patch (DENTI-PATCH); combination with prilocaine in an occlusive dressing (EMLA); combination with tetracaine (PLIAGIS)
- Mepivacaine (CARBAOCAINE, POLOCAINE, others)
- Methohexital (BREVITAL)
- Nitric oxide
- Nitrous oxide
- Oxygen
- Pramoxine (various preparations including creams, lotions, sprays, gel, wipes, and foams available for topical application)
- Prilocaine (CITANEST)
- Procaine (NOVOCAINE)
- Proparacaine (ALCAINE, OPHTHAINE, others)
- Propofol (DIPRIVAN)

(continues)

This chapter will be most useful after having a basic understanding of the material in Chapter 19, General Anesthetics and Therapeutic Gases and Chapter 20, Local Anesthetics in *Goodman & Gilman's The Pharmacological Basis of Therapeutics*, 12th Edition. In addition to the material presented here, the chapters in the 12th Edition include:

- Details of the general principles of surgical anesthesia
- A detailed discussion of the mechanisms of anesthesia
- The chemical structures of parenteral, inhalational, and local anesthetics
- A detailed discussion of therapeutic gases
- Figure 20-3 which is a depiction of the local anesthetic receptor site
- Table 20-1 Susceptibility to Block Types of Nerve Fibers
- A detailed discussion of the mechanisms of action of local anesthetics
- A detailed discussion of the various ways that local anesthetics are administered

LEARNING OBJECTIVES

- ☑ Learn the mechanisms of action of parenteral, inhalational, and local anesthetics.
- ☑ Understand the ways that anesthetics (parenteral, inhalational, and local) are used to facilitate surgical and other painful medical procedures.
- ☑ Know the major pharmacological properties and toxicities of anesthetic drugs.

MECHANISMS OF ACTION OF ANESTHETIC AGENTS

DRUG CLASS	DRUG	MECHSM OF ACTION
Parenteral Anesthetics	Sodium thiopental Methohexital	Barbiturates act on $GABA_A$ receptors (see Chapter 9)
	Propofol Fospropofol	Sedative and hypnotic The action of propofol is mediated by its action on $GABA_A$ receptors to increase chloride conduction and hyperpolarize neurons; fospropofol is a prodrug of propofol and has a similar mechanism of action
	Etomidate	Modulator of $GABA_A$ receptors
	Ketamine	Inhibits NMDA receptors (see Chapter 5)
Inhalational Anesthetics	Halothane Isoflurane Enflurane Desflurane Sevoflurane	See Side Bar MECHANISMS OF GENERAL ANESTHESIA
	Nitrous oxide	Potent and selective inhibitor of NMDA-activated currents

(Continued)

Anesthetic Agents and Therapeutic Gases

CHAPTER 11

DRUG CLASS	DRUG	MECHANISM OF ACTION
Anesthetic Adjuncts	Xenon	Potent and selective inhibitor of NMDA-activated currents
	Benzodiazepines	See Chapter 9
	Dexmedetomidine	Selective α_2-adrenergic receptor agonist that produces sedation and analgesia, but not general anesthesia
	Analgesics	See Chapter 10
	Neuromuscular blocking agents	See Chapter 6
Therapeutic Gases	Oxygen	Increases tissue oxygenation Hyperbaric oxygen is administered at greater than atmospheric pressure to improve oxygenation of damaged tissues
	Carbon dioxide	Product of metabolism Hypocarbia constricts cerebral vessels
	Nitric oxide	Critical endogenous cell signaling molecule that activates soluble guanylate cyclase (see Chapter 1)
	Helium	Inert gas with low density, low solubility, and high thermal conductivity
Local Anesthetics	Lidocaine Bupivicaine Articaine Chloroprocaine Mepivacaine Prilocaine Ropivacaine Procaine Tetracaine Dibucaine Dyclonine Pramoxine Benzocaine Proparacaine Cocaine	Local anesthetics act at the nerve cell membrane to prevent the generation and conduction of nerve impulses They do this by direct interaction with voltage-gated Na$^+$ channels (see Figure 11-4) to decrease or prevent the large transient flux of Na$^+$ that normally is produced by a slight depolarization of the membrane (see Chapters 5 and 6)

DRUGS INCLUDED IN THIS CHAPTER (Cont.)

Ropivacaine (NAROPIN, others)
Sevoflurane (ULTRANE, others)
Tetracaine (PONTOCAINE)
Thiopental Sodium (PENTOTHAL, others)
Xenon

MECHANISMS OF GENERAL ANESTHESIA[a]

Cellular mechanisms
- Inhalational anesthetics can hyperpolarize neurons.
- Inhalational and parenteral anesthetics have effects on synaptic transmission and lesser effects on action-potential generation or propagation.

Molecular mechanisms
- Increase sensitivity of the GABA$_A$ receptor to GABA, thus enhancing inhibitory neurotransmission.
- Ketamine, nitrous oxide, and xenon inhibit NMDA receptors, which are glutamate-gated cation channels.
- Halogenated inhalational anesthetics, xenon, and nitrous oxide activate K$^+$ channels known as two-pore domain channels located in pre-and postsynaptic sites.

[a]Details can be found in Chapter 19 of *Goodman and Gilman's The Pharmacological Basis of Therapeutics*, 12th Edition.

COMPONENTS OF THE ANESTHETIC STATE

- Amnesia
- Immobility in response to noxious stimuli
- Analgesia
- Unconsciousness

CASE 11-1

A 32-year-old woman is about to be anesthetized for her first time for a surgical procedure.

a. **What is anesthesia? What are important general issues concerning anesthesia to be aware of?**

General anesthetics depress the CNS to a sufficient degree to permit the performance of surgery and other noxious or unpleasant procedures. The components of anesthesia are shown in the Side Bar COMPONENTS OF THE ANESTHETIC STATE. The general principles of anesthesia are listed in the Side Bar GENERAL PRINCIPLES OF SURGICAL ANESTHESIA.

(Continued)

SECTION II

GENERAL PRINCIPLES OF SURGICAL ANESTHESIA[a]

- Minimize potential deleterious direct and indirect effects of anesthetic agents and techniques
- Sustain physiologic homeostasis, including preventing excessive blood loss, tissue ischemia, reperfusion of ischemic tissues, fluid shifts, exposure to cold environment, and impaired coagulation
- Improve postoperative outcomes by choosing techniques that block or treat components of the surgical stress response

[a]Details can be found in Chapter 19 of *Goodman and Gilman's The Pharmacological Basis of Therapeutics*, 12th Edition.

Neuropharmacology

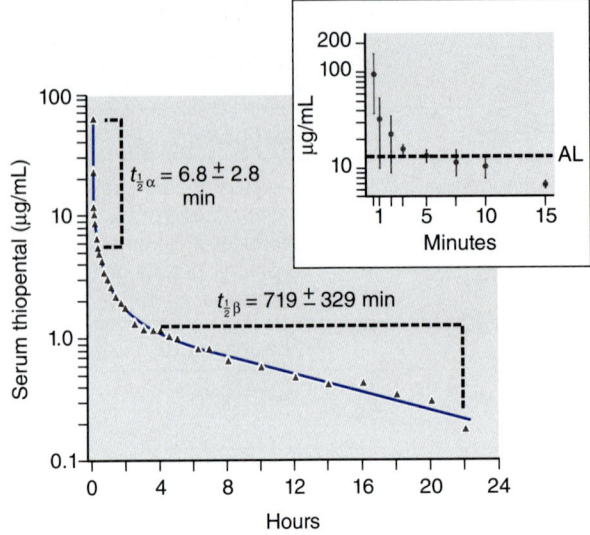

FIGURE 11-1 Thiopental serum levels after a single intravenous induction dose. Thiopental serum levels after a bolus can be described by 2 time constants, $t_{1/2}\alpha$ and $t_{1/2}\beta$. The initial fall is rapid ($t_{1/2\alpha} <10$ minutes) and is due to redistribution of drug from the plasma and the highly perfused brain and spinal cord into less well-perfused tissues such as muscle and fat. During this redistribution phase, serum thiopental concentration falls to levels at which patients awaken (AL, awakening level; see inset—the average thiopental serum concentration in 12 patients after a 6 mg/kg intravenous bolus of thiopental). Subsequent metabolism and elimination is much slower and is characterized by a half-life ($t_{1/2}\beta$) of more than 10 hours. (Adapted with permission from Burch PG, and Stanski DR, The role of metabolism and protein binding in thiopental anesthesia. *Anesthesiology, 1983;58:146-152.* Copyright Lippincott Williams & Wilkins. http://lww.com.)

Inevitably, anesthetics also suppress normal homeostatic reflexes. The most prominent physiological effect of anesthesia induction, associated with the majority of both intravenous and inhalational agents, is a decrease in systemic arterial blood pressure. Airway maintenance is essential following induction of anesthesia, as nearly all general anesthetics reduce or eliminate both ventilatory drive and the reflexes that maintain airway patency. Therefore, ventilation generally must be assisted or controlled for at least some period during surgery.

Patients commonly develop hypothermia (body temperature <36°C) during surgery. Prevention of hypothermia has emerged as a major goal of anesthetic care.

Nausea and vomiting in the postoperative period continue to be significant problems following general anesthesia and are caused by an action of anesthetics on the chemoreceptor trigger zone and the brainstem vomiting center.

Pain control can be complicated in the immediate postoperative period. The respiratory suppression associated with opioids can be problematic among postoperative patients who still have a substantial residual anesthetic effect. Regional anesthetic techniques are an important part of a perioperative multimodal approach that employs local anesthetic wound infiltration, epidural, spinal, and plexus blocks. Nonsteroidal anti-inflammatory drugs, opioids, α_2-adrenergic receptor agonists, and NMDA-receptor antagonists are commonly used as analgesics.

b. **What are the different types of anesthesia?**

The type of anesthesia generally depends on the type of surgery being performed and whether the surgical procedure is being performed on an outpatient basis. There are parenteral, inhalational, and local anesthetics. These are discussed in the following cases.

c. **What are the mechanisms of general anesthesia?**

The mechanisms by which general anesthetics produce their effects have remained one of the great mysteries of pharmacology. The current thinking on the cellular and

(Continued)

molecular mechanisms of anesthesia is shown in the Side Bar MECHANISMS OF ANESTHESIA.

In principle, general anesthetics could interrupt nervous system function at a myriad of anatomic sites, including peripheral sensory neurons, the spinal cord, the brainstem, and the cerebral cortex. Delineation of the precise anatomic sites of action is difficult because many anesthetics diffusely inhibit electrical activity in the central nervous system (CNS).

CASE 11-2

The patient in Case 11-1 will be given a parenteral anesthetic as an inducing agent.

a. **Why give an inducing agent?**

   Inhalational anesthetics are often irritating and onset of anesthesia can be variable. Consequently, anesthesia is usually begun with a parenteral agent that has a rapid and predictable onset. The commonly used parenteral anesthetics and their pharmacological properties are shown in Table 11-1.

b. **What are factors that control onset and termination of effect of a parenteral anesthetic?**

   Hydrophobicity is the key factor governing the pharmacokinetics of parenteral anesthetics. After a single intravenous bolus, these drugs preferentially partition into the highly perfused and lipophilic tissues of the brain and spinal cord where they produce anesthesia within a single circulation time. Subsequently blood levels fall rapidly, resulting in drug redistribution out of the CNS back into the blood. The anesthetic then diffuses into less perfused tissues such as muscle and viscera, and at a slower rate into the poorly perfused but very hydrophobic adipose tissue. Termination of anesthesia after single boluses of parenteral anesthetics primarily reflects redistribution out of the CNS rather than metabolism (see Figure 11-1). After redistribution, anesthetic blood levels fall according to a complex interaction between the metabolic rate and the amount and lipophilicity of the drug stored in

(Continued)

TABLE 11-1 Pharmacological Properties of Parenteral Anesthetics

DRUG	FORMULATION	IV INDUCTION DOSE (mg/kg)	MINIMAL HYPNOTIC LEVEL (µg/mL)	INDUCTION DOSE DURATION (min)	$t_{1/2\beta}$ (HOURS)	CL (mL · min^{-1}· kg^{-1})	PROTEIN BINDING (%)	V_{ss} (L/kg)
Thiopental	25 mg/mL in aqueous solution + 1.5 mg/mL Na$_2$CO$_3$; pH = 10-11	3-5	15.6	5-8	12.1	3.4	85	2.3
Methohexital	10 mg/mL in aqueous solution + 1.5 mg/mL Na$_2$CO$_3$; pH = 10-11	1-2	10	4-7	3.9	10.9	85	2.2
Propofol	10 mg/mL in 10% soybean oil, 2.25% glycerol, 1.2% egg PL, 0.005% EDTA or 0.025% Na-MBS; pH = 4.5-7	1.5-2.5	1.1	4-8	1.8	30	98	2.3
Etomidate	2 mg/mL in 35% PG; pH = 6.9	0.2-0.4	0.3	4-8	2.9	17.9	76	2.5
Ketamine	10, 50, or 100 mg/mL in aqueous solution; pH = 3.5-5.5	0.5-1.5	1	10-15	3.0	19.1	27	3.1

$t_{1/2\beta,\beta}$ phase half-life; CL, clearance; V_{ss}, volume of distribution at steady state; EDTA, ethylenediaminetetraacetic acid; Na-MBS, Na-metabisulfite; PG, propylene glycol; PL, phospholipid.

SECTION II Neuropharmacology

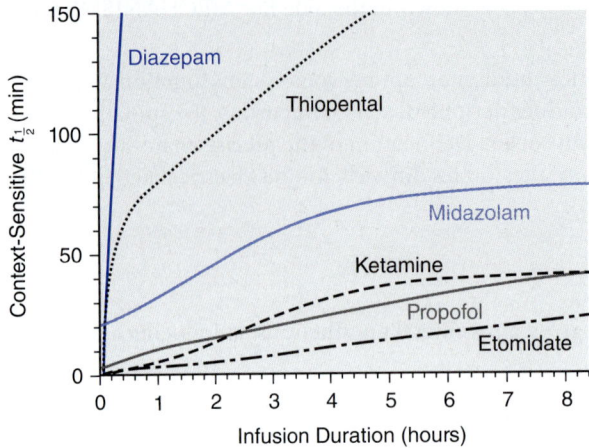

FIGURE 11-2 Context-sensitive half-time of general anesthetics. The duration of action of single intravenous doses of anesthetic/hypnotic drugs is similarly short for all and is determined by redistribution of the drugs away from their active sites (see Figure 11-1). However, after prolonged infusions, drug half-lives and durations of action are dependent on a complex interaction between the rate of redistribution of the drug, the amount of drug accumulated in fat, and the drug's metabolic rate. This phenomenon has been termed the context-sensitive half-time; that is, the $t_{1/2}$ of a drug can be estimated only if one knows the context—the total dose and over what time period it has been given. Note that the half-times of some drugs such as etomidate, propofol, and ketamine increase only modestly with prolonged infusions; others (eg, diazepam and thiopental) increase dramatically. *(Reproduced with permission from Reves JG, Glass PSA, Lubarsky DA, et al: Intravenous anesthetics, in Miller RD et al, (eds): Miller's Anesthesia, 7th ed. Philadelphia: Churchill Livingstone, 2010, p 718. Copyright © Elsevier.)*

the peripheral compartments. Thus, parenteral anesthetic half-lives are "context-sensitive," and the degree to which a $t_{1/2}$ is contextual varies greatly from drug to drug, as might be predicted based on their differing hydrophobicities and metabolic clearances (see Table 11-1 and Figure 11-2). For example, after a single bolus of thiopental, patients usually emerge from anesthesia within 10 minutes; however, a patient may require more than a day to awaken from a prolonged thiopental infusion.

c. **What are the differences between the parenteral anesthetic agents?**

Each of these drugs will produce anesthesia and the choice of which agent to use is usually based on its pharmacological properties. Table 11-1 lists the pharmacological properties of the parenteral anesthetic agents. Most individual variability in sensitivity to parenteral anesthetics can be accounted for by pharmacokinetic factors. For example, in patients with lower cardiac output, the relative perfusion of the brain and the fraction of anesthetic dose delivered to the brain are higher; thus, patients in septic shock or with cardiomyopathy usually require lower doses of anesthetic. The elderly also typically require a smaller anesthetic dose, primarily because of a smaller initial volume of distribution.

CASE 11-3

For the patient in Case 11-1, after induction of her anesthesia with a parenteral agent she is to be maintained with an inhalational anesthetic.

a. **What are the choices of inhalational anesthetic agents to maintain anesthesia?**

Table 11-2 lists the widely varying physical properties of the inhalational agents in clinical use. These properties are important because they govern the pharmacokinetics of the inhalational agents. Ideally, an inhalational agent would produce a rapid induction of anesthesia and a rapid recovery following discontinuation.

(Continued)

TABLE 11-2 Properties of Inhalational Anesthetic Agents

ANESTHETIC AGENT	MAC[a] (vol %)	MAC$_{awake}$[b] (vol %)	EC$_{50}$[c] FOR SUPPRESSION OF MEMORY (vol %)	VAPOR PRESSURE (mm Hg at 20°C)	PARTITION COEFFICIENT AT 37°C			RECOVERED AS METABOLITES (%)
					Blood:Gas	Brain:Blood	Fat:Blood	
Halothane	0.75	0.41	—	243	2.3	2.9	51	20
Isoflurane	1.2	0.4	0.24	250	1.4	2.6	45	0.2
Enflurane	1.6	0.4	—	175	1.8	1.4	36	2.4
Sevoflurane	2	0.6	—	160	0.65	1.7	48	3
Desflurane	6	2.4	—	664	0.45	1.3	27	0.02
Nitrous oxide	105	60.0	52.5	Gas	0.47	1.1	2.3	0.004
Xenon	71	32.6	—	Gas	0.12	—	—	0

[a]MAC (minimum alveolar concentration) values are expressed as vol %, the percentage of the atmosphere that is anesthetic. A value of MAC greater than 100% means that hyperbaric conditions would be required.
[b]MAC$_{awake}$ is the concentration at which appropriate responses to commands are lost.
[c]EC$_{50}$ is the concentration that produces memory suppression in 50% of patients. —, Not available.

b. How is potency measured for inhalational anesthetics?

The potency of general anesthetic agents usually is measured by determining the concentration of general anesthetic that prevents movement in response to surgical stimulation. For inhalational anesthetics, anesthetic potency is measured in minimum alveolar concentration (MAC) units, with 1 MAC defined as the minimum alveolar concentration that prevents movement in response to surgical stimulation in 50% of subjects.

c. What are the pharmacokinetic principles of inhalational anesthetics?

In considering the pharmacokinetics of anesthetics, one important parameter is the speed of anesthetic induction. Anesthesia is produced when anesthetic partial pressure in the brain is equal to or greater than MAC. Because the brain is well perfused, anesthetic partial pressure in brain becomes equal to the partial pressure in alveolar gas (and in blood) over the course of several minutes. Therefore, anesthesia is achieved shortly after alveolar partial pressure reaches MAC. While the rate of rise of alveolar partial pressure will be slower for anesthetics that are highly soluble in blood and other tissues, this limitation on speed of induction can be overcome largely by delivering higher inspired partial pressures of the anesthetic.

Elimination of inhalational anesthetics is largely the reverse process of uptake. For agents with low blood and tissue solubility, recovery from anesthesia should mirror anesthetic induction, regardless of the duration of anesthetic administration. For inhalational agents with high blood and tissue solubility, recovery will be a function of the duration of anesthetic administration. This occurs because the accumulated amounts of anesthetic in the fat reservoir will prevent blood (and therefore alveolar) partial pressures from falling rapidly. Patients will be arousable when alveolar partial pressure reaches MAC$_{awake}$, a partial pressure somewhat lower than MAC (see Table 11-2).

d. What governs the speed of induction of an inhalational anesthetic?

It is essential to understand that inhalational anesthetics distribute between tissues (or between blood and gas) such that equilibrium is achieved when the partial pressure of anesthetic gas is equal in all tissues. When a person has breathed an inhalational anesthetic for a sufficiently long time that all tissues are equilibrated with the anesthetic, the partial pressure of the anesthetic in all tissues will be equal to the partial pressure of the anesthetic in inspired gas. Note, however, that while

(Continued)

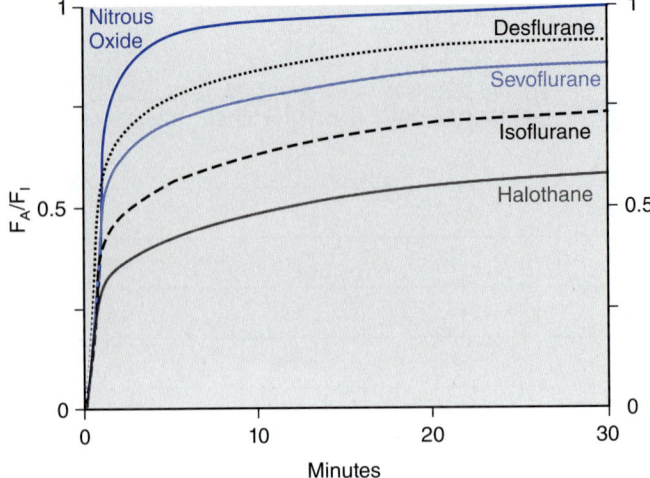

FIGURE 11-3 Uptake of inhalational general anesthetics. The rise in end-tidal alveolar (F_A) anesthetic concentration toward the inspired (F_I) concentration is most rapid with the least soluble anesthetics, nitrous oxide and desflurane, and slowest with the most soluble anesthetic, halothane. All data are from human studies. *(Reproduced with permission from Eger EI, II: Inhaled anesthetics: Uptake and distribution, in Miller RD et al, (eds): Miller's Anesthesia, 7th ed. Philadelphia: Churchill Livingstone, 2010, p 540. Copyright © Elsevier.)*

the partial pressure of the anesthetic may be equal in all tissues, the concentration of anesthetic in each tissue will be different. Indeed, anesthetic partition coefficients are defined as the ratio of anesthetic concentration in 2 tissues when the partial pressures of anesthetic are equal in the 2 tissues. Blood:gas, brain:blood, and fat:blood partition coefficients for the various inhalational agents are listed in Table 11-2. These partition coefficients show that inhalational anesthetics are more soluble in some tissues (eg, fat) than they are in others (eg, blood), and that there is significant range in the solubility of the various inhalational agents in such tissues.

For example, desflurane has a very low blood:gas partition coefficient (0.42) and also is not very soluble in fat or other peripheral tissues (see Table 11-2). For this reason, the alveolar (and blood) concentration rapidly rises to the level of inspired concentration (see Figure 11-3). Indeed, within 5 minutes of administration, the alveolar concentration reaches 80% of the inspired concentration. This provides for a very rapid induction of anesthesia and for rapid changes in depth of anesthesia following changes in the inspired concentration. Emergence from anesthesia also is very rapid with desflurane. The time to awakening following desflurane is shorter than with halothane or sevoflurane and usually does not exceed 5 to 10 minutes in the absence of other sedative agents.

CASE 11-4

During anesthesia for the patient in Case 11-1, she will require endotracheal intubation.

a. **What drugs are chosen for this?**

   Endotracheal intubation frequently requires the administration of a neuromuscular blocking drug to relax the muscles of the jaw. The pharmacology of these drugs is discussed in Chapter 6.

b. **Why was the patient in Case 11-1 administered a benzodiazepine sedative prior to her surgery?**

   As adjuncts, benzodiazepines are used for anxiolysis, amnesia, and sedation prior to induction of anesthesia or for sedation during procedures not requiring general anesthesia. The benzodiazepine most frequently used in the perioperative period is midazolam followed distantly by diazepam, and lorazepam. The pharmacology of these drugs is discussed in Chapter 9.

(Continued)

Anesthetic Agents and Therapeutic Gases

CHAPTER 11

USES OF LOCAL ANESTHETICS[a]

- Topical
- Local infiltration
- Field block
- Nerve block
- Intravenous regional anesthesia
- Spinal anesthesia
- Epidural anesthesia

[a]Details of each can be found in Chapter 20 of *Goodman and Gilman's The Pharmacological Basis of Therapeutics,* 12th Edition.

c. **Why will this patient require an analgesic prior to surgery, during the surgery, and during the immediate postoperative period?**

With the exception of ketamine, neither parenteral nor currently available inhalational anesthetics are effective analgesics. Thus, analgesics typically are administered with general anesthetics to reduce anesthetic requirement and minimize hemodynamic changes produced by painful stimuli. Opioids are the primary analgesics used during the perioperative period because of the rapid and profound analgesia they produce. During the perioperative period, opioids often are given at induction to preempt responses to predictable painful stimuli (eg, endotracheal intubation and surgical incision). Subsequent doses either by bolus or by infusion are titrated to the surgical stimulus and the patient's hemodynamic response.

CASE 11-5

A 33-year-old man is about to undergo a dental procedure. His dentist says that the local anesthetic he will be using contains epinephrine and asks if there is any history of a heart condition or high blood pressure.

a. **What is the mechanism of action of local anesthetics?**

Local anesthetics act at the cell membrane to prevent the generation and the conduction of nerve impulses. Local anesthetics block conduction by decreasing or preventing the large transient increase in the permeability of excitable membranes to Na^+ that normally is produced by a slight depolarization of the membrane. This action of local anesthetics is due to their direct interaction with voltage-gated Na^+ channels (see Figure 11-4). As the anesthetic action progressively develops in a nerve, the threshold for electrical excitability gradually increases, the rate of rise of the action potential declines, impulse conduction slows, and the safety factor for conduction decreases. These factors decrease the probability of propagation of the action potential, and nerve conduction eventually fails.

b. **Why would the local anesthetic contain epinephrine?**

The duration of action of a local anesthetic is proportional to the time of contact with nerve. Consequently, maneuvers that keep the drug at the nerve prolong the period of anesthesia. In clinical practice, a vasoconstrictor, usually epinephrine, is often added to local anesthetics. The vasoconstrictor performs a dual service. By decreasing the rate of absorption, it not only localizes the anesthetic at the desired site, but also allows the rate at which it is destroyed in the body to keep pace with the rate at which it is absorbed into the circulation. This reduces its systemic toxicity.

c. **Are their any concerns about the use of epinephrine with local anesthetics?**

Some of the vasoconstrictor agents used with local anesthetics may be absorbed systemically, occasionally to an extent sufficient to cause untoward reactions. There also may be delayed wound healing, tissue edema, or necrosis after local anesthesia. These effects seem to occur partly because sympathomimetic amines increase the oxygen consumption of the tissue; this, together with the vasoconstriction, leads to hypoxia and local tissue damage. The use of vasoconstrictors in local anesthetic preparations for anatomical regions with limited collateral circulation could produce irreversible hypoxic damage, tissue necrosis, and gangrene, and therefore are contraindicated. It should be stressed that untoward cardiovascular effects of local anesthetic agents may result from their inadvertent intravascular administration, especially if epinephrine also is present.

CASE 11-6

A 54-year-old man is having a procedure for which he has been told he will receive spinal anesthesia.

a. **What is spinal anesthesia?**

Spinal anesthesia occurs following the injection of local anesthetic into the cerebrospinal fluid (CSF) in the lumbar space. For a number of reasons, including the

(Continued)

SECTION II Neuropharmacology

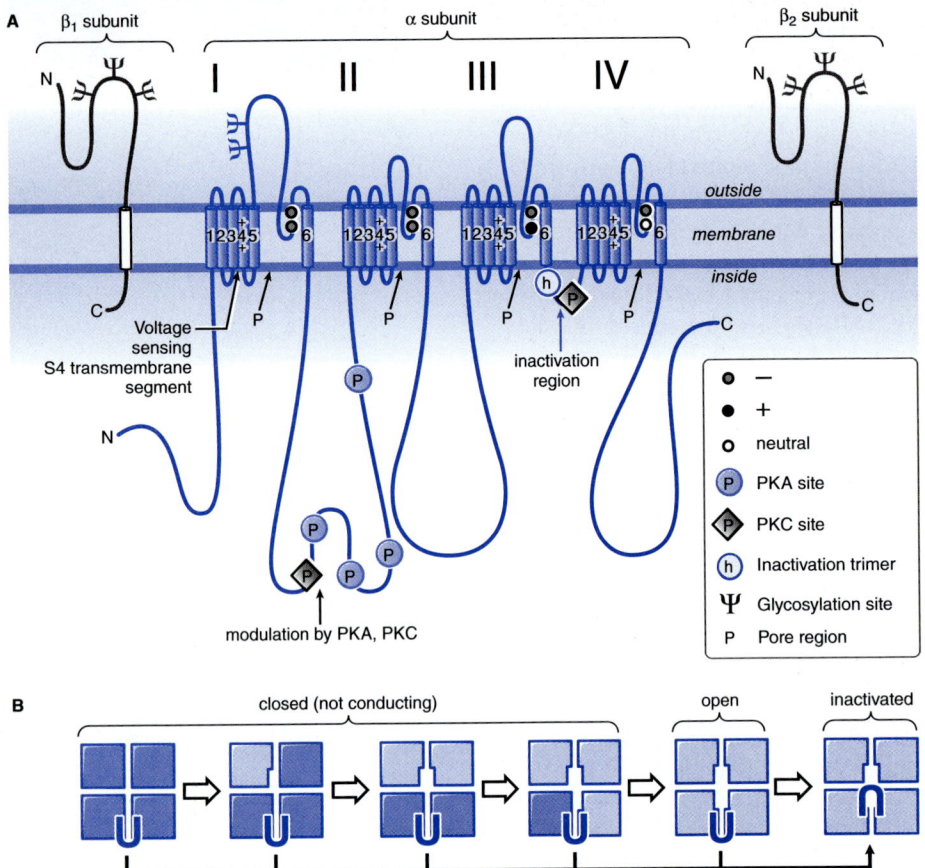

FIGURE 11-4 Structure and function of voltage-gated Na⁺ channels. **A.** A two-dimensional representation of the α (center), β₁ (left), and β₂ (right) subunits of the voltage-gated Na⁺ channel from mammalian brain. The polypeptide chains are represented by continuous lines with length approximately proportional to the actual length of each segment of the channel protein. Cylinders represent regions of transmembrane α helices. Ψ indicates sites of demonstrated N-linked glycosylation. Note the repeated structure of the 4 homologous domains (I-IV) of the α subunit. **Voltage Sensing**. The S4 transmembrane segments in each homologous domain of the α subunit serve as voltage sensors. (+) represents the positively charged amino acid residues at every third position within these segments. Electrical field (negative inside) exerts a force on these charged amino acid residues, pulling them toward the intracellular side of the membrane; depolarization allows them to move outward. **Pore**. The S5 and S6 transmembrane segments and the short membrane-associated loop between them (P loop) form the walls of the pore in the center of an approximately symmetrical square array of the 4 homologous domains (see panel B). The amino acid residues indicated by circles in the P loop are critical for determining the conductance and ion selectivity of the Na⁺ channel and its ability to bind the extracellular pore-blocking toxins tetrodotoxin and saxitoxin. **Inactivation**. The short intracellular loop connecting homologous domains III and IV serves as the inactivation gate of the Na⁺ channel. It is thought to fold into the intracellular mouth of the pore and occlude it within a few milliseconds after the channel opens. Three hydrophobic residues (isoleucine–phenylalanine–methionine; IFM) at the position marked **h** appear to serve as an inactivation particle, entering the intracellular mouth of the pore and binding to an inactivation gate receptor there. **Modulation**. The gating of the Na⁺ channel can be modulated by protein phosphorylation. Phosphorylation of the inactivation gate between homologous domains III and IV by PKC slows inactivation. Phosphorylation of sites in the intracellular loop between homologous domains I and II by either PKC or PKA reduces Na⁺ channel activation. (*Adapted with permission from Catterall W, From ionic currents to molecular mechanisms: the structure and function of voltage-gated sodium channels. Neuron, 2000;26:13-25. Copyright © Elsevier.*) **B.** The 4 homologous domains of the Na⁺ channel α subunit are illustrated as a square array, as viewed looking down on the membrane. The sequence of conformational changes that the Na⁺ channel undergoes during activation and inactivation is diagrammed. Upon depolarization, each of the 4 homologous domains sequentially undergoes a conformational change to an activated state. After all 4 domains have activated, the Na⁺ channel can open. Within a few milliseconds after opening, the inactivation gate between domains III and IV closes over the intracellular mouth of the channel and occludes it, preventing further ion conductance.

ability to produce anesthesia of a considerable fraction of the body with a dose of local anesthetic that produces negligible plasma levels, spinal anesthesia remains one of the most popular forms of anesthesia.

Currently in the United States, the drugs most commonly used in spinal anesthesia are lidocaine, tetracaine, and bupivacaine. General guidelines are to use lidocaine for short procedures, bupivacaine for intermediate to long procedures, and tetracaine for long procedures.

(*Continued*)

b. What problems might occur with spinal anesthesia?

Persistent neurological deficits following spinal anesthesia are extremely rare. Thorough evaluation of a suspected deficit should be performed in collaboration with a neurologist. Neurological sequelae can be both immediate and late. Possible causes include introduction of foreign substances (such as disinfectants or talc) into the subarachnoid space, infection, hematoma, or direct mechanical trauma.

A more common sequela following any lumbar puncture, including spinal anesthesia, is a postural headache with classic features. The incidence of headache decreases with increasing age of the patient and decreasing needle diameter. Headache following lumbar puncture must be thoroughly evaluated to exclude serious complications such as meningitis. Treatment usually is conservative, with bed rest and analgesics.

c. What are the other ways that local anesthetics can be administered?

Other ways that local anesthetics are used during surgical procedures are shown in the Side Bar USES OF LOCAL ANESTHETICS. The details of each of these can be found in Chapter 20 of *Goodman and Gilman's The Pharmacological Basis of Therapeutics*, 12th Edition.

KEY CONCEPTS

- General anesthetics have low therapeutic indices and thus require administration by specially trained personnel.
- All general anesthetics produce a relatively similar anesthetic state, but they are quite dissimilar in their secondary actions (side effects) on other organ systems.
- After a single intravenous bolus, a parenteral anesthetic partitions into the highly perfused and lipophilic tissues of the brain and spinal cord where it produces anesthesia within a single circulation time.
- Termination of a parenteral anesthetic after a single bolus primarily reflects redistribution out of the CNS (see Figure 11-1).
- Parenteral anesthetics ultimately accumulate in fatty tissue prolonging recovery if multiple doses are given.
- Inhalation anesthetics have a low safety margin.
- A general anesthetic is rarely given as the sole agent; anesthetic adjuncts such as sedatives, analgesics, or neuromuscular blocking agents are used to augment specific components of anesthesia (Side Bar COMPONENTS OF ANESTHETIC STATE).
- Local anesthetics bind reversibly to a specific receptor site within the pore of Na^+ channels in nerves and block ion movement through the pore.
- The duration of action of a local anesthetic is proportional to the time of contact with the nerve; consequently, maneuvers (the addition of a vasoconstrictor agent such as epinephrine) that keep the drug at the nerve prolong the period of anesthesia.
- Local anesthetics are administered clinically in various ways including topical, infiltration, field blocks, nerve blocks, intravenous regional, spinal, and epidural.

SUMMARY QUIZ

QUESTION 11-1 Current evidence supports the view that most intravenous general anesthetics act predominantly through

a. 5-HT receptors.

b. D_2 dopamine receptors.

c. $GABA_A$ receptors.

SECTION II — Neuropharmacology

d. α_2-adrenergic receptors.

e. β_1-adrenergic receptors.

QUESTION 11-2 Termination of anesthesia after a single bolus of a parenteral anesthetic primarily reflects

a. redistribution out of the CNS.

b. metabolism by the liver.

c. excretion by the kidney.

d. enhanced protein plasma protein binding.

e. hydrolysis by plasma esterases.

QUESTION 11-3 A 23-year-old man is having outpatient surgery for a torn anterior cruciate ligament as the result of a skiing injury. He is most likely to receive which of the following drugs as a parenteral anesthetic?

a. Phenobarbital

b. Diazepam

c. Propranolol

d. Lidocaine

e. Propofol

QUESTION 11-4 A 35-year-old woman is anesthetized with desflurane for outpatient surgery. The induction with desflurane is rapid because desflurane is not very soluble in fat and because desflurane

a. has a high blood:gas partition coefficient.

b. is highly protein bound.

c. is metabolized rapidly to an active metabolite.

d. increases cerebral vascular resistance.

e. has a low blood:gas partition coefficient.

QUESTION 11-5 If the patient in Question 11-4 is anesthetized with equipment in which the CO_2 absorbent is not well hydrated, she is at risk of poisoning with

a. NO.

b. O_2.

c. CO.

d. H_2S.

e. He.

QUESTION 11-6 A 19-year-old woman is undergoing dental surgery. Immediately upon infiltration of the local anesthetic, tetracaine with epinephrine, she begins to wheeze and have an allergic reaction. The cause of her allergic reaction is likely

a. epinephrine.

b. sulfite.

c. tetracaine.

d. nickel.

e. penicillin.

QUESTION 11-7 A 44-year-old man is undergoing surgery on the fifth finger of his right hand. A local anesthetic without epinephrine is used because epinephrine in this setting may cause

a. methemoglobinemia.

b. renal impairment.

c. liver injury.

d. gangrene.

e. necrosis of the optic nerve.

QUESTION 11-8 While eating mussels, a 36-year-old woman develops numbness and tingling of her lips and tongue. She begins to have difficulty breathing and rapidly becomes unconscious. Her apparent respiratory paralysis is the result of

a. the block of Na^+ channels.

b. serotonin syndrome.

c. malignant hyperthermia.

d. depletion of norepinephrine.

e. inhibition of monoamine oxidase (MAO).

SUMMARY QUIZ ANSWER KEY

QUESTION 11-1 Answer is **c.** Current evidence supports the view that most intravenous general anesthetics act predominantly through $GABA_A$ receptors and perhaps through some interactions with other ligand-gated ion channels such as NMDA receptors and two-pore K^+ channels.

QUESTION 11-2 Answer is **a.** Termination of anesthesia after a single bolus of a parenteral anesthetic primarily reflects redistribution out of the CNS rather than metabolism (see Figure 11-1).

QUESTION 11-3 Answer is **e.** Propofol is the most commonly used parenteral anesthetic in the United States. Propofol is advantageous for procedures where rapid return to a preoperative mental status is desirable.

QUESTION 11-4 Answer is **e.** Desflurane has a very low blood:gas partition coefficient (0.42) and also is not very soluble in fat or other peripheral tissues (see Table 11-2). For this reason, the alveolar (and blood) concentration rapidly rises to the level of inspired concentration. Indeed, within 5 minutes of administration, the alveolar concentration reaches 80% of the inspired concentration (see Figure 11-3). This provides for a very rapid induction of anesthesia and for rapid changes in depth of anesthesia following changes in the inspired concentration. Emergence from anesthesia also is very rapid with desflurane for the same reasons.

QUESTION 11-5 Answer is **c.** Inhaled anesthetics are administered via a circle system circuit that permits unidirectional flow of gas. This system permits rebreathing of exhaled gases that contain CO_2. To prevent rebreathing of CO_2 (which can lead to hypercarbia), CO_2 absorbers are incorporated into the anesthesia delivery circuits. These CO_2 absorbers contained either $Ca(OH)_2$ or $Ba(OH)_2$ and smaller quantities of more potent alkalis, NaOH and KOH. Interaction of inhaled anesthetics with these strong alkalis results in the formation of CO. The amount of CO produced is insignificant as long as the CO_2 absorbent is sufficiently hydrated. With almost complete desiccation of the CO_2 absorbents, substantial quantities of CO can be produced. This effect is greatest with desflurane and can be prevented by the use of well-hydrated, fresh CO_2 absorbent.

QUESTION 11-6 Answer is **b.** Although allergic responses to agents of the amide type are uncommon, solutions of such agents may contain preservatives such as methylparaben that may provoke an allergic reaction. Local anesthetic preparations containing a vasoconstrictor, such as epinephrine, also may elicit allergic responses due to the sulfite added as an antioxidant for the catecholamine/vasoconstrictor.

QUESTION 11-7 Answer is **d.** Epinephrine-containing solutions should not be injected into tissues supplied by end arteries—for example, fingers and toes, ears, the nose, and the penis. The resulting vasoconstriction may cause gangrene. For the same

(Continued)

SECTION II Neuropharmacology

reason, epinephrine should be avoided in solutions injected intracutaneously. Since epinephrine also is absorbed into the circulation, its use should be avoided in those for whom adrenergic stimulation is undesirable.

QUESTION 11-8 Answer is **a.** This woman's symptoms are consistent with ingestion of saxitoxin in the mussels she is eating. Saxitoxin blocks the pores of the Na$^+$ channel (see Figure 11-4). Saxitoxin is elaborated by the dinoflagellates *Gonyaulax catenella* and *Gonyaulax tamarensis* and retained in the tissues of clams and other shellfish that eat these organisms. Given the right conditions of temperature and light, the *Gonyaulax* may multiply so rapidly as to discolor the ocean, causing the condition known as red tide. Shellfish feeding on *Gonyaulax* at this time become extremely toxic to humans and are responsible for periodic outbreaks of paralytic shellfish poisoning. Saxitoxin in nanomolar concentrations specifically blocks the outer mouth of the pore of Na$^+$ channels in the membranes of excitable cells. As a result, the action potential is blocked.

SUMMARY TABLE: ANESTHETIC AGENTS AND THERAPEUTIC GASES

CLASS AND SUBCLASSES	NAMES	CLINICAL USES	TOXICITIES COMMON	TOXICITIES UNIQUE: CLINICALLY IMPORTANT
Parenteral Anesthetics	Sodium thiopental Methohexital	Used for induction of general anesthesia Protectant against cerebral ischemia	Excitatory symptoms such as cough, hiccup, muscle tremors, twitching, and hypertonus upon induction Dose-dependent decrease in blood pressure	Respiratory depression Fatal attacks of porphyria in patients with acute intermittent porphyria or variegate porphyria
	Propofol Fospropofol	Induction and maintenance of anesthesia Fospropofol is a prodrug of propofol	Similar to thiopental Greater degree of hypotension than with thiopental	Slightly greater degree of respiratory depression than thiopental Propofol infusion syndrome (PRIS) characterized by metabolic acidosis, hyperlipidemia, rhabdomyolysis, and enlarged liver
	Etomidate	Induction of anesthesia in patients at risk for hypotension	Pain at injection site Myoclonic movements Nausea and vomiting	Respiratory depression is less than with thiopental
	Ketamine	Induction of anesthesia in patients at risk for hypotension and bronchospasm Profound analgesia and amnesia		Emergence delirium characterized by hallucinations, vivid dreams, and delusions
Inhalational Anesthetics	Halothane	Used for maintenance of general anesthesia Desflurane is a widely used anesthetic for outpatient surgery because of its rapid onset of action and rapid recovery Sevoflurane is also used for outpatient anesthesia because of its rapid recovery profile	Dose-dependent decrease in blood pressure Sinus bradycardia	Fulminant hepatic necrosis (halothane hepatitis) Increased intracranial pressure
	Isoflurane		Dose-dependent decrease in blood pressure	Concentration-dependent depression of ventilation Increased intracranial pressure

(Continued)

Anesthetic Agents and Therapeutic Gases — CHAPTER 11

CLASS AND SUBCLASSES	NAMES	CLINICAL USES	TOXICITIES COMMON	UNIQUE: CLINICALLY IMPORTANT
Inhalational Anesthetics (*Cont.*)	Enflurane		Dose-dependent decrease in blood pressure	Concentration-dependent depression of ventilation Increased intracranial pressure
	Desflurane		Dose-dependent decrease in blood pressure	Concentration-dependent depression of ventilation Increased intracranial pressure Carbon monoxide (CO) production with CO_2 absorbers that are not sufficiently hydrated
	Sevoflurane		Dose-dependent decrease in blood pressure	Carbon monoxide (CO) production with CO_2 absorbers that are not sufficiently hydrated A degradation product produced by the interaction of sevoflurane with the CO_2 absorbent soda lime has been associated with nephrotoxicity
	Nitrous oxide	Weak anesthetic agent with significant analgesic effects Used primarily as an adjunct to other inhalational or intravenous anesthetics		
	Xenon	Inert gas not approved in the United States Use is limited by availability		
Anesthetic Adjuncts	Benzodiazepines	See Chapter 9	See Chapter 9	See Chapter 9
	Dexmedetomidine	Short-term sedation in critically ill patients Sedation prior to and/or during surgical or other medical procedures in nonintubated patients	Hypotension and bradycardia	
	Analgesics	See Chapter 10	See Chapter 10	See Chapter 10
	Neuromuscular blocking agents	See Chapter 6	See Chapter 6	See Chapter 6
Therapeutic Gases	Oxygen	Treatment of tissue hypoxia	See Chapter 20 of *Goodman and Gilman's The Pharmacological Basis of Therapeutics*, 12th Edition	See Chapter 20 of *Goodman and Gilman's The Pharmacological Basis of Therapeutics*, 12th Edition
	Carbon dioxide	Used for insufflation during endoscopic procedures Used to flood surgical field during cardiac surgery, and to adjust pH during cardiac bypass surgery	See Chapter 20 of *Goodman and Gilman's The Pharmacological Basis of Therapeutics*, 12th Edition	See Chapter 20 of *Goodman and Gilman's The Pharmacological Basis of Therapeutics*, 12th Edition
	Nitric oxide	Used to treat persistent pulmonary hypertension in the newborn Selectively dilates pulmonary vasculature		

SECTION II: Neuropharmacology

CLASS AND SUBCLASSES	NAMES	CLINICAL USES	TOXICITIES COMMON	UNIQUE: CLINICALLY IMPORTANT
	Helium	Used for pulmonary function testing, the treatment of respiratory obstruction, laser airway surgery, as a label in imaging studies, and for gas mixtures used for diving at depth		
Local Anesthetics	Lidocaine	Used to provide local anesthesia Also used as an antiarrhythmic agent (see Chapter 18)	Drowsiness, tinnitus, dysgeusia, dizziness, twitching	Respiratory depression and arrest, seizures, coma
	Bupivicaine	Long-acting local anesthesia		More cardiotoxic than equieffective doses of lidocaine
	Articaine	Used for local anesthesia		
	Chloroprocaine			Prolonged sensory and motor block after epidural or subarachnoid administration of large doses
	Mepivacaine			Toxicity in neonate due to lower pH of neonatal blood
	Prilocaine			May cause methemoglobinemia
	Ropivacaine			
	Procaine		Hydrolyzed in vivo to para-aminobenzoic acid which inhibits the action of sulfonamides	
	Tetracaine			Potential for systemic toxicity because of slow metabolism
	Dibucaine			
	Dyclonine			
	Pramoxine			
	Benzocaine			May cause methemoglobinemia
	Proparacaine	Local anesthetic for ophthalmic use		
	Cocaine	Used for topical anesthesia of the upper respiratory tract	Potential for abuse (see Chapter 14)	

CHAPTER 12

Pharmacotherapy of the Epilepsies

This chapter will be most useful after having a basic understanding of the material in Chapter 21, Pharmacotherapy of the Epilepsies in *Goodman & Gilman's The Pharmacological Basis of Therapeutics*, 12th Edition. In addition to the material presented here, the 12th Edition includes:

- A detailed discussion of the nature and mechanisms of seizures, including models of epilepsy
- A discussion of the genetic approaches to the epilepsies
- The structures of the antiseizure drugs
- A detailed discussion of the general principles that determine the choice of drugs for therapy of the epilepsies

LEARNING OBJECTIVES

- ☑ Know the different seizure types and the mechanisms that are responsible for each type.
- ☑ Understand the mechanisms of action of the antiseizure drugs and how they are used to treat the different types of seizures.
- ☑ Describe the toxicities, adverse effects, and salient drug interactions of drugs used to treat the epilepsies.
- ☑ Know the general principles of drug therapy of the epilepsies.

DRUGS INCLUDED IN THIS CHAPTER

- Acetazolamide (DIAMOX, others)
- Carbamezepine (TEGRETOL, CARBATROL, others)
- Clonazepam (KLONOPIN, others)
- Clorazepate (TRANXENE, others)
- Ethosuximide (ZARONTIN, others)
- Felbamate (FELBATOL)—withdrawn from market
- Fosphenytoin (CEREBYX, others)
- Gabapentin (NEURONTIN, others)
- Lacosamide (VIMPAT)
- Lamotrigine (LAMICTAL, others)
- Levetiracetam (KEPPRA, others)
- Methsuximide (CELONTIN)
- Oxcarbazepine (TRILEPTAL, others)
- Phenobarbital (LUMINAL, others)
- Phenytoin (DILANTIN, others)
- Pregabalin (LYROCA, others)
- Rufinamide (BANZEL)
- Tiagabine (GABITRIL)
- Topiramate (TOPAMAX, others)
- Valproic acid (DEPAKENE, others)
- Vigabatrin (SABRIL)
- Zonisamide (ZONEGRAN, others)

MECHANISMS OF ACTION OF ANTISEIZURE DRUGS[a]

DRUG CLASS	DRUG	MECHANISMS OF ACTION
Hydantoins	Phenytoin Fosphenytoin	Enhance fast inactivation of voltage-gated Na^+ channels (see Figure 12-1)
Barbiturates	Phenobarbital	$GABA_A$ receptor allosteric modulator (see Figure 12-2) AMPA/kainate receptor antagonist
Iminostilbenes	Carbamazepine Oxycarbazepine	Enhance fast inactivation of voltage-gated Na^+ channels (see Figure 12-1) $GABA_A$ receptor allosteric modulator (see Figure 12-2)
Succinimides	Ethosuximide Methsuximide	T-type Ca^{2+} channel blocker (see Figure 12-3)
Valproic Acid	Valproic Acid	Enhance fast inactivation of voltage-gated Na^+ channel (see Figure 12-1) T-type Ca^{2+} channel blocker (see Figure 12-3)
Benzodiazepines	Clonazepam Clorazepate	$GABA_A$ receptor allosteric modulator (see Figure 12-2)
Other Antiseizure Drugs	Gabapentin Pregabalin	Ligand of α2δ subunit of T-type Ca^{2+} channel
	Acetazolamide	Inhibitor of brain carbonic anhydrase
	Lamotrigine	Enhances fast inactivation of voltage-gated Na^+ channel (see Figure 12-1) T-type Ca^{2+} channel blocker (see Figure 12-3)
	Levetiracetam	Binds to synaptic vesicle protein SV2A

(Continued)

SECTION II

Neuropharmacology

SUMMARY OF THE MECHANISMS OF ACTION OF ANTISEIZURE DRUGS

- Limit the sustained, repetitive firing of voltage-activated Na⁺ channels (see Figure 12-1)
- Enhanced γ-aminobutyric acid (GABA)-mediated synaptic inhibition either by a presynaptic or postsynaptic action (see Figure 12-2)
- Inhibition of voltage-activated Ca^{2+} channels responsible for T-type Ca^{2+} currents (see Figure 12-3)

DRUG CLASS	DRUG	MECHANISMS OF ACTION
	Tiagabine	GABA uptake inhibitor GABA-transaminase inhibitor (see Figure 12-2)
	Topiramate	Enhances fast inactivation of voltage-gated Na⁺ channel (see Figure 12-1) $GABA_A$ receptor allosteric modulator (see Figure 12-2) AMPA/kainate receptor antagonist Inhibitor of brain carbonic anhydrase
	Felbamate	Enhances fast inactivation of voltage-gated Na⁺ channel (see Figure 12-1) $GABA_A$ receptor allosteric modulator (see Figure 12-2) NMDA receptor antagonist
	Zonisamide	Inhibitor of T-type Ca^{2+} channel current (see Figure 12-3) Inhibitor of brain carbonic anhydrase
	Lacosamide	Enhances slow inactivation of voltage-gated Na⁺ channel (see Figure 12-1)
	Rufinamide	Enhances slow inactivation of voltage-gated Na⁺ channel (see Figure 12-1)
	Vigabatrin	GABA uptake inhibitor GABA-transaminase inhibitor (see Figure 12-2)

[a]More details available in Table 21-2 of *Goodman and Gilman's The Pharmacologicial Basis of Therapeutics*, 12th Edition.

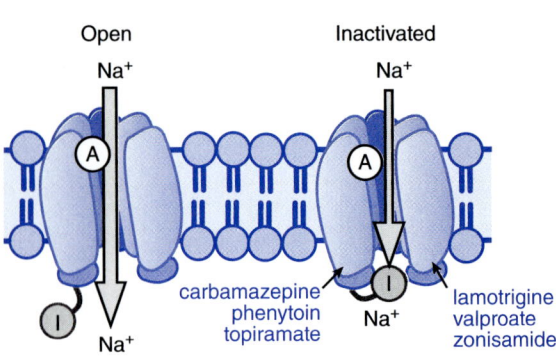

FIGURE 12-1 Antiseizure drug-enhanced Na⁺ channel inactivation. Some antiseizure drugs (shown in blue text) prolong the inactivation of the Na⁺ channels, thereby reducing the ability of neurons to fire at high frequencies. Note that the inactivated channel itself appears to remain open, but is blocked by the inactivation gate (I). A, activation gate.

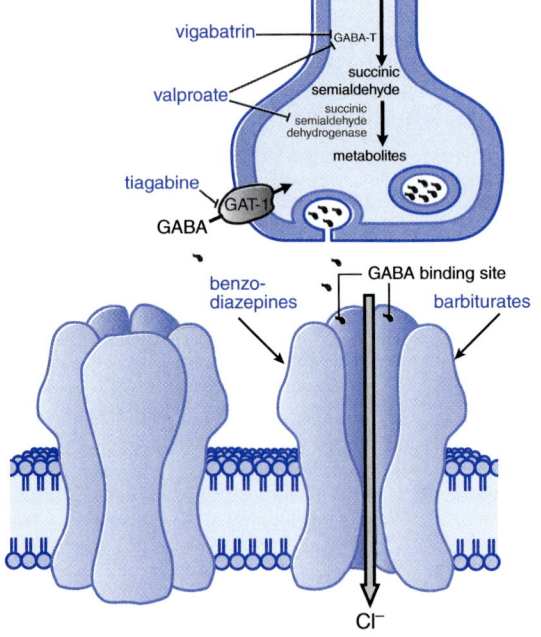

FIGURE 12-2 Enhanced GABA synaptic transmission. In the presence of GABA, the $GABA_A$ receptor (structure on left) is opened, allowing an influx of Cl^-, which in turn increases membrane polarization. Some antiseizure drugs (show in larger blue text) act by reducing the metabolism of GABA. Others act at the $GABA_A$ receptor, enhancing Cl^- influx in response to GABA. Gabapentin acts presynaptically to promote GABA release; its molecular target is currently under investigation. GABA molecules, GABA-T, GABA transaminase; GAT-1, GABA transporter.

Pharmacotherapy of the Epilepsies

CHAPTER 12

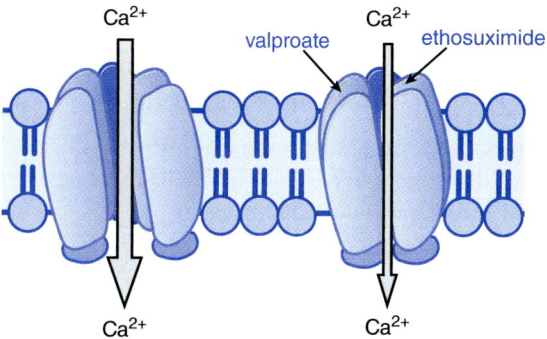

FIGURE 12-3 Antiseizure drug-induced reduction of current through T-type Ca^{2+} channels. Some antiseizure drugs (shown in blue text) reduce the flow of Ca^{2+} through T-type Ca^{2+} channels thus reducing the pacemaker current that underlies the thalamic rhythm in spikes and waves seen in generalized absence seizures.

GENERAL PRINCIPLES AND CHOICE OF DRUGS FOR THE THERAPY OF THE EPILEPSIES

- Early diagnosis and treatment of seizure disorders with a single appropriate agent offers the best prospect of achieving prolonged seizure-free periods with the lowest risk of toxicity.
- The efficacy combined with the unwanted effects of a given drug determine which particular drug is optimal for a given patient.
- Unless extenuating circumstances such as status epilepticus exist, only monotherapy should be initiated.
- Dosage is increased at appropriate intervals as required for control of seizures or as limited by toxicity.
- If compliance has been confirmed yet seizures persist, another drug should be substituted.
- If therapy with a second single drug is inadequate, combination therapy is warranted.
- It is wise to select 2 drugs that each act by distinct mechanisms.
- Side effects of each drug and the potential drug interactions also should be considered when using 2 drugs (see Table 12-1).
- Measurement of plasma drug concentration at appropriate intervals greatly facilitates the initial adjustment of dosage to minimize dose-related adverse effects without sacrificing seizure control.
- Once initiated, antiseizure drugs are typically continued for at least 2 years.
- When discontinuing, medications should be tapered slowly over a period of several months.

TABLE 12-1 Interactions of Anti-Seizure Drugs with Hepatic Microsomal Enzymes

DRUG	INDUCES CYP	INDUCES UGT	INHIBITS CYP	INHIBITS UGT	METABOLIZED BY CYP	METABOLIZED BY UGT
Carbamazepine	2C9/3A	Yes			1A2/2C8 2C9/3A4	No
Ethosuximide	No	No	No	No	?	?
Gabapentin	No	No	No	No	No	No
Lacosamide	No	No	No	No	2C19	?
Lamotrigine	No	Yes	No	No	No	Yes
Levetiracetam	No	No	No	No	No	No
Oxcarbazepine	3A4/5	Yes	2C19	Weak	No	Yes
Phenobarbital	2C/3A	Yes	Yes	No	2C9/19	No
Phenytoin	2C/3A	Yes	Yes	No	2C9/19	No
Pregabalin	No	No	No	No	No	No
Primidone	2C/3A	Yes	Yes	No	2C9/19	No
Rufinamide	3A4	2C9/19	No	?	No	Yes
Tiagabine	No	No	No	No	3A4	No
Topiramate	No	No	2C19	No		
Valproate	No	No	2C9	Yes	2C9/19	Yes
Vigabatrin	No	No	No	No	No	No
Zonisamide	No	No	No	No	3A4	Yes

CYP, cytochrome P450; UGT, uridine diphosphate-glucuronosyltransferase.

SECTION II: Neuropharmacology

CASE 12-1

A 12-year-old girl has her first tonic-clonic seizure while at school. Her seizure was preceded by lip smacking and lasted about 1 minute during which she lost consciousness.

a. During subsequent neurological tests, her parents ask for a classification of epileptic seizures so that they might understand where their child falls in the spectrum of epilepsies. What is a useful classification of epilepsies?

Table 12-2 classifies epileptic seizures into partial seizures and generalized seizures. The type of epileptic seizure is one determinant of the drug selected for therapy.

Apart from this epileptic seizure classification, an additional classification specifies epileptic syndromes, which refer to a cluster of symptoms frequently occurring together and include seizure types, etiology, age of onset, and other factors. More than 50 distinct epileptic syndromes have been identified and categorized into partial versus generalized epilepsies. The partial epilepsies may consist of any of the partial seizure types (see Table 12-2) and account for roughly 60% of all epilepsies. The etiology commonly consists of a lesion in some part of the cortex, such as a tumor, developmental malformation, or damage due to trauma or stroke. Such lesions often are evident on brain magnetic resonance imaging (MRI). Alternatively, the etiology may be genetic.

The generalized epilepsies are characterized most commonly by one or more of the generalized seizure types listed in Table 12-2 and account for ~40% of all epilepsies. The etiology is usually genetic. The most common generalized epilepsy is referred to as juvenile myoclonic epilepsy, accounting for ~10% of all epileptic syndromes. The age of onset is in the early teens, and the condition is characterized by myoclonic, tonic-clonic, and often absence seizures. Like most of the generalized-onset epilepsies, juvenile myoclonic epilepsy is a complex genetic disorder that is probably due to inheritance of multiple susceptibility genes; there is a familial clustering of cases, but the pattern of inheritance is not mendelian. The classification of epileptic syndromes guides clinical assessment and management, and in some instances, selection of antiseizure drugs.

b. What seizure type is this patient exhibiting?

Although it is difficult to make an absolute diagnosis without all of the clinical data, it would seem that this patient has had a complex partial seizure with a secondarily generalized tonic-clonic seizure.

c. Should antiseizure medication be started immediately in this patient?

Early diagnosis and treatment of seizure disorders with a single appropriate agent offers the best prospect of achieving prolonged seizure-free periods with the lowest risk of toxicity. An attempt should be made to determine the cause of the epilepsy with the hope of discovering a correctable lesion, either structural or metabolic. The efficacy combined with the unwanted effects of a given drug determines which particular drug is optimal for a given patient.

The first decision to make is whether and when to initiate treatment. For example, it may not be necessary to initiate antiseizure therapy after an isolated tonic-clonic seizure in a healthy young adult who lacks a family history of epilepsy and who has a normal neurological examination, a normal EEG, and a normal brain MRI scan. The odds of seizure recurrence in the next year (15%) are similar to the risk of a drug reaction sufficiently severe to warrant discontinuation of medication. On the other hand, a similar seizure occurring in an individual with a positive family history of epilepsy, an abnormal neurological examination, an abnormal EEG, and an abnormal MRI carries a risk of recurrence approximating 60%, odds that favor initiation of therapy.

d. What other general principles of the treatment of seizure disorders should be followed in this patient?

The general principles of therapy of the epilepsies are outlined in the Side Bar GENERAL PRINCIPLES AND CHOICE OF DRUGS FOR THE THERAPY OF THE EPILEPSIES.

Pharmacotherapy of the Epilepsies — CHAPTER 12

TABLE 12-2 Classification of Epileptic Seizures

SEIZURE TYPE	FEATURES	CONVENTIONAL ANTI-SEIZURE DRUGS	RECENTLY DEVELOPED ANTI-SEIZURE DRUGS
Partial Seizures			
Simple partial	Diverse manifestations determined by the region of cortex activated by the seizure (eg, if motor cortex representing left thumb, clonic jerking of left thumb results; if somatosensory cortex representing left thumb, paresthesia of left thumb results), lasting approximating 20-60 seconds. *Key feature is preservation of consciousness.*	Carbamazepine, phenytoin, valproate	Gabapentin, lacosamide, lamotrigine, levetiracetam, rufinamide, tiagabine, topiramate, zonisamide
Complex partial	Impaired consciousness lasting 30 seconds to 2 minutes, often associated with purposeless movements such as lip smacking or hand wringing.		
Partial with secondarily generalized tonic-clonic seizure	Simple or complex partial seizure evolves into a tonic-clonic seizure with loss consciousness and sustained contractions (tonic) of muscles throughout the body followed by periods of muscle contraction alternating with periods of relaxation (clonic), typically lasting 1-2 minutes.	Carbamazepine, phenobarbital, phenytoin, primidone, valproate	
Generalized Seizures			
Absence seizure	Abrupt onset of impaired consciousness associated with staring and cessation of ongoing activities typically lasting less than 30 seconds.	Ethosuximide, valproate, clonazepam	Lamotrigine
Myoclonic seizure	A brief (perhaps a second), shocklike contraction of muscles that may be restricted to part of one extremity or may be generalized.	Valproate, clonazepam	Levetiracetam
Tonic-clonic seizure	As described earlier in table for partial with secondarily generalized tonic-clonic seizures except that it is not preceded by a partial seizure.	Carbamazepine, phenobarbital, phenytoin, primidone, valproate	Lamotrigine, levetiracetam, topiramate

Modified with permission from Leppik IE, Kelly KM, deToledo-Morrell L et al. Basic research in epilepsy and aging. *Epilepsy Res*, 2006, 68 (Suppl 1): 21. Copyright© Elsevier.

CASE 12-2

The patient in Case 12-1 had a second tonic-clonic seizure and it was decided that she should be treated with phenytoin.

a. What is the mechanism of action of phenytoin?

The mechanisms of action of antiseizure drugs are listed in the Table MECHANISMS OF ACTION OF ANTISEIZURE DRUGS. Phenytoin limits the repetitive firing of action potentials evoked by a sustained depolarization of mouse spinal cord neurons maintained in vitro. This effect is mediated by a slowing of the rate of recovery of voltage-activated Na^+ channels from inactivation, an action that is both voltage- (greater effect if membrane is depolarized) and use-dependent (see Figure 12-1).

b. What is unique about the elimination of phenytoin?

Phenytoin is one of the few drugs for which the rate of elimination varies as a function of its concentration (ie, the rate is nonlinear). The plasma $t_{1/2}$ of phenytoin ranges between 6 and 24 hours at plasma concentrations below 10 μg/mL but increases with higher concentrations; as a result, plasma drug concentration increases disproportionately as dosage is increased, even with small adjustments for levels near the therapeutic range.

c. How should phenytoin treatment be monitored?

A good correlation usually is observed between the total concentration of phenytoin in plasma and its clinical effect. Thus, control of seizures generally is obtained

(Continued)

with total concentrations above 10 µg/mL, while toxic effects such as nystagmus develop at total concentrations around 20 µg/mL.

d. What untoward effects might this patient expect from long-term phenytoin treatment?

Toxic effects associated with chronic phenytoin treatment are primarily dose-related cerebellar-vestibular effects but also include other CNS effects, behavioral changes, increased frequency of seizures, GI symptoms, gingival hyperplasia, osteomalacia, and megaloblastic anemia. Hirsutism is an annoying untoward effect in young females. Usually, these phenomena can be diminished by proper adjustment of dosage. Serious adverse effects, including those on the skin, bone marrow, and liver, probably are manifestations of drug allergy. Although rare, they necessitate withdrawal of the drug.

Gingival hyperplasia occurs in ~20% of all patients during chronic therapy and is probably the most common manifestation of phenytoin toxicity in children and young adolescents. It may be more frequent in those individuals who also develop coarsened facial features. The overgrowth of gingival tissue appears to involve altered collagen metabolism. Toothless portions of the gums are not affected. The condition does not necessarily require withdrawal of medication and can be minimized by good oral hygiene.

A variety of endocrine effects have been reported. Inhibition of release of antidiuretic hormone (ADH) has been observed in patients with inappropriate ADH secretion. Hyperglycemia and glycosuria appear to be due to inhibition of insulin secretion. Osteomalacia, with hypocalcemia and elevated alkaline phosphatase activity, has been attributed to both altered metabolism of vitamin D and the attendant inhibition of intestinal absorption of Ca^{2+}.

Hypersensitivity reactions include morbilliform rash in 2 to 5% of patients and occasionally more serious skin reactions, including Stevens-Johnson syndrome and toxic epidermal necrolysis.

CASE 12-3

A 7-year-old boy is diagnosed with absence seizures. This patient has an older brother who also has absence seizures that progressed to tonic-clonic seizures within 1 year.

a. What is an absence seizure and what is thought to be the mechanism of seizure activity in this type of seizure?

In contrast to partial seizures, which arise from localized regions of the cerebral cortex, generalized-onset seizures arise from the reciprocal firing of the thalamus and cerebral cortex. The EEG hallmark of an absence seizure is generalized spike-and-wave discharges at a frequency of 3 per second (3 Hz).

These reverberatory, low-frequency rhythms are made possible by a combination of factors, including reciprocal excitatory synaptic connections between the neocortex and thalamus as well as intrinsic properties of neurons in the thalamus. One intrinsic property of thalamic neurons that is pivotally involved in the generation of the 3-Hz spike-and-wave discharges is a particular type of Ca^{2+} current, the low threshold ("T-type") current. T-type Ca^{2+} channels are activated at a much more negative membrane potential (hence "low threshold") than most other voltage-gated Ca^{2+} channels expressed in the brain.

b. What are the mechanisms of action of valproic acid?

The principal mechanism by which anti–absence-seizure drugs (ethosuximide, valproic acid) are thought to act is by inhibition of the T-type Ca^{2+} channels (see Figure 12-3). Thus, inhibiting voltage-gated ion channels is a common mechanism of action among antiseizure drugs, with anti–partial-seizure drugs inhibiting voltage-activated Na^+ channels and anti–absence-seizure drugs inhibiting voltage-activated Ca^{2+} channels (see Figures 12-1 and 12-3).

(Continued)

Pharmacotherapy of the Epilepsies — CHAPTER 12

c. Should therapy with valproic acid be monitored by plasma concentrations?

Valproate plasma concentrations associated with therapeutic effects are ~30 to 100 μg/mL. However, there is a poor correlation between the plasma concentration and efficacy.

d. What untoward effects might be expected with valproate therapy?

The most common side effects are transient GI symptoms, including anorexia, nausea, and vomiting in ~16% of patients. Effects on the CNS include sedation, ataxia, and tremor; these symptoms occur infrequently and usually respond to a decrease in dosage. Rash, alopecia, and stimulation of appetite have been observed occasionally and weight gain has been seen with chronic valproic acid treatment in some patients. Valproic acid has several effects on hepatic function. Elevation of hepatic transaminases in plasma is observed in up to 40% of patients and often occurs asymptomatically during the first several months of therapy.

A rare complication is a fulminant hepatitis that is frequently fatal. Pathological examination reveals a microvesicular steatosis without evidence of inflammation or hypersensitivity reaction. Children younger than 2 years with other medical conditions who were given multiple antiseizure agents were especially likely to suffer fatal hepatic injury. At the other extreme, there were no deaths reported for patients older than the age of 10 years who received only valproate.

Interactions of antiseizure drugs with hepatic microsomal enzymes can be found in Table 12-1. This knowledge will help predict drug interactions when using more than one antiseizure medication.

CASE 12-4

In the patient in Case 12-3, there was initial consideration of treatment with ethosuximide.

a. Why is valproate a better choice for this patient than ethosuximide?

Ethosuximide and valproate are considered equally effective in the treatment of absence seizures. Between 50 and 75% of newly diagnosed patients are free of seizures following therapy with either drug. If tonic-clonic seizures are present (as with the sibling of this patient) or emerge during therapy, valproate is the agent of first choice.

b. What is the mechanism of action of ethosuximide?

Ethosuximide reduces low threshold Ca^{2+} currents (T-type currents) in thalamic neurons (see Figure 12-3). The thalamus plays an important role in generation of 3-Hz spike-and-wave rhythms typical of absence seizures. Neurons in the thalamus exhibit large-amplitude T-type currents that underlie bursts of action potentials and likely play an important role in thalamic oscillatory activity such as 3-Hz spike-and-wave activity. At clinically relevant concentrations, ethosuximide inhibits the T-type current, as is evident in voltage-clamp recordings of acutely isolated, ventrobasal thalamic neurons from rats and guinea pigs.

c. What side effects might have been expected if this patient were treated with ethosuximide?

The most common dose-related side effects of ethosuximide are gastrointestinal complaints (nausea, vomiting, and anorexia) and CNS effects (drowsiness, lethargy, euphoria, dizziness, headache, and hiccough). Some tolerance to these effects develops. Parkinson-like symptoms and photophobia also have been reported. Restlessness, agitation, anxiety, aggressiveness, inability to concentrate, and other behavioral effects have occurred primarily in patients with a prior history of psychiatric disturbance.

Urticaria and other skin reactions, including Stevens-Johnson syndrome, as well as systemic lupus erythematosus, eosinophilia, leukopenia, thrombocytopenia, pancytopenia, and aplastic anemia also have been attributed to ethosuximide. The leukopenia may be transient despite continuation of the drug, but several deaths have resulted from bone marrow depression. Renal or hepatic toxicity has not been reported.

SECTION II

Neuropharmacology

CASE 12-5

A 3-year-old boy with the diagnosis of Lennox-Gastaut syndrome has been treated for 6 months with phenytoin. The phenytoin has been reducing the seizure frequency, but the decision is made to add lamotrigine to the regimen to further reduce seizure frequency.

a. What is Lennox-Gastaut syndrome?

Lennox-Gastaut syndrome is a disorder of childhood characterized by multiple seizure types, mental retardation, and refractoriness to antiseizure medication.

b. What is the mechanism of action of lamotrigine?

Lamotrigine blocks sustained repetitive firing of mouse spinal cord neurons and delays the recovery from inactivation of recombinant Na^+ channels, mechanisms similar to those of phenytoin and carbamazepine (see Figure 12-1). This may well explain lamotrigine's actions on partial and secondarily generalized seizures. Lamotrigine is effective against a broader spectrum of seizures than phenytoin and carbamazepine, suggesting that lamotrigine may have actions in addition to regulating recovery from inactivation of Na^+ channels. The mechanisms underlying its broad spectrum of actions are incompletely understood. One possibility involves lamotrigine's inhibition of glutamate release in rat cortical slices treated with veratridine, a Na^+ channel activator, raising the possibility that lamotrigine inhibits synaptic release of glutamate by acting at Na^+ channels themselves.

c. What precaution with the dose of lamotrigine should be taken with this patient?

Patients who are already taking a hepatic enzyme–inducing antiseizure drug (such as carbamazepine, phenytoin, phenobarbital, or primidone, but not valproate) should be given lamotrigine initially at 50 mg/d for 2 weeks. The dose is increased to 50 mg twice per day for 2 weeks and then increased in increments of 100 mg/d each week up to a maintenance dose of 300 to 500 mg/d divided into 2 doses.

d. What untoward effects might be expected from lamotrigine?

The most common adverse effects are dizziness, ataxia, blurred or double vision, nausea, vomiting, and rash when lamotrigine was added to another antiseizure drug. A few cases of Stevens-Johnson syndrome and disseminated intravascular coagulation have been reported. The incidence of serious rash in pediatric patients (~0.8%) is higher than in the adult population (0.3%).

CASE 12-6

A 23-year-old woman is diagnosed with simple partial seizures. Treatment with carbamazepine is initiated.

a. What is the mechanism of action of carbamazepine?

Like phenytoin, carbamazepine limits the repetitive firing of action potentials evoked by a sustained depolarization of mouse spinal cord or cortical neurons maintained in vitro. This appears to be mediated by a slowing of the rate of recovery of voltage-activated Na^+ channels from inactivation (see Figure 12-1).

The predominant pathway of metabolism in humans involves conversion to the 10,11-epoxide. This metabolite is as active as the parent compound in various animal models, and its concentrations in plasma and brain may reach 50% of those of carbamazepine, especially during the concurrent administration of phenytoin or phenobarbital. The 10,11-epoxide is metabolized further to inactive compounds, which are excreted in the urine principally as glucuronides.

b. How should the therapy with carbamazepine be monitored?

There is no simple relationship between the dose of carbamazepine and concentrations of the drug in plasma. Therapeutic concentrations are reported to be 6 to

(Continued)

12 μg/mL, although considerable variation occurs. Side effects referable to the CNS are frequent at concentrations more than 9 μg/mL.

c. What toxicity might be expected in this patient?

During long-term therapy, the more frequent untoward effects of the drug include drowsiness, vertigo, ataxia, diplopia, and blurred vision. The frequency of seizures may increase, especially with overdosage. Other adverse effects include nausea, vomiting, serious hematological toxicity (aplastic anemia, agranulocytosis), and hypersensitivity reactions (dangerous skin reactions, eosinophilia, lymphadenopathy, splenomegaly). A late complication of therapy with carbamazepine is retention of water, with decreased osmolality and concentration of Na^+ in plasma, especially in elderly patients with cardiac disease.

A transient, mild leukopenia occurs in ~10% of patients during initiation of therapy and usually resolves within the first 4 months of continued treatment; transient thrombocytopenia also has been noted. In ~2% of patients, a persistent leukopenia may develop that requires withdrawal of the drug.

d. Is carbamazepine used for other disorders?

Carbamazepine is the primary agent for treatment of trigeminal and glossopharyngeal neuralgias. It is also effective for lightning-type ("tabetic") pain associated with bodily wasting. Most patients with neuralgia benefit initially, but only 70% obtain continuing relief. Adverse effects require discontinuation of medication in 5 to 20% of patients. The therapeutic range of plasma concentrations for antiseizure therapy serves as a guideline for its use in neuralgia. Carbamazepine is also used in the treatment of bipolar affective disorders, as discussed further in Chapter 8.

KEY CONCEPTS

- Therapy of epilepsies is symptomatic in that available drugs inhibit seizures, but neither effective prophylaxis nor cure is available.
- Reducing the rate of recovery of Na^+ channels from inactivation would limit the ability of a neuron to fire at high frequencies, an effect that likely underlies the effects of carbamazepine, lamotrigine, phenytoin, topiramate, valproic acid, and zonisamide against partial seizures.
- The principal mechanism by which anti-absence-seizure drugs (ethosuximide, valproic acid) are thought to act is by inhibition of the T-type Ca^{2+} channel.
- Activation of the $GABA_A$ receptor inhibits the postsynaptic cell by increasing the flow of Cl^- ions into the cell, which tends to hyperpolarize the neuron.
- The antiseizure drug tiagabine inhibits the GABA transporter, GAT-1, and reduces neuronal and glial uptake of GABA.
- The goal of treating patients with epilepsy is to select the appropriate drug or combination of drugs that best controls seizures at an acceptable level of untoward effects.
- Measurement of drug concentrations in plasma facilitates optimizing antiseizure medication, especially when therapy is initiated, after dosage adjustments, in the event of therapeutic failure, when toxic effects occur, or when multiple-drug therapy is instituted.
- When initiating combination antiseizure therapy, it is wise to select 2 drugs that act by distinct mechanisms (eg, one that promotes Na^+ channel inactivation and another that enhances GABA-mediated synaptic inhibition).
- The goal of treating status epilepticus is rapid termination of behavioral and electrical seizure activity; the longer the episode is untreated, the more difficult it is to control and the greater the risk of permanent brain damage.

SECTION II   Neuropharmacology

SUMMARY QUIZ

QUESTION 12-1 A 28-year-old man is being treated with phenytoin for tonic-clonic seizures. His drug plasma concentration is in the low therapeutic range and he is still having occasional seizures. His dose is increased slightly. Within 2 weeks he is ataxic, lethargic, and has nystagmus. A repeat of his plasma concentration shows that he is now slightly above the upper limit of the therapeutic range. The reason for the dramatic rise in his plasma concentration following a modest increase in his dose is most likely because of

a. renal failure.
b. liver failure.
c. nonlinear elimination.
d. metabolic acidosis.
e. poor GI absorption of Ca^{2+}.

QUESTION 12-2 A 34-year-old woman is being treated with carbamazepine for complex partial seizures. Carbamazepine is metabolized to an active metabolite, the

a. 10,11-epoxide metabolite.
b. *N*-acetyl metabolite.
c. desmethyl metabolite.
d. hydroxyl metabolite.
e. para-hydroxy-phenyl metabolite.

QUESTION 12-3 A 19-year-old woman is being treated with ethosuximide, most likely for which type of seizure?

a. Simple partial
b. Complex partial
c. Tonic-clonic
d. Absence
e. Status epilepticus

QUESTION 12-4 A 29-year-old woman is being treated with valproic acid for simple partial seizures. She is at risk for developing a rise in her plasma

a. calcium.
b. hepatic transaminases.
c. blood urea nitrogen (BUN).
d. potassium.
e. glucose.

QUESTION 12-5 A 33-year-old man is taking valproic acid for tonic-clonic seizures. Lamotrigine is added to improve seizure control. The plasma concentrations of lamotrigine may be increased because valproate inhibits

a. hydroxylation.
b. glucuronidation.
c. acetylation.
d. urinary excretion.
e. biliary excretion.

QUESTION 12-6 A 44-year-old man has levetiracetam added to his therapy because he is refractory to his current antiseizure regimen. Levetiracetam acts by

a. inactivation of voltage-gated Na^+ channels.
b. enhanced GABA synaptic transmission.

(Continued)

c. an unknown mechanism.

d. reducing current through T-type Ca^{2+} channels.

e. antagonizing D_2 dopaminergic receptors.

QUESTION 12-7 A 20-year-old woman is taking topiramate as monotherapy for refractory generalized tonic-clonic seizures. She should be warned to increase her dose of

a. levothyroxine.

b. metoprolol.

c. insulin.

d. botox.

e. oral contraceptive.

QUESTION 12-8 A 32-year-old woman is being treated with vigabatrin because her complex seizures have been refractory to all other therapies. Vigabatrin is reserved for use in patients such as this although its availability is restricted due to

a. renal failure.

b. liver failure.

c. heart failure.

d. vision loss.

e. hearing loss.

SUMMARY QUIZ ANSWER KEY

QUESTION 12-1 Answer is **c**. Phenytoin is one of the few drugs for which the rate of elimination varies as a function of its concentration (ie, the rate is nonlinear). The plasma $t_{1/2}$ of phenytoin ranges between 6 and 24 hours at plasma concentrations below 10 μg/mL but increases with higher concentrations; as a result, plasma drug concentration increases disproportionately as dosage is increased, even with small adjustments for levels near the therapeutic range.

QUESTION 12-2 Answer is **a**. The predominant pathway of metabolism in humans involves conversion to the 10,11-epoxide. This metabolite is as active as the parent compound in various animal models, and its concentrations in plasma and brain may reach 50% of those of carbamazepine, especially during the concurrent administration of phenytoin or phenobarbital.

QUESTION 12-3 Answer is **d**. Ethosuximide is effective against absence seizures but not partial or tonic-clonic seizures.

QUESTION 12-4 Answer is **b**. Elevation of hepatic transaminases in plasma is observed in up to 40% of patients treated with valproic acid and often occurs asymptomatically during the first several months of therapy.

QUESTION 12-5 Answer is **b**. Lamotrigine is completely absorbed from the gastrointestinal tract and is metabolized primarily by glucuronidation. The plasma $t_{1/2}$ of a single dose is 24 to 30 hours. Administration of phenytoin, carbamazepine, or phenobarbital reduces the $t_{1/2}$ and plasma concentrations of lamotrigine. Conversely, addition of valproate markedly increases plasma concentrations of lamotrigine, likely by inhibiting glucuronidation.

QUESTION 12-6 Answer is **c**. The mechanism by which levetiracetam exerts its antiseizure effects is unknown. No evidence for an action on voltage-gated Na^+ channels, or either GABA- or glutamate-mediated synaptic transmission has emerged.

SECTION II — Neuropharmacology

QUESTION 12-7 Answer is **e**. Reduced estradiol plasma concentrations occur with concurrent topiramate, suggesting the need for higher doses of oral contraceptives when coadministered with topiramate.

QUESTION 12-8 Answer is **d**. Due to progressive and permanent bilateral vision loss, vigabatrin must be reserved for patients who have failed several alternative therapies; its availability is restricted under the conditions of the SHARE special distribution program.

SUMMARY TABLE: ANTISEIZURE DRUGS

CLASS AND SUBCLASSES	NAMES	CLINICAL USES	TOXICITIES COMMON	TOXICITIES UNIQUE: CLINICALLY IMPORTANT
Hydantoins	Phenytoin, Fosphenytoin	Used to treat partial and tonic-clonic seizures. Not active against absence seizures	Gingival hyperplasia, Ataxia	Cardiac arrhythmia, Osteomalacia, Megaloblastic anemia, Inhibition of insulin secretion, Skin hypersensitivity reactions including Stevens-Johnson syndrome
Barbiturates	Phenobarbital	Used to treat generalized tonic-clonic and partial seizures	See Chapter 9	See Chapter 9
Imminostilbenes	Carbamazepine	Used to treat generalized tonic-clonic and both simple and complex partial seizures	Drowsiness, ataxia, vertigo, diplopia, blurred vision, nausea, and vomiting. Transient leukopenia and thrombocytopenia	Acute intoxication results in stupor or coma, hyperirritability, convulsions, and respiratory depression. Aplastic anemia. Transient elevation of hepatic transaminases. May reduce plasma concentrations of oral contraceptives
	Oxcarbazepine	Used to treat partial seizures		Induction of CYP3A4 and reduction of plasma concentrations of oral contraceptives
Succinimides	Ethosuximide	Effective against absence seizures, but not tonic-clonic seizures	Nausea, vomiting, anorexia. Drowsiness, lethargy, euphoria, dizziness, headache, hiccough	Parkinson-like symptoms, photophobia, anxiety, aggression, and inability to concentrate. Hypersensitivity skin reactions including Stevens-Johnson syndrome. Transient leukopenia. Death from bone marrow depression has been reported
	Methsuximide	No longer in common use		
Valproic Acid	Valproic acid	Broad-spectrum antiseizure drug effective against absence, myoclonic, partial, and tonic-clonic seizures	Anorexia, nausea, and vomiting. Sedation, ataxia, and tremor	Inhibits drugs that are substrates for CYP2C9, including phenytoin and phenobarbital. Inhibits UGT and thus the metabolism of lamotrigine and lorazepam. Elevation of hepatic transaminases. Rarely may cause fulminant hepatitis

Pharmacotherapy of the Epilepsies — CHAPTER 12

CLASS AND SUBCLASSES	NAMES	CLINICAL USES	TOXICITIES COMMON	UNIQUE: CLINICALLY IMPORTANT
Benzodiazepines	Clonazepam	Used to treat absence seizures and myoclonic seizures in children	See Chapter 9	Tolerance to antiseizure effects develops after 1-6 months
	Clorazepate	Used in combination with other drugs to treat partial seizures	See Chapter 9	
Other Antiseizure Drugs	Gabapentin Pregabalin	Effective, when used with other drugs, against partial seizures	Somnolence, dizziness, ataxia, and fatigue	Pregnancy Category C
	Lamotrigine	Used as monotherapy and add-on therapy of partial and secondarily generalized tonic-clonic seizures in adults and Lennox-Gastaut syndrome in children and adults	Dizziness, ataxia, blurred of double vision, nausea, and vomiting	Stevens-Johnson syndrome and disseminated intravascular coagulation have been reported
	Levetriacetam	Used for refractory partial seizures or uncontrolled generalized tonic-clonic seizures. Adjunctive therapy for refractory generalized myoclonic seizures	Somnolence, asthenia, and dizziness	
	Tiagabine	Effective as add-on therapy of refractory partial seizures with or without secondary generalization	Dizziness, somnolence, and tremor	May be contraindicated in generalized absence epilepsy
	Topiramate	Used as initial monotherapy (in patients at least 10 years old) and as adjunctive therapy (for patients as young as 2 years of age) for partial onset or primary generalized tonic-clonic seizures, for Lennox-Gastaut syndrome in patients 2 years of age or older, and for migraine prophylaxis in adults	Somnolence, fatigue, weight loss, and nervousness	Renal calculi due to inhibition of carbonic anhydrase. Cognitive impairment
	Acetazolamide	Sometimes effective in absence seizures		Usefulness is limited by the rapid development of tolerance
	Felbamate	Withdrawn from the market because of cases of aplastic anemia		
	Zonisamide	Add-on therapy for patients with refractory partial seizures	Somnolence, ataxia, anorexia, nervousness, and fatigue	Renal calculi due to inhibition of carbonic anhydrase. Metabolic acidosis—more frequent and severe in younger patients
	Lacosamide	Add-on therapy for adults with refractory partial seizures		
	Rufinamide	Reduces tonic-clonic seizure frequency in children with Lennox-Gastaut syndrome		
	Vigabatrin	Adjunctive therapy for refractory partial complex seizures in adults. May also be of limited benefit in children with infantile spasms		Progressive and permanent bilateral vision loss. Vigabatrin reserved for use in patients who have failed other therapies

CHAPTER 13

Drug Therapy of Neurodegenerative Diseases

DRUGS INCLUDED IN THIS CHAPTER

- Amantadine (SYMMETREL)
- Apomorphine (APOKYN)
- Baclofen (LIORESAL)
- Carbidopa (LODOSYN)
- Carbidopa/levodopa (SINEMET, ATAMET, others; orally disintegrating tablet, PARCOPA)
- Dantrolene (DANTRIUM)
- Donepezil (ARICEPT)
- Entacapone (COMTAN; fixed combination with carbidopa/levodopa, STAVELO)
- Galantamine (NIVALIN, others)
- Levodopa (L-DOPA, LARODOPA)
- Memantine (NAMENDA)
- Pramipexole (MIRAPEX)
- Rasagiline (AZILECT)
- Riluzole (RILUTEK)
- Rivastigmine (EXELON)
- Ropinirole (REQUIP)
- Selegiline (ELDEPRYL; oral disintegrating tablet, EMSAM; transdermal patch, ZELAPAR)
- Tacrine (COGNEX)—discontinued in the United States
- Tetrabenazine (XENAZINENITOMAN)
- Tizanidine (ZANAFLEX)
- Tolcapone (TASMAR)

This chapter will be most useful after having a basic understanding of the material in Chapter 22, Treatment of Central Nervous System Degenerative Disorders in *Goodman & Gilman's The Pharmacological Basis of Therapeutics*, 12th Edition. In addition to the material presented here, the 12th Edition includes:

- A discussion of the selective vulnerabilities of specific CNS neurons
- A detailed discussion of the roll of genetics and environment in neurodegenerative disorders
- The common cellular mechanisms of neurodegeneration
- A detailed discussion of the neural mechanisms and neuroprotective mechanisms of parkinsonism
- A complete discussion of the genetics of Huntington's disease
- Chemical structures of the drugs used to treat and manage neurodegenerative disorders
- Figure 22-8 *Monosynaptic muscle stretch reflex with descending control via inhibitory interneurons*

LEARNING OBJECTIVES

☑ Understand the pathophysiology of neurodegenerative diseases, including Parkinson's disease (PD), Alzheimer's disease (AD), Huntington's disease (HD), and amyotrophic lateral sclerosis (ALS).

☑ Understand the role of drugs in the treatment and management of the symptoms of neurodegenerative diseases.

☑ Know the mechanisms of action and the adverse effects of drugs that are used to treat and manage neurodegenerative diseases.

MECHANISMS OF ACTION OF DRUGS USED TO TREAT AND MANAGE NEURODENERATIVE DISORDERS

DRUG CLASS	DRUG	MECHANISM OF ACTION
Drugs Used to Treat Parkinson's Disease	Levodopa	Decarboxylated in the brain to dopamine (DA)
	Carbidopa	Peripheral DOPA-decarboxylase inhibitor
	Carbidopa/levodopa combination	Combination prevents decarboxylation of levodopa in the periphery allowing more to be available to enter the brain
	Entacapone	Catechol-*O*-methyltransferase (COMT) inhibitor that blocks the peripheral conversion of levodopa to 3-*O*-methyDOPA
	Tolcapone	Catechol-*O*-methyltransferase (COMT) inhibitor that blocks the peripheral conversion of levodopa to 3-*O*-methyDOPA
	Ropinirole	DA receptor agonist
	Pramipexole	DA receptor agonist
	Selegiline	Selective monoamine oxidase B (MAO-B) inhibitor

(Continued)

Drug Therapy of Neurodegenerative Diseases

CHAPTER 13

DRUG CLASS	DRUG	MECHANISM OF ACTION
	Rasagiline	Selective monoamine oxidase B (MAO-B) inhibitor
	Amantadine	Antiviral agent that alters DA release in the striatum Blocks NMDA glutamate receptors
	Apomorphine	DA receptor agonist
Drugs Used to Treat Alzheimer's Disease	Donepezil	Reversible antagonist of cholinesterase
	Rivastigmine	Reversible antagonist of cholinesterase
	Galantamine	Reversible antagonist of cholinesterase
	Tacrine	Reversible antagonist of cholinesterase
	Memantine	Noncompetitive antagonist of the NMDA-type glutamate receptor
Drugs Used to Treat Huntington's Disease	Tetrabenazine	Inhibits the vesicular monoamine transporter 2 (VMAT2) and causes presynaptic depletion of catecholamines
Drugs Used to Treat ALS	Riluzole	Inhibits presynaptic release of glutamate, blocks postsynaptic NMDA- and kainate-type glutamate receptors, and inhibits voltage-dependent Na^+ channels
	Baclofen	$GABA_B$ receptor agonist muscle relaxant
	Tizanidine	α_2 adrenergic receptor agonist
	Dantrolene	Acts directly on muscle fibers to impair Ca^{2+} release from the sarcoplasmic reticulum

CASE 13-1

A 68-year-old man is diagnosed with Parkinson's disease (PD).

a. What is the pathophysiology of Parkinson's disease?

The dopaminergic deficit in PD arises from a loss of the neurons in the substantia nigra pars compacta that provide innervation to the striatum (caudate and putamen). The current understanding of the pathophysiology of PD is based on the finding that the striatal DA content is reduced in excess of 80%. This paralleled the loss of neurons from the substantia nigra, suggesting that replacement of DA could restore function.

b. How is dopamine synthesized in neurons?

DA, a catecholamine, is synthesized in the terminals of dopaminergic neurons from tyrosine and stored, released, and metabolized by processes described in Chapter 5 and summarized in Figure 13-1. The actions of DA in the brain are mediated by a family of DA receptor proteins. Two types of DA receptors are identified in the mammalian brain using pharmacological techniques: D_1 receptors, which stimulate the synthesis of the intracellular second messenger cyclic AMP; and D_2 receptors, which inhibit cyclic AMP synthesis as well as suppress Ca^{2+} currents and activate receptor-operated K^+ currents.

(Continued)

CARDINAL FEATURES OF PARKINSON DISEASE (PD)

- Bradykinesia (slowness and poverty of movement)
- Muscular rigidity
- Resting tremor (which usually abates during voluntary movement)
- Impairment of postural balance leading to disturbances of gait and falling

SECTION II Neuropharmacology

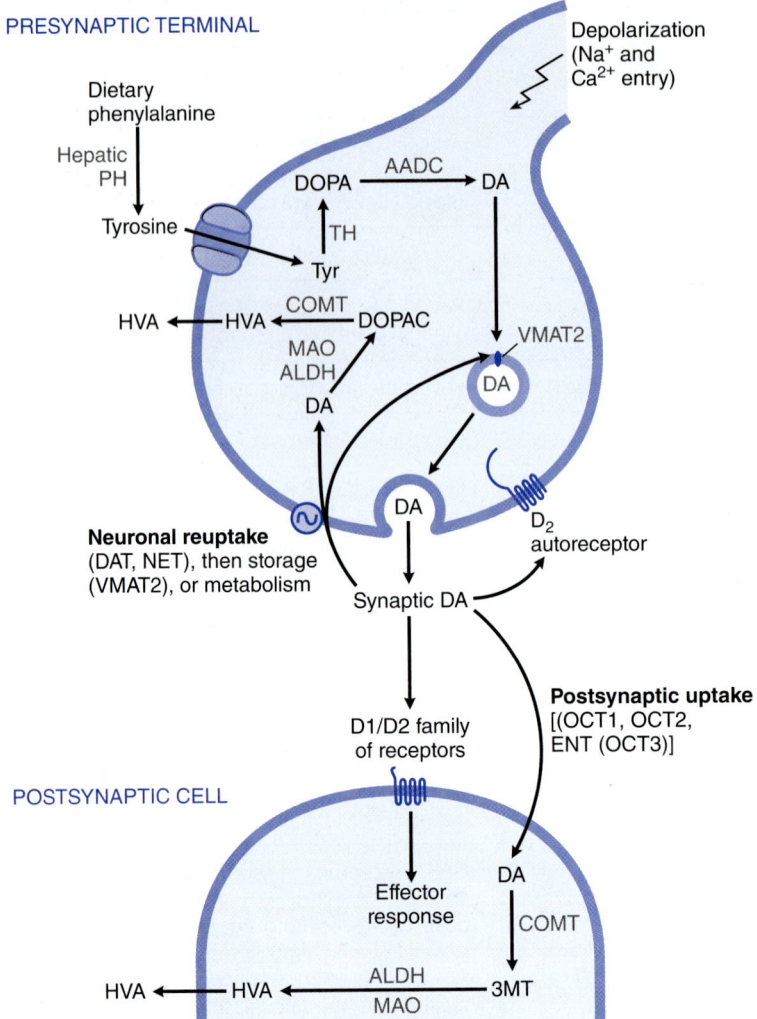

FIGURE 13-1 Dopaminergic nerve terminal. Dopamine (DA) is synthesized from tyrosine in the nerve terminal by the sequential actions of tyrosine hydrolase (TH) and aromatic amino acid decarboxylase (AADC). DA is sequestered by VMAT2 in storage granules and released by exocytosis. Synaptic DA activates presynaptic autoreceptors and postsynaptic D_1 and D_2 receptors. Synaptic DA may be taken up into the neuron via the DA and NE transporters (DAT, NET), or removed by postsynaptic uptake via OCT3 transporters. Cytosolic DA is subject to degradation by monoamine oxidase (MAO) and aldehyde dehydrogenase (ALDH) in the neuron, and by catechol-O-methyltransferase (COMT) and MAO/ALDH in non-neuronal cells; the final metabolic product is homovanillic acid (HVA). See structures in Figure 13-4. PH, phenylalanine hydroxylase.

c. **How is dopamine neurotransmission affected by Parkinson's disease?**

Considerable effort has been devoted to understanding how the loss of dopaminergic input to the neurons of the neostriatum gives rise to the clinical features of PD. The basal ganglia can be viewed as a modulatory side loop that regulates the flow of information from the cerebral cortex to the motor neurons of the spinal cord (see Figure 13-2). The neostriatum is the principal input structure of the basal ganglia and receives excitatory glutamatergic input from many areas of the cortex. Most neurons within the striatum are projection neurons that innervate other basal ganglia structures. A small but important subgroup of striatal neurons consists of interneurons that connect neurons within the striatum but do not project beyond its borders. Acetylcholine (ACh) and neuropeptides are used as transmitters by these striatal interneurons.

(Continued)

Drug Therapy of Neurodegenerative Diseases

CHAPTER 13

The key feature of this model of basal ganglia function, which accounts for the symptoms observed in PD as a result of loss of dopaminergic neurons, is the differential effect of DA on the direct and indirect pathways (see Figure 13-3). The dopaminergic neurons of the substantia nigra pars compacta (SNpc) innervate all parts of the striatum; however, the target striatal neurons express distinct types of DA receptors. The striatal neurons giving rise to the direct pathway express primarily the excitatory D_1 dopamine receptor protein, whereas the striatal neurons forming the indirect pathway express primarily the inhibitory D_2 type. Thus, DA released in the striatum tends to increase the activity of the direct pathway and reduce the activity of the indirect pathway, whereas the depletion that occurs in PD has the opposite effect. The net effect of the reduced dopaminergic input in PD is to increase markedly the inhibitory outflow from the SNpc and globus pallidus interna (GPi) to the thalamus and reduce excitation of the motor cortex.

d. What is the prognosis for this patient?

Progressive loss of dopamine (DA)-containing neurons is a feature of normal aging; however, most people do not lose the 70 to 80% of dopaminergic neurons required to cause symptomatic PD. Without treatment, PD progresses over 5 to 10 years to a rigid, akinetic state in which patients are incapable of caring for themselves. Death frequently results from complications of immobility, including aspiration pneumonia or pulmonary embolism. The availability of effective pharmacological treatment has radically altered the prognosis of PD; in most cases, good functional mobility can be maintained for many years. Life expectancy of adequately treated patients is increased substantially, but overall mortality remains higher than that of the general population. Commonly used medications for the treatment of PD are summarized in Table 13-1.

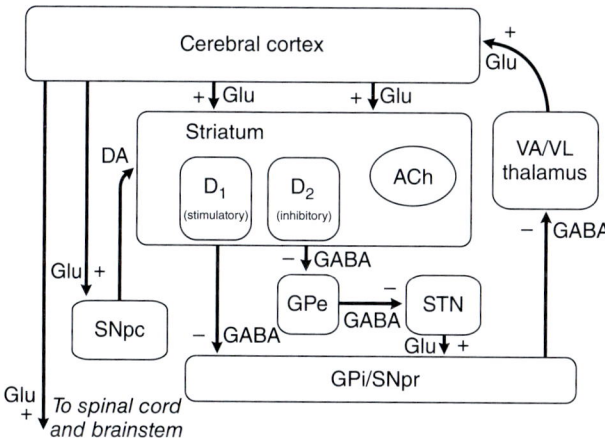

FIGURE 13-2 Schematic wiring diagram of the basal ganglia. The striatum is the principal input structure of the basal ganglia and receives excitatory glutamatergic input from many areas of cerebral cortex. The striatum contains projection neurons expressing predominantly D_1 or D_2 dopamine receptors, as well as interneurons that use acetylcholine (ACh) as a neurotransmitter. Outflow from the striatum proceeds along two routes. The direct pathway, from the striatum to the substantianigra pars reticulata (SNpr) and globus pallidus interna (GPi), uses the inhibitory transmitter GABA. The indirect pathway, from the striatum through the globus pallidus externa (GPe) and the subthalamic nucleus (STN) to the SNpr and GPi consists of two inhibitory GABAergic links and one excitatory glutamatergic projection (Glu). The substantia nigra pars compacta (SNpc) provides dopaminergic innervation to the striatal neurons, giving rise to both the direct and indirect pathways, and regulates the relative activity of these two paths. The SNpr and GPi are the output structures of the basal ganglia and provide feedback to the cerebral cortex through the ventroanterior and ventrolateralnuclei of the thalamus (VA/VL).

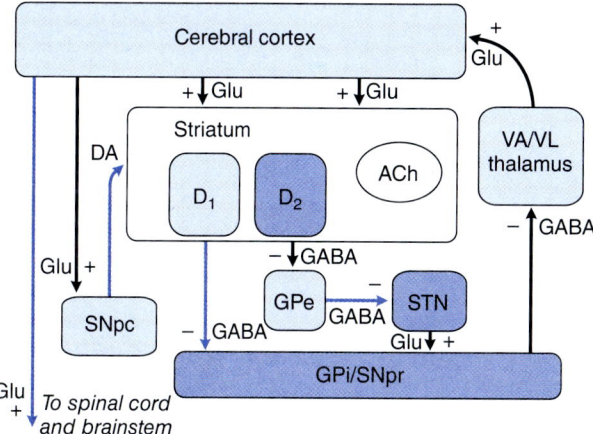

FIGURE 13-3 The basal ganglia in Parkinson's disease. The primary defect is destruction of the dopaminergic neurons of the SNpc. The striatal neurons that form the direct pathway from the striatum to the SNpr and GPi express primarily the *excitatory* D_1 dopamine receptor, whereas the striatal neurons that project to the GPe and form the indirect pathway express the *inhibitory* D_2 dopamine receptor. Thus, loss of the dopaminergic input to the striatum has a differential effect on the two outflow pathways; the direct pathway to the SNpr and GPi is less active (*structures in light blue*), whereas the activity in the indirect pathway is increased (*structures in dark blue*). The net effect is that neurons in the SNpr and GPi become more active. This leads to increased inhibition of the VA/VL thalamus and reduced excitatory input to the cortex. (See legend to Figure 13–2 for definitions of anatomical abbreviations.)

SECTION II — Neuropharmacology

CASE 13-2

The patient in Case 13-1 is early in the course of his Parkinson's disease

a. What are the treatment options at this stage of his disease?

Commonly used medications for the treatment of PD are summarized in Table 13-1. Pharmacological treatment of PD should be tailored to the individual patient. Drug therapy is not obligatory in early PD; many patients can be managed for a time with exercise and lifestyle interventions. For patients with mild symptoms, MAO-B inhibitors, amantadine, or (in younger patients) anticholinergics are reasonable choices. In most patients, treatment with a dopaminergic drug, either levodopa

(Continued)

TABLE 13-1 Commonly Used Medications for the Treatment of Parkinson's Disease

AGENT	TYPICAL INITIAL DOSE	DAILY DOSE RANGE	COMMENTS
Levodopa Formulations			
Carbidopa/levodopa	25 mg carbidopa + 100 mg levodopa ("25/100" tablet), 2-3x daily	200-1200 mg levodopa	
Carbidopa/levodopa sustained-release	50 mg carbidopa + 200 mg levodopa ("50/200 sustained-release" tablet) 2x daily	200-1200 mg levodopa	Bioavailability 75% of immediate-release form
Carbidopa-levodopa orally disintegrating tablets (PARCOPA)	25 mg carbidopa + 100 mg levodopa ("25/100" tablet), 2-3x daily	200-1200 mg levodopa	
COMT Inhibitors			
Entacapone	200 mg with each dose of levodopa/carbidopa	600-2000 mg	
Tolcapone	100 mg with carbidopa/levodopa	100-300 mg	May be hepatotoxic. Use only in patients not responding satisfactorily to other treatments. Requires monitoring of liver function
Carbidopa/levodopa/entacapone	12.5 mg carbidopa + 50 levodopa + 200 mg entacapone (STALEVO 50), 3x daily	150-1200 mg levodopa	
DA Agonists			
Apomorphine	2 mg subcutaneous	6-18 mg subcutaneous	Trimethobenzamide or other antiemetic is used to reduce nausea when initiating therapy
Bromocriptine	1.25 mg	2.5-15 mg daily	Ergot; long-term use is associated with cardiac valve fibrosis
Pramipexole	0.125 mg 3x daily	1.5-4.5 mg	
Ropinirole	0.25 mg 3x daily	1.5-24 mg	
Ropinirole sustained-release	2 mg per day	2-24 mg	
MAO Inhibitors			
Rasagiline	1 mg daily	0.5-1 mg	
Selegiline	5 mg 2x daily	2.5-10 mg	
Other Medications			
Trihexyphenidyl HCl	1 mg 2x daily	2-15 mg	
Amantadine	100 mg 2x daily	100-200 mg	

or a DA agonist, is eventually required. Large controlled clinical trials provide convincing evidence for a reduced rate of motor fluctuation in patients in which DA agonists are used as initial treatment. This benefit was, however, accompanied by an increased rate of adverse effects, especially somnolence and hallucinations. Practitioners prefer a DA agonist as initial therapy in younger patients in order to reduce the occurrence of motor complications. In older patients or those with substantial comorbidity, levodopa/carbidopa is generally better tolerated.

CASE 13-3

As this (the patient from Case 13-1) patient's disease progresses, it is recommended that he be treated with levodopa.

a. What is levodopa, and how is it used in the treatment of Parkinson's disease?

Levodopa, the metabolic precursor of DA, is the single most effective agent in the treatment of PD. Levodopa is itself largely inert; both its therapeutic and adverse effects result from the decarboxylation of levodopa to DA. The metabolism of levodopa is shown in Figure 13-4.

Entry of levodopa into the CNS across the blood-brain barrier is mediated by a membrane transporter for aromatic amino acids, and competition between dietary protein and levodopa may occur at this level. In the brain, levodopa is converted to DA by decarboxylation primarily within the presynaptic terminals of dopaminergic neurons in the stratium (see Figure 13-5). The DA produced in the presynaptic terminals is responsible for the therapeutic effectiveness of levodopa in PD; after release, it is either transported back into dopaminergic terminals by the presynaptic uptake mechanism or metabolized by the actions of MAO and catechol-O-methyl-transferase (COMT) (see Figure 13-4).

b. What other drugs should be administered with levodopa?

In clinical practice, levodopa is almost always administered in combination with a peripherally acting inhibitor of aromatic L-amino acid decarboxylase, such as carbidopa or benserazide (available outside the United States), drugs that do not penetrate well into the CNS. If levodopa is administered alone, the drug is largely decarboxylated by enzymes in the intestinal mucosa and other peripheral sites so that relatively little unchanged drug reaches the cerebral circulation and probably

(Continued)

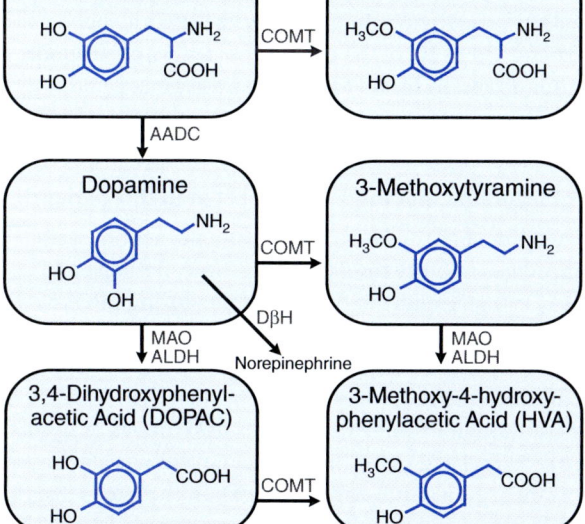

FIGURE 13-4 Metabolism of levodopa (L-DOPA). ALDH, aldehyde dehydrogenase; COMT, catechol-O-methyltransferase; DβH, dopamine β-hydroxylase; AADC, aromatic L-amino acid decarboxylase; MAO, monoamine oxidase.

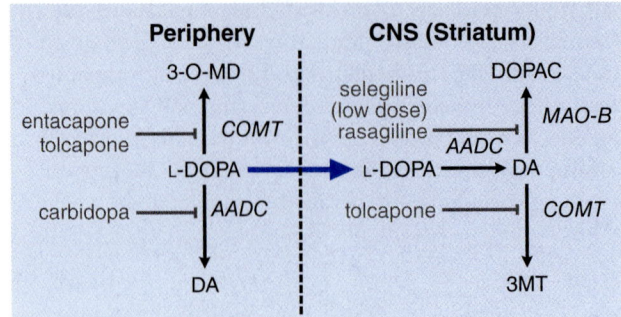

FIGURE 13-5 Pharmacological preservation of L-DOPA and striatal dopamine. The principal site of action of inhibitors of catechol-*O*-methyltransferase (COMT) (such as tolcapone and entacapone) is in the peripheral circulation. They block the *O*-methylation of levodopa (L-DOPA) and increase the fraction of the drug available for delivery to the brain. Tolcapone also has effects in the CNS. Inhibitors of MAO-B, such as low-dose selegiline and rasagiline, will act within the CNS to reduce oxidative deamination of DA, thereby enhancing vesicular stores. AADC, aromatic L-amino acid decarboxylase; DA, dopamine; DOPAC, 3,4-dihydroxyphenylacetic acid; MAO, monoamine oxidase; 3MT, 3-methoxyltyramine; 3-O-MD, 3-O-methyl DOPA.

less than 1% penetrates the CNS. In addition, DA release into the circulation by peripheral conversion of levodopa produces undesirable effects, particularly nausea. Inhibition of peripheral decarboxylase, with carbidopa, markedly increases the fraction of administered levodopa that remains unmetabolized and available to cross the blood-brain barrier (see Figure 13-5) and reduces the incidence of GI side effects.

Drugs for the treatment of PD include inhibitors of the enzyme COMT, which, together with MAO, metabolizes levodopa and DA. COMT transfers a methyl group from the donor *S*-adenosyl-L-methionine, producing the pharmacologically inactive compounds 3-*O*-methyl DOPA (from levodopa) and 3-methoxytyramine (from DA; see Figure 13-4). The principal therapeutic action of the COMT inhibitors is to block this peripheral conversion of levodopa to 3-*O*-methyl DOPA, increasing both the plasma $t_{1/2}$ of levodopa as well as the fraction of each dose that reaches the CNS.

Two COMT inhibitors presently are available for this use in the United States, tolcapone and entacapone. The action of entacapone is attributable principally to peripheral inhibition of COMT. The common adverse effects of these agents are similar to those of levodopa/carbidopa alone and include nausea, orthostatic hypotension, vivid dreams, confusion, and hallucinations. An important adverse effect associated with tolcapone is hepatotoxicity. Up to 2% of the patients treated with tolcapone have increased serum alanine aminotransferase and aspartate transaminase; and at least 3 fatal cases of fulminant hepatic failure in patients taking tolcapone have been observed, leading to the addition of a black box warning to the label.

c. **What are the adverse effects of levodopa that might be expected in this patient?**

A common problem is the development of the "wearing off" phenomenon: each dose of levodopa effectively improves mobility for a period of time, perhaps 1 to 2 hours, but rigidity and akinesia return rapidly at the end of the dosing interval. Increasing the dose and frequency of administration can improve this situation, but this often is limited by the development of dyskinesias, excessive and abnormal involuntary movements. Dyskinesias are observed most often when the plasma levodopa concentration is high, although in some individuals dyskinesias or dystonia may be triggered when the level is rising or falling. These movements can be as uncomfortable and disabling as the rigidity and akinesia of PD. In the later stages of PD, patients may fluctuate rapidly between being "off," having no beneficial effects from their medications, and being "on" but with disabling dyskinesias, a situation called the on/off phenomenon.

(Continued)

Drug Therapy of Neurodegenerative Diseases

CHAPTER 13

In addition to motor complications and nausea, several other adverse effects may be observed with levodopa treatment. A frequent and troubling adverse effect is the induction of hallucinations and confusion, especially in elderly patients or in patients with preexisting cognitive dysfunction. This adverse effect often limits the ability to treat parkinsonian symptoms adequately.

Peripheral decarboxylation of levodopa and release of DA into the circulation may activate vascular DA receptors and produce orthostatic hypotension. Administration of levodopa with nonspecific inhibitors of MAO, such as phenelzine and tranylcypromine, markedly accentuate the actions of levodopa and may precipitate life-threatening hypertensive crisis and hyperpyrexia; nonspecific MAO inhibitors should always be discontinued at least 14 days before levodopa is administered (note that this prohibition does not include the MAO-B subtype-specific inhibitors selegiline and rasagiline, which are often administered safely in combination with levodopa). Abrupt withdrawal of levodopa or other dopaminergic medications may precipitate the neuroleptic malignant syndrome of confusion, rigidity, and hyperthermia, a potentially lethal adverse effect.

d. What other drugs can be used for the treatment of PD?

An alternative to levodopa is the use of drugs that are direct agonists of striatal DA receptors, an approach that offers several potential advantages. Since enzymatic conversion of these drugs is not required for their activity, they do not depend on the functional capacities of the nigrostriatal neurons. The direct DA receptor agonists in clinical use have durations of action substantially longer than that of levodopa; they are often used in the management of dose-related fluctuations in motor state, and may be helpful in preventing motor complications. Finally, it has been suggested that DA receptor agonists may have the potential to modify the course of PD by reducing endogenous release of DA as well as the need for exogenous levodopa, thereby reducing free radical formation.

Two orally administered DA receptor agonists commonly used for treatment of PD are ropinirole and pramipexole.

Two isoenzymes of MAO oxidize monoamines. While both isoenzymes (MAO-A and MAO-B) are present in the periphery and inactivate monoamines of intestinal origin, the isoenzyme MAO-B is the predominant form in the striatum and is responsible for most of the oxidative metabolism of DA in the brain. Two selective MAO-B inhibitors are used for the treatment of PD: selegiline and rasagiline. Both agents exert modest beneficial effects on the symptoms of PD.

Selegiline has been used for many years as a symptomatic treatment for PD and is generally well tolerated in younger patients with early or mild PD. In patients with more advanced PD or underlying cognitive impairment, selegiline may accentuate the adverse motor and cognitive effects of levodopa therapy. Metabolites of selegiline include amphetamine and methamphetamine, which may cause anxiety, insomnia, and other adverse symptoms.

Unlike selegiline, rasagiline does not give rise to undesirable amphetamine metabolites. In randomized controlled clinical trials, rasagiline monotherapy was effective in early PD.

Amantadine, an antiviral agent used for the prophylaxis and treatment of influenza A (see Chapter 44), has antiparkinsonian activity. Amantadine appears to alter DA release in the striatum, has anticholinergic properties, and blocks NMDA glutamate receptors.

CASE 13-4

A 72-year-old woman is diagnosed with Alzheimer's disease (AD).

a. What is the pathophysiology of AD?

The pathological hallmarks of AD are amyloid plaques, which are extracellular accumulations of amyloid-β peptides (Aβ), and intracellular neurofibrillary tangles

(Continued)

SECTION II

Neuropharmacology

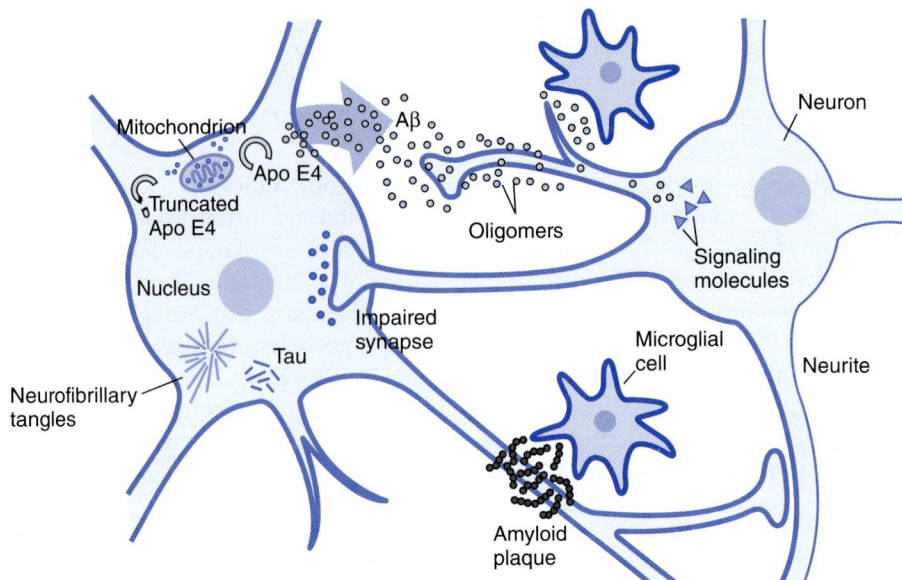

FIGURE 13-6 Molecular and cellular processes presumed to participate in AD pathogenesis. *(From Roberson ED, Mucke L. 100 years and counting: Prospects for defeating Alzheimer's disease.* Science, *2006, 314:781–784. Reprinted with permission from AAAS.)*

composed of the microtubule-associated protein tau (see Figure 13-6). While the development of amyloid plaques is an early and invariant feature of AD, tangle burden accrues over time in a manner that correlates more closely with the development of cognitive impairment. The current consensus is that Aβ accumulation is an upstream event that triggers tau pathology, resulting in impaired neuronal function and cell loss.

The most striking neurochemical disturbance in AD is a deficiency of acetylcholine (ACh). The anatomical basis of the cholinergic deficit is atrophy and degeneration of subcortical cholinergic neurons, particularly those in the basal forebrain (nucleus basalis of Meynert) that provide cholinergic innervation to the cerebral cortex. The selective deficiency of ACh in AD, as well as the observation that central cholinergic antagonists such as atropine can induce a confusional state that bears some resemblance to the dementia of AD, has given rise to the "cholinergic hypothesis," which proposes that a deficiency of ACh is critical in the genesis of the AD symptoms. Although viewing AD as a "cholinergic deficiency syndrome" akin to the "dopaminergic deficiency syndrome" of PD provides a useful framework, it is important to note that the deficit in AD is far more complex. AD involves multiple neurotransmitter systems, including glutamate, 5-HT, and neuropeptides, and there is destruction of not only cholinergic neurons but also the cortical and hippocampal targets that receive cholinergic input.

b. What treatment is available for the cognitive symptoms of AD?

Augmentation of the cholinergic transmission is currently the mainstay of AD treatment. Three drugs—donepezil, rivastigmine, and galantamine—are widely used for this purpose; a fourth drug, tacrine, was the first drug approved to treat AD but is rarely used now because it has much more extensive side effects compared to the newer agents (see Table 13-2).

All 4 agents are reversible antagonists of cholinesterases, enzymes that act to limit cholinergic neurotransmission by catalyzing the cleavage of acetylcholine in the synaptic cleft into choline and acetate (see Chapter 6).

Memantine is used either as an adjunct or as an alternative to cholinesterase inhibitors in AD and is also commonly used to treat other neurodegenerative dementias. Memantine is a noncompetitive antagonist of the NMDA-type glutamate receptor.

(Continued)

Drug Therapy of Neurodegenerative Diseases — CHAPTER 13

TABLE 13-2 Cholinesterase Inhibitors Used for the Treatment of Alzheimer's Disease

	DONEPEZIL	**RIVASTIGMINE**	**GALANTAMINE**	**TACRINE**[a]
Brand name	ARICEPT	EXELON, generic	RAZADYNE, generic	COGNEX
Enzymes inhibited[b]	AChE	AChE, BuChE	AChE	AChE, BuChE
Mechanism	Noncompetitive	Noncompetitive	Competitive	Noncompetitiv
Typical maintenance dose[c]	10 mg once daily	9.5 mg/24h (transdermal) 3-6 mg twice daily (oral)	8-12 mg twice daily (immediate-release) 16-24 mg/day (extended-release)	20 mg, four times daily
FDA-approved indications	Mild–severe AD	Mild–moderate AD, Mild–moderate PDD[d]	Mild–moderate AD	Mild–moderate AD
Metabolism[e]	CYP2D6, CYP3A4	Esterases	CYP2D6, CYP3A4	CYP1A2

[a] Tacrine was the first cholinesterase inhibitor approved for the treatment of AD, but is now rarely used because of hepatotoxicity and adverse effects.
[b] AChE (acetylcholinesterase) is the major cholinesterase in the brain; BuChE (butyrylcholinesterase) is a serum and hepatic cholinesterase that is upregulated in AD brain.
[c] Typical starting doses are one-half of the maintenance dose and are given for the first month of therapy.
[d] PDD, Parkinson's disease dementia.
[e] Drugs metabolized by CYP2D6 and CYP3A4 are subject to increased serum levels when co-administered with drugs known to inhibit these enzymes, such as ketoconazole and paroxetine. Similarly, tacrine levels are increased by co-administration with the CYP1A2 inhibitors theophylline, cimetidine, and fluvoxamine.

It interacts with the Mg^{2+} binding site of the channel to prevent excessive activation while sparing normal function. Memantine significantly reduces the rate of clinical deterioration in patients with moderate to severe AD.

c. What treatment is available for the behavioral symptoms of AD?

In addition to cognitive decline, behavioral and psychiatric symptoms in dementia (BPSD) are common, particularly in middle stages of the disease. These symptoms, including irritability and agitation, paranoia and delusional thinking, wandering, anxiety, and depression, are a major source of caregiver distress and often precipitate nursing home placement.

Atypical antipsychotics, such as respiridone, olanzepine, and quetiapin (see Chapter 8), are the most efficacious therapy for agitation and psychosis in AD. Risperidone and olanzapine are effective, but their use is often limited by adverse effects, including parkinsonism, sedation, and falls. In addition, the use of atypical antipsychotics in elderly patients with dementia-related psychosis has been associated with a higher risk of stroke and overall mortality, leading the FDA to order inclusion of a boxed warning in the prescribing information for all drugs in this class. Unfortunately, there are few effective alternatives.

Antidepressants (see Chapter 8) can be useful for BPSD, particularly when depression or anxiety contribute. Because of the adverse anticholinergic effects of tricyclic agents, serotonergic antidepressants are favored. These agents are generally well tolerated. Trazodone has modest benefits, but for the most part, selective serotonin reuptake inhibitors (SSRIs) are the preferred class of drugs.

The typical AD patient presenting in early stages of disease should probably be treated with a cholinesterase inhibitor. Patients and families should be counseled that a realistic goal of therapy is to induce a temporary reprieve from progression, or at least a reduction in the rate of decline, rather than long-term recovery of cognition. As the disease progresses, memantine can be added to the regimen. Behavioral symptoms are often treated with a serotonergic antidepressant or, if they are severe enough to warrant the risk of higher mortality, an atypical antipsychotic. Eliminating drugs likely to aggravate cognitive impairments, particularly

(Continued)

anticholinergics, benzodiazepines, and other sedative/hypnotics, from the patient's regimen is another important aspect of AD pharmacotherapy.

CASE 13-5

A 39-year-old man is diagnosed with Huntington's disease (HD).

a. What is the pathophysiology of Huntington's disease?

HD is characterized by prominent neuronal loss in the striatum (caudate/putamen) of the brain. Atrophy of these structures proceeds in an orderly fashion, first affecting the tail of the caudate nucleus and then proceeding anteriorly from mediodorsal to ventrolateral.

Selective vulnerability also appears to underlie the most conspicuous clinical feature of HD, the development of chorea. In most adult-onset cases, the medium spiny neurons that project to the GPi and SNpr (the indirect pathway) appear to be affected earlier than those projecting to the globus pallidus externa (GPe; the direct pathway; see Figure 13-5). The disproportionate impairment of the indirect pathway increases excitatory drive to the neocortex, producing involuntary choreiform movements (see Figure 13-7).

b. What drugs are available for the treatment of patients with Huntington disease?

Treatment for symptomatic HD emphasizes the selective use of medications. None of the currently available medications slows the progression of the disease.

Treatment is needed for patients who are depressed, irritable, paranoid, excessively anxious, or psychotic. Depression can be treated effectively with standard antidepressant drugs with the caveat that drugs with substantial anticholinergic profiles can exacerbate chorea. Fluoxetine (see Chapter 8) is effective treatment for both the depression and the irritability manifest in symptomatic HD. Carbamazepine (see Chapter 12) also has been found to be effective for depression. Paranoia, delusional states, and psychosis are treated with antipsychotic drugs, but usually at lower doses than those used in primary psychiatric disorders (see Chapter 8). These agents also reduce cognitive function and impair mobility and thus should be used in the lowest doses possible and should be discontinued when the psychiatric symptoms resolve.

(Continued)

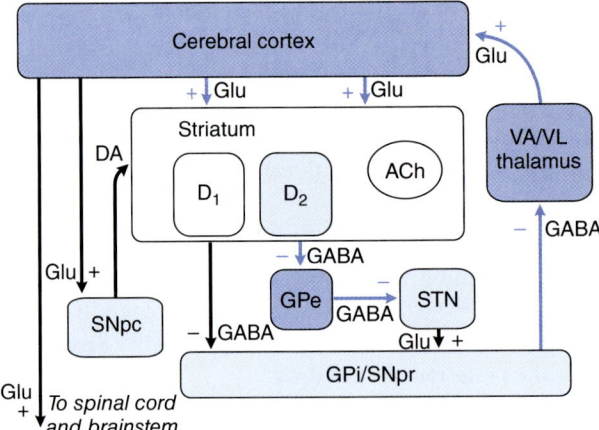

FIGURE 13-7 The basal ganglia in Huntington's disease. HD is characterized by loss of neurons from the striatum. The neurons that project from the striatum to the GPe and form the indirect pathway are affected earlier in the course of the disease than those which project to the GPi. This leads to a loss of inhibition of the GPe. The increased activity in this structure, in turn, inhibits the STN, SNpr, and GPi, resulting in a loss of inhibition to the VA/VL thalamus and increased thalamocortical excitatorydrive. Structures in light blue have reduced activity in HD, whereas structures in dark blue have increased activity. (See legend to Figure 13-2 for definitions of anatomical abbreviations.)

Drug Therapy of Neurodegenerative Diseases

CHAPTER 13

The movement disorder of HD per se only rarely justifies pharmacological therapy. For those with large-amplitude chorea causing frequent falls and injury, tetrabenazine has recently become available in the United States for the treatment of chorea associated with HD. Tetrabenazine and the related drug reserpine are inhibitors of the vesicular monoamine transporter 2 (VMAT2) and cause presynaptic depletion of catecholamines.

CASE 13-6

A 53-year-old man is diagnosed with amyotrophic lateral sclerosis (ALS).

a. What is ALS?

ALS (or Lou Gehrig disease) is a disorder of the motor neurons of the ventral horn of the spinal cord (lower motor neurons) and the cortical neurons that provide their afferent input (upper motor neurons). The disorder is characterized by rapidly progressive weakness, muscle atrophy and fasciculations, spasticity, dysarthria, dysphagia, and respiratory compromise. Sensory, autonomic, and oculomotor function is generally spared.

The pathology of ALS corresponds closely to the clinical features: There is prominent loss of the spinal and brainstem motor neurons that project to striated muscles (although the oculomotor neurons are spared), as well as loss of the large pyramidal motor neurons in layer V of the motor cortex, which are the origin of the descending corticospinal tracts.

ALS usually is progressive and fatal. Most patients die of respiratory compromise and pneumonia after 2 to 3 years, although some individuals have a more indolent course and survive for many years.

b. What treatment options are available for patients with ALS?

Riluzole is an agent with complex actions in the nervous system. It inhibits glutamate release, but it also blocks postsynaptic NMDA- and kainate-type glutamate receptors and inhibits voltage-dependent Na$^+$ channels.

In clinical trials riluzole has modest but genuine effects on the survival of patients with ALS. Meta-analyses of the available trials indicate that riluzole extends survival by 2 to 3 months.

Spasticity is an important component of the clinical features of ALS and the feature most amenable to present forms of treatment. Spasticity often leads to considerable pain and discomfort and further reduces mobility, which already is compromised by weakness. Spasticity is defined as an increase in muscle tone characterized by an initial resistance to passive displacement of a limb at a joint, followed by a sudden relaxation (the so-called clasped-knife phenomenon).

The best agent for the symptomatic treatment of spasticity in ALS is baclofen, a GABA$_B$ receptor agonist.

Tizanidine is an agonist of α_2 adrenergic receptors in the CNS. It reduces muscle spasticity and is assumed to act by increasing presynaptic inhibition of motor neurons.

Benzodiazepines (see Chapter 9) such as clonazepam are effective antispasticity agents, but they are sedating and may contribute to respiratory depression in patients with advanced ALS.

Dantrolene also is approved in the United States for the treatment of muscle spasm. In contrast to the other agents discussed, dantrolene acts directly on skeletal muscle fibers, impairing Ca^{2+} release from the sarcoplasmic reticulum. Because it can exacerbate muscular weakness, it is not used in ALS but is effective in treating spasticity associated with stroke or spinal cord injury and in treating malignant hyperthermia.

SECTION II — Neuropharmacology

KEY CONCEPTS

- Neurodegenerative disorders are characterized by progressive and irreversible loss of neurons from specific regions of the brain.
- Currently available therapies for neurodegenerative disorders alleviate the disease symptoms but do not alter the underlying neurodegenerative processes.
- The dopaminergic deficit in Parkinson's disease arises from a loss of the neurons in the substantia nigra pars compacta that provide innervation to the striatum.
- Drug therapy is not obligatory in early Parkinson's disease; pharmacological treatment of Parkinson's disease should be tailored to the individual patient.
- A realistic goal for the treatment of a patient with Alzheimer's disease is to induce a temporary reprieve from progression, or at least a reduction in the rate of decline, rather than long-term recovery of cognition.
- Huntington's disease is a dominantly inherited disorder characterized by prominent neuronal loss in the striatum of the brain and by the gradual onset of motor incoordination and cognitive decline in midlife.
- At present there is no effective treatment for Huntington's disease; therapy is aimed toward control of the motor and behavioral features of the disorder.
- Amyotrophic lateral sclerosis is a progressive degenerative disease of spinal motor neurons leading to weakness and eventually paralysis.
- The drug riluzole is the only treatment established to alter the course of amyotrophic lateral sclerosis; its effect is modest, prolonging survival by only a few months.

SUMMARY QUIZ

QUESTION 13-1 A 72-year-old man with Parkinson's disease is being treated with selegiline. Over the past 2 weeks he has noticed an increase in insomnia and anxiety. It is likely these symptoms are due to

a. dopamine.
b. ephedrine.
c. amphetamine.
d. serotonin.
e. caffeine.

QUESTION 13-2 A 75-year-old woman with Parkinson's disease is being treated with the combination of levodopa/carbidopa. Entacapone is added. This patient is treated with this combination of drugs to increase the amount of which of the following substance to reach the CNS?

a. Carbidopa
b. Levodopa
c. Entacapone
d. Acetylcholine
e. Dopamine

QUESTION 13-3 A 66-year-old woman with Alzheimer's disease is being treated with the cholinesterase inhibitor donepezil. The patient's family learns that donepezil is related to pesticides. When the family expresses concern they are told that donepezil may decrease the rate of cognition decline by increasing the concentration of which substance in the brain?

a. Acetylcholine
b. Serotonin

(Continued)

c. Dopamine
d. Epinephrine
e. Glutamate

QUESTION 13-4 A 73-year-old man with Alzheimer's disease is being treated with donepezil. Because his cognition is deteriorating, memantine is added. Memantine is a noncompetitive antagonist of the

a. dopamine D_2 receptor.
b. NMDA-type glutamate receptor.
c. β adrenergic receptor.
d. α adrenergic receptor.
e. $5-HT_2$ serotonergic receptor.

QUESTION 13-5 A 57-year-old man with amyotrophic lateral sclerosis is treated with riluzole. The patient's family is told that the drug may extend survival by

a. 2 to 3 days.
b. 2 to 3 months.
c. 2 to 3 years.
d. an indefinite period of time.
e. none of the above; because it is not thought to extend survival.

QUESTION 13-6 A 65-year-old man with Parkinson's disease is treated with pramipexole. This drug acts as an agonist at striatal

a. 5-HT serotonergic receptors.
b. D_1 dopaminergic receptors.
c. norepinephrine adrenergic receptors.
d. D_2 dopaminergic receptors.
e. opiate μ receptors.

SUMMARY QUIZ ANSWER KEY

QUESTION 13-1 Answer is **c.** Metabolites of selegiline include amphetamine and methamphetamine, which may cause anxiety, insomnia, and other adverse symptoms. Unlike selegiline, rasagiline does not give rise to undesirable amphetamine metabolites.

QUESTION 13-2 Answer is **b.** Drugs for the treatment of PD include inhibitors of the enzyme COMT, which, together with MAO, metabolize levodopa and DA. COMT transfers a methyl group from the donor S-adenosyl-L-methionine, producing the pharmacologically inactive compounds 3-O-methyl DOPA (from levodopa) and 3-methoxytyramine (from DA; see Figure 13-5). When levodopa is administered orally, nearly 99% of the drug is metabolized in the periphery and does not reach the brain. Most is converted by aromatic L-amino acid decarboxylase (AADC) to DA, which causes nausea and hypotension. Addition of an AADC inhibitor such as carbidopa reduces the peripheral formation of DA but increases the fraction of levodopa that is methylated by COMT. The principal therapeutic action of the COMT inhibitor entacapone is to block this peripheral conversion of levodopa to 3-O-methyl DOPA, increasing both the plasma $t_{1/2}$ of levodopa as well as the fraction of levodopa that reaches the CNS.

QUESTION 13-3 Answer is **a.** The most striking neurochemical disturbance in AD is a deficiency of acetylcholine. The anatomical basis of the cholinergic deficit is atrophy and degeneration of subcortical cholinergic neurons, particularly those in the basal forebrain (nucleus basalis of Meynert) that provides cholinergic innervation to the cerebral cortex.

(Continued)

SECTION II Neuropharmacology

Donepezil is a reversible antagonist of cholinesterases, enzymes that act to limit cholinergic neurotransmission by catalyzing the cleavage of acetylcholine in the synaptic cleft into choline and acetate (see Chapter 6). Cholinesterase inhibitors are the usual first-line therapy for symptomatic treatment of cognitive impairments in mild or moderate AD. Augmentation of the cholinergic transmission is currently the mainstay of AD treatment.

QUESTION 13-4 Answer is **b.** Memantine is used either as an adjunct or an alternative to cholinesterase inhibitors in AD, and is also commonly used to treat other neurodegenerative dementias. Memantine is a noncompetitive antagonist of the NMDA-type glutamate receptor. It interacts with the Mg^{2+}-binding site of the channel to prevent excessive activation while sparing normal function.

QUESTION 13-5 Answer is **b.** Riluzole is an agent with complex actions in the nervous system. It inhibits glutamate release, but it also blocks postsynaptic NMDA- and kainate-type glutamate receptors and inhibits voltage-dependent Na^+ channels. In clinical trials riluzole has modest but genuine effects on the survival of patients with ALS. Meta-analyses of the available trials indicate that riluzole extends survival by 2 to 3 months.

QUESTION 13-6 Answer is **d.** Two orally administered DA receptor agonists are commonly used for treatment of PD: ropinirole and pramipexole. Ropinirole and pramipexole have selective agonist activity at D_2 class sites (specifically at the D_2 and D_3 receptor) and little or no activity at D_1 class sites.

SUMMARY TABLE: DRUGS USED TO TREAT NEURODENERATIVE DISORDERS

CLASS AND SUBCLASSES	NAMES	CLINICAL USES	TOXICITIES COMMON	TOXICITIES UNIQUE: CLINICALLY IMPORTANT
Drugs Used to Treat Parkinson's Disease	Levodopa	Treatment of Parkinson's disease	Nausea	Hallucinations and confusion Orthostatic hypotension Contraindicated with nonspecific inhibitors of MAO Abrupt withdrawal may precipitate neuroleptic malignant syndrome
	Carbidopa/levodopa combination	Treatment of Parkinson's disease	Nausea	Hallucinations and confusion Orthostatic hypotension Contraindicated with nonspecific inhibitors of MAO Abrupt withdrawal may precipitate neuroleptic malignant syndrome
	Entacapone	Combined with levodopa/carbidopa to treat Parkinson's disease	Nausea	Vivid dreams, confusion, orthostatic hypotension
	Tolcapone	Combined with levodopa/carbidopa to treat Parkinson's disease	Nausea	Associated with hepatotoxicity Vivid dreams, confusion, orthostatic hypotension
	Ropinirole	Treatment of Parkinson's disease	Nausea Fatigue and somnolence	Hallucinations and confusion
	Pramipexole	Treatment of Parkinson's disease	Nausea Fatigue and somnolence	Hallucinations and confusion

Drug Therapy of Neurodegenerative Diseases — CHAPTER 13

CLASS AND SUBCLASSES	NAMES	CLINICAL USES	TOXICITIES COMMON	TOXICITIES UNIQUE: CLINICALLY IMPORTANT
	Selegiline	Selective inhibitor of MAO-B used to treat Parkinson's disease	Anxiety and insomnia due to its amphetamine and meth-amphetamine metabolites	May exacerbate the adverse motor and cognitive effects of levodopa. Contraindicated for use with meperidine. Used with caution in patients taking SSRIs
	Rasagiline	Selective inhibitor of MAO-B used to treat Parkinson's disease		May exacerbate the adverse motor and cognitive effects of levodopa. Contraindicated for use with meperidine. Used with caution in patients taking SSRIs
	Amantadine	Antiviral agent used to treat Parkinson's disease. Its effects are modest	Dizziness, lethargy, anti-cholinergic effects, and sleep disturbance	
	Apomorphine	Intermittent therapy of Parkinson's disease	Severe nausea and vomiting requiring pretreatment with an antiemetic not of the 5-HT_3 antagonist class	Hallucinations, dyskinesia, and abnormal behavior
Drugs Used to Treat Alzheimer's Disease	Donepezil	Used to treat Alzheimer's disease	GI distress, muscle cramping, abnormal dreams	See Chapter 6. Used with caution in patients with bradycardia or syncope
	Rivastigmine	Used to treat Alzheimer's disease	GI distress, muscle cramping, abnormal dreams	See Chapter 6. Used with caution in patients with bradycardia or syncope
	Galantamine	Used to treat Alzheimer's disease	GI distress, muscle cramping, abnormal dreams	See Chapter 6. Used with caution in patients with bradycardia or syncope
	Tacrine	Used to treat Alzheimer's disease	GI distress, muscle cramping, abnormal dreams	See Chapter 6. Used with caution in patients with bradycardia or syncope
	Memantine	Used as an adjunct or an alternative to treat Alzheimer's disease	Headache and dizziness	Dosage reduced in patients with renal impairment
Drugs Used to Treat Huntington's Disease	Tetrabenazine	Treatment of chorea associated with Huntington's disease		Depression. Hypotension
Drugs Used to Treat ALS	Riluzole	Treatment of amyotrophic lateral sclerosis (ALS). May prolong survival by 2-3 months	Nausea and diarrhea	Associated with hepatic injury
	Baclofen	Treatment of spasticity of ALS. Intrathecal administration may avoid sedation	Sedation	Abrupt withdrawal of intrathecal baclofen may cause rebound spasticity, rhabdomyolitis, and multiple organ failure
	Tizanidine	Treatment of spasticity of ALS	Drowsiness, asthenia, and dizziness	
	Dantrolene	Treatment of spasticity of ALS		Associated with hepatotoxicity

CHAPTER 14

Drug Addiction

This chapter will be most useful after having a basic understanding of the material in Chapter 24, Drug Addiction in *Goodman & Gilman's The Pharmacological Basis of Therapeutics*, 12th Edition. The specific pharmacology (including the mechanisms of action) of drugs mentioned in Chapter 14 is discussed in previous or subsequent chapters. The drugs presented in Chapter 14 are discussed in relation to their ability to produce tolerance, physical dependence, and addiction. No **Mechanisms of Action Table** nor **Clinical Summary Table** are included as a part of Chapter 14 because new drugs are not introduced. The few drugs that are used therapeutically to treat specific drug addictions are discussed in the narratives of the clinical cases. In addition to the material presented here, the 12th Edition includes:

- Table 24-2 Dependence among Users 1990 to 1992
- Figure 24-2 Cocaine-induced changes in CNS dopamine release
- Figure 24-3 Nicotine concentrations in blood resulting from five different nicotine delivery systems
- A detailed discussion of the variables affecting the onset and continuation of drug abuse and addiction
- A detailed discussion of the different types of tolerance

LEARNING OBJECTIVES

- ☑ Understand the pharmacological principles of tolerance, physical dependence, and withdrawal.
- ☑ Describe the characteristic withdrawal syndromes for the commonly abused drugs.
- ☑ Know the patterns of abuse behavior and the toxicity of the commonly abused drugs.
- ☑ Know the available pharmacological interventions for the acute treatment and long-term management of the commonly abused drugs.

CASE 14-1

A 56-year-old obese woman is being treated with immediate-release oxycodone for chronic back pain. She is also taking a muscle relaxant, cyclobenzaprine, and a short-acting benzodiazepine for sleep.

a. **What concerns are there with the use of an opiate-like immediate-release oxycodone for the treatment of chronic pain?**

Rapid-onset, short-duration opioids are excellent for acute short-term use, such as during the postoperative period. As tolerance and physical dependence develop, however, the patient may experience the early symptoms of withdrawal between doses, and during withdrawal, the threshold for pain decreases. The diversion of prescription opioids such as oxycodone and hydrocodone to illegal markets has become an important source of opiate abuse in the United States (see answer to Case 14-1c below).

The risk for addiction is highest in patients complaining of pain with no clear physical explanation or in patients with evidence of a chronic, non-life-threatening disorder. Examples are chronic headaches, backaches, abdominal pain, or peripheral neuropathy. Even in these cases, an opioid may be considered as a brief emergency treatment, but long-term treatment with opioids should be used only after other alternatives have been exhausted.

(Continued)

b. Over the past year this patient has doubled her dose of oxycodone. Why has she increased the dose of oxycodone?

While abuse and addiction are complex conditions combining many variables (see Table 14-1), there are a number of relevant pharmacological phenomena that occur independent of social and psychological dimensions. First are the changes in the way the body responds to a drug with repeated use. Tolerance, the most common response to repetitive use of the same drug, can be defined as the reduction in response to the drug after repeated administrations. Figure 14-1 shows an idealized dose-response curve for an administered drug. As the dose of the drug increases, the observed effect of the drug increases. With repeated use of the drug, however, the curve shifts to the right (tolerance). Thus, a higher dose is required to produce the same effect that was once obtained at a lower dose. As outlined in Table 14-2, there are many forms of tolerance, likely arising through multiple mechanisms.

Tolerance to some drug effects develops much more rapidly than to other effects of the same drug. For example, tolerance develops rapidly to the euphoria produced by opioids such as heroin, and addicts tend to increase their dose in order to reexperience that elusive "high." In contrast, tolerance to the gastrointestinal effects of opioids develops more slowly. The discrepancy between tolerance to euphorigenic effects (rapid) and tolerance to effects on vital functions (slow), such as respiration and blood pressure, can lead to potentially fatal overdoses in sedative abusers trying to reexperience the euphoria they recall from earlier use (see Case 14-5).

(Continued)

TABLE 14-1 Multiple Simultaneous Variables Affecting Onset and Continuation of Drug Abuse and Addiction

Agent (drug)
Availability
Cost
Purity/potency
Mode of administration
    Chewing (absorption *via* oral mucous membranes)
    Gastrointestinal
    Intranasal
    Subcutaneous and intramuscular
    Intravenous
    Inhalation
Speed of onset and termination of effects (pharmacokinetics: combination of agent and host)

Host (user)
Heredity
    Innate tolerance
    Speed of developing acquired tolerance
    Likelihood of experiencing intoxication as pleasure
Metabolism of the drug (nicotine and alcohol data already available)
Psychiatric symptoms
Prior experiences/expectations
Propensity for risk-taking behavior

Environment
Social setting
Community attitudes
    Peer influence, role models
Availability of other reinforcers (sources of pleasure or recreation)
Employment or educational opportunities
Conditioned stimuli: environmental cues become associated with drugs after repeated use in the same environment

SECTION II Neuropharmacology

TABLE 14-2 Types of Tolerance

Innate (pre-existing sensitivity or insensitivity)
Acquired
    Pharmacokinetic (dispositional or metabolic)
    Pharmacodynamic
    Learned tolerance
        Behavioral
        Conditioned
    Acute tolerance
    Reverse tolerance (sensitization)
    Cross-tolerance

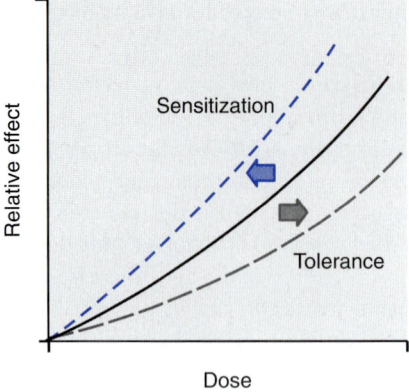

FIGURE 14-1 Shifts in a dose-response curve with tolerance and sensitization. With tolerance, there is a shift of the curve to the right such that doses higher than initial doses are required to achieve the same effects. With sensitization, there is a leftward shift of the curve such that for a given dose, there is a greater effect than seen after the initial dose.

c. What are the options for treatment of this patient?

For chronic administration, long-acting opioids are preferred. While methadone is long-acting because of its metabolism to active metabolites, the long-acting version of oxycodone has been formulated to release slowly, thereby changing a short-acting opioid into a long-acting one. Unfortunately, this mechanism can be subverted by breaking the tablet and making the full dose of oxycodone immediately available. This has led to diversion of oxycodone to illicit traffic because high-dose oxycodone produces euphoria that is sought by opiate abusers.

CASE 14-2

A 43-year-old man is admitted to the hospital because of a fractured hip. He has a long history of alcohol consumption. Recently he has begun taking a drink of alcohol in the morning.

a. Is it appropriate to assume that he has developed tolerance and physical dependence to alcohol?

Heavy consumers of alcohol not only acquire tolerance but also inevitably develop a state of physical dependence. This often leads to drinking in the morning to restore blood alcohol levels diminished during the night. Eventually, they may awaken during the night and take a drink to avoid the restlessness produced by falling alcohol levels.

b. What are the major signs and symptoms of alcohol withdrawal?

The alcohol-withdrawal syndrome (see Table 14-3) generally depends on the size of the average daily dose and usually is "treated" by resumption of alcohol ingestion. Withdrawal symptoms are experienced frequently but usually are not severe or life-threatening until they occur in conjunction with other problems, such as infection, trauma, malnutrition, or electrolyte imbalance. In the setting of such complications, the syndrome of delirium tremens becomes likely.

c. What is the appropriate treatment to prevent and treat alcohol withdrawal?

A patient who presents in a medical setting with an alcohol-withdrawal syndrome should be considered to have a potentially lethal condition. Although most mild cases of alcohol withdrawal never come to medical attention, severe cases require general evaluation; attention to hydration and electrolytes; vitamins, especially high-dose thiamine (see Chapter 9); and a sedating medication that has cross-tolerance with alcohol. To block or diminish the symptoms described in Table 14-3, a short-acting benzodiazepine such as oxazepam can be used at a dose of 15 to 30 mg every 6 to 8 hours according to the stage and severity of withdrawal; some authorities recommend

TABLE 14-3 Alcohol Withdrawal Syndrome

Alcohol craving
Tremor, irritability
Nausea
Sleep disturbance
Tachycardia
Hypertension
Sweating
Perceptual distortion
Seizures (6-48 hours after last drink)
Visual (and occasionally auditory or tactile) hallucinations (12-48 hours after last drink)
Delirium tremens (48-96 hours after last drink; rare in uncomplicated withdrawal)
    Severe agitation
    Confusion
    Fever, profuse sweating
    Tachycardia
    Nausea, diarrhea
    Dilated pupils

(Continued)

a long-acting benzodiazepine unless there is demonstrated liver impairment. Anticonvulsants such as carbamazepine have been shown to be effective in alcohol withdrawal, although they appear not to relieve subjective symptoms as well as benzodiazepines. After medical evaluation, uncomplicated alcohol withdrawal can be treated effectively on an outpatient basis. When there are medical problems, a history of seizures, or simultaneous dependence on other drugs, hospitalization is required.

d. What are the options for this patient if he desires treatment for his alcoholism upon discharge from the hospital?

Detoxification is only the first step of treatment. Complete abstinence is the objective of long-term treatment, and this is accomplished mainly by behavioral approaches. Medications that aid in the prevention of relapse are under development. Disulfiram (ANTABUSE; see Chapter 9) has been useful in some programs that focus behavioral efforts on ingestion of the medication. Disulfiram blocks aldehyde dehydrogenase, the second step in ethanol metabolism, resulting in the accumulation of acetaldehyde, which produces an unpleasant flushing reaction when alcohol is ingested. Knowledge of this unpleasant reaction helps the patient to resist taking a drink. Although quite effective pharmacologically, disulfiram has not been found to be effective in controlled clinical trials because so many patients failed to ingest the medication.

Naltrexone (REVIA; see Chapter 10), an opioid receptor antagonist that blocks the reinforcing properties of alcohol, is FDA-approved as an adjunct in the treatment of alcoholism. Chronic administration of naltrexone resulted in a decreased rate of relapse to alcohol drinking in the majority of published double-blind clinical trials. It works best in combination with behavioral treatment programs that encourage adherence to medication and abstinence from alcohol. A depot preparation of naltrexone with a duration of 30 days (VIVITROL) was approved by the FDA in 2006; it greatly improves medication adherence, the major problem with the use of medications in treating alcoholism.

Acamprosate (CAMPRAL; see Chapter 9), another FDA-approved medication for alcoholism, is a competitive inhibitor of the N-methyl-D-aspartate (NMDA)–type glutamate receptor. The drug appears to normalize the dysregulated neurotransmission associated with chronic ethanol intake and thereby to attenuate one of the mechanisms that lead to relapse.

CASE 14-3

A 75-year-old woman with early dementia has been taking alprazolam as a sleep aid for the past 10 years. She has consistently taken the same prescribed dose, but when her prescription expired she forgot to renew it.

a. Is she likely to have developed tolerance or physical dependence to the benzodiazepine?

When a benzodiazepine is taken for up to several weeks, there is little tolerance or physical dependence and no difficulty in stopping the medication when the condition no longer warrants its use. After several months, the proportion of patients who demonstrate physical dependence increases, and reducing the dose or stopping the medication abruptly produces withdrawal symptoms (see Table 14-4).

b. What symptoms might she experience as a result of abruptly stopping the benzodiazepine?

It can be difficult to distinguish withdrawal symptoms (see Table 14-4) from the reappearance of the anxiety symptoms for which the benzodiazepine was prescribed initially. Some patients may increase their dose over time because tolerance definitely develops to the sedative effects. Many patients and their physicians, however, contend that antianxiety benefits continue to occur long after tolerance develops to the sedating effects. Moreover, these patients continue to take the medication for years

(Continued)

TABLE 14-4 Benzodiazepine Withdrawal Symptoms

Following moderate dose usage
- Anxiety, agitation
- Increased sensitivity to light and sound
- Paresthesias, strange sensations
- Muscle cramps
- Myoclonic jerks
- Sleep disturbance
- Dizziness

Following high-dose usage
- Seizures
- Delirium

according to medical directions without increasing their dose and are able to function very effectively as long as they take the benzodiazepine. The degree to which tolerance develops to the anxiolytic effects of benzodiazepines is a subject of controversy.

c. How might this patient's withdrawal syndrome be treated?

If patients receiving long-term benzodiazepine treatment by prescription wish to stop their medication, the process may take months of gradual dose reduction. Withdrawal symptoms (see Table 14-4) may occur during this outpatient detoxification, but in most cases the symptoms are mild. If anxiety symptoms return, a nonbenzodiazepine such as buspirone may be prescribed, but this agent usually is less effective than benzodiazepines for treatment of anxiety in these patients. Some authorities recommend transferring the patient to a long $t_{1/2}$ benzodiazepine during detoxification; others recommend an anticonvulsant, carbamazepine or phenobarbital. Controlled studies comparing different treatment regimens are lacking. Since patients who have been on low doses of benzodiazepines for years usually have no adverse effects, the physician and patient should decide jointly whether detoxification and possible transfer to a new anxiolytic are worth the effort.

After detoxification, the prevention of relapse requires a long-term outpatient rehabilitation program similar to the treatment of alcoholism. No specific medications have been found to be useful in the rehabilitation of sedative abusers; but, of course, specific psychiatric disorders such as depression or schizophrenia, if present, require appropriate medications.

CASE 14-4

A 53-year-old man has been smoking since he was a teenager. He now desires to quit smoking.

a. What are the issues of nicotine addiction that should be considered in this patient?

The basic pharmacology of nicotine and agents for smoking cessation are discussed in Chapter 6. Because nicotine provides the reinforcement for cigarette smoking, the most common cause of preventable death and disease in the United States, it is arguably the most dangerous dependence-producing drug. The dependence produced by nicotine can be extremely durable, as exemplified by the high failure rate among smokers who try to quit. Although more than 80% of smokers express a desire to quit, only 35% try to stop each year, and fewer than 5% are successful in unaided attempts to quit.

Cigarette addiction is influenced by multiple variables. Nicotine itself produces reinforcement; users compare nicotine to stimulants such as cocaine or amphetamine, although its effects are of lower magnitude. While there are many casual users of alcohol and cocaine, few individuals who smoke cigarettes smoke a small enough quantity (≤5 cigarettes per day) to avoid dependence. Nicotine is absorbed readily through the skin, mucous membranes, and lungs. The pulmonary route produces discernible CNS effects in as little as 7 seconds. Thus, each puff produces some discrete reinforcement. With 10 puffs per cigarette, the 1-pack-per-day smoker reinforces the habit 200 times daily. The timing, setting, situation, and preparation all become associated repetitively with the effects of nicotine.

There is evidence for tolerance to the subjective effects of nicotine. Smokers typically report that the first cigarette of the day after a night of abstinence gives the "best" feeling. Smokers who return to cigarettes after a period of abstinence may experience nausea if they return immediately to their previous dose. Persons naive to the effects of nicotine will experience nausea at low nicotine blood levels, and smokers will experience nausea if nicotine levels are raised above their accustomed levels.

Negative reinforcement refers to the benefits obtained from the termination of an unpleasant state. In dependent smokers, the urge to smoke correlates with a low blood nicotine level, as though smoking were a means to achieve a certain nicotine

(Continued)

level and thus avoid withdrawal symptoms. Some smokers even awaken during the night to have a cigarette, which ameliorates the effect of low nicotine blood levels that could disrupt sleep. Thus, smokers may be smoking to achieve the reward of nicotine effects, to avoid the pain of nicotine withdrawal, or most likely a combination of the two. Nicotine withdrawal symptoms are listed in Table 14-5.

TABLE 14-5 Nicotine Withdrawal Symptoms

Irritability, impatience, hostility
Anxiety
Dysphoric or depressed mood
Difficulty concentrating
Restlessness
Decreased heart rate
Increased appetite or weight gain

b. What options are available to help him with his desire to quit smoking?

The nicotine withdrawal syndrome (see Table 14-5) can be alleviated by nicotine-replacement therapy, available with a prescription (eg, NICOTROL inhaler and nasal spray) or without (eg, NICORETTE gum and others; COMMIT lozenges and others; and NICODERM CQ transdermal patch and others). Figure 24-3 in *Goodman and Gilman's The Pharmacological Basis of Therapeutics*, 12th Edition shows the blood nicotine concentrations achieved by different methods of nicotine delivery. Because nicotine gum and a nicotine patch do not achieve the peak levels seen with cigarettes, they do not produce the same magnitude of subjective effects as smoking. These methods do, however, suppress the symptoms of nicotine withdrawal. Thus, smokers should be able to transfer their dependence to the alternative delivery system and gradually reduce the daily nicotine dose with minimal symptoms. Although this results in more smokers achieving abstinence, most resume smoking over the ensuing weeks or months. Comparisons with placebo treatment show large benefits of nicotine replacement at 6 weeks, but the effect diminishes with time. The nicotine patch produces a steady blood level and seems to have better patient compliance than that observed with nicotine gum. Verified abstinence rates at 12 months are reported to be in the range of 20%. The necessary goal of complete abstinence contributes to the poor success rate; when ex-smokers "slip" and begin smoking a little, they usually relapse quickly to their prior level of dependence.

The search for better medications to treat nicotine addiction has become an important goal of the pharmaceutical industry, and other types of medication have been tested in clinical trials. A sustained-release preparation of the antidepressant bupropion (ZYBAN; see Chapter 8) improves abstinence rates among smokers and remains a useful option. The cannabinoid CB_1 receptor inverse agonist rimonabant improves abstinence rates and reduces the weight gain seen frequently in ex-smokers. Unfortunately, the CB_1 inverse agonist mechanism led to a high frequency of depressive and neurologic symptoms, ending its development in the United States. Varenicline, a partial agonist at the $α_4β_2$ subtype of the nicotinic acetylcholine receptor, improves abstinence rates but has also been linked to risk of developing suicidal ideation. Varenicline partially stimulates nicotinic receptors, thereby reducing craving and preventing most withdrawal symptoms. It has high receptor affinity, thus blocking access to nicotine, so if the treated smoker relapses, there is little reward and abstinence is more likely to be maintained.

CASE 14-5

A 16-year-old woman is brought to the emergency room with a heroin overdose. This has occurred 8 hours after she was discharged from a detoxification center.

a. Why is heroin so addictive?

Injection of a heroin solution produces a variety of sensations described as warmth, taste, or high and intense pleasure ("rush") often compared with sexual orgasm. There are some differences among the opioids in their acute effects, with morphine producing more of a histamine-releasing effect and meperidine producing more excitation or confusion.

Thus, the popularity of heroin may be due to its availability on the illicit market and its rapid onset. After intravenous injection, the euphoric effects begin in less than a minute. Heroin has high lipid solubility, crosses the blood-brain barrier quickly, and is deacetylated to the active metabolites 6-monoacetyl morphine and morphine. After the intense euphoria, which lasts from 45 seconds

(Continued)

to several minutes, there is a period of sedation and tranquility ("on the nod") lasting up to an hour. The effects of heroin wear off in 3 to 5 hours, depending on the dose. Experienced users may inject 2 to 4 times per day. Thus, the heroin addict is constantly oscillating between being "high" and feeling the sickness of early withdrawal (see Figure 14-2). This produces many problems in the homeostatic systems regulated at least in part by endogenous opioids. For example, the hypothalamic-pituitary-gonadal axis and the hypothalamic-pituitary-adrenal axis are abnormal in heroin addicts. Women on heroin have irregular menses, and men have a variety of sexual performance problems. Mood also is affected. Heroin addicts are relatively docile and compliant after taking heroin, but during withdrawal, they become irritable and aggressive.

b. What is likely to have led to the overdose in this particular patient?

Based on patient reports, tolerance develops early to the euphoria-producing effects of opioids. There also is tolerance to the respiratory depressant, analgesic, sedative, and emetic properties. Heroin users tend to increase their daily dose, depending on their financial resources and the availability of the drug. If a supply is available, the dose can be increased progressively by 100-fold. Even in highly tolerant individuals, the possibility of overdose remains if tolerance is exceeded. Overdose is likely to occur when potency of the street sample is unexpectedly high, when the heroin is mixed with a far more potent opioid, such as fentanyl (SUBLIMAZE, others), or after release from a detoxification program (loss of tolerance) with the individual returning to her previously used dose of heroin, as occurred with this patient.

c. What treatment options are available to this patient?

Opioid withdrawal signs and symptoms (see Table 14-6) can be treated by 3 different approaches. The first and most commonly used approach depends on cross-tolerance and consists of transfer to a prescription opioid medication and then gradual dose reduction. The same principles of detoxification apply as for other types of physical dependence. It is convenient to change the patient from a short-acting opioid such as heroin to a long-acting one such as methadone. Detoxification and subsequent maintenance of opiate dependence with methadone is specifically limited to accredited opioid treatment programs (OTPs) and is regulated by Federal Opioid Treatment

(Continued)

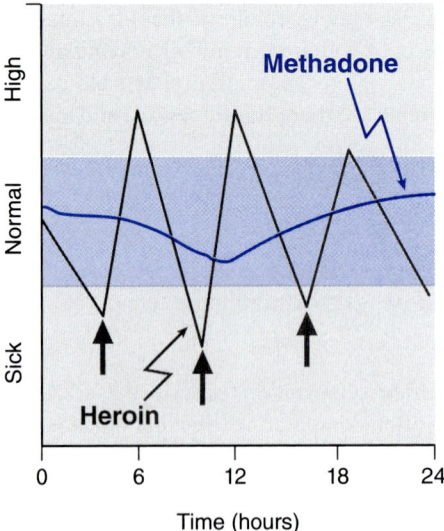

FIGURE 14-2 Differences in responses to heroin and methadone. A person who injects heroin (↑) several times per day oscillates (gray line) between being sick and being high. In contrast, the typical methadone patient (blue line) remains in the "normal" range (indicated in shaded blue) with little fluctuation after dosing once per day. The ordinate values represent the subject's mental and physical state, not plasma levels of the drug.

Drug Addiction — CHAPTER 14

TABLE 14-6 Characteristics of Opioid Withdrawal

SYMPTOMS	SIGNS
Regular withdrawal	
Craving for opioids	Pupillary dilation
Restlessness, irritability	Sweating
Increased sensitivity to pain	Piloerection ("gooseflesh") Tachycardia
Nausea, cramps	Vomiting, diarrhea
Muscle aches	Increased blood pressure
Dysphoric mood	Yawning
Insomnia, anxiety	Fever
Protracted withdrawal	
Anxiety Insomnia Drug craving	Cyclic changes in weight, pupil size, respiratory center sensitivity

Standards. The initial dose of methadone is typically 20 to 30 mg. This is a test dose to determine the level needed to reduce observed withdrawal symptoms. The first day's total dose then can be calculated depending on the response and then reduced by 20% per day during the course of detoxification.

A second approach to detoxification involves the use of oral clonidine (CATAPRES, others), a medication approved only for the treatment of hypertension. Clonidine is an α_2 adrenergic receptor agonist that decreases adrenergic neurotransmission from the locus ceruleus (see Chapter 7). Many of the autonomic symptoms of opioid withdrawal such as nausea, vomiting, cramps, sweating, tachycardia, and hypertension result from the loss of opioid suppression of the locus ceruleus system during the abstinence syndrome. Clonidine, acting upon distinct non-opioid receptors but by cellular mechanisms that mimic opioid effects, can alleviate many of the symptoms of opioid withdrawal, but not the generalized aches and opioid craving. When using clonidine to treat withdrawal, the dose must be titrated according to the stage and severity of withdrawal, beginning with 0.2 mg orally; postural hypotension is a common side effect. A similar drug, lofexidine (currently in clinical trials in the United States), has greater selectivity for α_{2A} adrenergic receptors and is associated with less of the hypotension that limits the usefulness of clonidine in this setting.

A third method of treating opioid withdrawal involves activation of the endogenous opioid system without medication. The techniques proposed include acupuncture and several methods of CNS activation using transcutaneous electrical stimulation. While attractive theoretically, this has not yet been found to be practical. Rapid antagonist-precipitated opioid detoxification under general anesthesia has received considerable publicity because it promises detoxification in several hours while the patient is unconscious and not experiencing withdrawal discomfort. A mixture of medications has been used, but morbidity and mortality as reported in the lay press are unacceptable, with no demonstrated advantage in long-term outcome.

The most successful treatment for heroin addiction consists of stabilization on methadone in accordance with state and federal regulations. Patients who relapse repeatedly during drug-free treatment can be transferred directly to methadone without requiring detoxification. The dose of methadone must be sufficient to prevent withdrawal symptoms for at least 24 hours. The introduction of buprenorphine, a partial agonist at μ-opioid receptors (see Chapter 10), represents a major

(Continued)

change in the treatment of opiate addiction. This drug produces minimal withdrawal symptoms when discontinued and has a low potential for overdose, a long duration of action, and the ability to block heroin effects. Treatment can take place in a qualified physician's private office rather than in a special center, as required for methadone. When taken sublingually, buprenorphine (SUBUTEX) is active, but it also has the potential to be dissolved and injected (abused). A buprenorphine-naloxone combination (SUBOXONE) is also available. When taken orally (sublingually), the naloxone moiety is not effective, but if the patient abuses the medication by injecting, the naloxone will block or diminish the subjective high that could be produced by buprenorphine alone.

Another pharmacological option is opioid antagonist treatment. Naltrexone (REVIA, others; see Chapter 10) is an antagonist with a high affinity for the μ-opioid receptor (MOR); it will competitively block the effects of heroin or other MOR agonists. Naltrexone has almost no agonist effects of its own and will not satisfy craving or relieve protracted withdrawal symptoms. For these reasons, naltrexone treatment does not appeal to the average heroin addict, but it can be used after detoxification for patients with high motivation to remain opioid-free. Physicians, nurses, and pharmacists who have frequent access to opioid drugs make excellent candidates for this treatment approach. A depot formulation of naltrexone that provides 30 days of medication after a single injection (VIVITROL) has been approved for the treatment of alcoholism. This formulation eliminates the necessity of daily medication and prevents relapse when the recently detoxified patient leaves a protected environment.

CASE 14-6

A 26-year-old man is brought to the emergency room as the result of a motor vehicle accident. A urine drug screen is positive for benzoylecgonine. A blood alcohol concentration is just below the legal limit for driving.

a. What does the urine drug screen indicate?

The major route for cocaine metabolism involves hydrolysis of each of its 2 ester groups. Benzoylecgonine, produced on loss of the methyl group, represents the major urinary metabolite and can be found in the urine for 2 to 5 days after a binge. As a result, the benzoylecgonine test is a valid method for detecting cocaine use; the metabolite remains detectable in the urine of heavy users for up to 10 days.

b. What are the effects of cocaine that may have led to the accident?

The general pharmacology and medicinal use of cocaine as a local anesthetic are discussed in Chapter 11. Cocaine produces a dose-dependent increase in heart rate and blood pressure accompanied by increased arousal, improved performance on tasks of vigilance and alertness, and a sense of self-confidence and well-being. Higher doses produce euphoria, which has a brief duration and often is followed by a desire for more drug. Repeated doses may lead to involuntary motor activity, stereotyped behavior, and paranoia. Irritability and increased risk of violence are found among heavy chronic users. Of particular concern in drivers who are taking cocaine is increased risk-taking and a sense of invincibility.

c. Why is cocaine addiction so difficult to treat?

A form of maladaptive memory begins with the administration of substances (eg, cocaine) or behaviors (eg, the thrill of gambling) that directly and intensely activate brain reward circuits. Activation of these circuits motivates normal behavior and most humans simply enjoy the experience without being compelled to repeat it. For some (~16% of those who try cocaine) the experience produces strong conditioned associations to environmental cues that signal the availability of the drug or the behavior. Thus, reflexive activation of reward circuits becomes involuntary and with a very rapid onset. The cues acquire strong salience that overwhelms other behaviors. The individual becomes drawn into compulsive repetition of the experience

(Continued)

Drug Addiction — CHAPTER 14

focusing on the immediate pleasure despite negative long-term consequences and neglect of important social responsibilities. Of course, underlying this behavior are poorly understood changes in neural circuits.

Since cocaine withdrawal (see Table 14-7) is generally mild, treatment of withdrawal symptoms usually is not required. The major problem in treatment is not detoxification but helping the patient to resist the urge to resume compulsive cocaine use. Rehabilitation programs involving individual and group psychotherapy based on the principles of alcoholics anonymous, and behavioral treatments based on reinforcing cocaine-free urine tests, result in significant improvement in the majority of cocaine users. Nonetheless, there is great interest in finding a medication that can aid in the rehabilitation of cocaine addicts.

d. What other medical conditions is this patient at risk of?

Other risks of cocaine, beyond the potential for addiction, include cardiac arrhythmias, myocardial ischemia, myocarditis, aortic dissection, cerebral vasoconstriction, and seizures. Death from trauma also is associated with cocaine use.

TABLE 14-7 Cocaine Withdrawal Symptoms and Signs

Dysphoria
Depression
Sleepiness
Fatigue
Cocaine craving
Bradycardia

CASE 14-7

A 35-year-old woman is an occasional user of cannabis.

a. What is the mechanism of action of cannabis?

The cannabis plant has been cultivated for centuries both for the production of hemp fiber and for its presumed medicinal and psychoactive properties. The smoke from burning cannabis contains many chemicals, including 61 different cannabinoids that have been identified. One of these, Δ-9-tetrahydrocannabinol (Δ-9-THC), produces most of the characteristic pharmacological effects of smoked marijuana.

Cannabinoid receptors CB_1 (mainly CNS) and CB_2 (peripheral) have been identified and cloned. An arachidonic acid derivative, anandamide, has been proposed as an endogenous ligand for CB receptors. While the physiological function of these receptors and their endogenous ligands are incompletely understood, they are likely to have important functions because they are dispersed widely with high densities in the cerebral cortex, hippocampus, striatum, and cerebellum.

b. What are the pharmacological effects of marijuana?

The pharmacological effects of Δ-9-THC vary with the dose, route of administration, experience of the user, vulnerability to psychoactive effects, and setting of use. Intoxication with marijuana produces changes in mood, perception, and motivation, but the effect most frequently sought is the "high" and "mellowing out." This effect is described as different from the high produced by a stimulant or opiate. Effects vary with dose, but typically last ~2 hours. During the high, cognitive functions, perception, reaction time, learning, and memory are impaired. Coordination and tracking behavior may be impaired for several hours beyond the perception of the high, with obvious implications for the operation of a motor vehicle and performance in the workplace or at school.

Marijuana also produces complex behavioral changes such as giddiness and increased hunger. There are unsubstantiated claims of increased pleasure from sex and increased insight during a marijuana high. Unpleasant reactions such as panic or hallucinations and even acute psychosis may occur; several surveys indicate that 50 to 60% of marijuana users have reported at least one anxiety experience. These reactions are seen commonly with higher doses and with oral ingestion rather than smoked marijuana, because smoking permits the titration of dose according to the effects. While there is no convincing evidence that marijuana can produce a lasting schizophrenia-like syndrome, association studies suggest a correlation of early marijuana use with an increased risk of later developing schizophrenia. Numerous clinical reports suggest that marijuana use may precipitate a recurrence of psychosis in people with a history of schizophrenia.

TABLE 14-8 Marijuana Withdrawal Syndrome

Restlessness
Irritability
Mild agitation
Insomnia
Sleep EEG disturbance
Nausea, cramping

SECTION II Neuropharmacology

KEY CONCEPTS

- Tolerance to a drug is the reduction in response to the drug with repeated use.
- Physical dependence is a state that develops as a result of tolerance to a drug produced by a resetting of homeostatic mechanisms in response to repeated drug use.
- Withdrawal symptoms are characteristic for a given category of drugs and tend to be opposite to the original effects produced by the drug before tolerance developed.
- Addiction is usually characterized by compulsive drug-taking.
- Tolerance, physical dependence, and withdrawal are biological phenomena and in themselves do not imply that the individual is involved in misuse or addictive behavior.
- Fear of producing a medical addict often results in needless suffering among patients with pain due to limited use of appropriate medications.
- Opioids should never be withheld from patients with cancer out of fear of producing addiction.
- Abuse of combinations of drugs is common; alcohol is so widely available that it is often combined with all categories of abused drugs.
- Patients with a history of alcohol- or other drug-abuse problems have an increased risk for the development of benzodiazepine abuse and should rarely, if ever, be treated with benzodiazepines on a chronic basis.
- Smokers may be smoking to achieve the reward of nicotine effects, to avoid the pain of nicotine withdrawal, or most likely a combination of the two.
- The management of drug abuse and addiction must be individualized according to the drugs involved and the associated psychosocial problems of the individual patient.

SUMMARY QUIZ

QUESTION 14-1 A 24-year-old woman has increased her dosage of hydrocodone to achieve the same analgesic effect. This is a demonstration of

a. physical dependence.

b. first-pass metabolism.

c. tolerance.

d. an adverse effect.

e. addiction.

QUESTION 14-2 A 28-year-old man has been taking the same dose of oxycodone for several weeks as the result of a knee injury. He has not needed to increase his dose of oxycodone to achieve analgesia. He develops irritability and muscle aches upon abruptly stopping his oxycodone. This is a demonstration of

a. physical dependence.

b. first-pass metabolism.

c. tolerance.

d. an adverse effect.

e. addiction.

QUESTION 14-3 A 47-year-old man has consumed approximately 1 bottle of whiskey daily for the past 5 years. He is brought to the emergency room one evening because he is belligerent. In the emergency room he does not appear sedated despite a blood

(Continued)

alcohol concentration of 275 mg/dL. Within minutes of his blood being drawn he develops a respiratory arrest and is intubated successfully. Because of tolerance to alcohol's sedative effect the therapeutic index of alcohol in this patient is

a. increased.
b. decreased.
c. unchanged.
d. irrelevant.
e. negative reinforcement.

QUESTION 14-4 A 33-year-old woman who smokes 1 pack of cigarettes per day has recently begun getting up at 3 AM to smoke a cigarette. This is a demonstration of

a. positive reinforcement.
b. negative reinforcement.
c. insomnia.
d. depression.
e. increased therapeutic index of nicotine.

QUESTION 14-5 A 34-year-old man is a recreational user of cocaine. He is also a regular consumer of alcohol. The effect of alcohol on cocaine metabolism is demonstrated by the presence in the urine of

a. benzoylecgonine.
b. methanol.
c. benzocaine.
d. cocaethylene.
e. methylecgonine.

QUESTION 14-6 A 19-year-old woman is brought to the emergency room because of fearful hallucinations and suicidal thoughts after consuming methylenedioxymethamphetamine (MDMA). MDMA is thought to interact with

a. α_2 adrenergic receptors.
b. β_1 adrenergic receptors.
c. D_2 dopaminergic receptors.
d. μ opioid receptors.
e. $5\text{-}HT_2$ serotonergic receptors.

QUESTION 14-7 A 48-year-old woman is undergoing chemotherapy for advanced breast cancer. To allay her nausea and vomiting, she is given

a. diphenhydramine.
b. pseudoephedrine.
c. Δ-9-THC.
d. LSD.
e. 10, 11-epoxycarbamezepine.

SUMMARY QUIZ ANSWER KEY

QUESTION 14-1 Answer is **c.** Tolerance, the most common response to repetitive use of the same drug, can be defined as the reduction in response to the drug after repeated administrations. Figure 14-1 shows an idealized dose-response curve for an administered drug. As the dose of the drug increases, the observed effect of the drug increases. With repeated use of the drug, however, the curve shifts to the right (tolerance). Thus, a higher dose is required to produce the same effect that was once obtained at a lower dose.

SECTION II Neuropharmacology

QUESTION 14-2 Answer is **a.** The appearance of a withdrawal syndrome when administration of the drug is terminated is the only actual evidence of physical dependence. Withdrawal signs and symptoms occur when drug administration in a physically dependent person is terminated abruptly.

QUESTION 14-3 Answer is **b.** Experience with alcohol can produce greater tolerance (acquired tolerance) such that extremely high blood levels (300-400 mg/dL) can be found in alcoholics who do not appear grossly sedated. In these cases, the lethal dose of alcohol does not increase proportionately to the sedating dose, and thus the margin of safety (therapeutic index) is decreased. The concept of therapeutic index is introduced in Chapter 3.

QUESTION 14-4 Answer is **b.** Negative reinforcement refers to the benefits obtained from the termination of an unpleasant state. In dependent smokers, the urge to smoke correlates with a low blood nicotine level, as though smoking were a means to achieve a certain nicotine level and thus avoid withdrawal symptoms (see Table 14-5). Some smokers even awaken during the night to have a cigarette, which ameliorates the effect of low nicotine blood levels that could disrupt sleep. Thus, smokers may be smoking to achieve the reward of nicotine effects, to avoid the pain of nicotine withdrawal, or most likely a combination of the two.

QUESTION 14-5 Answer is **d.** Ethanol is frequently abused with cocaine, as it reduces the irritability induced by cocaine. Dual addiction to alcohol and cocaine is common. When cocaine and alcohol are taken concurrently, cocaine may be transesterified to cocaethylene, which is equipotent to cocaine in blocking DA reuptake.

QUESTION 14-6 Answer is **e.** The phenethylamine hallucinogens include mescaline, dimethoxymethamphetamine (DOM), methylenedioxyamphetamine (MDA), and MDMA, have a relatively high affinity for 5-HT_2 receptors (see Chapter 7), but they differ in their affinity for other subtypes of 5-HT receptors. There is a good correlation between the relative affinity of these compounds for 5-HT_2 receptors and their potency as hallucinogens in humans.

QUESTION 14-7 Answer is **c.** Marijuana has medicinal effects, including antiemetic properties that relieve side effects of anticancer chemotherapy. An oral capsule containing Δ-9-THC (dronabinol; MARINOL, others) is approved for anorexia associated with weight loss in patients with HIV infection and for cancer chemotherapy-induced nausea and vomiting.

SECTION III

Modulation of Cardiovascular Function

15. Drug Therapy of Hypertension, Edema, and Disorders of Sodium and Water Balance 268

16. Drug Therapy of Myocardial Ischemia 289

17. Pharmacotherapy Therapy of Heart Failure 301

18. Antiarrhythmic Drugs 312

19. Drug Therapy of Thromboembolic Disorders 323

20. Drug Therapy of Dyslipidemias 334

CHAPTER 15

Drug Therapy of Hypertension, Edema, and Disorders of Sodium and Water Balance

DRUGS INCLUDED IN THIS CHAPTER

- Acetazolamide (DIAMOX, others)
- β Adrenergic receptor antagonists (many; Table 15-1; see Chapter 7)
- Aliskiren (TEKTURNA)
- Amiloride (MIDAMOR, others)
- Amiloride/hydrochlorothiazide (generic)
- Amlodipine (NORVASC)
- Bendroflumethiazide (NATURETIN)
- Benzapril (LOTENSIN, others)
- Bumetanide (BUMEX, others)
- Candesartan cilexetil (ATACAND)
- Captopril (CAPOTEN, others)
- Chlorothiazide (DIURIL)
- Chlorthalidone (HYGROTON)
- Clevidipine (CLEVIPREX)
- Clonidine (CATAPRES, others)
- Conivaptan (VAPRISOL)
- Desmopressin acetate (1-deamino-8-D-arginine vasopressin, DDAVP, others)
- Diazoxide
- Dichlorphenamide (DARAMIDE)
- Diltiazem (CARDIZEM)
- Doxazosin (CARDURA, others)
- Enalapril (VASOTEC, others)
- Enalaprilat (VASOTEC INJECTION, others)
- Eplerenone (INSPRA, others)
- Ethacrynic acid (EDECRIN, others)
- Felodipine (PLENDIL)
- Fenoldopam (CORLOPAM)
- Fosinopril (MONOPRIL, others)
- Furosemide (LASIX, others)
- Glycerin (OSMOGLYN)
- Guanabenz (WYTENSIN)
- Guanadrel
- Guanfacine (INTUNIV, TENEX)
- Human recombinant ANP (carperitide, available only in Japan)
- Human recombinant BNP (nesiritide, NATRECOR)

(continues)

This chapter will be most useful after having a basic understanding of the material in the section on hypertension in Chapter 27 Drug Therapy of Myocardial Ischemia and Hypertension in *Goodman & Gilman's The Pharmacological Basis of Therapeutics*, 12th Edition (pp 765-785), as well as material in Chapter 25 Regulation of Renal Volume and Vascular Volume and Chapter 26 Renin and Angiotensin. In addition to the material presented here, the 12th Edition contains:

- The molecular structures of drugs used to treat hypertension, edema, and other disorders of Na^+ and water balance
- Figure 25-1 The anatomy and nomenclature of the nephron
- Figure 25-5 Changes in the extracellular fluid volume and weight with diuretic therapy
- An extensive discussion of the functions and effects of the renin-angiotensin system in Chapter 26

LEARNING OBJECTIVES

- ☑ Understand the mechanisms of action of drugs used to treat hypertension, edema, and other disorders of Na^+ and water balance.
- ☑ Know the untoward effects of drugs used to treat hypertension, edema, and other disorders of Na^+ and water balance.
- ☑ Know which patients should be treated and when treatment should be initiated.
- ☑ Know which drugs are most effective in treating individual hypertensive patients with specific comorbidities, including diabetes mellitus, congestive heart failure, and renal disease.
- ☑ Know which drugs can be used in combination.
- ☑ Know how to set treatment goals based on target blood pressures and other clinical measures.

MECHANISMS OF ACTION OF DIURETICS

DRUG CLASS	DRUG	MECHANISM OF ACTION
Inhibitors of Carbonic Anhydrase	Acetazolamide Dichlorphenamide Methazolamide	Inhibit carbonic anhydrase (CA) in the proximal tubule resulting in abolition of $NaHCO_3$ reabsorption Inhibition of CA in the collecting duct is a secondary site of action
Osmotic Diuretics	Glycerin Isosorbide Mannitol Urea	Act at the loop of Henle (primary site of action) to diminish passive reabsorption of NaCl by reducing medullary tonicity Act in the proximal tubule (secondary site) by increasing the osmolality of tubular fluid thereby reducing luminal Na^+ concentration and Na^+ reabsorption

(Continued)

Drug Therapy of Hypertension and Na+ Balance Disorders

CHAPTER 15

DRUG CLASS	DRUG	MECHANISM OF ACTION
Inhibitors of the Na+-K+-2Cl- Symporter (Loop Diuretics, High-Ceiling Diuretics)	Furosemide Bumetanide Ethacrynic acid Torsemide	Inhibit activity of the Na+-K+-2Cl- symporter in the thick ascending limb of the loop of Henle Highly efficacious diuretics because ~25% of the filtered Na+ load is normally reabsorbed by the thick ascending limb
Inhibitors of the Na+-Cl- symporter (Thiazide and Thiazide-Like Diuretics)	Bendroflumethiazide Chlorothiazide Hydrochlorothiazide Hydroflumethiazide Methyclothiazide Polythiazide Trichlormethiazide Chlorthalidone Indapamide Metolazone Quinethazone	Inhibit activity of Na+-Cl- symporter in the distal collecting tubule Less efficacious than loop diuretics because ~90% of the filtered Na+ load is reabsorbed before reaching the distal collecting tubule
Inhibitors of Renal Epithelial Na+ Channels (K+-Sparing Diuretics)	Triamterene Amiloride	Inhibit renal epithelial Na+ channels in the late distal tubule and collecting duct Cause small increases in NaCl excretion and are antikaliuretic
Mineralocorticoid Receptor Antagonists (Aldosterone Antagonists, K+-sparing Diuretics)	Spironolactone Eplerenone	Competitively inhibit aldosterone binding to the mineralocorticoid receptor which blocks the synthesis of aldosterone-induced proteins (AIPs) in epithelial cells in the late distal tubule and collecting duct
Diuretic Atrial Natriuretic Peptides (Inhibitors of the Cyclic Nucleotide-Gated Nonspecific Cation Channel)	Human recombinant ANP (carperitide, available only in Japan) Human recombinant BNP (nesiritide)	Activate natriuretic peptide receptors on the surface of epithelial cells in the inner medullary collecting duct which stimulates the formation of cyclic GMP that subsequently inhibits the cyclic nucleotide-gated nonspecific cation channel (CNGC); the CNGC is the primary channel for Na+ entry in these cells

DRUGS INCLUDED IN THIS CHAPTER (Cont.)

- Hydralazine (APRESOLINE)
- Hydrochlorothiazide (HYDRODIURIL)
- Hydroflumethiazide (SALURON)
- Indapamide (LOZOL)
- Irbesartan (AVAPRO)
- Isosorbide (ISMOTIC)
- Isradipine (DYNACIRC)
- Lisinopril (PRINIVIL, ZESTRIL, others)
- Losartan (COZAAR)
- Mannitol (OSMITROL, others)
- Methazolamide (GLAUCTABS)
- Methyclothiazide (ENDURON)
- Methyldopa (ALDOMET, others)
- Metolazone (MYKROX, ZAROXOLYN)
- Minoxidil (LONITEN)
- Moexipril (UNIVASC, others)
- Nicardipine (CARDENE)
- Nifedipine (PROCARDIA ER)
- Nisoldipine (SULAR)
- Nitroprusside
- Olmesartan medoxomil (BENICAR)
- Perindopril (ACEON)
- Polythiazide (RENESE)
- Prazosin (MINIPRESS, others)
- Quinapril (ACCUPRIL, others)
- Quinethazone (HYDROMOX)
- Ramipril (ALTACE, others)
- Reserpine
- Spironolactone (ALDACTONE, others)
- Telmisartan (MICARDIS)
- Terazosin (HYTRIN and others)
- Terlipressin (LUCASSIN)
- Tolvaptan (SAMSCA)
- Torsemide (DEMADEX, others)
- Trandolapril (MAVIK, others)
- Triamterene (DYRENIUM)
- Triamterene/hydrochlorothiazide (DYAZIDE, MAXZIDE, others)
- Trichlormethiazide (NAQUA)
- Urea (UREAPHIL, currently not available in the United States)
- Valsartan (DIOVAN)
- Vasopressin (8-L-arginine vasopressin, PITRESSIN, others)
- Verapamil (CALAN, others)

CASE 15-1

A 43-year-old man has a blood pressure of 138/88 taken during his annual examination. He has no other health problems and his blood laboratory results are in the normal range. He is modestly overweight and has a family history of cardiovascular disease.

a. What, if any, are the therapeutic options for this patient?

This patient is considered to have prehypertension (see Table 15-1). It is appropriate to recommend nonpharmacological approaches to reduce his risk of developing hypertension. The lifestyle modifications that could lower this patient's blood pressure include:

- Reduction in body weight
- Restricting sodium consumption (the Dietary Approaches to Stop Hypertension [DASH] diet may be particularly useful)

(Continued)

SECTION III

Modulation of Cardiovascular Function

OVERVIEW OF NEPHRON ANATOMY, NOMENCLATURE, AND FUNCTION (see Figure 25-1 in *Goodman & Gilman's The Pharmacological Basis of Therapeutics*, 12th Edition)

- The basic urine-forming unit of the kidney is the nephron.
- The nephron consists of a filtering apparatus, the glomerulus, connected to a long tubule portion that reabsorbs substances the body must conserve, and leaves behind and/or secretes substances that must be eliminated.
- The nephron can be divided into 4 major anatomical and functional regions:
  - The proximal tubule
  - The loop of Henle (which consists of the proximal straight tubule, the intermediate tubule, the thick ascending limb)
  - The distal convoluted tubule
  - The collecting duct
- Normally ~65% of filtered Na^+ is reabsorbed in the proximal tubule; this part of the tubule is highly permeable to water.
- Approximately 25% of filtered Na^+ is reabsorbed in the loop of Henle.
- The distal convoluted tubule actively transports NaCl and is impermeable to water.
- The fine control of ultrafiltrate composition and volume takes place in the collecting duct.
- The transport that occurs in a specific segment of the nephron is primarily determined by the transporters present in the epithelial cells and the whether they are located on the luminal or basolateral membrane.

PRINCIPLES OF DIURETIC ACTION

- Diuretics increase the rate of urine flow.
- Clinically useful diuretics also increase the rate of Na^+ excretion (natriuresis), as well as an anion such as Cl^-.
- Most diuretics are used to reduce extracellular fluid volume by decreasing total NaCl content.

TABLE 15-1 Criteria for Hypertension in Adults

CLASSIFICATION	BLOOD PRESSURE (mm Hg)	
	SYSTOLIC	DIASTOLIC
Normal	<120	and <80
Prehypertension	120-139	or 80-89
Hypertension, stage 1	140-159	or 90-99
Hypertension, stage 2	≥160	or ≥100

- Restriction of ethanol intake to modest levels
- Increased physical activity

b. A year later at his next annual examination, the patient's blood pressure is 142/91. What, if any, are the therapeutic options for this patient?

This patient's prehypertension has progressed to stage 1 hypertension (see Table 15-1). In addition to emphasizing the importance of the lifestyle modifications listed above, this patient should be started on antihypertensive drug therapy.

c. What are the considerations in choosing an appropriate antihypertensive drug therapy for this patient?

Choice of an antihypertensive drug should be driven by the likely benefit in an individual patient, taking into account concomitant diseases such as diabetes mellitus, problematic adverse effects of specific drugs, and cost. National guidelines recommend diuretics as preferred initial therapy for most patients with uncomplicated stage 1 hypertension who are unresponsive to nonpharmacological measures. Patients also are commonly treated with other drugs (see Table 15-2): β receptor antagonists, ACE inhibitors/AT_1-receptor antagonists, and Ca^{2+} channel blockers.

(Continued)

TABLE 15-2 Classification of Antihypertensive Drugs by Their Primary Site or Mechanism of Action

Diuretics
1. Thiazides and related agents (hydrochlorothiazide, chlorthalidone, chlorothiazide, indapamide, methylclothiazide, metolazone)
2. Loop diuretics (furosemide, bumetanide, torsemide, ethacrynic acid)
3. K^+-sparing diuretics (amiloride, triamterene, spironolactone)

Sympatholytic drugs (see Chapter 7)
1. β receptor antagonists (metoprolol, atenolol, betaxolol, bisoprolol, carteolol, esmolol, nadolol, nebivolol, penbutolol, pindolol, propranolol, timolol)
2. α receptor antagonists (prazosin, terazosin, doxazosin, phenoxybenzamine, phentolamine)
3. Mixed α-β receptor antagonists (labetalol, carvedilol)
4. Centrally acting adrenergic agents (methyldopa, clonidine, guanabenz, guanfacine)
5. Adrenergic neuron blocking agents (guanadrel, reserpine)

Ca^{2+} channel blockers (verapamil, diltiazem, nisoldipine, felodipine, nicardipine, isradipine, amlodipine, clevidipine, nifedipine[a])

Angiotensin-converting enzyme inhibitors (captopril, enalapril, lisinopril, quinapril, ramipril, benazepril, fosinopril, moexipril, perindopril, trandolapril)

AngII receptor antagonists (losartan, candesartan, irbesartan, valsartan, telmisartan, eprosartan, olmesartan)

Direct renin inhibitor (aliskiren)

Vasodilators
1. Arterial (hydralazine, minoxidil, diazoxide, fenoldopam)
2. Arterial and venous (nitroprusside)

[a]Extended-release nifedipine is approved for hypertension.

Drug Therapy of Hypertension and Na+ Balance Disorders — CHAPTER 15

d. He is prescribed hydrochlorothiazide (12.5 mg daily). What is the mechanism of action of this drug in reducing blood pressure?

The initial action of the thiazide diuretics is to decrease extracellular volume by interacting with a thiazide-sensitive NaCl cotransporter expressed in the distal convoluted tubule in the kidney (see Figure 15-1), which enhances Na$^+$ excretion in the urine, leading to a fall in cardiac output and a consequent reduction in mean arterial pressure. However, the hypotensive effect is maintained during long-term therapy due to decreased vascular resistance; cardiac output returns to pretreatment values and extracellular volume returns almost to normal due to compensatory responses such as activation of the renin-angiotensin system (RAS; Figure 15-2). The explanation for the long-term vasodilation induced by these drugs is unknown. Hydrochlorothiazide may open Ca^{2+}-activated K$^+$ channels, leading to hyperpolarization of vascular smooth muscle cells, which leads in turn to closing of L-type Ca^{2+} channels and lower probability of opening, resulting in decreased Ca^{2+} entry and reduced vasoconstriction. Hydrochlorothiazide also inhibits vascular carbonic anhydrase, which hypothetically may alter smooth muscle cell cytosolic pH and thereby cause opening of Ca^{2+}-activated K$^+$ channels with the consequences noted. The major action of thiazide diuretics on the NaCl cotransporter—expressed predominantly in the distal convoluted tubules and not in vascular smooth muscle or the heart—has contributed to repeated suggestions that these drugs decrease peripheral resistance as an indirect effect of negative sodium balance. That thiazides lose efficacy in treating hypertension in patients with co-existing renal insufficiency is compatible with this hypothesis.

> **PRINCIPLES OF DIURETIC ACTION (Cont.)**
> - With chronic diuretic administration, renal compensatory mechanisms adjust Na$^+$ excretion to match Na$^+$ intake (see Figure 25-5 in *Goodman & Gilman's The Pharmacological Basis of Therapeutics*, 12th Edition).
> - Diuretics are classified based on their mechanism of action and their site of action in the nephron (Table 15-3 and Figure 15-1).

TABLE 15-3 Excretory and Renal Hemodynamic Effects of Diuretics[a]

DIURETIC MECHANISM (PRIMARY SITE OF ACTION)	CATIONS					ANIONS			URIC ACID		RENAL HEMODYNAMICS			
	Na$^+$	K$^+$	H^{+b}	Ca^{2+}	Mg^{2+}	Cl$^-$	HCO$_3^-$	H$_2$PO$_4^-$	ACUTE	CHRONIC	RBF	GFR	FF	TGF
Inhibitors of CA (proximal tubule)	+	++	−	NC	V	(+)	++	++	I	−	−	−	NC	+
Osmotic diuretics (loop of Henle)	++	+	I	+	++	+	+	+	+	I	+	NC	−	I
Inhibitors of Na$^+$-K$^+$-2Cl$^-$ symport (thick ascending limb)	++	++	+	++	++	++	+^{c}	+^{c}	+	−	V(+)	NC	V(−)	−
Inhibitors of Na$^+$-Cl$^-$ symport (distal convoluted tubule)	+	++	+	V(−)	V(+)	+	+^{c}	+^{c}	+	−	NC	V(−)	V(−)	NC
Inhibitors of renal epithelial Na$^+$ channels (late distal tubule, collecting duct)	+	−	−	−	−	+	(+)	NC	I	−	NC	NC	NC	NC
Antagonists of mineralocorticoid receptors (late distal tubule, collecting duct)	+	−	−	I	−	+	(+)	I	I	−	NC	NC	NC	NC

[a] Except for uric acid, changes are for acute effects of diuretics in the absence of significant volume depletion, which would trigger complex physiological adjustments.

[b] H$^+$, titratable acid and NH$_4^+$.

[c] In general, these effects are restricted to those individual agents that inhibit carbonic anhydrase. However, there are notable exceptions in which symport inhibitors increase bicarbonate and phosphate (eg, metolazone, bumetanide).

++, +, (+), −, NC, V, V(+), V(−), and I indicate marked increase, mild to moderate increase, slight increase, decrease, no change, variable effect, variable increase, variable decrease, and insufficient data, respectively. For cations and anions, the indicated effects refer to absolute changes in fractional excretion.

RBF, renal blood flow; GFR, glomerular filtration rate; FF, filtration fraction; TGF, tubuloglomerular feedback; CA, carbonic anhydrase.

SECTION III Modulation of Cardiovascular Function

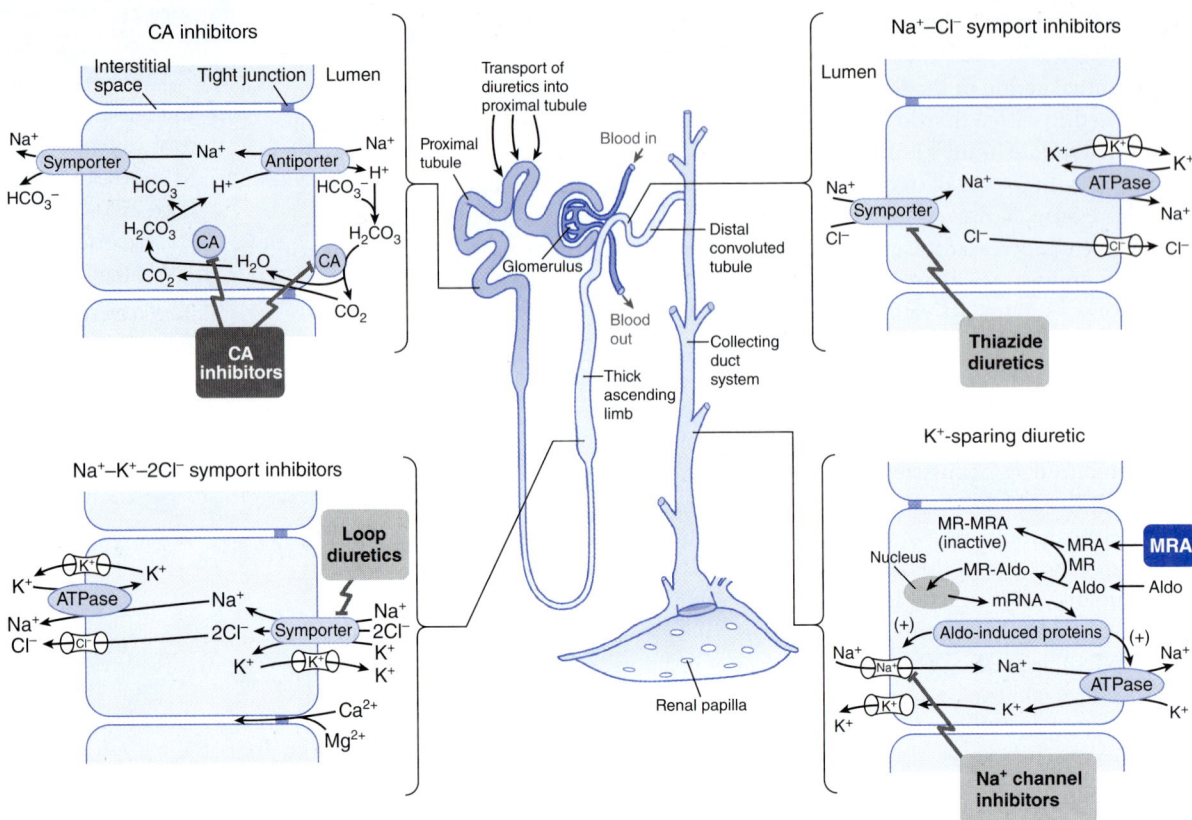

FIGURE 15-1 Summary of the site and mechanism of action of diuretics. Three important features of this summary figure are worth special note. 1. Transport of solute across epithelial cells in all nephron segments involves highly specialized proteins, which for the most part are apical and basolateral membrane integral proteins. 2. Diuretics target and block the action of epithelial proteins involved in solute transport. 3. The site and mechanism of action of a given class of diuretics are determined by the specific protein inhibited by the diuretic. Aldo, aldosterone; CA, carbonic anhydrase; MR, mineralocorticoid receptor; MRA, mineralocorticoid receptor antagonist.

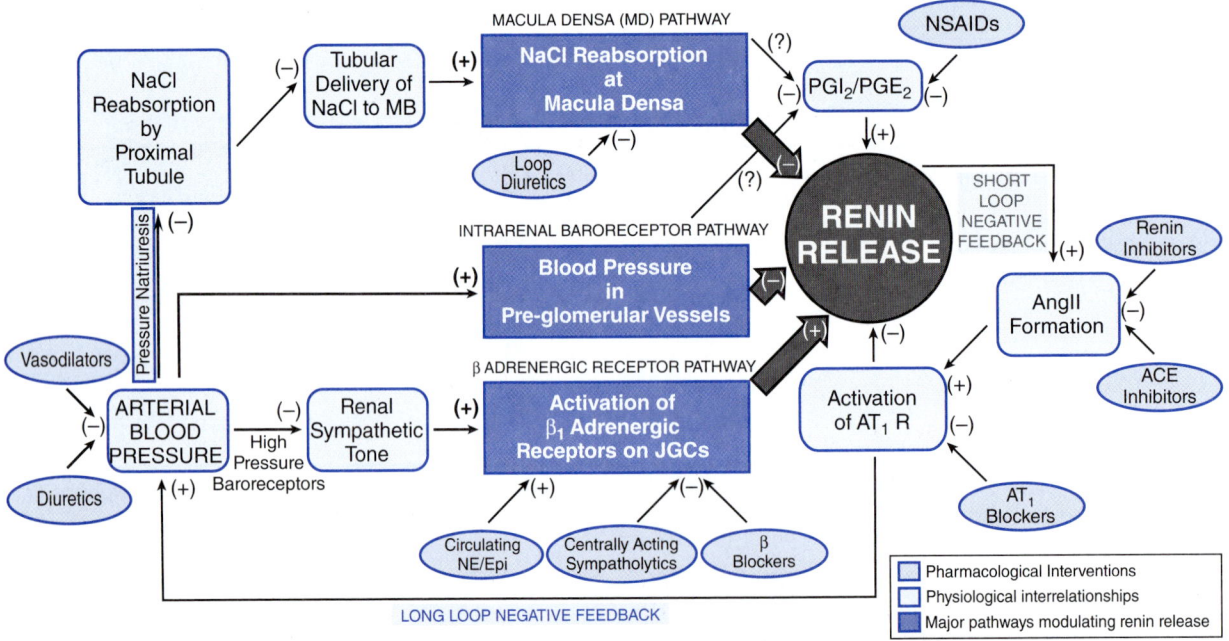

FIGURE 15-2 Schematic portrayal of the 3 major physiological pathways regulating renin release. ACE, angiotensin-converting enzyme; AngII, angiotensin II; $AT_1 R$, angiotensin subtype 1 receptor; JGCs, juxtaglomerular cells; MD, macula densa; NE/Epi, norepinephrine/epinephrine; NSAIDs, nonsteroidal anti-inflammatory drugs; PGI_2/PGE_2, prostaglandins I_2 and E_2.

Drug Therapy of Hypertension and Na+ Balance Disorders — CHAPTER 15

MECHANISMS OF ACTION OF INHIBITORS OF THE RENIN-ANGIOTENSIN SYSTEM (RAS; see Table 15-4)

DRUG CLASS	DRUG	MECHANISM OF ACTION
Angiotensin Converting Enzyme Inhibitors (ACEIs)	Captopril Enalapril Enalaprilat Lisinopril Benzapril Fosinopril Trandolapril Quinapril Ramipril Moexipril Perindopril	Prevent the conversion of AngI to active AngII by inhibiting angiotensin converting enzyme (ACE), thus blocking AngII's pressor responses and cardiovascular structural effects (see Figures 15-2, 15-3, and 15-4) Note: Many of the drugs are ester-containing prodrugs that have better bioavailability than the active molecules (see Figure 26-9 from *Goodman & Gilman's The Pharmacological Basis of Therapeutics*, 12th Edition for structures of drugs and prodrugs)
Angiotensin Receptor Blockers (ARBs)	Candesartan cilexetil Irbesartan Losartan Olmesartan medoxomil Telmisartan Valsartan	Competitive (but insurmountable) inhibitors of angiotensin AT_1 receptors (see Figures 15-2 and 15-4) that block AngII's pressor responses and cardiovascular structural effects (see Figure 15-3) Note: Some of the drugs are prodrugs that have better bioavailability than the active molecules (see Figure 26-10 from *Goodman & Gilman's The Pharmacological Basis of Therapeutics*, 12th Edition for structures of drugs and prodrugs)
Direct Renin Inhibitors (DRIs)	Aliskiren	Competitive inhibitor of renin preventing the conversion of angiotensinogen to AngI (see Figures 15-2 and 15-4)

CASE 15-2

A 68-year-old woman is being treated with 25 mg of hydrochlorothiazide for her hypertension. During her most recent checkup, her blood pressure was 161/93 and she was also diagnosed with type 2 diabetes.

a. **What changes should be made in her treatment?**

This patient has stage 2 hypertension (see Table 15-1) and an important comorbidity, type 2 diabetes mellitus. The risk of cardiovascular disease, disability, and death in hypertensive patients is increased markedly by concomitant cigarette smoking, diabetes, or elevated low-density lipoprotein; the coexistence of hypertension with

(Continued)

TABLE 15-4 Effects of Anti-hypertensive Agents on Components of the RAS

	DIRECT RENIN INHIBITORS	ACE-INHIBITORS	ARBs	DIURETICS	Ca^{2+} CHANNEL BLOCKERS	β BLOCKERS
PRC	↑	↑	↑	↑	↔	↓
PRA	↓	↑	↑	↑	↔	↓
AngI	↓	↑	↑	↑	↔	↓
AngII	↓	↓	↑	↑	↔	↓
ACE	↔	↓	↔			
Bradykinin	↔	↑	↔			
AT_1 receptors	↔	↔	inhibition			
AT_2 receptors	↔	↔	stimulation			

PRC, plasma renin concentration; PRA, plasma renin activity; ACE, angiotensin converting enzyme; ARB, angiotensin receptor blocker.

SECTION III — Modulation of Cardiovascular Function

DIURETIC THERAPY

- Diuretics are used to treat hypertension (see Table 15-2), edema, or volume overload associated with various disease states (see Figure 15-5).
- Restriction of dietary Na^+ intake is also important in reducing hypertension and edema, but compliance can be problematic.
- The pathophysiological mechanisms of edema formation and the effects of diuretics and dietary Na^+ restriction are shown in Figure 15-5.
- An algorithm for treating edema in patients caused by renal, hepatic, or cardiac disorders is shown in Figure 15-6.
- Diuretic resistance to a less effective diuretic such as a thiazide may require substituting with a more efficacious drug such as a loop diuretic, but resistance to loop diuretics can also occur.
- NSAID coadministration, which reduces the production of prostaglandins (especially PGE_2), is a common cause of diuretic resistance that can be prevented.
- There are several options available to overcome resistance to loop diuretics:
  - Bed rest to increase renal circulation
  - Increasing dose of the diuretic to the ceiling dose
  - Administering smaller doses more frequently
  - Continuous intravenous infusion
  - Combination therapy with 2 diuretics with different sites of action (eg, a thiazide and loop diuretic), although patients should be monitored to avoid serious complications such as hyponatremia, hypokalemia, and volume depletion
  - Reducing salt intake
  - Administering diuretics shortly before food intake to ensure effective concentrations of diuretic in the tubule lumen when salt load is highest

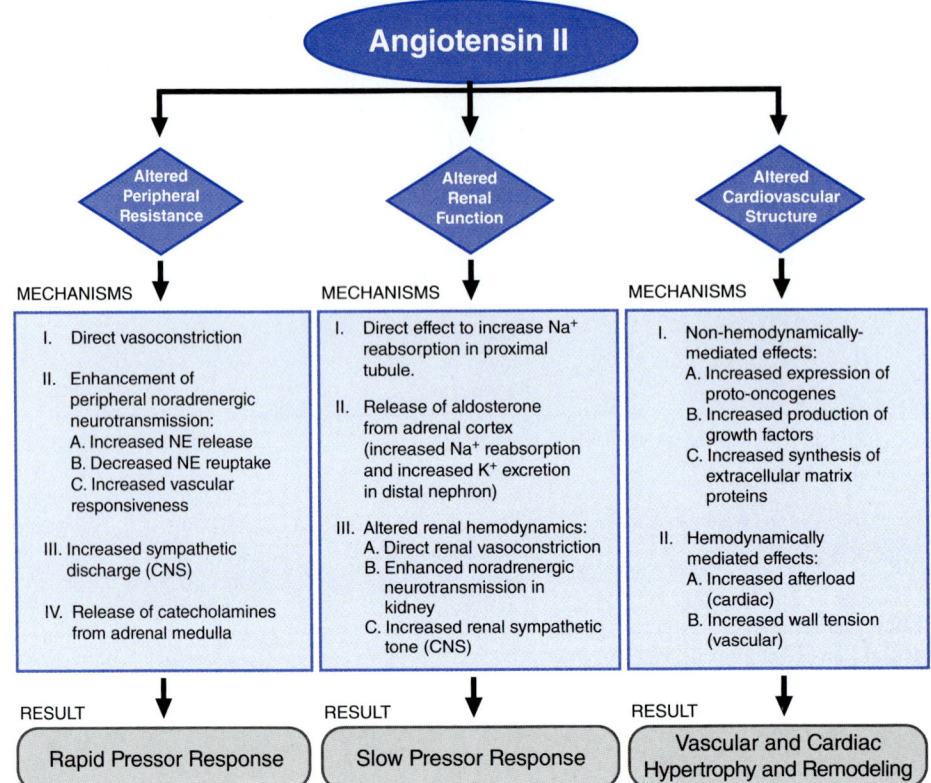

FIGURE 15-3 Summary of the 3 major effects of AngII and the mechanisms that mediate them. NE, norepinephrine.

these risk factors increases cardiovascular morbidity and mortality to a degree that is compounded by each additional risk factor. Because the purpose of treating hypertension is to decrease cardiovascular risk, other dietary and pharmacological interventions may be required to treat these comorbid conditions. ACE inhibitors/AT_1-receptor antagonists should be first-line drugs in the treatment of diabetics with hypertension in view of these drugs' well-established benefits in slowing the development and progression of diabetic glomerulopathy.

b. How would this patient's treatment differ if she did not have diabetes?

Patients with uncomplicated stage 2 hypertension will likely require a diuretic and another drug from a different class. Subsequently, doses can be titrated upward and additional drugs added to achieve goal blood pressures (blood pressure <140/90 mm Hg in uncomplicated patients). Some of these patients may require four different drugs to reach the goal.

c. This patient is prescribed enalapril in addition to her hydrochlorothiazide. What adverse effects are possible that the patient should be counseled to be aware of?

There are several cautions in the use of ACE inhibitors such as enalapril in patients with hypertension. Following the initial dose of an ACE inhibitor, there may be a considerable fall in blood pressure in some patients; this response to the initial dose is a function of plasma renin activity prior to treatment. The potential for a large initial drop in blood pressure is the reason for using a low dose to initiate therapy, especially in patients who may have a very active RAS supporting blood pressure, such as patients with diuretic-induced volume contraction or congestive heart failure.

(Continued)

Drug Therapy of Hypertension and Na⁺ Balance Disorders

CHAPTER 15

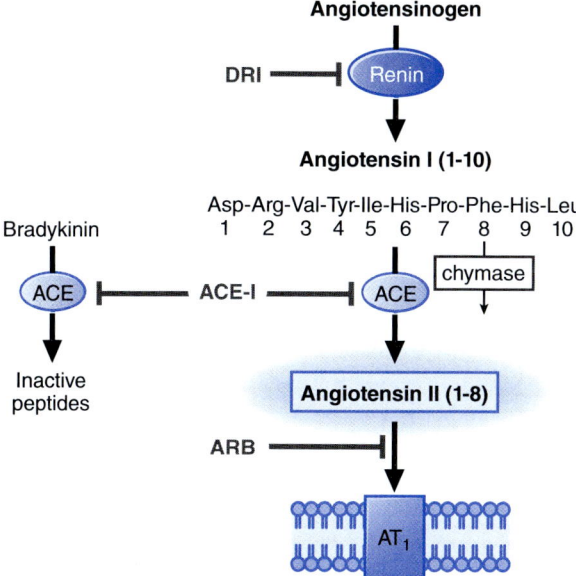

FIGURE 15-4 Inhibitors of the RAS. ACE-I, angiotensin-converting enzyme inhibitor; ARB, angiotensin receptor blocker; DRI, direct renin inhibitor.

PHYSIOLOGICAL FACTORS AND PHARMACOLOGICAL AGENTS REGULATING RENIN RELEASE (see Figure 15-2)

- Physiological factors
  - Arterial blood pressure (intrarenal baroreceptor pathway)
  - Dietary salt intake (macula densa pathway)
  - Activation of the sympathetic nervous system (β adrenergic receptor pathway)
  - Prostaglandins (PGI_2/PGE_2)
  - Activation of juxtaglomerular angiotensin AT_1 receptors
- Pharmacological agents
  - Loop diuretics
  - Nonsteroidal anti-inflammatory agents (NSAIDs)
  - ACE inhibitors, ARBs, and renin inhibitors
  - Centrally acting sympatholytic drugs
  - β Adrenergic blockers

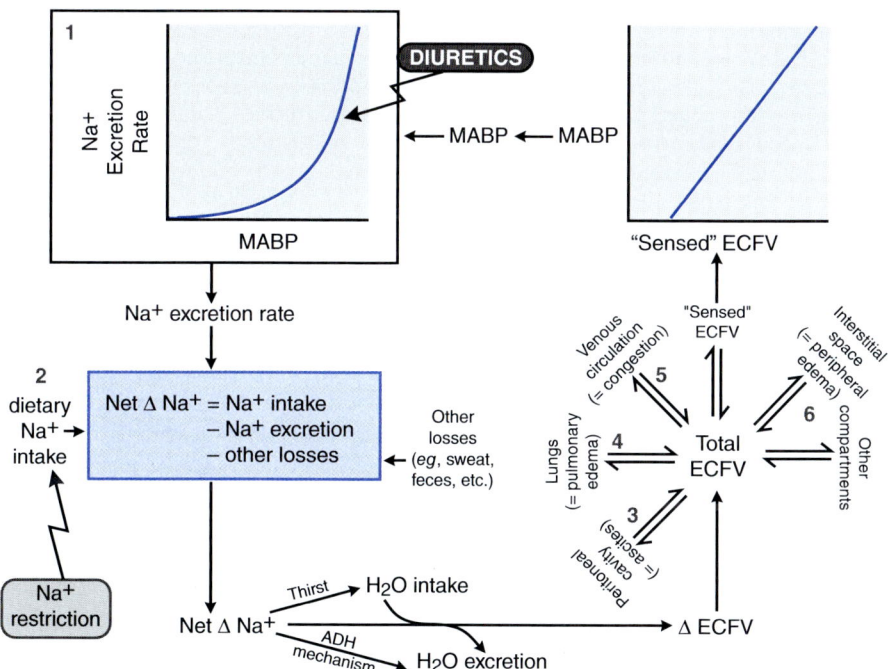

FIGURE 15-5 Interrelationships among renal function, Na⁺ intake, water homeostasis, distribution of extracellular fluid volume, and mean arterial blood pressure. Pathophysiological mechanisms of edema formation. 1. Rightward shift of renal pressure natriuresis curve. 2. Excessive dietary Na⁺ intake. 3. Increased distribution of extracellular fluid volume (ECFV) to peritoneal cavity (eg, liver cirrhosis with increased hepatic sinusoidal hydrostatic pressure) leading to ascites formation. 4. Increased distribution of ECFV to lungs (eg, left-sided heart failure with increased pulmonary capillary hydrostatic pressure) leading to pulmonary edema. 5. Increased distribution of ECFV to venous circulation (eg, right-sided heart failure) leading to venous congestion. 6. Peripheral edema caused by altered Starling forces causing increased distribution of ECFV to interstitial space (eg, diminished plasma proteins in nephrotic syndrome, severe burns, and liver disease).

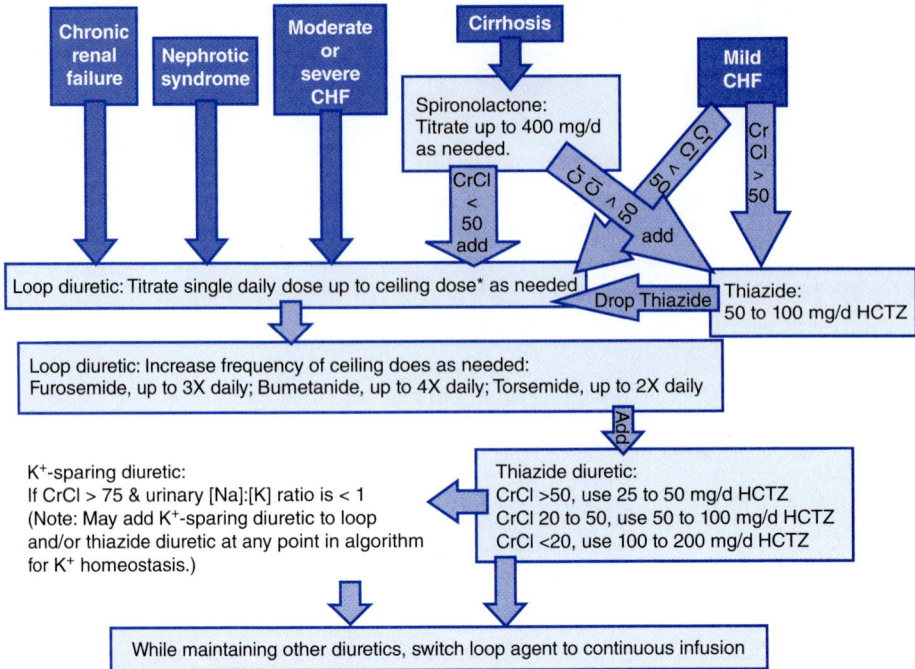

FIGURE 15-6 "Brater's algorithm" for diuretic therapy of chronic renal failure, nephrotic syndrome, congestive heart failure, and cirrhosis. Follow algorithm until adequate response is achieved. If adequate response is not obtained, advance to the next step. For illustrative purposes, the thiazide diuretic used in Brater's algorithm is hydrochlorothiazide (HCTZ). An alternative thiazide-type diuretic may be substituted with appropriate dosage adjustment so as to be pharmacologically equivalent to the recommended dose of HCTZ. *Do not combine two K^+-sparing diuretics because of the risk of hyperkalemia.* CrCl indicates creatinine clearance in mL/min, and ceiling dose refers to the smallest dose of diuretic that produces a near-maximal effect. Ceiling doses of loop diuretics and dosing regimens for continuous intravenous infusions of loop diuretics are disease-state-specific. Doses are for adults only.

With continuing treatment, there usually is a progressive fall in blood pressure that in most patients does not reach a maximum for several weeks.

ACE inhibitors not only prevent conversion of angiotensin I (AngI) to AngII, but also block degradation of bradykinin and substance P. The increase in bradykinin and substance P can give rise to a common (5-20% of patients) adverse effect, dry cough, and may also contribute to the less frequent (0.1-0.5%) occurrence of angioedema. Angioedema is a rare but serious and potentially fatal adverse effect of the ACE inhibitors. Patients starting treatment with these drugs should be explicitly warned to discontinue their use with the advent of any signs of angioedema; once ACE inhibitors are stopped, angioedema disappears within hours. AngII receptor antagonists have a reduced risk of dry cough and angioedema and can be used as alternative RAS inhibitors in patients who cannot tolerate the dry cough or who develop angioedema.

The attenuation of aldosterone production by ACE inhibitors also influences K^+ homeostasis. There is only a very small and clinically unimportant rise in serum K^+ when these agents are used alone in patients with normal renal function. However, substantial retention of K^+ can occur in some patients with renal insufficiency or diabetes. Furthermore, the potential for developing hyperkalemia should be considered when ACE inhibitors are used with other drugs that can cause K^+ retention, including the K^+-sparing diuretics (amiloride, triamterene, and spironolactone), NSAIDs, K^+ supplements, and β receptor antagonists. Some patients with diabetic nephropathy may be at greater risk of hyperkalemia.

Drug Therapy of Hypertension and Na+ Balance Disorders

CHAPTER 15

MECHANISMS OF ACTION OF SYMPATHOLYTIC AGENTS USED IN TREATING HYPERTENSION

DRUG CLASS	DRUG	MECHANISM OF ACTION
β Adrenergic Receptor Antagonists	Many (see Table 15-2 and Chapter 7)	Blocking β adrenergic receptors in the heart results in reduction in cardiac output by lowering myocardial contractility and heart rate, thus lowering arterial blood pressure Blockade of β adrenergic receptors in the juxtaglomerular complex reduces renin secretion, thereby reducing plasma AngII Some of the β adrenergic blockers have additional effects on lowering blood pressure through effects on blocking α_2 adrenergic receptors (labetalol, carvedilol), or increasing NO production (nebivolol)
α_1 Adrenergic Receptor Antagonists	Prazosin Terazosin Doxazosin	Block α_2 adrenergic receptors in arteriolar and venous vascular smooth muscle reduces arteriolar resistance and increases venous capacitance, respectively
Centrally Acting Adrenergic Agents—Methyldopa	Methyldopa	Converted to α-methylnorepinephrine and stored in central adrenergic neurons; it inhibits adrenergic neuronal outflow from the brainstem to the peripheral sympathetic nervous system
Centrally Acting Adrenergic Agents—α_2 Adrenergic Receptor Antagonists	Clonidine Guanabenz Guanfacine	Stimulate the α_{2A} subtype of α_2 adrenergic receptors in the brainstem, reducing sympathetic outflow from the CNS
Adrenergic Neuron Blocking Agents	Guanadrel Reserpine	Guanadrel acts as a false (inactive) neurotransmitter in postganglionic adrenergic neurons Reserpine acts at central and peripheral adrenergic neurons to delete catecholamines

MECHANISMS OF ACTION OF L-TYPE CA^{2+} CHANNEL BLOCKERS

DRUG CLASS	DRUG	MECHANISM OF ACTION
Dihydropyridines	Nisoldipine Felodipine Nicardipine Isradipine Amlodipine Clevidipine Nifedipine	Inhibit L-type voltage-gated Ca^{2+} channels in arteriolar vascular smooth resulting in smooth muscle relaxation
Nondihydropyridines	Verapamil Diltiazem	Inhibit L-type voltage-gated Ca^{2+} channels in arteriolar vascular smooth resulting in smooth muscle relaxation The nondihydropyridine calcium channel blockers also inhibit L-type Ca^{2+} channels in heart, thereby lowering cardiac output by effects on SA node (bradycardia) and reduced contractility

CASE 15-3

A 31-year-old woman is being treated for mild hypertension with valsartan and hydrochlorothiazide. She is in good health and becomes pregnant.

a. Are the drugs she is taking for her hypertension safe in pregnancy?

All of the thiazide-like drugs cross the placenta, but they have not been shown to have direct adverse effects on the fetus. However, ACE inhibitors, AT$_1$-receptor antagonists, and the direct renin inhibitor, aliskiren, are teratogenic and should be discontinued as soon as pregnancy is detected.

b. What changes in her drug therapy should be made?

This woman had chronic hypertension prior to her pregnancy, but is considered low risk because she had mild hypertension with no evidence of organ damage. To minimize risk to the fetus, she should not receive an antihypertensive drug unless

(Continued)

SECTION III Modulation of Cardiovascular Function

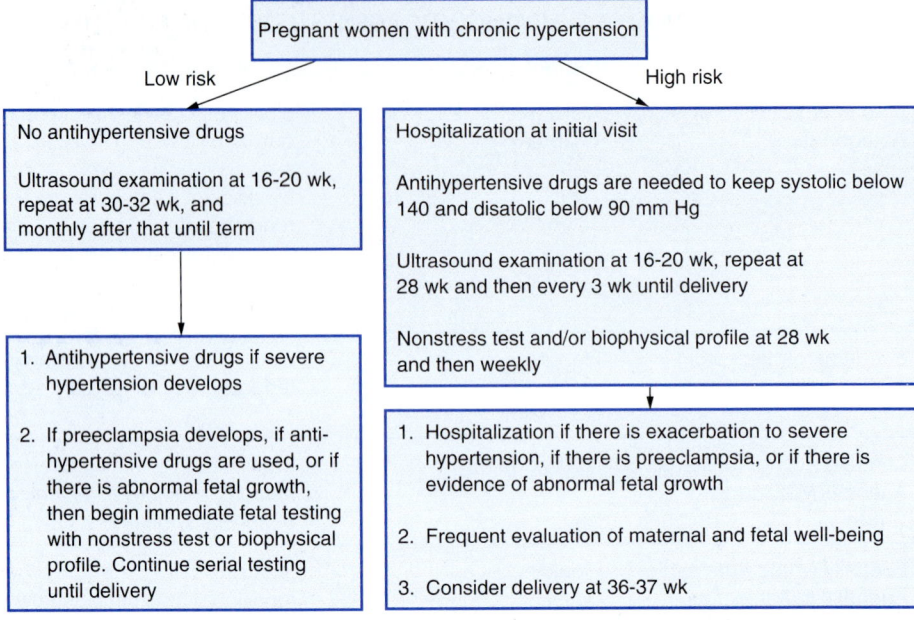

FIGURE 15-7 Algorithm for the management of pregnant women with chronic hypertension. (*Reproduced with permission from Sibai BM. Chronic hypertension in pregnancy. Obstet Gynecol. 2002;100:369-377.*)

her systolic blood pressure exceeds 160 mm Hg or her diastolic pressure exceeds 110 mm Hg (see Figure 15-7). If her blood pressure exceeds these values, methyldopa is the drug of choice because of its record of safety and efficacy. Hydralazine and a β-adrenergic blocker such as labetalol can also be used. Patients at high risk or who develop hypertension during pregnancy should be managed according to the algorithm shown in Figure 15-7.

MECHANISMS OF ACTION OF DIRECT VASODILATORS

DRUG CLASS	DRUG	MECHANISM OF ACTION
Arterial vasodilators	Hydralazine	Hydralazine directly relaxes arteriolar smooth muscle, but the mechanism is unclear
	Minoxidil	Minoxidil is bioactivated to form minoxidil sulfate which relaxes arteriolar smooth muscle by activating ATP-modulated K$^+$ channels (K$_{ATP}$ channels)
	Diazoxide	Diazoxide activates vascular smooth muscle K$^+$ channels
	Fenoldopam	Fenoldopam is a short-acting D1 dopamine receptor agonist that has minimal adrenergic effects
Arterial and venous vasodilators	Nitroprusside	Acts as a nonselective vasodilator by releasing NO through a mechanism(s) that is unclear

CASE 15-4

A 68-year-old man has taken diltiazem for his hypertension and his chronic angina for more than 5 years. He suffers a mild myocardial infarction and during his stay in the hospital, he is taken off diltiazem and placed on a regimen that includes captopril, carvedilol, and aspirin.

a. What is the rationale for taking this patient off diltiazem?

Diltiazem is a calcium channel blocker that is effective in treating hypertension and stable angina because of its effects on relaxing vascular smooth muscle, thus reducing arterial blood pressure and dilating coronary arteries. Its calcium channel blocking activity also reduces cardiac output by slowing heart rate and lowering cardiac contractility. Because of its negative inotropic effects, it can impair cardiac output during and after a myocardial infarction.

(Continued)

Drug Therapy of Hypertension and Na+ Balance Disorders — CHAPTER 15

b. **What is the rationale for placing this patient on captopril during his stay in the hospital?**

The beneficial effects of ACE inhibitors in acute myocardial infarction are particularly large in hypertensive and diabetic patients. Unless contraindicated (eg, cardiogenic shock or severe hypotension), ACE inhibitors should be started immediately during the acute phase of myocardial infarction and can be administered along with thrombolytics, aspirin, and β adrenergic receptor antagonists. In high-risk patients (eg, large infarct, systolic ventricular dysfunction), ACE inhibition should be continued long term. One of the benefits of long-term ACE inhibitor therapy is to inhibit AngII-stimulated remodeling of the cardiovascular system, which causes hypertrophy of vascular and cardiac cells and increased synthesis and deposition of collagen by cardiac fibroblasts (see Figure 15-3). This remodeling process is thought to be an important feature in the development of chronic heart failure. Current recommendations are to use ACE inhibitors as first-line agents for the treatment of heart failure and to reserve ARBs for treatment of heart failure in patients who cannot tolerate or have an unsatisfactory response to ACE inhibitors.

c. **Within an hour of starting the patient on captopril, he begins to notice swelling in his nose, throat, mouth, glottis, larynx, lips, and tongue. What is likely to be causing this adverse effect and how can it be reversed?**

The patient is experiencing angioedema, which is caused by an increase in circulating bradykinin. A small number of patients receiving ACE inhibitors experience angioedema that results from inhibition of ACE, the enzyme that degrades bradykinin and substance P. To reverse the drug's effect, the ACE inhibitor should be stopped, and the angioedema will disappear within hours. While the effects of the angioedema are diminishing, the patient's airway should be protected, and if necessary, epinephrine, an antihistamine, and/or a glucocorticoid should be administered. African Americans have a 4.5 times greater risk of ACE inhibitor–induced angioedema than Caucasians. Although rare, angioedema of the intestine (visceral angioedema) characterized by emesis, watery diarrhea, and abdominal pain also has been reported. As an alternative to an ACE inhibitor in this patient, an ARB such as valsartan can be substituted. The incidence of angioedema with ARBs is much lower than with ACE inhibitors. Valsartan is approved for heart failure and to reduce cardiovascular mortality in clinically stable patients with left ventricular failure or left ventricular dysfunction following myocardial infarction.

d. **What is the rationale for starting this patient on carvedilol?**

β Adrenergic receptor antagonists that do not have intrinsic sympathomimetic activity (ie, partial agonists) improve mortality in myocardial infarction patients. They should be started early and continued indefinitely in patients who can tolerate them. Carvedilol is a mixed α–β receptor antagonist that is approved for use in patients with left ventricular dysfunction.

MECHANISMS OF ACTION OF VASOPRESSIN RECEPTOR AGONISTS AND ANTAGONISTS (see Figure 15-8)

DRUG CLASS	DRUG	MECHANISM OF ACTION
Vasopressin Agonist—V_1 Receptor Agonists	Vasopressin Terlipressin	Activate V_1 receptors in GI and vascular smooth muscle to cause contraction
Vasopressin Agonist—V_2 Receptor Agonist	Desmopressin	Activate V_2 receptors in collecting duct to increase water permeability (antidiuresis) Activate extrarenal V_2 receptors on vascular endothelium to release procoagulant factor VIII and von Willebrand factor
Vasopressin Antagonists—Selective V_2 Receptor (V_2R) Antagonists ("Aquaretics")	Tolvaptan	Inhibit V_2 receptors in collecting duct to increase free water excretion without excretion of electrolytes
Vasopressin Antagonists—Nonselective $V_{1a}R$/V_2R Antagonist ("Aquaretics")	Conivaptan	Inhibit V_2 receptors in collecting duct to increase free water excretion without excretion of electrolytes Inhibition of V_{1a} receptors in mesangial cells and vascular smooth muscle cells of vasa recta and efferent arteriole acts to increase inner medullary blood flow

SECTION III
Modulation of Cardiovascular Function

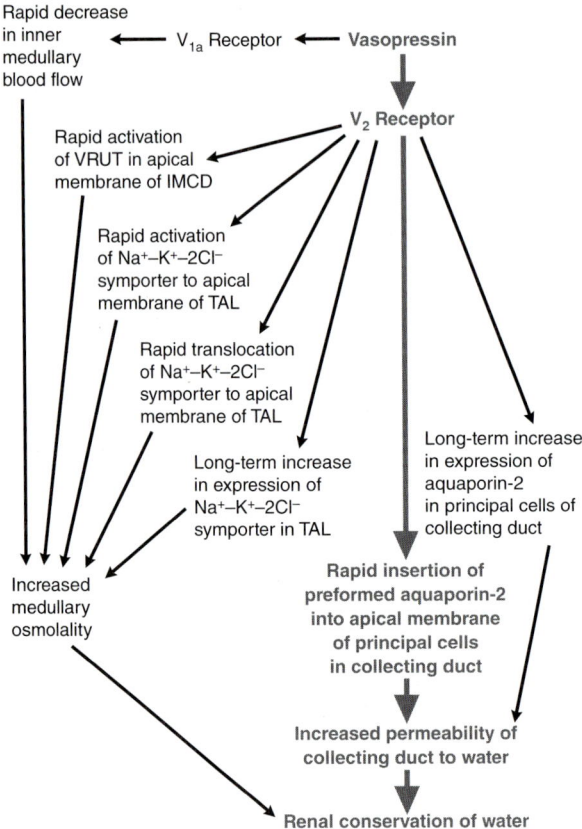

FIGURE 15-8 Mechanisms by which vasopressin increases the renal conservation of water. Gray and black arrows denote major and minor pathways, respectively. IMCD, inner medullary collecting duct; TAL, thick ascending limb; VRUT, vasopressin-regulated urea transporter.

CASE 15-5

A 74-year-old male patient with heart failure is hospitalized because of significant pulmonary edema that is impairing his breathing. He is receiving valsartan and furosemide.

a. What are the mechanisms of action of these agents?

Valsartan is an angiotensin receptor blocker (ARB) that lowers blood pressure and prevents vascular and cardiac remodeling by blocking the effects of AngII on AT_1 receptors (see Figure 15-3). It has been shown to reduce morbidity and mortality in patients with heart failure. Furosemide is a highly efficacious diuretic that inhibits the Na^+-K^+-$2Cl^-$ symporter in the thick ascending limb of the loop of Henle; hence, it is termed a loop diuretic.

b. What additional agent(s) might be added to improve natriuresis and improve hemodynamics?

An agent that might be useful in this patient is nesiritide which is recombinant human B-type natriuretic peptide (BNP). BNP is an endogenous peptide released by cardiac ventricular muscle when it is stretched. BNP activates natriuretic peptide receptors on the surface of epithelial cells in the inner medullary collecting duct which stimulates the formation of cyclic GMP that subsequently inhibits the cyclic nucleotide-gated nonspecific cation channel (CNGC); the CNGC is the primary channel for Na^+ entry in these cells. BNP also relaxes vascular smooth muscle and lowers vascular resistance.

Eplerenone might also be useful in this patient. It is a diuretic that acts on the mineralocorticoid receptor to blocks the synthesis of aldosterone-induced proteins (AIPs) in epithelial cells in the late distal tubule and collecting duct. It has been

(Continued)

Drug Therapy of Hypertension and Na⁺ Balance Disorders

shown to reduce morbidity and mortality in patients when added to other agents in patients with moderate to severe heart failure. However, because it is a K⁺-sparing diuretic, it could cause hyperkalemia when used in combination with valsartan.

c. After several days in the hospital, the patient still has significant edema, but he has become hyponatremic. What agent might be useful in causing diuresis without loss of Na⁺?

A vasopressin receptor antagonist such as tolvaptan or conivaptan might be used to induce diuresis without significant loss of Na⁺. These agents are referred to as aquaretics because they can increase renal-free water excretion without corresponding loss of Na⁺ as with diuretics such as furosemide.

Tolvaptan is a selective oral V_2R antagonist that is approved for clinically significant hypervolemic and euvolemic hyponatremia. The drug is labeled with a black box warning against too rapid correction of hyponatremia (can have serious and fatal consequences) and the recommendation to initiate therapy in a hospital setting capable of close monitoring of serum Na⁺. Tolvaptan is contraindicated in patients receiving drugs that inhibit CYP3A4.

Conivaptan is a nonselective $V_{1a}R/V_2R$ antagonist that is FDA approved for the treatment of hospitalized patients with euvolemic hyponatremia and hypervolemic hyponatremia. The drug is available only for intravenous infusion. In CHF patients, conivaptan increases renal free water excretion without a change in systemic vascular resistance.

KEY CONCEPTS

- Nonpharmacological approaches to treat moderately elevated blood pressure may be sufficient in many patients and can augment the effects of antihypertensive drugs.
- Choice of antihypertensive drugs for individual patients may be complex and should be driven by the likely benefit to patient, taking into consideration the patient's concomitant diseases, adverse effects of specific drugs, and cost.
- Diuretics are preferred as initial therapy for most patients with uncomplicated stage 1 hypertension who are unresponsive to nonpharmacological approaches, although patients are also commonly treated with other drugs: β receptor antagonists, ACE inhibitors/AT_1 receptor antagonists, and Ca^{2+} channel blockers.
- Patients with congestive heart failure should ideally be treated with a diuretic, β receptor antagonist, ACE inhibitor/AT_1 receptor antagonist, and (in selected patients) spironolactone.
- ACE inhibitors or AT_1 receptor antagonists should be first-line drugs in the treatment of diabetics with hypertension.
- To achieve stringent control of hypertension, many patients require 2, 3, or 4 appropriately selected drugs used at optimal doses.

SUMMARY QUIZ

QUESTION 15-1 A 46-year-old man with uncomplicated stage 1 hypertension is placed on lisinopril and hydrochlorothiazide. After several weeks, the patient develops a dry cough. What is the underlying cause of the cough?

a. Bradykinins that accumulate because of the effects of lowering blood pressure.
b. Bradykinins that accumulate because of the effects of lisinopril.
c. The diuresis caused by hydrochlorothiazide dries out mucus membranes in the upper respiratory tract.
d. The dry cough is unrelated to the pharmacological effects of either drug.

SECTION III

Modulation of Cardiovascular Function

QUESTION 15-2 A 55-year-old woman who begins taking amlodipine to lower her blood pressure develops edema in her ankles after several weeks of taking the drug. What is causing the edema?
a. The reduced blood pressure is causing reduced water excretion by the kidneys.
b. Amlodipine has direct effects on the kidney to reduce water excretion.
c. Amlodipine increases capillary hydrostatic pressure by dilating precapillary arterioles without dilating postcapillary vessels.
d. The edema is unrelated to the pharmacological effects of the drug.

QUESTION 15-3 An elderly man with stage 2 hypertension is taking valsartan and hydrochlorothiazide. He also takes ibuprofen for his arthritis. He monitors his blood pressure daily, and tells you that his blood pressure is often greater than 140/90. What is likely causing these high blood pressure readings?
a. The valsartan-hydrochlorothiazide combination is known to be ineffective.
b. The ibuprofen is reducing the effectiveness of the antihypertensives.
c. He is probably not using the blood pressure cuff correctly.
d. He is probably not taking his antihypertensive drugs as prescribed.

QUESTION 15-4 A patient with long-standing hypertension is taking aliskiren, amlodipine, and triamterene. What adverse effects might occur with this drug combination?
a. There is a risk of hyperkalemia with this drug combination.
b. There is a risk of hypokalemia with this drug combination.
c. There is a risk of hypernatremia with this drug combination.
d. There is a risk of hyponatremia with this drug combination.

QUESTION 15-5 A 71-year-old man with chronic renal failure with edema has been titrated up to the maximal single daily dose of bumetanide, but he still has significant edema. What option should initially be considered to reduce the edema?
a. Increase the single dose of bumetanide above the ceiling dose.
b. Increase the frequency of dosing of bumetanide.
c. Add a K^+-sparing diuretic.
d. Add a thiazide diuretic.
e. Begin IV infusion of bumetanide.

SUMMARY QUIZ ANSWER KEY

QUESTION 15-1 Answer is **b**. Between 5 and 20% of patients taking ACE inhibitors develop dry cough which some patients cannot tolerate. The cough is caused by the accumulation of bradykinin and substance P that is a direct result of inhibiting ACE, which is the enzyme that degrades these endogenous peptides. For patients who cannot tolerate the cough, ARBs are a good option because there is a much lower incidence of this adverse effect.

QUESTION 15-2 Answer is **c**. The calcium channel blockers are selective for inhibiting arteriolar smooth muscle compared to venous smooth muscle. This can result in an increase in capillary hydrostatic pressure which forces fluid into the interstitial space. To alleviate the edema, calcium channel blockers are often administered with a thiazide diuretic to prevent the edema. This combination also has additive antihypertensive effects since thiazides lower blood pressure through a different mechanism.

Drug Therapy of Hypertension and Na+ Balance Disorders

CHAPTER 15

QUESTION 15-3 Answer is **b**. It is most likely that ibuprofen is opposing the actions of the antihypertensive drugs. NSAIDs are known to reduce the effectiveness of many antihypertensive drugs, especially those that inhibit the renin-angiotensin system (see Figure 15-2). It is also possible that the patient is not adherent to his antihypertensive medications, or his salt intake is excessive. Another possibility is that other drugs, including over-the-counter drugs or herbal preparations, are the cause. For example, NSAIDs, sympathomimetic decongestants, cyclosporine, erythropoietin, ephedra (ma huang), and licorice are known to reduce the effectiveness of many antihypertensive drugs. Before changing medications or altering dosing it is important to identify and eliminate, if possible, causes of the resistant hypertension.

QUESTION 15-4 Answer is **a**. Both aliskiren, a direct renin inhibitor, and triamterene, a K+-sparing diuretic, can increase plasma K+ concentrations. When used in combination they can be additive in their effects and can cause hyperkalemia.

QUESTION 15-5 Answer is **b**. Patients with chronic renal failure and other disease states often require aggressive diuretic therapies to control edema. Figure 15-6 illustrates "Brater's algorithm" for diuretic therapy in various disease states including chronic renal failure. According to the algorithm, the next step after titrating the single daily dose of a loop diuretic up to the ceiling dose is to increase the frequency of dosing. In the case of bumetanide, the algorithm recommends increasing the frequency of the ceiling dose to 4X daily. Nothing is gained by increasing a single dose above the ceiling dose (the dose that gives near maximal effect for a given disease state). A K+-sparing diuretic can be added to the loop diuretic to maintain K+ homeostasis and may improve therapeutic response. The next step in the algorithm is to add a thiazide diuretic which may result in a synergistic interaction. The last step in the algorithm is to switch to continuous infusion of the loop diuretic while maintaining the other diuretics.

SUMMARY TABLE: DRUGS USED IN THE TREATMENT OF HYPERTENSION, EDEMA, AND DISORDERS OF NA+ AND WATER BALANCE

CLASS AND SUBCLASSES	NAMES	CLINICAL USES	TOXICITIES COMMON	TOXICITIES UNIQUE; CLINICALLY IMPORTANT
Diuretics—Inhibitors of Carbonic Anhydrase	Acetazolamide	Edema when used in combination with other diuretics Prophylaxis and treatment of high-altitude sickness Familial periodic paralysis Correcting metabolic alkalosis, especially diuretic-induced H+ excretion	Most adverse effects, contraindications, and drug interactions are secondary to urinary alkalinization or metabolic acidosis	Sulfonamide-related toxicities, including bone marrow suppression, skin toxicities, renal lesions, and allergic reactions At high doses, drowsiness and paresthesias
	Dorzolamide brinzolamide	Open-angle glaucoma and other situations that require lowering intraocular pressure		
Diuretics—Osmotic Diuretics	Glycerin Isosorbide Mannitol Urea (currently not available in the United States)	Treatment of dialysis disequilibrium syndrome by increasing the osmolality of the extracellular fluid By increasing plasma osmotic pressure they are used to reduce intraocular pressure and reduce cerebral edema	Headache, nausea, and vomiting caused by hyponatremia due to extraction of water from intracellular compartments	Can cause pulmonary edema in patients with heart failure Contraindicated in patients who are anuric due to severe renal disease

SECTION III — Modulation of Cardiovascular Function

CLASS AND SUBCLASSES	NAMES	CLINICAL USES	TOXICITIES COMMON	TOXICITIES UNIQUE; CLINICALLY IMPORTANT
Diuretics—Inhibitors of Na^+-K^+-$2Cl^-$ Symport (Loop Diuretics, High-Ceiling Diuretics)	Furosemide Bumetanide Ethacrynic acid Torsemide	Hypertension (although short $t_{1/2}$ limits use) Chronic congestive heart failure to reduce venous and pulmonary congestion Acute pulmonary edema Edema of nephrotic syndrome, chronic kidney disease, and liver cirrhosis	Overzealous use of loop diuretics can cause serious depletion of total-body Na^+ If dietary K^+ intake is not sufficient, hypokalemia may develop increasing the risk of arrhythmias	Ototoxicity (including hearing loss and vertigo) is usually reversible Irreversible ototoxicity can occur at high doses, with rapid IV administration, and during concomitant therapy with other drugs known to be ototoxic Hyperuricemia, hyperglycemia, and dyslipidemia Contraindicated in severe hyponatremia and volume depletion, hypersensitivity to sulfonamides (only the sulfonamide-based agents)
Diuretics—Inhibitors of Na^+-Cl^- Symport (Thiazide and Thiazide-Like Diuretics)	Bendroflumethiazide Chlorothiazide Hydrochlorothiazide Hydroflumethiazide Methyclothiazide Polythiazide Trichlormethiazide Chlorthalidone Indapamide Metolazone Quinethazone	Widely used for the treatment of hypertension either alone or in combination with other antihypertensive drugs (can have additive or synergistic effects when used in combination with other classes) Best initial therapy for uncomplicated hypertension Edema associated with heart failure, hepatic cirrhosis, and renal disease (except when GFR is <30-40 mL/min) Ca^{2+} nephrolithiasis Treatment of nephrogenic diabetes insipidus by increasing proximal tubular water reabsorption (secondary to volume contraction) and by blocking the ability of the distal convoluted tubule to form dilute urine	If dietary K^+ intake is not sufficient, hypokalemia may develop increasing the risk of arrhythmias Hypokalemia can increase risk of fatal arrhythmias when used in combination with quinidine (see Chapter 18)	Most serious adverse effects of thiazides are related to abnormalities of fluid and electrolyte balance (extracellular volume depletion, hypotension, hypokalemia, hyponatremia, hypochloremia, metabolic alkalosis, hypomagnesemia, hypercalcemia, and hyperuricemia) Thiazide diuretics have caused fatal or near-fatal hyponatremia Impaired glucose tolerance, dyslipidemias Contraindicated in patients with sulfonamide hypersensitivity
Diuretics—Inhibitors of Renal Epithelial Na^+ Channels (K^+-sparing Diuretics)	Triamterene and fixed dose combination triamterene/hydrochloro-thiazide	Used in combination with thiazide and loop diuretics to augment diuresis and antihypertensive effects and offset the kaliuretic effects of the thiazide and loop diuretics	Nausea, vomiting, diarrhea, and headache	Life-threatening hyperkalemia, thus contraindicated in patients with hyperkalemia or those at risk of hyperkalemia
	Amiloride and fixed dose combination amiloride/hydrochlorothiazide	Used in combination with thiazide and loop diuretics to augment diuresis and antihypertensive effects, and offset the kaliuretic effects of the thiazide and loop diuretics	Nausea, vomiting, leg cramps, and dizziness	Life-threatening hyperkalemia, thus contraindicated in patients with hyperkalemia or those at risk of hyperkalemia

Drug Therapy of Hypertension and Na+ Balance Disorders — CHAPTER 15

CLASS AND SUBCLASSES	NAMES	CLINICAL USES	TOXICITIES — COMMON	TOXICITIES — UNIQUE; CLINICALLY IMPORTANT
Diuretics—Mineralocorticoid Receptor Antagonists (Aldosterone Antagonists, K+-Sparing Diuretics)	Spironolactone Eplerenone	Similar to other K+-sparing diuretics, spironolactone is often co-administered with thiazide or loop diuretics to treat edema and hypertension Spironolactone is the diuretic of choice in patients with hepatic cirrhosis When added to standard therapy, morbidity and mortality are reduced in patients with heart failure (see Chapter 17)	Can bind to other steroid receptors and may cause gynecomastia, impotence, decreased libido, hirsutism, and menstrual irregularities Can induce diarrhea and other gastric disturbances Can cause CNS effects such drowsiness, ataxia, and headache	Life-threatening hyperkalemia, thus contraindicated in patients with hyperkalemia or those at risk of hyperkalemia Contraindicated in patients with peptic ulcers
Diuretics—Atrial Natriuretic Peptides (Inhibitors of the Cyclic Nucleotide-Gated Nonspecific Cation Channel)	Human recombinant ANP (carperitide, available only in Japan) Human recombinant BNP (nesiritide)	Use is limited to patients with acutely decompensated congestive heart failure who are short of breath at rest to improve hemodynamics (should not be used in place of diuretics)		
Angiotensin Converting Enzyme Inhibitors (ACEIs)	Captopril Enalapril Enalaprilat Lisinopril Benzapril Fosinopril Trandolapril Quinapril Ramipril Moexipril Perindopril	Treatment of hypertension as monotherapy or in combination with a Ca^{2+} channel blocker, β adrenergic blocker, or diuretic Prevention or delay of heart failure in patients with systolic dysfunction Prevention of cardiovascular events in patients with acute myocardial infarction and in patients who are high risk of cardiovascular events Prevention or delay of renal disease in patients with type 1 diabetes mellitus	Hypotension, especially in patients with elevated plasma renin activity Dry cough (5-20% of patients) due to accumulation of bradykinin, substance P and/or prostaglandins in the lungs	May cause hyperkalemia in patients taking K+-sparing diuretics, K+ supplements, β receptor blockers, or NSAIDs Acute renal failure in patients with reduced renal perfusion Patients who are pregnant should discontinue ACEIs due to teratogenic potential Angioedema (0.1-0.5% of patients)
Angiotensin Receptor Blockers (ARBs)	Candesartan cilexetil Irbesartan Losartan Olmesartan medoxomil Telmisartan Valsartan	Treatment of hypertension as monotherapy or in combination with a Ca^{2+} channel blocker, β adrenergic blocker, or diuretic Irbesartan and losartan are approved for diabetic nephropathy Losartan is approved for stroke prophylaxis Valsartan is approved for heart failure and to reduce cardiovascular events in patients with left ventricular dysfunction following myocardial infarction	Hypotension in patients whose blood pressure is highly dependent on the RAS or with combination therapy with other antihypertensive drugs Incidence of cough is lower than ACEIs	Hyperkalemia in patients with renal disease or those taking K+-sparing diuretics or K+ supplements Acute renal failure in patients with reduced renal perfusion Incidence of angioedema is lower than ACEIs Patients who are pregnant should discontinue ARBs due to teratogenic potential

SECTION III — Modulation of Cardiovascular Function

CLASS AND SUBCLASSES	NAMES	CLINICAL USES	TOXICITIES COMMON	TOXICITIES UNIQUE; CLINICALLY IMPORTANT
Direct Renin Inhibitors (DRIs)	Aliskiren	Treatment of hypertension as monotherapy or in combination with other antihypertensive agents, particularly with ACE inhibitors or ARBs (which increase plasma renin activity; see Table 15-2) Cardioprotective and renoprotective in combination therapy Recommended in patients intolerant to other antihypertensive drugs or for further blood pressure control	Mild GI symptoms at high doses Incidence of cough and angioedema less than with ACE inhibitors	Not recommended in pregnant patients
β Adrenergic Receptor Antagonists	Many (see Table 15-2 and Chapter 7)	Effective therapy for all grades of hypertension as monotherapy or in combination with other agents Highly preferred for hypertensive patients with conditions such as MI, ischemic heart disease, or congestive heart failure	Should be avoided in patients with reactive airway disease (asthma) or with SA or AV nodal dysfunction or in combination with other drugs that inhibit AV conduction, such as verapamil	Risk of hypoglycemic reactions may be increased in diabetics taking insulin Sudden discontinuation can cause rebound hypertension; dosage should be tapered gradually over 10-14 days prior to discontinuation
α_1 Adrenergic Receptor Antagonists	Prazosin Terazosin Doxazosin	Not recommended as monotherapy for hypertensive patients Used primarily in conjunction with diuretics, β blockers, and other antihypertensive agents Useful for hypertensive patients with benign prostatic hyperplasia because they also improve urinary symptoms	First-dose phenomenon (in up to 50% of patients) in which symptomatic orthostatic hypotension occurs within 30-90 minutes (or longer) of the initial dose of the drug or after a dosage increase	Patients with pheochromocytoma can have a vasoconstrictor response to epinephrine resulting from activation of unblocked vascular α_2 adrenergic receptors
Centrally Acting Adrenergic Agents—Methyldopa	Methyldopa	Current use largely limited to treatment of hypertension in pregnancy, where it has a record for safety	Transient sedation Diminution in psychic energy may persist, depression occurs occasionally Dryness of the mouth Diminished libido Parkinsonian signs Hyper-prolactinemia that may cause gynecomastia and galactorrhea	May precipitate severe bradycardia and sinus arrest Hepatotoxicity, sometimes associated with fever >20% of patients who receive methyldopa for a year develop a positive Coombs test and 1-5% of these patients will develop a hemolytic anemia that requires prompt discontinuation of the drug
Centrally Acting Adrenergic Agents—α_2 Adrenergic Receptor Antagonists	Clonidine Guanabenz Guanfacine	No fixed place for these drugs in the treatment of hypertension because of CNS effects and lack of evidence demonstrating reduction in risk of adverse cardiovascular events	Sedation and xerostomia are prominent Postural hypotension and erectile dysfunction may be prominent	Symptomatic bradycardia and sinus arrest in patients with dysfunction of the SA node and AV block in patients with AV nodal disease; sudden discontinuation may cause a withdrawal syndrome consisting of headache, apprehension, tremors, abdominal pain, sweating, tachycardia, rebound hypertension

Drug Therapy of Hypertension and Na⁺ Balance Disorders — CHAPTER 15

CLASS AND SUBCLASSES	NAMES	CLINICAL USES	TOXICITIES COMMON	TOXICITIES UNIQUE; CLINICALLY IMPORTANT
Adrenergic Neuron Blocking Agents	Guanadrel (not marketed in the United States) Reserpine	Rarely used because of adverse effects	Undesirable effects that are related to sympathetic blockade, including hypotension during standing and exercise, general feeling of fatigue and lassitude CNS effects with reserpine include sedation and inability to perform complex tasks	Occasional psychotic depression that can lead to suicide with reserpine Reserpine must be discontinued at first sign of depression; reserpine-induced depression may last several months after drug is discontinued
L-type Ca^{2+} Channel Blockers—Dihydropyridines	Nisoldipine Felodipine Nicardipine Isradipine Amlodipine Clevidipine Nifedipine	Used alone or in combination with other antihypertensive drugs May be more efficacious than other agents as monotherapy in elderly subjects and in African Americans, population groups in which the low renin status is more prevalent May be a preferred treatment in patients with isolated systolic hypertension Parenteral administration of the short-acting clevidipine may be useful in treating severe or perioperative hypertension	Reflex tachycardia	
L-type Ca^{2+} Channel Blockers—Nondihydropyridines	Verapamil Diltiazem	Used alone or in combination with other antihypertensive drugs May be more efficacious than other agents as monotherapy in elderly subjects and in African Americans, population groups in which the low renin status is more prevalent May be a preferred treatment in patients with isolated systolic hypertension	Direct negative chrontropic and inotropic effects Concurrent use of a β receptor antagonist may magnify negative chronotropic effects of these drugs or cause heart block in susceptible patients	May worsen symptoms in patients with heart failure due to direct negative inotropic effects
Arterial Vasodilators	Hydralazine Minoxidil Diazoxide Fenoldopam	Hydralazine no longer a first-line drug; may have utility in the treatment of severe hypertension, in some patients with CHF, and in hypertensive emergencies in pregnant women (especially preeclampsia) Systemic minoxidil best reserved for severe hypertension that responds poorly to other antihypertensive medications, especially in male patients with renal insufficiency	Hydralazine causes symptoms of severe vasodilation, including headache, nausea, flushing, hypotension, palpitations, tachycardia, dizziness, and angina pectoris Minoxidil has strong antinatriuretic effects, causes reflex increases in sympathetic cardiac effects, and hypertrichosis	Hydralazine can cause autoimmune reactions, including drug-induced lupus syndrome, serum sickness, hemolytic anemia, vasculitis, and rapidly progressive glomerulonephritis
Arterial and Venous Vasodilators	Nitroprusside	Used primarily to treat hypertensive emergencies, also in situations when short-term reduction of cardiac preload and/or afterload is desired	Excessive vasodilation	At high doses, conversion to cyanide can be toxic but prevented by coadministration of sodium thiosulfate

SECTION III — Modulation of Cardiovascular Function

CLASS AND SUBCLASSES	NAMES	CLINICAL USES	TOXICITIES COMMON	TOXICITIES UNIQUE; CLINICALLY IMPORTANT
Vasopressin Agonist—V_1 Receptor Agonists	Vasopressin Terlipressin	Used to induce GI smooth muscle contraction to treat postoperative ileus, abdominal distension, and dispel intestinal gas prior to abdominal x-ray imaging. Used to vasoconstrict splachnic and portal arteries to reduce bleeding associated with various abdominal procedures, hemorrhagic disorders such as esophageal varices, and surgeries in patients with portal hypertension. Terlipressin is preferred for bleeding esophageal varices because of increased safety, and is effective in treating patients with hepatorenal syndrome	V_1-mediated effects include cutaneous vasoconstriction, nausea, belching, cramps, and an urge to defecate. Major V_2 receptor-mediated adverse effect of vasopressin is water intoxication; must not be administered to patients with primary or psychogenic polydipsia	Vasoconstriction of coronary and peripheral arteries. Vasopressin should be administered only at low doses and with extreme caution in individuals suffering from vascular disease, especially coronary artery disease. Arrhythmia and decreased cardiac output. Peripheral vasoconstriction and gangrene with large doses of vasopressin
Vasopressin Agonist—V_2 Receptor Agonist	Desmopressin (DDAVP)	Drug of choice for treatment of central diabetes insipidus to control polyuria and polydypsia. Reduces bleeding time by increasing release of vWF and factor VIII in patients with certain bleeding disorders. Primary nocturnal enuresis. Relieves post-lumbar puncture headache	Mild facial flushing and headache. Major adverse effect is water intoxication; patients receiving desmopressin to maintain hemostasis should be advised to reduce fluid intake. Must not be administered to patients with primary or psychogenic polydipsia. Tachyphylaxis to desmopressin's procoagulant effects usually occurs after several days owing to depletion of factor VIII and vWF	May cause transient thrombo-cytopenia in individuals with type IIb vWD and is contraindicated in such patients
Vasopressin Antagonists—Selective V_2 Receptor (V_2R) Antagonists ("Aquaretics")	Tolvaptan	Used in disease states with water excess and hyponatremia (chronic heart failure, cirrhosis, nephrosis) to increase renal free water without changing electrolyte excretion. Used in patients with euvolemic or hypervolemic hyponatremia associated with SIADH	GI effects, hyperglycemia, and pyrexia	Metabolized by CYP3A4 (drug-drug interactions). Less common adverse effects: life-threatening thrombosis, ventricular fibrillation, urethral and vaginal hemorrhage, respiratory failure, diabetic ketoacidosis, ischemic colitis, increase in prothrombin time, rhabdomyolysis
Vasopressin Antagonists—Nonselective V_{1a}R/V_2R Antagonist ("Aquaretics")	Conivaptan	Treatment of hospitalized patients with euvolemic hyponatremia and hypervolemic hyponatremia	Infusion site reaction (drug should only be infused into large veins and infusion sites changed daily). Headache, hypertension, hypotension, hypokalemia, and pyrexia	Metabolized by CYP3A4 (drug-drug interactions)

Drug Therapy of Myocardial Ischemia

CHAPTER 16

This chapter will be most useful after having a basic understanding of the material related to angina at the beginning of Chapter 27, Treatment of Myocardial Ischemia and Hypertension in *Goodman & Gilman's The Pharmacological Basis of Therapeutics*, 12th Edition. In addition to the material presented here, the 12th Edition contains:

- Table 27-1 Organic Nitrates Available for Clinical Use, which provides information about the preparations, usual doses, and routes of administration of organic nitrates
- The molecular structures of drugs used to treat myocardial ischemia

LEARNING OBJECTIVES

- ☑ Understand the mechanisms of action of drugs used to treat myocardial ischemia and relieve symptoms of angina.
- ☑ Understand the goals of treatment based on a knowledge of the underlying cause(s) of angina.
- ☑ Know which drugs are most effective in treating different types of angina.
- ☑ Know which drugs are used in combination to treat angina.
- ☑ Know the untoward effects and contraindications of the major classes of drugs used to treat angina.
- ☑ Know the role of drug-eluting stents to treat patients with acute coronary syndromes.

DRUGS INCLUDED IN THIS CHAPTER

- Antithrombin agents (see Chapter 19)
- Antiplatelet drugs (see Chapter 19)
- β Adrenergic receptor antagonists (see Chapter 7)
- Numerous dihydropyridines (nifedipine [ADALAT, PROCARDIA, others], amlodipine [NORVASC, others], felodipine [PLENDIL, others], isradipine [DYNACIRC, others], nicardipine [CARDENE, others], nisoldipine, nimodipine, clevidipine, others)
- Diltiazem (CARDIZEM, DILACOR-XR, others)
- Isosorbide dinitrate (ISDN; ISORDIL, SORBITRATE, DILATRATE-SR, others)
- Isosorbide-5-mononitrate (ISMN; IMDUR, ISMO, others)
- Nitroglycerin (glyceryl trinitrate; NITRO-BID, NITROSTAT, NITROL, NITRO-DUR, others)
- Paclitaxel drug-eluting stents
- Ranolazine (RANEXA)
- Sildenafil (VIAGRA, REVATIO)
- Sirolimus drug-eluting stents
- Tadalafil (CIALIS, ADCIRCA)
- Thrombolytic agents (see Chapter 19)
- Vardenafil (LEVITRA)
- Verapamil (CALAN, ISOPTIN, others)

SYMPTOMS OF MYOCARDIAL ISCHEMIA

- Angina pectoris, the primary symptom of ischemic heart disease, is caused by transient episodes of myocardial ischemia that are due to an imbalance in the myocardial oxygen supply–demand relationship (see Figure 16-1).
- Angina pectoris is a heavy, pressing substernal discomfort (rarely described as "pain") often radiating to the
  - ▸ Left shoulder
  - ▸ Flexor aspect of the left arm
  - ▸ Jaw
  - ▸ Epigastrium

(continued)

MECHANISMS OF ACTION OF DRUGS USED TO TREAT MYOCARDIAL ISCHEMIA

DRUG CLASS	DRUG	MECHANISM OF ACTION
Organic Nitrates (Nitrovasodilators, NO Donors)	Nitroglycerin (glyceryl trinitrate) Isosorbide dinitrate (ISDN) Isosorbide-5-mononitrate (ISMN)	Prodrugs that are the source of NO that increase intracellular cGMP and cause relaxation of large veins (reduced preload reduces myocardial O_2 demand), relaxation of arteriolar resistance vessels (reduced afterload reduces myocardial O_2 demand), and relaxation of coronary vessels (improved myocardial O_2 supply)
β Adrenergic Receptor Antagonists	see Chapter 7	Block myocardial β adrenergic receptors to slow heart rate (improved myocardial O_2 supply and reduced O_2 demand) and reduce ventricular contractility (reduced O_2 demand)

(Continued)

SECTION III — Modulation of Cardiovascular Function

SYMPTOMS OF MYOCARDIAL ISCHEMIA (Cont.)

- A significant number of patients note discomfort in a different location or of a different character:
  - Women, the elderly, and diabetics are more likely to experience myocardial ischemia with atypical symptoms.
  - Some patients experience myocardial ischemia with no symptoms of angina (silent ischemia), but with electrocardiographic, echocardiographic, or radionuclide evidence of ischemia.

DRUG CLASS	DRUG	MECHANISM OF ACTION
Ca^{2+} Channel Antagonists (Ca^{2+} Entry Blockers)	Verapamil Diltiazem Numerous dihydropyridines (nifedipine, amlodipine, felodipine, isradipine, nicardipine, nisoldipine, nimodipine, clevidipine, others)	Blocking voltage-sensitive L-type Ca^{2+} channels relaxes coronary arteries (improved myocardial O_2 supply) and relaxes peripheral arteriole resistance vessels (reduced afterload reduces myocardial O_2 demand)
Antiplatelet Drugs	see chapter 19	Inhibiting platelet aggregation at site of ruptured coronary atherosclerotic plaque prevents occlusion of coronary blood flow
Statins	see chapter 20	Correct dyslipidemias that lead to coronary atherosclerosis and stabilize coronary plaques
Na^+ Channel Blocker (Late Inward Na^+ Current Blocker)	Ranolazine	Blocks late inward Na^+ current in cardiac myocytes that leads to increased ventricular diastolic wall tension (reduced O_2 demand)

CLASSIFICATION OF MYOCARDIAL ISCHEMIA

TYPE OF MYOCARDIAL ISCHEMIA	ETIOLOGY	THERAPIES
Typical angina (stable angina, exertional angina, exercise-induced angina)	Decreased coronary vessel radius due to coronary atherosclerosis results in ischemia when combined with exertion	Therapy is directed at reducing myocardial O_2 demand (nitrates and β adrenergic antagonists; see Figure 16-1)
Unstable angina and non-ST-segment-elevation myocardial infarction (acute coronary syndrome)	Acute or subacute worsening of anginal symptoms caused by decreased coronary flow due to thrombosis at the site of ruptured coronary plaque with partial or total occlusion of the vessel	Therapies directed at decreasing myocardial oxygen demand (nitrates and β adrenergic antagonists) have limited efficacy Additional therapies are directed at the atherosclerotic plaque and consequences or prevention of its rupture including: • antiplatelet agents • antithrombin agents • thrombolytic agents • angioplasty and mechanotherapy with intracoronary stents (see Side Bar DRUG-ELUTING INTRACORONARY STENTS) • coronary bypass surgery in selected patients Reduce coronary vasospasm with IV nitroglycerin, and possibly a Ca^{2+} channel blocker to increase O_2 supply (see Figure 16-1)
Acute myocardial infarction	Ischemia with loss of myocardial tissue caused by blockage of one or more coronary vessels	Therapy is directed at reducing the size of the infarct, preserving viable tissue by reducing O_2 demand of the myocardium, and preventing ventricular remodeling Nitroglycerin to relieve ischemic pain but should not be used if hypotension limits the administration of β blockers Reperfusion therapies are critical with angioplasty and stents having better outcomes than thrombolytic therapy
Variant or Prinzmetal angina	Intermittent decrease in flow due to localized coronary vasospasm	Increase myocardial O_2 supply with coronary vasodilators (see Figure 16-1); Ca^{2+} channel blockers reduce mortality and the incidence of MI Long-acting nitrates can occasionally be effective alone but additional Ca^{2+} channel blocker therapy is usually required

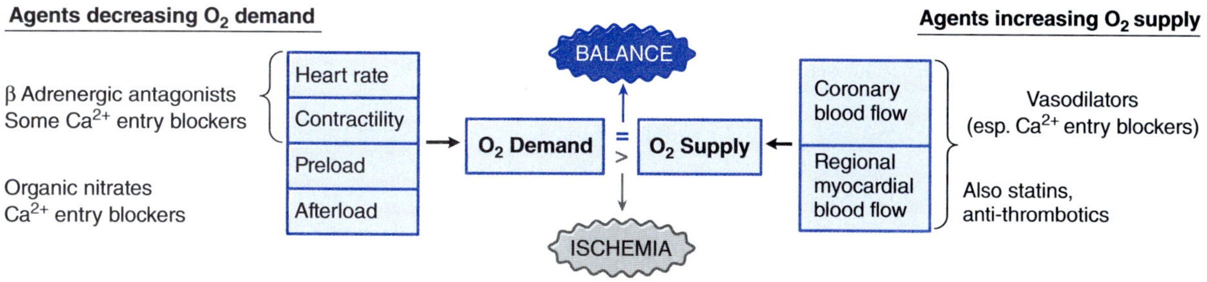

Drug Therapy of Myocardial Ischemia

CHAPTER 16

FIGURE 16-1 Pharmacological modification of the major determinants of myocardial O_2 supply. When myocardial O_2 requirements exceed O_2 supply, an ischemic episode results. This figure shows the primary hemodynamic sites of actions of pharmacological agents that can reduce O_2 demand (*left side*) or enhance O_2 supply (*right side*). Some classes of agents have multiple effects. Stents, angioplasty, and coronary bypass surgery are mechanical interventions that increase O_2 supply. Both pharmacotherapy and mechanotherapy attempt to restore a dynamic balance between O_2 demand and O_2 supply.

CASE 16-1

A 52-year-old man who suffers from angina when he climbs stairs or participates in similar activities receives a prescription for nitroglycerin (glyceryl trinitrate). He is instructed to take a tablet 1 or 2 minutes before he expects to climb stairs to prevent the angina.

a. What is the mechanism of action of nitroglycerin that prevents angina from developing in this patient?

Nitroglycerin and the other organic nitrates used to treat angina are prodrugs that are sources of nitric oxide (NO). NO activates the soluble isoform of guanylyl cyclase, thereby increasing intracellular levels of cyclic GMP and leading to the relaxation of smooth muscle cells in a broad range of tissues. The NO-dependent relaxation of vascular smooth muscle leads to vasodilation. Low concentrations of nitroglycerin preferentially dilate veins more than arterioles. This venodilation decreases venous return, leading to a fall in left and right ventricular chamber size and end-diastolic pressures, but usually results in little change in systemic vascular resistance. Systemic arterial pressure may fall slightly, and heart rate is unchanged or may increase slightly in response to a decrease in blood pressure. Nitroglycerin can dilate epicardial stenoses and reduce the resistance to flow through such areas resulting in an increase in blood flow that would be distributed preferentially to ischemic myocardial regions as a consequence of vasodilation induced by autoregulation.

By their effects on the systemic circulation, the organic nitrates also can reduce myocardial O_2 demand (see Figure 16-1). The major determinants of myocardial O_2 consumption include left ventricular wall tension, heart rate, and myocardial contractility. Ventricular wall tension is affected by a number of factors that may be considered under the categories of preload and afterload. Organic nitrates decrease both preload and afterload as a result of respective dilation of venous capacitance and arteriolar resistance vessels. The ability of nitrates to dilate epicardial coronary arteries, even in areas of atherosclerotic stenosis, is modest, and the preponderance of evidence continues to favor a reduction in myocardial work, and thus in myocardial O_2 demand, as their primary effect in chronic stable angina.

b. How and when should the nitroglycerin be administered to prevent anginal pain?

Anginal pain may be prevented when the drug is used prophylactically immediately prior to exercise or stress. The smallest effective dose should be prescribed. Sublingual organic nitrates should be taken at the time of an anginal attack or in anticipation of exercise or stress. Such intermittent treatment provides reproducible cardiovascular effects. Peak concentrations of nitroglycerin are found in plasma within 4 minutes of sublingual administration; the drug has a $t_{1/2}$ of 1 to 3 minutes because of rapid and complete first-pass metabolism by the liver. The onset of action of nitroglycerin may be even more rapid if it is delivered as a sublingual spray rather than as a sublingual tablet.

(Continued)

INTERACTIONS OF NITRATES WITH PHOSPHODIESTERASE 5 (PDE5) INHIBITORS

- Erectile dysfunction is common in patients with coronary artery disease; thus many men desiring therapy for erectile dysfunction may be receiving antianginal therapy.

- The PDE5 inhibitors (sildenafil, tadalafil, and vardenafil) block the cyclic GMP-specific PDE5 family of phosphodiesterases which are widely expressed in vascular smooth muscle, including the smooth muscle of the corpus cavernosum and penile arteries.

- The accumulation of cyclic GMP in vascular smooth muscle that occurs with NO stimulation of guanylyl cyclase can be enhanced by inhibiting PDE5 activity.

- Given alone, the PDE5 inhibitors cause modest drops in blood pressure, but in men who are taking organic nitrate vasodilators, a fall in blood pressure of more than 25 mm Hg can occur.

- Because of the possibility of extreme hypotension, PDE5 inhibitors are contraindicated for patients receiving any form of nitrate and should not be prescribed to such patients.

- Patients should be questioned about the use of PDE5 inhibitors within the past 24 hours before nitrates are administered; a period longer than 24 hours may be needed to avoid drug interactions, especially with tadalafil which has the longest half-life.

SECTION III — Modulation of Cardiovascular Function

Frequently repeated or continuous exposure to high doses of organic nitrates leads to a marked attenuation in the magnitude of most of their pharmacological effects. The magnitude of tolerance is a function of dosage and frequency of use. In patients who require constant administration of an organic nitrate to prevent symptoms of angina, tolerance can develop rapidly. An effective approach to preventing tolerance or restoring responsiveness is to interrupt therapy for 8 to 12 hours each day, which allows the return of efficacy. It is usually most convenient to omit dosing at night in patients with exertional angina either by adjusting dosing intervals of oral or buccal preparations or by removing cutaneous nitroglycerin.

Patients should be instructed to seek medical attention immediately if 3 tablets taken over a 15-minute period do not relieve a sustained attack because this situation may be indicative of myocardial infarction (MI), unstable angina, or another cause of the pain. Patients also should be advised that there is no virtue in trying to avoid taking sublingual nitroglycerin for anginal pain.

c. What are the expected adverse effects of nitroglycerin therapy?

Untoward responses to the therapeutic use of organic nitrates are almost all secondary to actions on the cardiovascular system. Headache is common and can be severe. It usually decreases over a few days if treatment is continued and often can be controlled by decreasing the dose. Transient episodes of dizziness, weakness, and other manifestations associated with postural hypotension may develop, particularly if the patient is standing immobile, and may progress occasionally to loss of consciousness, a reaction that appears to be accentuated by alcohol. It also may be seen with very low doses of nitrates in patients with autonomic dysfunction. Even in severe nitrate syncope, positioning and other measures that facilitate venous return are the only therapeutic measures required. All the organic nitrates occasionally can produce drug rash.

d. What drug combinations should be avoided?

Erectile dysfunction is a frequently encountered problem whose risk factors parallel those of coronary artery disease. Thus many men desiring therapy for erectile dysfunction already may be receiving (or may require, especially if they increase physical activity) antianginal therapy. The combination of a phosphodiesterase 5 (PDE5) inhibitor (sildenafil, tadalafil, vardenafil) used for erectile dysfunction with organic nitrate vasodilators can cause extreme hypotension (see Side Bar INTERACTIONS OF NITRATES WITH PHOSPHODIESTERASE 5 (PDE5) INHIBITORS). PDE5 inhibitors should not be prescribed to patients receiving any form of nitrate and patients should be questioned about the use of PDE5 inhibitors within 24 hours before nitrates are administered. A period of longer than 24 hours may be needed following administration of a PDE5 inhibitor for safe use of nitrates, especially with tadalafil because of its prolonged $t_{1/2}$. In the event that patients develop significant hypotension following combined administration of a PDE5 inhibitor and a nitrate, fluids and α adrenergic receptor agonists, if needed, should be used for support.

CASE 16-2

A 67-year-old woman with mild heart failure (LVEF = 45%) has anginal pain with exercise and is prescribed a β adrenergic blocker.

a. How does therapy with a β adrenergic blocker prevent anginal pain?

The effectiveness of β adrenergic receptor antagonists in the treatment of exertional angina is attributable primarily to a fall in myocardial O_2 consumption at rest and during exertion, although there also is some tendency for increased flow toward ischemic regions. The decrease in myocardial O_2 consumption is due to a negative chronotropic effect (particularly during exercise), a negative inotropic effect, and a reduction in arterial blood pressure (particularly systolic pressure) during exercise (see Figure 16-1). The reduction in arterial blood pressure is secondary to a drop in cardiac output due to the negative chronotropic and inotropic effects of β blockers.

(Continued)

b. What is the rationale underlying the choice of a β adrenergic blocker for this patient?

Because there is a proven mortality benefit from the use of β adrenergic receptor antagonists in patients with heart disease, this class of drugs represents the first line of therapy. β Adrenergic receptor antagonists are effective in reducing the severity and frequency of attacks of exertional angina and are recommended for patients with mild heart failure (LVEF ≥40%; Table 16-1). Moreover, several β adrenergic receptor antagonists have been shown to reduce mortality in patients with congestive heart failure and treatment of patients with heart failure with β adrenergic antagonist drugs has become standard therapy for many such patients (see Chapters 12 and 28 in *Goodman & Gilman's The Pharmacological Basis of Therapeutics*, 12th Edition). Most β adrenergic receptor antagonists appear to be equally effective in the treatment of exertional angina. Timolol, metoprolol, atenolol, and propranolol have been shown to exert cardioprotective effects.

(Continued)

TABLE 16-1 Recommended Drug Therapy for Angina in Patients with Other Medical Conditions

CONDITION	RECOMMENDED TREATMENT (AND ALTERNATIVES) FOR ANGINA	DRUGS TO AVOID
Medical Conditions		
Systemic hypertension	β receptor antagonists (Ca^{2+} channel antagonists)	
Migraine or vascular headaches	β receptor antagonists (Ca^{2+} channel antagonists)	
Asthma or chronic obstructive pulmonary disease with bronchospasm	Verapamil or diltiazem	β receptor antagonists
Hyperthyroidism	β receptor antagonists	
Raynaud's syndrome	Long-acting, slow-release Ca^{2+} antagonists	β receptor antagonists
Insulin-dependent diabetes mellitus	β receptor antagonists (particularly if prior MI) or long-acting, slow-release Ca^{2+} channel antagonists	
Non-insulin-dependent diabetes mellitus	β receptor antagonists or long-acting, slow-release Ca^{2+} channel antagonists	
Depression	Long-acting, slow-release Ca^{2+} channel antagonists	β receptor antagonists
Mild peripheral vascular disease	β receptor antagonists or Ca^{2+} channel antanogists	
Severe peripheral vascular disease with rest ischemia	Ca^{2+} channel antagonists	β receptor antagonists
Cardiac Arrhythmias and Conduction Abnormalities		
Sinus bradycardia	Dihydropyridine Ca^{2+} channel antagonists	β receptor antagonists, diltiazem, verapamil
Sinus tachycardia (not due to heart failure)	β receptor antagonists	
Supraventricular tachycardia	Verapamil, diltiazem, or β receptor antagonists	
Atrioventricular block	Dihydropyridine Ca^{2+} channel antagonists	β receptor antagonists, diltiazem, verapamil
Rapid atrial fibrillation (with digitalis)	Verapamil, diltiazem, or β receptor antagonists	
Ventricular arrhythmias	β receptor antagonists	

(Continued)

CONDITION	RECOMMENDED TREATMENT (AND ALTERNATIVES) FOR ANGINA	DRUGS TO AVOID
Left Ventricular Dysfunction		
Congestive heart failure		
Mild (LVEF ≥40%)	β receptor antagonists	
Moderate to severe (LVEF <40%)	Amlodipine or felodipine (nitrates)	
Left-sided valvular heart disease		
Mild aortic stenosis	β receptor antagonists	
Aortic insufficiency	Long-acting, slow-release dihydropyridines	
Mitral regurgitation	Long-acting, slow-release dihydropyridines	
Mitral stenosis	β receptor antagonists	
Hypertrophic cardiomyopathy	β receptor antagonists, nondihydropyridine Ca^{2+} channel antagonists	Nitrates, dihydropyridine Ca^{2+} channel antagonists

Reproduced with permission from Gibbons RJ, Chatterjee K, Daley J et al. ACC/AHA/ACP-ASIM Guidelines for the management of patients with chronic stable angina: A report of the American College of Cardiology / American Heart Association Task Force on Practice Guidelines (Committee on Management of Patients With Chronic Stable Angina). *J Am Coll Cardiol* 1999;33:2092-197. Copyright © 1999 by the American College of Cardiology Foundation.

c. **If the patient's angina is not adequately controlled by monotherapy with a β adrenergic receptor antagonist, what other classes of antianginal drugs could be added to the β adrenergic blocker therapy in this patient?**

The concurrent use of organic nitrates and β adrenergic receptor antagonists can be very effective in the treatment of typical exertional angina. The additive efficacy primarily is a result of the blockade by one drug of a reflex effect elicited by the other. β Adrenergic receptor antagonists can block the baroreceptor-mediated reflex tachycardia and positive inotropic effects that are sometimes associated with nitrates, whereas nitrates, by increasing venous capacitance, can attenuate the increase in left ventricular end-diastolic volume associated with β receptor blockade. Concurrent administration of nitrates also can alleviate the increase in coronary vascular resistance associated with blockade of β adrenergic receptors.

When angina is not controlled adequately by a β receptor antagonist plus nitrates, additional improvement sometimes can be achieved by the addition of a Ca^{2+} channel blocker, especially if there is a component of coronary vasospasm. The differences among the chemical classes of Ca^{2+} channel blockers can lead to important adverse or salutary drug interactions with β receptor antagonists (see text in Chapter 27 in *Goodman & Gilman's The Pharmacological Basis of Therapeutics*, 12th Edition).

CASE 16-3

A man with hypertension and occasional symptoms of angina with exercise is prescribed amlodipine.

a. **What is the mechanism of action of amlodipine that is beneficial in treating hypertension and angina?**

Amlodipine inhibits L-type voltage-sensitive Ca^{2+} channels in vascular smooth muscle, especially in arterial beds. The basis for the use of Ca^{2+} channel antagonists in hypertension comes from the understanding that hypertension generally is the result of increased peripheral vascular resistance. All of the Ca^{2+} channel blockers lower blood pressure by relaxing arteriolar smooth muscle and decreasing

(Continued)

peripheral vascular resistance. Ca²⁺ channel blockers are effective when used alone or in combination with other drugs for the treatment of hypertension.

The utility of Ca²⁺ channel antagonists in the treatment of exertional, or exercise-induced, angina results from an increase in coronary blood flow owing to coronary arterial dilation, from a decrease in myocardial O_2 demand (secondary to a decrease in arterial blood pressure, heart rate, or contractility), or both (see Figure 16-1). Amlodipine, as with other dihydropyridine Ca²⁺ channel blockers, has potent vasodilator activity but minimal effects on cardiac contractility, SA nodal activity, or AV nodal activity at concentrations that cause vasodilation (Table 16-2). In contrast to the dihydropyridines, verapamil and diltiazem have direct negative inotropic and chronotropic effects (see Table 16-2).

b. What are the potential side effects of the Ca²⁺ channel antagonists?

The profile of adverse reactions to the Ca²⁺ channel blockers varies among the drugs in this class. Patients receiving immediate-release short-acting formulations of nifedipine develop headache, flushing, dizziness, and peripheral edema; these preparations are not appropriate in the long-term treatment of angina or hypertension. Dizziness and flushing are much less of a problem with sustained-release formulations and with the dihydropyridines having a long $t_{1/2}$ and relatively constant concentrations of drug in plasma. Peripheral edema may occur in some patients with Ca²⁺ channel blockers and most likely results from increased hydrostatic pressure in the lower extremities owing to precapillary dilation and reflex postcapillary constriction. Some other adverse effects of these drugs are due to actions in nonvascular smooth muscle such as the lower esophageal sphincter (which can cause or aggravate gastroesophageal reflux), constipation (a common side effect of verapamil, but less frequent with other Ca²⁺ channel blockers), and urinary retention (a rare adverse effect).

c. What are the important contraindications for the use of Ca²⁺ channel blockers?

The use of intravenous verapamil with an intravenous β adrenergic receptor antagonist is contraindicated because of the increased propensity for AV block and/or severe depression of ventricular function. Patients with ventricular dysfunction, SA or AV nodal conduction disturbances, and systolic blood pressures below 90 mm Hg should not be treated with verapamil or diltiazem, particularly intravenously (see Table 16-1).

TREATMENT OF CLAUDICATION AND PERIPHERAL VASCULAR DISEASE

- Most patients with peripheral artery disease also have coronary artery disease and the therapeutic approaches overlap.
- Reductions in cardiovascular morbidity and mortality in patients with peripheral arterial disease have been documented with antiplatelet therapy, ACE inhibitors, and treatment of hyperlipidemia.
- Risk factor and lifestyle modifications (physical exercise, rehabilitation, and smoking cessation) remain cornerstones of therapy for patients with claudication.
- Pentoxifylline and cilostazol are drugs used specifically for lower extremity claudication.
  - Pentoxifylline is a rheological modifier that increases the deformability of red blood cells.
  - Cilostazol is PDE3 inhibitor that inhibits platelet aggregation and vasodilation by increasing intracellular cyclic AMP in many cells, including platelets.

TABLE 16-2 Ca²⁺ Channel Blockers: Chemical Structures and Some Relative Cardiovascular Effects[a]

CHEMICAL STRUCTURE GENERIC NAME (TRADE NAME)	VASODILATION (CORONARY FLOW)	SUPPRESSION OF CARDIAC CONTRACTILITY	SUPPRESSION OF AUTOMATICITY (SA NODE)	SUPPRESSION OF CONDUCTION (AV NODE)
Amlodipine (NORVASC, others)	5	1	1	0
Felodipine (PLENDIL, others)	5	1	1	0

SECTION III Modulation of Cardiovascular Function

CHEMICAL STRUCTURE GENERIC NAME (TRADE NAME)	VASODILATION (CORONARY FLOW)	SUPPRESSION OF CARDIAC CONTRACTILITY	SUPPRESSION OF AUTOMATICITY (SA NODE)	SUPPRESSION OF CONDUCTION (AV NODE)
Isradipine (DYNACIRC, others)	NR	NR	NR	NR
Nicardipine (CARDENE, others)	5	0	1	0
Nifedipine (ADALAT, PROCARDIA, others)	5	1	1	0
Diltiazem (CARDIZEM, DILACOR-XR, others)	3	2	5	4
Verapamil (CALAN, ISOPTIN, others)	4	4	5	5

^aRelative effects are ranked from *no effect* (0) to *prominent* (5). NR, not ranked.

CASE 16-4

A 58-year-old man with a long history of exertional angina begins to develop more frequent episodes of anginal pain that are also more intense. His cardiologist tells him he has unstable angina.

a. What is the medical therapy for patients with unstable angina?

The term unstable angina pectoris has been used to describe a broad spectrum of clinical entities characterized by an acute or subacute worsening in a patient's anginal symptoms. More recently, efforts have been directed toward identifying patients with unstable angina on the basis of their risks for subsequent adverse outcomes such as MI or death. The term acute coronary syndrome has been useful in this context. Common to most clinical presentations of acute coronary syndrome is disruption of a coronary plaque, leading to local platelet aggregation and thrombosis at the arterial wall, with subsequent partial or total occlusion of the vessel.

The principal therapeutic goal in unstable angina is to increase myocardial blood flow. Medical therapy for unstable angina involves the administration of aspirin,

(Continued)

which reduces mortality, nitrates, β adrenergic receptor blocking agents, and heparin, which are effective in controlling ischemic episodes and angina. Because vasospasm occurs in some patients with unstable angina, Ca^{2+} channel blockers may offer an additional approach to the treatment of unstable angina. However, there is insufficient evidence to assess whether such treatment decreases mortality except when the underlying mechanism is vasospasm. In contrast, therapy directed toward reduction of platelet function and thrombotic episodes clearly decreases morbidity and mortality in patients with unstable angina (see Chapters 34 and 30 in *Goodman & Gilman's The Pharmacological Basis of Therapeutics*, 12th Edition), and administration of statins to treat dyslipidemias (see Chapter 20) also can reduce the risk of adverse cardiac events.

b. **What other therapies might be considered to relieve angina symptoms in this patient?**

Percutaneous coronary interventions (PCI) such as angioplasty and coronary artery stent deployment, or (less commonly) emergency coronary bypass surgery, can complement pharmacological treatment. In some subsets of patients, percutaneous or surgical revascularization may have a survival advantage over medical treatment alone. Intracoronary stents can ameliorate angina and reduce adverse events in patients with acute coronary syndromes. However, the long-term efficacy of intracoronary stents is limited by subacute luminal restenosis within the stent, which occurs in a substantial minority of patients. The development of drug-eluting stents to prevent the smooth muscle proliferation that is responsible for restenosis has had an important impact on clinical practice. Two drugs are currently being used in intravascular stents: paclitaxel and sirolimus (see Side Bar DRUG-ELUTING INTRACORONARY STENTS).

Stent-induced damage to the vascular endothelial cell layer can lead to thrombosis; patients typically are treated with antiplatelet agents, including clopidogrel (for up to 6 months) and aspirin (indefinitely), sometimes in conjunction with intravenous heparin and/or GPIIb/IIIa inhibitors (see Chapter 19) administered at the time of the revascularization procedure. The inhibition of cellular proliferation by paclitaxel and sirolimus not only affects vascular smooth muscle cell proliferation but also attenuates the formation of an intact endothelial layer within the stented artery. Therefore, antiplatelet therapy (typically with clopidogrel) is continued for several months after intracoronary stenting with drug-eluting stents.

DRUG-ELUTING INTRACORONARY STENTS

- Intracoronary stents can ameliorate angina and reduce adverse events in patients with acute coronary syndromes.
- Luminal subacute restenosis caused by smooth muscle proliferation within the lumen of the stented artery reduces the long-term efficacy of stents in a substantial minority of patients.
- Drug-eluting stents containing either paclitaxel or sirolimus can reduce the rate of restenosis compared to "bare metal" stents.
- Long-term (6 months) therapy with clopidogrel and lifelong therapy with aspirin may be needed to prevent stent thrombosis in patients receiving drug-eluting stents, but these long-term antiplatelet therapies can increase the risk of bleeding (see Chapter 19).

CASE 16-5

A 42-year-old woman develops symptoms of angina at rest. She has not had angina before and has no history of cardiovascular disease. After an exercise stress test and other tests, she is diagnosed as having variant angina.

a. **What is variant angina and what is the main therapeutic goal in treating it?**

In variant angina, focal or diffuse coronary vasospasm episodically reduces coronary flow. Patients also may display a mixed pattern of angina with the addition of altered vessel tone on a background of atherosclerotic narrowing. The principal therapeutic aim in variant or Prinzmetal angina is to prevent coronary vasospasm and improve O_2 delivery to ischemic myocardium.

b. **What are the treatment options to relieve this patient's symptoms of angina?**

Whereas long-acting nitrates alone are occasionally efficacious in abolishing episodes of variant angina, additional therapy with Ca^{2+} channel blockers usually is required. Ca^{2+} channel blockers, but not nitrates, have been shown to influence mortality and the incidence of MI favorably in variant angina; they should generally be included in therapy. β Receptor antagonists should be used with caution if the underlying pathophysiology is coronary vasospasm.

SECTION III

Modulation of Cardiovascular Function

KEY CONCEPTS

➡ In typical stable angina, the primary therapeutic goal is to reduce myocardial O_2 demand, typically with an organic nitrate, a β receptor antagonist, a Ca^{2+} channel blocker, or a combination of these 3 classes of drugs.

➡ The therapeutic goal in treating vasospastic angina is to prevent coronary vasospasm and maintain myocardial O_2 supply using a Ca^{2+} channel blocker, an organic nitrate, or a combination of these 2 classes of drugs.

➡ Acute coronary syndromes are caused by disruption of an atherosclerotic coronary plaque causing local platelet aggregation and thrombosis that partially or totally occludes the coronary vessel.

➡ The primary therapeutic goal in treating acute coronary syndromes is to prevent the disruption of coronary blood flow by inhibiting platelet aggregation and thrombosis, and secondarily reducing myocardial O_2 demand.

➡ In addition to pharmacological therapy, long-term prevention of angina in patients with acute coronary syndrome may require angioplasty, intracoronary stents, or in some patients, coronary bypass surgery.

SUMMARY QUIZ

QUESTION 16-1 The antianginal drug of choice to use in a patient with vasospastic angina who has sinus bradycardia is

a. propranolol.
b. verapamil.
c. diltiazem.
d. amlodipidine.
e. nitroglycerin.

QUESTION 16-2 A patient with chronic exertional angina is refractory to combination therapy with a β blocker, organic nitrate, and Ca^{2+} channel blocker. Which of the following drugs may be useful in reducing the symptoms of angina in this patient?

a. A PDE5 inhibitor
b. Aspirin
c. Heparin
d. A statin
e. Ranolazine

QUESTION 16-3 The mechanism underlying the life-threatening interaction of organic nitrates and PDE5 inhibitors is that

a. PDE5 inhibitors block the degradation of organic nitrates in the liver.
b. PDE inhibitors block the degradation of cyclic GMP in vascular smooth muscle.
c. PDE inhibitors enhance the conversion of organic nitrates to NO.
d. PDE5 inhibitor degradation is blocked by organic nitrates.
e. PDE5 inhibitor excretion is blocked by organic nitrates.

QUESTION 16-4 This combination of antianginal drugs should be avoided to circumventan adverse drug interaction:

a. Nitroglycerin and a β adrenergic receptor antagonist
b. Nitroglycerin and verapamil
c. Verapamil and a β adrenergic receptor antagonist
d. Amlodipine and a β adrenergic receptor antagonist
e. Ranolazine and a β adrenergic receptor antagonist

QUESTION 16-5 The main advantage of isosorbide-5-mononitrate (ISMN) over nitroglycerin for treatment of chronic angina is that

a. it is less expensive than nitroglycerin.
b. tolerance does not develop to its antianginal effects.
c. it can be used in combination with β adrenergic receptor blockers.
d. it can be used in combination with Ca^{2+} channel blockers.
e. it does not undergo rapid first-pass metabolism allowing once- or twice-daily oral administration.

SUMMARY QUIZ ANSWER KEY

QUESTION 16-1 Answer is **d.** Amlodipine is the drug of choice to use in this patient. β Adrenergic blockers, verapamil, and diltiazem will all slow his heart rate by inhibiting SA nodal activity, which will exacerbate his sinus bradycardia. Although nitroglycerin will not inhibit SA nodal activity, it is not as effective as a dihydropyridine in preventing the symptoms of angina in a patient with vasospastic angina.

QUESTION 16-2 Answer is **e.** Ranolazine is an antianginal agent reserved for use in patients who are refractory to treatment with other antianginal agents. It has a unique mechanism of action that reduces myocardial O_2 demand without affecting hemodynamics. It appears to act by blocking the late inward Na^+ current (late I_{Na}) in ventricular myocytes, which in turn reduces intracellular concentrations of Na^+ during diastole. Lowering intracellular Na^+ facilitates efflux of Ca^{2+} from myocytes through the Na^+-Ca^{2+} exchanger. The reduction in intracellular Ca^{2+} facilitates relaxation of ventricular myocytes and reduces O_2 demand. Ranolazine would be added to the antianginal therapy this patient is receiving.

QUESTION 16-3 Answer is **b.** PDE5 inhibitors inhibit the degradation of cyclic GMP in vascular smooth muscle cells which increases the intracellular concentration of cyclic GMP. This causes vascular smooth muscle to relax which results in a lowering of blood pressure. The organic nitrates act by stimulating the synthesis of cyclic GMP in vascular smooth muscle which also leads to a lowering of blood pressure. When an organic nitrate is used within 24 hours of a PDE5 inhibitor, there can be a dangerous drop in blood pressure because these different agents cause an additive or synergistic increase in vascular smooth muscle cyclic GMP concentrations.

QUESTION 16-4 Answer is **c.** Because verapamil and β blockers have additive effects on inhibiting SA node and AV conduction, the combination should be avoided to prevent severe bradycardia and conduction block. These agents can also have additive effects on decreasing left ventricular function which could seriously impair cardiac output in a patient with heart failure.

QUESTION 16-5 Answer is **e.** Isosorbide-5-mononitrate does not undergo significant first-pass hepatic metabolism allowing it to be administered orally once or twice daily depending on the formulation. However, cutaneous administration of nitroglycerin using ointments or transdermal patches can also be administered for long-lasting effect (see Table 27-1 in *Goodman & Gilman's The Pharmacological Basis of Therapeutics*, 12th Edition). With any sustained administration of an organic nitrate, tolerance will develop rapidly and it is important to interrupt therapy for 8 to 12 hours each day, which allows the return of efficacy. It is usually most convenient to omit dosing at night in patients with exertional angina either by adjusting dosing intervals of oral or buccal preparations or by removing cutaneous nitroglycerin. However, patients whose anginal pattern suggests its precipitation by increased left ventricular filling pressures (ie, occurring in association with orthopnea or paroxysmal nocturnal dyspnea) may benefit from continuing nitrates at night and omitting them during a quiet period of the day. To avoid tolerance with isosorbide-5-mononitrate, an eccentric twice-daily dosing schedule appears to maintain efficacy. Some patients develop an increased frequency of nocturnal angina when a nitrate-free interval is employed using nitroglycerin patches; such patients may require another class of antianginal agent during this period.

SECTION III — Modulation of Cardiovascular Function

SUMMARY TABLE: DRUGS USED IN THE TREATMENT OF ANGINA AND ERECTILE DYSFUNCTION

CLASS AND SUBCLASSES	NAMES	CLINICAL USES	TOXICITIES — COMMON	TOXICITIES — UNIQUE; CLINICALLY IMPORTANT
Organic Nitrate Vasodilators (Nitrovasodilators, NO Donors)	Nitroglycerin (glyceryl trinitrate) Isosorbide dinitrate (ISDN) Isosorbide-5-mononitrate (ISMN)	Treatment of angina (reduce preload and relax large coronary vessels)	Headache (can be severe), transient episodes of dizziness, and postural hypotension, all of which are secondary to effects on the cardiovascular system. Occasional drug rash	Tolerance can develop rapidly but can be avoided by interrupting therapy for 8-12 hours each day. PDE5 inhibitors (for erectile dysfunction) can cause extreme hypotension in patients taking organic nitrates and are contraindicated. See Table 16-1
Phosphodiesterase 5 Inhibitors (PDE5 Inhibitors)	Sildenafil Tadalafil Vardenafil	Treatment of erectile dysfunction. Less commonly used to treat pulmonary artery hypertension	Headache, flushing, rhinitis, dyspepsia owing to relaxation of smooth muscle (all of these are predictable based on their effects on PDE5). Sildenafil and vardenafil can produce visual disturbances and one-sided hearing loss	Extreme hypotension when administered in combination with organic nitrates. PDE5 inhibitors should not be prescribed to patients receiving nitrates. Nitrates should not be administered within 24 hours (or longer) after use of a PDE5 inhibitor
β Adrenergic Receptor Antagonists	Propranolol Timolol Metoprolol Atenolol Many others (see Chapter 7)	Treatment of angina (slow heart rate, decrease contractility). Other indications are described in Chapter 7	See Chapter 7	See Table 16-1 and Chapter 7
Ca^{2+} Channel Antagonists (Ca^{2+} Entry blockers)—Phenylalkylamine	Verapamil	Treatment of angina (reduce afterload, relax coronary vessels, slow heart rate, decrease contractility). Treatment of hypertension (see Chapter 15)	Constipation, headache, flushing, dizziness, and peripheral edema	IV administration with IV β blocker is contraindicated because of risk of AV block and/or severe depression of ventricular function. Avoid in patients with ventricular dysfunction, SA or AV nodal conduction disturbances, or systolic blood pressures below 90 mm Hg. See Table 16-1. Blocks the P-glycoprotein transporter
Ca^{2+} Channel Antagonists (Ca^{2+} Entry Blockers)—Benzothiazepine	Diltiazem	Treatment of angina (reduce afterload, relax coronary vessels, slow heart rate, decrease contractility). Treatment of hypertension (see Chapter 15)	Headache, flushing, dizziness, and peripheral edema	Avoid in patients with ventricular dysfunction, SA or AV nodal conduction disturbances, or systolic blood pressures <90 mm Hg. See Table 16-1
Ca^{2+} Channel Antagonists (Ca^{2+} Entry Blockers)—Dihydropyridines	Amlodipine Clevidipine Felodipine Isradipine Nicardipine Nifedipine Nimodipine Nisoldipine	Treatment of angina (reduce afterload, relax coronary vessels). Treatment of hypertension (see Chapter 15)	Headache, flushing, dizziness, and peripheral edema	May aggravate anginal symptoms in some patients when used without a β blocker because of reflex tachycardia. See Table 16-1
Na^+ Channel Blocker (Late Inward Na^+ Current Blocker)	Ranolazine	Treatment of angina (reduces ventricular diastolic wall tension, reducing O_2 demand); used in patients refractory to other antianginal therapy	Prolongs QTc interval	Avoid using with other drugs that prolong QT interval. Contraindicated in patients with hepatic cirrhosis

CHAPTER 17

Pharmacotherapy of Heart Failure

This chapter will be most useful after having a basic understanding of the material in Chapter 28, Pharmacotherapy of Heart Failure in *Goodman & Gilman's The Pharmacological Basis of Therapeutics*, 12th Edition. In particular, the reader is directed to the following table:

- Table 28-3, Vasodilator Drugs Used to Treat Heart Failure, which shows drugs used as vasodilators to treat heart failure including their mechanism of action and their effects on preload and afterload

LEARNING OBJECTIVES

- ☑ Know the stages of heart failure and the treatments that are recommended at each stage.
- ☑ Understand the rationale for the use of drugs that prevent and slow the progression of heart failure.
- ☑ Understand the mechanism of action of inotropic drugs and how they are used to maintain left ventricular function.
- ☑ Identify the major side effects and adverse drug reactions of the drugs used to treat heart failure.

DRUGS IN THIS CHAPTER

- Bisoprolol (ZEBETA)
- Candesartan (ATACAND)
- Captopril (CAPOTEN, others)
- Carvedilol (COREG, others)
- Digoxin (LANOXIN, others)
- Dobutamine (DOBUTREX, others)
- Dopamine
- Enalapril (VASOTEC, others)
- Eplerenone (INSPRA, others)
- Furosemide (LASIX, others)
- Hydralazine (APRESOLINE)
- Hydralazine and isosorbide dinitrate (BIDIL)
- Inamrinone (INOCOR)
- Isosorbide dinitrate (ISORDIL, SORBITRATE, others)
- Labetalol (NORMODYNE, TRANDATE, others)
- Lisinopril (PRINIVIL, ZESTRIL, others)
- Losartan (COZAAR)
- Metoprolol (LOPRESSOR, TOPROL XL, others)
- Milrinone (PRIMACOR IV)
- Minoxidil (LONITEN)
- Nesiritide (NATRECOR)
- Nitroglycerin (trinitroglycerin, NITROSTAT, NITRO-BID, others)
- Nitroprusside (NITROPRESS, others)
- Spironolactone (ALDACTONE)
- Thiazide diuretics (many, see Chapter 15)
- Valsartan (DIOVAN)

MECHANISMS OF ACTIONS OF DRUGS USED TO TREAT HEART FAILURE (SEE FIGURE 17-1)

DRUG CLASS	DRUG	MECHANISM OF ACTION
Angiotensin-Converting Enzyme (ACE) Inhibitors	Captopril, enalapril, lisinopril, others (see Chapter 15)	Prevent the conversion of AngI to active AngII by inhibiting angiotensin converting enzyme (ACE)
Angiotensin Receptor (AT_1) Blockers (ARBs)	Losartan, candesartan, valsartan, others (see Chapter 15)	Competitive (but insurmountable) inhibitors of angiotensin AT_1 receptors
Specific β Adrenergic Receptor Antagonists	Metoprolol, carvedilol, labetalol, bisoprolol, others (see Chapter 7)	Block β adrenergic receptors in the heart, thereby protecting the heart from the cytotoxic effects of high circulating catecholamines. Blockade of β adrenergic receptors in the juxtaglomerular complex reduces renin secretion, thereby reducing plasma AngII
Na^+/K^+-ATPase Inhibitors (Cardiac Glycosides)	Digoxin	Inhibit the Na^+/K^+-ATPase in cardiac myocytes which ultimately increases accumulation of intracellular Ca^{2+} by slowing Ca^{2+} efflux through the Na^+-Ca^{2+} exchanger (see Figure 17-2)
Diuretics (various mechanisms, see Chapter 15)	Thiazides, loop diuretics (furosemide, others), K^+-sparing diuretics (see Chapter 15)	Reduce extracellular fluid volume and ventricular filling pressure by increasing water and sodium excretion
Vasodilators (various mechanisms, Table 17-1)	Hydralazine, organic nitrates, others (see Chapter 15)	Reduce afterload and preload (filling pressure)

(Continued)

SECTION III

Modulation of Cardiovascular Function

CHARACTERISTICS AND CAUSES OF HEART FAILURE

- Congestive heart failure (CHF) is a complex clinical syndrome characterized by:
  - Impaired ventricular performance caused by the inability of the left ventricle to adequately fill (diastolic dysfunction) or empty (systolic dysfunction)
  - Exercise intolerance
  - A high incidence of ventricular arrhythmias
  - Shortened life expectancy
- There is no single definitive diagnostic test for CHF
- Pathophysiological mechanisms that lead to congestive heart failure include activation of the sympathetic nervous system and renin-angiotensin-aldosterone axis (see Figure 17-1)
- Many diseases can lead to heart failure, with the most common in the United States being:
  - Coronary artery disease
  - Hypertension
  - Diabetes mellitus
  - Drug abuse

SYMPTOMS OF HEART FAILURE

- Fatigue
- Shortness of breath
- Rapid heart rate
- Fluid retention resulting in peripheral and pulmonary edema (congestion)

COMORBIDITIES COMMON IN HEART FAILURE

- Coronary artery disease (CAD)
- Atrial fibrillation (AF)
- Myocardial infarction (MI)
- Sudden cardiac death

DRUG CLASS	DRUG	MECHANISM OF ACTION
Aldosterone antagonists	Spironolactone, eplerenone	Block the pathophysiological effects of aldosterone that occur with activation of the renin-angiotensin-aldosterone system (see Table 28-2 in *Goodman & Gilman's The Pharmacological Basis of Therapeutics*, 12th Edition)
β Adrenergic and Dopaminergic Receptor Agonists	Dobutamine, dopamine	Provide short-term increase in cardiac contractility in patients with severely decompensated CHF Dopamine also increases renal blood flow and increases diuresis
Type III Phosphodiesterase (PDE3) Inhibitors ("Inodilators")	Milrinone, inamrinone	Inhibit degradation of cAMP in cardiac and smooth muscle myocytes which increases cardiac contractility and relaxes vascular smooth muscle
Natriuretic Peptide Receptor Agonist	Nesiritide (Human recombinant B-type natriuretic peptide; BNP)	Stimulates natriuretic peptide receptors which increases synthesis of cGMP in target tissues causing natriuresis and vascular smooth muscle relaxation

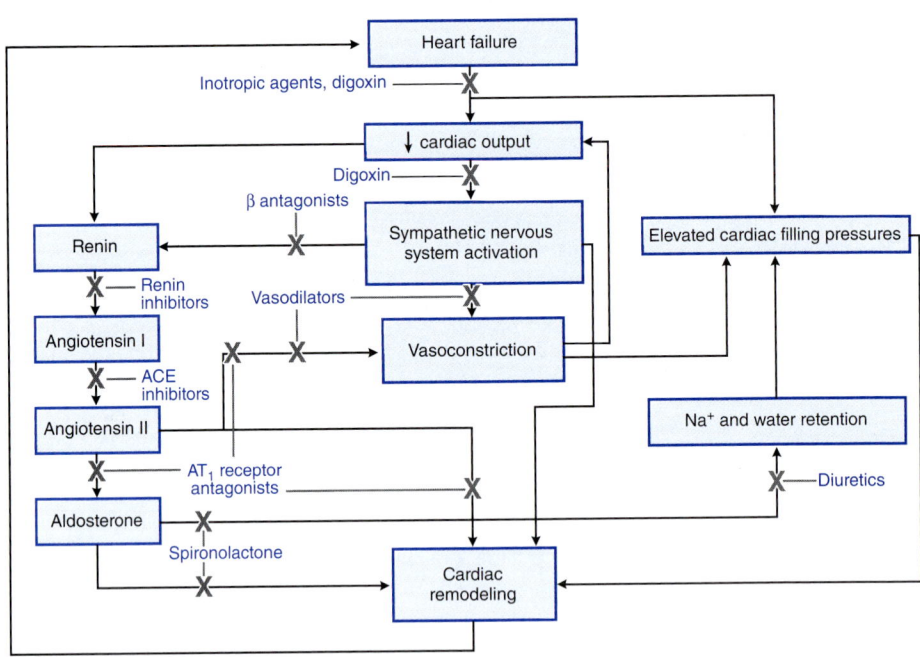

FIGURE 17-1 Pathophysiologic mechanisms of heart failure and major sites of drug action. Congestive heart failure is accompanied by compensatory neurohormonal responses, including activation of the sympathetic nervous and renin–angiotensin–aldosterone axis. Increased ventricular afterload, due to systemic vasoconstriction and chamber dilation, causes depression in systolic function. In addition, increased afterload and the direct effects of angiotensin and norepinephrine on the ventricular myocardium cause pathologic remodeling characterized by progressive chamber dilation and loss of contractile function. Key congestive heart failure medications and their targets of action are presented. ACE, angiotensin-converting enzyme; AT_1 receptor, type 1 angiotensin receptor.

Pharmacotherapy of Heart Failure
CHAPTER 17

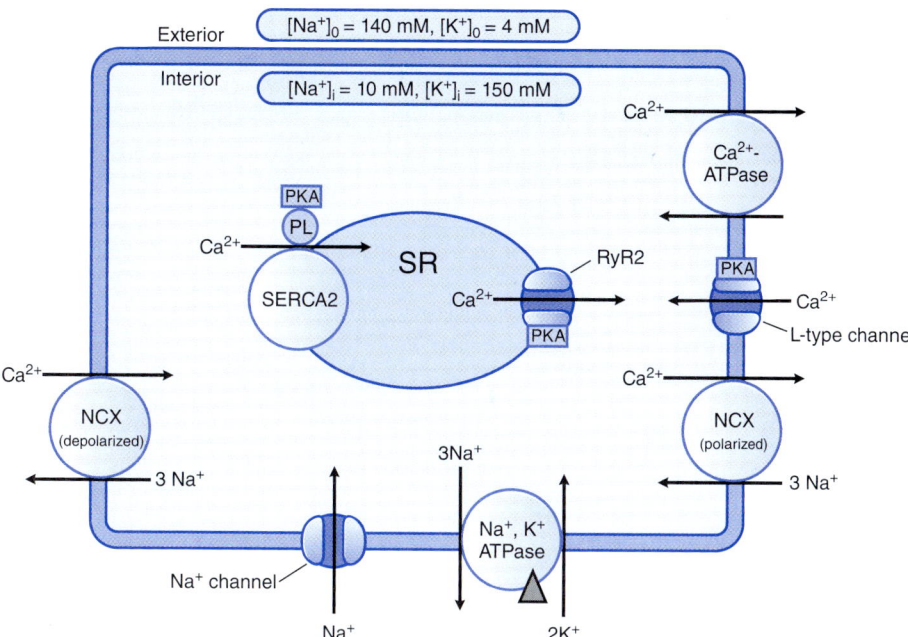

FIGURE 17-2 Sarcolemmal exchange of Na^+ and Ca^{2+} during cell depolarization and repolarization. Na^+ and Ca^{2+} enter the cardiac myocyte via the Na^+ channel and the L-type Ca^{2+} channel during each cycle of membrane depolarization, triggering the release, through the ryanodine receptor (RyR), of larger amounts of Ca^{2+} from internal stores in the sarcoplasmic reticulum (SR). The resulting increase in intracellular Ca^{2+} interacts with troponin C and activates interactions between actin and myosin that result in sarcomere shortening. The electrochemical gradient for Na^+ across the sarcolemma is maintained by active transport of Na^+ out of the cell by the sarcolemmal Na^+,K^+-ATPase. The bulk of cytosolic Ca^{2+} is pumped back into the SR by a Ca^{2+}-ATPase, SERCA2. The remainder is removed from the cell by either a sarcolemmal Ca^{2+}-ATPase or a high-capacity Na^+-Ca^{2+} exchanger, NCX. NCX exchanges 3 Na^+ for every Ca^{2+}, using the electrochemical potential of Na^+ to drive Ca^{2+} extrusion. The direction of Na^+-Ca^{2+} exchange may reverse briefly during depolarization, when the electrical gradient across the sarcolemma is transiently reversed. β Adrenergic agonists and PDE inhibitors, by increasing intracellular cyclic AMP levels, activate PKA, which phosphorylates phospholamban (PL), the α subunit of the L-type Ca^{2+} channel, and regulatory components of the RyR, as well as TnI, the inhibitory subunit of troponin (not shown). As a result, the probabilities of opening of the L-type Ca^{2+} channel and the RyR2 Ca^{2+} channel are doubled; SERCA2 is uninhibited and accumulates Ca^{2+} into the SR faster, more avidly, and to a higher concentration; and relaxation occurs at slightly higher $[Ca^{2+}]_i$ due to slightly reduced sensitivity of the troponin complex to Ca^{2+}. The net effect of these phosphorylations is a positive inotropic effect: a faster rate of tension development to a higher level of tension, followed by a faster rate of relaxation. ▲ indicates site of cardiac glycoside binding. See the text in Chapter 28, Pharmacotherapy of Heart Failure in *Goodman & Gilman's The Pharmacological Basis of Therapeutics*, 12th Edition for the mechanism of positive inotropic effect of cardiac glycosides.

CASE 17-1

A 64-year-old man who suffered a myocardial infarction at the age of 56 complains of difficulty sleeping because he wakes up feeling out of breath. Chest sounds reveal crackles and rales. He has difficulty walking more than 150 feet before having to stop to catch his breath. He is taking a β adrenergic blocker (metoprolol) and an ACE inhibitor (captopril). He also takes ibuprofen every day to relieve pain in his knees.

a. What Stage of heart failure is this patient in?

This patient is in Stage C (structural disease with current symptoms, see Figure 17-3). His prior myocardial infarction caused structural damage to his heart which is now impairing left ventricular function enough to cause symptoms of heart failure.

b. What is causing this patient's symptoms?

This patient has developed pulmonary edema (congestion) because he is retaining Na^+ and water due to activation of the renin-angiotensin-aldosterone axis. The patient has difficulty breathing at night when lying down because the pulmonary edema worsens and impairs ventilation and gas exchange. Heart failure patients with pulmonary congestion often sleep more comfortably if their head and upper body are elevated with a couple of pillows. The symptoms of exercise intolerance and shortness of breath are also the result of the patient's heart failure.

(Continued)

RATIONALE FOR PHARMACOLOGICAL THERAPY OF HEART FAILURE (See Figure 17-3)

- The goal of therapy for patients who are at risk of developing heart failure (Stages A and B) is to slow or stop the progression of the disease, decrease morbidity and mortality, and improve quality of life through the use of inhibitors of the renin-angiotensin-aldosterone system (ACE inhibitors and ARBs) and β adrenergic receptor blockers.

- ACE inhibitors, ARBs, and β blockers are also used in patients who have structural disease with symptoms of heart failure (Stages C and D), but additional therapies are added to treat symptoms of edema (diuretics), improve hemodynamics (inotropes and vasodilators), and facilitate natriuresis (dopamine and nesiritide).

SECTION III — Modulation of Cardiovascular Function

TABLE 17-1 Vasodilator Drugs Used to Treat Heart Failure

DRUG CLASS	EXAMPLES	MECHANISM OF VASODILATING ACTION	PRELOAD REDUCTION	AFTERLOAD REDUCTION
Organic nitrates	Nitroglycerin, isosorbide dinitrate	NO-mediated vasodilation	+++	+
NO donors	Nitroprusside	NO-mediated vasodilation	+++	+++
ACE inhibitors	Captopril, enalapril, lisinopril	Inhibition of AngII generation, ↓ BK degradation	++	++
AngII receptor blockers	Losartan, candesartan	AT_1 receptors blockade	++	++
PDE inhibitors	Milrinone, inamrinone	Inhibition of cyclic AMP degradation	++	++
K^+ channel agonist	Hydralazine	Unknown	+	+++
	Minoxidil	Hyperpolarization of vascular smooth muscle cells	+	+++
α_1 antagonists	Doxazosin, prazosin	Selective α_1 adrenergic receptor blockade	+++	++
Nonselective α antagonists	Phentolamine	Nonselective α adrenergic receptor blockade	+++	+++
β/α_1 antagonists	Carvedilol, labetalol	Selective α_1 adrenergic receptor blockade	++	++
Ca^{2+} channel blockers	Amlodipine, nifedipine, felodipine	Inhibition of L-type Ca^{2+} channels	+	+++
β agonists	Isoproterenol	Stimulation of vascular β_2 adrenergic receptors	+	++

AngII, angiotensin II; AT_1, type 1 angiotensin II receptor; NO, nitric oxide; ACE, angiotensin converting enzyme; PDE, cyclic nucleotide phosphodiesterase; BK, bradykinin.

c. **Why is he taking a β blocker and an ACE inhibitor?**

β Blocker therapy is recommended in patients who have had a myocardial infarction (see Chapter 16) because it reduces mortality. Certain β blockers are also recommended in many heart failure patients who can tolerate them because it blocks the deleterious effects of catecholamines and may lower the risk of arrhythmias. ACE inhibitors are recommended in patients with Stage B and C heart failure to slow disease progression by inhibiting the effects of angiotensin II.

d. **What drugs, if any, should be added, changed, or withdrawn?**

To relieve the symptoms of edema, diuretics are typically added to the medications of patients in Stage C heart failure. The patient should also be counseled to reduce sodium intake since that will also contribute to fluid retention. NSAIDs such as ibuprofen may also contribute to sodium and fluid retention and should be avoided, if possible. There is evidence that NSAIDs such as ibuprofen may increase the risk of cardiovascular events such as stroke in patients who have had an MI.

CASE 17-2

You are counseling a 34-year-old woman who is moderately overweight, and has mild hypertension and type II diabetes. Her father had his first myocardial infarction when he was 45 and died of a subsequent myocardial infarction when he was 52.

a. **Is this patient at risk to develop heart failure and what can she do to lower her risks?**

This woman has several risk factors for developing heart failure, including obesity, hypertension, diabetes, and her family history of cardiovascular disease. She may also have dyslipidemia. She is in Stage A of heart failure (high risk of developing heart failure but no symptoms). She has no control over her genetics, but she can reduce her risk of developing heart failure by controlling her weight, blood pressure, and diabetes.

b. **What medications are recommended for this patient?**

This patient may be able to reduce all of her controllable risks by adopting a healthier life-style (ie, regular exercise and adopting a healthier diet). If lifestyle

(Continued)

Pharmacotherapy of Heart Failure

CHAPTER 17

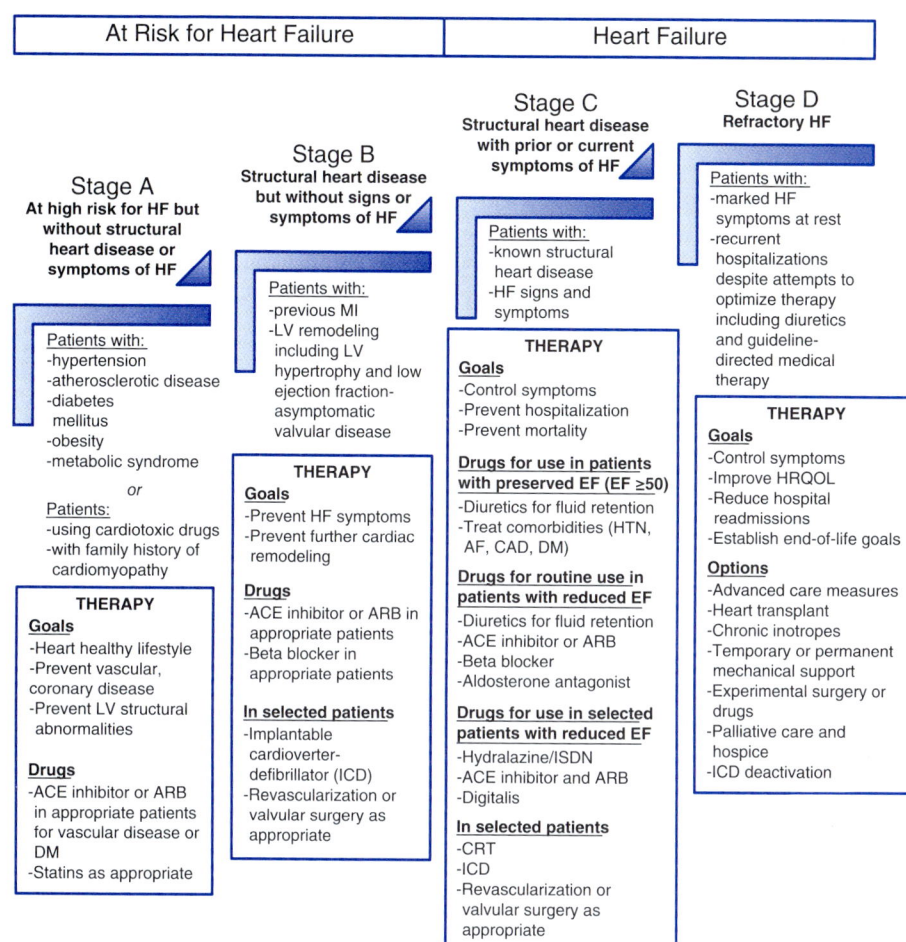

FIGURE 17-3 Stages in the development of HF and recommended therapy by stage. ACE indicates angiotensin-converting enzyme; AF, atrial fibrillation; ARB, angiotensin-receptor blocker; CAD, coronary artery disease; CRT, cardiac resynchronization therapy; DM, diabetes mellitus; EF, ejection fraction; GDMT, guideline-directed medical therapy; HF, heart failure; HRQOL, health-related quality of life; HTN, hypertension; ICD, implantable cardioverter-defibrillator; LV, left ventricular; and MI, myocardial infarction. Preserved EF is defined as an EF ≥ 50%. Reduced EF is defined as an EF ≤ 40%. *(Modified from Yancy CW et al. Circulation. 2013;128:e240-e327.)*

modifications do not fully control her diabetes and hypertension, antidiabetic (see Chapter 30) and antihypertensive therapies (see Chapter 15) are recommended. The antihypertensives that would be most appropriate in this patient are ACE inhibitors or AT_1 blockers (see Chapter 15). If she has dyslipidemia that is not controlled by diet and exercise, a lipid-lowering drug is recommended (see Chapter 20).

CASE 17-3

You are reviewing the medications of a 67-year-old man who has recently developed mild pulmonary congestion and peripheral edema. He has a history of mild heart failure, hypertension, and he occasionally suffers from angina. The drugs he is prescribed to take on a daily basis are aspirin, furosemide, lisinopril, lovastatin, metoprolol, and verapamil. He is also on a low-salt diet.

a. **What are the possible reasons for the pulmonary congestion and peripheral edema?**

Despite being on an ACE inhibitor (lisinopril), a β blocker (metoprolol), and a loop diuretic (furosemide), this patient is decompensating and retaining fluid. It's possible the patient's heart failure is worsening, or the patient is not adhering to the low-salt diet or is not taking his diuretic as prescribed.

(Continued)

SECTION III

Modulation of Cardiovascular Function

BIDIL AND THE AFRICAN-AMERICAN HEART FAILURE TRIAL

The African-American Heart Failure Trial showed significantly reduced mortality and morbidity in self-described African-American patients with heart failure (predominantly NYHA Class III) taking standard therapy with hydralazine and isosorbide dinitrate (ISDN). This lead to the development of the fixed-dose combination agent, BiDil (hydralazine and ISDN).

- The mechanism for the greater efficacy of this drug combination may be due to lower vascular responsiveness to nitric oxide (NO) in African-Americans.
- BiDil was the first race-based drug to be approved by the FDA.
- BiDil is recommended for patients self-described as African-Americans, with moderate to severe symptoms of CHF who are already on optimal therapy with ACE inhibitors, β blockers, and diuretics.

b. **What can be done to relieve this patient's symptoms?**

It is important to first eliminate any possible causes of the edema or worsening of heart failure. One drug that might be worsening the patient's heart failure is verapamil, a calcium channel blocker that can lower left ventricular function. It should be possible to adequately control the patient's hypertension using lisinopril, metoprolol, and furosemide. If a calcium channel blocker is needed to control the patient's angina, a dihydropyridine calcium channel blocker (see Chapter 15) with minimal effects on left ventricular function is recommended. It is also important to determine whether the patient is adhering to a low-salt diet and is taking his diuretic and other drugs as prescribed.

CASE 17-4

A 72-year-old African-American woman with mild heart failure comes in for her annual check-up. During her examination, she complains of occasional dizziness, especially when she stands up quickly. She is taking an ACE inhibitor, thiazide diuretic, and β blocker. Her lung sounds are normal and there is no evidence of peripheral edema.

a. **What might be the reason for this patient's complaint?**

She has orthostatic hypotension which might be due to taking multiple drugs that can lower her blood pressure. Although all of these drugs are appropriate in a patient with mild heart failure, it may be necessary to reduce the dosing of one or more, especially the diuretic since she has no evidence of congestion.

b. **Are there other heart failure therapies that might be appropriate for this patient?**

If her symptoms worsen and are not well controlled by the ACE inhibitor and β blocker, it might be worth adding BiDil (see Side Bar BIDIL AND THE AFRICAN-AMERICAN HEART FAILURE TRIAL). However, her symptoms of mild heart failure appear to be well managed so changes in her medications are not appropriate except for reducing or eliminating the diuretic.

CASE 17-5

A 72-year-old man with atrial fibrillation is hospitalized because of severe pulmonary and peripheral edema that is not adequately treated by his current medications that include losartan, carvedilol, and furosemide. During his stay in the hospital, his edema is controlled by aggressive intravenous (IV) furosemide administration and a strict low-salt diet. He is also started on digoxin and spironolactone.

a. **What is the rationale for adding digoxin?**

Digoxin is a mild inotrope that was once used in most patients with congestive heart failure. Clinical trials have shown that it does not reduce mortality but does reduce hospitalization rates of patients with moderate to severe heart failure when added to standard therapy. By increasing the inotropic state of the ventricles, it will improve kidney function and reduce the risk of rehospitalization due to edema. This patient will also benefit from digoxin because he has atrial fibrillation, which can lead to ventricular tachycardia. Digoxin will increase vagal tone to the heart and thereby slow or block conduction of impulses passing through the AV node and protect the ventricles from atrial-induced tachycardia.

b. **What are the risks of digoxin therapy in this patient?**

Digoxin has a narrow therapeutic index, with toxicity possible at therapeutic doses. Life-threatening toxicities include ventricular arrhythmias and sinus bradycardia.

c. **What are the symptoms of digoxin toxicity?**

The symptoms of digoxin toxicity include cardiac rhythm disturbances, neurological effects, including various visual disturbances, and gastrointestinal symptoms. Severe toxicity can be treated with a neutralizing antidigoxin antisera Fab fragment (DIGIBIND).

(Continued)

Pharmacotherapy of Heart Failure — CHAPTER 17

d. **What is the rationale for adding spironolactone?**

Spironolactone is an aldosterone antagonist that reduces mortality and heart failure-related hospitalizations in patients with moderate to severe heart failure by inhibiting the deleterious effects of aldosterone on kidney and cardiac function (see Table 28-2 in *Goodman & Gilman's The Pharmacological Basis of Therapeutics*, 12th Edition).

e. **What are the side effects of spironolactone?**

Treatment with spironolactone is generally well tolerated, but there is a risk of severe hyperkalemia, especially in combination with an ACE inhibitor and in patients with renal impairment. Gynecomastia is a common side effect of spironolactone that is not common with the more aldosterone-specific antagonist, eplerenone.

CASE 17-6

A 72-year-old woman who had a coronary artery bypass graft when she was 60, and has had symptoms of heart failure for the past 6 years is hospitalized with decompensated heart failure. Her medications prior to hospitalization included losartan, metoprolol, aldosterone, furosemide, and digoxin.

a. **What medications should be considered to restore left ventricular function?**

A parenteral inotrope such as dobutamine, dopamine, or a type 3 phosphodiesterase (PDE3) inhibitor is often needed for patients in Stage D heart failure to maintain LVF. These agents are much more powerful inotropes than digoxin. The choice of an agent depends on whether the patient is hypotensive, has signs of renal insufficiency, or has become refractory to another inotrope.

b. **What are the mechanisms by which inotropic agents exert their effects on the heart?**

All inotropic agents act by increasing Ca^{2+} delivery to the contractile apparatus in ventricular myocytes, but through different mechanisms.

Digoxin (a cardiac glycoside) is a weak orally administered inotrope that acts by inhibiting myocardial Na^+, K^+-ATPase. Inhibition of this pump reduces the ability of the myocyte to remove Ca^{2+} through the Na^+-Ca^{2+} exchanger (NCX). This results in more intracellular Ca^{2+}, more Ca^{2+} being taken up by the sarcoplasmic reticulum (SR), and more Ca^{2+} release from the SR during subsequent excitation-contraction cycles (see Figure 28-5 in *Goodman & Gilman's The Pharmacological Basis of Therapeutics*, 12th Edition).

Dobutamine and dopamine are β adrenergic agonists that are administered parenterally and are reserved for patients in Stage D heart failure. At the doses used clinically to maintain cardiac output in patients with heart failure, their primary mechanism is through stimulation of myocardial β adrenergic receptors. Activation of β adrenergic receptors causes an increase in cAMP, which activates protein kinase A (PKA). Activation of PKA results in phosphorylation of the L-type Ca^{2+} channel which increases Ca^{2+} entry into cardiac myocytes. PKA also phosphorylates proteins on the sarcoplasmic reticulum (SR) membrane that increase SR uptake of Ca^{2+} and subsequent release of Ca^{2+} from the SR.

Dobutamine is administered as a continuous IV infusion ($t_{1/2}$ of ~2 minutes) to patients in end-stage systolic dysfunction (Stage D) to maintain cardiac output. It is a strong positive inotrope because of its myocardial $β_1$ receptor agonism. It also reduces load on the heart because of its $β_2$ adrenergic vasodilating effects in skeletal muscle blood vessels. Tachyphylaxis due to β adrenergic receptor desensitization begins to develop at 2 hours and becomes significant after 72 hours which may require adding or switching to a PDE3 inhibitor to maintain cardiac output. Some patients in Stage D heart failure may benefit from concurrent administration of a β blocker, but this can reduce the efficacy of dobutamine.

Dopamine is preferred over dobutamine in patients with cardiogenic shock or compromised renal function because of its ability to increase mean arterial pressure and

(*Continued*)

SECTION III — Modulation of Cardiovascular Function

NESIRITIDE

Nesiritide is recombinant B-type natriuretic peptide (BNP) approved for acute treatment of patients with decompensated heart failure.

- BNP is normally released by the ventricles when exposed to high filling pressures that stretch the cardiac muscle fibers
- BNP is administered by continuous IV infusion and lowers preload and afterload without increasing heart rate, and improves renal function
- Hypotension is a major adverse effect of BNP and should not be used in patients with low blood pressure

stimulate natriuresis. The hemodynamic effects of dopamine are dose-dependent due to its ability activate a spectrum of receptors in the vasculature with different affinities (see Chapter 7). At the high doses of dopamine used in patients with heart failure, there is an increase in cardiac contractility (activation of heart β_1 receptors), systolic blood pressure is increased (activation of peripheral arterial α adrenergic receptors), venous return is increased (activation of venous α adrenergic receptors), and natriuresis is stimulated.

Milrinone and inamrinone are used for short-term parenteral inotropic support in patients in Stage D heart failure. These agents inhibit type 3 cyclic nucleotide phosphodiesterase (PDE3). Because PDE3 hydrolyzes cAMP in cardiac and vascular smooth muscle cells, inhibition of this enzyme increases cAMP in these cells. In cardiac myocytes, inhibition of PDE3 enhances Ca^{2+} delivery to the contractile proteins through the same PKA-mediated pathway as β adrenergic agonists. In vascular smooth muscle cells, increases in cAMP result in PKA phosphorylation of substrates that cause relaxation and vasodilation. The PDE3 inhibitors are sometimes referred to as inodilators because of their combined inotropic and vasodilating effects. However, they also increase heart rate and predispose patients to ventricular arrhythmias. Because tachyphylaxis does not occur with the PDE3 inhibitors, they can be used to temporarily replace dobutamine for chronic inotrope therapy.

c. What is the preferred parenteral inotrope if this patient is normotensive?

Dobutamine is preferred in normotensive patients, but because of tachyphylaxis, switching to a PDE3 inhibitor will be required after ~72 hours of dobutamine administration.

d. Which inotropic agent is used if the patient is hypotensive?

Dopamine at high doses will increase blood pressure because of its α adrenergic vasoconstrictor effects on peripheral arterials.

PHARMACOLOGY OF INOTROPIC DRUGS

DRUG	MAP	PCWP	SVR	CO	PATIENT POPULATION
Digoxin	⇔	⇔/⇓	⇔	⇔/⇑	AFib or symptomatic patients on maximal β blocker and ACE-I therapy
Dopamine (high dose)	⇑⇑	⇑/⇔	⇑⇑	⇑	Preferred in patients with septic/cardiogenic shock or renal dysfunction
Dobutamine	⇑/⇓	⇓	⇔/⇓	⇑⇑	Preferred β agonist for end-stage systolic dysfunction
Milrinone, inamrinone	⇑/⇓	⇓	⇓⇓	⇑⇑	Preferred in patients on β blocker therapy

AFib: atrial fibrillation; CO: cardiac output; MAP: Mean arterial pressure; PCWP: Pulmonary capillary wedge pressure; SVR: Systemic vascular resistance

KEY CONCEPTS

- Contemporary approaches to treating heart failure recognize that it is a progressive disorder that can be "staged."
- ACE inhibitors and ARBs are first-line drugs used at all stages to prevent and slow the progression of heart failure by inhibiting the renin-angiotensin-aldosterone system.
- β Blockers are first-line drugs used after structural heart disease occurs to prevent the cardiotoxic and arrhythmogenic effects of high catecholamine levels.
- Diuretics are used symptomatically to reduce edema and fluid volume.
  - Diuretics do not reduce mortality.

(Continued)

Pharmacotherapy of Heart Failure — CHAPTER 17

- ➤ Vasodilators are used in selected patients in combination with the first-line drugs to reduce the load on the heart.
- ➤ Inotropic agents are used at late stages of heart failure to improve symptoms by maintaining adequate cardiac output.
  - ➤ Inotropes do not reduce mortality or slow progression of heart failure.

SUMMARY QUIZ

QUESTION 17-1 You are counseling a heart failure patient who is receiving a new prescription for digoxin to treat their atrial fibrillation. Which of the following are common side effects that might indicate digoxin toxicity?

a. Blood in the urine
b. Muscle cramps and joint pain
c. GI disturbances and yellow-green vision changes
d. Photosensitivity and skin discoloration

QUESTION 17-2 A 32-year-old woman has chronic hypertension and a family history of cardiomyopathy. She has no history herself of heart problems and no symptoms of heart failure. Which drug is most appropriate to prevent or slow the development of heart failure in this patient?

a. Lisinopril
b. Verapamil
c. Digoxin
d. Dobutamine

QUESTION 17-3 A 74-year-old man who self-describes himself as being African-American is taking metoprolol, losartan, furosemide, and digoxin to treat his heart failure. However, he still has some symptoms of heart failure. The most appropriate drug to add to this patient's drugs is

a. captopril.
b. diltiazem.
c. nesiritide.
d. BiDil (a combination of hydralazine and isosorbide dinitrate).

QUESTION 17-4 You are reviewing the discharge instructions of a 52-year-old man who was hospitalized with a mild myocardial infarction. He has recovered well and will be able to return to work next week. Before his hospitalization, he was taking lovastatin, enalapril, and low-dose aspirin. The following drug should be added to these drugs because clinical trials have demonstrated that it will help reduce his risk of death:

a. diltiazem.
b. hydrochlorothiazide.
c. carvedilol.
d. digoxin.

QUESTION 17-5 A patient who has recently been hospitalized with severe heart failure and has been receiving IV dobutamine starts to have worsening symptoms. What drug should be used to replace the dobutamine?

a. Norepinephrine
b. Epinephrine
c. Isoproteronol
d. Milrinone

SECTION III Modulation of Cardiovascular Function

SUMMARY QUIZ ANSWER KEY

QUESTION 17-1 Answer is **c**. GI disturbances such as nausea are some of the first indications of digoxin toxicity. Yellow-green vision changes are also a common manifestation of cardiac glycoside toxicity.

QUESTION 17-2 Answer is **a**. This patient has multiple risk factors for development of heart failure including hypertension and a family history of cardiomyopathy. She is in Stage A of heart failure (see Figure 17-3). She should be started on an ACE inhibitor such as lisinopril to control her blood pressure and to reduce her risk of developing structural heart disease (ie, slow or prevent progression to Stage B).

QUESTION 17-3 Answer is **d**. This patient is taking appropriate medications for his heart failure, including first-line medications, an ARB (losartan), and a β blocker (metoprolol), which have been shown to reduce morbidity and mortality in heart failure. The loop diuretic (furosemide) and mild inotrope (digoxin) will help with symptoms, but do not reduce mortality. Evidence from clinical trials shows that BiDil (hydralazine and isosorbide dinitrate) can reduce mortality in African-Americans with heart failure who are being maximally treated with first-line agents but who are still symptomatic.

QUESTION 17-4 Answer is **c**. Carvedilol or another appropriate β blocker (metoprolol or bisoprolol) should be initiated before discharge to reduce mortality in patients who have had a myocardial infarction. The β blocker should be started with a low dose and gradually increased over the course of 6 to 8 weeks until the target dose or maximally tolerated dose is reached.

QUESTION 17-5 Answer is **d**. The PDE3 inhibitors, milrinone and inamrinone, are used to substitute for dobutamine when tachyphylaxis develops to the β receptor agonist. They act by increasing intracellular myocardial and vascular smooth muscle cAMP independent of β receptor activation and are not associated with tachyphylaxis. However, they are associated with life-threatening cardiac arrhythmias and their use is restricted to short-term inotropic support. Milrinone is preferred to inamrinone because of its greater selectivity for PDE3, short $t_{1/2}$, and favorable side effect profile.

SUMMARY: DRUGS USED TO TREAT HEART FAILURE

CLASS AND SUBCLASSES	NAMES	CLINICAL USES	TOXICITIES COMMON	TOXICITIES UNIQUE; CLINICALLY IMPORTANT
Angiotensin-Converting Enzyme (ACE) Inhibitors	Captopril Enalapril, Lisinopril Others (see Chapter 15)	First-line agents used in all stages of heart failure to slow disease progression and reduce mortality	Hypotension and renal insufficiency Dry cough due to increased levels of kinins	Angioneurotic edema (due to increased production of kinins) Teratogenic
Angiotensin Receptor (AT_1) Blockers (ARBs)	Losartan Candesartan Valsartan Others (see Chapter 15)	Same as ACE inhibitors; indicated in patients who cannot tolerate the side effects of increased levels of kinins associated with ACE inhibitors	Hypotension and renal insufficiency	Teratogenic
β Adrenergic Receptor Blockers	Metoprolol Carvedilol Bisoprolol	First-line agents used in Stages B, C, and D to slow disease progression and reduce mortality	Bradycardia, hypotension Can impair LV function and exacerbate heart failure symptoms Should be avoided in patients with reactive airway disease (asthma) or with SA or AV nodal dysfunction or in combination with other drugs that inhibit AV conduction, such as verapamil	Risk of hypoglycemic reactions may be increased in diabetics taking insulin

Pharmacotherapy of Heart Failure — CHAPTER 17

CLASS AND SUBCLASSES	NAMES	CLINICAL USES	TOXICITIES	
			COMMON	UNIQUE; CLINICALLY IMPORTANT
Na^+, K^+-ATPase Inhibitor	Digoxin	Indicated in patients with LV dysfunction in atrial fibrillation, or patients who remain symptomatic despite maximal therapy with ACE inhibitors and β blockers	GI disturbances Neurological disturbances (confusion, hallucinations, other), visual (yellow-green) disturbances Ventricular bradycardia, AV block, supraventricular tachycardia	Can exacerbate supraventricular arrhythmias and lead to ventricular arrhythmias
Aldosterone Receptor Antagonists	Spironolactone Eplerenone	Indicated for patients with low LV ejection fraction When added to standard therapy, morbidity and mortality are reduced in patients with heart failure	Hyperkalemia Can induce diarrhea and other gastric disturbances Can cause CNS effects such drowsiness, ataxia, and headache	Gynecomastia (less frequently with eplerenone) Life-threatening hyperkalemia, thus contraindicated in patients with hyperkalemia or those at risk of hyperkalemia Contraindicated in patients with peptic ulcers
Vasodilators	Hydralazine Organic nitrates Others (see Table 17-1 and Chapter 15)	To reduce preload (filling pressure) and afterload (mean arterial pressure)	Hypotension	Depends on agent (see Chapter 15)
Diuretics (Many Subclasses)	Many agents (see Chapter 15)	To reduce fluid retention, especially in patients with peripheral and pulmonary edema	Hypokalemia, hyponatremia, and other electrolyte effects, depending on agent (see Chapter 15)	Depends on agent (see Chapter 15)
β Adrenergic Receptor Agonists	Dopamine Dobutamine	Inotropic agents Indicated in patients with end-stage heart failure (Stage D) requiring chronic inotropic therapy to maintain LV function	Arrhythmogenic, increased mortality	Tachyphylaxis develops rapidly requiring short-term substitution with PDE3 inhibitors
Phosphodiesterase Type III (PDE3) Inhibitors	Milrinone Inamrinone	Parenteral short-term agents used in end-stage heart failure patients who have become tolerant to β adrenergic agonists	Arrhythmogenic, increased mortality	
Natriuretic Peptide Receptor Agonist	Nesiritide	Indicated in acutely decompensated end-stage heart failure patients to increase natriuresis, and reduce preload and afterload	Hypotension	

CHAPTER 18

Antiarrhythmic Drugs

This chapter will be most useful after having a basic understanding of the material in Chapter 29, Anti-Arrhythmic Drugs in *Goodman & Gilman's The Pharmacological Basis of Therapeutics*, 12th Edition. In particular, the reader is directed to the following tables, and to animations available in the online version of *Goodman & Gilman's The Pharmacological Basis of Therapeutics*:

- Table 29-1 Drug-Induced Cardiac Arrhythmias, which shows drugs known to cause arrhythmias (ie, proarrhythmias), the likely arrhythmogenic mechanism, the treatment, and the clinical features of the proarrhythmia
- Table 29-4 Patient-Specific Anti-arrhythmic Drug Contraindications, which shows conditions and contraindicated drugs
- Several animations in the online version of *Goodman & Gilman's The Pharmacological Basis of Therapeutics* illustrate the electrophysiology of cardiac cells and the mechanism of action of antiarrhythmic drugs

LEARNING OBJECTIVES

☑ Know the principles of cardiac electrophysiology especially the ion channels, exchangers, and pumps that are targets of antiarrhythmic drugs.
☑ Understand the mechanisms that cause cardiac arrhythmias.
☑ Know the common and important tachyarrhythmias and their mechanisms.
☑ Understand the mechanisms and classification of antiarrhythmic drugs.
☑ Know the principles of antiarrhythmic drug pharmacotherapy.
☑ Know the pharmacological, pharmacokinetic, and adverse effects of specific antiarrhythmic agents.

DRUGS IN THIS CHAPTER

- Adenosine (ADENOCARD)
- Amiodarone (CORDARONE)
- Digoxin (LANOXIN; see Chapter 17)
- Diltiazem (CARDIZEM)
- Disopyramide (NORPACE)
- Dofetilide (TIKOSYN)
- Dronedarone (MULTAQ)
- Esmolol (BREVIBLOC)
- Flecainide (TAMBOCOR)
- Ibutilide (CORVERT)
- Lidocaine (XYLOCAINE)
- Mexiletine (MEXITIL)
- Procainamide (PRONESTYL)
- Propafenone (RYTHMOL)
- Propranolol (INDERAL; see Chapter 7)
- Quinidine (QUINIDEX)
- Sotalol (BETAPACE)
- Verapamil (CALAN; see Chapter 16)

THE CARDIAC ACTION POTENTIAL

- In fast-conducting cardiac myocytes and cells of the conducting system, Phase 0 depolarization is caused by the opening of voltage-gated Na^+ channels.
- In slow-conducting cells of the sinoatrial (SA) node and atrioventricular (AV) node, which have relatively few voltage-gated Na^+ channels, Phase 0 depolarization is caused by opening of voltage-gated L-type Ca^{2+} channels.
- Phase 3 repolarization is primarily caused by K^+ movement out of the cell through voltage-gated K^+ channels.
- Figure 18-1 shows action potentials from different regions of the heart, the ion currents that contribute to these action potentials, and the corresponding effects of the ion currents on the electrocardiogram (ECG).

MECHANISMS OF ACTION OF DRUGS USED TO TREAT CARDIAC ARRHYTHMIAS

ANTIARRHYTHMIC DRUG CLASS	DRUG	PRIMARY MECHANISM OF ACTION*
Class IA	Quinidine, procainamide, disopyramide	Na^+ channel blocker, prolongs action potential duration (APD)
Class IB	Lidocaine, mexiletine	Na^+ channel blocker, rapid dissociation
Class IC	Flecainide, propafenone	Na^+ channel blocker, slow dissociation
Class II	Propranolol, sotalol, esmolol	β Adrenergic blocker
Class III	Amiodarone, sotalol, ibutilide, dofetilide, dronedarone	Prolongs APD (primarily by K^+ channel blockade)
Class IV	Verapamil, diltiazem	Ca^{2+} channel blocker (nondihydropyridine)
Miscellaneous	Adenosine	Adenosine receptor agonist
Miscellaneous	Digoxin	Na^+, K^+-ATPase inhibitor

*Note: Most antiarrhythmic drugs have multiple mechanisms of action (Table 18-1).

Antiarrhythmic Drugs

CHAPTER 18

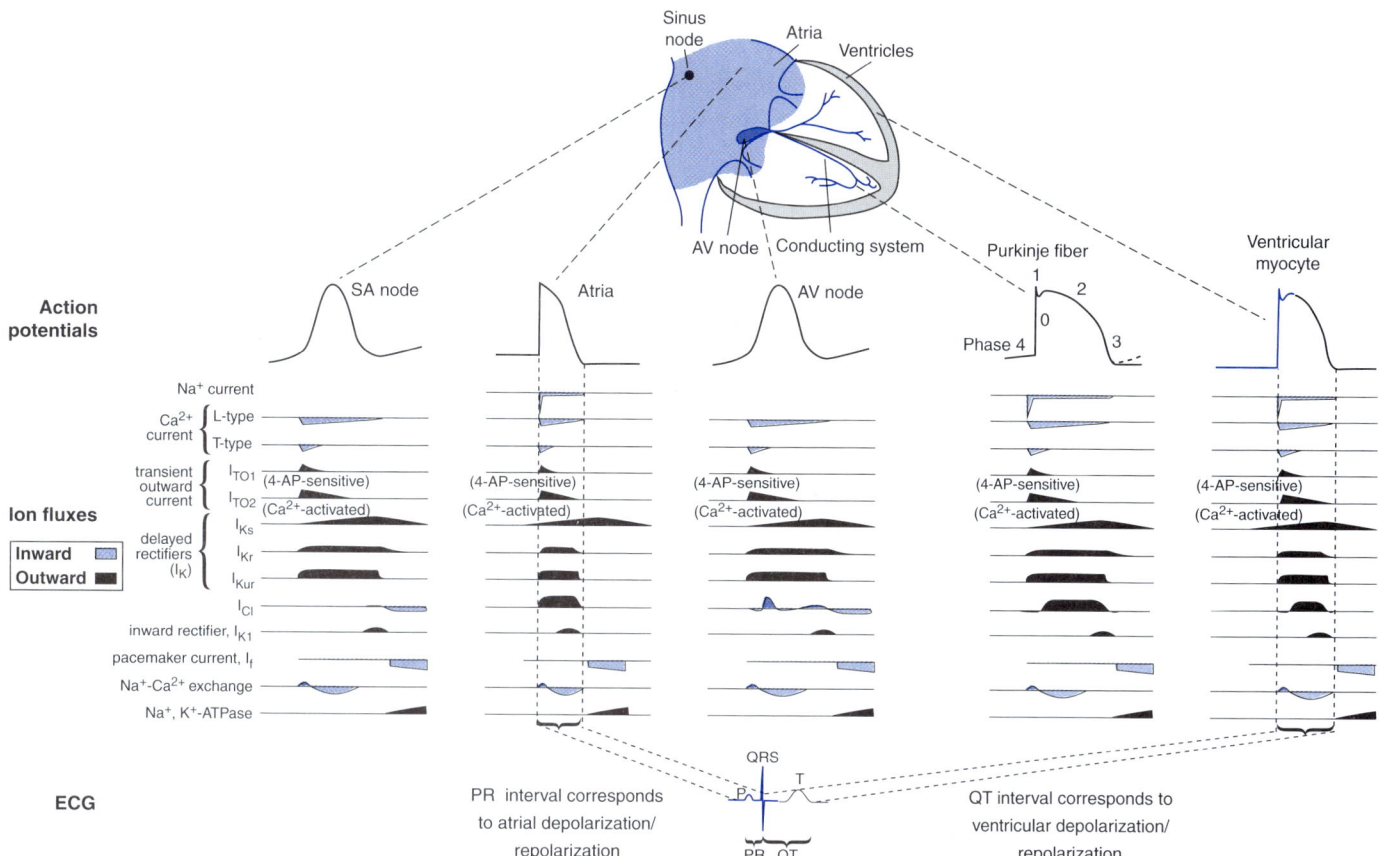

FIGURE 18-1 Action potentials that occur during normal impulse propagation and the time course of the ion currents that generate them.

CASE 18-1

A 53-year-old woman visits the emergency department after losing consciousness while working in her garden. She says she has recently had episodes of dizziness and fainting. Her ECG looks unremarkable except that the QT interval is prolonged.

a. **What are the possible causes of her recent fainting spells?**

The prolonged QT interval suggests that her fainting spells may be due to torsade de pointes (TdP) (see Side Bar LONG QT AND TORSADE DE POINTES). Because her syncope has started fairly recently, it is likely that the TdP might be due to a drug that prolongs action potential duration. Drugs that can prolong QT include Class IA and Class III antiarrhythmic drugs (see MECHANISMS OF ACTION OF DRUGS USED TO TREAT CARDIAC ARRHYTHMIAS), as well as many other drugs, including antibiotics (erythromycin, sparfloxacin), antipsychotics (chlorpromazine, haloperidol), and antiemetics (domperidone, droperidol). Another possible cause is hypokalemia, especially if she has been taking diuretics that cause loss of K^+. She might also have a form of hereditary long QT that has become manifested due to a QT-prolonging drug or hypokalemia. It is important to determine the drugs that this patient is currently taking and whether any of them have been started recently. It would also be useful to know whether there is a family history of sudden cardiac death which might indicate she has a hereditary form of long QT syndrome.

(Continued)

MECHANISMS OF CARDIAC TACHYARRHYTHMIAS

- Three arrhythmogenic mechanisms are thought to underlie most tachyarrhythmias:
  - Enhanced automaticity resulting from enhanced phase 4 spontaneous depolarization (see Figure 29-10, *Goodman & Gilman*, 12th Edition)
  - Triggered automaticity, including abnormal rhythms associated with delayed afterdepolarizations (DADs) resulting from Ca^{2+} overload, and those associated with early afterdepolarizations (EADs) caused by prolongation of the action potential (see Figure 29-6, *Goodman & Gilman*, 12th Edition)
  - Reentry, which involves the formation of a self-perpetuating circuit caused by anisotropic conduction around an anatomic or functional barrier (see Figures 29-7 and 29-8, *Goodman & Gilman's The Pharmacological Basis of Therapeutics*, 12th Edition)
- Understanding the underlying arrhythmogenic mechanism can facilitate the choice of antiarrhythmic drugs (see Table 18-1)

SECTION III — Modulation of Cardiovascular Function

TABLE 18-1 A Mechanistic Approach to Antiarrhythmic Therapy

ARRHYTHMIA	COMMON MECHANISM	ACUTE THERAPY[a]	CHRONIC THERAPY[a]
Premature atrial, nodal, or ventricular depolarizations	Unknown	None indicated	None indicated
Atrial fibrillation	Disorganized "functional" reentry Continual AV node stimulation and irregular, often rapid, ventricular rate	1. Control ventricular response: AV node block[b] 2. Restore sinus rhythm: DC cardioversion	1. Control ventricular response: AV nodal block[b] 2. Maintain normal rhythm: K$^+$ channel block, Na$^+$ channel block, Na$^+$ channel block with $\tau_{recovery}$ >1 second
Atrial flutter	Stable reentrant circuit in the right atrium Ventricular rate often rapid and irregular	Same as atrial fibrillation	Same as atrial fibrillation AV nodal blocking drugs especially desirable to avoid ↑ ventricular rate Ablation in selected cases[c]
Atrial tachycardia	Enhanced automaticity, DAD-related automaticity, or reentry in atrium	Same as atrial fibrillation	Same as atrial fibrillation Ablation of tachycardia "focus"[c]
AV nodal reentrant tachycardia (PSVT)	Reentrant circuit within or near AV node	*Adenosine AV nodal block Less commonly: ↑ vagal tone (digitalis, edrophonium, phenylephrine)	*AV nodal block Flecainide Propafenone *Ablation[c]
Arrhythmias associated with WPW syndrome: 1. AV reentry (PSVT)	Reentry	Same as AV nodal reentry	K$^+$ channel block Na$^+$ channel block with $\tau_{recovery}$ >1 second *Ablation[c]
2. Atrial fibrillation with atrioventricular conduction via accessory pathway	Very rapid rate due to nondecremental properties of accessory pathway	*DC cardioversion *Procainamide	K$^+$ channel block Na$^+$ channel block with $\tau_{recovery}$ >1 second (AV nodal blockers can be harmful)
VT in patients with remote myocardial infarction	Reentry near the rim of the healed myocardial infarction	Lidocaine Amiodarone Procainamide *DC cardioversion	*ICD[d] Amiodarone K$^+$ channel block Na$^+$ channel block
VT in patients without structural heart disease	DADs triggered by ↑ sympathetic tone	Adenosine[e] Verapamil[e] β Blockers[e] DC cardioversion	Verapamil[e] β Blockers[e]
VF	Disorganized reentry	*DC cardioversion Lidocaine *Amiodarone Procainamide	*ICD[d] Amiodarone K$^+$ channel block Na$^+$ channel block
Torsades de pointes, congenital or acquired (often drug related)	EAD-related triggered activity	Pacing Magnesium Isoproterenol	β Blockade Pacing

*Indicates treatment of choice.

[a]Acute drug therapy is administered intravenously; chronic therapy implies long-term oral use.

[b]AV nodal block can be achieved clinically by adenosine, Ca^{2+} channel block, β adrenergic receptor blockade, or increased vagal tone (a major anti-arrhythmic effect of digitalis glycosides).

[c]Ablation is a procedure in which tissue responsible for the maintenance of a tachycardia is identified by specialized recording techniques and then selectively destroyed, usually by high-frequency radio waves delivered through a catheter placed in the heart.

[d]ICD, implanted cardioverter–defibrillator: a device that can sense VT or VF and deliver pacing and/or cardioverting shocks to restore normal rhythm.

[e]These may be harmful in reentrant VT and so should be used for acute therapy only if the diagnosis is secure. DAD, delayed afterdepolarization; EAD, early afterdepolarization; WPW, Wolff–Parkinson–White syndrome; PSVT, paroxysmal supraventricular tachycardia; VT, ventricular tachycardia; VF, ventricular fibrillation.

b. **What are your therapeutic options?**

If the fainting is thought to be due to TdP, it is important to first identify the cause of this arrhythmia and remove it, if possible. Drugs are the most likely cause so it is important to review the patient's medications, particularly ones that she has started taking recently. If she is hypokalemic, this should be corrected with supplemental K^+. If she is taking a diuretic, her dosing could be reduced or she should be changed to a potassium-sparing diuretic. If the patient is suspected of carrying one of the mutations that results in hereditary long QT syndrome, genetic testing that involves sequencing all of these genes may facilitate appropriate choice of therapy. For instance, patients with hereditary long QT whose TdP is brought on by exercise and activation of the sympathetic nervous system may benefit from β-adrenergic blockers.

CASE 18-2

A 47-year-old man with uncomplicated atrial fibrillation is prescribed diltiazem.

a. **What is the mechanistic rationale for using diltiazem to treat atrial fibrillation?**

Diltiazem inhibits L-type voltage-gated Ca^{2+} channels in the SA and AV nodes of the heart. By inhibiting these channels in the AV node, conduction of impulses through the AV node is slowed or blocked. This protects the ventricular rate of depolarization from being controlled by the aberrantly high rate of depolarization of the atria.

b. **What effect will diltiazem have on the ECG of this patient?**

In a patient with atrial fibrillation, the ventricular rate can be rapid and irregular. This will result in an ECG in which the RR intervals are relatively short and variable. Diltiazem is expected to slow ventricular rate and reduce irregular ventricular depolarizations which will be seen on the ECG as a prolongation of RR intervals and an increase in the regularity of RR intervals. In a patient without atrial fibrillation, diltiazem will increase the PR interval (which reflects the time an impulse takes to travel through the AV node) and increase the RR interval secondary to slowing the spontaneous depolarization of the SA node.

c. **What are the other effects and potential risks of using diltiazem?**

Because diltiazem blocks L-type Ca^{2+} channels in the heart and in arterial smooth muscle cells, the drug has negative inotropic effects on the heart and lowers blood pressure because of its vasodilating effects. In patients with poor ventricular function or low blood pressure, this agent could further reduce cardiac output and lower mean arterial pressure.

d. **If diltiazem is not well tolerated by this patient, what other classes of drugs might be useful in treating this patient's atrial fibrillation?**

Other classes of drugs that could be used for ventricular rate control include β adrenergic blockers. To treat the arrhythmogenesis of atrial fibrillation, antiarrhythmic drugs that block Na^+ channels and/or K^+ channels in atrial myocytes might be useful (see Table 18-1).

e. **What other class of drugs are indicated in patients with uncomplicated atrial fibrillation?**

Patients with atrial fibrillation are at significantly increased risk of stroke and other thromboembolic events due to stasis of blood in the atria. To reduce the risk of blood clots, patients with sustained uncomplicated atrial fibrillation typically take oral anticoagulants such as warfarin, dabigatran, rivaroxaban, or apixaban (see Chapter 19).

LONG QT AND TORSADE DE POINTES

- A prolongation of the QT interval on the ECG is an indication that repolarization of ventricular myocytes is slowed.

- Because the outward repolarizing currents (the delayed rectifier currents) are carried by various voltage-gated K^+ channels, drugs that inhibit these channels can prolong QT interval.

- Mutations in genes that regulate these K^+ channels can lead to hereditary long QT syndrome (LQT).

- Patients with drug-induced LQT (DILQT) or hereditary LQT are at risk of developing a life-threatening polymorphic ventricular tachycardia known as torsade de pointes (TdP; "twisting of the points" in French) which can progress to ventricular fibrillation.

- TdP is so-named because the QRS complexes progressively increase and decrease in size giving the illusion of a picket fence that is being twisted around a central axis (see Figure 29-9 in *Goodman & Gilman's The Pharmacological Basis of Therapeutics*, 12th Edition).

- Treatment of patients who develop TdP include removing the underlying cause, if known, and intravenous magnesium sulfate to terminate the arrhythmia.

SECTION III   Modulation of Cardiovascular Function

CASE 18-3

A 59-year-old man suddenly loses consciousness in a shopping mall. A security guard at the mall cannot detect a pulse and uses an automated external defibrillator (AED) to resuscitate the man. He regains consciousness and is taken by ambulance to a nearby hospital. In the emergency department waiting room, he loses consciousness again. His ECG shows that he is in ventricular fibrillation.

a. What treatment will this patient receive in the ED?

Ventricular fibrillation is a life-threatening arrhythmia and must be treated aggressively to restore normal sinus rhythm. The patient should be defibrillated and should be administered an intravenous antiarrhythmic drug such as amiodarone, lidocaine, or procainamide to prevent recurrence. Of these 3 drugs, IV amiodarone is the drug of choice for this indication (see Table 18-1).

b. What is the mechanistic rationale for the drug(s) used for the acute treatment of patients in ventricular fibrillation?

Ventricular fibrillation is characterized by disorganized reentry in the ventricular myocardium. Amiodarone, lidocaine, and procainamide all block the voltage-gated Na^+ channel and increase the threshold voltage required to open the channel. Moreover, all 3 agents exhibit state-dependent block of the Na^+ channel (Table 18-2), with amiodarone binding the Inactive (I) state, procainamide binding the Open (O) state, and lidocaine binding both the Inactive and Open states (I>O). By blocking the Na^+ channel in the Open and Inactive states, the drugs will preferentially block rapidly depolarizing myocytes, leaving those myocytes depolarizing at normal rates relatively unaffected. Thus, any reentrant circuits formed in the ventricles following the electrical defibrillation will be selectively inhibited, thereby preventing recurrence of the tachyarrhythmia. In addition to blocking the Na^+ channel, amiodarone and procainamide also have antiarrhythmic effects through their actions on blocking outward K^+ currents.

c. What treatments might be used in the long-term to prevent another episode of ventricular fibrillation in this patient?

The treatment of choice for long-term prevention of ventricular fibrillation is an implantable cardioverter-defibrillator (ICD; see Table 18-1). Such a device can be programmed to detect ventricular tachyarrhythmias and deliver a shock and/or pacing to maintain normal sinus rhythm. As an alternative or in addition to an ICD, drug therapy that includes a Na^+ and/or K^+ channel blocker could be used. Amiodarone is a drug of choice for chronic therapy because it has both Na^+ and K^+ channel blocking activities and has minimal negative inotropic effects.

CASE 18-4

A 38-year-old man complains of not having the energy to participate in strenuous sports that are part of his active lifestyle. He had been a competitive amateur cyclist but now has difficulty training. An ECG indicates he has atrial fibrillation.

a. What are the risks and benefits of starting this patient on antiarrhythmic drug therapy?

The risks of therapy include proarrhythmias as well as extracardiac side effects associated with long-term drug therapy. Pharmacological therapy that alleviates the patient's atrial fibrillation may improve quality of life and reduce the risk of stroke, but may not reduce mortality.

b. What are the treatment options?

Because of the patient's age and good health, nonpharmacological therapies should be considered including ablation and DC cardioversion (see Table 18-1). These have the potential to provide permanent or long-term termination of the arrhythmia. Antiarrhythmic drugs carry significant risks, and it might be safer to avoid any drug therapy, except for anticoagulant therapy, to reduce the risk of stroke.

TABLE 18-2 Major Electrophysiologic Actions of Anitarrhythmic Drugs

DRUG	Na+ CHANNEL BLOCK $\tau_{RECOVERY}$[1], SECONDS	STATE DEPENDENCE[1]	↑APD	Ca^{2+} CHANNEL BLOCK	AUTONOMIC EFFECTS	OTHER EFFECTS
Lidocaine	0.1	I > O				
Phenytoin	0.2	I				
Mexiletine[a]	0.3					
Procainamide	1.8	O	✓		Ganglionic blockade (especially intravenous)	✓: Metabolite prolongs APD
Quinidine	3	O	✓	(x)	α Blockade, vagolytic Anticholinergic	
Disopyramide[b]	9	O	✓		Anticholinergic	
Propafenone[b]	11	O ≈ I	✓		β Blockade (variable clinical effect)	
Flecainide[a]	11	O	(x)	(x)		
β Blockers: Propanolol[b]					β Blockade	Na+ channel block *in vitro*
Sotalol[b]			✓		β Blockade	
Amiodarone, Dronedarone	1.6	I	✓	(x)	Noncompetitive β blockade	Antithyroid action
Dofetilide			✓			
Ibutilide			✓			
Verapamil[a]				✓		
Diltiazem[a]				✓		
Digoxin					✓: Vagal stimulation	✓: Inhibition of Na+, K+-ATPase
Adenosine				✓	✓: Adenosine receptor Activation	✓: Activation of outward K+ current
Magnesium				?✓		Mechanism not well understood

✓Indicates an effect that is important in mediating the clinical action of a drug. (x)Indicates a demonstrable effect whose relationship to drug action in patients is less well established.
[a]Indicates drugs prescribed as racemates, and the enantiomers are thought to exert similar electrophysiologic effects.
[b]Indicates racemates for which clinically relevant differences in the electrophysiologic properties of individual enantiomers have been reported (see text). One approach to classifying drugs is:

Class	Major action
I	Na+ channel block
II	β blockade
III	action potential prolongation (usually by K+ channel block)
IV	Ca^{2+} channel block

Drugs are listed here according to this scheme. It is important to bear in mind, however, that many drugs exert multiple effects that contribute to their clinical actions. It is occasionally clinically useful to subclassify Na+ channel blockers by their rates of recovery from drug-induced block ($\tau_{recovery}$) under physiologic conditions. Because this is a continuous variable and can be modulated by factors such as depolarization of the resting potential, these distinctions can become blurred: class Ib, $\tau_{recovery}$ <1 s; class Ia, $\tau_{recovery}$ 1–10 s; class Ic, $\tau_{recovery}$ >10 s. These class and subclass effects are associated with distinctive ECG changes, characteristic "class" toxicities, and efficacy in specific arrhythmia syndromes.
[1]These data are dependent on experimental conditions, including species and temperature. O, open-state blocker; I, inactivated-state blocker; APD, action potential duration.

SECTION III — Modulation of Cardiovascular Function

CASE 18-5

A 12-year-old girl is brought to the ED with intermittent symptoms of dizziness and syncope. Her ECG shows that she has paroxysmal supraventricular tachycardia (PSVT).

a. What is the most likely arrhythmogenic mechanism causing the PSVT?

The most common mechanism causing PSVT is a reentrant circuit within or near the AV node (see Figures 29-7 and 29-8, in *Goodman & Gilman's The Pharmacological Basis of Therapeutics*, 12th Edition).

b. What is the drug of choice to rapidly terminate the PSVT?

Adenosine (IV) is the drug of choice to rapidly terminate PSVT because of its ability to inhibit conduction through the AV node (see Table 18-1). It acts through purinergic receptors to hyperpolarize AV nodal cells and has a very short half-life (<10 seconds). Other drugs that block AV nodal conduction include Ca^{2+} channel blockers (diltiazem and verapamil) and β adrenergic blockers, but adenosine is the drug of first choice because of its short half-life. Drugs that increase vagal tone (digitalis, edrophonium, phenylephrine) are less commonly used AV nodal blockers.

c. What can be done to prevent recurrence of PSVT in this patient?

Oral AV nodal blocking agents are the drugs of choice to prevent recurrence of PSVTs (see Table 18-1). Flecainide and propafenone are also useful drugs because of their ability to alter the electrophysiological properties of the fast-conducting tissue in the reentrant circuit. Selective ablation of tissue that is critical to the maintenance of the reentrant circuit (eg, an accessory pathway) is a treatment of choice because it can result in a permanent cure.

CASE 18-6

A 62-year-old man who had a myocardial infarction 3 years ago now complains of episodes of light-headedness. His cardiologist determines that his symptoms are the result of nonsustained ventricular tachycardia (VT), and that he has developed moderate systolic heart failure.

a. What is the likely cause of this patient's ventricular tachycardia?

This patient's VT is likely due to a reentrant circuit near the site of the healed infarction (see Table 18-1).

b. What are the treatment options for this patient?

The treatment of choice for this patient is an ICD that can sense when the patient has VT or ventricular fibrillation and can pace or cardiovert the heart into normal sinus rhythm (see Table 18-1). Alternatively or in addition to the ICD, this patient might receive an antiarrhythmic drug. Because this patient has heart failure, antiarrhythmic drugs that decrease left ventricular function (eg, disopyramide and flecainide) should be avoided. Drugs that would be appropriate are amiodarone, dronedarone, and K^+ channel blockers such as dofetilide.

c. The patient's cardiologist prescribes amiodarone. What are the toxicities that might be seen with long-term therapy?

As with most antiarrhythmic agents, there are risks of long-term therapy with amiodarone that must be considered and mitigated, if possible. Although amiodarone is effective in treating a wide range of arrhythmias and is one of the few antiarrhythmic agents that has been shown to reduce mortality in clinical trials, it is associated with a large number of extracardiac toxicities. Serious toxicities (some of which are life threatening) include pulmonary toxicity, hepatotoxicity, effects on thyroid function, neuromuscular symptoms, dermatological reactions, and effects on vision. The risk of these toxicities is increased because the mean elimination half-life of amiodarone is more than 50 days.

Antiarrhythmic Drugs

CHAPTER 18

KEY CONCEPTS

➡ Antiarrhythmic drugs act by altering cardiac ion fluxes, directly or indirectly.

➡ Most antiarrhythmic drugs have multiple mechanisms of action.

➡ Antiarrhythmic drugs can cause arrhythmias and can have other life-threatening side effects.

➡ In choosing an antiarrhythmic drug therapy, the risks of therapy, as well as possible benefits, should be considered; patients who are asymptomatic may derive little benefit from taking a drug that carries significant risks.

SUMMARY QUIZ

QUESTION 18-1 An 84-year-old woman being treated for hypertension, mild heart failure (NYHA class II), and persistent atrial fibrillation is taking several different medications: aspirin, sotalol, diltiazem, metoprolol, captopril, chlorothiazide, and warfarin. Over the past several weeks, she has begun to complain that she is no longer able to take her dog for long walks because she tires easily. She also complains of shortness of breath. The drug-drug interactions most likely contributing to the patient's recent symptoms are

a. sotalol and diltiazem.
b. diltiazem and metoprolol.
c. sotalol and metoprolol.
d. all of the above.

QUESTION 18-2 A 68-year-old man who had a myocardial infarction a year earlier shows premature ventricular beats on his ECG during a routine physical examination. He has not had any symptoms related to this arrhythmia such as dizziness or syncope. What is the best drug therapy for this patient to treat his arrhythmia?

a. No drug therapy
b. An AV nodal blocker
c. A Na^+ channel blocker
d. A K^+ channel blocker
e. A Ca^{2+} blocker

QUESTION 18-3 A 72-year-old patient with heart failure and atrial fibrillation is receiving digoxin. The mechanistic rationale for using digoxin to treat the patient's arrhythmia is that

a. digoxin inhibits Ca^{2+} channels in the AV node.
b. digoxin inhibits atrial depolarizations by its effects on Na^+ channels.
c. digoxin increases vagal tone.
d. digoxin slows repolarization in cardiac myocytes.

QUESTION 18-4 What is the rationale for the use of lidocaine in treating a patient with ventricular tachycardia?

a. It blocks Ca^{2+} channels in ventricular myocytes.
b. It blocks Na^+ channels in ventricular myocytes.
c. It blocks K^+ channels in ventricular myocytes.
d. It blocks β adrenergic receptors in ventricular myocytes.
e. It activates purinergic receptors in the AV node.

PRINCIPLES IN THE CLINICAL USE OF ANTIARRHYTHMIC DRUGS

Antiarrhythmic drugs can be very efficacious in terminating or preventing cardiac arrhythmias, but often carry significant risks, even when used at therapeutic concentrations. The fundamental principles of antiarrhythmic therapy should be applied to optimize benefits and minimize risks:

1. Identify and remove precipitating factors.
   ▸ Electrolyte disturbances (especially hypokalemia)
   ▸ Myocardial ischemia
   ▸ Drugs that can cause arrhythmias, including many that prolong QT interval

2. Establish the goals of treatment.
   ▸ Some arrhythmias should not be treated, as illustrated by the CAST clinical trial.
   ▸ Some patients with arrhythmias may be asymptomatic and it may be difficult to establish the benefit of antiarrhythmic drug therapy.
   ▸ Choice of therapy should be based on the goals of treatment.

3. Minimize risks.
   ▸ A common risk of antiarrhythmic drugs is proarrhythmias (see Table 29-1 in *Goodman & Gilman's The Pharmacological Basis of Therapeutics*, 12th Edition).
   ▸ Monitoring of drug concentrations in the plasma may minimize some adverse effects.
   ▸ Some antiarrhythmic drugs may be contraindicated in specific patients (see Table 29-4 in *Goodman & Gilman's The Pharmacological Basis of Therapeutics*, 12th Edition), including many patients who are at higher risk of arrhythmias.

4. The electrophysiology of the heart is a "Moving Target" and can change in response to external factors.
   ▸ Changes in autonomic tone
   ▸ Myocardial ischemia
   ▸ Myocardial stretch as can occur in heart failure
   ▸ Serum electrolyte disturbances

SECTION III — Modulation of Cardiovascular Function

QUESTION 18-5 What is the mechanism of action of sotalol in preventing ventricular and atrial arrhythmias?

a. It blocks Ca^{2+} channels in ventricular myocytes.
b. It blocks Na^+ channels in ventricular myocytes.
c. It blocks K^+ channels in ventricular myocytes.
d. It blocks β adrenergic receptors in ventricular myocytes.
e. It blocks K^+ channels and β adrenergic receptors in ventricular myocytes.

SUMMARY QUIZ ANSWER KEY

QUESTION 18-1 Answer is **d**. All of the indicated drug combinations would be expected to have additive effects in slowing heart rate and depressing left ventricular function. Because this person has mild heart failure, drugs that depress left ventricular function can exacerbate her heart failure causing or worsening symptoms of fatigue and shortness of breath.

QUESTION 18-2 Answer is **a**. Because this patient has a benign arrhythmia and is asymptomatic, no drug therapies are recommended because the risks of therapy outweigh any benefits. Although a Na^+ channel blocker such as flecainide might be very efficacious in preventing PVCs in this patient, the CAST study showed a significant increase in mortality in patients taking this and other Class IC drugs who have had a recent MI and who have a reduced ejection fraction.

QUESTION 18-3 Answer is **c**. Digoxin inhibits the Na^+,K^+-ATPase in cardiac muscle and in other excitable tissue, including neurons. It has effects on the central nervous system that result in an increase in vagal tone, which inhibits conduction of impulses through the AV node. By inhibiting the AV node, the ventricles are protected from the high rate of impulses generated in the atria during atrial fibrillation.

QUESTION 18-4 Answer is **b**. By blocking voltage-gated Na^+ channels in ventricular myocytes, the myocytes are less likely to depolarize and conduction of impulses through the ventricular myocardium is slowed.

QUESTION 18-5 Answer is **e**. Sotalol is a racemic mixture that has both β adrenergic blocking and K^+ channel blocking activities. Both enantiomers have comparable K^+ channel blocking activity, but the L-enantiomer contributes most of the β adrenergic blocking activity.

SUMMARY: ANTIARRHYTHMIC DRUGS

CLASS AND SUBCLASSES	NAMES	CLINICAL USES	TOXICITIES COMMON	TOXICITIES UNIQUE; CLINICALLY IMPORTANT
Class IA Antiarrhythmics—Sodium Channel Blockers (Prolong QT Interval; Slow to Intermediate Kinetics)	Procainamide	Acute and chronic treatment of ventricular tachycardia; Acute and chronic treatment of ventricular fibrillation (VF); Acute and chronic treatment of supraventricular arrhythmias	40% of patients discontinue within 6 months of therapy due to side effects: hypotension, nausea; Torsade de pointes (TdP)	Lupus-like syndrome (25-50% with chronic) that can be fatal; starts with rash and mild arthralgia
	Quinidine	Chronic treatment of atrial flutter/fibrillation (AF); Chronic treatment of ventricular tachycardia and VF	Diarrhea (30-50% of patients); diarrhea-induced hypokalemia may potentiate TdP; Thrombocytopenia; Cinchonism: CNS, hypotension, syncope, GI	Marked long QT (2-8% of patients) with increased risk of TdP at therapeutic or subtherapeutic concentrations

Antiarrhythmic Drugs — CHAPTER 18

CLASS AND SUBCLASSES	NAMES	CLINICAL USES	TOXICITIES COMMON	TOXICITIES UNIQUE; CLINICALLY IMPORTANT
	Disopyramide	Chronic treatment of atrial flutter/AF Chronic treatment of ventricular tachycardia and VF	Anticholinergic effects	Can worsen heart failure Long QT (TdP)
Class IB Antiarrhythmics—Sodium Channel Blockers (Little Effect on ECG; Fast Kinetics)	Lidocaine	Chronic treatment of ventricular tachycardia and VF	CNS: seizures and tinnitus	CNS: tremor, hallucinations, drowsiness, coma Severe interactions with other antiarrhythmics
	Mexiletine	Chronic treatment of ventricular tachycardia and VF	Tremor and nausea	Severe interactions with other antiarrhythmics
Class IC Antiarrhythmics—Sodium Channel Blockers (Prolong PR and Broaden QRS Intervals; Slow Kinetics)	Flecainide	Chronic treatment of AV nodal reentry in patients w/o structural heart disease Chronic treatment of life-threatening ventricular arrhythmias	Blurred vision Can worsen heart failure	Life-threatening CAST proarrhythmia in patients with MI
	Propafenone	Chronic treatment of AV nodal reentry (PSVTs) and AF Chronic treatment of ventricular arrhythmias (modest efficacy)	β Adrenergic blocking effects (worsening of heart failure and bronchospasm)	Can increase frequency or severity of ventricular tachycardias
Class II Antiarrhythmics—β Adrenergic Receptor Antagonists	Propranolol (and others, see Chapter 7)	Chronic prevention of TdP Rate control in AF	β Adrenergic blocking effects (worsening of heart failure and bronchospasm; see Chapter 7)	See Chapter 7
	Sotalol	Chronic treatment of ventricular tachycardia Chronic treatment of atrial flutter/AF	β Adrenergic blocking effects	Prolongs QT interval increasing risk of TdP
	Esmolol	Rapid, short-term control of ventricular rate in patients with AF or atrial flutter in perioperative and post-operative settings	β Adrenergic blocking effects (dissipate rapidly when drug is removed)	Because of short half-life (9 min), should only be used for short-term use
Class III Antiarrhythmics—Increase Refractory Period (Prolong QT)	Amiodarone	Drug of choice for acute treatment of VF (IV administration) Acute and chronic treatment of ventricular tachycardia Chronic treatment of AF and VF	Hypotension and depressed ventricular function with IV	Pulmonary fibrosis with chronic therapy which can be fatal (requires periodic monitoring of lung function) Many other AEs: corneal microdeposits, hepatotoxicity, neuropathies photosensitivity, thyroid dysfunction Note: Tissue half-life of several months
	Dronedarone	Chronic treatment of atrial flutter/AF	GI disturbances Less than amiodarone	Increases mortality in patients with severe heart failure
	Sotalol	Chronic treatment of ventricular tachycardia Chronic treatment of atrial flutter/AF	β adrenergic blocking effects	Prolongs QT interval increasing risk of TdP

SECTION III Modulation of Cardiovascular Function

CLASS AND SUBCLASSES	NAMES	CLINICAL USES	TOXICITIES COMMON	UNIQUE; CLINICALLY IMPORTANT
	Dofetilide	Chronic treatment of AF		Prolongs QT interval increasing risk of TdP
	Ibutilide	Acute treatment of AF		Prolongs QT interval increasing risk of TdP
Class IV Antiarrhythmics—Ca^{2+} Channel Blockers (Nondihydropyridine; Inhibit SA and AV Nodes; Prolong PR)	Diltiazem	Acute and chronic treatment of AV nodal reentry (PSVTs) Acute and chronic control of ventricular rate in atrial flutter/AF	Hypotension	Sinus bradycardia or AV block in combination with β blockers
	Verapamil	Acute and chronic treatment of AV nodal reentry (PSVTs) Acute and chronic control of ventricular rate in atrial flutter/AF	Constipation	Sinus bradycardia or AV block in combination with β blockers Worsening of heart failure
Miscellaneous Antiarrhythmics—Adenosine Receptor Agonist	Adenosine	Drug of choice for acute treatment of AV nodal reentry (IV administration)	Asystole (<5 seconds) Dyspnea	Short half-life (<5 seconds) minimizes toxicities
Miscellaneous Antiarrhythmics—Unknown Mechanism	Magnesium sulfate	Acute treatment of TdP		
Miscellaneous Antiarrhythmics—Na^+, K^+-ATPase Inhibitor That Increases Vagal Tone	Digoxin	Ventricular rate control in atrial fibrillation Modest positive inotrope (see Chapter 17)	GI, vision, cognitive dysfunction	Arrhythmias Sinus bradycardia and AV block Severe toxicities can be treated with antibody (DIGIBIND)

Drug Therapy of Thromboembolic Disorders

CHAPTER 19

This chapter will be most useful after having a basic understanding of the material in Chapter 30, Blood Coagulation and Anticoagulant, Fibrinolytic, and Antiplatelet Drugs in *Goodman & Gilman's The Pharmacological Basis of Therapeutics*, 12th Edition. In particular, the reader is directed to the following table and to animations available in the online version of *Goodman & Gilman's The Pharmacological Basis of Therapeutics*:

- Table 30-3 Absolute and Relative Contraindications to Fibrinolytic Therapy.
- Several animations in the online version of *Goodman & Gilman's The Pharmacological Basis of Therapeutics* illustrate the mechanism of action of many anticoagulant, fibrinolytic, and antiplatelet drugs.

LEARNING OBJECTIVES

- ☑ Know the classes of drugs that inhibit platelet function, their mechanisms of action, and their role in the prevention and treatment of acute coronary syndromes, strokes, and transient ischemic attacks.
- ☑ Know the classes of drugs used as anticoagulants, their mechanisms of action, their indications in preventing and treating venous thromboembolism, pulmonary embolism, and strokes.
- ☑ Know how anticoagulant drug therapy is monitored.
- ☑ Know the mechanism of action of fibrinolytic agents, and their indications in treating ischemic stroke and myocardial infarction.
- ☑ Know the major toxicities and contraindications of each class of drug.

DRUGS INCLUDED IN THIS CHAPTER

- Abciximab (REOPRO)
- Apixaban (ELIQUIS)
- Argatroban (ARGATROBAN)
- Aspirin (acetylsalicylic acid, ASA)
- Bivalirudin (ANGIOMAX)
- Clopidogrel (PLAVIX)
- Dabigatran (PRADAXA)
- Drotrecogin alfa (XIGRIS)
- Eptifibatide (INTEGRILIN)
- Fondaparinux (ARIXTRA)
- Heparin
- Low-Molecular-Weight Heparins (LMWHs; enoxaparin [LOVENOX], dalteparin [FRAGMIN], tinzaparin [INNOHEP], ardeparin [NORMIFLO], nadroparin [FRAXIPARIN])
- Prasugrel (EFFIENT)
- Rivaroxaban (XARELTO)
- Ticlopidine (TICLID)
- Tirofiban (AGGRASTAT)
- Tissue plasminogen activator (t-PA; alteplase [ACTIVASE], reteplase [RETEVASE], tenecteplase [TNKASE])
- Warfarin (COUMADIN)

MECHANISMS OF ACTION OF DRUGS COMMMONLY USED TO PREVENT OR TREAT THROMBOEMBOLISM

DRUG CLASS	DRUG	MECHANISM OF ACTION
Antiplatelet Agent	Aspirin	Irreversibly inhibits platelet COX-1
	Thienopyridines: ticlopidine, clopidogrel, prasugrel	Irreversibly inhibits platelet ADP receptors (P2Y$_{12}$)
	Abciximab, eptifibatide, tirofiban	Inhibits activated GPIIb/IIIa on platelets
Parenteral Anticoagulant	Heparin, low-molecular-weight heparins (LMWHs), fondaparinux	Inhibits thrombin or factor Xa by activating antithrombin
	Bivalirudin, argatroban	Directly inhibits thrombin
	Activated protein C (drotrecogin alfa)	Degrades factors Va and VIIa
Oral Anticoagulant	Warfarin (and other coumarins)	Vitamin K antagonist (inhibits synthesis of vitamin K-dependent clotting factors)
	Dabigatran	Directly inhibits thrombin
	Rivaroxaban, apixaban	Directly inhibits factor Xa
Fibrinolytic Agent	t-PA (alteplase) and its derivatives (reteplase, tenecteplase)	Activates plasminogen

SECTION III — Modulation of Cardiovascular Function

COMMON INDICATIONS FOR THE USE OF ANTIPLATELET DRUGS

- Prevention of platelet thrombi after coronary angioplasty
- Secondary prevention of myocardial infarction, transient ischemic attacks (TIAs), and stroke
- Primary prevention of myocardial infarction, TIAs, and stroke in high-risk patients

CASE 19-1

A 62-year-old man with a history of angina calls 911 complaining of crushing chest pain. The 911 operator sends an ambulance and instructs the patient to chew an aspirin while waiting for the ambulance to arrive.

a. Why did the 911 operator have the patient take an aspirin?

The patient's history of angina suggests he has coronary artery disease and an elevated risk of an MI, and his symptoms of crushing chest pain indicate he may be having a myocardial infarction. In a patient with long-standing coronary artery disease, coronary vessel wall damage resulting from a ruptured atherosclerotic plaque can expose collagen, vWF, and other subendothelial prothrombotic substances to the blood (see Figures 19-1 and 19-2); these subendothelial substances will bind and activate circulating platelets. The activated platelets will release a number of mediators, including thromboxane A2 (TXA_2), which will activate other platelets in the blood vessel and stimulate the platelets to aggregate at the site of the vessel wall damage. Aspirin can inhibit platelet production of TXA_2 by irreversibly inhibiting platelet COX-1. By chewing an aspirin to increase absorption in the GI tract, the patient will rapidly inhibit platelet activation and aggregation, and slow the development of a platelet thrombus that may lead to the occlusion of a major coronary vessel.

b. When the patient arrives at the hospital, he is diagnosed as having a myocardial infarction and undergoes percutaneous angioplasty to clear the clot in his coronary artery. He also receives a stent to keep the vessel patent. What drugs will this patient likely receive while in the hospital to prevent recurrence of a thrombus in the stented coronary vessel?

The patient will receive aggressive antiplatelet and anticoagulant therapy in the hospital to reduce the likelihood of platelet and fibrin clots in the stented coronary vessel. To prevent platelet thrombi, he would continue to receive aspirin as well as more efficacious antiplatelet inhibitors, including an ADP receptor antagonist (ie, clopidogrel or prasugrel) and possibly a GPIIb/IIIa inhibitor (ie, abciximab,

(Continued)

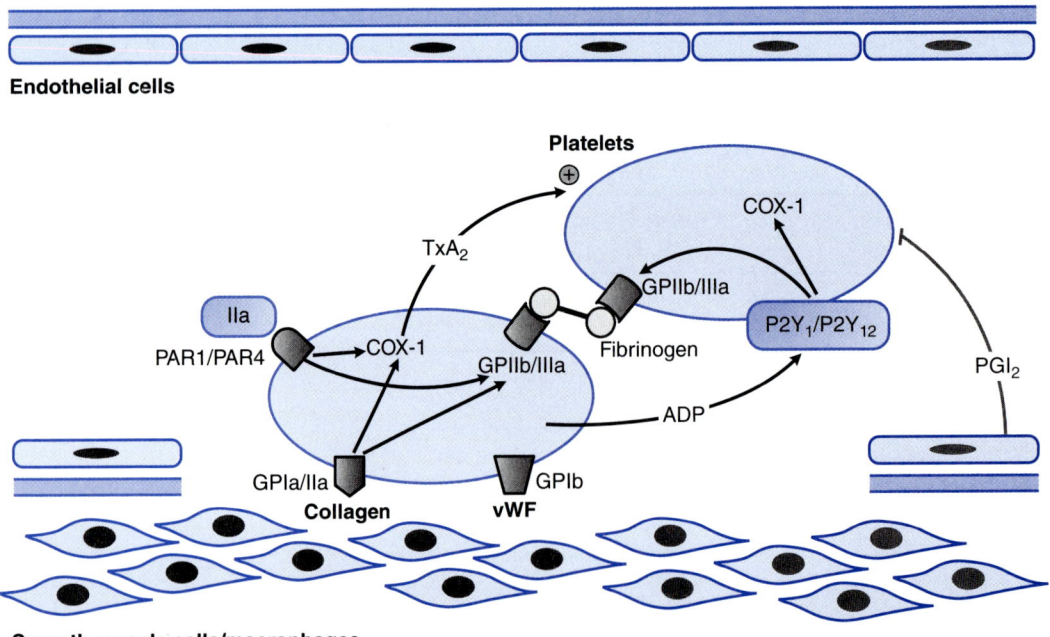

FIGURE 19-1 Platelet adhesion and aggregation. GPIa/IIa and GPIb are platelet receptors that bind to collagen and von Willebrand factor (vWF), causing platelets to adhere to the subendothelium of a damaged blood vessel. PAR1 and PAR4 are protease-activated receptors that respond to thrombin (IIa); $P2Y_1$ and $P2Y_{12}$ are receptors for ADP; when stimulated by agonists, these receptors activate the fibrinogen-binding protein GPIIb/IIIa and cyclooxygenase-1 (COX-1) to promote platelet aggregation and secretion. Thromboxane A_2 (TxA_2) is the major product of COX-1 involved in platelet activation. Prostaglandin I_2 (prostacyclin, PGI_2), synthesized by endothelial cells, inhibits platelet activation.

Drug Therapy of Thromboembolic Disorders

CHAPTER 19

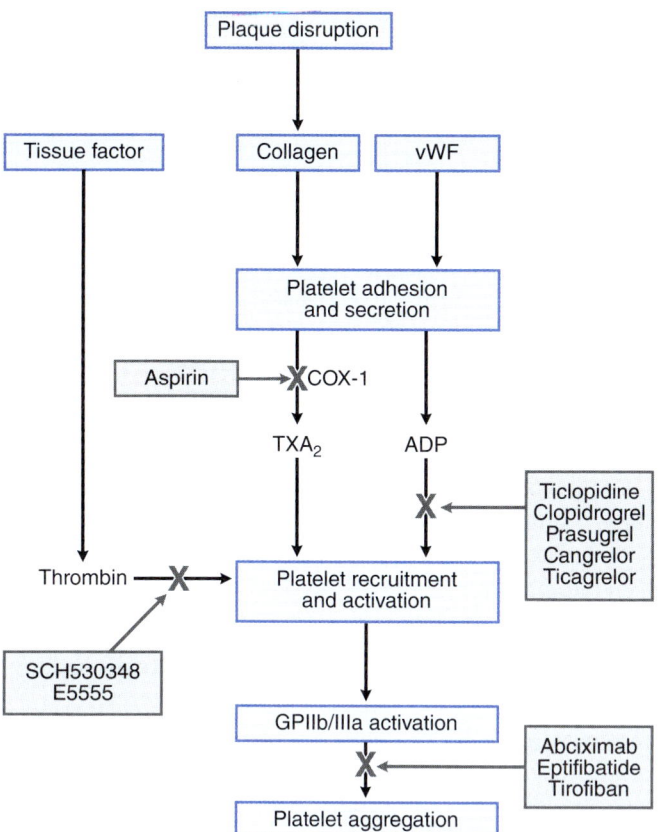

FIGURE 19-2 Sites of action of antiplatelet drugs. Aspirin inhibits thromboxane A_2 (TxA_2) synthesis by irreversibly acetylating cyclooxygenase-1 (COX-1). Reduced TxA_2 release attenuates platelet activation and recruitment to the site of vascular injury. Ticlopidine, clopidogrel, and prasugrel irreversibly block $P2Y_{12}$, a key ADP receptor on the platelet surface; cangrelor and ticagrelor are reversible inhibitors of $P2Y_{12}$. Abciximab, eptifibatide, and tirofiban inhibit the final common pathway of platelet aggregation by blocking fibrinogen and von Willebrand factor (vWF) from binding to activated glycoprotein (GP) IIb/IIIa. SCH530348 (now known as vorapaxar [ZANTIVITY]) and E5555 (also known as atopaxar) inhibit thrombin-mediated platelet activation by targeting protease-activated receptor-1 (PAR-1), the major thrombin receptor on platelets.

BIOACTIVATION OF THIENOPYRIDINES (TICLOPIDINE, CLOPIDOGREL, AND PRASUGREL)

- All thienopyridines are prodrugs that require bioactivation by CYPs and/or esterases
- There is wide interindividual variability in antiplatelet effects of clopidogrel because the prodrug is primarily activated by CYP2C19 which has a loss-of-function polymorphism (*CYP2C19*2*) and several reduced-function polymorphisms (*CYP2C19*3, *4, *5*)
- Prasugrel has rapid and nearly complete absorption and activation compared with only 15% activation of absorbed clopidogrel
- Prasugrel is more efficacious and predictable than clopidogrel but is also associated with higher rates of fatal and life-threatening bleeding

COMMON INDICATIONS FOR THE USE OF ANTICOAGULANTS

- Treatment of venous thrombosis and pulmonary embolism
- Prevention of thromboembolism in patients with unstable angina or acute myocardial infarction
- Prevention of thromboembolism in patients with atrial fibrillation
- Prevention of postoperative deep vein thrombosis in patients undergoing abdominothoracic surgery, and knee and hip replacements
- Cardiopulmonary bypass surgery to prevent clotting of the oxygenator

eptifibatide, or tirofiban). To inhibit the formation of fibrin clots, the patient would receive heparin or an LMWH. He would also be started on an oral anticoagulant (ie, warfarin) before discharge but kept on the heparinoid until his INR (see Side Bar LABORATORY MONITORING OF ANTICOAGULANT THERAPY) is within the therapeutic range.

c. **What drugs is this patient likely to receive after being discharged from the hospital?**

To prevent reocclusion of the stented coronary artery, he will need to take low-dose aspirin, an ADP receptor antagonist (clopidogrel or prasugrel), and warfarin. He will also be started on a β adrenergic antagonist to reduce his risk of heart failure and ventricular arrhythmias.

CASE 19-2

A 78-year-old man receives a total knee replacement. He lives by himself about an hour's drive from the nearest medical facility. Upon discharge, he is given a prescription for lovenox.

a. **What is the rationale for the use of this agent?**

Patients having major orthopedic surgeries such as total knee replacement or hip replacement are at risk of fibrin clot formation because of the surgery which activates the clotting cascade (see Figure 19-3) and subsequent immobilization which

(Continued)

SECTION III Modulation of Cardiovascular Function

promotes blood stasis. To minimize the risk of fibrin clot formation that could lead to pulmonary embolism or stroke, such patients receive an LMWH such as lovenox. Because this agent has very predictable pharmacokinetics, it does not require laboratory monitoring, and it can be self-administered by subcutaneous injection, and is thus well suited for this patient who lives a considerable distance from the nearest medical facility.

b. What is the mechanism of action of lovenox?

Lovenox is one of several LMWH agents and has the same mechanism of action as heparin and other heparinoids such as fondaparinux. Heparin and all of the heparinoids contain a pentasaccharide structure (see Figure 19-4) that binds and activates antithrombin, an endogenous anticoagulant (see Figure 30-5 in *Goodman & Gilman's The Pharmacological Basis of Therapeutics,* 12th Edition). Once activated, antithrombin inhibits the clotting factors thrombin (factor IIa) and factor Xa (see Figure 19-3). Inhibition of thrombin blocks the conversion of fibrinogen to insoluble fibrin, whereas inhibition of factor Xa inhibits conversion of the inactive prothrombin (factor II) zymogen to active thrombin (factor IIa). Because of the smaller size of the LMWHs compared to standard heparin, the LMWH-antithrombin complexes are more specific inhibitors of factor Xa than thrombin (see Figure 30-5 in *Goodman & Gilman's The Pharmacological Basis of Therapeutics,* 12th Edition).

c. What are the important drug toxicities that this patient should be cautioned to watch for?

As with all anticoagulants, bleeding is the most important and common toxicity. Heparin-induced thrombocytopenia (HIT) is also possible with the LMWHs, but this adverse effect is much less common than with standard heparin.

CASE 19-3

A 32-year-old woman in good health is discovered to have atrial fibrillation during a routine checkup. She does not recall having any symptoms of arrhythmia such as dizziness or fainting, although she is not able to exercise for as long as she could a few years ago. Her cardiologist prescribes warfarin.

(Continued)

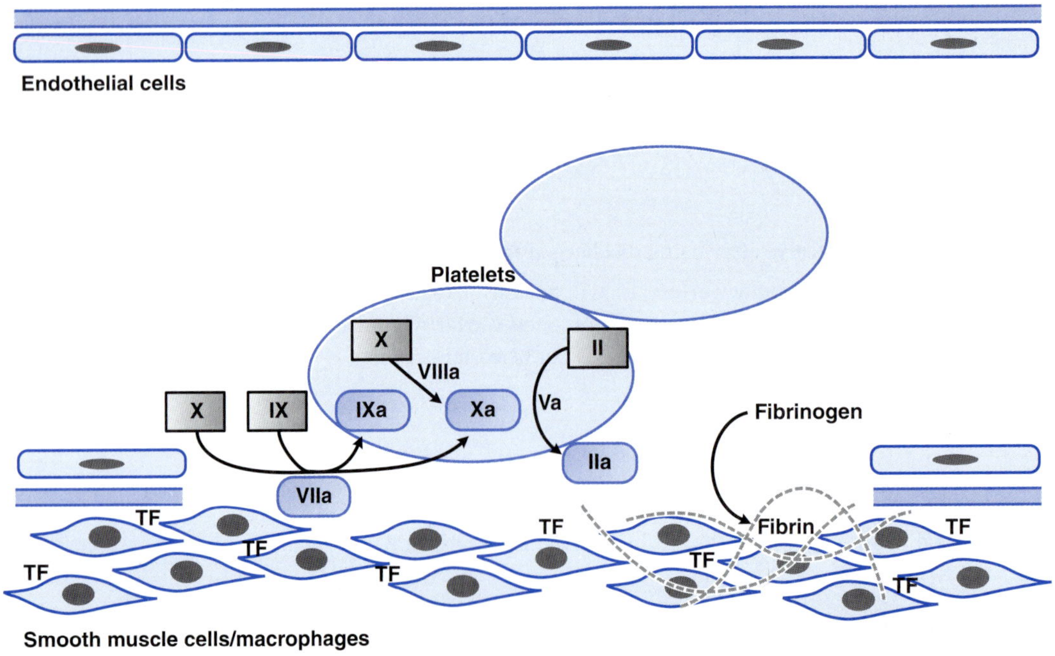

FIGURE 19-3 Major reactions of blood coagulation. Shown are interactions among proteins of the "extrinsic" (tissue factor and factor VII), "intrinsic" (factors IX and VIII), and "common" (factors X, V, and II) coagulation pathways that are important *in vivo*. Boxes enclose the coagulation factor zymogens (indicated by Roman numerals); the rounded boxes represent the active proteases. TF, tissue factor. Activated coagulation factors are followed by the letter "a": II, prothrombin; IIa, thrombin.

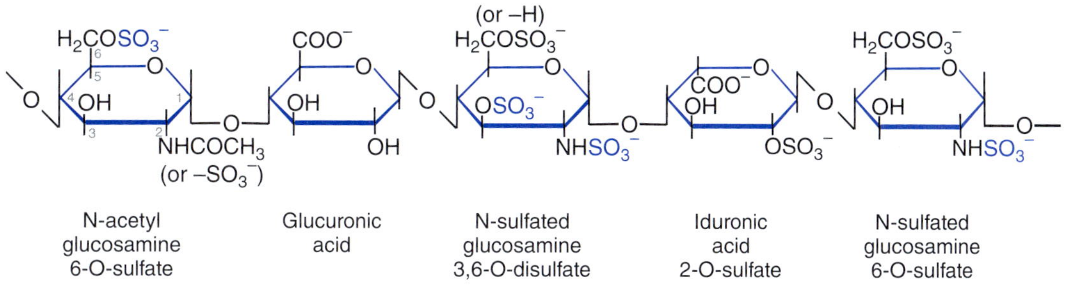

Drug Therapy of Thromboembolic Disorders CHAPTER 19

FIGURE 19-4 The antithrombin-binding pentasaccharide structure of heparin. Sulfate groups required for binding to antithrombin are indicated in blue.

a. **What is the rationale for using warfarin in this patient?**

Patients with atrial fibrillation are at high risk of developing fibrin clots that can lead to transient ischemic attacks (TIAs), strokes, and pulmonary embolism. Because the atria do not contract properly in patients with atrial fibrillation, blood can pool in the atria increasing the chance a fibrin thrombus will form. Warfarin is an oral anticoagulant that can reduce the risk of fibrin clot formation.

b. **What is the mechanism of action of warfarin?**

Warfarin is classified as a vitamin K antagonist. It blocks the enzyme that converts the oxidized form of vitamin K to the reduced form (see Figure 19-5). The reduced form of vitamin K is a cofactor required in the post-translational modification of clotting factors II, VII, IX, and X. This post-translational modification, γ-carboxylation

(Continued)

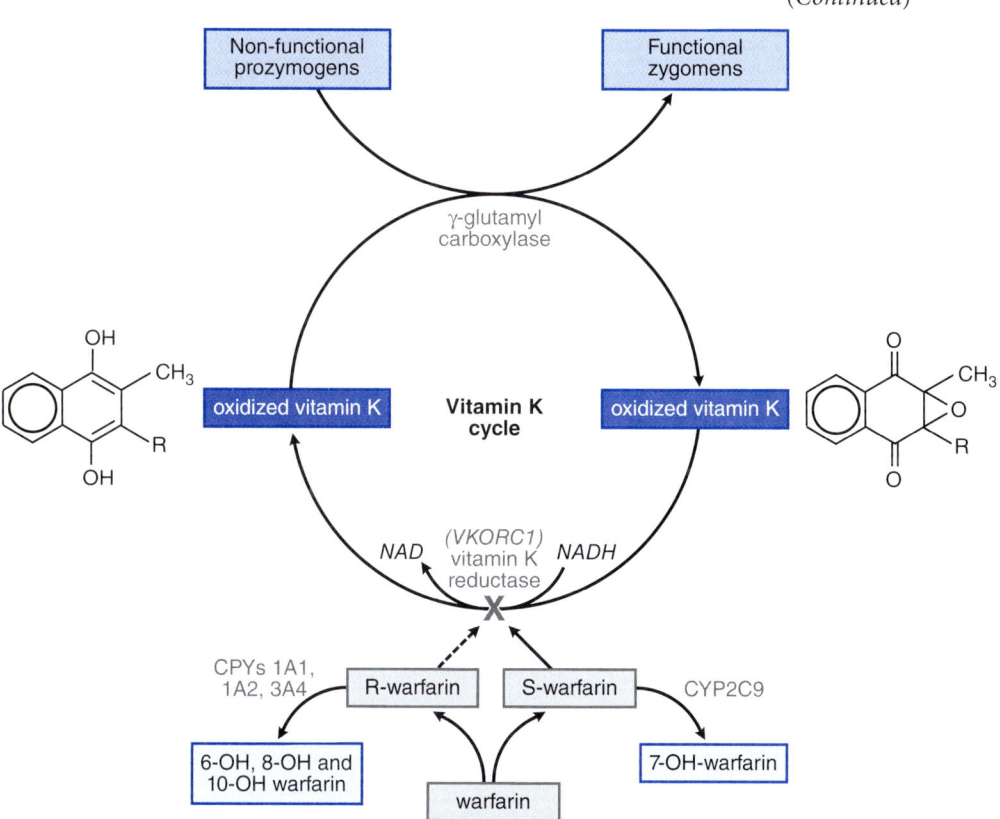

FIGURE 19-5 The vitamin K cycle and mechanism of action of warfarin. In the racemic mixture of S- and R-enantiomers, S-warfarin is more active. By blocking vitamin K epoxide reductase encoded by the *VKORC1* gene, warfarin inhibits the conversion of oxidized vitamin K epoxide into its reduced form, vitamin K hydroquinone. This inhibits vitamin K-dependent γ-carboxylation of factors II, VII, IX, and X because reduced vitamin K serves as a cofactor for a γ-glutamyl carboxylase that catalyzes the γ-carboxylation process, thereby converting prozymogens to zymogens capable of binding Ca^{2+} and interacting with anionic phospholipid surfaces. S-warfarin is metabolized by *CYP2C9*. Common genetic polymorphisms in this enzyme can influence warfarin metabolism. Polymorphisms in the C1 subunit of vitamin K reductase (VKORC1) also can affect the susceptibility of the enzyme to warfarin-induced inhibition, thereby influencing warfarin dosage requirements.

of specific glutamic acids, is required for biological activity of these clotting factors. Thus, warfarin blocks the final step in the synthesis of these key coagulation factors. Therapeutic doses of warfarin reduce by 30 to 50% the total amount of each vitamin K-dependent clotting factor, and reduce the level of γ-carboxylation (and biological activity) by 10 to 40%.

c. **What kinds of laboratory monitoring are required for patients receiving warfarin and why?**

Because many factors can alter the anticoagulant activity of warfarin (see Side Bar FACTORS LEADING TO ALTERED ANTICOAGULANT ACTIVITY OF WARFARIN), it is necessary to regularly monitor anticoagulant status using the laboratory test called the prothrombin time (PT) assay. The PT is normalized based on the activity of one of the assay reagents to give a value known as the INR (international normalized ratio). Dose adjustments of warfarin are used to maintain a patient's INR within a narrow range of values. For most indications, the target INR is 2 to 3, but a higher target INR (2.5-3.5) is indicated in patients with high-risk mechanical heart valves. INR values that are too high indicate the patient is receiving too much warfarin and is at risk of major bleeding events. INR values that are below the desired range indicate the warfarin dosing is too low and the patient is at greater risk of stroke and pulmonary emboli. Patients who are initiated on warfarin therapy require laboratory monitoring every few days, but once a stable therapeutic INR is achieved, the frequency of monitoring can be reduced to once every few weeks.

d. **What are the risks and toxicities associated with warfarin therapy?**

As with all anticoagulant agents, the most common risk is bleeding. The risk of major bleeding is less than 3% in patients who are maintained within a therapeutic target INR of 2 to 3. The risk of intracranial bleeding increases markedly with INR more than 4. In patients whose INR is more than or equal to 5, vitamin K_1 administration may be required to restore clotting function. Warfarin administration during pregnancy causes birth defects and abortion; heparin, LMWHs, or fondaparinux should be used instead of warfarin in pregnant women. Less common toxicities of warfarin include skin necrosis, purple toe syndrome, and other toxicities that are described in Chapter 30 of *Goodman & Gilman's The Pharmacological Basis of Therapeutics*, 12th Edition.

e. **What counseling should this patient receive?**

Because this patient is of child-bearing age, she needs to be warned that warfarin causes birth defects and abortion. She should be changed to a heparinoid if there is a possibility she is pregnant or will become pregnant. All patients receiving warfarin should be educated to report any changes in medications (including nonprescription drugs) or food supplements because of the large number of drug–drug and food–drug interactions possible with warfarin that alter the pharmacokinetics and efficacy of warfarin's anticoagulant properties (see Side Bar FACTORS LEADING TO ALTERED ANTICOAGULANT ACTIVITY OF WARFARIN). Dietary changes can also affect warfarin efficacy by altering the intake of vitamin K. For instance, changing to a diet that is rich in green leafy vegetables (which are high in vitamin K) can lower the patient's INR. The patient should report any change in medications, dietary supplements, or significant change in diet so that more frequent INR testing can be done and the results used to adjust warfarin dosing.

f. **Are there other oral anticoagulants that this patient might be prescribed instead of warfarin?**

Because this patient has nonvalvular atrial fibrillation, alternative oral anticoagulants that could be considered include the oral direct thrombin inhibitor dabigatran etexilate, or one of the oral direct factor Xa inhibitors, rivaroxaban or apixaban. An advantage of these agents over warfarin is that they do not require routine laboratory monitoring of anticoagulant status because they have predictable pharmacokinetics and few drug–drug or food–drug interactions.

Drug Therapy of Thromboembolic Disorders — CHAPTER 19

CASE 19-4

While shopping in the grocery store, a 61-year-old man develops symptoms of weakness on one side of his body and his wife notices that he has trouble speaking. Suspecting that he is having a stroke, they go to the nearest hospital which is a 20-minute drive from the store. At the hospital it is determined that the patient has had an ischemic stroke and alteplase is administered.

a. What is the rationale for administering alteplase to this patient?

Alteplase is a fibrinolytic ("clot-buster") agent that breaks down fibrin clots. In this patient, who has an ischemic stroke, alteplase lyses the fibrin clots that are occluding blood vessels in the patient's brain, thus restoring blood flow to the ischemic regions and preventing irreversible damage.

b. What is the mechanism of action of alteplase?

Alteplase is the recombinant form of tissue plasminogen activator (t-PA; see Figure 19-6). Alteplase and its genetically engineered derivatives, reteplase and tenecteplase, are serine proteases that cleave plasminogen to plasmin, thus activating plasmin's proteolytic activity (see Figure 19-6). Plasmin is the endogenous protease that is responsible for digesting fibrin clots (see Figure 30-3 in *Goodman & Gilman's The Pharmacological Basis of Therapeutics*, 12th Edition).

c. What must be considered before using alteplase to treat a patient with symptoms of stroke?

During the initial workup of this patient, it must be determined that this patient is having an acute ischemic stroke rather than a hemorrhagic stroke since the symptoms are similar. Administering a fibrinolytic agent to a patient with a hemorrhagic stroke would be catastrophic. It is also important to determine the time the patient first experienced symptoms because fibrinolytic therapy is maximally effective within the first 3 hours following the development of symptoms. Because of the risk of major bleeding that can occur with fibrinolysis of physiological clots, there are a number of contraindications to fibrinolytic therapy (see Table 30-3 in *Goodman & Gilman's The Pharmacological Basis of Therapeutics*, 12th Edition).

(Continued)

FACTORS LEADING TO ALTERED ANTICOAGULANT ACTIVITY OF WARFARIN

- Warfarin has a narrow therapeutic index requiring regular laboratory monitoring (INR, see Side Bar LABORATORY MONITORING OF ANTICOAGULANT THERAPY) to maintain adequate anticoagulation and minimize risk of bleeding
- Warfarin has more than 200 drug–drug and food–drug interactions than can alter dosing
- Common factors that can alter warfarin's anticoagulant effects:
  - Changes in diet, particularly increases or decreases in vitamin K-rich foods or supplements
  - Changes in diet or intestinal flora that affect gut bacteria synthesis of vitamin K
  - Reduction in absorption of drug from the GI tract
  - Increased clearance of drug resulting from induction of hepatic enzymes, especially CYP2C9
  - Low concentrations of coagulation factors due to hepatic disease, congestive heart failure, and other disease states

(continues)

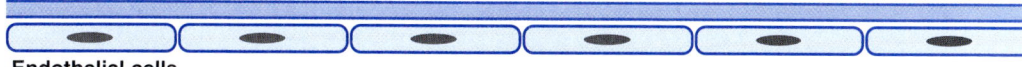

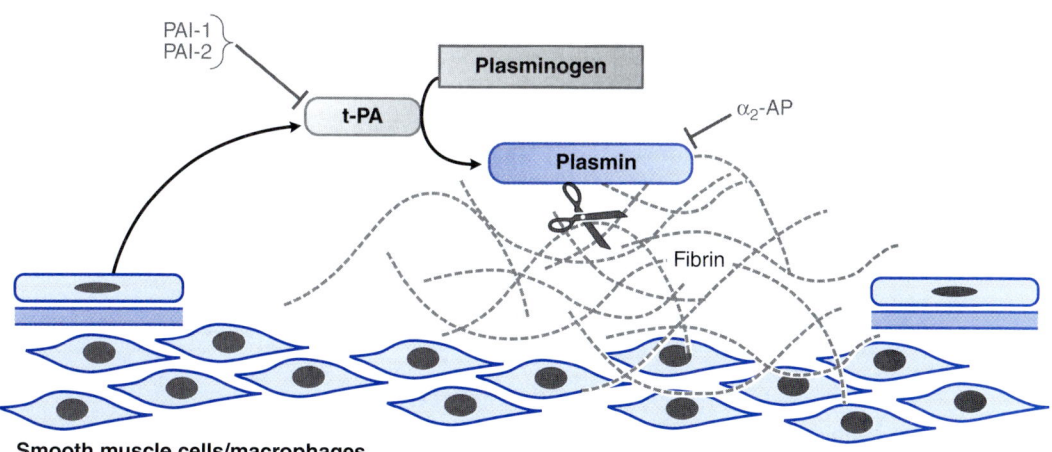

FIGURE 19-6 Fibrinolysis. Endothelial cells secrete tissue plasminogen activator (t-PA) at sites of injury. t-PA binds to fibrin and converts plasminogen to plasmin, which digests fibrin. Plasminogen activator inhibitors-1 and -2 (PAI-1, PAI-2) inactivate t-PA; α_2-antiplasmin (α_2-AP) inactivates plasmin.

SECTION III — Modulation of Cardiovascular Function

FACTORS LEADING TO ALTERED ANTICOAGULANT ACTIVITY OF WARFARIN (Cont.)

- Increased levels of coagulation factors during pregnancy (although warfarin should not be used in most pregnancies because of its teratogenic effects)
- Genetic polymorphisms that alter warfarin pharmacokinetics and pharmacodynamics also lead to large differences in dosing requirements
  - Polymorphisms in *CYP2C9* that reduce the rate of metabolism of warfarin and require dose reduction compared to wild-type (see Table 30-2 in *Goodman & Gilman's The Pharmacological Basis of Therapeutics*, 12th Edition)
  - Polymorphisms in *VKORC1* (vitamin K epoxide reductase complex, subunit 1) that reduce the activity of the gene product and require dose reduction compared to wild-type (see Table 30-2 in *Goodman & Gilman's The Pharmacological Basis of Therapeutics*, 12th Edition)

LABORATORY MONITORING OF ANTICOAGULANT THERAPY

- Prothrombin time (PT, with values converted to the INR) is used to monitor warfarin therapy but is not required for the direct inhibitors of thrombin or factor Xa
- aPTT is used to monitor standard heparin therapy but is not required for LMWH or fondaparinux; it is also used for monitoring bivalirudin and argatroban
- Activated clotting time is used to monitor anticoagulant status in patients receiving high-dose heparin
- Chromogenic factor Xa activity assays (also termed antifactor Xa assays) can be used to monitor heparin and LMWH efficacy

---

d. What is the most important toxicity associated with alteplase?

Major bleeding is the most important toxicity associated with alteplase and other fibrinolytic agents, hence the many contraindications listed in Table 30-3 in *Goodman & Gilman's The Pharmacological Basis of Therapeutics*, 12th Edition. Major bleeding is caused by the lysis of fibrin at sites of vascular injury and by systemic activation of plasmin that results in degradation of fibrinogen and clotting factors.

e. Are there other indications for fibrinolytic agents?

Fibrinolytic agents are also indicated for the treatment of acute myocardial infarction although coronary angioplasty, when feasible, is the treatment of choice. Fibrinolytic therapy is also indicated for the treatment of pulmonary embolism associated with deep vein thrombosis.

KEY CONCEPTS

- Antiplatelet drugs are used to prevent platelet activation and aggregation in arterial blood vessels.
- Combination therapy with antiplatelet drugs from different classes can be additive or synergistic.
- Anticoagulants are used to prevent the formation of fibrin clots.
- Anticoagulant drugs either reduce the activation of thrombin (directly or indirectly) or inhibit thrombin (directly or indirectly).
- Fibrinolytic drugs act by increasing the amounts of plasmin, the protease that breaks down fibrin.
- Fibrinolytic drugs are most effective in breaking down clots when used soon after fibrin clots are formed.
- Bleeding is the most common adverse effect of antiplatelet agents, anticoagulants, and fibrinolytic agents; the therapeutic benefit should outweigh risk of major bleeding.
- Combination therapy with antiplatelet agents and anticoagulants may be indicated to prevent thrombus formation, but the risk of bleeding is increased.

SUMMARY QUIZ

QUESTION 19-1 A patient diagnosed with acute coronary syndrome is prescribed clopidogrel. What is the mechanism of action of this agent?

a. It vasodilates coronary arteries.
b. It irreversibly blocks ADP receptors.
c. It blocks thrombin receptors on platelets.
d. It inhibits thrombin.

QUESTION 19-2 Following a trans-Pacific flight from Australia, a 57-year-old man develops deep vein thrombosis in his right leg. He receives heparin to treat the DVT but after 6 days of heparin therapy he develops heparin-induced thrombocytopenia (HIT). What drug is he likely to receive instead of heparin?

a. Argatroban
b. Warfarin
c. Activated protein C (drotrecogin alpha)
d. Dabigatran
e. Rivaroxaban

(Continued)

Drug Therapy of Thromboembolic Disorders — CHAPTER 19

QUESTION 19-3 A 52-year-old woman with atrial fibrillation is prescribed apixaban. What is the mechanism of action of this oral anticoagulant?

a. It indirectly inhibits thrombin by activating antithrombin.
b. It directly inhibits thrombin.
c. It indirectly inhibits factor Xa by activating antithrombin.
d. It directly inhibits factor Xa.
e. It blocks the synthesis of active clotting factors.

QUESTION 19-4 There is significant patient-to-patient variability in the dose of clopidogrel required to achieve therapeutic inhibition of platelet function, but not for prasugrel. What is the reason for this variability in clopidogrel, but not prasugrel?

a. There are many significant food–drug interactions that affect the pharmacodynamics of clopidogrel.
b. There are many significant drug–drug interactions that affect the pharmacokinetics of clopidogrel.
c. The are genetic polymorphisms in the enzymes that activate clopidogrel to its active form.
d. There are genetic polymorphisms in the enzymes that degrade clopidogrel to its inactive form.

QUESTION 19-5 A patient who is hospitalized for an acute myocardial infarction receives abciximab. What is the mechanism of action and rationale for using this drug?

a. Abciximab degrades fibrin clots in the occluded coronary arteries.
b. Abciximab inhibits the formation of fibrin clots.
c. Abciximab blocks ADP receptors on platelets.
d. Abciximab inhibits the activity of COX1 in platelets.
e. Abciximab blocks interactions of platelet GPIIb/IIIa with fibrinogen.

SUMMARY QUIZ ANSWER KEY

QUESTION 19-1 Answer is **b**. Clopidogrel and the other thienopyridines (ticlopidine, prasugrel) irreversibly block $P2Y_{12}$ (ADP) receptors on platelets, which inhibits platelet activation and aggregation. A patient with acute coronary syndrome is at high risk of acute myocardial infarction caused by platelet thrombus formation at the site of ruptured coronary artery plaques (see Chapter 16). Antiplatelet therapy will reduce the risk of myocardial infarction in such patients.

QUESTION 19-2 Answer is **a**. The patient is most likely to receive argatroban which is a parenterally administered small molecule direct thrombin inhibitor. Alternatives to argatroban for patients with HIT include bivalirudin or fondaparinux. Warfarin should not be used initially to replace heparin because there is a risk of developing venous limb gangrene, but can be started after the patient has been stably anticoagulated with argatroban and his platelet count has increased. Activated protein C would not be an effective anticoagulant in this setting. The oral anticoagulants dabigatran (oral direct thrombin inhibitor) and rivaroxaban (oral direct factor Xa inhibitor) are theoretically good alternatives to heparin in patients with DVTs, but have not yet been tested clinically for this indication.

QUESTION 19-3 Answer is **d**. Apixaban is an oral direct inhibitor of factor Xa. Inhibition of factor Xa blocks the conversion of prothrombin (factor II) to thrombin (factor IIa) (see Figure 19-3). The anticoagulant drugs that indirectly inhibit thrombin and factor Xa by activating antithrombin are the heparinoids. The anticoagulant drug that blocks the synthesis of active clotting factors is warfarin.

QUESTION 19-4 Answer is **c**. There is wide interindividual variability in antiplatelet effects of clopidogrel because the prodrug is primarily activated by CYP2C19 which

(Continued)

SECTION III — Modulation of Cardiovascular Function

has a loss-of-function polymorphism (CYP2C19*2) and several reduced-function polymorphisms (CYP2C19*3, *4, *5). In contrast, prasugrel is activated by esterases which are not limiting and do not have polymorphisms that affect prasugrel activation.

QUESTION 19-5 Answer is **e**. Abciximab is a humanized monoclonal antibody that binds to the glycoprotein IIb/IIIa (GPIIb/IIIa) complex on the surface of activated platelets (see Figure 19-1). When platelets are activated, GPIIb/IIIa undergoes a conformational change that allows the complex to bind to fibrinogen in the blood and von Willebrand factor on the surface of subendothelial cells. This is a key step in anchoring platelets to the wall of the damaged blood vessel and in forming platelet aggregates. Abciximab blocks these interactions, thus preventing the formation of platelet thrombi even though platelets are activated by mediators such as ADP and TxA_2. Other agents that also block GPIIb/IIIa interactions with fibrinogen include eptifibatide and tirofiban.

SUMMARY TABLE: DRUGS USED IN THE PREVENTION AND TREATMENT OF THROMBOEMBOLIC DISORDERS

CLASS AND SUBCLASSES	NAMES	CLINICAL USES	TOXICITIES COMMON	TOXICITIES UNIQUE; CLINICALLY IMPORTANT
Antiplatelet—Irreversible COX-1 Inhibitor	Aspirin (ASA)	Prophylaxis of pathological arterial thromboses including MI, stroke, and peripheral vascular thromboses	GI bleeding	
Antiplatelet—Irreversible ADP Receptor ($P2Y_{12}$) Antagonist	Ticlopidine	Secondary prevention and treatment of MI and stroke	Nausea, vomiting, diarrhea, bleeding	Severe neutropenia; Fatal agranulocytosis with thrombocytopenia; Thrombotic thrombocytopenic purpura-hemolytic uremic syndrome (TTP-HUS)
	Clopidogrel	Secondary prevention of stroke, MI; Peripheral artery disease, acute coronary syndrome; Used with ASA for prevention of recurrent ischemia in unstable angina, after angioplasty with stent placement	Bleeding; increased risk for bleeding if urgent surgery required due to irreversible inhibition of platelets	Thrombocytopenia and leukopenia (much less often than with ticlopidine); Wide inter-individual variability because of *CYP2C19* polymorphisms
	Prasugrel	Same as clopidogrel; more efficacious and predictable antiplatelet effects than clopidogrel because of high degree of bioactivation	Bleeding; increased risk for bleeding if urgent surgery required due to irreversible inhibition of platelets	Contraindicated in patients with a history of cerebrovascular disease because of increased risk of life-threatening bleeding; Dose reduction in patients weighing <60 kg, >75 years of age, or renal impairment
Antiplatelet—GPIIb/IIIa Inhibitor	Abciximab	Percutaneous angioplasty in patients with coronary thromboses; administered with aspirin and heparin	Bleeding, major bleeding in 1-10% of patients depending on intensity of heparin anticoagulation	Thrombocytopenia in ~2% of patients
	Eptifibatide	Acute coronary syndrome and coronary angioplasty; administered with aspirin and heparin	Bleeding, major bleeding in 10% of patients (with heparin)	Thrombocytopenia in 0.5-1% of patients
	Tirofiban	Non-Q-wave myocardial infarction, unstable angina; used with heparin	Bleeding (similar to eptifibatide)	

Drug Therapy of Thromboembolic Disorders — CHAPTER 19

CLASS AND SUBCLASSES	NAMES	CLINICAL USES	TOXICITIES COMMON	TOXICITIES UNIQUE; CLINICALLY IMPORTANT
Anticoagulant (parenteral)—Heparinoid	Heparin	Prevent or treat venous thromboembolism; immediate anticoagulant effects when given IV	Bleeding, with major bleeding in 1-5% in patients receiving IV heparin; must be monitored by aPTT	Heparin-induced thrombocytopenia (HIT); allergic reactions
	LMWHs (enoxaparin, dalteparin, tinzaparin, ardeparin, nadroparin)	Same as heparin; preferred over heparin because of more predictable PK, no monitoring required, less risk of HIT	Bleeding, but monitoring not usually required because of predictable dosing	Heparin-induced thrombocytopenia (HIT), but less common than heparin
	Fondaparinux	Same as heparin; preferred over heparin because of more predictable PK, no monitoring, much less risk of HIT than heparin or LMWHs	Bleeding	Should not be used in renal patients because drug is excreted in urine
Anticoagulant (parenteral)—Direct Thrombin Inhibitor	Desirudin, bivalirudin, argatroban	As an alternative to heparinoids, especially in patients with HIT	Bleeding	Lepirudin and desirudin are excreted by the kidneys and can cause bleeding in renal failure patients. Patients may develop antibodies to these proteins
Anticoagulant (parenteral)—Activated Protein C	Drotrecogin alpha	Severe sepsis	Bleeding	
Anticoagulant (oral)—Vitamin K Antagonist	Warfarin	Prevent progression or recurrence of acute DVT or pulmonary embolism following heparin therapy. Prevent venous thromboembolism in at-risk patients including those with acute MI, prosthetic heart valve, atrial fibrillation, or undergoing orthopedic or gynecological surgery	Bleeding, with risk of major bleeding <3% in patients with target INR of 2-3; risk of intracranial bleeding increases with INR >4	Contraindicated during pregnancy due to birth defects and abortion (use a heparinoid anticoagulant instead). Skin necrosis (rare). Purple toe syndrome. Antidote to warfarin overdose is vitamin K
Anticoagulant (oral)—Direct Thrombin Inhibitor	Dabigatran etexilate	Alternative to warfarin for chronic anticoagulation in nonvalvular atrial fibrillation. Prevention of venous thromboembolism and stroke after knee, hip surgery	Bleeding (routine laboratory monitoring is unnecessary)	No currently available antidote (as there is for warfarin)
Anticoagulant (oral)—Direct Factor Xa Inhibitor	Rivaroxaban, apixaban	Alternative to warfarin for chronic anticoagulation in nonvalvular atrial fibrillation. Prevention of venous thromboembolism and stroke after knee, hip surgery	Bleeding (routine laboratory monitoring is unnecessary)	No currently available antidote
Fibrinolytic—tPA	Alteplase, reteplase, tenecteplase	Treatment of choice for patients with acute ischemic stroke who present within 3 hours of symptoms. Treatment of myocardial infarction when coronary angioplasty is not feasible	Bleeding, hemorrhagic stroke, serious bleeding in 2-4% of patients with heparin	Contraindications are risk of life-threatening hemorrhage (see Table 30-3 in *Goodman & Gilman's The Pharmacological Basis of Therapeutics*, 12th Edition)

CHAPTER 20

Drug Therapy of Dyslipidemias

DRUGS INCLUDED IN THIS CHAPTER

- Atorvastatin (LIPITOR)
- Bezafibrate (not marketed in the United States)
- Cholestyramine (QUESTRAN, CHOLYBAR, others)
- Ciprofibrate (not marketed in the United States)
- Clofibrate (no longer available)
- Colesevelam (WELCHOL)
- Colestipol (COLESTID, others)
- Ezetimibe (ZETIA)
- Ezetimibe/simvastatin (VYTORIN)
- Fenofibrate (TRICOR, TRIGLIDE)
- Fluvastatin (LESCOL)
- Gemfibrozil (LOPID)
- Lovastatin (MEVACOR)
- Niacin (NIACOR, NIASPAN, others)
- Pitavastatin (LIVALO)
- Pravastatin (PRAVACHOL)
- Rosuvastatin (CRESTOR)
- Simvastatin (ZOCOR)

This chapter will be most useful after having a basic understanding of the material in Chapter 31, Drug Therapy for Hypercholesterolemia and Dyslipidemia in *Goodman & Gilman's The Pharmacological Basis of Therapeutics*, 12th Edition. In addition to the material presented here, the 12th Edition contains:

- Table 31-1 Characteristics of Plasma Lipoproteins which lists the major classes of lipoproteins and their properties
- Table 31-2 Apolipoproteins which describes the properties and functions of apolipoproteins that have well-defined roles in plasma protein metabolism
- Table 31-6 Assessing 10-Year Risk of CVD Events which provides an algorithm for estimating a patient's risk of a cardiovascular disease (CVD) event (ie, myocardial infarction [MI], stroke, transient ischemic attack [(TIA)], peripheral vascular disease, heart failure)
- Table 31-8 Clinical Identification of the Metabolic Syndrome which provides levels of the five CHD risk factors that define metabolic syndrome
- Table 31-9 Guidelines Based on the LDL-C and Total Cholesterol:HDL-C Ratio for Treatment of Low HDL-C Patients which provides an algorithm for treating patients with low high-density lipoprotein cholesterol (HDL-C) levels
- Table 31-10 Dose (mg) of Stains Required to Achieve Various Reductions in Low-Density-Lipoprotein Cholesterol From Baseline which provides an algorithm for initiating dosing of statins based on baseline low-density lipoprotein cholesterol (LDL-C) levels
- The molecular structures of drugs used to treat dyslipidemias

LEARNING OBJECTIVES

☑ Understand the mechanisms of action of drugs used to treat dyslipidemia.
☑ Know the untoward effects of drugs used to treat dyslipidemias.
☑ Know which patients with dyslipidemias should be treated and when treatment should be initiated.
☑ Know which drugs are most effective in treating patients with different dyslipidemias.
☑ Know which drugs can be used in combination to treat dyslipidemias.
☑ Know the effects of treatment on lowering the 10-year risk of a CVD event, and how to set treatment goals based on primary and secondary prevention of a CVD event.

MECHANISMS OF ACTION OF DRUGS USED TO TREAT DYSLIPIDEMIAS

DRUG CLASS	DRUG	MECHANISM OF ACTION
HMG-CoA Reductase Inhibitors (Statins)	Atorvastatin, simvastatin, rosuvastatin calcium, lovastatin, pravastatin sodium, fluvastatin sodium, pitavastatin calcium	Competitive inhibitors of HMG-CoA reductase, the rate-limiting step in liver cholesterol biosynthesis; inhibition of hepatic cholesterol synthesis increases expression of the LDL receptor on hepatocytes which increases the removal LDL from the blood
Bile Acid–Binding Resins (Bile Acid Sequestrants)	Cholestyramine, colestipol, colesevelam	Highly positively charged bile acid sequestrants that bind bile acids in the GI system, thereby depleting the pool of bile acids and stimulating hepatic bile acid production which leads to reduced hepatic cholesterol content

(Continued)

Drug Therapy of Dyslipidemias

CHAPTER 20

DRUG CLASS	DRUG	MECHANISM OF ACTION
Nicotinic Acid (Niacin)	Niacin	Binds a GPCR (GPR109A) for niacin in adipose tissue that leads to the inhibition of triglyceride lipolysis by hormone-sensitive lipase, which reduces transport of free fatty acids to the liver and decreases hepatic triglyceride synthesis
Fibric acid (Fibrates)	Gemfibrozil, fenofibrate, ciprofibrate (not marketed in the United States), bezafibrate (not marketed in the United States), clofibrate (no longer available)	Unclear, but likely involves activation of PPARα in liver and brown adipose tissue which stimulates fatty acid oxidation, increases lipoprotein lipase, and reduces expression of apoC-III
Cholesterol Absorption Inhibitors	Ezetimibe	Inhibits cholesterol absorption at the brush border of the small intestine by inhibiting sterol transport protein Niemann-PickC1-Like1 (NPC1L1) in jejunal enterocytes

CASE 20-1

A 58-year-old man sees his physician for a routine checkup. He is in good health with no symptoms or complaints. He does not have a family history of premature heart disease, although his paternal grandfather suffered a nonfatal heart attack when he was 67. Just prior to the checkup, he provides fasting blood samples for lipid profiles. His plasma cholesterols are: total cholesterol, 203 mg/dL; HDL cholesterol, 52 mg/dL; LDL cholesterol, 130 mg/mL; VLDL cholesterol, 21 mg/dL. His triglycerides are 148 mg/dL. His fasting serum glucose is in the normal range and his blood pressure is 128/75. He is not currently taking any medications, has never smoked, and usually has 1 or 2 glasses of wine with dinner, but consumes no other alcoholic beverages.

a. **What is this patient's 10-year risk of a CVD event?**

Table 31-6 in *Goodman & Gilman's The Pharmacological Basis of Therapeutics*, 12th Edition provides an algorithm for estimating the 10-risk of coronary vascular disease (CVD) events based on data from the Framingham Heart Study. The risk prediction for a CVD event will exceed the risk of a coronary heart disease (CHD) event. For this patient, the risk factors and CVD points associated with each risk

(Continued)

TRADITIONAL MAJOR RISK FACTORS FOR CORONARY HEART DISEASE

- Elevated LDL-C (>160 mg/dL; see Tables 20-1 and 20-2)
- Reduced HDL-C (<40 mg/dL; see Table 20-2)
- Cigarette smoking (within the preceding 30 days)
- Hypertension (blood pressure ≥140/90 mm Hg or use of antihypertensive medication, regardless of blood pressure)
- Type 2 diabetes mellitus
- Advancing age (men >45 years of age or women >55 years of age)
- Family history of premature coronary heart disease (CHD) events (men <55 years; women <65 years) in a first-degree relative
- Obesity (body mass index [BMI] >25 kg/m² and waist circumference >40 in [men] or >35 in [women])

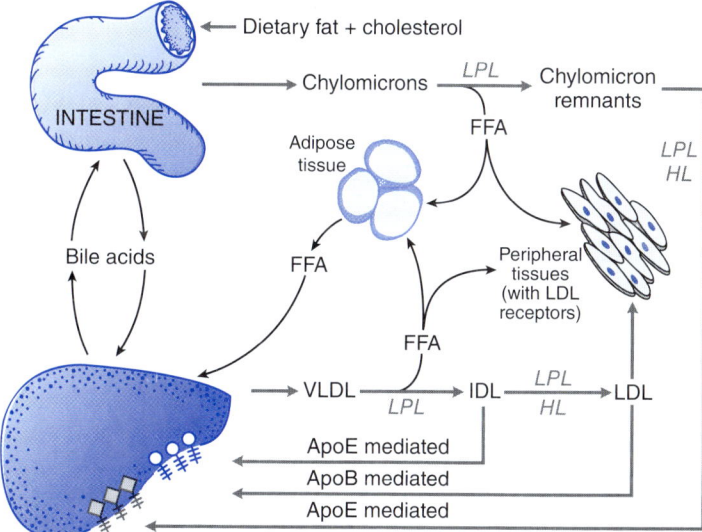

FIGURE 20-1 The major pathways involved in the metabolism of chylomicrons synthesized by the intestine and VLDL synthesized by the liver. Chylomicrons are converted to chylomicron remnants by the hydrolysis of their triglycerides by LPL. Chylomicron remnants are rapidly cleared from the plasma by the liver. "Remnant receptors" include the LDL receptor–related protein (LRP), LDL receptors, and perhaps other receptors. Free fatty acid (FFA) released by LPL is used by muscle tissue as an energy source or taken up and stored by adipose tissue. HL, hepatic lipase; IDL, intermediate-density lipoproteins; LDL, low-density lipoproteins; LPL, lipoprotein lipase; VLDL, very-low-density lipoproteins.

HIGH-RISK DYSLIPIDEMIAS (SEE TABLE 20-2)

- High total cholesterol (≥240 mg/dL)
- High LDL-C (>160 mg/dL)
- Low HDL-C (<40 mg/dL)
- Severe hypertriglyceridemia (≥500 mg/dL)

335

SECTION III — Modulation of Cardiovascular Function

PRIMORDIAL PREVENTION GUIDELINES (TO PREVENT DEVELOPMENT OF CVD RISK FACTORS)

- 150 min/wk of moderate intensity exercise (walking 20-30 min/d)
- Reducing total calories from fat to less than 30%, with saturated and transfat to less than 7%
- Consuming less than 300 mg cholesterol/d
- Eat a variety of oily fish at least twice a week
- Eat oils/foods rich in α-linolenic acid
- Restricting sugary beverages to less than 36 oz/wk for a person consuming 2000 Kcal daily

factor are: age (10 points); HDL (−1 point); total cholesterol (2 points); systolic blood pressure (0 points); smoker (0 points), diabetic (0 points). The total number of CVD points is 11, placing his 10-year risk of a CVD event at 11.2%.

b. What, if anything, can be done to reduce this patient's risk of a CVD event?

This patient's largest CVD risk is his age, which is not a modifiable risk factor. Another risk factor which cannot be modified is his sex; a woman of the same age with all the same lipid, blood pressure, and history would have a 10-year risk of a CVD event of 6.3%. Based on Table 31-6 in *Goodman & Gilman's The Pharmacological Basis of Therapeutics*, 12th Edition, the modifiable risk factors for this patient are his blood lipids and his systolic blood pressure. With optimal blood lipids and systolic blood pressure, his CVD points would be reduced to 6 points and his 10-year risk of a CVD event would be reduced to 4.7%.

c. What are the treatment options to maximally reduce this patient's 10-year CVD risk?

The first option is for the patient to adopt changes in exercise and diet (see Side Bar PRIMORDIAL PREVENTION GUIDELINES). Such lifestyle changes can be effective in lowering blood pressure and improving blood lipid profiles. If lifestyle changes do not adequately improve blood lipid profiles, it may be prudent to start the patient on drugs that lower serum cholesterol (based on Table 20-1). To reach optimal levels of total cholesterol and LDL-C in this patient (<200 mg/dL and <100 mg/dL, respectively; see Table 20-2), the lowest dose of a statin drug should be sufficient (see Table 31-10 in *Goodman & Gilman's The Pharmacological Basis of Therapeutics*, 12th Edition).

(Continued)

TABLE 20-1 Treatment Based on LDL-C Levels (2004 Revision of NCEP Adult Treatment Panel III Guidelines)

RISK CATEGORY	LDL-C GOAL (mg/dL)	NON-HDL-C GOAL (mg/dL)	THERAPEUTIC LIFESTYLE CHANGE	THRESHOLD FOR DRUG THERAPY (mg/dL)
Very high risk Atherosclerosis-induced CHD plus one of: • multiple risk factors • diabetes mellitus • a poorly controlled single factor • acute coronary syndrome • metabolic syndrome	<70[a]	<100	No threshold (initiate change)	No threshold (initiate therapy)
High risk CHD or CHD Equivalent	<100[a]	<130	No threshold	No threshold
Moderately high risk 2+ risk factors 10-year risk: <10–20%	<130 (optional <100)	<160	No threshold	≥130 (100-129)[b]
Moderate risk 2+ risk factors 10-year risk <10%	<130	<160	No threshold	>160
0–1 risk factor	<160	<160	No threshold	≥190 (optional: 160–189)[c]

[a] If pretreatment LDL-C is near or below LDL-C goal value, then a statin dose sufficient to lower LDL-C by 30-40% should be prescribed.

[b] Patients in this category include those with a 10-year risk of 10-20% and one of the following: age >60 years, three or more risk factors, a severe risk factor, triglycerides >200 mg/dL and HDL-C <40 mg/dL, metabolic syndrome, highly sensitive C-reactive protein (CRP) >3 mg/L, and coronary calcium score (age/gender adjusted) >75th percentile.

[c] Patients include those with any severe single risk factor, multiple major risk factors, 10-year risk >8%.

After attaining the LDL-C goal, additional therapy may be necessary to reach the non-HDL-C goal. CHD, coronary heart disease; CHD equivalent, peripheral vascular disease, abdominal aortic aneurysm, symptomatic carotid artery disease, >20% 10-year CHD risk, or diabetes mellitus; HDL-C, high-density-lipoprotein cholesterol; LDL-C, low-density-lipoprotein cholesterol; NCEP, National Cholesterol Education Program.

TABLE 20-2 Classification of Plasma Lipid Levels (mg/dL)[a]

Total cholesterol	
<200	Desirable
200-239	Borderline high
≥240	High

HDL-C	
<40	Low (consider <50 mg/dL as low for women)
>60	High

LDL-C	
<70	Optimal for very high risk (minimal goal for CHD equivalent patients)
<100	Optimal
100-129	Near optimal
130-159	Borderline high
160-189	High
≥190	Very high

Triglycerides	
<150	Normal
150-199	Borderline high
200-499	High
≥500	Very high

[a]2001 National Cholesterol Education Program guidelines. HDL-C, high-density-lipoprotein cholesterol; LDL-C, low-density-lipoprotein cholesterol. From The Expert Panel, 2002.

d. What is the mechanism(s) by which statins reduce CVD risk?

The statins competitively inhibit 3-hydroxy-3-methylglutaryl-coenzyme A (HMG-CoA) reductase, the early rate-limiting step in hepatic cholesterol biosynthesis. They are the most effective and best-tolerated agents for treating dyslipidemias. By inhibiting hepatocyte cholesterol synthesis, the statins induce an increase in the expression of LDL receptors on hepatocytes. The greater number of LDL receptors on the surface of hepatocytes facilitates the removal of LDL from the blood, which lowers LDL-C levels. High levels of LDL-C are associated with a high risk of CVD.

There is also evidence that statin-induced increases in hepatocyte LDL receptors also enhance the removal of circulating LDL precursors, VLDL, and IDL (see Figure 20-1). Statin-mediated reduction in hepatic cholesterol synthesis also reduces hepatic production of VLDL, which can reduce serum triglyceride levels.

In addition to lowering LDL-C, a number of other potential cardioprotective effects have been ascribed to the statins (see Potential Cardioprotective Effects Other than LDL Lowering, p. 894, in *Goodman & Gilman's The Pharmacological Basis of Therapeutics*, 12th Edition).

SECTION III Modulation of Cardiovascular Function

CASE 20-2

A 52-year-old woman with a history of angina, hypertension (blood pressure of 140/80 mm Hg), and type 2 diabetes suffers an acute myocardial infarction and receives angioplasty and a stent to open a blocked coronary artery. She has been taking medications for her hypertension and diabetes, but no other medications. She smokes a pack of cigarettes each day. Before she is discharged from the hospital, her fasting blood lipids are measured: total cholesterol, 240 mg/dL; HDL-C, 30 mg/dL; LDL-C, 160 mg/dL; triglycerides, 220 mg/dL.

a. What is the 10-year risk this woman will have a CVD event?

Based on Table 31-6 in *Goodman & Gilman's The Pharmacological Basis of Therapeutics*, 12th Edition, this patient's risk factors and CVD points are: age (7 points), HDL-C (2 points), total cholesterol (4 points), SBP (5 points), smoker (3 points), and diabetes (4 points). Her total number of CVD points is 25 placing her 10-year risk of a CVD event at greater than 30%.

b. What are the recommended treatment options to reduce the risk of another myocardial infarction or other CVD event in this patient?

Patients such as this woman who have had a CVD event are at the greatest risk of another CVD event and need to be treated aggressively to reduce their risk (see Table 20-1). She should be counseled to adopt a healthy diet and to begin a moderate exercise program (see Side Bar PRIMORDIAL PREVENTION GUIDELINES). Her hypertension and diabetes medications should also be reviewed and adjusted to optimize systolic blood pressure and blood glucose.

Her dyslipidemias should be treated aggressively with goals of reducing her LDL-C to less than 70 mg/dL (see Table 20-1) and TC:HDL-C ratio to less than 3.5 (see Table 31-9 in *Goodman & Gilman's The Pharmacological Basis of Therapeutics*, 12th Edition). To reach the goal of reducing her LDL-C to less than 70 mg/L (ie, 44%), she should be started on a statin dosage that achieves this goal (see Table 31-10 in *Goodman & Gilman's The Pharmacological Basis of Therapeutics*, 12th Edition).

c. She is started on rosuvastatin 10 mg daily. When should she take this dose?

Rosuvastatin has a $t_{1/2}$ of 20 to 30 hours and can be taken at any time of the day. Statins with a short $t_{1/2}$ (<4 hours) such as fluvastatin, lovastatin, simvastatin, and others (see text) should be taken in the evening since hepatic cholesterol synthesis is maximal between midnight and 2:00 AM.

d. What are the common adverse effects of statins?

Myopathy and rhabdomyolysis are the major adverse effects of statins and can result in death (1 death per million 30-day prescriptions). The risk of myopathy is increased with dose and plasma concentrations. Concomitant use of drugs that diminish statin catabolism or interfere with hepatic uptake is associated with 50 to 60% of all cases of myopathy and rhabdomyolysis. The most common statin interactions are with some of the fibrates such as gemfibrozil. Gemfibrozil interferes with hepatocyte uptake of statins by OATP1B1 and its catabolism by glucuronidation. Fibrates such as fenofibrate do not interfere with statin glucuronidation, and are not associated with myopathy when used concomitantly.

Hepatotoxicity has also been associated with statin use and is dose-related. Serious hepatotoxicity occurs at a rate of 1 case per million person-years of use. Because there is some risk of liver damage with statins, it is reasonable to measure serum alanine aminotransferase (ALT) at baseline and subsequently when clinically indicated.

CASE 20-3

A 64-year-old man with highly elevated total cholesterol and LDL-C is not responding adequately to high-dose statin therapy.

(Continued)

a. **What additional drug therapies are available to lower this patient's serum cholesterol?**

When used in combination with statins, other lipid-lowering drugs such as the bile acid–binding resins, niacin, fibrate, and ezetimibe can produce greater reductions in LDL-C than can be achieved with statins alone (see text: Statins in Combination With Other Lipid-Lowering Drugs in *Goodman & Gilman's The Pharmacological Basis of Therapeutics*, 12th Edition). Triple therapy with resins, niacin, and statins can reduce LDL-C by up to 70%. Vytorin, a fixed combination of simvastatin and ezetimibe, can reduce LDL-C levels by 60%.

b. **What are the considerations in using multiple agents to treat dyslipidemias?**

There can be adverse drug interactions that occur when statins are combined with other lipid-lowering agents, as well adverse effects due solely to each of the individual agents. Cholestyramine and colestipol bind to many drugs and interfere with their absorption, including some of the statins. Thus, it is wise to administer all drugs either 1 hour before or 3 to 4 hours after a dose of cholestyramine, colestipol, or other bile acid–binding resins. Patients taking cholestyramine and colestipol often complain of bloating and dyspepsia.

The occurrence of myopathy increases when statin doses of greater than 25% of the maximal dose (eg, 20 mg of simvastatin or atorvastatin) are used with niacin.

There is also an increased risk of myopathy with combination therapy using a statin and fibrate (gemfibrozil or fenofibrate), but this combination is usually safe if the fibrate is used at its usual maximal dose and a statin at no more than 25% of its maximal dose. Fenofibrate is least likely to interfere with statin metabolism and appears to be the safest drug to use with statins. Combined statin-fibrate therapy should be avoided in patients with compromised renal function.

CASE 20-4

A 30-year-old woman makes her first visit to the doctor in 10 years. Her fasting plasma lipids are: total cholesterol, 210 mg/dL; LDL-C, 140 mg/dL; HDL-C, 40 mg/dL; and triglycerides, 180 mg/dL. Her fasting glucose is 110 mg/dL, her waist circumference is 40 in, and her blood pressure is 125/80 mm Hg. This patient has 3 or more risk factors that identify her as having metabolic syndrome.

a. **What are this patient's CHD risk factors that are part of the constellation known as metabolic syndrome?**

The CHD risk factors that identify this patient as having metabolic syndrome are her abdominal obesity, high levels of triglycerides, low HDL-C, and high fasting glucose (see Table 31-8 in *Goodman & Gilman's The Pharmacological Basis of Therapeutics*, 12th Edition). There is an increased CHD risk associated with the insulin-resistant, prediabetic state known as metabolic syndrome.

b. **What should be the focus of treatment in this patient?**

Treatment should focus on weight loss and increased physical activity to reduce obesity. In addition, reducing or eliminating alcohol intake and reducing as much fat as possible from the diet can reduce triglyceride levels. Drug therapy should focus on reducing LDL-C, non–HDL-C, and triglycerides, and increasing HDL-C. The LDL-C therapy goal should be less than 70 mg/dL (see Table 20-1).

c. **What drug therapies are most effective in treating patients with high triglycerides and low HDL-C levels associated with the metabolic syndrome?**

The fibrates play an important role in such patients. It is important to monitor LDL levels when using fibrates in these patients as LDL levels may rise. If LDL levels rise, it might be necessary to add a low-dose statin. Many such patients are treated first with a statin; then a fibrate is added. It is important to monitor for myopathy when using a statin-fibrate combination (see answer to Case 20-3, question b).

(Continued)

Niacin is indicated for hypertriglyceridemia and elevated LDL-C, and is especially useful in patients with both hypertriglyceridemia and low HDL-C levels. However, niacin can cause hyperglycemia and, if used in patients with known or suspected diabetes, blood glucose levels should be monitored weekly until proven to be stable.

Bile acid resins can cause an increase in hepatic triglyceride synthesis, which is of consequence in patients with baseline triglyceride levels of greater than 250 mg/dL.

d. Because this patient is of childbearing age, what considerations must be made in choosing an appropriate drug therapy?

The safety of statins during pregnancy has not been established. Women of childbearing age who take statins should use highly effective contraception (see Chapter 28); women who wish to become pregnant or who are nursing children should not take statins. Fibrates should not be used by children or pregnant women. Niacin, at doses used in humans, has been associated with birth defects in experimental animals and should not be taken by pregnant women. The safety of ezetimibe during pregnancy has not been established; combination products containing ezetimibe and a statin should not be used by women in childbearing years. The bile acid sequestrants are not absorbed systemically but should be used with caution since there have not been studies in women. No adverse effects of colesevelam have been seen in animal reproduction studies and it is classified as pregnancy risk factor B. Also, regular prenatal vitamin supplementation may be inadequate as these agents can interfere with vitamin absorption.

CASE 20-5

A male patient's LDL-C levels remain high even with maximal dosing (80 mg daily) of simvastatin. He is changed to a combination tablet (VYTORIN) containing 80 mg simvastatin and 10 mg ezetimibe.

a. What is the rational for this drug combination?

Statins, which inhibit cholesterol biosynthesis, increase intestinal cholesterol absorption. Ezetimibe, which inhibits intestinal cholesterol absorption, enhances cholesterol biosynthesis. Dual therapy with these 2 classes of drugs prevents both the enhanced cholesterol synthesis induced by ezetimibe and the increase in cholesterol absorption induced by statins. This combination provides additive reductions in LDL-C levels irrespective of the statin employed.

b. What is the molecular target of ezetimibe?

Ezetimibe inhibits luminal cholesterol uptake by jejunal enterocytes, by inhibiting the transport protein NPC1L. Ezetimibe does not affect intestinal triglyceride absorption. In human subjects, ezetimibe reduced cholesterol absorption by 54%, precipitating a compensatory increase in cholesterol synthesis that can be inhibited with a cholesterol synthesis inhibitor such as a statin.

c. How does ezetimibe reduce plasma LDL-C?

Inhibiting intestinal cholesterol absorption causes a reduction in the incorporation of cholesterol into chylomicrons. The reduced cholesterol content of chylomicrons diminishes the delivery of cholesterol to the liver by chylomicron remnants. Reduced delivery of intestinal cholesterol to the liver by chylomicron remnants stimulates expression of the hepatic genes regulating LDL receptor expression and cholesterol biosynthesis. The greater expression of hepatic LDL receptors enhances LDL-C clearance from the plasma. Indeed, ezetimibe reduces LDL-C levels by 15 to 20%.

d. Why not use ezetimibe for monotherapy?

The maximal efficacy of ezetimibe for lowering LDL-C is 15 to 20% when used as monotherapy. This reduction is equivalent to, or less than, that attained with 10- to 20-mg doses of most statins. Consequently, the role of ezetimibe as monotherapy in patients with elevated LDL-C levels appears to be limited to the small group of statin-intolerant patients.

Drug Therapy of Dyslipidemias

CHAPTER 20

KEY CONCEPTS

- Patients with any type of dyslipidemia are at increased risk of CHD and CVD events.
- In the absence of vascular disease, type 2 diabetes mellitus, or metabolic syndrome, the need for cholesterol-lowering drugs in many patients will be alleviated by maintaining ideal body weight, eating a diet low in saturated fat and cholesterol, and regular exercise.
- Lifestyle changes are a cornerstone of managing dyslipidemias.
- Dyslipidemic patients with a risk for a CVD should be treated to achieve target lipid values.
- Statins should be the first-line choice when choosing a lipid-lowering drug.
- Initiate treatment with statin doses adequate to reduce the patient's lipid values to target goals.
- Patients should be counseled regarding the rare but serious side effects of hepatotoxicity and rhabdomyolysis.
- For patients with low HDL-C levels, treatment should be based on both LDL-C levels and the ratio of total cholesterol:HDL-C (see Table 31-9 in *Goodman & Gilman's The Pharmacological Basis of Therapeutics*, 12th Edition).

SUMMARY QUIZ

QUESTION 20-1 A patient is prescribed fenofibrate as part of his therapy to raise his/her HDL-C levels. Fenofibrate most likely acts by

a. inhibiting HMG-CoA reductase.
b. binding cell membrane receptors that leads to lowering of adipocyte hormone–sensitive lipase activity.
c. sequestering bile acids in the small intestine.
d. binding PPARα receptors in liver and brown adipose tissue.
e. inhibiting cholesterol uptake from the small intestine.

QUESTION 20-2 A patient is prescribed niacin to reduce his/her triglyceride and LDL-C levels. The side effect(s) of niacin that most commonly limits patient compliance include

a. bloating.
b. flushing and dyspepsia.
c. tinnitus.
d. dry cough.
e. chills.

QUESTION 20-3 A patient is prescribed lovastatin to lower total cholesterol and LDL-C. For maximal effect, he should take his medication

a. before breakfast.
b. with breakfast.
c. an hour after breakfast.
d. with his evening meal.
e. at bedtime.

SECTION III — Modulation of Cardiovascular Function

QUESTION 20-4 A patient taking digoxin for his heart failure is started on lovastatin and cholestyramine to lower his/her LDL-C levels. The dose of digoxin

a. should be increased.

b. should be decreased.

c. should be taken 1 hour before or 3 to 4 hours after a dose of cholestyramine.

d. should be eliminated to prevent serious drug interactions.

e. will not be affected as there are no known drug interactions among these drugs.

QUESTION 20-5 A patient is being started on statin therapy. What should be considered in choosing which statin to use?

a. Efficacy in reducing LDL-C

b. Cost

c. Safety

d. All of the above

e. None of the above

SUMMARY QUIZ ANSWER KEY

QUESTION 20-1 Answer is **d.** The effects of fenofibrate and other fibrates on blood lipids are mediated by their interaction with the peroxisome proliferator–activated receptors (PPARs). Fibrates bind to PPARα, which is expressed primarily in the liver and brown adipose tissue and to a lesser extent in the kidney, heart, and skeletal muscle. Fibrates reduce triglycerides through PPARα-mediated stimulation of fatty acid oxidation, increased LPL synthesis, and reduced expression of apoC-III. An increase in LPL would enhance the clearance of triglyceride-rich lipoproteins. A reduction in hepatic production of apoC-III, which serves as an inhibitor of lipolytic processing and receptor-mediated clearance, would enhance the clearance of VLDL. Fibrate-mediated increases in HDL-C are due to PPARα stimulation of apoA-I and apoA-II expression, which increases HDL levels. Most fibric acid agents have potential antithrombotic effects, including inhibition of coagulation and enhancement of fibrinolysis. These salutary effects also could alter cardiovascular outcomes by mechanisms unrelated to any hypolipidemic activity.

QUESTION 20-2 Answer is **b.** Two of niacin's side effects, flushing and dyspepsia, limit patient compliance. The cutaneous effects include flushing and pruritus of the face and upper trunk, skin rashes, and acanthosis nigricans. Flushing and associated pruritus are prostaglandin-mediated. Flushing is worse when therapy is initiated or the dosage is increased but ceases in most patients after 1 to 2 weeks of a stable dose. Taking an aspirin each day alleviates the flushing in many patients. Flushing recurs if only 1 or 2 doses are missed, and the flushing is more likely to occur when niacin is consumed with hot beverages (coffee, tea) or with ethanol-containing beverages. Flushing is minimized if therapy is initiated with low doses (100-250 mg twice daily) and if the drug is taken after breakfast or supper. Dry skin, a frequent complaint, can be dealt with by using skin moisturizers, and acanthosis nigricans can be dealt with by using lotions or creams containing salicylic acid. Dyspepsia and rarer episodes of nausea, vomiting, and diarrhea are less likely to occur if the drug is taken after a meal. Patients with any history of peptic ulcer disease should not take niacin because it can reactivate ulcer disease. The most common, medically serious side effects are hepatotoxicity, manifested as elevated serum transaminases, and hyperglycemia.

QUESTION 20-3 Answer is **d.** Lovastatin is slightly more effective if taken with the evening meal than if it is taken at bedtime, although bedtime dosing is preferable to missing doses. Hepatic cholesterol synthesis is maximal between midnight and 2:00 AM. Thus, statins with $t_{1/2}$ 4 hours or less (all but atorvastatin and rosuvastatin) should be taken in the evening.

QUESTION 20-4 Answer is **c.** Cholestyramine and colestipol bind and interfere with the absorption of many drugs, including some thiazides, furosemide, propranolol,

Drug Therapy of Dyslipidemias
CHAPTER 20

L-thyroxine, digoxin, warfarin, and some of the statins. The effect of cholestyramine and colestipol on the absorption of most drugs has not been studied. For this reason, it is wise to administer all drugs either 1 hour before or 3 to 4 hours after a dose of cholestyramine or colestipol. Colesevelam does not appear to interfere with the absorption of fat-soluble vitamins or of drugs such as digoxin, lovastatin, warfarin, metoprolol, quinidine, and valproic acid. The effect of colesevelam on the absorption of other drugs has not been tested, but it seems prudent to recommend that patients take other medications 1 hour before or 3 to 4 hours after a dose of colesevelam.

QUESTION 20-5 Answer is **d**. The choice of statins should be based on efficacy (reduction of LDL-C), cost, and safety. Three drugs (lovastatin, simvastatin, and pravastatin) have been used safely in clinical trials involving thousands of subjects for 5 or more years. The documented safety records of these statins should be considered, especially when initiating therapy in younger patients. Once drug treatment is initiated, it is almost always lifelong.

SUMMARY: DRUGS USED IN THE TREATMENT OF DYSLIPIDEMIAS

CLASS AND SUBCLASSES	NAMES	CLINICAL USES	TOXICITIES COMMON	TOXICITIES UNIQUE; CLINICALLY IMPORTANT
HMG-CoA Reductase Inhibitors (Statins)	Atorvastatin Simvastatin Rosuvastatin Lovastatin Pravastatin Fluvastatin Pitavastatin	The most effective and best-tolerated agents to treat dyslipidemias, especially elevated LDL-C	*The safety of statins during pregnancy has not been established;* women wishing to conceive and nursing mothers should not take statins; during their childbearing years, women taking statins should use highly effective contraception	Hepatotoxicity (1 case per million person-years of use); it is reasonable to measure liver enzymes (ALT) at baseline and thereafter when clinically indicated. Myopathy and rhabdomyolysis (1 death per million) prescriptions (30-day supply); risk increases with statin dose and other factors including concomitant administration with drugs that interfere with statin catabolism or hepatic uptake; gemfibrozil is the drug most commonly associated with statin-induced myopathy
Bile Acid–Binding Resins (Bile Acid Sequestrants)	Cholestyramine Colestipol Colesevelam	Probably the safest lipid-lowering drugs because they are not absorbed systemically. Recommended for patients 11-20 y of age. Often used as second agents with statins	Bloating and dyspepsia. Constipation. Colesevelam may be less likely to cause dyspepsia, bloating, and constipation. Cholestyramine and colestipol bind and interfere with the absorption of many drugs; it is wise to administer all drugs either 1 h before or 3-4 h after a dose of a bile acid resin	Rare instances of hyperchloremic acidosis because these are administered as chloride salts. Severe hypertriglyceridemia is a contraindication to the use of cholestyramine and colestipol because these resins increase triglyceride levels
Nicotinic Acid	Niacin	Favorably affects all lipid parameters, it is the best agent for increasing HDL-C, and also lowers triglycerides, and reduces LDL-C	Flushing, pruritus, and dyspepsia limit patient compliance. Rarer episodes of nausea, vomiting, and diarrhea. *Should not be taken by pregnant women*	Hepatotoxicity, manifested as elevated serum transaminases. Hyperglycemia and niacin-induced insulin resistance; in patients with known or suspected diabetes, blood glucose levels should be monitored at least weekly until proven to be stable. Concurrent use of niacin and a statin can cause myopathy; the statin should be administered at no more than 25% of its maximal dose; patients should be instructed to discontinue therapy if flu-like muscle aches occur. Patients with any history of peptic ulcer disease should not take niacin. Gout is a relative contraindication

SECTION III: Modulation of Cardiovascular Function

CLASS AND SUBCLASSES	NAMES	CLINICAL USES	TOXICITIES COMMON	TOXICITIES UNIQUE; CLINICALLY IMPORTANT
Fibric Acid (Fibrates)	Gemfibrozil Clofibrate (no longer available) Fenofibrate Ciprofibrate (not marketed in the United States) Bezafibrate (not marketed in the United States)	Usually the drugs of choice for treating severe hypertriglyceridemia, the chylomicronemia syndrome, hyperlipidemic subjects with type III hyperlipoproteinemia as well as subjects with severe hypertriglyceridemia (triglycerides >1000 mg/dL) who are at risk for pancreatitis Fibrates appear to have an important role in subjects with high triglycerides and low HDL-C levels associated with the metabolic syndrome or type 2 diabetes mellitus	Gastrointestinal side effects occur in up to 5% of patients *Fibrates should not be used by children or pregnant women*	A myopathy syndrome occasionally occurs in subjects taking clofibrate, gemfibrozil, or fenofibrate Myopathy may occur in up to 5% of patients treated with a combination of gemfibrozil and higher doses of statins Fenofibrate-statin combinations are less likely to cause myopathy than combination therapy with gemfibrozil and statins Renal failure and hepatic dysfunction are relative contraindications to the use of fibrates
Cholesterol Absorption Inhibitor	Ezetimibe	Monotherapy in patients with elevated LDL-C levels who are statin-intolerant		Bile acid sequestrants inhibit absorption of ezetimibe, and the 2 agents should not be administered together
	Ezetimibe/simvastatin	Combination with statin provides additive reductions in LDL-C, greater than that can be achieved with any statin as monotherapy	*Combination products containing ezetimibe and a statin should not be used by women in childbearing years in the absence of contraception*	

Inflammation, Immunomodulation, and Hematopoiesis

SECTION IV

21. Histamine, Bradykinin, and Their Antagonists 346
22. Prostaglandins, NSAIDs, and Pharmacotherapy of Gout 356
23. Immunotherapeutic Agents... 375
24. Pulmonary Pharmacology.. 389
25. Hematopoietic Agents 405

CHAPTER 21

Histamine, Bradykinin, and Their Antagonists

DRUGS INCLUDED IN THIS CHAPTER

- Acrivastine (SEMPREX-D*)
- Aprotinin (TRAYSYLOL)
- Azelastine (ASTELIN)
- Brompheniramine maleate (BROMPHEN, others)
- Carbinoxamine (RONDEC*, others)
- Cetirizine (ZYRTEC)
- Chlorpheniramine (CHLOR-TRIMETON, others)
- Clemastine fumarate (TAVIST, others)
- Cyclizine (MAREZINE)
- Cyproheptadine (PERIACTIN)
- Desloratadine (CLARINEX, AERIUS)
- Dimenhydrinate (combination of diphenhydramine and 8-chlorotheophylline; DRAMAMINE, others)
- Diphenhydramine (BENADRYL, others)
- Doxepin (SINEQUAN)
- Ebastine (EBASTEL)
- Fexofenadine (ALLEGRA, TELFAST)
- Hydroxyzine (ATARAX, others)
- Hydroxyzine (VISTARIL)
- Icatibant (FIRAZYR)
- Ketotifen fumarate (ZADITOR)
- Levocabastine (LIVOSTIN)
- Levocetirizine (XYZAL)
- Loratadine (CLARITIN)
- Meclizine (ANTIVERT, others)
- Mizolastine (MIZOLLEN)
- Olopatadine (PATANOL, PATANASE, others)
- Phenindamine (NOLAHIST)
- Promethazine (PHENERGAN, others)
- Pyrilamine (POLY–HISTINE-D*)
- Tripelennamine (PBZ)

*Trade-name drug that contains other medications.

This chapter will be most useful after having a basic understanding of the material in Chapter 32, Histamine, Bradykinin, and Their Antagonists in *Goodman & Gilman's The Pharmacological Basis of Therapeutics*, 12th Edition. In addition to the material presented here, the 12th Edition contains:

- Table 32-1 Characteristics of Histamine Receptors, which shows the biochemical properties, tissue distribution, and representative agonists and antagonists of the 4 histamine receptors (H_1, H_2, H_3, and H_4)
- Table 32-2 Preparations and Dosage of Representative H_1-Receptor Antagonists
- The molecular structures of histamine and drugs that are agonists and antagonists of the various histamine receptors

LEARNING OBJECTIVES

- ☑ Understand the role of histamine and bradykinin in different physiological and pathophysiological processes.
- ☑ Understand the mechanisms of action of drugs that act as antagonists of the H_1 receptor.
- ☑ Know the therapeutic utility of H_1-receptor antagonists, alone and in combination with other agents.
- ☑ Know the important adverse effects of H_1-receptor antagonists, and the difference between first- and second-generation H_1 antihistamines with regard to adverse effects.

MECHANISMS OF ACTION OF HISTAMINE RECEPTOR AND BRADYKININ ANTAGONISTS

DRUG CLASS	DRUG	MECHANISM OF ACTION
First-Generation H_1-Receptor Antagonists	Doxepin Carbinoxamine Clemastine fumarate Diphenhydramine Dimenhydrinate (combination of diphenhydramine and 8-chlorotheophylline) Pyrilamine Tripelennamine Chlorpheniramine Brompheniramine maleate Hydroxyzine Cyclizine Meclizine Promethazine Cyproheptadine Phenindamine	Act as inverse agonists to reduce the constitutive activity of H_1 receptors and compete with histamine at H_1 receptors on target tissues, including smooth muscle, capillaries, peripheral nerve endings, and some exocrine glands First-generation H_1 antagonists can cross the blood-brain barrier and both stimulate and depress the CNS, though central depression is more common Many first-generation H_1 antagonists have anticholinergic effects mediated through muscarinic receptors (see Chapter 6)

(Continued)

Histamine, Bradykinin, and Their Antagonists

CHAPTER 21

DRUG CLASS	DRUG	MECHANISM OF ACTION
Second-Generation H_1-Receptor Antagonists	Olopatadine Acrivastine Cetirizine Levocetirizine Azelastine Levocabastine Ketotifen fumarate Loratadine Desloratadine Ebastine Mizolastine Fexofenadine	Act as inverse agonists to reduce the constitutive activity of H_1 receptors and compete with histamine at H_1 receptors on target tissues, including smooth muscle, capillaries, peripheral nerve endings, and some exocrine glands
H_2-Receptor Antagonists	See Chapter 32	Inhibit H_2 receptors in the GI system which reduces gastric secretion (see Chapter 32)
H_3-Receptor Antagonists	No agents are currently available (several are currently in clinical trials)	Inhibit H_3 receptors which are presynaptic autoreceptors on histaminergic neurons in the CNS and enterochromaffin-like cells of the stomach
H_4 receptor antagonists	No agents are currently available	Inhibit H_4 receptor which is expressed on cells with inflammatory or immune functions
Kallikrein Inhibitor	Aprotinin (no longer available)	Inhibit the proteinase activity of kallikreins, thus inhibiting the production of kallidin and bradykinin from kininogens (see Figure 32-4 in *Goodman & Gilman's The Pharmacological Basis of Therapeutics*, 12th Edition)
Kinin Receptor Antagonists	Icatibant (only approved in Europe)	Inhibit B_1 and B_2 (bradykinin) receptors

TRIPLE RESPONSE OF LEWIS

Intradermal injection of histamine elicits a characteristic phenomenon known as the triple response first described in 1927 by Lewis. The triple response consists of:

- A localized red spot extending for a few millimeters around the site of injection that appears within a few seconds and reaches a maximum in ~1 minute
  - The initial red spot results from the direct vasodilatory effect of histamine (H_1 receptor–mediated NO production)
- A brighter red flush, or "flare," extending ~1 cm beyond the original red spot and developing more slowly
  - The flare is due to histamine-induced stimulation of axon reflexes that cause indirect vasodilation
- A wheal that is discernible in 1 to 2 minutes and occupies the same area as the original small red spot at the injection site
  - The wheal reflects histamine's capacity to increase capillary permeability (edema formation)

FIRST-GENERATION VERSUS SECOND-GENERATION H_1 ANTIHISTAMINES

- Side effects are most prominent with first-generation H_1 antihistamines, which cross the blood-brain barrier and cause sedation.
- Some of the first-generation H_1-receptor antagonists also have anticholinergic properties that can be responsible for symptoms such as dryness of the mouth and respiratory passages, urinary retention or frequency, and dysuria (see Chapter 6).
- The significant sedative effects of some first-generation antihistamines have led to their use in treating insomnia, although better drugs are available (see Chapter 9).
- Some first-generation H_1 antagonists (eg, dimenhydrinate, cyclizine, meclizine, and promethazine) can prevent motion sickness, although scopolamine is more effective.
  - Antiemetic effects of these H_1 antihistamines can be beneficial in treating vertigo or postoperative emesis.

(continues)

CASE 21-1

A 24-year-old woman has seasonal allergies in the summer due to various pollens and grasses. Her symptoms include a runny nose and itchy, watery eyes. At the beginning of the summer she takes over-the-counter (OTC) diphenhydramine for relief of symptoms.

a. What is the mechanism of action of diphenhydramine in treating this patient's symptoms?

Diphenhydramine is a first-generation H_1-receptor antagonist. H_1 antagonists are most useful in acute types of allergy that present with symptoms of rhinitis, urticaria, and conjunctivitis. Their effect is confined to the suppression of symptoms attributable to the histamine released by the antigen-antibody reaction. These drugs relieve the sneezing, rhinorrhea, and itching of eyes, nose, and throat. A gratifying response is obtained in most patients, especially at the beginning of the season when pollen counts are low; however, the drugs are less effective when the allergens are most abundant, when exposure to them is prolonged, and when nasal congestion is prominent.

(Continued)

SECTION IV

Inflammation, Immunomodulation, and Hematopoiesis

FIRST-GENERATION VERSUS SECOND-GENERATION H1 ANTIHISTAMINES (Cont.)

- Many H_1 antihistamines (both first and second generation) are metabolized by CYPs; thus, inhibitors of CYP activity can increase H_1 antihistamine levels, leading to toxicity.
- Certain H_1 antihistamines, especially first-generation drugs, are possible teratogens or cause symptomatic effects in infants resulting from secretion of the drug into breast milk.
  - ▶ Cetirizine and loratadine are preferred in pregnant women if H_1 antihistamines are required, but if they are not effective, diphenhydramine can be used safely in pregnant (but not breast-feeding) women.

b. She finds the diphenhydramine causes her to be drowsy. Why does this agent cause drowsiness?

The first-generation H_1 antagonists can cross the blood-brain barrier and can both stimulate and depress the CNS. The most frequent side effect in first-generation H_1 antagonists is sedation and usually accompanies therapeutic doses of the older H_1 antagonists. Diminished alertness, slowed reaction times, and somnolence are common manifestations of the central CNS depression caused by these agents. Concurrent ingestion of alcohol or other CNS depressants produces an additive effect that impairs motor skills. Patients vary in their susceptibility and responses to individual drugs. The ethanolamines, which include diphenhydramine, are particularly prone to causing sedation. Because of the sedation that occurs with first-generation antihistamines, these drugs cannot be tolerated or used safely by many patients except at bedtime. Even then, patients may experience an antihistamine "hangover" in the morning, resulting in sedation with or without psychomotor impairment. CNS stimulation occasionally is encountered in patients given conventional doses of first-generation H_1 antagonists; they become restless, nervous, and unable to sleep. Central excitation also is a striking feature of overdose, which commonly results in convulsions, particularly in infants. Other untoward central actions caused by first-generation H_1 antagonists include dizziness, tinnitus, lassitude, incoordination, fatigue, blurred vision, diplopia, euphoria, nervousness, insomnia, and tremors.

c. What alternatives does she have to treat her allergy symptoms without getting drowsy?

The second-generation H_1 antagonists (eg, levocetirizine, cetirizine, loratadine, desloratadine, fexofenadine) are largely devoid of these side effects because they do not penetrate the central nervous system (CNS). Thus, they usually are the drugs of choice for the treatment of allergic disorders.

d. She plans to get pregnant and is concerned about whether she can treat her allergies when she is pregnant. What are her options?

Caution should be used in treating pregnant or lactating women with certain H_1 antihistamines, especially first-generation drugs, because of their possible teratogenic effects or symptomatic effects on infants resulting from secretion of the drug into breast milk. Cetirizine and loratadine are preferred if H_1 antihistamines are required, but if they are not effective, diphenhydramine can be used safely in pregnant (but not breast-feeding) women.

CASE 21-2

A 32-year-old man visits his dermatologist because he is very sensitive to mosquito bites. When bitten by a mosquito, he immediately experiences redness at the site of the bite. The redness gradually grows to about the size of a dime and a small itchy bump forms.

a. What is causing the progression in this patient's symptoms following a mosquito bite?

The mosquito bite is causing the release of histamine from mast cells in the skin that results in a classic "triple response" (see Side Bar TRIPLE RESPONSE OF LEWIS) of redness, flare, and wheal characteristic of intradermal injection of histamine.

b. What can be done to treat this patient's mosquito bites?

H_1 antihistamines can effectively attenuate or block all of the reactions to the mosquito bite. Topical preparations of H_1 antihistamines are available (see Table 32-2 in *Goodman & Gilman's The Pharmacological Basis of Therapeutics*, 12th Edition) that can be applied to the mosquito bite to relieve itching and reduce the redness and wheal. However, there is a possibility of producing allergic dermatitis due to the development of drug allergy with topical application of H_1 antagonists. The patient may also benefit from taking an oral antihistamine if he receives a number of bites, although relief of symptoms may take 1 hour or longer.

(Continued)

Histamine, Bradykinin, and Their Antagonists

CHAPTER 21

CASE 21-3

A 57-year-old woman with a history of allergies to seafood suddenly develops swelling of her lips and face while dining in a restaurant. She also begins to feel light-headed, and her tongue and mouth begin to itch.

a. **What is likely causing this woman's symptoms?**

Her symptoms are consistent with an allergic (ie, immediate hypersensitivity) reaction, perhaps due to the presence of seafood in something she has just eaten at the restaurant. The principal target cells of immediate hypersensitivity reactions are mast cells and basophils. As part of the allergic response to an antigen, immunoglobulin E (IgE) antibodies are generated and bind to the surfaces of mast cells and basophils via specific high-affinity F_c receptors. Antigen bridges the IgE molecules and via FcεRI activates signaling pathways in mast cells or basophils involving tyrosine kinases and subsequent phosphorylation of multiple protein substrates within 5 to 15 seconds of contact with antigen. These events trigger the exocytosis of the contents of secretory granules, which contain histamine. After its release from storage granules, histamine plays a central role in immediate hypersensitivity and allergic responses. The actions of histamine on bronchial smooth muscle and blood vessels account for many, but not all, of the symptoms of the allergic response. A broad spectrum of other inflammatory mediators is released on mast cell activation including platelet-activating factor (PAF) and metabolites of arachidonic acid such as leukotrienes C_4 and D_4, which contract the smooth muscles of the bronchial tree. Kinins also are generated during some allergic responses.

The effects of histamine in an allergic reaction are largely mediated by its activation of H_1 receptors which are distributed widely in the periphery. Histamine characteristically dilates resistance vessels, increases capillary permeability, and lowers systemic blood pressure. Vasodilation is the most important vascular effect of histamine in humans. Activation of either the H_1 or H_2 receptor can elicit maximal vasodilation, but the responses differ. H_1 receptors have a higher affinity for histamine and cause Ca^{2+}-dependent activation of endothelial NOS (eNOS) in endothelial cells; NO diffuses to vascular smooth muscle, increasing cyclic guanosine monophosphate (cyclic GMP) (see Table 32–1 in *Goodman & Gilman's The Pharmacological Basis of Therapeutics*, 12th Edition) and causes relaxation that results in a relatively rapid and short-lived vasodilation. By contrast, activation of H_2 receptors on vascular smooth muscle stimulates the cyclic AMP–PKA pathway, causing dilation that develops more slowly and is more sustained. As a result, H_1 antagonists effectively counter small dilator responses to low concentrations of histamine but only blunt the initial phase of larger responses to higher concentrations of the amine. Histamine's effect on small vessels results in efflux of plasma protein and fluid into the extracellular spaces and an increase lymph flow, causing edema. H_1 receptors on endothelial cells are the major mediators of this response. Increased capillary permeability results from histamine activation of H_1 receptors on postcapillary venules, which causes contraction of the endothelial cells, disrupts interendothelial junctions, and exposes the basement membrane, which is freely permeable to plasma proteins and fluid.

b. **The woman recognizes the symptoms of an allergic reaction and takes some diphenhydramine, which she always carries with her (as well as an EPI-PEN autoinjector). The swelling in her throat continues and she begins having difficulty breathing so she self-administers epinephrine using the EPI-PEN. Why did she need epinephrine in addition to diphenhydramine?**

During hypersensitivity reactions, histamine is one of the many potent autacoids released, and its relative contribution to the ensuing symptoms varies widely. Edema formation and itch are effectively suppressed by H_1 antagonists such as diphenhydramine, but other effects, such as hypotension, are less well antagonized. This may be explained by the participation of other types of H receptors and by effects of other mast cell mediators, chiefly eicosanoids (see Chapter 22).

(Continued)

Bronchoconstriction, which is causing the patient's difficulty in breathing, is reduced little, if at all by antihistamines. The beneficial effects of β adrenergic agonists such as epinephrine in allergic states such as asthma and anaphylaxis are due mainly to relaxing bronchial smooth muscle. After she self-administers her epinephrine, the patient should seek medical attention immediately. The EPI-PEN is designed to be an effective, but short-term measure to allow the user time to reach an emergency room where additional epinephrine and other drugs such as corticosteroids may be needed to treat the anaphylactic reaction.

CASE 21-4

A patient who is prone to motion sickness will be taking a small ferry to reach an island destination on her vacation travels.

a. She would like to take something to prevent the motion sickness on the ferry ride. What are her options?

Many of the first-generation H_1 antagonists have antimuscarinic actions in the CNS that can be used to treat motion sickness (see Chapter 9). Cyclizine and meclizine are used primarily to prevent motion sickness and vertigo although promethazine and diphenhydramine are more effective. None of these agents are as effective as the antimuscarinic agent scopolamine, which is the most effective drug for the prophylaxis and treatment of motion sickness. However, the H_1 antagonists are useful for milder cases of motion sickness and have fewer adverse effects. Promethazine is the most potent and effective of the H_1 antagonists in preventing motion sickness, and its additional antiemetic properties may be valuable in reducing vomiting.

b. When should she take the medication?

Whenever possible, the various drugs should be administered ~1 hour before the anticipated motion. Treatment after the onset of nausea and vomiting rarely is beneficial.

c. What side effects should she expect with the H_1 antagonists used for motion sickness?

Sedation is to be expected with all of these agents.

CASE 21-5

A 23-year old woman has a 2-year old son and both she and her son have symptoms of a cold, including cough, runny nose, sneezing, and watery eyes. She finds an OTC cough and cold medication at the grocery store that is advertised to be effective in relieving their symptoms.

a. When she gets home from the store she reads the label more carefully and sees that promethazine is one of the active ingredients in the cough and cold medication she purchased. She also reads a warning "Do Not Use in Children 4 Years and Younger." What is the reason for this warning?

Use of OTC cough and cold medicines (containing mixtures of antihistamines, decongestants, antitussives, expectorants) in young children has been associated with serious side effects and deaths. In 2008, the Food and Drug Administration (FDA) recommended that they not be used in children younger than 2 years, and drug manufacturers affiliated with the Consumer Healthcare Products Association voluntarily relabeled products "do not use" for children younger than 4 years. The FDA is reviewing the safety of these medicines in children aged 2 to 11 years.

b. What value does promethazine have in this cold medication?

H_1 antagonists are without value in combating the causes of the common cold. The weak anticholinergic effects of the older agents may tend to lessen rhinorrhea, but this drying effect may do more harm than good, as may their tendency to induce somnolence.

Histamine, Bradykinin, and Their Antagonists

CHAPTER 21

KEY CONCEPTS

- H_1 antagonists are most useful in acute types of allergy that present with symptoms of rhinitis, urticaria, and conjunctivitis.
  - Their effect is confined to the suppression of symptoms attributable to the histamine released by the antigen-antibody reaction.
- In the treatment of systemic anaphylaxis, where autacoids other than histamine are important, the mainstay of therapy is epinephrine; histamine antagonists have only a subordinate and adjuvant role.
- Histamine antagonists have limited efficacy in treating bronchial asthma and are not used as sole therapy.
- Because of their effects on the CNS, the first-generation H_1 antagonists also have therapeutic value in suppressing motion sickness or for sedation.
- Second-generation drugs are usually the drugs of choice for the treatment of allergic disorders as they are largely devoid of sedating side effects because they do not penetrate the CNS and do not have antimuscarinic properties.

SUMMARY QUIZ

QUESTION 21-1 This antihistamine has antiemetic effects useful in treating vertigo or postoperative emesis.

a. Cetirizine
b. Loratadine
c. Fexofenadine
d. Promethazine
e. None of the above

QUESTION 21-2 This antihistamine is approved for use in children.

a. Cetirizine
b. Meclizine
c. Promethazine
d. Diphenhydramine
e. None of the above

QUESTION 21-3 The H_1 antihistamines are highly effective in treating this histamine-mediated process in humans.

a. Gastric secretions
b. Anaphylactic bronchospasm
c. Allergic urticaria
d. Bronchial asthma
e. Severe angioedema

QUESTION 21-4 The antihistamine of choice in treating seasonal allergy symptoms in a pregnant woman is

a. cetirizine.
b. meclizine.
c. promethazine.
d. dimenhydrinate.
e. none of the above.

QUESTION 21-5 The antihistamine of choice in preventing motion sickness is

a. cetirizine.
b. loratadine.
c. fexofenadine.
d. promethazine.
e. none of the above.

SUMMARY QUIZ ANSWER KEY

QUESTION 21-1 Answer is **d.** The antiemetic effects of some first-generation H_1 antagonists (eg, dimenhydrinate, cyclizine, meclizine, and promethazine) can be beneficial in treating vertigo or postoperative emesis. Dimenhydrinate and meclizine often are of benefit in vestibular disturbances such as Ménière disease and in other types of true vertigo. Only promethazine is useful in treating the nausea and vomiting subsequent to chemotherapy or radiation therapy for malignancies; however, other, more effective antiemetic drugs (eg, 5-HT_3 antagonists) are available (see Chapter 33).

QUESTION 21-2 Answer is **a.** The second-generation H_1 antagonists—loratadine, desloratadine, fexofenadine, cetirizine, levocetirizine, and azelastine (intranasal)—have been approved by the FDA for use in children and are available in appropriate lower-dose formulations (eg, chewable or rapidly dissolving tablets, syrup). First-generation antihistamines are not recommended for use in children because their sedative effects can impair learning and school performance.

QUESTION 21-3 Answer is **c.** H_1 antagonists are most useful in acute types of allergy that present with symptoms of rhinitis, urticaria, and conjunctivitis. Their effect is confined to the suppression of symptoms attributable to the histamine released by the antigen-antibody reaction. In bronchial asthma, histamine antagonists have limited efficacy and are not used as sole therapy. In the treatment of systemic anaphylaxis, where autacoids other than histamine are important, the mainstay of therapy is epinephrine; histamine antagonists have only a subordinate and adjuvant role. The same is true for severe angioedema, in which laryngeal swelling constitutes a threat to life.

QUESTION 21-4 Answer is **a.** Caution should be used in treating pregnant or lactating women with certain H_1 antihistamines, especially first-generation drugs, because of their possible teratogenic effects or symptomatic effects on infants resulting from secretion of the drug into breast milk. Cetirizine and loratadine are preferred if H_1 antihistamines are required, but if they are not effective, diphenhydramine can be used safely in pregnant (but not breast-feeding) women.

QUESTION 21-5 Answer is **d.** Some first-generation H_1 antagonists are useful for preventing motion sickness and have fewer adverse effects than scopolamine, the most effective drug for the prophylaxis and treatment of motion sickness. These antihistamines include dimenhydrinate and the piperazines (eg, cyclizine, meclizine). Promethazine, a phenothiazine, is more potent and more effective than the other antihistamines; its additional antiemetic properties may be of value in reducing vomiting, but its pronounced sedative action usually is disadvantageous.

Histamine, Bradykinin, and Their Antagonists — CHAPTER 21

SUMMARY: HISTAMINE RECEPTOR AND BRADYKININ ANTAGONISTS

CLASS AND SUBCLASSES	NAMES	CLINICAL USES	TOXICITIES — COMMON	TOXICITIES — UNIQUE; CLINICALLY IMPORTANT
First-Generation H_1-Receptor Antagonists—Tricyclic Dibenzoxepins	Doxepin	Treatment of allergic disorders, relieving the symptoms of seasonal rhinitis and conjunctivitis Limited benefit in bronchial asthma Useful adjuncts to epinephrine in the treatment of systemic anaphylaxis or severe angioedema Used to treat certain allergic dermatoses	Can cause drowsiness and is associated with anticholinergic effects Even small doses (eg, 20 mg) may cause disorientation and confusion, but better tolerated by patients with depression than those who are not depressed Loss of appetite, nausea, vomiting, epigastric distress, and constipation or diarrhea (taking the drug with meals may reduce incidence of GI effects)	Not recommended for use in children because their sedative effects can impair learning and school performance OTC cough and cold medicines (containing mixtures of antihistamines, and other drugs) have been associated with serious side effects and deaths in young children Do not use in children <4 years of age
First-Generation H_1-Receptor Antagonists—Ethanolamines	Carbinoxamine Clemastine fumarate Diphenhydramine Dimenhydrinate (combination of diphenhydramine and 8-chlorotheophylline)	Treatment of allergic disorders, relieving the symptoms of seasonal rhinitis and conjunctivitis Limited benefit in bronchial asthma Useful adjuncts to epinephrine in the treatment of systemic anaphylaxis or severe angioedema Used to treat certain allergic dermatoses Diphenhydramine can be used safely in pregnant (but not breast-feeding) women Dimenhydrinate can prevent motion sickness	Possess significant antimuscarinic activity and have a pronounced tendency to induce sedation About half of those treated acutely with conventional doses experience somnolence and cannot be tolerated or used safely by many patients except at bedtime; patients may experience an antihistamine "hangover" in the morning, resulting in sedation with or without psychomotor impairment GI side effects	Not recommended for use in children because their sedative effects can impair learning and school performance OTC cough and cold medicines (containing mixtures of antihistamines, and other drugs) have been associated with serious side effects and deaths in young children Do not use in children <4 years of age
First-Generation H_1-Receptor Antagonists—Ethylenediamines	Pyrilamine Tripelennamine	Treatment of allergic disorders, relieving the symptoms of seasonal rhinitis and conjunctivitis Limited benefit in bronchial asthma Useful adjuncts to epinephrine in the treatment of systemic anaphylaxis or severe angioedema Used to treat certain allergic dermatoses	Central effects are relatively feeble, but somnolence occurs in a fair proportion of patients GI side effects are quite common	Not recommended for use in children because their sedative effects can impair learning and school performance OTC cough and cold medicines (containing mixtures of antihistamines, and other drugs) have been associated with serious side effects and deaths in young children Do not use in children <4 years of age

SECTION IV — Inflammation, Immunomodulation, and Hematopoiesis

CLASS AND SUBCLASSES	NAMES	CLINICAL USES	TOXICITIES – COMMON	TOXICITIES – UNIQUE; CLINICALLY IMPORTANT
First-Generation H_1-Receptor Antagonists—Alkylamines	Chlorpheniramine Brompheniramine maleate	Treatment of allergic disorders, relieving the symptoms of seasonal rhinitis and conjunctivitis • Limited benefit in bronchial asthma • Useful adjuncts to epinephrine in the treatment of systemic anaphylaxis or severe angioedema • Used to treat certain allergic dermatoses	Less prone to produce drowsiness and are more suitable for daytime use, but a significant proportion of patients experience sedation • Side effects involving CNS stimulation are more common than first-generation agents from other chemical structure groups • GI side effects	Not recommended for use in children because their sedative effects can impair learning and school performance • OTC cough and cold medicines (containing mixtures of antihistamines, and other drugs) have been associated with serious side effects and deaths in young children • Do not use in children <4 years of age
First-Generation H_1-Receptor Antagonists—Piperazines	Hydroxyzine Cyclizine Meclizine	Treatment of allergic disorders, relieving the symptoms of seasonal rhinitis and conjunctivitis • Limited benefit in bronchial asthma • Useful adjuncts to epinephrine in the treatment of systemic anaphylaxis or severe angioedema • Hydroxyzine is a long-acting compound widely used for skin allergies; its considerable CNS-depressant activity may contribute to its prominent antipruritic action • Cyclizine and meclizine are used primarily to prevent motion sickness and vertigo although promethazine and diphenhydramine are more effective	Considerable CNS-depressant activity and antimuscarinic effects • Loss of appetite, nausea, vomiting, epigastric distress, and constipation or diarrhea (taking the drug with meals may reduce incidence of GI effects)	Not recommended for use in children because their sedative effects can impair learning and school performance • OTC cough and cold medicines (containing mixtures of antihistamines, and other drugs) have been associated with serious side effects and deaths in young children • Do not use in children <4 years of age
First-generation H_1-Receptor Antagonists—Phenothiazines	Promethazine	Treatment of allergic disorders, relieving the symptoms of seasonal rhinitis and conjunctivitis • Limited benefit in bronchial asthma • Useful adjuncts to epinephrine in the treatment of systemic anaphylaxis or severe angioedema • Used to treat certain allergic dermatoses • Promethazine is the most effective H_1 antagonist in combating motion sickness because of its antimuscarinic effects	Considerable CNS-depressant activity and antimuscarinic effects • Loss of appetite, nausea, vomiting, epigastric distress, and constipation or diarrhea (taking the drug with meals may reduce incidence of GI effects)	Not recommended for use in children because their sedative effects can impair learning and school performance • OTC cough and cold medicines (containing mixtures of antihistamines, and other drugs) have been associated with serious side effects and deaths in young children • Do not use in children <4 years of age
First-Generation H_1-Receptor Antagonists—Piperidines	Cyproheptadine Phenindamine	Treatment of allergic disorders, relieving the symptoms of seasonal rhinitis and conjunctivitis • Limited benefit in bronchial asthma • Useful adjuncts to epinephrine in the treatment of systemic anaphylaxis or severe angioedema • Used to treat certain allergic dermatoses	Cause drowsiness, have significant anticholinergic effects • Can increase appetite and cause weight gain	Not recommended for use in children because their sedative effects can impair learning and school performance • OTC cough and cold medicines (containing mixtures of antihistamines, and other drugs) have been associated with serious side effects and deaths in young children • Do not use in children <4 years of age

Histamine, Bradykinin, and Their Antagonists — CHAPTER 21

CLASS AND SUBCLASSES	NAMES	CLINICAL USES	TOXICITIES COMMON	UNIQUE; CLINICALLY IMPORTANT
Second-Generation H_1-Receptor Antagonists—Tricyclic Dibenzoxepins	Olopatadine	Usually drugs of choice for treatment of allergic disorders, relieving the symptoms of seasonal rhinitis and conjunctivitis Limited benefit in bronchial asthma Useful adjuncts to epinephrine in the treatment of systemic anaphylaxis or severe angioedema Used to treat certain allergic dermatoses	Somewhat higher incidence of drowsiness than the other second-generation H_1 antagonists	
Second-Generation H_1-Receptor Antagonists—Alkylamines	Acrivastine	Usually drugs of choice for treatment of allergic disorders, relieving the symptoms of seasonal rhinitis and conjunctivitis Limited benefit in bronchial asthma Useful adjuncts to epinephrine in the treatment of systemic anaphylaxis or severe angioedema Used to treat certain allergic dermatoses	Lack significant anticholinergic actions; penetrate poorly into the CNS, and low incidence of side effects	
Second-Generation H_1-Receptor Antagonists—Piperazines	Cetirizine Levocetirizine	Usually drugs of choice for treatment of allergic disorders, relieving the symptoms of seasonal rhinitis and conjunctivitis Limited benefit in bronchial asthma Useful adjuncts to epinephrine in the treatment of systemic anaphylaxis or severe angioedema Used to treat certain allergic dermatoses Cetirizine is a preferred drug in pregnant or breast-feeding women if H_1 antihistamines are required	Lack significant anticholinergic actions; penetrate poorly into the CNS, and low incidence of side effects	
Second-Generation H_1-Receptor Antagonists—Phthalazines	Azelastine	Usually drugs of choice for treatment of allergic disorders, relieving the symptoms of seasonal rhinitis and conjunctivitis Limited benefit in bronchial asthma Useful adjuncts to epinephrine in the treatment of systemic anaphylaxis or severe angioedema Used to treat certain allergic dermatoses	Lack significant anticholinergic actions; penetrate poorly into the CNS, and low incidence of side effects	
Second-Generation H_1-Receptor Antagonists—Piperidines	Levocabastine Ketotifen fumarate Loratadine Desloratadine Ebastine Mizolastine Fexofenadine	Usually drugs of choice for treatment of allergic disorders, relieving the symptoms of seasonal rhinitis and conjunctivitis Limited benefit in bronchial asthma Useful adjuncts to epinephrine in the treatment of systemic anaphylaxis or severe angioedema Used to treat certain allergic dermatoses Loratadine is a preferred drug in pregnant or breast-feeding women if H_1 antihistamines are required	Lack significant anticholinergic actions; penetrate poorly into the CNS, and low incidence of side effects	
H_2-Receptor Antagonists	See Chapter 32	Inhibit gastric secretion	See Chapter 32	See Chapter 32
Kinin Receptor Antagonists—B_2 (Bradykinin) Antagonist	Icatibant	Treatment of acute episodes of swelling in patients with hereditary angioedema		

CHAPTER 22

Prostaglandins, NSAIDs, and Pharmacotherapy of Gout

DRUGS INCLUDED IN THIS CHAPTER

- Acetaminophen (TYLENOL, others)
- Allopurinol (ZYLOPRIM, ALOPRIM, others)
- Alprostadil (CAVERJECT, EDEX, MUSE, PROSTIN VR PEDIATRIC)
- Aspirin (acetylsalicylic acid, ASA)
- Balsalazide (COLAZOL, others)
- Bimatoprost (LUMIGAN)
- Bromfenac (XIBROM)
- Carboprost tromethamine (HEMABATE)
- Celecoxib (CELEBREX)
- Colchicine
- Diclofenac (CATAFLAM, ZIPSOR, FLECTOR, VOLTAREN, SOLAREZE, CAMBIA, others)
- Diflunisal
- Dinoprostone (CERVIDIL, PREPIDIL)
- Etodolac (LODINE)
- Febuxostat (ULORIC)
- Fenoprofen (NALFON 200, others)
- Flurbiprofen (ANSAID, OCUFEN, others)
- Ibuprofen (ADVIL, MOTRIN, NEOPROFEN, CALDOLOR, others)
- Iloprost (VENTAVIS)
- Indomethacin (INDOCIN, others)
- Ketoprofen
- Ketorolac (ACULAR, others)
- Latanoprost (XALATAN)
- Meclofenamate (MECLOMEN)
- Mefenamic acid (PONSTEL)
- Meloxicam (MOBIC, others)
- Mesalamine (ASACOL, LIALDA, APRISO, DIPENTUM, CANASA)
- Misoprostol (CYTOTEC)
- Nabumetone (RELAFEN)
- Naproxen (ALEVE, NAPROSYN, others)
- Nepafenac (NEVANAC)
- Olsalazine
- Oxaprozin (DAYPRO)

(continues)

This chapter will be most useful after having a basic understanding of the material in Chapter 33, Lipid-Derived Autacoids: Eicosanoids and Platelet-Activating Factor, and Chapter 34, Anti-inflammatory, Antipyretic, and Analgesic Agents: Pharmacotherapy of Gout in *Goodman & Gilman's The Pharmacological Basis of Therapeutics*, 12th Edition. In addition to the material presented here, the 12th Edition contains:

- Table 33-1 Eicosanoid Receptors that lists the major classes of eicosanoid receptors and their signaling characteristics
- The molecular structures of lipid-derived autacoids, nonsteroidal anti-inflammatory drugs (NSAIDs), and drugs used to treat gout

LEARNING OBJECTIVES

- ☑ Understand the mechanisms of action of drugs used as prostaglandin agonists.
- ☑ Understand the mechanisms of action of the NSAIDs.
- ☑ Understand the mechanisms of action of the drugs used in the pharmacotherapy of gout.
- ☑ Know the untoward effects of prostaglandin agonists, NSAIDs, and the drugs used in the pharmacotherapy of gout.
- ☑ Know the therapeutic utility of prostaglandin agonists, NSAIDs, and the drugs used in the pharmacotherapy of gout.
- ☑ Know which drugs can be used in combination, and those that should not be used concomitantly to treat inflammatory disorders, fever, pain, arthritis, and gout.

MECHANISMS OF ACTION OF PROSTAGLANDINS AND THEIR ANALOGS

DRUG CLASS	DRUG	MECHANISM OF ACTION
PGE_1	Alprostadil	Activates EP prostaglandin receptors in vascular smooth muscle causing vasodilation The ductus arteriosus in neonates is highly sensitive to relaxation by PGE_1
PGE_1 Analog	Misoprostol	Activates EP prostaglandin receptors in the stomach, increasing mucous secretion and reducing acid secretion and pepsin content
PGE_2	Dinoprostone	Activates EP prostaglandin receptors in the uterus and cervix, promoting uterine contractions, cervical ripening, and cervical dilation
$PGF_{2\alpha}$ Analog	Carboprost tromethamine Latanoprost Bimatoprost Travoprost	Activates FP prostaglandin receptors in the uterus and cervix, promoting uterine contractions, cervical ripening, and cervical dilation Activates FP prostaglandin receptors in the eye, causing a decrease in intraocular pressure by increasing aqueous humor outflow via the uveoscleral and trabecular meshwork pathway

(Continued)

Prostaglandins, NSAIDs, and Pharmacotherapy of Gout

CHAPTER 22

DRUG CLASS	DRUG	MECHANISM OF ACTION
PGI$_2$	Prostacyclin	Activates IP prostaglandin receptors in pulmonary artery smooth muscle, causing vasodilation
PGI$_2$ Analog	Iloprost Treprostinil	Activates IP prostaglandin receptors in pulmonary artery smooth muscle, causing vasodilation

MECHANISMS OF ACTION OF NSAIDs

DRUG CLASS	DRUG	MECHANISM OF ACTION
NSAID—Irreversible COX-1 and COX-2 inhibitor	Aspirin	Covalently acetylates COX-1 and COX-2 impeding the ability of these enzymes to make prostaglandins (see Figure 22-1) Does not inhibit the LOX pathway of arachidonic acid metabolism (see Figure 22-2)
Traditional NSAID (tNSAID)	Salsalate Salicylate Diflunisal Mesalamine Sulfasalazine Balsalazide Olsalazine Acetaminophen Indomethacin Sulindac Etodolac Tolmetin Ketorolac Diclofenac Bromfenac Nepafenac Mefenamic acid Meclofenamate Ibuprofen Naproxen Fenoprofen Ketoprofen Flurbiprofen Oxaprozin Piroxicam Meloxicam Nabumetone	Reversible, competitive, active site inhibitors of COX-1 and COX-2 (see Figure 22-1), though each agent varies in COX isoform selectivity (eg, meloxicam, diclofenac, and etodolac are more COX-2 selective; see Figure 22-4) Does not inhibit the LOX pathway of arachidonic acid metabolism (see Figure 22-2)
NSAID—Selective COX-2 Inhibitor ("coxib")	Celecoxib	Selective inhibition of COX-2, preserving COX-1 synthesis of cytoprotective PGE$_2$ and PGI$_2$ by gastric epithelium

DRUGS INCLUDED IN THIS CHAPTER (Cont.)

- Piroxicam (FELDENE, others)
- Probenecid (PROBALAN)
- Prostacyclin (epoprostenol, FLOLAN)
- Rasburicase (ELITEK)
- Salicylate (DOAN'S, MOMENTUM, others)
- Salsalate
- Sulfasalazine (AZULFIDINE, others)
- Sulindac (CLINORIL, others)
- Tolmetin (TOLECTIN, others)
- Travoprost (TRAVATAN)
- Treprostinil (REMODULIN)

THE INFLAMMATORY RESPONSE

- Inflammation can be evoked by a wide variety of noxious agents (eg, infections, antibodies, physical injuries).
- The classic inflammatory symptoms include calor (warmth), dolor (pain), rubor (redness), and tumor (swelling).
- Many mediators are involved in the inflammatory response:
  - Histamine (see Chapter 21)
  - Bradykinin (see Chapter 21)
  - 5-hydroxytryptamine (5-HT, serotonin)
  - Prostanoids produced by cyclooxygenase-1 (COX-1) and cyclooxygenase-2 (COX-2) (see Figure 22-1), in particular, PGE$_2$ and PGI$_2$
  - Leukotrienes (LTs; see Figure 22-2)
  - Platelet-activating factor (PAF; see Figure 22-3)
  - Other soluble mediators including complement factor C5a, proinflammatory cytokines (TNF, IL-1, IL-2, IL-6, IL-8; see Chapters 23 and 25), and growth factors (GM-CSF; see Chapter 25)
- COX-2, which is rapidly induced during inflammation, is the major source of proinflammatory prostanoids.
- COX-1 plays a dominant role in producing proinflammatory prostanoids during the initial phase of an acute inflammatory response.

SECTION IV — Inflammation, Immunomodulation, and Hematopoiesis

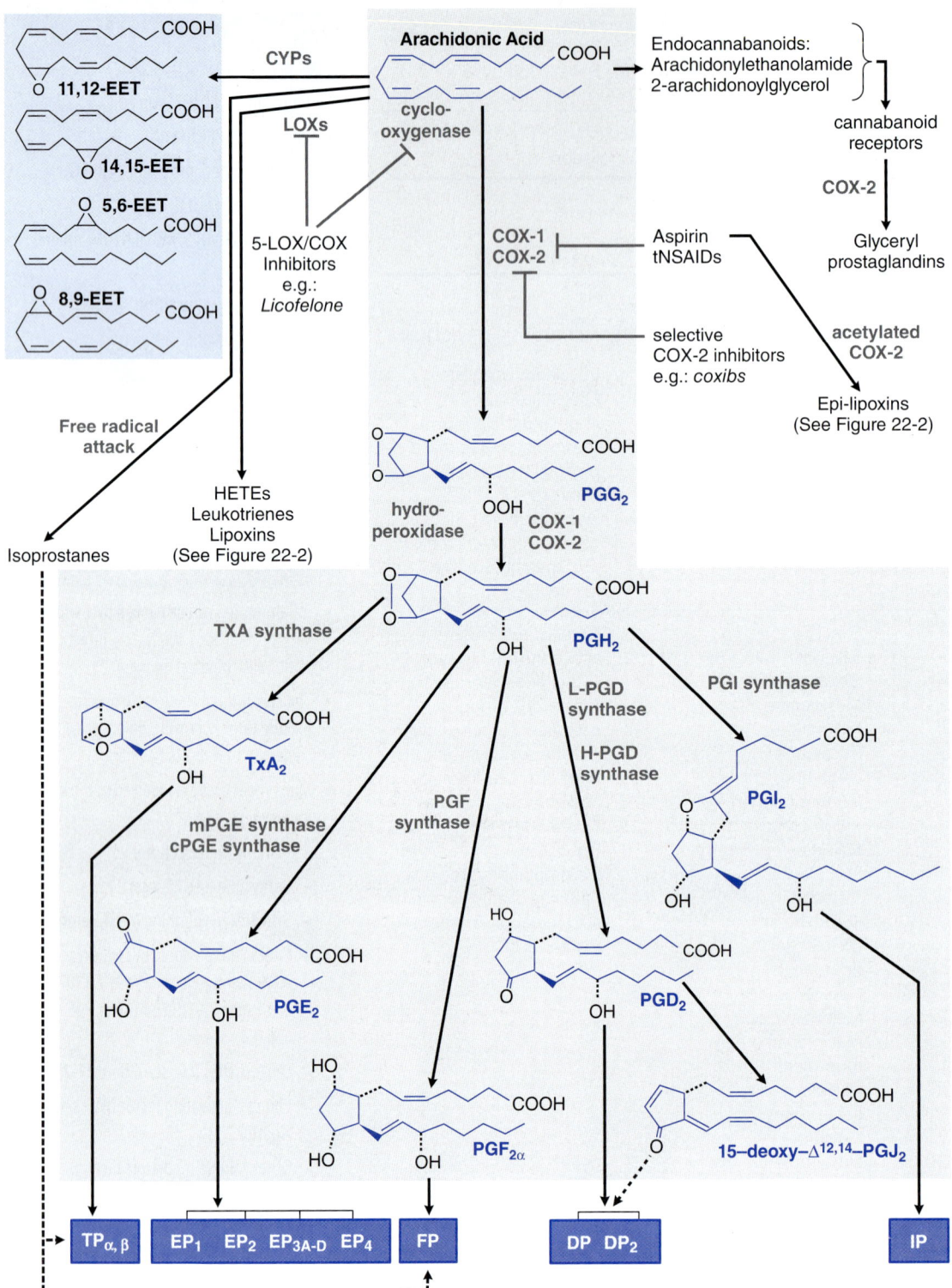

FIGURE 22-1 Metabolism of arachidonic acid (AA). The cyclooxygenase (COX) pathway is highlighted in gray. The lipoxygenase (LOX) pathways are expanded in Figure 22-2. Cyclic endoperoxides (PGG_2 and PGH_2) arise from the sequential COX and hydroperoxidase actions of COX-1 or COX-2 on AA released from membrane phospholipids. Subsequent products are generated by tissue-specific synthases and transduce their effects via membrane-bound receptors (blue boxes). Dashed lines indicate putative ligand–receptor interactions. Epoxyeicosatrienoic acids (EETs; shaded in blue) and isoprostanes are generated via CYP activity and nonenzymatic free radical attack, respectively. COX-2 can use modified arachidonoylglycerol, an endocannabinoid, to generate the glyceryl prostaglandins. Aspirin and tNSAIDs are nonselective inhibitors of COX-1 and COX-2, but do not affect LOX activity. Epi-lipoxins are generated by COX-2 following its acetylation by aspirin (see Figure 22-2). Dual 5-LOX–COX inhibitors interfere with both pathways.

Prostaglandins, NSAIDs, and Pharmacotherapy of Gout   CHAPTER 22

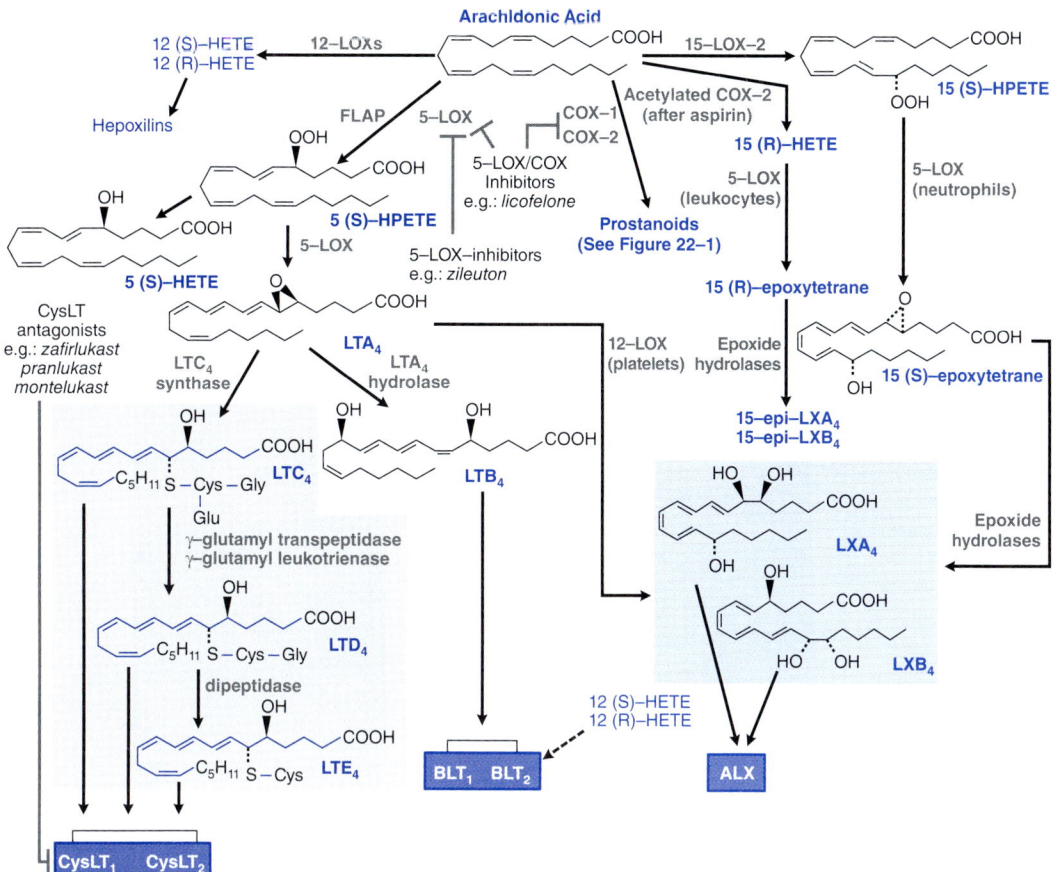

FIGURE 22-2 Lipoxygenase pathways of arachidonic acid metabolism. 5-LOX–activating protein (FLAP) presents arachidonic acid to 5-LOX, leading to the generation of the LTs. CysLTs are shaded in gray. Lipoxins (shaded in blue) are products of cellular interaction via a 5-LOX–12-LOX pathway or via a 15-LOX–5-LOX pathway. Biological effects are transduced via membrane-bound receptors dark (blue boxes). The dashed line indicates putative ligand–receptor interactions. Zileuton inhibits 5-LOX but not the COX pathways (expanded in Figure 22-1). Dual 5-LOX–COX inhibitors interfere with both pathways. CysLT antagonists prevent activation of the CysLT1 receptor.

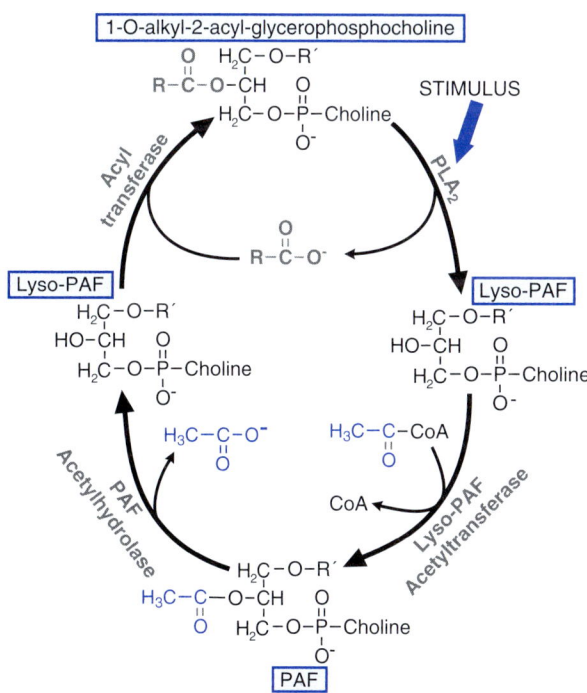

FIGURE 22-3 Synthesis and degradation of platelet-activating factor (PAF). RCOO⁻ is a mixture of fatty acids but is enriched in arachidonic acid that may be metabolized to eicosanoids. CoA, coenzyme A.

SECTION IV Inflammation, Immunomodulation, and Hematopoiesis

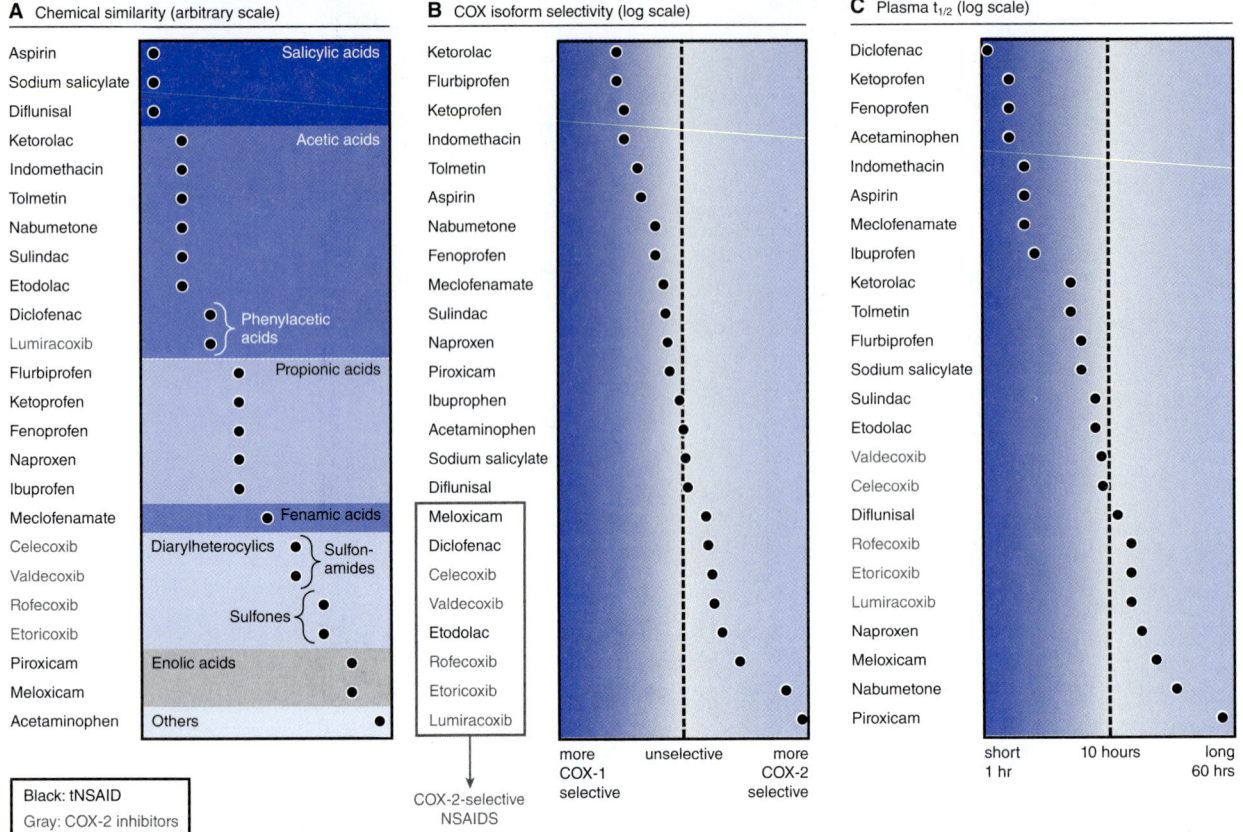

FIGURE 22-4 Classification of NSAIDs by chemical similarity (panel A), cyclooxygenase (COX) isoform selectivity (panel B), and plasma $t_{1/2}$ (panel C). tNSAIDs, traditional nonsteroidal anti-inflammatory drugs.

TABLE 22-1 Classification and Comparison of Nonsteroidal Analgesics

CLASS/DRUG (SUBSTITUTION)	PHARMACOKINETICS		DOSING[d]		COMMENTS	COMPARED TO ASPIRIN
Salicylates						
Aspirin (acetyl ester)	Peak C_p[a] Protein binding Metabolites[b] $t_{1/2}$[c], therapeutic $t_{1/2}$, toxic dose	1 hour 80-90% Salicyluric acid 2-3 hours 15-30 hours	Antiplatelet Pain/fever Rheumatic fever Children	40-80 mg/day 325-650 mg every 4-6 hours 1 g every 4-6 hours 10 mg/kg every 4-6 hours	Permanent platelet COX-1 inhibition (acetylation) Main side effects: GI, increased bleeding time, hypersensitivity Avoid in children with acute febrile illness	
Diflunisal (defluoro-phenyl)	Peak C_p Protein binding Metabolites $t_{1/2}$	2-3 hours 99% Glucuronide 8-12 hours	250-500 mg every 8-12 hours		Not metabolized to salicylic acid Competitive COX inhibitor Excreted into breast milk	Analgesic and anti-inflammatory effects 4-5 times more potent Antipyretic effect weaker Fewer platelet and GI side effects

(Continued)

Prostaglandins, NSAIDs, and Pharmacotherapy of Gout — CHAPTER 22

CLASS/DRUG (SUBSTITUTION)	PHARMACOKINETICS		DOSING[d]		COMMENTS	COMPARED TO ASPIRIN
Para-aminophenol derivative						
Acetaminophen	Peak C_p Protein binding Metabolites $t_{1/2}$	30-60 minutes 20-50% Glucuronide conjugates (60%); sulfuric acid conjugates (35%) 2 hours	10-15 mg/kg every 4 hours (maximum of 5 doses/24 hours)		Weak nonspecific COX inhibitor at common doses Potency may be modulated by peroxides Overdose leads to production of toxic metabolite and liver necrosis	Analgesic and antipyretic effects equivalent Anti-inflammatory, GI, and platelet effects less than aspirin at 1000 mg/day
Acetic acid derivatives						
Indomethacin (methylated indole)	Peak C_p Protein binding Metabolites $t_{1/2}$	1-2 hours 90% O-demethylation (50%); unchanged (20%) 2.5 hours	25 mg 2-3 times/day; 75-100 mg at night		Side effects (3-50% of patients): frontal headache, neutropenia, thrombocytopenia; 20% discontinue therapy	10-40x more potent; intolerance limits dose
Sulindac (sulfoxide prodrug)	Peak C_p Metabolites $t_{1/2}$	1-2 hours; 8 hours for sulfide metabolite; extensive enterohepatic circulation Sulfone and conjugates (30%); sulindac and conjugates (25%) 7 hours; 18 hours for metabolite	150-200 mg twice/day		20% suffer GI side effects; 10% get CNS side effects	Efficacy comparable
Etodolac (pyranocarboxylic acid)	Peak C_p Protein binding Metabolites $t_{1/2}$	1 hour 99% Hepatic metabolites 7 hours	200-400 mg 3-4 times/day		Some COX-2 selectivity *in vitro*	100 mg etodolac has similar efficacy to 650 mg of aspirin, but may be better tolerated
Tolmetin (heteroaryl acetate derivative)	Peak C_p Protein binding Metabolites $t_{1/2}$	20-60 99% Oxidized to carboxylic acid/other derivatives, then conjugated 5 hours	400-600 mg 3 times/day	20 mg/kg/day in 3-4 divided doses for children (anti-inflammatory)	Food delays and decreases peak absorption May persist longer in synovial fluid to give a biological efficacy longer than its plasma $t_{1/2}$	Efficacy similar; 25-40% develop side effects; 5-10% discontinue drug
Ketorolac (pyrrolizine carboxylate)	Peak C_p Protein binding Metabolites $t_{1/2}$	30-60 99% glucuronide conjugate (90%) 4-6 hours	<65 years: 20 mg (orally), then 10 mg every 4-6 hours (not to exceed 40 mg/24 hours); >65 years: 10 mg every 4-6 hours (not to exceed 40 mg/24 hours)		Commonly given parenterally (60 mg IM followed by 30 mg every 6 hours, or 30 mg IV every 6 hours) Available as ocular preparation (0.25%); 1 drop every 6 hours	Potent analgesic, poor anti-inflammatory

(Continued)

SECTION IV — Inflammation, Immunomodulation, and Hematopoiesis

CLASS/DRUG (SUBSTITUTION)	PHARMACOKINETICS		DOSING[d]		COMMENTS	COMPARED TO ASPIRIN
Diclofenac (phenylacetate derivatives)	Peak C_p Protein binding Metabolites $t_{1/2}$	2-3 hours 99% Glucuronide and sulfide (renal 65%, bile 35%) 1-2 hours	50 mg 3 times/day or 75 mg twice/day		Available as topical gel, ophthalmic solution, and oral tablets combined with misoprostol First-pass effect; oral bioavailability, 50%	More potent; 20% develop side effects, 2% discontinue use, 15% develop elevated liver enzymes
Fenamates (*N*-phenyl-anthranilates)						
Mefenamic acid	Peak C_p Protein binding Metabolites $t_{1/2}$	2-4 hours High Conjugates of 3-hydroxy and 3-carboxyl metabolites (20% recovered in feces) 3-4 hours	500-mg load, then 250 mg every 6 hours		Isolated cases of hemolytic anemia May have some central action	Efficacy similar; GI side effects (25%)
Meclofenamate	Peak C_p Protein binding Metabolites $t_{1/2}$	0.5-2 hours 99% Hepatic metabolism; fecal and renal excretion 2-3 hours	50-100 mg 4-6/day (maximum of 400 mg/day)			Efficacy similar; GI side effects (25%)
Flufenamic acid	Not available in the U.S.					
Propionic acid derivatives					Intolerance of one does not preclude use of another propionate derivative	Usually better tolerated
Ibuprofen	Peak C_p Protein binding Metabolites $t_{1/2}$	15-30 minutes 99% Conjugates of hydroxyl and carboxyl metabolites 2-4 hours	Analgesia Anti-inflammatory	200-400 mg every 4-6 hours 300 mg/6-8 hours or 400-800 mg 3-4 times/day	10-15% discontinue due to adverse effects Children's dosing Antipyretic: 5-10 mg/kg every 6 hours (max: 40 mg/kg/day) Anti-inflammatory: 20-40 mg/kg/day in 3-4 divided doses	Equipotent
Naproxen	Peak C_p Protein binding Metabolites $t_{1/2}$	1 hour 99% (less in elderly) 6-demethyl and other metabolites 14 hours	250 mg 4 times/day or 500 mg twice/day Children: anti-inflammatory	5 mg/kg twice/day	Peak anti-inflammatory effects may not be seen until 2-4 weeks of use Decreased protein binding and delayed excretion increase risk of toxicity in elderly	More potent *in vitro*; usually better tolerated; variably prolonged $t_{1/2}$ may afford cardioprotection in some individuals
Fenoprofen	Peak C_p Protein binding Metabolites $t_{1/2}$	2 hours 99% Glucuronide, 4-OH metabolite 2 hours	200 mg 4-6 times/day; 300-600 mg 3-4 times/day			15% experience side effects; few discontinue use

(Continued)

Prostaglandins, NSAIDs, and Pharmacotherapy of Gout — CHAPTER 22

CLASS/DRUG (SUBSTITUTION)	PHARMACOKINETICS		DOSING[d]		COMMENTS	COMPARED TO ASPIRIN
Ketoprofen	Peak C_p Protein binding Metabolites $t_{1/2}$	1-2 hours 98% Glucuronide conjugates 2 hours	Analgesia Anti-inflammatory	25 mg 3-4 times/day 50-75 mg 3-4 times/day		30% develop side effects (usually GI, usually mild)
Flurbiprofen	Peak C_p Protein binding Metabolites $t_{1/2}$	1-2 hours 99% Hydroxylates and conjugates 6 hours	200-300 mg/day in 2-4 divided doses		Available as a 0.03% ophthalmic solution	
Oxaprozin	Peak C_p Protein binding Major metabolites $t_{1/2}$	3-4 hours 99% Oxidates and glucuronide conjugates 40-60 hours	600-1800 mg/day		Long $t_{1/2}$ allows for daily administration; slow onset of action; inappropriate for fever/acute analgesia	
Enolic acid derivatives						
Piroxicam	Peak C_p Protein binding Metabolites $t_{1/2}$	3-5 hours 99% Hydroxylates and then conjugated 45-50 hours	20 mg/day		May inhibit activation of neutrophils, activity of proteoglycanase, collagenases	Equipotent; perhaps better tolerated 20% develop side effects; 5% discontinue drug
Meloxicam	Peak C_p Protein binding Metabolites $t_{1/2}$	5-10 hours 99% Hydroxylation 15-20 hours	7.5-15 mg/day			Some COX-2 selectivity, especially at lower doses
Nabumetone (naphthyl alkanone)	Peak C_p Protein binding Major metabolites $t_{1/2}$	3-6 hours 99% O-demethylation, then conjugation 24 hours	500-1000 mg 1-2 times/day		A prodrug, rapidly metabolized to 6-methoxy-2-naphthyl acetic acid; pharmacokinetics reflect active compound	Shows some COX-2 selectivity (active metabolite does not) Fewer GI side effects than many NSAIDs
Diaryl heterocyclic NSAIDs (COX-2 selective)					Evidence for cardiovascular adverse events	Decrease in GI side effects and in platelet effects
Celecoxib [diaryl substituted pyrazone; (sulfonamide derivative)]	Peak C_p Protein binding Metabolites $t_{1/2}$	2-4 hours 97% Carboxylic acid and glucuronide conjugates 6-12 hours	100 mg 1-2 times/day		Substrate for CYP2C9; inhibitor of CYP2D6 Coadministration with inhibitors of CYP2C9 or substrates of CYP2D6 should be done with caution	See the text for an overview of COX-2 inhibitors
Parecoxib Etoricoxib Lumaricoxi	Not approved for use in the U.S.					

[a]Time to peak plasma drug concentration (C_p) after a single dose. In general, food delays absorption but does not decrease peak concentration.
[b]The majority of NSAIDs undergo hepatic metabolism, and the metabolites are excreted in the urine. Major metabolites or disposal pathways are listed.
[c]Typical $t_{1/2}$ is listed for therapeutic doses; if $t_{1/2}$ is much different with the toxic dose, this is also given.
[d]Limited dosing information given. For additional information, refer to the product information literature.
CNS, central nervous system; COX, cyclooxygenase; GI, gastrointestinal; IM, intramuscularly; IV, intravenously.

SECTION IV

Inflammation, Immunomodulation, and Hematopoiesis

MAJOR THERAPEUTIC USES OF NSAIDs

- All NSAIDs, including COX-2 Inhibitors, are anti-inflammatory, analgesic, and anti-pyretic, except for acetaminophen, which is largely devoid of anti-inflammatory activity.
  - Used as anti-inflammatory agents in the treatment of musculoskeletal disorders (the primary clinical application of NSAIDs)
    - Rheumatoid arthritis
    - Osteoarthritis
    - Ankylosing spondylitis
    - Gout
  - Used as analgesics to treat pain of low to moderate intensity
    - NSAIDs lack the unwanted adverse CNS effects of opiates (respiratory depression and development of physical dependence).
    - Coadministration of NSAIDs with opioids can reduce the dose of opiate and the likelihood of adverse CNS effects.
    - NSAIDs are particularly effective in treating dental pain, postoperative pain, pain arising from inflammation, and menstrual cramps (the latter due to release of prostaglandins from the endometrium).
    - NSAIDs are commonly used as first-line agents in treating migraine attacks and can be combined with second-line agents such as the triptans, or with antiemetics for relief of nausea.
    - NSAIDs lack efficacy in treating neuropathic pain or pain arising from the hollow viscera.
  - Can reduce fever in most situations, but antipyretic effects may obscure the course of illness
    - Antipyretic therapy is reserved for patients with deleterious fever and those who experience relief when fever is lowered.
- Used in neonates to close inappropriately patent ductus arteriosus, which is very sensitive to the dilating effects of PGE_1.
- Low-dose aspirin reduces the risk of serious cardiovascular events in high-risk patients, probably by irreversibly inhibiting thromboxane A_2 (TxA_2) production by platelets (see Chapter 19).

TABLE 22-2 Common and Shared Side Effects of NSAIDs

SYSTEM	MANIFESTATIONS
GI	Abdominal pain Nausea Diarrhea Anorexia Gastric erosions/ulcers[a] Anemia[a] GI hemorrhage[a] Perforation/obstruction[a]
Platelets	Inhibited platelet activation[a] Propensity for bruising[a] Increased risk of hemorrhage[a]
Renal	Salt and water retention Edema, worsening of renal function in renal/cardiac and cirrhotic patients Decreased effectiveness of antihypertensive medications Decreased effectiveness of diuretic medications Decreased urate excretion (especially with aspirin) Hyperkalemia
Cardiovascular	Closure of ductus arteriosus Myocardial infarction[b] Stroke[b] Thrombosis[b]
CNS	Headache Vertigo Dizziness Confusion Hyperventilation (salicylates)
Uterus	Prolongation of gestation Inhibition of labor
Hypersensitivity	Vasomotor rhinitis Angioneurotic edema Asthma Urticaria Flushing Hypotension Shock

[a]Side effects decreased with COX-2-selective NSAIDs.
[b]With the exception of low-dose aspirin.

CASE 22-1

A 24-year-old woman experiences severe menstrual cramping each month. The cramping and pain are relieved when she takes ibuprofen.

a. What is causing this patient's menstrual cramping?

The release of PGs by the endometrium during menstruation may cause severe cramps and other symptoms of primary dysmenorrhea.

b. What is the mechanism of action of ibuprofen in relieving this patient's pain and cramping?

Ibuprofen and other NSAIDs are effective in treating menstrual cramping because of their ability to inhibit synthesis of PGs by the endometrium through their inhibitory effects on COX-1 and COX-2. The selective COX-2 inhibitors also are efficacious in this condition.

(Continued)

Prostaglandins, NSAIDs, and Pharmacotherapy of Gout

CHAPTER 22

c. **If this patient becomes pregnant, are there any hazards to her or the fetus in using NSAIDs for relief of headaches and musculoskeletal pains?**

The use of NSAIDs and aspirin late in pregnancy may increase the risk of postpartum hemorrhage. Therefore, pregnancy, especially close to term, is a relative contraindication to the use of all NSAIDs. In addition, their use must be weighed against potential fetal risk, even in cases of premature labor, and especially in cases of pregnancy-induced hypertension. NSAID use is associated with closure of the ductus arteriosus and impaired fetal circulation in utero, particularly in fetuses older than 32 weeks' gestation.

CASE 22-2

A 64-year-old man who suffered a myocardial infarction 2 years earlier is taking 80 mg of aspirin each day on the recommendation of his family physician. His doctor has advised him that this will reduce his chances of another myocardial infarction or stroke.

a. **What is the mechanism of aspirin's cardioprotective effect in this patient?**

This effect is due to irreversible acetylation of platelet COX-1, which permanently and completely suppresses platelet thromboxane A_2 (TxA_2) formation, with the consequent inhibition of platelet function (see Figure 19-1). Platelets, which being anucleate, have a markedly limited capacity for protein synthesis. Thus, the consequences of inhibition of platelet COX-1 (COX-2 is not expressed in mature platelets) last for the lifetime of the platelet. Inhibition of platelet COX-1–dependent TxA_2 formation, therefore, is cumulative with repeated doses of aspirin (at least as low as 30 mg/d) and takes ~8 to 12 days—the platelet turnover time—to recover fully once therapy has been stopped. Low-dose aspirin therapy does not significantly impair synthesis of PGI_2 by vascular endothelium, in part because of the ability of endothelial cells to continuously express COX-1 and COX-2. Thus, daily low-dose aspirin blocks the formation of TxA_2, which promotes platelet aggregation, while leaving intact the synthesis of PGI_2, which inhibits platelet function (see Figure 19-1).

Aspirin reduces the risk of serious vascular events in high-risk patients (eg, those with previous myocardial infarction) by 20 to 25%. Low-dose (<100 mg/d) aspirin, which is relatively (but not exclusively) selective for COX-1, is as effective as higher doses (eg, 325 mg/d).

b. **What are the hazards of daily aspirin therapy?**

Because of impairment of platelet function, the most serious hazard to daily aspirin therapy is an increased risk of hemorrhage. Placebo-controlled trials reveal that aspirin increases the incidence of serious GI bleeds, reflecting suppression not just of platelet thromboxane, but also reduction in gastroepithelial PGE_2 and PGI_2. It also increases the incidence of intracranial bleeds. Although benefit from aspirin outweighs these risks in the case of secondary prevention of cardiovascular disease, the issue is much more nuanced in patients who have never had a serious atherothrombotic event (primary prevention); here, prevention of myocardial infarction by aspirin is numerically balanced by the serious GI bleeds it precipitates

Daily aspirin therapy can also increase the risk of gastric ulcers. COX-1 is expressed as the dominant, constitutive isoform in gastric epithelial cells and is thought to be the major source of cytoprotective PG formation. Inhibition of COX-1 at this site is thought to account largely for the gastric adverse events that complicate therapy with tNSAIDs.

c. **What concomitantly administered drugs might impair the cardioprotective effects of aspirin?**

Many patients combine either tNSAIDs or COX-2 inhibitors with cardioprotective, low-dose aspirin. Epidemiological studies suggest that this combination therapy increases significantly the likelihood of GI adverse events over either class of NSAID alone.

(Continued)

MECHANISMS OF GASTRIC DAMAGE BY NSAIDs

- Inhibition of COX-1 in gastric epithelial cells depresses mucosal cytoprotective PGs, especially PGE_2 and PGI_2.
  - ▸ COX-2 inhibition in gastric epithelial cells may also contribute to some loss of cytoprotective PGs.
- Local irritation of gastric mucosa by orally administered NSAIDs.
- Enhanced generation of lipoxygenase (LOX) products (eg, LTs; see Figure 22-2) may contribute to ulcerogenicity in patients treated with NSAIDs.

CARDIOVASCULAR HAZARD WITH COX-2–SELECTIVE NSAIDs

- Inhibition of COX-2 in the vasculature reduces vascular PGI_2 (prostacyclin) production which is antithrombotic and antiatherogenic.
- Inhibition of COX-2 in the kidney reduces renal PGI_2 and PGE_2 production which results in hypertension and edema due to the contribution of these PGs in maintaining arterial pressure homeostasis.
- In addition to the COX-2-selective ("coxib") drug celecoxib, several traditional NSAIDs (tNSAIDs) exhibit relative selectivity for COX-2 (eg, etodolac, diclofenac, meloxicam; see Figure 22-4) and are likely to have similar cardiovascular risks as the coxibs.
- The COX-2-selective NSAIDs (including the tNSAIDs with relative selectivity for COX-2) should not be used in patients with ischemic heart disease or stroke, and should be used with caution in patients with risk factors for heart disease.
  - ▸ For all such COX-2-selective NSAIDs, it is advisable to use the lowest possible dose for the shortest possible time.

Prior occupancy of the active site of platelet COX-1 by the commonly consumed tNSAID ibuprofen impedes access of aspirin to its target Ser 529 and prevents irreversible inhibition of platelet function. Whether this interaction is clinically important has yet to be definitively answered.

CASE 22-3

A 23-year-old male college student suffering from a cold started taking several different over-the-counter (OTC) cold/flu medications 2 days ago to relieve symptoms. He is feeling better and decides to attend an end-of-term party with his classmates where they will be celebrating with beer and other alcoholic beverages.

a. Is this student at risk of any serious drug interactions when taking multiple OTC cold/flu medications?

A large number of nonprescription multisymptom cold/flu medications contain acetaminophen to reduce fever and relieve the muscle aches that are common symptoms of colds and the flu. Severe liver damage can occur with more than 4000 mg of acetaminophen in a 24-hour period. Taking the maximum recommended daily dose of a single multisymptom cold/flu medication will typically be 2400 mg or less of acetaminophen, but taking maximal doses of multiple cold/flu medication, or a cold/flu medication in combination with acetaminophen could result in a total dose that is more than 4000 mg of acetaminophen. In 2009, a Food and Drug Administration (FDA) advisory panel recommended a lower maximum daily dose of acetaminophen of 2600 mg and a decrease in the maximum single dose from 1000 to 650 mg.

b. Are there any risks with consuming alcohol while taking OTC cold/flu medications?

The chances of severe liver damage are increased when alcohol is consumed while taking acetaminophen. Conditions of cytochrome P450 (CYP) induction (eg, heavy alcohol consumption) or glutathione (GSH) depletion (eg, fasting or malnutrition) increase the susceptibility to hepatic injury with acetaminophen, which has been documented, albeit uncommonly, with doses in the therapeutic range. The maximum daily dose of acetaminophen is 2000 mg/d for chronic alcoholics.

c. What are the symptoms of acetaminophen toxicity?

Symptoms that occur during the first 2 days of acute poisoning by acetaminophen reflect gastric distress (eg, nausea, abdominal pain, anorexia) and belie the potential seriousness of the intoxication (see Case 3-5 in Chapter 3). Plasma transaminases become elevated, sometimes markedly so, beginning ~12 to 36 hours after ingestion. Clinical indications of hepatic damage manifest within 2 to 4 days of ingestion of toxic doses, with right subcostal pain, tender hepatomegaly, jaundice, and coagulopathy. Renal impairment or frank renal failure may occur. Liver enzyme abnormalities typically peak 72 to 96 hours after ingestion. The onset of hepatic encephalopathy or worsening coagulopathy beyond this time indicates a poor prognosis. Biopsy of the liver reveals centrilobular necrosis with sparing of the periportal area. In nonfatal cases, the hepatic lesions are reversible over a period of weeks or months.

CASE 22-4

A 72-year-old woman has developed arthritis in her hands and has difficulty opening jars and other common tasks because of the pain. She asks her doctor to recommend a drug to relieve the pain so she can complete her normal tasks.

a. What are the considerations in choosing a drug to relieve this patient's symptoms?

NSAIDs are the drugs of choice for treating the symptoms of arthritis because of their analgesic and anti-inflammatory effects. Choice and dosing of an NSAID are usually guided by multiple considerations, including patient age, coincident diseases or allergies, the drug's safety and interaction profile, and cost considerations. Drugs with a longer duration of action may be preferable for management of arthritic pain.

(Continued)

Prostaglandins, NSAIDs, and Pharmacotherapy of Gout CHAPTER 22

The choice among tNSAIDs for the treatment of chronic arthritic conditions is largely empirical. Substantial differences in response have been noted among individuals treated with the same tNSAID and within an individual treated with different tNSAIDs, even when the drugs are structurally related. It is reasonable to give a drug for a week or two as a therapeutic trial and to continue it if the response is satisfactory. Initially, all patients should be asked about previous hypersensitivity to aspirin or any member of the NSAID class. Thereafter, low doses of the chosen agent should be prescribed to determine initial patient tolerance. Older patients may require lower doses than younger patients to reduce the risk of toxicity. Regulatory agencies stress use of the lowest effective dose for the shortest possible duration of treatment. Alterations in dosing may take several days (>3-4 $t_{1/2}$) to translate into clinically detectable changes. Delayed distribution into the synovial compartment may extend this interval. Indeed, some NSAIDs that are short-lived in plasma are sustained in synovial fluid and may afford sufficient relief even when administered at intervals longer than their plasma $t_{1/2}$ life. If the patient does not achieve therapeutic benefit from 1 NSAID, another may be tried. For mild arthropathies, the scheme outlined earlier in this paragraph, together with rest and physical therapy, probably will be sufficiently effective. When the patient has sleeping problems because of pain or morning stiffness, a larger proportion of the daily dose may be given at night.

b. **What are the expected adverse effects of NSAIDs for treatment of osteoarthritis and when would these effects occur?**

Table 22-2 lists the common and shared side effects of NSAIDs. The most common side effects associated with these drugs are gastrointestinal, including anorexia, nausea, dyspepsia, abdominal pain, and diarrhea. These symptoms may be related to the induction of gastric or intestinal ulcers, which is estimated to occur in 15 to 30% of regular users. Ulceration may range from small superficial erosions to full-thickness perforation of the muscularis mucosa. There may be single or multiple ulcers, and ulceration may be uncomplicated or complicated by bleeding, perforation, or obstruction. Blood loss can be gradual, leading to anemia over time, or acute and life-threatening. The risk is further increased in patients with *Helicobacter pylori* infection, heavy alcohol consumption, or other risk factors for mucosal injury, including the concurrent use of glucocorticoids.

Some adverse effects may manifest in the first weeks of therapy; however, the risk of gastric ulceration and bleeding accumulates with the duration of dosing. Combination therapy with more than 1 NSAID is to be avoided.

c. **What is the mechanism underlying the gastric adverse effects of NSAIDs, and what can be done to minimize these effects in the treatment of arthritis?**

Gastric damage by NSAIDs can be brought about by at least 2 distinct mechanisms (see Side Bar MECHANISMS OF GASTRIC DAMAGE BY NSAIDs). Inhibition of COX-1 in gastric epithelial cells depresses mucosal cytoprotective PGs, especially PGI_2 and PGE_2. These eicosanoids inhibit acid secretion by the stomach, enhance mucosal blood flow, and promote the secretion of cytoprotective mucus in the intestine. Inhibition of PGI_2 and PGE_2 synthesis may render the stomach more susceptible to damage and can occur with oral, parenteral, or transdermal administration of aspirin or NSAIDs. There is some evidence that COX-2 also contributes to constitutive formation of these PGs by human gastric epithelium.

Another mechanism by which NSAIDs or aspirin may cause ulceration is by local irritation from contact of orally administered drug with the gastric mucosa. Local irritation allows back diffusion of acid into the gastric mucosa and induces tissue damage. However, the incidence of GI adverse events is not significantly reduced by formulations that reduce drug contact with the gastric mucosa, such as enteric coating or efferent solutions, suggesting that the contribution of direct irritation to the overall risk is minor. It also is possible that enhanced generation of LOX products (eg, LTs) contributes to ulcerogenicity in patients treated with NSAIDs.

(Continued)

SECTION IV — Inflammation, Immunomodulation, and Hematopoiesis

A number of risk factors for GI complications have been determined in epidemiological studies. Patients at high risk for GI complications should be prescribed a gastroprotective agent. Coadministration of the PGE_1 analog, misoprostol, or proton pump inhibitors (PPIs, see Chapter 32) in conjunction with NSAIDs can be beneficial in the prevention of duodenal and gastric ulceration. For instance, diclofenac is available in combination with misoprostol, a PGE_1 analog (ARTHROTEC). This combination retains the efficacy of diclofenac while reducing the frequency of GI ulcers and erosions. Patients at high risk for GI complications also are potential candidates for a COX-2–selective NSAID (see Chapter 32).

d. What are the considerations in choosing a COX-2–selective NSAID to reduce GI complications?

COX-2–selective NSAIDs were developed to improve the GI safety of anti-inflammatory therapy in patients at elevated risk for GI complications. However, placebo-controlled trials with 3 structurally distinct COX-2–selective NSAIDs revealed an increase in the incidence of myocardial infarction, stroke, and thrombosis. The risk appears to also extend to those of the older tNSAIDs, which are quite selective for COX-2 (see Side Bar CARDIOVASCULAR HAZARD WITH COX-2–SELECTIVE NSAIDs). Regulatory agencies in the United States, European Union, and Australia have concluded that all NSAIDs (with the exception of aspirin, see Case 22-2) have the potential to increase the risk of heart attack and stroke.

PHARMACOTHERAPY OF RHEUMATOID ARTHRITIS

- Rheumatoid arthritis is an autoimmune disease (see Chapter 23).
- The goal of therapy is symptomatic relief of pain with NSAIDs, and reduction in disease activity and retardation of arthritic tissue destruction using DMARDs (see Table 22-3 and Chapter 23).

PHARMACOTHERAPY OF GOUT

- Gout results from the precipitation of urate crystals in tissues and the subsequent inflammatory response.
- Acute gout usually causes painful distal arthritis, but can also cause joint destruction, subcutaneous deposits (tophi), and renal calculi and damage.
- Hyperuricemia is a necessary condition for gout, but does not inevitably lead to gout.
- In most patients with gout, hyperuricemia is the result of underexcretion of urate, rather than overproduction.
- The aims of treatment are to:
  ▸ Decrease the symptoms of an acute attack
  ▸ Decrease the risk of recurrent attacks
  ▸ Lower serum urate levels
- The agents used to treat gout are:
  ▸ Drugs that relieve inflammation and pain (NSAIDs, colchicine, glucocorticoids)
  ▸ Drugs that prevent the inflammatory responses to urate crystals (colchicine and NSAIDs)
  ▸ Drugs that inhibit urate formation (allopurinol, febuxostat)
  ▸ Drugs that augment urate excretion (probenecid)

TABLE 22-3 Disease-Modifying Anti-Rheumatic Drugs

DRUG	CLASS OR ACTION	REFERENCE (CHAPTER NUMBER)
Small molecules		
Methotrexate	Anti-folate	45
Leflunomide	Pyrimidine synthase inhibitor	45
Hydroxychloroquine	Anti-malarial	35
Minocycline	5-lipoxygenase inhibitor, tetracycline antibiotic	This chapter, 41
Sulfasalazine	Salicylate	This chapter, 33
Azathioprine	Purine synthase inhibitor	45
Cyclosporine	Calcineurin inhibitor	23
Cyclophosphamide	Alkylating agent	45
Biologicals		
Adalimumab	Ab, TNF-α antagonist	23
Golimumab	Ab, TNF-α antagonist	23
Infliximab	IgG-TNF receptor fusion protein (anti-TNF)	23
Certolizumab	Fab fragment toward TNF-α	23
Abatacept	T-cell co-stimulation inhibitor (binds B7 protein on antigen-presenting cell)	23
Rituximab	Ab toward CD20 (cytotoxic toward B cells)	46
Anakinra	IL-1-receptor antagonist	23, 46

IL, interleukin; TNF, tumor necrosis factor.

Prostaglandins, NSAIDs, and Pharmacotherapy of Gout

CHAPTER 22

CASE 22-5

A 6-year-old girl catches a viral infection that some of her classmates at kindergarten have recently had. She develops a fever and headache. Her parents are concerned and want to give her something to relieve her symptoms.

a. What are the considerations in choosing an NSAID for this patient?

Therapeutic indications for NSAID use in children include fever, mild pain, postoperative pain, and inflammatory disorders, such as juvenile arthritis and Kawasaki disease. The choice of drugs for children is considerably restricted; only drugs that have been extensively tested in children should be used (acetaminophen, ibuprofen, and naproxen).

b. Why is aspirin to be avoided in this patient?

Because of the possible association with Reye syndrome, aspirin and other salicylates are contraindicated in children and young adults aged younger than 20 years with viral illness–associated fever. Reye syndrome, a severe and often fatal disease, is characterized by the acute onset of encephalopathy, liver dysfunction, and fatty infiltration of the liver and other viscera. The etiology and pathophysiology are not clear, nor is it clear whether a causal relationship between aspirin and Reye syndrome exists. However, the epidemiologic evidence for an association between aspirin use and Reye syndrome seemed sufficiently compelling that labeling of aspirin and aspirin-containing medications to indicate Reye syndrome as a risk in children was first mandated in 1986 and extended to bismuth subsalicylate in 2004. Since then, the use of aspirin in children has declined dramatically, and Reye syndrome has almost disappeared. Acetaminophen has not been implicated in Reye syndrome and is the drug of choice for antipyresis in children, teens, and young adults.

(Continued)

MECHANISMS OF ACTION OF DRUGS USED TO TREAT GOUT

DRUG CLASS	DRUG	MECHANISM OF ACTION
NSAID	See Side Bar MECHANISMS OF ACTION OF NSAIDS	Inhibits COX-1 and COX-2 impeding the ability of these enzymes to make prostaglandins (see Figure 22-1) which are involved in inflammation and pain
Glucocorticoid	See Chapter 29	See Chapter 29
Microtubule Disruptor	Colchicine	A variety of pharmacological effects, many of which involve inhibition of microtubule and spindle formation, including antimitotic effects (neutrophils and GI epithelium), inhibition of neutrophil motility, inhibition of neutrophil and mast cell release of mediators, and inhibition of endothelial cell expression of adhesion molecules
Xanthine Oxidase Inhibitor	Allopurinol Febuxostat	Prevents the synthesis of urate from hypoxanthine and xanthine by inhibiting xanthine oxidase Allopurinol is a substrate for xanthine oxidase and its product, oxypurinol, is a noncompetitive inhibitor of the reduced form of the enzyme Febuxostat forms a stable enzyme-inhibitor complex with both the reduced and oxidized form of the enzyme
Recombinant Urate Oxidase	Rasburicase	Catalyzes the enzymatic oxidation of uric acid into the soluble and inactive metabolite, allantoin
Uricosuric Agents	Probenecid	Inhibits URAT-1, the primary organic anion transporter involved in reabsorption of urate in the kidney, thus increasing the rate of excretion of urate

SECTION IV Inflammation, Immunomodulation, and Hematopoiesis

CASE 22-6

A 50-year-old man has occasional episodes of gout that are painful and debilitating. He requires drugs to treat the symptoms of acute gout attacks and to prevent recurrent attacks.

a. What causes this patient's painful episodes of gout?

Gout results from the precipitation of urate crystals in the tissues and the subsequent inflammatory response. Acute gout usually causes an exquisitely painful distal monoarthritis, but it also can cause joint destruction, subcutaneous deposits (tophi), and renal calculi and damage. Gout affects ~0.5 to 1% of the population of Western countries. It is the most common form of inflammatory arthritis in the elderly.

The pathophysiology of gout is not fully understood. Hyperuricemia, while a prerequisite, does not inevitably lead to gout. Uric acid, the end product of purine metabolism, is relatively insoluble compared to its hypoxanthine and xanthine precursors, and normal serum urate levels (~5 mg/dL, or 0.3 mM) approach the limit of solubility. In most patients with gout, hyperuricemia arises from underexcretion rather than overproduction of urate.

b. What is the therapeutic rationale for the drugs used to treat gout in this patient?

The aims of treatment are to decrease the symptoms of an acute attack, decrease the risk of recurrent attacks, and lower serum urate levels (see Side Bar PHARMACOTHERAPY OF GOUT). The drugs that relieve the symptoms of an acute attack (inflammation and pain) are NSAIDs, colchicine, and glucocorticoids (see Chapter 29). The drugs that decrease the risk of recurrent attacks by preventing inflammatory responses to urate crystals are colchicine and NSAIDs. The drugs that inhibit urate crystal formation by lowering serum urate levels act by reducing urate formation (allopurinol, febuxostat) or augmenting urate excretion (probenecid).

c. This patient is prescribed colchicine. What is the mechanism of action of this drug?

Colchicine is thought to alleviate inflammation rapidly through multiple mechanisms, including the inhibition of neutrophil chemotaxis and activation. Symptoms usually resolve within 2 to 3 days, but adverse GI events are frequent, and toxicity may include bone marrow depression. The therapeutic index of colchicine is narrow—especially in the elderly.

d. How does probenecid increase the excretion of uric acid?

Probenecid and other uricosuric agents increase the rate of uric acid excretion by inhibiting its tubular reabsorption. They compete with uric acid for organic acid transporters, primarily URAT-1, which mediate urate exchange in the proximal tubule. Certain drugs, particularly thiazide diuretics (see Chapter 15), and immunosuppressant agents (especially cyclosporine, see Chapter 23) may impair urate excretion and thereby increase the risk of gout attacks. Probenecid generally is well tolerated but causes mild GI irritation in some patients.

KEY CONCEPTS

➤ NSAIDs are effective in reducing inflammation (except for acetominophen, which lacks appreciable anti-inflammatory activity), most forms of low to moderate pain, and fever.

➤ NSAIDs inhibit the formation of prostaglandins by inhibiting COX-1 and/or COX-2.

➤ GI disturbances are the most common adverse effects of NSAIDs, except the COX-2-selective inhibitors which have reduced effects on prostaglandin production by gastric epithelium.

(Continued)

Prostaglandins, NSAIDs, and Pharmacotherapy of Gout

CHAPTER 22

➡ All NSAIDs except aspirin increase the risk of cardiovascular events (myocardial infarction, stroke, and thrombosis).

➡ Patients at risk of cardiovascular disease should not be treated with COX-2–selective inhibitors.

➡ For patients treated with COX-2–selective inhibitors, treatment should be with the lowest dose possible for the shortest time possible.

➡ Pharmacotherapy of gout includes treatment of pain and inflammation, and reduction in tissue urate crystals.

SUMMARY QUIZ

QUESTION 22-1 Which NSAID has the least anti-inflammatory efficacy?

a. Aspirin
b. Acetaminophen
c. Ibuprofen
d. Naproxen
e. Celecoxib

QUESTION 22-2 Which NSAID permanently inactivates TxA_2 synthesis by platelets?

a. Aspirin
b. Acetaminophen
c. Ibuprofen
d. Naproxen
e. Celecoxib

QUESTION 22-3 What is the primary mechanism of action of allopurinol in treating gout?

a. It is an analgesic agent.
b. It is an anti-inflammatory agent.
c. It blocks inflammatory responses to urate crystals.
d. It inhibits urate formation.
e. It augments urate excretion.

QUESTION 22-4 The cardiovascular risk associated with celecoxib results from

a. inhibition of prostaglandin production in the gastric epithelium.
b. inhibition of platelet thromboxane production.
c. effects on myocardial ion channels.
d. inhibition of prostaglandin in the kidney.
e. enhanced prostacyclin production by vascular endothelium.

QUESTION 22-5 Diclofenac has a $t_{1/2}$ in plasma of 1 to 2 hours, yet its therapeutic effects in treating rheumatoid arthritis last for much longer. This prolongation of therapeutic effect is due to

a. irreversible inhibition of COX-1 and COX-2.
b. its relative selectivity for COX-2.
c. its accumulation in synovial fluid.
d. the formation of a long-lived active metabolite.
e. CNS effects unrelated to inhibition of prostaglandin synthesis.

SECTION IV: Inflammation, Immunomodulation, and Hematopoiesis

SUMMARY QUIZ ANSWER KEY

QUESTION 22-1 Answer is **b**. Acetaminophen, is antipyretic and analgesic, but is largely devoid of anti-inflammatory activity.

QUESTION 22-2 Answer is **a**. Aspirin is an irreversible inhibitor of COX-1. Because platelets are anucleate and have minimal capacity for synthesis of new protein, inhibition of platelet COX-1 lasts for the lifetime of the platelet (8-12 days).

QUESTION 22-3 Answer is **d**. Allopurinol inhibits xanthine oxidase and prevents the synthesis of urate from hypoxanthine and xanthine.

QUESTION 22-4 Answer is **d**. Inhibition of PG production in the kidney, which increases the likelihood of hypertension and edema, occurs with celecoxib, as well as nonselective COX inhibitors. The lack of an effect on COX-1 production in platelets and the inhibition of prostacyclin synthesis by COX-2 in vascular endothelium increase the risk of thrombosis resulting in myocardial infarction and ischemic stroke.

QUESTION 22-5 Answer is **c**. Diclofenac accumulates in synovial fluid after oral administration which likely explains why its duration of therapeutic effect is considerably longer than its plasma $t_{1/2}$. The selectivity of diclofenac for COX-2 resembles that of celecoxib, but this does not explain its prolonged duration of therapeutic effect.

SUMMARY: PROSTAGLANDINS, NSAIDs, AND PHARMACOTHERAPY OF GOUT

CLASS AND SUBCLASSES	NAMES	CLINICAL USES	TOXICITIES COMMON	TOXICITIES UNIQUE; CLINICALLY IMPORTANT
PGE_1	Alprostadil	Second-line treatment for erectile dysfunction (see PDE5 inhibitors, Chapter 16) Temporary maintenance of patent ductus arteriosus in neonates with congenital heart disease	When used in neonates for maintenance of patent ductus arteriosus, apnea occurs in ~10%, particularly in those <2 kg at birth	
PGE_1 Analog	Misoprostol	Prevention of NSAID-induced gastric ulcers (see Chapter 32)		
PGE_2	Dinoprostone	Induction of mid-trimester abortion Induction of labor at term, and facilitation of labor		
$PGF_{2\alpha}$ Analog	Carboprost tromethamine	Induction of mid-trimester abortion Induction of labor at term, and facilitation of labor Control of postpartum hemorrhage not responding to conventional methods		
$PGF_{2\alpha}$ Analog—Long-acting	Latanoprost Bimatoprost Travoprost	Treatment of open-angle glaucoma (see Chapter 47)		
PGI_2	Prostacyclin (epoprostenol)	Long-term treatment of pulmonary hypertension		
PGI_2 Analog	Iloprost Treprostinil	Long-term treatment of pulmonary hypertension		

Prostaglandins, NSAIDs, and Pharmacotherapy of Gout — CHAPTER 22

CLASS AND SUBCLASSES	NAMES	CLINICAL USES	TOXICITIES COMMON	TOXICITIES UNIQUE; CLINICALLY IMPORTANT
NSAID—Irreversible COX-1 Inhibitor	Aspirin (acetylsalicylic acid, ASA)	Antiplatelet (irreversible COX-1 inhibition) Pain/fever Anti-inflammatory (See Side Bar MAJOR THERAPEUTIC USES OF NSAIDs)	GI effects (see Side Bar MECHANISMS OF GASTRIC DAMAGE BY NSAIDs) Increased bleeding time Hypersensitivity (see Table 22-2)	Increased risk of GI bleeding and intracranial bleeding Associated with Reye syndrome (see Case 22-5) (see Table 22-2 for additional toxicities)
NSAID—Traditional (tNSAID)	Salsalate Salicylate Diflunisal Mesalamine Sulfasalazine Balsalazide Olsalazine Acetaminophen Indomethacin Sulindac Etodolac Tolmetin Ketorolac Diclofenac Bromfenac Nepafenac Mefenamic acid Meclofenamate Ibuprofen Naproxen Fenoprofen Ketoprofen Flurbiprofen Oxaprozin Piroxicam Meloxicam Nabumetone	Pain (efficacy depends on agent) Fever (efficacy depends on agent) Anti-inflammatory (efficacy depends on agent) (See Table 22-1 and Side Bar MAJOR THERAPEUTIC USES OF NSAIDs)	GI (see Side Bar MECHANISMS OF GASTRIC DAMAGE BY NSAIDs) (See Table 22-2 for additional toxicities)	Increased risk of cardiovascular disease (see Table 22-2 for additional toxicities)
NSAID—COX-2–Selective ("coxibs")	Celecoxib	Pain Fever Inflammation	(See Table 22-2; decreased GI side effects and platelet effects compared to tNSAIDs)	Increased risk of cardiovascular disease (see Table 22-2 and Side Bar CARDIOVASCULAR HAZARD WITH COX-2–SELECTIVE NSAIDs)
Microtubule Disruptor	Colchicine	Acute gout attacks Prevention of acute gout (off-label)	GI (nausea, vomiting, diarrhea, and abdominal pain)	Acute intoxication causes hemorrhagic gastropathy Life-threatening (especially in combination with P-gp or CYP3A4 inhibitors): myelosuppression, leukopenia, granulocytopenia, thrombopenia, aplastic anemia, and rhabdomyolysis
Xanthine Oxidase Inhibitor	Allopurinol	Gout Hyperuricemia secondary to malignancies Calcium oxalate calculi	Occasionally induces drowsiness Hypersensitivity reaction (may occur after months of therapy) Fever, malaise, and myalgias	Serious hypersensitivity reactions preclude further use Cutaneous reaction Toxic epidermal necrolysis Stevens-Johnson syndrome

SECTION IV Inflammation, Immunomodulation, and Hematopoiesis

CLASS AND SUBCLASSES	NAMES	CLINICAL USES	TOXICITIES COMMON	UNIQUE; CLINICALLY IMPORTANT
	Febuxostat	Hyperuricemia with gout attacks	Liver function abnormalities, nausea, joint pain, rash	Increase in gout flares with initiation of therapy caused by mobilization of urate from tissue deposits Possible increased cardiovascular risk Contraindicated in patients on azathioprine, mercaptopurine, or theophylline (drugs metabolized by xanthine oxidase)
Recombinant Urate Oxidase	Rasburicase	Initial management of elevated plasma uric acid levels in pediatric patients with leukemia, lymphoma, and solid tumor malignancies who are receiving anticancer therapy expected to result in tumor lysis and significant hyperuricemia	Vomiting, fever, nausea, headache, abdominal pain, constipation, diarrhea, and mucositis	Hemolysis in G6PD-deficient patients, methemoglobinemia, acute renal failure, anaphylaxis Efficacy may be hampered by antibodies produced against the drug
Uricosuric Agents	Probenecid	Gout	Mild GI irritation Hypersensitivity reactions (2-4%) usually are mild	Probenecid should not be used in gouty patients with nephrolithiasis or with overproduction of uric acid Liberal fluid intake should be maintained throughout therapy to minimize the risk of renal stones Substantial overdosage results in CNS stimulation, convulsions, and death from respiratory failure

CHAPTER 23

Immunotherapeutic Agents

This chapter will be most useful after having a basic understanding of the material in Chapter 35, Immunosuppressants, Tolerogens, and Immunostimulants in *Goodman & Gilman's The Pharmacological Basis of Therapeutics*, 12th Edition. In addition to the material presented here, the 12th Edition contains:

- Figure 35-3 Generation of monoclonal antibodies that illustrates the method used to generate monoclonal antibodies
- The molecular structures of immunotherapeutic drugs
- A Case Study: Immunotherapy for Multiple Sclerosis that includes Table 35-3 Pharmacotherapy of Multiple Sclerosis listing specific pharmacotherapies for treating multiple sclerosis (MS)

LEARNING OBJECTIVES

- ☑ Understand the mechanisms of action of drugs used to suppress the immune response in organ transplantation and autoimmune diseases.
- ☑ Understand the mechanisms of action of drugs used to stimulate the immune system.
- ☑ Know the untoward effects of immunotherapeutic drugs.
- ☑ Know the drugs used at each step in organ transplantation.
- ☑ Know the drugs used in treating different autoimmune disorders.
- ☑ Know which immunotherapeutic drugs are used in combination with other drugs.

DRUGS INCLUDED IN THIS CHAPTER

- Abatacept (ORENCIA)
- Adalimumab (HUMIRA)
- Aldesleukin (PROLEUKIN)
- Alefacept (AMEVIVE)
- Alemtuzumab (CAMPATH)
- Anakinra (KINERET)
- Azathioprine (IMURAN, others)
- Bacillus Calmette–Guerin (BCG; TICE BCG, THERACYS)
- Basiliximab (SIMULECT)
- Belatacept (NULOJIX)
- Canakinumab (ILARIS)
- Cyclosporine (NEORAL, SANDIMMUNE, GENGRAF, others)
- Daclizumab (ZENAPAX)
- Efalizumab (RAPTIVA)
- Etanercept (ENBREL)
- Everolimus
- Glatiramer acetate (GA; COPAXONE)
- Immune globulin preparations such as ATG (see Table 23-1)
- Infliximab (REMICADE)
- Interferon-α-2b (IFN-α-2b; INTRON A)
- Interferon-β-1a (IFN-β-1a; AVONEX, REBIF)
- Interferon-β-1b (IFN-β-1b; BETASERON)
- Interferon-γ-1b (IFN-γ-1b; ACTIMMUNE)
- Lenalidomide (REVLIMID)
- Mitoxantrone (NOVANTRONE, others)
- MPA (MYFORTIC)
- Muromonab-CD3 (OKT3, ORTHOCLONE OKT3)
- Mycophenolate mofetil (MMF, CELL-CEPT)
- Natalizumab (TYSABRI)
- Rilonacept (IL-1 TRAP)
- Sirolimus (rapamycin; RAPAMUNE)
- Some cancer chemotherapeutic agents (see Chapter 45)
- Tacrolimus (PROGRAF, FK506)
- Tacrolimus (PROGRAF, PROTOPIC, others)
- Thalidomide (THALOMID)

MECHANISMS OF ACTION OF DRUGS USED AS IMMUNOSUPPRESSANTS

DRUG CLASS	DRUG	MECHANISM OF ACTION
Glucocorticoids	See Chapter 29	Regulate gene expression in lymphocytes and other inflammatory cells by binding glucocorticoid response elements in DNA
Calcineurin Inhibitors	Cyclosporine Tacrolimus	Inhibit the protein phosphatase activity of calcineurin, thus blocking expression of NFAT-regulated cytokines (see Figure 23-1)
Antiproliferative/ Antimetabolic Agents	Sirolimus (rapamycin) Everolimus Azathioprine Some cancer chemotherapeutic agents (see Chapter 45) Mycophenolate mofetil (MMF) MPA	Sirolimus and everolimus inhibit mTOR kinase activity blocking cell-cycle progression of lymphocytes (see Figure 23-1) Azathioprine is converted to 6-mercaptopurine which is incorporated into DNA as 6-thio-GTP impairing proliferation of lymphocytes MMF is a prodrug that is converted to mycophenolic acid (MPA) which in turn inhibits lymphocyte guanine nucleotide synthesis

(Continued)

375

SECTION IV

Immunomodulatory Agents

THE IMMUNE RESPONSE

- The immune system is composed of 2 complementary mechanisms, described as innate and adaptive immunity, capable of discriminating self from nonself (microbes and tumors).
- Characterisitics of innate (natural) immunity:
  - Does not require priming
  - Broadly reactive
  - Relatively low affinity
  - The most active component of the immune system early on in an immune response
  - Major effectors include complement, granulocytes, monocytes/macrophages, natural killer cells, mast cells, and basophils
- Characterisitics of adaptive (learned) immunity:
  - Antigen-specific
  - Depends on antigen priming
  - Can be very high affinity
  - Becomes the more dominant component of the immune response over time
  - Important in normal immune response to infection and tumors
  - Mediates transplant (allograft) rejection and autoimmunity
  - Major effectors include B and T lymphocytes
    - B lymphocytes make antibodies (immunoglobulins)
    - T lymphocytes function as helper, cytolytic, and regulatory (suppressor) cells
- Once activated by specific antigen recognition via cell surface receptors, B and T lymphocytes differentiate and divide, leading to release of soluble mediators (cytokines and lymphokines)

DRUG CLASS	DRUG	MECHANISM OF ACTION
Biological Immunosuppressants—Polyclonal Antibodies	Immune globulin preparations such as antithymocyte globulin (ATG; see Table 23-1)	Immune globulin preparations (polyclonal antibodies raised in animals against human thymocytes) are cytotoxic to lymphocytes and impair lymphocyte function by binding to cell surface proteins
Biological immunosuppressants—Anti-CD3 Monoclonal Antibody (mAb)	Muromonab-CD3	mAb that binds the CD3 cell surface protein on T lymphocytes causing its internalization, thus preventing antigen recognition and depleting T cells from the bloodstream
Biological Immunosuppressants—Anti–IL-2 receptor (anti-CD25) mAbs	Daclizumab Basiliximab	Anti-IL-2 (anti-CD25) recombinant mAbs that bind IL-2 receptors on activated T cells
Biological Immunosuppressants—Anti-CD52 mAb	Alemtuzumab	Humanized mAb that targets CD52 on lymphocytes, monocytes, macrophages, and natural killer cells, causing apoptosis
Biological Immunosuppressants—Anti-TNF Reagents	Infliximab Etanercept Adalimumab Golimumab Certolizumab pegol	Infliximab, adalimumab, and golimumab are anti–TNF-α (anti–tumor necrosis factor-α) mAbs that bind TNF-α, thus blocking this cytokine binding to its receptor Certolizumab is a Fab fragment of an anti–TNF-α mAb Etanercept is a fusion receptor protein containing the ligand-binding portion of human TNF-α receptor fused to the Fc portion of human IgG_1; it binds TNF-α and prevents it from binding its receptor
Biological Immunosuppressants—IL-1 Inhibitors	Anakinra Canakinumab Rilonacept	Anakinra is a recombinant, nonglycosylated form of the naturally occurring IL-1 receptor antagonist (IL-IRA) that blocks IL-1 inflammatory activity Canakinumab is an anti–IL-1β mAb that blocks this proinflammatory cytokine Rilonacept is a fusion protein that blocks IL-1 activity by binding it
Biological Immunosuppressants—Lymphocyte Function-associated Antigen-1 (LFA-1) and LFA-3 Inhibitors	Efalizumab Alefacept	Efalizumab is a humanized mAb that binds LFA-1 and prevents T-cell adhesion, trafficking, and activation by inhibiting interaction of LFA-1 with intercellular adhesion molecule (ICAM) Alefacept is a human LFA-3-IgG fusion protein that binds CD2 on T cells preventing their activation by LFA-3

Immunotherapeutic Agents

CHAPTER 23

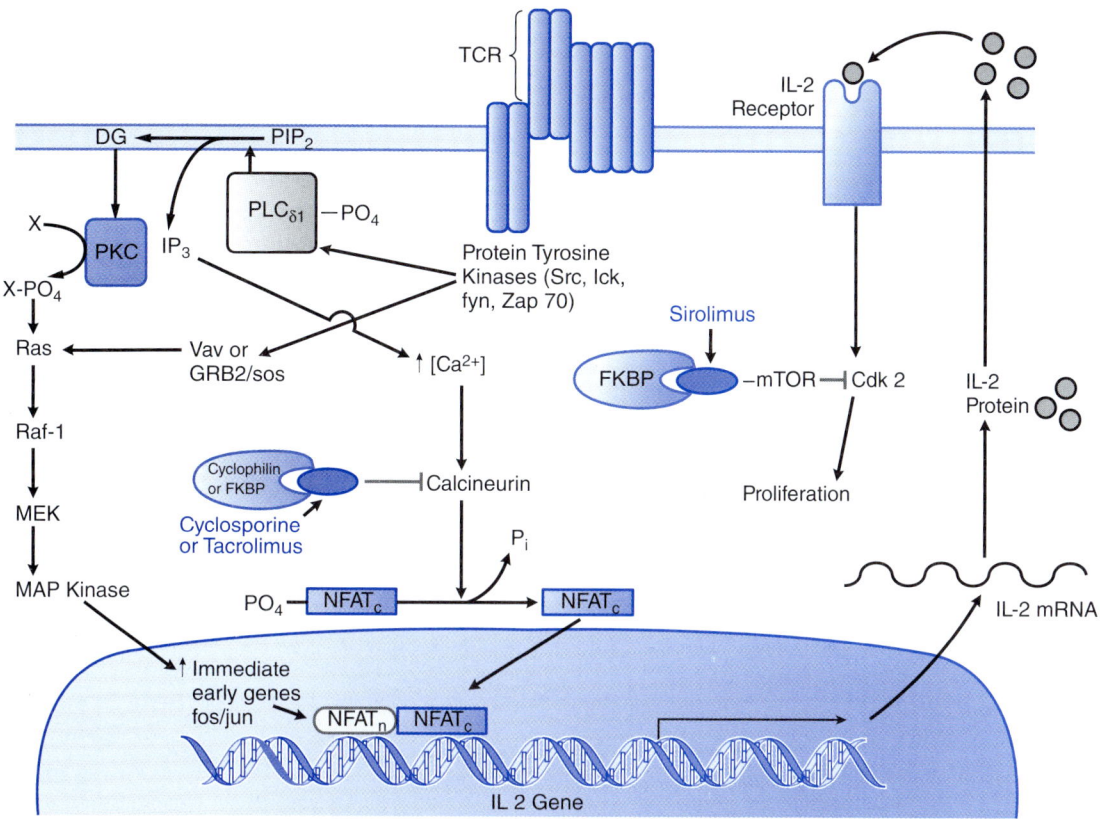

FIGURE 23-1 Mechanisms of action of cyclosporine, tacrolimus, and sirolimus on T lymphocytes. Both cyclosporine and tacrolimus bind to immunophilins (cyclophilin and FK506-binding protein [FKBP], respectively), forming a complex that binds the phosphatase calcineurin and inhibits the calcineurin-catalyzed dephosphorylation essential to permit movement of the nuclear factor of activated T cells (NFAT) into the nucleus. NFAT is required for transcription of interleukin-2 (IL-2) and other growth- and differentiation-associated cytokines (lymphokines). Sirolimus (rapamycin) works at a later stage in T-cell activation, downstream of the IL-2 receptor. Sirolimus also binds FKBP, but the FKBP-sirolimus complex binds to and inhibits the mammalian target of rapamycin (mTOR), a kinase involved in cell-cycle progression (proliferation). TCR, T-cell receptor. (Reproduced with permission from Pattison JM et al. Mechanisms of allograft rejection. In Neilson EG, Couser WG, eds. Immunologic Renal Diseases. Philadelphia, PA: Lippincott-Raven; 1997. http://lww.com.)

TABLE 23-1 Selected Immune Globulin Preparations

GENERIC NAME	COMMON SYNONYMS	ORIGIN	BRAND NAME
Antithymocyte globulin	ATG	Rabbit	THYMOGLOBULIN
Botulism immune globulin intravenous	BIG-IV	Human	BABYBIG
Cytomegalovirus immune globulin intravenous	CMV-IGIV	Human	CYTOGAM
Hepatitis B immune globulin	HBIG	Human	HEPAGAM B, HYPERHEP B S/D, NABI-HB
Immune globulin intramuscular	Gamma globulin, IgG, IGIM	Human	GAMASTAN S/D
Immune globulin intravenous	IVIG	Human	CARIMUNE NF, FLEBOGAMMA 5%, GAMMAGARD LIQUID, GAMUNEX, IVEEGAM EN, OCTAGAM, PRIVIGEN

(Continued)

USES OF IMMUNOTHERAPEUTIC DRUGS

- Immunosuppressants are used to dampen the immune response in organ transplant and autoimmune disease.

- Tolerogens are used to induce a state of antigen-specific nonresponsiveness in organ transplantation and autoimmune diseases while maintaining immune functions that protect against opportunistic infections and secondary tumors.

- Immunostimulants are used to augment the immune system in some patients with infections, cancers, and immunodeficiency.

SECTION IV

Immunomodulatory Agents

GENERAL PRINCIPLES OF ORGAN TRANSPLANT THERAPY

- Carefully prepare patient and select best available match for organ donor.
- Use a multitiered approach to immunosuppressive drug therapy with coadministration of several agents, each directed at a different molecular target in the allograft response.
- To gain early engraftment or to treat established rejection, use greater immunosuppression than used to maintain long-term immunosuppression.
- Carefully investigate each episode of transplant dysfunction to identify cause(s).
- An immunosuppressant drug should be reduced or withdrawn if its toxicity exceeds its benefit.

ADVERSE EFFECTS OF IMMUNOSUPPRESSANTS

- General suppression of the immune system increases the risk of opportunistic infections and secondary tumors.
- Calcineurin inhibitors are nephrotoxic.
- Glucocorticoids are diabetogenic and have many other adverse effects (see Chapter 29).
- Using drugs that have synergistic effects can reduce the doses needed for therapeutic efficacy and limit specific toxicities.

GENERIC NAME	COMMON SYNONYMS	ORIGIN	BRAND NAME
Immune globulin subcutaneous	IGSC	Human	VIVAGLOBIN
Lymphocyte immune globulin	ALG, antithymocyte globulin (equine), ATG (equine)	Equine	ATGAM
Rabies immune globulin	RIG	Human	HYPERRAB S/D, IMOGAM RABIES–HT
Rho(D) immune globulin intramuscular	Rho[D] IGIM	Human	HYPERRHO S/D, RHOGAM
Rho(D) immune globulin intravenous	Rho[D] IGIV	Human	RHOPHYLAC, WINRHO SDF
Rho(D) immune globulin microdose	Rho[D] IG microdose	Human	HYPERRHO S/D MICRODOSE, MICRHOGAM
Tetanus immune globulin	TIG	Human	BAYTET
Vaccinia immune globulin intravenous	VIGIV	Human	Generic

CASE 23-1

A 38-year-old male patient requires a kidney transplant because his kidneys have failed as the result of congenital renal disease. His biological daughter has agreed to donate one of her kidneys.

a. What is typically done prior to an organ transplant such as this?

Organ transplantation therapy is organized around 5 general principles (see Side Bar GENERAL PRINCIPLES OF ORGAN TRANSPLANT THERAPY). The first principle is careful patient preparation and selection of the best available ABO blood type–compatible human leukocyte antigen (HLA) match for organ donation. Because the organ donor in this case is the patient's daughter, the match is likely to be excellent. By having a good match, the possibility of acute immune rejection is significantly reduced.

b. What drugs are used prophylactically to prevent organ transplant rejection?

Biological agents for induction therapy in the prophylaxis of rejection currently are used in ~70% of de novo transplant patients and have been propelled by several factors, including the introduction of the relatively safe anti–IL-2R antibodies and the emergence of antithymocyte globulin (ATG) as a safer and more effective alternative to lymphocyte immune globulin or muromonab-CD3. Induction therapy with biological agents is used to delay the use of the nephrotoxic calcineurin inhibitors or to intensify the initial immunosuppressive therapy in patients at high risk of rejection (ie, repeat transplants, broadly presensitized patients, African American patients, or pediatric patients).

Biologicals for induction can be divided into 2 groups: the depleting agents and the immune modulators. The depleting agents consist of lymphocyte immune globulin, ATG, and muromonab-CD3 mAb (the latter also produces immune modulation); their efficacy derives from their ability to deplete the recipient's CD3-positive cells at the time of transplant and antigen presentation. ATG is the most frequently used depleting agent. Lymphocyte immune globulin and OKT3 are rarely used because of poorer efficacy and acute side effects, respectively. Alemtuzumab, a humanized anti-CD52 monoclonal antibody that produces prolonged lymphocyte depletion, is increasingly used off-label as induction therapy in transplantation.

(Continued)

The second group of biological agents used for induction are the immune modulators, specifically the anti–IL-2R mAbs. These agents do not deplete T lymphocytes, with the possible exception of T regulatory cells, but rather block IL-2–mediated T-cell activation by binding to the α chain of IL-2R. These agents include anakinra, canakinumab, and rilonacept.

c. What is the approach to using immunosuppressants in organ transplants?

Immunosuppressive drugs are used to dampen the immune response in organ transplantation. A multitiered approach to immunosuppressive drug therapy is employed. Several agents, each of which is directed at a different molecular target within the allograft response (see MECHANISMS OF ACTION OF DRUGS USED AS IMMUNOSUPPRESSANTS), are used simultaneously. Synergistic effects permit use of the various agents at relatively low doses, thereby limiting specific toxicities while maximizing the immunosuppressive effect. Therapy typically involves a calcineurin inhibitor, glucocorticoids, and mycophenolate, each directed at a discrete site in T-cell activation. Glucocorticoids, azathioprine, cyclosporine, tacrolimus, mycophenolate, sirolimus, and various monoclonal and polyclonal antibodies all are approved for use in transplantation.

Greater immunosuppression is required to gain early engraftment and/or to treat established rejection than to maintain long-term immunosuppression. Maintenance immunosuppression consists of a calcineurin inhibitor (cyclosporine or tacrolimus), glucocorticoids, and an antimetabolite (azathioprine or mycophenolate). Mycophenolate has largely replaced azathioprine as part of the standard immunosuppressive regimen after transplant.

d. What are the risks of immunosuppressant drugs?

Immunosuppressant therapies require lifelong use and nonspecifically suppress the entire immune system, exposing patients to considerably higher risks of infection and cancer. The calcineurin inhibitors and glucocorticoids, in particular, are nephrotoxic and diabetogenic, respectively, thus restricting their usefulness in a variety of clinical settings. To minimize risks after engraftment is achieved, lower-dose maintenance drug protocols are employed. In addition, a drug should be reduced or withdrawn if its toxicity exceeds its benefit.

e. What might cause organ transplant dysfunction?

There can be many causes of transplant dysfunction, including rejection, drug toxicity, and infection. These various problems can and often do coexist. Organ-specific problems (eg, obstruction in the case of kidney transplants) also must be considered. A general principle of organ transplantation is to investigate each episode of transplant dysfunction to identify the cause(s) and adjust therapy.

CASE 23-2

A 62-year-old woman suffers from severe rheumatoid arthritis. Her pharmacotherapy includes several agents that are also commonly used for organ transplant pharmacotherapy.

a. What is the therapeutic rationale in using immunosuppressant drugs to treat this patient's arthritis?

Rheumatoid arthritis is an autoimmune disease driven largely by activated T cells, giving rise to T cell–derived cytokines, such as IL-1 and TNF-α. Nonsteroidal anti-inflammatory drugs (NSAIDs) are widely used in patients with rheumatoid arthritis to relieve symptoms of pain and reduce inflammation (see Chapter 22), but they have minimal effect on disease progression and joint deformity. DMARDs (disease-modifying antirheumatic drugs), on the other hand, reduce the disease activity of rheumatoid arthritis and retard the progression of arthritic tissue destruction. These include a diverse group of small molecule nonbiologicals and biological agents (mainly antibodies or binding proteins), as summarized in Table 22-3,

(Continued)

SECTION IV

Immunomodulatory Agents

INDUCTION OF IMMUNOLOGICAL TOLERANCE BY COSTIMULATORY BLOCKADE

- Immunological tolerance is the state of nonresponsiveness of the immune system to a specific antigen or group of antigens.
- Antigen-specific tolerance would theoretically eliminate the risk of opportunistic infections and secondary tumors that occur with immunosuppression.
- Induction of antigen-specific immune responses by T lymphocytes requires 2 signals (referred to as costimulation; see Figure 23-2):
  - An antigen-specific signal via the T-cell receptor
  - A costimulatory signal provided by the interaction of molecules such as CD28 on the T lymphocyte and CD80 and CD86 on the antigen-presenting cell (APC)
- After a T cell is activated, it expresses additional costimulatory molecules.
  - CD152 is the CD40 ligand, which interacts with CD40 as a costimulatory pair.
  - CD154 (CTLA4) interacts with CD80 and CD86 to dampen or downregulate an immune response.
- Tolerance can be achieved by blocking costimulatory interactions.
  - Abatacept and belatacept are fusion proteins that contain a portion of CTLA4 fused to IgG_1.
  - These agents bind CD80 and CD86 on APCs and block interactions with CD28 on T cells.

Disease-Modifying Antirheumatic Drugs. Many of the agents listed in Table 22-3 include the immunosuppressants covered in this chapter, including cyclosporine, azathioprine, TNF-α antagonists (infliximab, adalimumab, etanercept), IL-1 receptor antagonists (anakinra), and costimulatory blockers (abatacept).

Cyclosporine is used in severe cases of rheumatoid arthritis that have not responded to methotrexate. It can be combined with methotrexate, but the levels of both drugs must be monitored closely. Azathioprine is used in patients with severe rheumatoid arthritis. Lower initial doses of azathioprine are used for rheumatoid arthritis than used to prevent organ rejection. Biological DMARDs remain reserved for patients with persistent moderate or high disease activity and indicators of poor prognosis such as functional impairment, radiographic bony erosions, extra-articular disease, and rheumatoid factor positivity. Therapy is tailored to the individual patient, and the use of these agents must be weighed against their potentially serious adverse effects. Infliximab is approved in the United States for treating the symptoms of rheumatoid arthritis and is typically used in combination with methotrexate in patients who do not respond to methotrexate alone. Etanercept is approved for treatment of rheumatoid arthritis in patients who have not responded to other treatments and can be used in combination with methotrexate in patients who have not responded adequately to methotrexate alone.

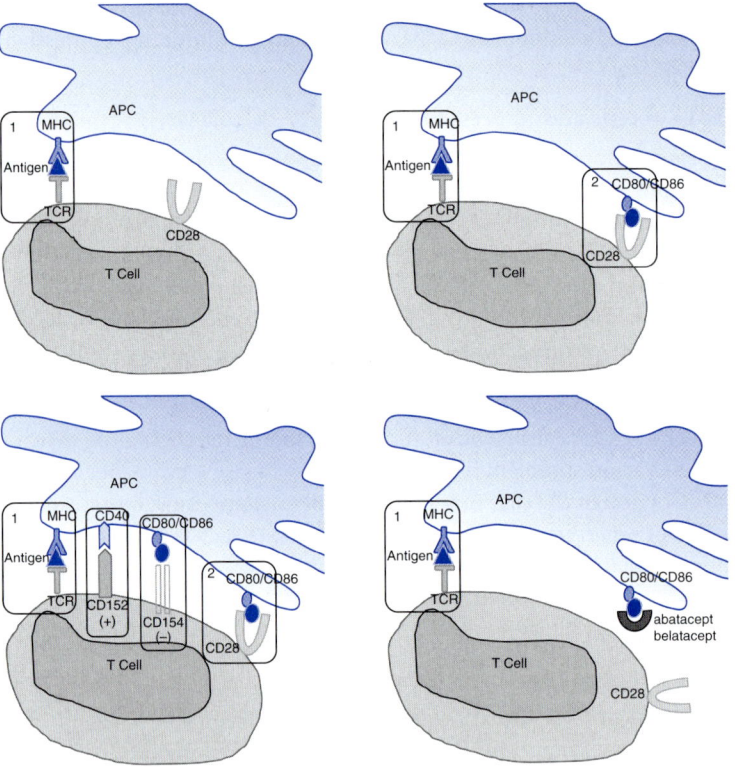

FIGURE 23-2 T-Cell Activation. Two signals are required for T-cell activation. The upper left panel shows Signal 1, stimulation via the T-cell receptor (TCR) by the MHC-antigen complex on the antigen presenting cell (APC). The upper right panel depicts Signal 2, co-stimulatory interactions between CD28 on the T cell (co-stimulatory receptor) and the co-stimulatory ligand on the APC, CD80/CD86. Signal 1 in the absence of Signal 2 does not result in T-cell activation. The lower left panel shows additional co-stimulatory interactions that occur after T-cell activation. CD152 interaction with CD40 on the APC enhances T-cell activation (+), whereas CD154 interaction with CD80/86 attenuates (-) T-cell activation. The lower right panel shows the mechanism of action of abatacept and belatacept, fusion proteins that contain the CTLA4 domain of CD154. These agents block co-stimulation of T cells by binding CD80/CD86.

Immunotherapeutic Agents — CHAPTER 23

CASE 23-3

A 24-year-old woman who has had symptoms of abdominal pain, diarrhea, and blood in the stool is diagnosed with Crohn's disease.

a. What is the pathophysiology of Crohn's disease and what agents are typically used to initiate therapy?

Crohn's disease is an inflammatory bowel disease that is associated with activation of the immune system. Drugs used to treat mild to moderately active Crohn's disease include sulfasalazine (an intestinal anti-inflammatory), budesonide (an enteric glucocorticoid with local anti-inflammatory effects), and oral corticosteroids (see Chapter 33).

b. What is the rationale for using TNF-α antagonists in the treatment of Crohn's disease?

Patients with Crohn's disease have elevated levels of TNF-α in their stools. As a result, a number of anti-TNF agents are used for the treatment of this disorder, including infliximab, adalimumab, and certolizumab pegol. Because these agents are associated with significant risks, they are reserved for patients with moderate to severe Crohn's disease who have failed to respond to conventional therapy. Also see Case 33-6.

MECHANISMS OF ACTION OF TOLEROGENS

DRUG CLASS	DRUG	MECHANISM OF ACTION
Selective T-Cell Costimulation Blocker	Belatacept	Contains the CD80- and CD86-binding region of CTLA4 (a CD28 homolog), and competitively inhibits CD28 co-stimulatory interactions of T cells with APCs
Selective T-Cell Costimulation Blocker	Abatacept	Contains a congener of the CD80- and CD86-binding region of CTLA4 (a CD28 homolog), and competitively inhibits CD28 co-stimulatory interactions of T cells with APCs

MECHANISMS OF ACTION OF IMMUNOSTIMULANT AND IMMUNOMODULATORY DRUGS

DRUG CLASS	DRUG	MECHANISM OF ACTION
Immunostimulant—Thalidomide and Its Analogs	Thalidomide Lenalidomide	Multiple mechanisms of action (see Chapter 46); mechanisms of action as an immunostimulatory drug are unclear
Immunostimulant—BCG	Bacillus Calmette–Guerin (BCG)	Attenuated, live culture of the BCG of *Mycobacterium bovis* that induces a granulomatous reaction at the site of administration; mechanisms of action as an immunostimulatory drug are unclear
Immunostimulants—Recombinant Cytokines, α and γ IFNs	Interferon-α-2b (IFN-α-2b) Interferon-γ-1b (IFN-γ-1b)	Bind to specific cell-surface receptors that initiate a series of intracellular events: induction of certain enzymes, inhibition of cell proliferation, and enhancement of immune activities, including increased phagocytosis by macrophages and augmentation of specific cytotoxicity by T lymphocytes
Immunostimulants—Recombinant Cytokines, Interleukin-2 (IL-2)	Aldesleukin	Simulates the biological effects of native IL-2: enhancement of lymphocyte proliferation and growth of IL-2–dependent cell lines, enhancement of lymphocyte-mediated cytotoxicity and killer cell activity, and induction of IFN-γ activity
Immunostimulants—Passive Immunization	See Table 23-1	Used to provide nonspecific or highly specific immunoglobulins to patients with immunodeficiencies, when there is inadequate time for active immunization, or when an existing disease can be ameliorated by passive antibodies
Immunomodulators—Recombinant Cytokines, β_1 IFNs	Interferon-β-1a (IFN-β-1a) Interferon-β-1b (IFN-β-1b)	IFN-β-1a and IFN-β-1b have antiviral and immunomodulatory properties: suppress proliferation of T lymphocytes, inhibit their movement into the CNS from the periphery, and shift the cytokine profile from pro- to anti-inflammatory types

(Continued)

SECTION IV — Immunomodulatory Agents

DRUG CLASS	DRUG	MECHANISM OF ACTION
Immunomodulators—Universal Altered Peptide Ligands (APLs)	Glatiramer acetate (GA)	Induces T-helper type 2 cells that enter the CNS; mediates bystander suppression at sites of inflammation
Immunomodulators—Anthracenedione-Derivative	Mitoxantrone	Intercalates DNA and suppresses cellular and humoral immune response
Immunomodulators—mAb	Natalizumab	mAb directed against the adhesion molecule $α_4$ integrin, antagonizes interactions of $α_4$-containing integrin heterodimers on the surface of activated lymphocytes and monocytes, thereby blocking their movement out of the bloodstream

CASE 23-4

A 31-year-old woman is diagnosed with relapsing-remitting multiple sclerosis (MS).

a. What is the pathophysiology of MS?

MS is a demyelinating inflammatory disease of the CNS white matter that displays a triad of pathogenic findings: mononuclear cell infiltration, demyelination, and scarring (gliosis). The peripheral nervous system is uninvolved. The disease, which may be episodic or progressive, occurs in early to middle adulthood with prevalence increasing from late adolescence to 35 years of age and then declining. The cause is unknown, but there is a strong genetic component, with a number of immune-related genetic variants, many of which are shared with different autoimmune diseases. In addition, MS patients have activated T cells that are reactive to different myelin antigens, and autoantibodies to myelin proteins can be eluted from CNS plaque tissue.

b. What is the rationale for using β-1 interferons in treating this patient's symptoms?

The β-1 interferons (IFN-β-1a, IFN-β-1b) are immunomodulatory and suppress the proliferation and activation of T lymphocytes by interfering with costimulatory molecules, inhibit T-cell movement into the CNS from the periphery, and shift the cytokine profile from pro- to anti-inflammatory types. These agents reduce the recurrence of relapsing-remitting attacks by one-third and reduce disease progression.

KEY CONCEPTS

- Immunosuppressant drugs are essential in preventing grant rejection in organ transplantation.
- Immunosuppressant drugs also have application in reducing symptoms and disease progression in a variety of autoimmune diseases.
- Immunosuppressant drugs with different mechanisms of action are typically used in combination to achieve greater efficacy and reduce dosing to reduce risk of drug-specific toxicities.
- General suppression of the immune system increases the risk of secondary infections and cancer.
- Many immunosuppressants must be used chronically over the life of the patient, which increases the risk of adverse effects.

SUMMARY QUIZ

QUESTION 23-1 Cyclosporine was one of the first immunosuppressants to be used for organ transplant therapy. The mechanism of action of cyclosporine is to

a. intercalate DNA in proliferating T cells.

(Continued)

b. block purine metabolism in proliferating T cells.
c. block CD52 on the surface of activated T cells.
d. block the protein phosphatase activity of calcineurin.
e. block the protein kinase activity of mTOR.

QUESTION 23-2 Tacrolimus is one of the most effective immunosuppressant drugs in routine use. The mechanism of action of tacrolimus is to

a. intercalate DNA in proliferating T cells.
b. block guanine nucleotide synthesis in proliferating T cells.
c. block CD52 on the surface of activated T cells.
d. block the protein phosphatase activity of calcineurin.
e. block the protein kinase activity of mTOR.

QUESTION 23-3 Sirolimus is used in combination with other drugs in patients receiving organ transplants. The mechanism of action of sirolimus is to

a. intercalate DNA in proliferating T cells.
b. block guanine nucleotide synthesis in proliferating T cells.
c. block CD52 on the surface of activated T cells.
d. block the protein phosphatase activity of calcineurin.
e. block the protein kinase activity of mTOR.

QUESTION 23-4 Mycophenolate mofetil (MMF) is typically used in combination with other agents for immunosuppression pharmacotherapy. The mechanism of action of mycophenolate is to

a. intercalate DNA in proliferating T cells.
b. block guanine nucleotide synthesis in proliferating T cells.
c. block CD52 on the surface of activated T cells.
d. block the protein phosphatase activity of calcineurin.
e. block the protein kinase activity of mTOR.

QUESTION 23-5 Adalimumab is a monoclonal antibody used in a variety of autoimmune diseases. The molecular target of adalimumab is

a. CD3 on T lymphocytes.
b. IL-2 receptor on T cells.
c. CD52 on lymphocytes, monocytes, macrophages, and natural killer cells.
d. TNF-α.
e. IL-1.

SUMMARY QUIZ ANSWER KEY

QUESTION 23-1 Answer is **d.** Cyclosporin targets intracellular signaling pathways induced as a consequence of T-cell receptor activation. The drug binds to an immunophilin known as cyclophilin which subsequently interacts with calcineurin to inhibit its protein phosphatase activity (see Figure 23-1). Calcineurin-catalyzed dephosphorylation of the protein nuclear factor of activated T lymphocytes (NFAT) is required for movement of NFAT into the nucleus. NFAT, in turn, is required to induce a number of cytokine genes, including that for interleukin-2 (IL-2), a prototypic T-cell growth and differentiation factor.

QUESTION 23-2 Answer is **d.** Although structurally unrelated to cyclosporine, tacrolimus inhibits T-cell signal transduction by almost the same mechanism. Tacrolimus binds the immunophilin FK506-binding protein-12 (FKBP-12), which is structurally

(Continued)

SECTION IV — Immunomodulatory Agents

related to cyclophilin, the target of cyclosporine. A complex of tacrolimus-FKBP-12, Ca^{2+}, calmodulin, and calcineurin then forms and the protein phosphatase activity of calcineurin is inhibited (see Figure 23-1). The inhibition of calcineurin prevents dephosphorylation and nuclear translocation of NFAT and inhibits T-cell activation. Thus, although the intracellular receptors differ, cyclosporine and tacrolimus target the same pathway for immunosuppression. Because of perceived slightly greater efficacy and ease of blood level monitoring, tacrolimus has become the preferred calcineurin inhibitor in most transplant centers

QUESTION 23-3 Answer is **e**. Sirolimus inhibits T-lymphocyte activation and proliferation downstream of the IL-2 receptor and other T-cell growth factor receptors (see Figure 23-1). Like cyclosporine and tacrolimus, the therapeutic action of sirolimus requires formation of a complex with an immunophilin, in this case FKBP-12. However, the sirolimus–FKBP-12 complex does not affect calcineurin activity. It binds to and inhibits a protein kinase, designated mTOR, which is a key enzyme in cell-cycle progression. Inhibition of mTOR blocks cell-cycle progression at the G1 → S phase transition. In animal models, sirolimus not only inhibits transplant rejection, graft-versus-host disease, and a variety of autoimmune diseases, but its effect also lasts several months after discontinuing therapy, suggesting a tolerizing effect. A newer indication for sirolimus is the avoidance of calcineurin inhibitors, even when patients are stable, to protect kidney function.

QUESTION 23-4 Answer is **b**. MMF is a prodrug that is rapidly hydrolyzed to the active drug, MPA, a selective, noncompetitive, reversible inhibitor of inosine monophosphate dehydrogenase (IMPDH), an important enzyme in the de novo pathway of guanine nucleotide synthesis. B and T lymphocytes are highly dependent on this pathway for cell proliferation, while other cell types can use salvage pathways; MPA therefore selectively inhibits lymphocyte proliferation and functions, including antibody formation, cellular adhesion, and migration. MMF is typically used in combination with glucocorticoids and a calcineurin inhibitor but not with azathioprine.

QUESTION 23-5 Answer is **d**. Adalimumab is one of several anti-TNF agents used to treat autoimmune diseases. TNF is a proinflammatory cytokine that has been implicated in the pathogenesis of several immune-mediated intestinal, skin, and joint diseases. Other anti-TNF agents include infliximab (a monoclonal antibody), golimumab (a monoclonal antibody), certolizumab (a Fab fragment directed toward TNF-α), and etanercept (a fusion protein that contains the ligand-binding portion of a human TNF-α receptor fused to the Fc portion of human IgG_1). Adalimumab is approved for use in rheumatoid arthritis, ankylosing spondylitis, Crohn's disease, juvenile idiopathic arthritis, plaque psoriasis, and psoriatic arthritis. All anti-TNF agents increase the risk for serious infections, lymphomas, and other malignancies.

SUMMARY TABLE: IMMUNOMODULATORY DRUGS

CLASS AND SUBCLASSES	NAMES	CLINICAL USES	TOXICITIES COMMON	TOXICITIES UNIQUE; CLINICALLY IMPORTANT
Glucocorticoids	See Chapter 29	Commonly combined with other immunosuppressive agents to prevent and treat transplant rejection. Treatment of many autoimmune disorders. Used to limit allergic reactions that occur with other immunosuppressive agents and to block first-dose cytokine storm caused by treatment with muromonab-CD3 and to a lesser extent ATG	Extensive use of steroids often results in disabling and life-threatening adverse effects, including growth retardation in children, avascular necrosis of bone, osteopenia, increased risk of infection, poor wound healing, cataracts, hyperglycemia, and hypertension	See Chapter 29

(Continued)

Immunotherapeutic Agents — CHAPTER 23

CLASS AND SUBCLASSES	NAMES	CLINICAL USES	TOXICITIES COMMON	TOXICITIES UNIQUE; CLINICALLY IMPORTANT
Calcineurin Inhibitors	Cyclosporine Tacrolimus	Indicated for the prophylaxis of solid-organ allograft rejection. Tacrolimus has become the preferred calcineurin inhibitor in most transplant centers. Severe cases of rheumatoid arthritis and psoriasis in which other therapies have failed	Nephrotoxicity (occurs in the majority of patients), neurotoxicity (eg, tremor, headache, motor disturbances, seizures), GI complaints, hypertension, hyperkalemia, hyperglycemia, and diabetes (combined use of calcineurin inhibitors and glucocorticoids is particularly diabetogenic). Increased risk of secondary tumors and opportunistic infections	Because of its potential for nephrotoxicity, tacrolimus blood levels and renal function should be monitored closely, especially when tacrolimus is used with other potentially nephrotoxic drugs. Coadministration with cyclosporine results in additive or synergistic nephrotoxicity; therefore, a delay of at least 24 h is required when switching a patient from cyclosporine to tacrolimus. Great care must be taken to differentiate renal toxicity from rejection in kidney transplant patients
Antiproliferative/ Antimetabolic Agents	Sirolimus (rapamycin) Everolimus Azathioprine Mycophenolate mofetil (MMF) MPA	Sirolimus and everolimus are indicated for prophylaxis of organ transplant rejection usually in combination with a reduced dose of calcineurin inhibitor and glucocorticoids. Sirolimus has been used with glucocorticoids and mycophenolate in patients experiencing or at high risk for calcineurin inhibitor–associated nephrotoxicity. Azathioprine is indicated as an adjunct for prevention of organ transplant rejection (but not with MMF) and in severe rheumatoid arthritis	Sirolimus and everolimus in renal transplant patients is associated with a dose-dependent increase in serum cholesterol and triglycerides. Azathioprine is associated with bone marrow suppression, including leukopenia (common), thrombocytopenia (less common), and/or anemia (uncommon), hepatotoxicity, alopecia, GI toxicity, pancreatitis. MMF principal toxicities are GI and hematologic. Increased risk of neoplasms and infections	If azathioprine and allopurinol are used concurrently, the azathioprine dose must be decreased to 25-33% of the usual dose; it is best not to use these 2 drugs together. Coadministration of azathioprine with other myelosuppressive agents or ACE inhibitors include leukopenia, thrombocytopenia, and anemia. MMF is teratogenic; women of childbearing age must use effective contraception
Biological Immunosuppressants— Polyclonal Antibodies	Immune globulin preparations such as ATG (see Table 23-1)	ATG is used for induction immunosuppression, although the only approved indication is in the treatment of acute renal transplant rejection in combination with other immunosuppressive agents	Polyclonal antibodies are xenogeneic proteins that can elicit major side effects, including fever and chills with the potential for hypotension. Increased risk of infection and malignancy	Serum sickness and glomerulonephritis can occur; anaphylaxis is a rare event. Hematologic complications include leukopenia and thrombocytopenia
Biological Immunosuppressants— Anti-CD3 Monoclonal Antibody (mAb)	Muromonab-CD3	Indicated for treatment of acute organ transplant rejection. Rarely used for induction and rejection therapy because of toxicity and the availability of ATG and alemtuzumab	Major side effect is the "cytokine release syndrome" caused by release of proinflammatory cytokines by activated T cells. Clinical manifestations include high fever, chills/rigor, headache, tremor, nausea, vomiting, diarrhea, abdominal pain, malaise, myalgias, arthralgias, and generalized weakness. Increased risk of infections and neoplasms	Potentially fatal pulmonary edema, acute respiratory distress syndrome, cardiovascular collapse, cardiac arrest, and arrhythmias. Administration of glucocorticoids before the injection of muromonab-CD3 prevents the release of cytokines and is standard procedure. A fully competent resuscitation facility must be immediately available for patients receiving their first several doses of this therapy

(Continued)

SECTION IV Immunomodulatory Agents

CLASS AND SUBCLASSES	NAMES	CLINICAL USES	TOXICITIES COMMON	TOXICITIES UNIQUE; CLINICALLY IMPORTANT
Biological Immunosuppressants—Anti–IL-2 Receptor (Anti-CD25) Monoclonal Antibodies (mAbs)	Daclizumab Basiliximab	Used for prophylaxis of acute organ rejection in adult patients	No cytokine-release syndrome has been observed with these antibodies, but anaphylactic reactions can occur Lymphoproliferative disorders and opportunistic infections may occur, but the incidence appears remarkably low	
Biological Immunosuppressants—Anti-CD52 Monoclonal Antibody (mAb)	Alemtuzumab	Approved for use in chronic lymphocytic leukemia Some use in renal transplantation because it produces prolonged T- and B-cell depletion and allows drug minimization, but large controlled studies of efficacy or safety are not available		
Biological Immunosuppressants—Anti-TNF Reagents	Infliximab Etanercept Adalimumab Golimumab Certolizumab pegol	Used in treating several immune-mediated intestinal, skin, and joint diseases including rheumatoid arthritis, Crohn's disease, ankylosing spondylitis, juvenile idiopathic arthritis, plaque psoriasis, psoriatic arthritis, and ulcerative colitis	About 1 of 6 patients receiving infliximab experiences an infusion reaction characterized by fever, urticaria, hypotension, and dyspnea within 1-2 h	Increase the risk for serious infections, lymphomas, and other malignancies Patients should be closely monitored for the signs and symptoms of infection during and after treatment including the possible development of tuberculosis in patients who tested negative prior to initiating therapy Fatal lymphomas and other malignancies have been reported in children, adolescent and young adult patients treated with TNF blockers
Biological Immunosuppressants—IL-1 Inhibitors	Anakinra Canakinumab Rilonacept	Anakinra is used alone or in combination with anti-TNF agents for management of joint disease in rheumatoid arthritis Canakinumab approved for treating cryopyrin-associated periodic syndromes (CAPS)		
Biological Immunosuppressants—Lymphocyte Function-Associated Antigen-1 (LFA-1) and LFA-3 Inhibitors	Efalizumab Alefacept	Pretransplant therapy, treatment of psoriasis	Risk of posttransplant lymphoproliferative diseases (PTLD) with higher-dose efalizumab	Progressive multifocal leukoencephalopathy (PML) also has occurred during therapy with efalizumab

(Continued)

Immunotherapeutic Agents   CHAPTER 23

CLASS AND SUBCLASSES	NAMES	CLINICAL USES	TOXICITIES COMMON	TOXICITIES UNIQUE; CLINICALLY IMPORTANT
Selective T-Cell Costimulation Blocker	Belatacept	Prevention of rejection in renal transplantation	Increased risk of infections (such as PML) and malignancies (including PTLD predominantly involving the CNS) Common adverse effects are anemia, diarrhea, peripheral edema, constipation, hypertension, pyrexia, graft dysfunction, cough, nausea, vomiting, headache, hypokalemia, hyperkalemia, and leukopenia	Risk of PTLD is significantly increased in patients without immunity to Epstein-Barr virus (EBV), thus contraindicated in patients who are EBV seronegative or unknown serostatus
Selective T-Cell Costimulation Blocker	Abatacept	Treatment of moderate to severe rheumatoid arthritis, juvenile idiopathic arthritis	Increased risk of infections (especially in combination with TNF antagonists) and malignancies	Increased risk of serious adverse events in patients with COPD
Immunostimulant—Thalidomide and Its Analogs	Thalidomide Lenalidomide	Thalidomide is indicated for treatment of erythema nodosum leprosum (see Chapter 42) and multiple myeloma, and has orphan drug status for mycobacterial infections, Crohn's disease, HIV-associated wasting, Kaposi sarcoma, lupus, myelofibrosis, brain malignancies, leprosy, graft-versus-host disease, and aphthous ulcers Lenalidomide is approved for treating transfusion-dependent anemia due to low- or intermediate-risk 5q minus cytogenetic myelodysplastic syndromes	Lenalidomide causes significant neutropenia and thrombocytopenia in almost all patients, which requires weekly blood counts and dosing adjustments	Teratogenic and should never be taken by women who are pregnant or who could become pregnant while taking the drug Lenalidomide is associated with a significant risk for deep vein thrombosis
Immunostimulant—BCG	Bacillus Calmette–Guerin (BCG)	Indicated for the treatment and prophylaxis of carcinoma in situ of the urinary bladder and for prophylaxis of primary and recurrent stage Ta and/or T1 papillary tumors after transurethral resection	Hypersensitivity, shock, chills, fever, malaise, and immune complex disease	
Immunostimulants—Recombinant Cytokines, α Interferons	Interferon-α-2b (IFN-α-2b)	Indicated in the treatment of a variety of tumors, including hairy cell leukemia, malignant melanoma, follicular lymphoma, and AIDS-related Kaposi sarcoma, and is also indicated for infectious diseases, chronic hepatitis B, and condylomata acuminata	Flu-like symptoms, including fever, chills, and headache	Risk of developing pulmonary hypertension Risk of cardiovascular (hypotension, arrhythmias, and rarely, cardiomyopathy, myocardial infarction) and CNS (depression, confusion) effects

(Continued)

SECTION IV Immunomodulatory Agents

CLASS AND SUBCLASSES	NAMES	CLINICAL USES	TOXICITIES COMMON	TOXICITIES UNIQUE; CLINICALLY IMPORTANT
Immunostimulants—Recombinant Cytokines, γ Interferons	Interferon-γ-1b (IFN-γ-1b)	Indicated to reduce frequency and severity of serious infections associated with chronic granulomatous disease and to delay time to progression in severe malignant osteopetrosis	Fever, headache, rash, fatigue, GI distress, anorexia, weight loss, myalgia, and depression	May increase mortality in patients with idiopathic pulmonary fibrosis
Immunostimulants—Recombinant Cytokines, Interleukin-2	Aldesleukin	Indicated for the treatment of adults with metastatic renal cell carcinoma and melanoma	Increased risk of disseminated infection due to impaired neutrophil function	Associated with serious cardiovascular toxicity resulting from capillary leak syndrome (loss of vascular tone and leak of plasma proteins and fluid into the extravascular space); hypotension, reduced organ perfusion, and death may occur
Immunostimulants—Passive Immunization	See Table 23-1	Indicated when an individual is deficient in antibodies because of a congenital or acquired immunodeficiency, when an individual with a high degree of risk is exposed to an agent and there is inadequate time for active immunization (eg, measles, rabies, hepatitis B), or when a disease is already present but can be ameliorated by passive antibodies (eg, botulism, diphtheria, tetanus) Intravenous immunoglobulin (IVIG) also used for a variety of autoimmune and inflammatory diseases	Plasma-derived products carry the theoretical risk of transmission of infectious disease	
Immunomodulators—Recombinant Cytokines, β-1 Interferons	Interferon-β-1a (IFN-β-1a) Interferon-β-1b (IFN-β-1b)	Treatment of relapsing-remitting MS (RRMS) to resolve acute attacks, reduce the frequency of clinical exacerbations, and slow progression of disability	Flu-like symptoms (fever, chills, myalgia) and injection-site reactions	
Immunomodulators—Universal Altered Peptide Ligands (APLs)	Glatiramer acetate (GA)	Treatment of RRMS to reduce the frequency of clinical exacerbations and slow progression of disability		
Immunomodulators—Anthracenedione Derivative	Mitoxantrone	Treatment of worsening forms of RRMS and secondary progressive MS (SPMS) to reduce frequency of relapses and slow progression	Cardiac toxicity; generally can be tolerated only up to an accumulated dose of 100-140 mg/m^2	FDA recommends that LVEF be evaluated before initiating therapy, prior to each dose, and annually after patients have finished treatment to detect late-occurring cardiac toxicity
Immunomodulators-Monoclonal Antibody (mAb)	Natalizumab	Treatment of RRMS to reduce frequency of episodes and slow progression of disability Treatment of moderate to severe Crohn's disease	Headache, joint pain, injection site reaction, edema, and infusion reaction	Increases the risk of developing progressive multifocal leukoencephalopathy (PML)

CHAPTER 24

Pulmonary Pharmacology

This chapter will be most useful after having a basic understanding of the material in Chapter 36, Pulmonary Pharmacology in *Goodman & Gilman's The Pharmacological Basis of Therapeutics*, 12th Edition. In addition to the material presented here, the 12th Edition contains:

- A description of the pathogenesis of asthma, including Figure 36-1: Cellular mechanisms of asthma
- A description of the pathogenesis of chronic obstructive pulmonary disease (COPD), including Figure 36-2: Cellular mechanisms in chronic obstructive pulmonary disease
- A description of the various routes of drug delivery to the lungs, including Figure 36-3: Schematic representation of the deposition of inhaled drugs
- The molecular structures of some of the drugs used to treat asthma, COPD, and other pulmonary diseases

LEARNING OBJECTIVES

- ☑ Understand the mechanisms of action of bronchodilator drugs used to relax airway smooth muscle and drugs used to prevent bronchoconstriction.
- ☑ Understand the anti-inflammatory mechanism of action of corticosteroids, and the role of inhaled and oral corticosteroids in the pharmacotherapy of asthma.
- ☑ Understand the mechanism of action of mucolytic agents.
- ☑ Understand the mechanisms of action of antitussive drugs.
- ☑ Understand the mechanisms of action of drugs used to treat pulmonary artery hypertension (PAH).
- ☑ Know the untoward effects of the various bronchodilator drugs, corticosteroids, antitussive drugs, and drugs used to treat PAH.
- ☑ Know which patients should be treated and when treatment should be initiated in patients with asthma, COPD, and PAH.
- ☑ Know which drugs are most effective in treating patients with asthma, COPD, and PAH.
- ☑ Know which drugs can be used in combination to treat asthma, COPD, and PAH.

DRUGS INCLUDED IN THIS CHAPTER

- Albuterol (salbutamol; VENTOLIN, PROVENTIL, ACCUNEB, others)
- Ambrisentan (LETAIRIS)
- Arformoterol (BROVENA)
- Beclomethasone dipropionate (QVAR)
- Benzonatate (TESSALON, others)
- Bosentan (TRACLEER)
- Budesonide (PULMICORT, others)
- Budesonide/formoterol (SYMBICORT)
- Ciclesonide (ALVESCO, OMNARIS)
- Codeine
- Dextromethorphan
- DNAase (dornase alfa, PULMOZYME)
- Doxapram (DOPRAM, others)
- Epoprostenol (prostacyclin, PGI_2; FLOLAN, others)
- Flunisolide (AEROBID)
- Fluticasone (AEROSPAN, FLOVENT)
- Fluticasone/salmeterol (ADVAIR)
- Formoterol (FORADIL, others)
- Guaifenesin
- Hydrocortisone
- Iloprost (VENTAVIS)
- Indacaterol (ARCAPTA NEOHALER)
- Ipratropium bromide (ATROVENT, others)
- Ipratropium/albuterol (COMBIVENT, DUONEB, others)
- Levalbuterol (XOPENEX)
- Metaproterenol (ALUPENT, METAPREL)
- Methylprednisolone
- Mometasone (ASMANEX)
- Montelukast (SINGULAIR)
- *N*-acetylcysteine (MUCOMYST, others)
- Omalizumab
- Pirbuterol (MAXAIR)
- Prednisolone
- Prednisone
- Salmeterol (SEREVENT)

(continues)

MECHANISMS OF ACTION OF DRUGS USED TO TREAT PULMONARY DISORDERS

DRUG CLASS	DRUG	MECHANISM OF ACTION
β_2 Adrenergic Agonists—Short-Acting (3-6 h)	Albuterol (salbutamol) Levalbuterol Metaproterenol Pirbuterol Terbutaline	β_2 Agonists produce bronchodilation by directly stimulating β_2 receptors in airway smooth muscle (see Figure 24-1), resulting in bronchodilation and a rapid decrease in airways resistance. In addition, β_2 agonists act indirectly by inhibiting the release of bronchoconstrictor mediators from inflammatory cells and of bronchoconstrictor neurotransmitters from airway nerves (see Side Bar INDIRECT ACTIONS OF β_2 AGONISTS TO CAUSE BRONCHODILATION)

(Continued)

SECTION IV

Inflammation, Immunomodulation, and Hematopoiesis

DRUGS INCLUDED IN THIS CHAPTER (Cont.)

- Sildenafil (REVATIO)
- Tadalafil (ADCIRCA)
- Terbutaline (BRETHINE, others)
- Tiotropium bromide (SPIRIVA)
- Treprostinil (REMODULIN, TYVASO)
- Triamcinolone (AZMACORT, others)
- Zafirlukast (ACCOLATE)
- Zileuton (ZYFLO)

DRUG CLASS	DRUG	MECHANISM OF ACTION
β_2 Adrenergic Agonists—Long-Acting (Long-Acting β Agonists [LABAs]; duration >12 h)	Salmeterol Formoterol Arformoterol Indacaterol	β_2 Agonists produce bronchodilation by directly stimulating β_2 receptors in airway smooth muscle (see Figure 24-1), resulting in bronchodilation and a rapid decrease in airways resistance. In addition, β_2 agonists act indirectly by inhibiting the release of bronchoconstrictor mediators from inflammatory cells and of bronchoconstrictor neurotransmitters from airway nerves (see Side Bar INDIRECT ACTIONS OF β_2 AGONISTS TO CAUSE BRONCHODILATION)
Methylxanthines	Theophylline	Mechanisms are uncertain, but nonselective PDE inhibition is likely to be important in bronchodilator effects; adenosine receptor antagonism may be an important mechanism in nonbronchodilator effects (see Figure 24-2)
Muscarinic Cholinergic Antagonists	Ipratropium bromide Tiotropium bromide	Competitively inhibit acetylcholine at muscarinic receptors on bronchial smooth muscle (see Chapter 6)
Corticosteroids—Inhaled Corticosteroids (ICSs)	Beclomethasone dipropionate Triamcinolone Flunisolide Budesonide Fluticasone Mometasone Ciclesonide	Glucocorticoid receptor agonists that reduce inflammation by altering expression of proinflammatory genes and other genes, primarily in airways cells (see Figures 24-3 and 24-4, and Chapter 29)
Corticosteroids—Systemic	Hydrocortisone Methylprednisolone Prednisolone Prednisone	Glucocorticoid receptor agonists that reduce inflammation by altering expression of proinflammatory genes and other genes in a variety of cells (see Figures 24-3 and 24-4; and Chapter 29)
Antileukotrienes—5'-Lipoxygenase (5-LOX) Inhibitors	Zileuton	Inhibit the formation of cysteinyl-leukotrienes (LTs), thus blocking the effects of LTs on airways cells (see Figure 24-5 and Chapter 22)
Antileukotrienes—Leukotriene Antagonists	Montelukast Zafirlukast	Inhibit the binding of cysteinyl-leukotrienes (LTs) to CysLT1 receptors on airways cells (see Figure 24-5 and Chapter 22)
Anti-IgE Monoclonal Antibodies	Omalizumab	Humanized monoclonal antibody that blocks the binding of IgE to high-affinity IgE receptors (FcϵR1) on mast cells and thus prevents their activation by allergens; also blocks IgE binding to low-affinity receptors on inflammatory cells thus reducing chronic inflammation
Mucolytics	N-acetylcysteine DNAase (dornase alfa)	N-acetylcysteine reduces disulfide bridges that bind glycoproteins to other proteins. DNAse reduces mucus viscosity in sputum of patients with cystic fibrosis
Expectorants	Guaifenesin	Appear to act by reducing release and/or production of mucins, thus thinning mucus and enhancing mucociliary clearance

(Continued)

Pulmonary Pharmacology

CHAPTER 24

DRUG CLASS	DRUG	MECHANISM OF ACTION
Antitussives	Codeine Dextromethorphan Benzonatate	Codeine and other opiates are agonists at μ opioid receptors in the central nervous system (CNS) medullary cough center, and may have additional peripheral action on cough receptors in the proximal airways (see Chapter 10) Dextromethorphan is a centrally active *N*-methyl-D-aspartate (NMDA) receptor antagonist Benzonatate acts peripherally by anesthetizing the stretch receptors located in the respiratory passages, lungs, and pleura
Ventilatory Stimulants	Doxapram	Stimulates carotid chemoreceptors, and at higher doses it stimulates medullary respiratory centers
Prostacyclin (PGI_2) and Its Analogs	Epoprostenol Treprostinil Iloprost	Bind IP receptors on pulmonary vascular smooth muscle cells, causing an increase in cyclic adenosine monophosphate (cAMP) and smooth muscle relaxation (see Chapter 22)
Endothelin-1 Receptor Antagonists	Bosentan Ambrisentan	Bosentan is an antagonist of both ET_A and ET_B receptors on vascular smooth muscle cells, inhibiting ET-1–induced pulmonary vasoconstriction Ambrisentan is a selective ET_A receptor antagonist
Phosphodiesterase-5 (PDE5) Inhibitors	Sildenafil Tadalafil	Inhibiting PDE5 activity in vascular smooth muscle causes an increase in cyclic guanosine monophosphate (cGMP) leading to vasodilation

INDIRECT ACTIONS OF $β_2$ AGONISTS TO CAUSE BRONCHODILATION

- Prevention of mediator release from human lung mast cells (via $β_2$ receptors)
- Prevention of microvascular leakage and thus the development of bronchial mucosal edema after exposure to mediators, such as histamine and leukotriene D_4
- Increase in mucus secretion from submucosal glands and ion transport across airway epithelium; these effects may enhance mucociliary clearance, and thereby reverse the defective mucus clearance found in asthma
- Reduction in neurotransmission in human airway cholinergic nerves by an action at presynaptic $β_2$ receptors to inhibit acetylcholine release, which may contribute to their bronchodilator effect by reducing reflex cholinergic bronchoconstriction

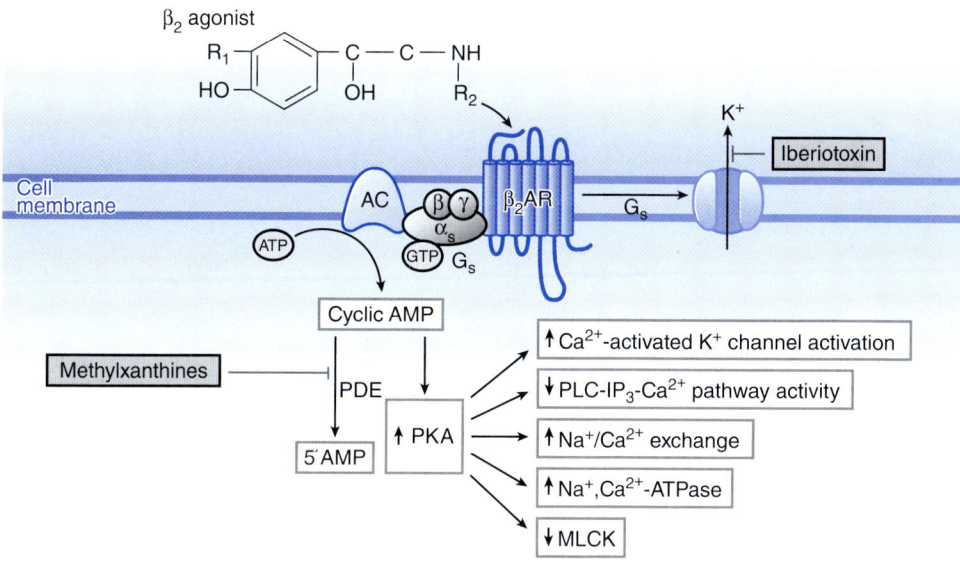

FIGURE 24-1 Molecular actions of $β_2$ agonists to induce relaxation of airway smooth muscle cells. Activation of $β_2$ receptors ($β_2$AR) results in activation of adenylyl cyclase (AC) via a stimulatory G protein intracellular cyclic adenosine monophosphate (cAMP) and activation of protein kinase A (PKA). PKA phosphorylates a variety of target substrates, resulting in opening of Ca^{2+}-activated K^+ channels (K_{Ca}), thereby facilitating hyperpolarization, decreased phosphoinositide (PI) hydrolysis, increased Na^+/Ca^{2+} exchange, increased Na^+,Ca^{2+}-ATPase activity, and decreased myosin light chain kinase (MLCK) activity. $β_2$ Receptors may also couple to K_{Ca} via G_s. PDE, cyclic nucleotide phosphodiesterase.

SECTION IV — Inflammation, Immunomodulation, and Hematopoiesis

SIDE EFFECTS OF β_2 AGONISTS

- Muscle tremor (direct effect on skeletal muscle β_2 receptors)
- Tachycardia (direct effect on atrial β_2 receptors, reflex effect from increased peripheral vasodilation via β_2 receptors)
- Hypokalemia (direct β_2 effect on skeletal muscle uptake of K^+)
- Restlessness
- Hypoxemia (increased $\dot{V}/\dot{Q}$ mismatch due to reversal of hypoxic pulmonary vasoconstriction)

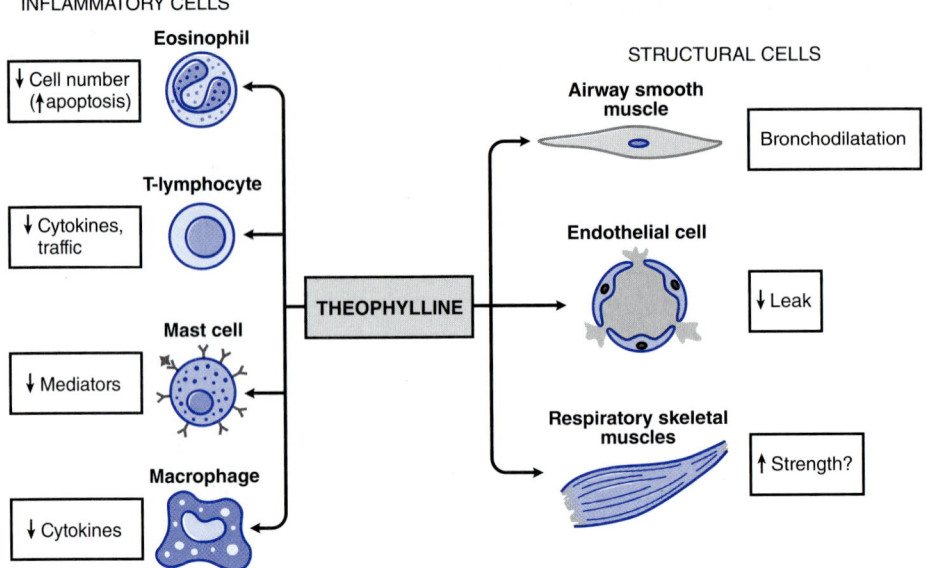

FIGURE 24-2 Theophylline affects multiple cells types in the airway.

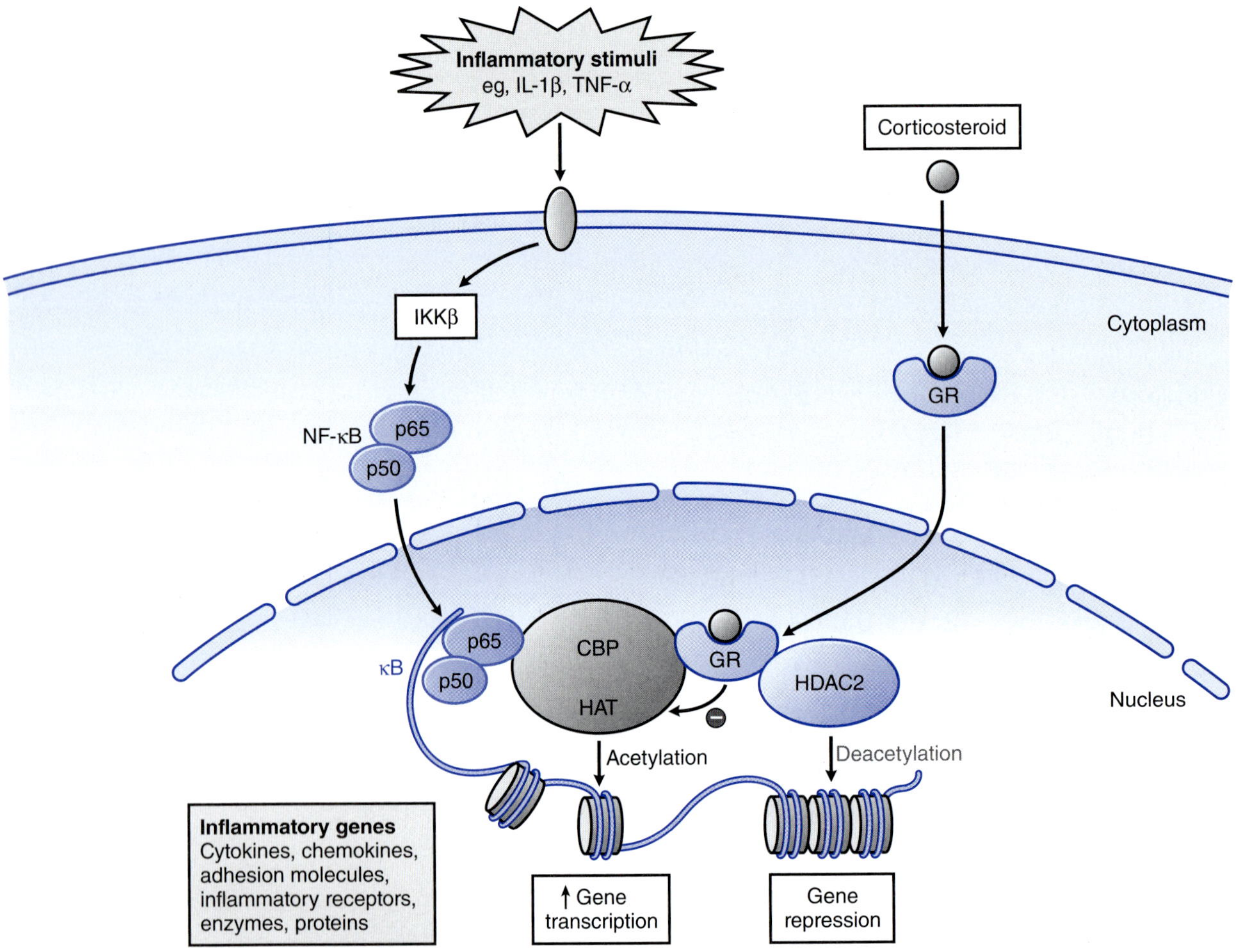

FIGURE 24-3 Mechanism of anti-inflammatory action of corticosteroids in asthma. Inflammatory genes are activated by inflammatory stimuli (IL-1β, TNF-α, etc), resulting in activation of IKKβ (inhibitor of I-κB kinase-β), which activates the transcription factor nuclear factor κB (NF-κB). A dimer of p50 and p65 NF-κB proteins translocates to the nucleus and binds to specific κB recognition sites and also to coactivators, such as CREB-binding protein (CBP), which have intrinsic histone acetyltransferase (HAT) activity. This results in acetylation of core histones and consequent increased expression of genes encoding multiple inflammatory proteins. Cytosolic glucocorticoid receptors (GR) bind corticosteroids; the receptor-ligand complexes translocate to the nucleus and bind to coactivators to inhibit HAT activity in 2 ways: directly and, more importantly, by recruiting histone deacetylase-2 (HDAC2), which reverses histone acetylation, leading to the suppression of activated inflammatory genes.

Pulmonary Pharmacology

CHAPTER 24

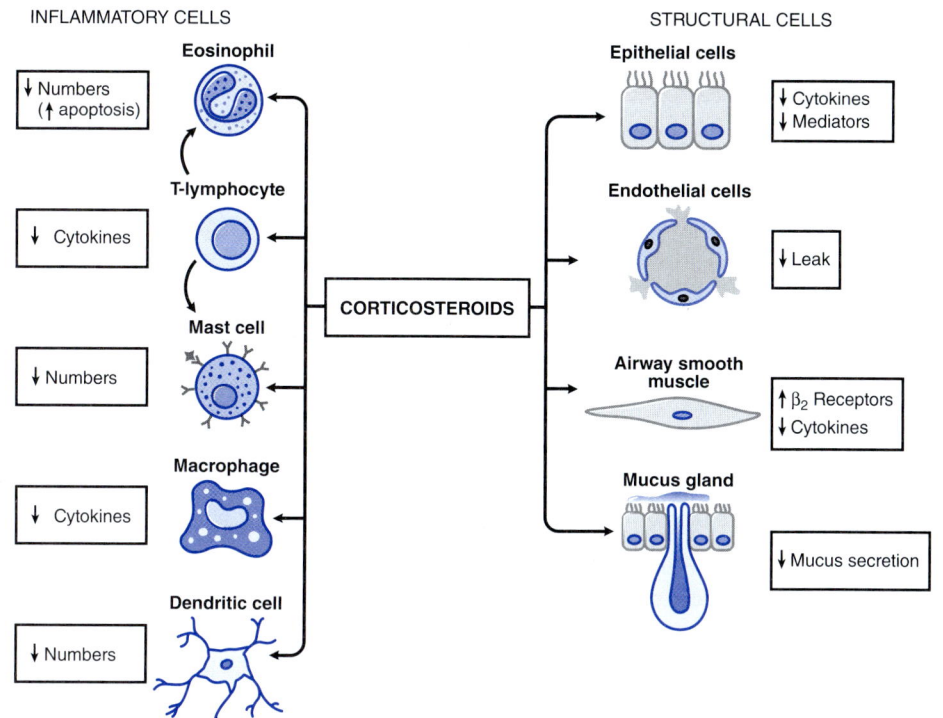

FIGURE 24-4 Effect of corticosteroids on inflammatory and structural cells in the airways.

SIDE EFFECTS OF INHALED CORTICOSTEROIDS

- Local side effects
  - Dysphonia
  - Oropharyngeal candidiasis
  - Cough
- Systemic side effects
  - Adrenal suppression and insufficiency
  - Growth suppression
  - Bruising
  - Osteoporosis
  - Cataracts
  - Glaucoma
  - Metabolic abnormalities (glucose, insulin, triglycerides)
  - Psychiatric disturbances (euphoria, depression)
  - Pneumonia

CASE 24-1

An 8-year-old boy has occasional episodes of mild asthma while playing basketball with his friends.

a. What are the symptoms of asthma and some of the underlying pathogenic events that cause these symptoms?

Asthma is characterized by variable airflow obstruction caused by airway smooth muscle contraction. It is a chronic inflammatory disease of the airways that is characterized by activation of mast cells, infiltration of eosinophils and T helper 2 (T_H2) lymphocytes. Mast cell activation by allergens and physical stimuli releases bronchoconstrictor mediators, such as histamine, leukotriene D_4, and prostaglandin D_2, which cause bronchoconstriction, microvascular leakage, and plasma exudation. Increased numbers of mast cells in airway smooth muscle are a characteristic of asthma.

The mechanism of chronic inflammation in asthma is still not well understood. It may initially be driven by allergen exposure, but it appears to become autonomous so that asthma is essentially incurable. Asthma usually starts in early childhood, and then may disappear during adolescence and reappear in adulthood. Asthma severity usually does not change so that patients with mild asthma rarely progress to severe asthma, and patients with severe asthma usually have this from the onset, although some patients, particularly with late-onset asthma, show a progressive loss of lung function like patients with COPD.

b. What treatment, if any, should this patient receive to relieve symptoms during an asthma attack?

Inhaled short-acting β_2 agonists are the most widely used and effective bronchodilators in the treatment of asthma due to their functional antagonism of bronchoconstriction. When inhaled from pressurized metered-dose inhalers (pMDIs) or dry powder inhalers (DPI), they are convenient, easy to use, rapid in onset, and without significant systemic side effects. In addition to their acute bronchodilator effect, these agents are effective in protecting against various challenges, such as exercise, cold air, and allergens.

(Continued)

SECTION IV — Inflammation, Immunomodulation, and Hematopoiesis

c. What are the mechanisms of action of β_2 agonists in treating asthma?

β_2 Agonists produce bronchodilation by directly stimulating β_2 receptors in airway smooth muscle (see Figure 24-1). β_2 Agonists act as functional antagonists and reverse bronchoconstriction irrespective of the contractile agent. This is an important property for the treatment of asthma because many bronchoconstrictor mechanisms (neurotransmitters and mediators) are likely to be contributory. β_2 Agonists may also indirectly cause bronchodilation by inhibiting the release of bronchoconstrictor mediators from inflammatory cells and of bronchoconstrictor neurotransmitters from airway nerves (see Side Bar INDIRECT ACTIONS OF β_2 AGONISTS TO CAUSE BRONCHODILATION). Although these additional effects of β_2 agonists may be relevant to the prophylactic use of these drugs against various challenges, their rapid bronchodilator action is probably attributable to a direct effect on airway smooth muscle.

d. If the asthma attacks occur more frequently, what changes in therapy might be appropriate for this patient?

Short-acting inhaled β_2 agonists, such as albuterol, should be used "as required" by symptoms and not on a regular basis in the treatment of mild asthma; increased use indicates the need for more effective anti-inflammatory therapy, that is, corticosteroids. Inhaled corticosteroids (ICSs) are recommended as first-line therapy for all patients with persistent asthma. They should be started in any patient who needs to use a β_2 agonist inhaler for symptom control more than twice weekly. They are effective in mild, moderate, and severe asthma and in children as well as adults. ICS may be used in children in the same way as in adults; at doses of 400 µg/d or less, there is no evidence of significant growth suppression. The dose of ICSs should be the minimal dose that controls asthma; once control is achieved, the dose should be slowly reduced.

CASE 24-2

A 72-year-old woman has chronic difficulty in breathing. She has smoked a pack of cigarettes every day for the last 55 years and was diagnosed as having COPD 15 years ago.

a. What is COPD and how does it differ from asthma?

Chronic obstructive pulmonary disease (COPD) involves inflammation of the respiratory tract with a pattern that differs from that of asthma. In COPD, there is a predominance of neutrophils, macrophages, and cytotoxic T lymphocytes (Tc1 cells). The inflammation predominantly affects small airways, resulting in progressive small airway narrowing and fibrosis (chronic obstructive bronchiolitis) and destruction of the lung parenchyma with destruction of the alveolar walls (emphysema). These pathological changes result in airway closure on expiration, leading to air trapping and hyperinflation, particularly on exercise (dynamic hyperinflation). This accounts for shortness of breath on exertion and exercise limitation that are characteristic symptoms of COPD.

In contrast to asthma, the airflow obstruction of COPD tends to be progressive. The inflammation in the peripheral lung of COPD patients is mediated by multiple inflammatory mediators and cytokines, although the pattern of mediators differs from that of asthma. In marked contrast to asthma, the inflammation in patients with COPD is largely corticosteroid-resistant, and there are currently no effective anti-inflammatory treatments for this disease. In addition to pulmonary disease, many patients with COPD have systemic manifestations (skeletal muscle wasting, weight loss, depression, osteoporosis, anemia) and comorbid diseases (ischemic heart disease, hypertension, congestive heart failure, diabetes). Whether these are due to spillover of inflammatory mediators from the lung or due to common causal mechanisms (such as smoking) is not yet clear, but it may be important to treat the systemic components in the overall management of COPD.

b. What treatments are available for this patient?

Bronchodilators are the mainstay of treatment in COPD and act to reduce air trapping by dilating peripheral airways. Anticholinergic drugs (ipratropium bromide and

(Continued)

Pulmonary Pharmacology

CHAPTER 24

tiotropium bromide) are the bronchodilators of choice in COPD, and are as effective as or even superior to β_2 agonists. Their relatively greater effect in COPD than in asthma may be explained by an inhibitory effect on vagal tone, which, although not necessarily increased in COPD, may be the only reversible element of airway obstruction and one that is exaggerated by geometric factors in the narrowed airways of COPD. Anticholinergic drugs reduce air trapping and improve exercise tolerance in COPD patients. Once-daily tiotropium is more effective than ipratropium 4 times daily. When given long term, tiotropium improves lung function and health status and reduces exacerbations and all-cause mortality, although there is no effect on disease progression. As a result, tiotropium is becoming the bronchodilator of choice for patients with COPD.

The long-acting inhaled β_2 agonists (LABAs) salmeterol, formoterol, and arformoterol are also used in COPD therapy. These drugs have a bronchodilator action of more than 12 hours and also protect against bronchoconstriction for a similar period. LABAs are effective bronchodilators that may be used alone or in combination with anticholinergics or ICSs. LABAs improve symptoms and exercise tolerance by reducing both air trapping and exacerbations.

Combination inhalers of an anticholinergic and β_2 agonist, such as ipratropium/albuterol, are widely used in patients with COPD. Several studies have demonstrated additive effects of these 2 drugs, thus providing an advantage over increasing the dose of β_2 agonist in patients who have side effects.

Combination inhalers that contain a LABA and a corticosteroid (eg, fluticasone/salmeterol, budesonide/formoterol) are also used in the treatment of COPD. These combination inhalers are more effective in patients with COPD than monotherapy with either a LABA or an ICS. Although patients with COPD occasionally respond to steroids alone, these patients are likely to have concomitant asthma. Corticosteroids have no objective short-term benefit on airway function in patients with true COPD, although these agents often produce subjective benefit because of their euphoric effect. Corticosteroids do not appear to have any significant anti-inflammatory effect in COPD.

Theophylline, an agent with multiple sites of action (see Figure 24-2), is sometimes used as a bronchodilator in COPD, but inhaled anticholinergics and β_2 agonists are preferred. Theophylline tends to be added to these inhaled bronchodilators in more severe patients and has been shown to give additional clinical improvement when added to a long-acting β_2 agonist.

c. What side effects are to be expected with inhaled anticholinergic drugs?

Inhaled anticholinergic drugs are generally well tolerated. On stopping inhaled anticholinergics, a small rebound increase in airway responsiveness has been described, but the clinical relevance of this is uncertain. Systemic side effects after ipratropium bromide and tiotropium bromide are uncommon during normal clinical use because there is little systemic absorption. A significant unwanted effect is the unpleasant bitter taste of inhaled ipratropium, which may contribute to poor compliance. Nebulized ipratropium bromide may precipitate glaucoma in elderly patients due to a direct effect of the nebulized drug on the eye. This may be prevented by nebulization with a mouthpiece rather than a face mask. Tiotropium causes dryness of the mouth in 10 to 15% of patients, but this usually disappears during continued therapy. Urinary retention is occasionally seen in elderly patients.

CASE 24-3

A 46-year-old woman has suffered from severe asthma since she was a girl. She complains of difficulty breathing nearly all of the time and occasionally has asthma attacks that are very severe.

a. What pharmacotherapeutic options are appropriate in this patient to improve her symptoms?

Because asthma is a chronic inflammatory disease, ICSs are considered as first-line therapy in all but the mildest of cases. Corticosteroids inhibit the expression of

(Continued)

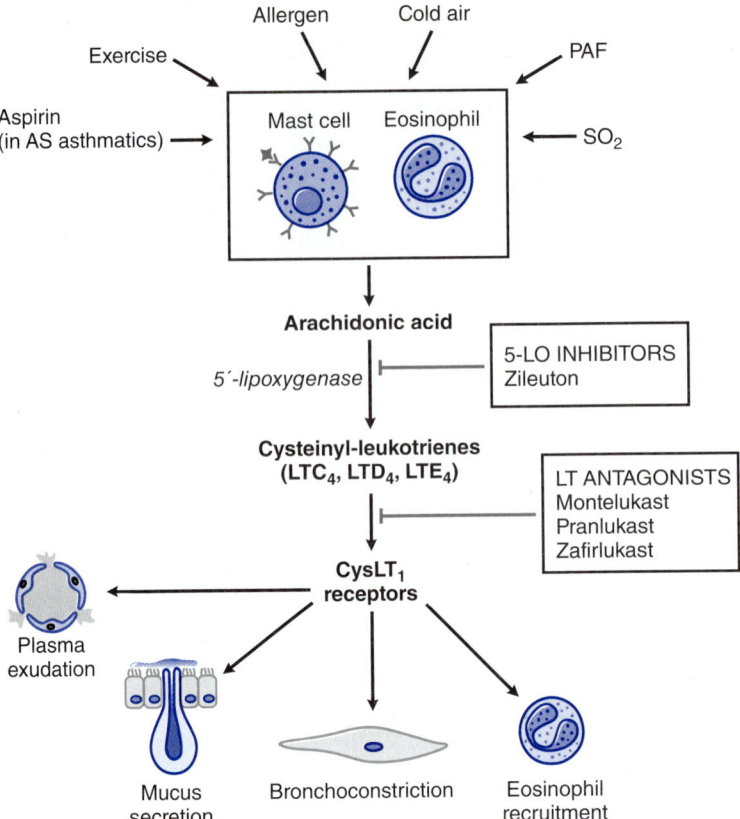

FIGURE 24-5 Effects of cysteinyl-leukotrienes on the airways and their inhibition by antileukotrienes. AS, aspirin-sensitive; 5-LO, 5′-lipoxygenase; LT, leukotriene; PAF, platelet-activating factor.

multiple inflammatory genes in airway epithelial cells, probably the most important action of ICSs in suppressing asthmatic inflammation (see Figure 24-3). Corticosteroids also increase the transcription of several anti-inflammatory genes. Steroids have inhibitory effects on many inflammatory and structural cells that are activated in asthma and prevent the recruitment of inflammatory cells into the airways (see Figure 24-4).

For most patients, ICSs should be used twice daily, a regimen that improves compliance once control of asthma has been achieved (which may require 4-times daily dosing initially or a course of oral steroids if symptoms are severe). Administration once daily of some steroids (eg, budesonide, mometasone, and ciclesonide) is effective when doses of 400 μg or less are needed. The dose of ICS should be the minimal dose that controls asthma; once control is achieved, the dose should be slowly reduced. ICSs have rapid anti-inflammatory effects, reducing airway hyperresponsiveness and inflammatory mediator concentrations within a few hours. However, it may take several weeks or months to achieve maximal effects on airway hyperresponsiveness, presumably reflecting the slow healing of the damaged inflamed airway. It is important to recognize that corticosteroids suppress inflammation in the airways but do not cure the underlying disease; when steroids are withdrawn, there is a recurrence of the same degree of airway hyperresponsiveness.

For this patient's acute severe asthma attacks, inhaled short-acting β_2 agonists are the bronchodilators of choice. The LABAs, salmeterol, formoterol, and arformoterol, are important in controlling asthma in patients with chronic symptoms. These drugs have a bronchodilator action of more than 12 hours and also protect against bronchoconstriction for a similar period. They improve asthma control (when given twice daily) compared with regular treatment with short-acting β_2 agonists (4-6 times daily).

(Continued)

Pulmonary Pharmacology

CHAPTER 24

Combination inhalers that contain a LABA and a corticosteroid (eg, fluticasone/salmeterol, budesonide/formoterol) are widely used in the treatment of persistent asthma. In asthma, there is a strong scientific rationale for combining a LABA with a corticosteroid because these treatments have complementary synergistic actions. The combination inhaler is more convenient for patients, simplifies therapy, and improves compliance with ICSs because the patients perceive clinical benefit, but there may be an additional advantage because delivering the 2 drugs in the same inhaler ensures they are delivered simultaneously to the same cells in the airways, allowing the beneficial molecular interactions between LABA and corticosteroids to occur. It is likely that these inhalers will become the preferred therapy for all patients with persistent asthma.

In asthmatic patients, anticholinergic drugs are less effective as bronchodilators than β_2 agonists and offer less efficient protection against bronchial challenges. These drugs may be more effective in older patients with asthma in whom there is an element of fixed airway obstruction. Anticholinergics are currently used as an additional bronchodilator in asthmatic patients not controlled on a LABA. Nebulized anticholinergic drugs are effective in acute severe asthma, but less effective than β_2 agonists. Nevertheless, in the acute and chronic treatment of asthma, anticholinergic drugs may have an additive effect with β_2 agonists and should therefore be considered when control of asthma is not adequate with nebulized β_2 agonists.

Theophylline can play a role as add-on therapy to ICS, although it is less effective as an add-on than a LABA. Although LABAs are more effective as an add-on therapy, theophylline is considerably less expensive and may be the only affordable add-on treatment when the costs of medication are limiting.

In patients with mild to moderate asthma, antileukotrienes (see Figure 24-5) cause a significant improvement in lung function and asthma symptoms, with a reduction in the use of rescue-inhaled β_2 agonists. Antileukotrienes are indicated as an add-on therapy in patients who are not well controlled on ICS therapy. The added benefit is small, equivalent to doubling the dose of ICS, and less effective than adding a LABA. In patients with severe asthma who are not controlled on high doses of ICS and LABA, antileukotrienes do not appear to provide any additional benefit.

Omalizumab, a humanized monoclonal antibody that blocks the binding of IgE to its receptors, is used for the treatment of patients with severe asthma. The antibody is administered by subcutaneous injection every 2 to 4 weeks, and the dose is determined by the titer of circulating IgE. Omalizumab reduces the requirement for oral and ICSs and markedly reduces asthma exacerbations. Because of its very high cost, this treatment is generally used only in patients with very severe asthma who are poorly controlled even on oral corticosteroids and in those with very severe concomitant allergic rhinitis.

b. Are there side effects or concerns with long-term use of ICSs and LABAs?

Suppression of the hypothalamic-pituitary-adrenal (HPA) axis by a negative feedback effect of corticosteroids on the pituitary gland (see Chapter 29) can occur with long-term use of oral corticosteroids and high daily doses of ICSs (ie, >2000 µg beclomethasone dipropionate or its equivalent daily). Systemic side effects of ICSs (see Side Bar SIDE EFFECTS OF INHALED CORTICOSTEROIDS) include dermal thinning and skin capillary fragility (relatively common in elderly patients after high-dose inhaled steroids). Other side effects, such as cataract formation, glaucoma, and osteoporosis, are reported but often in patients who are also receiving courses of oral steroids. Budesonide, fluticasone, mometasone, and ciclesonide have a lower oral bioavailability than beclomethasone dipropionate because they are subject to greater first-pass hepatic metabolism; this results in reduced systemic absorption from the fraction of the inhaled drug that is swallowed. Ciclesonide is a prodrug that is converted to the active metabolite by esterases in the lung, giving it a low oral bioavailability and a high therapeutic index.

ICSs may have local side effects due to the deposition of inhaled steroid in the oropharynx (see Side Bar SIDE EFFECTS OF INHALED CORTICOSTEROIDS). The most

(Continued)

common problem is hoarseness and weakness of the voice (dysphonia) due to atrophy of the vocal cords following laryngeal deposition of steroid; it may occur in up to 40% of patients and is noticed particularly by patients who need to use their voices during their work (lecturers, teachers, and singers). Oropharyngeal candidiasis occurs in ~5% of patients. There is no evidence for increased lung infections, including tuberculosis, in patients with asthma. When high doses of an ICS are required, a large volume spacer is recommended to reduce oropharyngeal deposition and systemic absorption.

Side effects are not common with inhaled LABA therapy. Muscle tremor is the most common side effect, and there are several other side effects related to stimulation of extrapulmonary β_2 receptors (see Side Bar SIDE EFFECTS OF β_2 AGONISTS). Tolerance to nonairway β_2 receptor–mediated responses, such as tremor and cardiovascular and metabolic responses, is readily induced in asthmatic patients, but tolerance to the bronchodilator effects of β_2 agonists has not usually been found. The reason for the relative resistance of airway smooth muscle β_2 responses to desensitization may reflect the large receptor reserve in airway smooth muscle compared to other tissues. The safety of LABAs in asthma remains controversial based on large-scale studies of asthma patients prescribed salmeterol and formoterol that showed an excess of respiratory deaths and near deaths. However, concomitant treatment with an ICS appears to obviate such risk, so it is recommended that LABAs should only be used when ICSs are also prescribed (preferably in the form of a combination inhaler so that the LABA can never be taken without the ICSs). All LABAs approved in the United States carry a black box warning cautioning against overuse.

CASE 24-4

A 76-year-old woman who complains of difficulty breathing due to pulmonary congestion is diagnosed with pulmonary artery hypertension (PAH).

a. What drugs should be considered in treating this patient's PAH?

PAH involves dysfunction of pulmonary vascular endothelial and smooth muscle cells, and results from an imbalance in vasoconstrictor and vasodilator mediators (see Figure 24-6). In PAH, there is an increase in the vasoconstrictor mediators endothelin-1 (ET-1), thromboxane A_2, and serotonin, and a decrease in the vasodilating mediators prostacyclin (PGI_2), NO, and VIP. Vasodilators are the mainstay of drug therapy for PAH (see Figure 24-6). However, the vasodilators used to treat systemic hypertension are problematic; they lower systemic blood pressure, which may result in reduced pulmonary perfusion.

Intravenous epoprostenol (prostacyclin, PGI_2) is effective in lowering pulmonary arterial pressures, improving exercise performance, and prolonging survival in primary PAH (PPAH), but must be administered by continuous IV infusion because of its short plasma $t_{1/2}$; this is inconvenient and therapy is very expensive. More stable prostacyclin analogs (treprostinil and iloprost) can be administered by other routes, including inhalation.

Bosentan and ambrisentan are oral endothelin receptor antagonists used for the treatment of PPAH. These agents differ in their selectivity for ET receptors. Stimulation of ET_A receptors by ET-1 contracts vascular smooth muscle cells and causes proliferation mainly, whereas ET_B receptors mediate the release of prostacyclin and NO from endothelial cells (see Figure 24-6). Bosentan is an antagonist of both ET_A and ET_B receptors, and is efficacious orally in reducing symptoms and improving mortality in PPAH. Ambrisentan is a selective ET_A receptor antagonist. The theoretical advantage of blocking only ET_A receptors is that ET_B receptors may continue to stimulate release of PGI_2 and NO, giving a greater therapeutic effect. However, the clinical efficacy of ambrisentan is similar to that of bosentan, as are its adverse effects.

The oral phosphodiesterase-5 (PDE5) inhibitors, sildenafil and tadalafil, are effective in improving symptoms of PAH because of their ability to induce vasodilation by elevating intracellular cyclic guanosine monophosphate (cGMP) concentrations in pulmonary artery smooth muscle (see Figure 24-6).

(Continued)

Pulmonary Pharmacology
CHAPTER 24

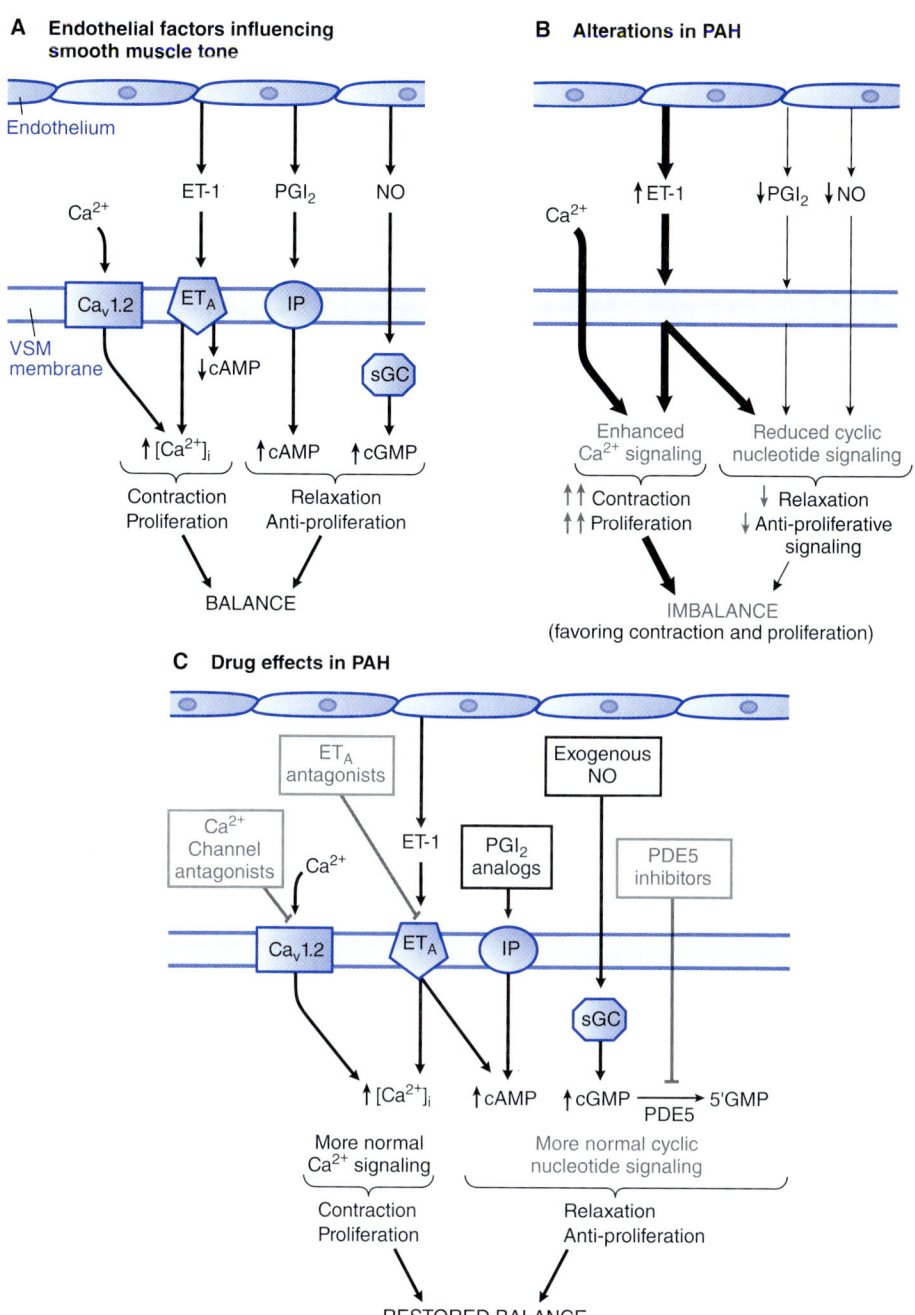

FIGURE 24-6 Interactions of endothelium and vascular smooth muscle in pulmonary artery hypertension (PAH). **A.** In normal pulmonary artery, there is a balance between constrictor and relaxant influences that may be viewed as competition between Ca^{2+} signaling pathways and cyclic nucleotide signaling pathways in vascular smooth muscle (VSM). Endothelin (ET-1) binds to the ET_A receptor on VSM cells and activates the G_q-PLC-IP_3 pathway to increase cytosolic Ca^{2+}; ET-1 may also couple to G_i to inhibit cyclic adenosine monophosphate (cAMP) production. In depolarizing VSM cells, Ca^{2+} may enter via the L-type Ca^{2+} channel ($Ca_v1.2$). Endothelial cells also produce relaxant factors, prostacyclin (PGI_2) and NO. NO stimulates the soluble guanylyl cyclase (cGC), causing accumulation of cyclic guanosine monophosphate (cGMP) in VSM cells; PGI_2 binds to the IP prostanoid receptor and stimulates the G_s-adenylyl cyclase pathway to enhance cAMP accumulation; elevation of these cyclic nucleotides promotes VSM relaxation (see Chapter 1). **B.** In PAH, ET-1 production is enhanced, production of PGI_2 and NO is reduced, and the balance is shifted toward constriction and proliferation of vascular smooth muscle. **C.** In treating PAH, ET_A receptor antagonists can reduce the constrictor effects of ET-1, and Ca^{2+} channel antagonists can further reduce Ca^{2+}-dependent contraction. Exogenous PGI_2 and NO can be supplied to promote vasodilation (relaxation of VSM); inhibition of PDE5 can enhance the relaxant effect of NO by inhibiting the degradation of cGMP, thereby promoting intracellular accumulation of cGMP and relaxation of VSM. Thus, these drugs can reduce Ca^{2+} signaling and enhance cyclic nucleotide signaling, restoring the balance between the forces of contraction/proliferation and relaxation/antiproliferation. Remodeling and deposition of extracellular matrix by adjacent fibroblasts is influenced positively and negatively by the same contractile and relaxant signaling pathways, respectively.

SECTION IV

Inflammation, Immunomodulation, and Hematopoiesis

b. What are the side effects associated with each of these agents?

Common side effects of IV epoprostenol are headache, flushing, diarrhea, nausea, and jaw pain. Inhaled iloprost is associated with the vasodilator effects of prostacyclin, including syncope. It may also cause cough and bronchoconstriction because it sensitizes airway sensory nerves.

The endothelin receptor antagonists are generally well tolerated and have similar side effect profiles. Adverse effects include abnormal liver function tests, anemia, headaches, peripheral edema, and nasal congestion. Given the risk of serious liver injury, liver aminotransferases should be monitored monthly. All endothelin receptor antagonists carry a risk of testicular atrophy and infertility. Bosentan is potentially teratogenic.

The PDE5 inhibitors, side effects are due in part to systemic hypotension (headache and flushing). Other side effects include dyspepsia and visual disturbances. Because of the risk of severe hypotension, concurrent administration with nitrovasodilators should be avoided (see Chapter 16).

CASE 24-5

A 54-year-old male patient complains of chronic cough. He is not a smoker, does not have asthma, but has a history of gastroesophageal reflux disease (GERD).

a. What treatments are most appropriate to reduce this patient's chronic cough?

Cough is a defensive reflex and its suppression may be inappropriate because it could mask the underlying cause. Whenever possible, treat the underlying cause, not the cough. A likely cause in this patient is GERD. Gastroesophageal reflux is a common cause of cough through a reflex mechanism and occasionally as a result of acid aspiration into the lungs. This cough may respond to suppression of gastric acid with an H_2 receptor antagonist or a proton pump inhibitor (see Chapter 32), although even large doses may not always be effective. Some patients have a chronic cough with no obvious cause, and this chronic idiopathic cough may be due to airway sensory neural hyperesthesia.

Over-the-counter cough medications containing dextromethorphan are largely ineffective, although they are widely used. Prescription cough suppressants include opiates such as codeine, and benzonatate, a local anesthetic.

KEY CONCEPTS

- Bronchodilators are key drugs in the treatment of asthma and COPD.
- When there is a choice of inhaled or oral route for a pulmonary drug (eg, β_2 agonist or corticosteroid), the inhaled route is always preferable, and the oral route should be reserved for the few patients unable to use inhalers (eg, small children, patients with physical problems such as severe arthritis of the hands).
- Inhaled β_2 agonists are functional antagonists of bronchoconstriction and reverse bronchoconstriction irrespective of the contractile agent.
- An inhaled β_2 agonist is the bronchodilator treatment of choice in asthma because β_2 agonists are the most effective bronchodilators and have minimal side effects when used correctly.
- Inhaled anticholinergic drugs are less effective as bronchodilators than β_2 agonists in patients with asthma, but may be as effective or superior to β_2 agonists in patients with COPD.
- ICSs are recommended as first-line therapy for all patients with persistent asthma (ie, patients who require inhaled β_2 agonists more than twice a week) because asthma is a chronic inflammatory disease.
- ICSs have limited therapeutic value in patients with COPD except in patients with concomitant asthma or severe COPD.

Pulmonary Pharmacology

CHAPTER 24

SUMMARY QUIZ

QUESTION 24-1 A 20-year-old woman has occasional asthma symptoms during the winter when she goes snowshoeing. The medication of choice to relieve her asthma symptoms is inhaled

a. albuterol.
b. salmeterol.
c. tiotropium bromide.
d. iloprost.
e. budesonide.

QUESTION 24-2 A 54-year-old man who had occupational exposure to asbestos has developed COPD and emphysema. The medication of choice to improve his breathing is inhaled

a. albuterol.
b. salmeterol.
c. tiotropium bromide.
d. iloprost.
e. budesonide.

QUESTION 24-3 An asthma patient with persistent asthma is prescribed a combination inhaler, budesonide/formoterol (SYMBICORT). The mechanisms of action of the 2 drugs in this formulation are

a. a long-acting β_2 adrenergic agonist and an anticholinergic.
b. a corticosteroid and a phosphodiesterase inhibitor.
c. an endothelin receptor antagonist and a prostacyclin receptor agonist.
d. a long-acting β_2 adrenergic agonist and a corticosteroid.
e. a corticosteroid and an anticholinergic.

QUESTION 24-4 The mechanistic rationale for using sildenafil to treat PAH is that it

a. increases cGMP synthesis in pulmonary artery smooth muscle.
b. enhances the effects of endothelin-1 in pulmonary artery smooth muscle.
c. enhances the effects of NO in pulmonary artery smooth muscle.
d. enhances the effects of prostacyclin in pulmonary artery smooth muscle.
e. inhibits the effects of endothelin-1 in pulmonary artery smooth muscle.

QUESTION 24-5 The mechanistic rationale for using inhaled ipratropium to treat COPD is that it

a. activates β_2 adrenergic receptor bronchial smooth muscle.
b. binds glucocorticoid receptors in inflammatory cells of the airways.
c. blocks ET-1 binding to ET_A and ET_B receptors in bronchial smooth muscle.
d. blocks binding of acetylcholine to muscarinic cholinergic receptors in bronchial smooth muscle.
e. inhibits the hydrolysis of cyclic nucleotides in bronchial smooth muscle.

SUMMARY QUIZ ANSWER KEY

QUESTION 24-1 Answer is **a**. To relieve occasional asthma symptoms such as those induced by cold air and exercise, the medication of choice is a short-acting β_2 agonist (eg, albuterol) delivered by inhalation.

QUESTION 24-2 Answer is **c**. In COPD, inhaled anticholinergic drugs such as tiotropium are the bronchodilators of choice in most patients. Clinical studies have shown

(Continued)

SECTION IV

Inflammation, Immunomodulation, and Hematopoiesis

that long-term use of tiotropium improves lung function and health status, and reduces exacerbations and all-cause mortality, although there is no effect on disease progression.

QUESTION 24-3 Answer is **d**. Budesonide is an ICS that has beneficial anti-inflammatory effects in asthma, and formoterol is a LABA that has bronchodilator and bronchoprotective effects. These agents have both complementary and synergistic effects in patients with persistent asthma. The combination inhaler is more convenient for patients, simplifies therapy, and improves compliance with ICS because the patients perceive clinical benefit. In addition, delivering the 2 drugs in the same inhaler ensures they are delivered simultaneously to the same cells in the airways, allowing the beneficial molecular interactions between LABA and corticosteroids to occur.

QUESTION 24-4 Answer is **c**. Sildenafil relaxes pulmonary artery smooth muscle by blocking the hydrolysis of cGMP by PDE5 (see Figure 24-6). Much of the cGMP in vascular smooth muscle is synthesized by soluble guanylate cyclase which is activated by nitric oxide (NO). Thus, sildenafil enhances the vasodilating effects of NO produced endogenously by vascular endothelium.

QUESTION 24-5 Answer is **d**. Ipratropium is a competitive antagonist of endogenous acetylcholine (ACh) binding to muscarinic cholinergic receptors in bronchial smooth muscle (see Chapter 6). Activation of muscarinic receptors on bronchial smooth muscle causes contraction and bronchoconstriction. Multiple and diverse stimuli cause reflex increases in parasympathetic activity that contribute to bronchoconstriction. The effects of ACh on the respiratory system include not only bronchoconstriction but also increased tracheobronchial secretion and stimulation of the chemoreceptors of the carotid and aortic bodies. Thus antimuscarinic drugs antagonizes these various pulmonary effects of acetylcholine released by parasympathetic neurons.

Acetylcholine may also be released from other airway cells, including epithelial cells. The synthesis of acetylcholine in epithelial cells is increased by inflammatory stimuli (such as TNF-α), which increase the expression of choline acetyltransferase, which could contribute to cholinergic effects in airway diseases. Muscarinic receptors are expressed in airway smooth muscle of small airways that do not appear to be innervated by cholinergic nerves; these receptors may be a mechanism of cholinergic narrowing in peripheral airways that could be relevant in COPD, responding to locally synthesized, non-neuronal ACh.

SUMMARY TABLE: DRUGS USED IN THE TREATMENT OF ASTHMA, COPD, AND OTHER PULMONARY DISORDERS

CLASS AND SUBCLASSES	NAMES	CLINICAL USES	TOXICITIES COMMON	TOXICITIES UNIQUE; CLINICALLY IMPORTANT
β_2 Adrenergic Agonists—Short-Acting (3-6 h)	Albuterol (salbutamol) Levalbuterol Metaproterenol Pirbuterol Terbutaline	The most widely used and effective bronchodilators in the treatment of asthma due to their functional antagonism of bronchoconstriction Effective in protecting against various challenges, such as exercise, cold air, and allergens Bronchodilators of choice in treating acute severe asthma	Side effects are not common with inhaled therapy, but quite common with oral or IV administration (see Side Bar SIDE EFFECTS OF β_2 AGONISTS)	Tolerance develops to the bronchoprotective effects of high-dose inhaled β_2 agonists, but not the bronchodilating effects Short-acting inhaled β_2 agonists should only be used on demand for symptom control, and if they are required frequently (more than twice weekly), an ICS is needed
β_2 Adrenergic Agonists—Long-Acting (Long-Acting β Agonists [LABAs] duration >12 h)	Salmeterol Formoterol Arformoterol Indacaterol	Improve asthma control (when given twice daily) compared with regular treatment with short-acting β_2 agonists (4-6 times daily) In COPD, LABAs are effective bronchodilators that may be used alone or in combination with an anticholinergic or ICS	Side effects are not common with inhaled therapy, but quite common with oral or IV administration (see Side Bar SIDE EFFECTS OF β_2 AGONISTS)	In asthma patients, LABAs should never be used alone because they do not treat the underlying chronic inflammation; rather, LABAs should always be used in combination with ICS (preferably in a fixed-dose combination inhaler) All LABAs approved in the United States carry a black box warning cautioning against overuse in asthma

(Continued)

Pulmonary Pharmacology — CHAPTER 24

CLASS AND SUBCLASSES	NAMES	CLINICAL USES	TOXICITIES — COMMON	TOXICITIES — UNIQUE; CLINICALLY IMPORTANT
Methylxanthines	Theophylline	Should be reserved for use as add-on maintenance therapy in asthma patients receiving high- or low-dose ICS or maximal β_2 agonist alone who require additional bronchodilator effect. Added to inhaled anticholinergics and β_2 agonists (LABAs) in patients with severe COPD	Headache, nausea, and vomiting (due to inhibition of PDE4), abdominal discomfort, and restlessness. Increased acid secretion (due to PDE inhibition) and diuresis (due to inhibition of adenosine A_1 receptors)	At high concentrations, cardiac arrhythmias. At very high concentrations, seizures. Low doses (5-10 mg/L) largely avoid side effects
Muscarinic Cholinergic Antagonists	Ipratropium bromide, Tiotropium bromide	Used as an additional bronchodilator in asthmatic patients not controlled on a LABA. In acute and chronic asthma therapy, may have an additive effect with β_2 agonists. In COPD, may be as effective as or even superior to β_2 agonists	Inhaled anticholinergic drugs are generally well tolerated with few systemic effects. Tiotropium causes dryness of the mouth in 10-15% of patients, but this usually disappears during continued therapy	Unpleasant bitter taste of inhaled ipratropium which may contribute to poor compliance. Bronchoconstriction may occur with ipratropium
Corticosteroids—Inhaled Corticosteroids (ICSs)	Beclomethasone dipropionate, Triamcinolone, Flunisolide, Budesonide, Fluticasone, Mometasone, Ciclesonide	ICSs are considered as first-line therapy in all but the mildest of asthma patients and should be started in any patient who needs to use a β_2 agonist inhaler for symptom control more than twice weekly. ICSs are much less effective in COPD and should only be used in patients with severe disease who have frequent exacerbations	See Chapter 29 and Side Bar SIDE EFFECTS OF INHALED CORTICOSTEROIDS. Budesonide, fluticasone, mometasone, and ciclesonide are subject to greater first-pass hepatic metabolism than beclomethasone dipropionate, thus have reduced adverse systemic effects	See Chapter 29 and Side Bar SIDE EFFECTS OF INHALED CORTICOSTEROIDS. All currently available ICSs are absorbed from the lung into the systemic circulation, so that some systemic absorption is inevitable. To reduce likelihood of systemic effects, use the lowest dose of inhaled steroid needed to control the asthma, and use a large-volume spacer to reduce oropharyngeal deposition
Corticosteroids—Systemic	Hydrocortisone, Methylprednisolone, Prednisolone, Prednisone	IV steroids are indicated in acute asthma if lung function is <30% of predicted and there is no improvement with β_2 agonist. Short courses of oral steroids (30-40 mg prednisolone daily for 1-2 weeks) are indicated for exacerbations of asthma. Oral corticosteroids remain the mainstay of treatment of several pulmonary diseases, such as sarcoidosis, interstitial lung diseases, and pulmonary eosinophilic syndromes	Adrenal suppression by a negative feedback effect on the pituitary gland. Significant adrenal suppression after short courses of corticosteroid therapy is not usually a problem, but prolonged suppression may occur after several months or years. Long-term oral corticosteroid side effects include fluid retention, increased appetite, weight gain, osteoporosis, capillary fragility, hypertension, peptic ulceration, diabetes, cataracts, and psychosis (see Chapter 29 for other toxicities and precautions)	Steroid doses after prolonged oral therapy must be reduced slowly; symptoms of "steroid withdrawal syndrome" include lassitude, musculoskeletal pains, and, occasionally, fever (see Chapter 29 for other toxicities and precautions)
Antileukotrienes—5'-Lipoxygenase (5-LOX) Inhibitors	Zileuton	Antileukotrienes are indicated as an add-on therapy in asthma patients who are not well controlled on ICSs		Associated with rare cases of hepatic dysfunction; thus liver-associated enzymes should be monitored

(Continued)

SECTION IV Inflammation, Immunomodulation, and Hematopoiesis

CLASS AND SUBCLASSES	NAMES	CLINICAL USES	TOXICITIES	
			COMMON	UNIQUE; CLINICALLY IMPORTANT
Antileukotrienes—Leukotriene Antagonists	Montelukast Zafirlukast	Antileukotrienes are indicated as an add-on therapy in asthma patients who are not well controlled on ICSs Cys-LT1 receptor antagonists have no role in the therapy of COPD		Associated with rare cases of hepatic dysfunction; thus liver-associated enzymes should be monitored Cases of Churg-Strauss syndrome have been reported
Anti-IgE Monoclonal Antibodies	Omalizumab	Used for the treatment of patients with severe asthma who are poorly controlled even on oral corticosteroids and in patients with very severe concomitant allergic rhinitis		Major side effect is an anaphylactic response, which is uncommon (<0.1%)
Mucolytics	N-acetylcysteine DNAase (dornase alfa)	Used to reduce mucus viscosity N-acetylcysteine is not recommended for COPD DNAse is indicated in patients with cystic fibrosis if there is significant symptomatic and lung function improvement after a trial of therapy		
Expectorants	Guaifenesin	Enhance clearance of mucus		
Antitussives	Codeine Dextromethorphan Benzonatate	Cough suppression (Note: Cough is a defensive reflex; *whenever possible, treat the underlying cause, not the cough*) Many over-the-counter cough medications containing dextromethorphan are largely ineffective	Codeine and other opiates are associated with sedation and constipation (see Chapter 10) Benzonatate is associated with dizziness and dysphagia	Dextromethorphan can cause hallucinations at higher doses and has significant abuse potential Seizures and cardiac arrest have occurred with acute ingestion of benzonatate Severe allergic reactions in patients taking benzonatate who are allergic to *p*-aminobenzoic acid
Ventilatory Stimulants	Doxapram	Increase ventilatory rate (Note: The use of doxapram to treat ventilatory failure in COPD has now largely been replaced by noninvasive ventilation)	Nausea, sweating, anxiety, and hallucinations At higher doses, increased pulmonary and systemic blood pressures	Should be used with caution if hepatic or renal function is impaired In COPD, the infusion of doxapram is restricted to 2 h
Prostacyclin (PGI_2) and Its Analogs	Epoprostenol (prostacyclin, PGI_2) Treprostinil Iloprost	Continuous IV epoprostenol is effective in lowering pulmonary arterial pressures, improving exercise performance, and prolonging survival in primary pulmonary artery hypertension (PPAH) Treprostinil and iloprost can be given by inhalation	Vasodilator effects (headache, flushing, syncope) diarrhea, nausea, and jaw pain Inhaled iloprost may cause cough and bronchoconstriction	
Endothelin-1 Receptor Antagonists	Bosentan Ambrisentan	Oral bosentan is efficacious in reducing symptoms and improving mortality in PPAH	Bosentan is generally well tolerated; adverse effects include abnormal liver function tests, anemia, headaches, peripheral edema, and nasal congestion	Risk of serious liver injury; liver aminotransferases should be monitored monthly Risk of testicular atrophy and infertility Bosentan is potentially teratogenic
Phosphodiesterase-5 (PDE5) Inhibitors	Sildenafil Tadalafil	Effective in lowering pulmonary resistance and improving exercise tolerance in patients with PAH	Headache, flushing, dyspepsia, and visual disturbances	Should not be used in patients receiving nitrovasodilators due to risk of severe hypotension (see Chapter 16)

Hematopoietic Agents

CHAPTER 25

This chapter will be most useful after having a basic understanding of the material in Chapter 37, Hematopoietic Agents: Growth Factors, Minerals, and Vitamins in *Goodman & Gilman's The Pharmacological Basis of Therapeutics*, 12th Edition. In addition to the material presented here, the 12th Edition contains:

- A description of hematopoietic cell growth and differentiation and the role of hematopoietic growth factors in these processes
- A discussion of iron metabolism and storage in the body
- A discussion of factors that cause iron deficiency anemia
- A discussion of vitamin deficiencies that can lead to anemia
- Table 37-3 Iron Requirements for Pregnancy
- Table 37-2 The Body Content of Iron
- Table 37-5 Average Response to Oral Iron
- The molecular structures of vitamin B_{12} and folic acid, and their congeners

LEARNING OBJECTIVES

☑ Understand the mechanisms of action of drugs, minerals, and vitamins used to stimulate hematopoiesis.

☑ Know the untoward effects of drugs used to stimulate hematopoiesis.

☑ Know the clinical application of hematopoietic growth factors and how efficacy of therapy is monitored.

☑ Know how mineral and vitamin deficiencies can lead to specific anemia, how these are diagnosed, and how they are treated with individual agents or combinations of agents.

☑ Know when iron and vitamin supplementation should be used prophylactically.

DRUGS INCLUDED IN THIS CHAPTER

- Copper sulfate (cupric sulfate)
- Cyanocobalamin (vitamin B_{12}; CALOMIST, NASCOBAL)
- Darbepoetin alfa (ARANESP)
- Eltrombopag (PROMACTA)
- Epoetin alfa (recombinant erythropoietin; EPOGEN, PROCRIT, EPREX)
- Ferrous fumarate (HEMCYTE, FEOSTAT, others)
- Ferrous gluconate (FERGON, others)
- Ferrous succinate, aspartate, and other ferrous salts
- Ferrous sulfate (FEOSOL, others)
- Ferumoxytol (FERAHEME)
- Folic acid (pteroylglutamic acid [PteGlu], L-methylfolate)
- Folinic acid (leucovorin calcium, citrovorum factor)
- G-CSF (recombinant G-CSF, filgrastim; NEUPOGEN)
- GM-CSF (recombinant GM-CSF, sargramostim; LEUKINE)
- Hydroxocobalamin (vitamin B_{12})
- IL-11 (recombinant IL-11; oprelvekin; [NEUMEGA])
- Iron dextran (DEXFERRUM, INFED, IMFERON)
- Iron sucrose (VENOFER)
- Pegylated recombinant G-CSF (pegfilgrastim; NEULASTA)
- Polysaccharide-ferrihydrite complex (NIFEREX, others)
- Pyridoxine
- Riboflavin
- Romiplostim (NPLATE)
- Sodium ferric gluconate (FERRLECIT)

MECHANISMS OF ACTION OF HEMATOPOIETIC AGENTS

DRUG CLASS	DRUG	MECHANISM OF ACTION
Erythropoiesis-Stimulating Agents (ESAs)	Epoetin alfa Darbepoetin alfa	Stimulate proliferation and maturation of committed erythroid progenitors to increase red blood cell (RBC) production (see Table 25-1 and Figure 25-1)
Myeloid Growth Factors	GM-CSF (sargrastim) G-CSF (filgrastim) Pegylated recombinant G-CSF (pegfilgrastim)	Stimulate proliferation and differentiation of 1 or more myeloid cell lines, and enhance the function of mature granulocytes and monocytes (see Table 25-1 and Figures 25-1 and 25-2)
Thrombopoietic Growth Factors	IL-11 (oprelvekin)	Enhance megakaryocyte maturation and increases peripheral blood platelet counts
	Romiplostim Eltrombopag	Activate thrombopoietin receptor which stimulates megakaryopoiesis

(Continued)

SECTION IV

Inflammation, Immunomodulation, and Hematopoiesis

DRUG CLASS	DRUG	MECHANISM OF ACTION
Iron Supplements—Oral	Ferrous sulfate Ferrous fumarate Ferrous succinate, aspartate, and other ferrous salts Ferrous gluconate Polysaccharide-ferrihydrite complex	Provide additional dietary iron needed to correct iron-deficiency anemia
Iron Supplements—Parenteral	Iron dextran Sodium ferric gluconate Ferumoxytol Iron sucrose	Provide iron needed to correct iron deficiency anemia when oral iron therapy fails
Copper Supplement	Copper sulfate (cupric sulfate)	Corrects copper deficiencies that interfere with absorption of iron and release of iron from reticuloendothelial cells that result in anemia
Vitamins—Pyridoxine	Pyridoxine Riboflavin	Pyridoxine improves hematopoiesis in patients with hereditary sideroblastic anemia and idiopathic acquired sideroblastic anemia
Vitamins—Vitamin B_{12}	Cyanocobalamin (vitamin B_{12}) Hydroxocobalamin (vitamin B_{12})	Cofactor required for normal synthesis of purines and pyrimidines needed for DNA synthesis, especially in rapidly dividing cells of the hematopoietic system (see Figure 25-3)
Vitamins—Folic Acid and Derivatives	Folic acid (pteroylglutamic acid [PteGlu], L-methylfolate) Folinic acid (leucovorin calcium, citrovorum factor)	Cofactor required for normal synthesis of purines and pyrimidines needed for DNA synthesis, especially in rapidly dividing cells of the hematopoietic system (see Figure 25-3)

CASE 25-1

A 64-year-old woman with chronic kidney disease has a low hematocrit and is started on therapy with epoetin alfa.

a. What is the mechanism of action of epoetin alfa?

Recombinant human erythropoietin (epoetin alfa) is nearly identical to the endogenous hormone except that the carbohydrate modification pattern of epoetin alfa differs slightly from the native protein; this difference apparently does not alter kinetics, potency, or immunoreactivity of the drug.

The endogenous protein is heavily glycosylated and expressed primarily in peritubular interstitial cells of the kidney. After secretion, erythropoietin binds to a receptor on the surface of committed erythroid progenitors in the marrow and is internalized. With anemia or hypoxemia, synthesis rapidly increases by 100-fold or more, serum erythropoietin levels rise, and marrow progenitor cell survival, proliferation, and maturation are dramatically stimulated (see Figure 25-1). This finely tuned feedback loop can be disrupted by kidney disease, marrow damage, or a deficiency in iron or an essential vitamin. With an infection or an inflammatory state, erythropoietin secretion, iron delivery, and progenitor proliferation all are suppressed by inflammatory cytokines. There is a clear dose–response relationship between the epoetin alfa dose and the rise in hematocrit in anephric patients, with eradication of their anemia at higher doses.

More recently, a novel erythropoiesis-stimulating protein, darbepoetin alfa, has been approved for clinical use in patients with indications similar to those

(Continued)

Hematopoietic Agents

CHAPTER 25

TABLE 25-1 Hematopoietic Growth Factors

ERYTHROPOIETIN (EPO)
- Stimulates proliferation and maturation of committed erythroid progenitors to increase red cell production

STEM CELL FACTOR (SCF, c-kit ligand, Steel factor) and FLT-3 LIGAND (FL)
- Act synergistically with a wide range of other colony-stimulating factors and interleukins to stimulate pluripotent and committed stem cells
- FL also stimulates both dendritic and NK cells (anti-tumor response)
- SCF also stimulates mast cells and melanocytes

INTERLEUKINS

IL-1, IL-3, IL-5, IL-6, IL-9, and IL-11
- Act synergistically with each other and SCF, GM-CSF, G-CSF, and EPO to stimulate BFU-E, CFU-GEMM, CFU-GM, CFU-E, and CFU-Meg growth
- Numerous immunologic roles, including stimulation of B cell and T cell growth

IL-5
- Controls eosinophil survival and differentiation

IL-6
- IL-6 stimulates human myeloma cells to proliferate
- IL-6 and IL-11 stimulate BFU-Meg to increase platelet production

IL-1, IL-2, IL-4, IL-7, and IL-12
- Stimulate growth and function of T cells, B cells, NK cells, and monocytes
- Co-stimulate B, T, and LAK cells

IL-8 and IL-10
- Numerous immunological activities involving B and T cell functions
- IL-8 acts as a chemotactic factor for basophils and neutrophils

GRANULOCYTE-MACROPHAGE COLONY–STIMULATING FACTOR (GM-CSF)
- Acts synergistically with SCF, IL-1, IL-3, and IL-6 to stimulate CFU-GM, and CFU-Meg to increase neutrophil and monocyte production
- With EPO may promote BFU-E formation
- Enhances migration, phagocytosis, superoxide production, and antibody-dependent cell-mediated toxicity of neutrophils, monocytes, and eosinophils
- Prevents alveolar proteinosis

GRANULOCYTE COLONY–STIMULATING FACTOR (G-CSF)
- Stimulates CFU-G to increase neutrophil production
- Enhances phagocytic and cytotoxic activities of neutrophils

MONOCYTE/MACROPHAGE COLONY–STIMULATING FACTOR (M-CSF, CSF-1)
- Stimulates CFU-M to increase monocyte precursors
- Activates and enhances function of monocyte/macrophages

MACROPHAGE COLONY–STIMULATING FACTOR (M-CSF)
- Stimulates CFU-M to increase monocyte/macrophage precursors
- Acts in concert with tissues and other growth factors to determine the proliferation, differentiation, and survival of a range of cells of the mononuclear phagocyte system

THROMBOPOIETIN (TPO, *Mpl* ligand)
- Stimulates the self-renewal and expansion of hematopoietic stem cells
- Stimulates stem cell differentiation into megakaryocyte progenitors
- Selectively stimulates megakaryocytopoiesis to increase platelet production
- Acts synergistically with other growth factors, especially IL-6 and IL-11

BFU, burst-forming unit; CFU, colony-forming unit; E, erythrocyte; G, granulocyte; M, macrophage; Meg, megakaryocyte; NK cells, natural killer cells; LAK cells, lymphokine-activated killer cells.

---

for epoetin alfa. It is a genetically modified form of erythropoietin in which 4 amino acids have been mutated such that additional carbohydrate side chains are added during its synthesis, prolonging the circulatory survival of the drug up to 24 to 26 hours.

b. What are other indications for erythropoiesis-stimulating agents (ESAs)?

Epoetin alfa also is effective in the treatment of anemia associated with surgery, AIDS, cancer chemotherapy, prematurity, and certain chronic inflammatory conditions. Darbepoetin alfa also has been approved for use in patients with anemia associated with chronic kidney disease and is under review for several other indications.

(Continued)

SECTION IV Inflammation, Immunomodulation, and Hematopoiesis

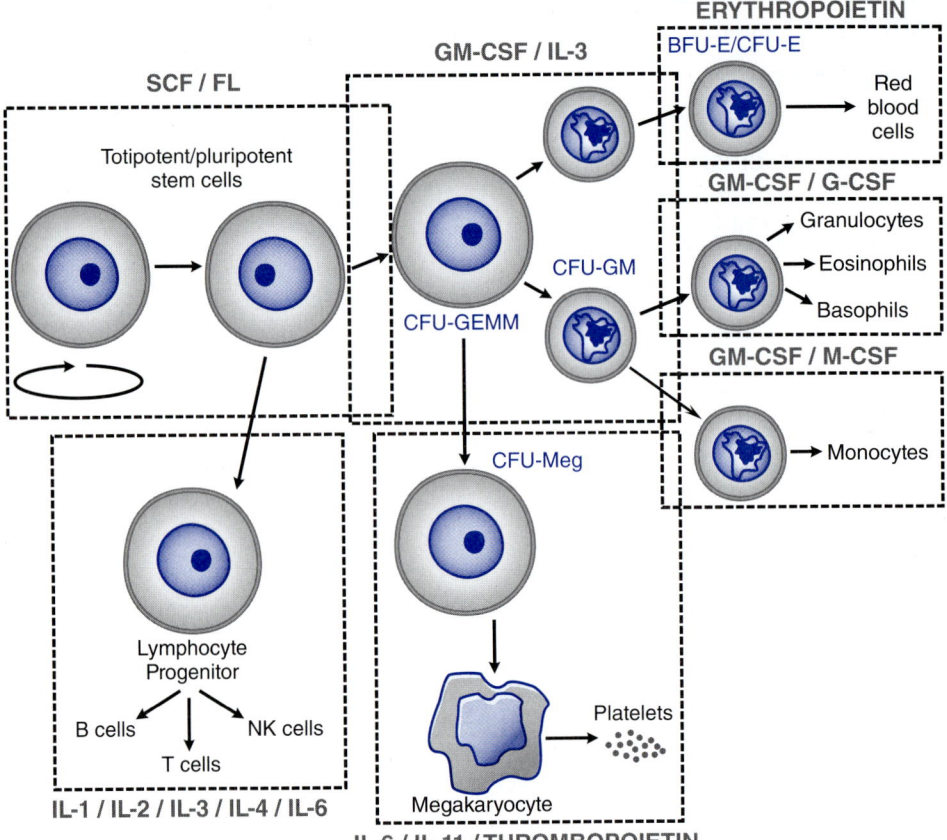

FIGURE 25-1 Sites of action of hematopoietic growth factors in the differentiation and maturation of marrow cell lines. A self-sustaining pool of marrow stem cells differentiates under the influence of specific hematopoietic growth factors to form a variety of hematopoietic and lymphopoietic cells. Stem cell factor (SCF), ligand (FL), interleukin-3 (IL-3), and granulocyte-macrophage colony-stimulating factor (GM-CSF), together with cell–cell interactions in the marrow, stimulate stem cells to form a series of burst-forming units (BFU) and colony-forming units (CFU): CFU-GEMM (granulocyte, erythrocyte, monocyte, and megakaryocyte), CFU-GM (granulocyte and macrophage), CFU-Meg (megakaryocyte), BFU-E (erythrocyte), and CFU-E (erythrocyte). After considerable proliferation, further differentiation is stimulated by synergistic interactions with growth factors for each of the major cell lines—granulocyte colony–stimulating factor (G-CSF), monocyte/macrophage-stimulating factor (M-CSF), thrombopoietin, and erythropoietin. Each of these factors also influences the proliferation, maturation, and, in some cases, the function of the derivative cell line (see Table 25-1).

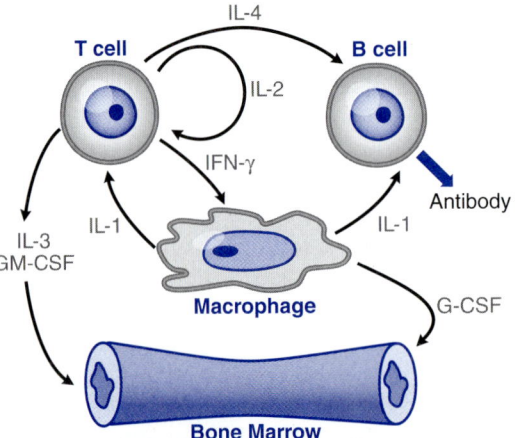

FIGURE 25-2 Cytokine–cell interactions. Macrophages, T cells, B cells, and marrow stem cells interact via several cytokines (IL-1, IL-2, IL-3, IL-4, IFN [interferon]-γ, GM-CSF, and G-CSF) in response to a bacterial or a foreign antigen challenge. See Table 25-1 for the functional activities of these various cytokines.

Hematopoietic Agents

CHAPTER 25

Highly competitive athletes have used epoetin alfa to increase their hemoglobin levels ("blood doping") and improve performance. Unfortunately, this misuse of the drug has been implicated in the deaths of several athletes and is strongly discouraged.

c. What are the therapeutic considerations to optimize therapy with epoetin alfa?

During erythropoietin therapy, absolute or functional iron deficiency may develop. Functional iron deficiency (ie, normal ferritin levels but low transferrin saturation) presumably results from the inability to mobilize iron stores rapidly enough to support the increased erythropoiesis. Virtually all patients eventually will require supplemental iron to increase or maintain transferrin saturation to levels that will adequately support stimulated erythropoiesis.

Resistance to epoetin alfa therapy is common in patients who develop an inflammatory illness or become iron deficient, so close monitoring of general health and iron status is essential. Less common causes of resistance include occult blood loss, folic acid deficiency, carnitine deficiency, inadequate dialysis, aluminum toxicity, and osteitis fibrosa cystica secondary to hyperparathyroidism.

d. What are the possible toxicities and hazards of therapy with epoetin alfa?

The most common side effect of epoetin alfa therapy is aggravation of hypertension, which occurs in 20 to 30% of patients and most often is associated with a rapid rise in hematocrit. Blood pressure usually can be controlled either by increasing antihypertensive therapy, ultrafiltration in dialysis patients, or by reducing the epoetin alfa dose to slow the hematocrit response. ESAs should not be used in patients with preexisting uncontrolled hypertension.

Headache, tachycardia, edema, shortness of breath, nausea, vomiting, diarrhea, injection site stinging, and flu-like symptoms (eg, arthralgias and myalgias) also have been reported in conjunction with epoetin alfa therapy.

During hemodialysis, patients receiving epoetin alfa or darbepoetin may require increased anticoagulation. Serious thromboembolic events have been reported, including migratory thrombophlebitis, microvascular thrombosis, pulmonary embolism, and thrombosis of the retinal artery and temporal and renal veins. The risk of thrombotic events, including vascular access thromboses, was higher in adults with ischemic heart disease or congestive heart failure receiving epoetin alfa therapy with the goal of reaching a normal hematocrit (42%) than in those with a lower-target hematocrit of 30%. The higher risk of cardiovascular events from erythropoietic therapies may be associated with higher hemoglobin or higher rates of rise in hemoglobin. The hemoglobin level should be managed to avoid exceeding a target level of 12 g/dL.

ESA use is associated with increased rates of cancer recurrence and decreased on-study survival in patients in whom the drugs are administered for cancer-induced or for chemotherapy-induced anemia. The cause(s) of this effect is presently unclear, but some studies suggest that tumor cells bearing the erythropoietin receptor are more likely to be affected by the use of ESAs.

CASE 25-2

A 42-year-old man with leukemia will undergo autologous peripheral blood stem cell transplant following high-dose chemotherapy.

a. What is the rationale for using myeloid growth factors in this procedure?

The myeloid growth factors (see Figure 25-1 and Table 25-1) are glycoproteins that stimulate the proliferation and differentiation of 1 or more myeloid cell lines. They also enhance the function of mature granulocytes and monocytes. Recombinant forms of several growth factors have been produced, including granulocyte-macrophage colony-stimulating factor (GM-CSF), granulocyte colony-stimulating factor (G-CSF), interleukin-3 (IL-3), macrophage colony-stimulating factor (M-CSF; also known as colony-stimulating factor, CSF-1), and stem cell factor (SCF).

(Continued)

SECTION IV
Inflammation, Immunomodulation, and Hematopoiesis

Recombinant human GM-CSF (sargramostim) and recombinant human G-CSF (filgrastim) are used in patients undergoing autologous bone marrow and peripheral blood stem cell transplant following high-dose chemotherapy to stimulate the proliferation, differentiation, and function of myeloid cell lines that are required to fight infection. Sargramostim and filgrastim shorten the duration of severe neutropenia and reduce transplant morbidity secondary to bacterial and fungal infections without a change in long-term survival or risk of inducing an early relapse of the malignant process.

b. **What is the difference in the effects of GM-CSF versus G-CSF?**

GM-CSF is capable of stimulating the proliferation, differentiation, and function of a number of the myeloid cell lineages (see Figure 25-1). It acts synergistically with other growth factors, including erythropoietin, at the level of the burst-forming unit (BFU). GM-CSF stimulates the colony-forming units (CFUs) CFU-GEMM, CFU-GM, CFU-M, CFU-E, and CFU-Meg to increase cell production. It also enhances the migration, phagocytosis, superoxide production, and antibody-dependent cell-mediated toxicity of neutrophils, monocytes, and eosinophils.

The activity of G-CSF is restricted to neutrophils and their progenitors, stimulating their proliferation, differentiation, and function. It acts primarily on the CFU-G, although it also can play a synergistic role with IL-3 and GM-CSF in stimulating other cell lines. G-CSF enhances phagocytic and cytotoxic activities of neutrophils. Unlike GM-CSF, G-CSF has little effect on monocytes, macrophages, and eosinophils, and reduces inflammation by inhibiting IL-1, tumor necrosis factor, and interferon γ. G-CSF also mobilizes primitive hematopoietic cells, including hematopoietic stem cells, from the marrow into the peripheral blood. This observation has virtually transformed the practice of stem cell transplantation, such that more than 90% of all such procedures today use G-CSF–mobilized peripheral blood stem cells (PBSCs) as the donor product.

c. **What are other indications for G-CSF?**

G-CSF also is effective in the treatment of severe congenital neutropenias. In patients with cyclic neutropenia, G-CSF therapy will increase the level of neutrophils and shorten the length of the cycle sufficiently to prevent recurrent bacterial infections. Filgrastim therapy can improve neutrophil counts in some patients with myelodysplasia or marrow damage (moderately severe aplastic anemia or tumor infiltration of the marrow). The neutropenia of AIDS patients receiving zidovudine also can be partially or completely reversed. Filgrastim is routinely used in patients undergoing peripheral blood stem cell (PBSC) collection for stem cell transplantation. It promotes the release of CD34[+] progenitor cells from the marrow, reducing the number of collections necessary for transplant. Moreover, filgrastim-mobilized PBSCs appear more capable of rapid engraftment. PBSC-transplanted patients require fewer days of platelet and red blood cell transfusions and a shorter duration of hospitalization than do patients receiving autologous bone marrow transplants.

INTERACTIONS OF VITAMIN B$_{12}$ AND FOLATE IN INTRACELLULAR METABOLISM (See Figure 25-3)

- Conversion of homocysteine to methionine
- Conversion of serine to glycine
- Synthesis of thymidylate
- Histidine metabolism
- Synthesis of purines
- Utilization or generation of formate

CASE 25-3

A 54-year-old woman diagnosed with metastatic breast cancer is undergoing chemotherapy. After the first course of chemotherapy, her platelet count drops to very low levels. To avoid using platelet transfusions in this patient, she is given a daily injection of oprelvekin following her second course of chemotherapy.

a. **What is the mechanism of action of oprelvekin?**

Oprelvekin is a recombinant version of IL-11, a cytokine that stimulates hematopoiesis and enhances megakaryocyte maturation (see Figure 25-1 and Table 25-1). Oprelvekin is approved for use in patients undergoing chemotherapy for non-myeloid malignancies that displayed severe thrombocytopenia (platelet count

(Continued)

Hematopoietic Agents

<20,000/μL) on a prior cycle of the same chemotherapy, and it is administered daily until the platelet count returns to greater than 100,000/μL. Administration of the recombinant cytokine is associated with less severe thrombocytopenia and reduced use of platelet transfusions in patients who previously demonstrated significant chemotherapy-induced thrombocytopenia.

b. What are the side effects of oprelvekin?

The major complications of oprelvekin therapy are fluid retention and associated cardiac symptoms, such as tachycardia, palpitation, edema, and shortness of breath; this is a significant concern in elderly patients and often requires concomitant therapy with diuretics. Fluid retention reverses upon drug discontinuation, but volume status should be carefully monitored in elderly patients, those with a history of heart failure, or those with preexisting fluid collections in the pleura, pericardium, or peritoneal cavity. Also reported are blurred vision, injection-site rash or erythema, and paresthesias.

TABLE 25-2 Daily Iron Intake and Absorption

SUBJECT	IRON REQUIREMENT (mg/kg)	AVAILABLE IRON (mg/kg) POOR DIET–GOOD DIET	SAFETY FACTOR AVAILABLE/REQUIREMENT
Infant	67	33-66	0.5-1
Child	22	48-96	2-4
Adolescent (male)	21	30-60	1.5-3
Adolescent (female)	20	30-60	1.5-3
Adult (male)	13	26-52	2-4
Adult (female)	21	18-36	1-2
Mid-to-late pregnancy	80	18-36	0.22-0.45

TABLE 25-3 Recommended Dietary Allowances (RDAs) For Iron For Nonvegetarians[a] (Food and Nutrition Board at the Institute of Medicine, 2001)

AGE	MALE (mg)	FEMALE (mg)	PREGNANCY (mg)	LACTATION (mg)
Birth to 6 months	0.27[b]	0.27[b]		
7-12 mo	11	11		
1-3 y	7	7		
4-8 y	10	10		
9-13 y	8	8		
14-18 y	11	15	27	10
19-50 y	8	18	27	9
51+ y	8	8		

[a] The RDAs for vegetarians are 1.8 times higher than for people who eat meat.
[b] For infants from birth to 6 months, the Food and Nutrition Board established an Adequate Intake (AI; established when evidence is insufficient to develop an RDA) for iron that is equivalent to the mean intake of iron in healthy, breast-fed infants.

CHAPTER 25

CAUSES OF VITAMIN B_{12} DEFICIENCY (See Figure 25-4)

- Deficiency of vitamin B_{12} can result from a congenital or acquired defect in any one of the following:
  - Inadequate dietary supply
  - Inadequate secretion of gastric intrinsic factor (classic pernicious anemia)
  - Ileal disease
  - Congenital absence of transcobalamin II (TcII)
  - Rapid depletion of hepatic stores by interference with reabsorption of vitamin B_{12} excreted in bile

GENERAL PRINCIPLES OF VITAMIN B_{12} THERAPY

1. Vitamin B_{12} should be given prophylactically only when there is a reasonable probability that a deficiency exists or will exist:
   - Dietary deficiency in the strict vegetarian
   - The predictable malabsorption of vitamin B_{12} in patients who have had a gastrectomy
   - Certain diseases of the small intestine
   - When GI function is normal, an oral prophylactic supplement of vitamins and minerals, including vitamin B_{12}, may be indicated; otherwise, the patient should receive monthly injections of cyanocobalamin

2. The relative ease of treatment with vitamin B_{12} should not prevent a full investigation of the etiology of the deficiency.
   - The initial diagnosis usually is suggested by a macrocytic anemia or an unexplained neuropsychiatric disorder.
   - Full understanding of the etiology of vitamin B_{12} deficiency involves studies of dietary supply, GI absorption, and transport.

3. Therapy always should be as specific as possible.
   - The use of shotgun vitamin therapy in the treatment of vitamin B_{12} deficiency can be dangerous; there is the danger that sufficient folic acid will be given to result in a hematologic recovery

(continues)

SECTION IV — Inflammation, Immunomodulation, and Hematopoiesis

GENERAL PRINCIPLES OF VITAMIN B_{12} THERAPY (Cont.)

that can mask continued vitamin B_{12} deficiency and permit neurological damage to develop or progress.

4. A classic therapeutic trial with small amounts of vitamin B_{12} can help confirm the diagnosis, but acutely ill elderly patients may not be able to tolerate the delay in the correction of a severe anemia.
   - Such patients require supplemental blood transfusions and immediate therapy with folic acid and vitamin B_{12} to guarantee rapid recovery.
5. Long-term therapy with vitamin B_{12} must be evaluated at intervals of 6 to 12 months in patients who are otherwise well
   - If there is an additional illness or a condition that may increase the requirement for the vitamin (eg, pregnancy), reassessment should be performed more frequently.

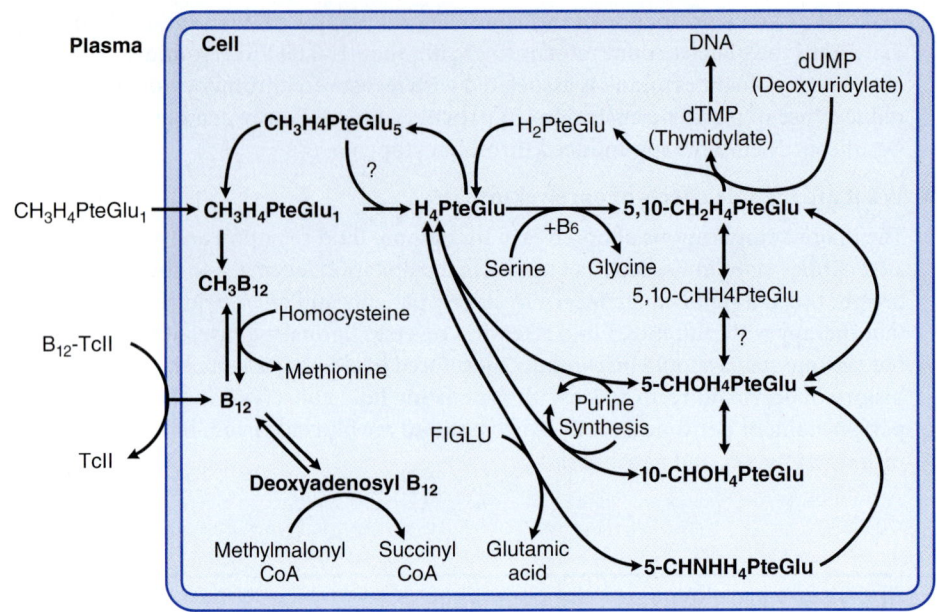

FIGURE 25-3 Interrelationships and metabolic roles of vitamin B_{12} and folic acid. See Side Bar INTERACTIONS OF VITAMIN B_{12} AND FOLATE IN INTRACELLULAR METABOLISM. FIGLU, formiminoglutamic acid, which arises from the catabolism of histidine; TcII, transcobalamin II; $CH_3H_4PteGlu_1$, methyltetrahydrofolate.

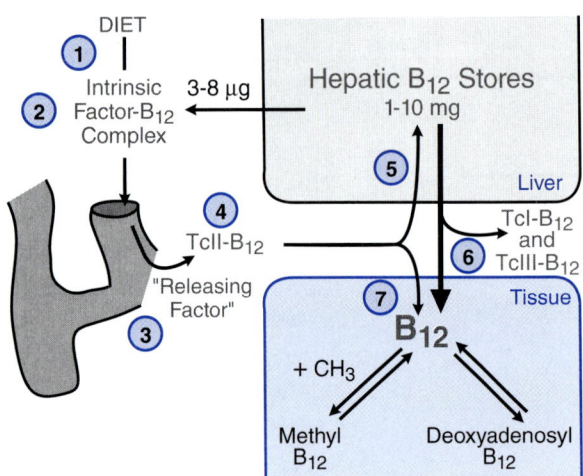

FIGURE 25-4 The absorption and distribution of vitamin B_{12}. Deficiency of vitamin B_{12} can result from a congenital or acquired defect in any one of the following: (1) inadequate dietary supply; (2) inadequate secretion of intrinsic factor (classic pernicious anemia); (3) ileal disease; (4) congenital absence of transcobalamin II (TcII); or (5) rapid depletion of hepatic stores by interference with reabsorption of vitamin B_{12} excreted in bile. The utility of measurements of the concentration of vitamin B_{12} in plasma to estimate supply available to tissues can be compromised by liver disease and (6) the appearance of abnormal amounts of transcobalamins I and III (TcI and III) in plasma. Finally, the formation of methylcobalamin requires (7) normal transport into cells and an adequate supply of folic acid as $CH_3H_4PteGlu_1$.

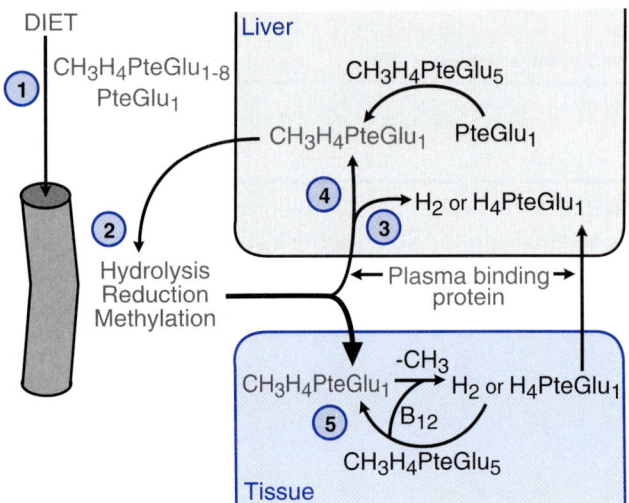

FIGURE 25-5 Absorption and distribution of folate derivatives. Dietary sources of folate polyglutamates are hydrolyzed to the monoglutamate, reduced, and methylated to $CH_3H_4PteGlu_1$ during gastrointestinal transport. Folate deficiency commonly results from (1) inadequate dietary supply and (2) small intestinal disease. In patients with uremia, alcoholism, or hepatic disease there may be defects in (3) the concentration of folate binding proteins in plasma and (4) the flow of $CH_3H_4PteGlu_1$ into bile for reabsorption and transport to tissue (the folate enterohepatic cycle). Finally, vitamin B_{12} deficiency will (5) "trap" folate as $CH_3H_4PteGlu_1$, thereby reducing the availability of $H_4PteGlu_1$ for its essential roles in purine and pyrimidine synthesis.

Hematopoietic Agents CHAPTER 25

CASE 25-4

A 22-year-old woman is pregnant with her first child. She is in good health, but her pediatrician prescribes an oral iron supplement.

a. What is the rationale for supplemental iron in this patient?

In developed countries, the normal adult diet contains ~6 mg of iron per 1000 calories, providing an average daily intake for adult men of between 12 and 20 mg, and for adult women a daily intake of between 8 and 15 mg. Normal iron absorption is ~1 mg/d in adult men and 1.4 mg/d in adult women; 3 to 4 mg of dietary iron is the most that can normally be absorbed.

Pregnancy and lactation impose a greater requirement for iron with the growth of the fetus and expansion of red cell mass (see Tables 25-2 and 25-3). A recent study found that 18% of pregnant women in the United States had iron deficiency, with 6.9% in the first trimester, 14.3% in the second trimester, and 29.7% in the third trimester. Iron deficiency during pregnancy increases the risk of maternal and infant mortality, premature birth, low birth weight, and impaired cognitive and behavioral development of the infant. Infants, especially those born preterm, with low birth weight, or whose mothers have iron deficiency, are at risk of iron deficiency due to their rapid growth.

Whereas iron balance in adult men and nonmenstruating women is reasonably secure, pregnancy and infancy represent periods of negative iron balance, and menstruating women also are at risk of iron deficiency. The difference between dietary supply and requirements is reflected in the size of iron stores, which are low or absent when iron balance is precarious and high when iron balance is favorable (see Table 37-2, *Goodman and Gilman's The Pharmacological Basis of Therapeutics*, 12th Edition). Thus in infants after the third month of life and in pregnant women after the first trimester, stores of iron are negligible. Menstruating women have approximately one-third the stored iron found in adult men, indicative of the extent to which the additional average daily loss of ~0.5 mg of iron affects iron balance.

b. What are the effects of iron deficiency in infants and children?

Iron deficiency in infants and young children can lead to behavioral disturbances and can impair development, which may not be fully reversible. Iron deficiency in children also can lead to an increased risk of lead toxicity secondary to pica and an increased absorption of heavy metals. Premature and low-birth-weight infants are at greatest risk for developing iron deficiency, especially if they are not breast-fed and/or do not receive iron-fortified formula. During adolescence there is a rapid growth combined with irregular dietary habits and the risk of iron deficiency increases again. Adolescent girls are at greatest risk; the dietary iron intake of most girls ages 11 to 18 years is insufficient to meet their requirements.

c. What are some of the considerations in optimizing the effects of oral medicinal iron?

To prevent iron deficiency in pregnant women, doses of 15 to 30 mg of iron per day are adequate to meet the daily requirement of the last 2 trimesters. Orally administered ferrous sulfate is the treatment of choice for iron deficiency. Ferrous salts are absorbed about 3 times as well as ferric salts, and the discrepancy becomes even greater at high dosages. Variations in the particular ferrous salt have relatively little effect on bioavailability; the sulfate, fumarate, succinate, gluconate, aspartate, other ferrous salts, and polysaccharide-ferrihydrite complex are all absorbed to approximately the same extent.

The effective dose of all of these preparations is based on iron content. It is essential that the coating of the tablet dissolve rapidly in the stomach because iron usually is absorbed in the upper small intestine. Bioavailability of iron ingested with food is probably one-half or one-third of that seen in the fasting subject. It is always preferable to administer iron in the fasting state, even if the dose must be reduced because of GI side effects. Antacids also reduce iron absorption if given concurrently.

(Continued)

> **COMMON CAUSES OF FOLATE DEFICIENCY (see FIGURE 25-5)**
>
> - Inadequate dietary supply.
> - Small intestinal disease.
> - In patients with uremia, alcoholism, or hepatic disease there may be defects in:
>   - The concentration of folate binding proteins in plasma
>   - The flow of $CH_3H_4PteGlu_1$ into bile for reabsorption and transport to tissue (the folate enterohepatic cycle)
> - Vitamin B_{12} deficiency will "trap" folate as $CH_3H_4PteGlu$, thereby reducing the availability of $H_4PteGlu_1$ for its essential roles in purine and pyrimidine synthesis.

SECTION IV

Inflammation, Immunomodulation, and Hematopoiesis

GENERAL PRINCIPLES OF FOLIC ACID THERAPY

1. Prophylactic administration of folic acid should be undertaken for clear indications.
   - Dietary supplementation is necessary when there is a requirement that may not be met by a "normal" diet.
   - The daily ingestion of a multivitamin preparation containing 400 to 500 µg of folic acid has become standard practice before and during pregnancy to reduce the incidence of neural tube defects and for as long as a woman is breast-feeding.
   - In women with a history of a pregnancy complicated by a neural tube defect, an even larger dose of 4 mg/d has been recommended (MRC Vitamin Study Research Group).
   - Patients on total parenteral nutrition should receive folic acid supplements as part of their fluid regimen because liver folate stores are limited.
   - Adult patients with a disease state characterized by high cell turnover (eg, hemolytic anemia) generally require larger doses, 1 mg of folic acid given once or twice a day.
   - The 1-mg dose also has been used in the treatment of patients with elevated levels of homocysteine.
2. As with vitamin B_{12} deficiency, any patient with folate deficiency and a megaloblastic anemia should be evaluated carefully to determine the underlying cause of the deficiency state including:
   - The effects of medications
   - The amount of alcohol intake
   - The patient's history of travel
   - The function of the GI tract
3. Therapy always should be as specific as possible.
   - Multivitamin preparations should be avoided unless there is good reason to suspect deficiency of several vitamins.
4. The potential danger of mistreating a patient who has vitamin B_{12} deficiency with folic acid must be kept in mind.
   - The administration of large doses of folic acid can result in an apparent improvement in the megaloblastic anemia, inasmuch as PteGlu is converted

Clinically, the effectiveness of iron therapy is best evaluated by tracking the reticulocyte response and the rise in the hemoglobin or the hematocrit. An increase in the reticulocyte count is not observed for at least 4 to 7 days after beginning therapy. A measurable increase in the hemoglobin level takes even longer.

CASE 25-5

During his annual visit to his family physician, a 68-year-old man complains of numbness in his hands, occasional tremors and loss of balance, and some loss of memory. He is found to be anemic with abnormally large red cells and other blood cell anomalies. He is a strict vegetarian and does not eat eggs or dairy products.

a. **What might be contributing to this patient's condition?**

This patient has symptoms consistent with deficiency of either vitamin B_{12} or folic acid. An early sign of deficiency is megaloblastic anemia. Abnormal macrocytic red blood cells are produced, and the patient becomes severely anemic. These vitamins are key cofactors in the biochemical pathways that are critical for normal synthesis of purines and pyrimidines (see Figure 25-3). A deficiency of either vitamin impairs DNA synthesis in any cell in which chromosomal replication and division are taking place. In addition, a deficiency of either vitamin B_{12} or folate leads to the decreased synthesis of methionine and S-adenosylmethionine, which interferes with protein biosynthesis, a number of methylation reactions, and the synthesis of polyamines. Because tissues with the greatest rate of cell turnover show the most dramatic effects with alterations in these pathways, the hematopoietic system is especially sensitive to deficiencies of these vitamins. Neurological lesions are also common with vitamin B_{12} deficiency, although the mechanisms are not well understood. Neurological signs and symptoms include paresthesia of the hands and feet, decreased vibration and position senses with resultant unsteadiness, decreased deep tendon reflexes, and in the later stages of vitamin B_{12} deficiency, confusion, moodiness, loss of memory, and even a loss of central vision. The patient may exhibit delusions, hallucinations, or even overt psychosis. Because the neurological damage can be dissociated from the changes in the hematopoietic system, vitamin B_{12} deficiency must be considered in elderly patients with dementia or psychiatric disorders, even if they are not anemic.

b. **Why might this patient be at risk for vitamin B_{12} or folic acid deficiency?**

This patient is a strict vegetarian and may be lacking these vitamins because of his diet (see Side Bars COMMON CAUSES OF FOLATE DEFICIENCY and CAUSES OF VITAMIN B_{12} DEFICIENCY). Vegetable products are free of vitamin B_{12} unless they are contaminated with microorganisms that grow in soil, sewage, water, or the intestinal lumen of animals that synthesize the vitamin. Despite this, strict vegetarians rarely develop vitamin B_{12} deficiency because some vitamin B_{12} is available from legumes, which are contaminated with bacteria capable of synthesizing vitamin B_{12}, and because vegetarians often fortify their diets with a wide range of vitamins and minerals.

Although this patient could be deficient in vitamin B_{12} because of diet, vitamin B_{12} deficiency in adults is rarely the result of a deficient diet per se; rather, it usually reflects a defect in one or another aspect of the complex sequence of steps in vitamin B_{12} absorption that is depicted in Figure 25-4. Achlorhydria and decreased secretion of intrinsic factor by parietal cells secondary to gastric atrophy or gastric surgery is a common cause of vitamin B_{12} deficiency in adults. Antibodies to parietal cells or intrinsic factor complex also can play a prominent role in producing a deficiency. A number of intestinal diseases can interfere with absorption, including pancreatic disorders (loss of pancreatic protease secretion), bacterial overgrowth, intestinal parasites, sprue, and localized damage to ileal mucosal cells by disease or as a result of surgery.

This patient is not likely to be deficient in dietary intake of folic acid because of his vegetarian diet since many food sources are rich in folate, especially fresh green vegetables,

(Continued)

yeast, and some fruits. (Liver is also rich in folate but would not be part of a vegetarian diet.) Generally, a standard US diet provides 50 to 500 µg of absorbable folate per day (the recommended daily intake for the normal adult is 400 µg), although individuals with high intakes of fresh vegetables and meats will ingest as much as 2 mg/d.

Folate deficiency is a common complication of diseases of the small intestine that interfere with the absorption of folate from food and the recirculation of folate through the enterohepatic cycle (see Figure 25-5). Because most absorption occurs in the proximal portion of the small intestine, it is not unusual for folate deficiency to occur when the jejunum is diseased. Both nontropical and tropical sprues are common causes of folate deficiency and megaloblastic anemia. In acute or chronic alcoholism, daily intake of folate in food may be severely restricted, and the enterohepatic cycle of the vitamin may be impaired by toxic effects of alcohol on hepatic parenchymal cells; this is the most common cause of folate-deficient megaloblastic erythropoiesis.

c. **What treatment is indicated for this patient?**

The general principles of therapy are described in the Side Bars GENERAL PRNCIPLES OF VITAMIN B_{12} THERAPY and GENERAL PRNCIPLES OF FOLIC ACID THERAPY. Because this patient has symptoms of neurological damage, effective therapy must not wait for detailed diagnostic tests. Inasmuch as the patient requires therapy before the exact cause of the disease has been defined, it is important to avoid the potential problem of a combined deficiency of vitamin B_{12} and folic acid. When the patient is deficient in both, therapy with only 1 vitamin will not provide an optimal response. Long-standing nontropical sprue is 1 example of a disease in which combined deficiency of B_{12} and folate is common. Once the megaloblastic erythropoiesis has been confirmed and sufficient blood collected for later measurements of vitamin B_{12} and folic acid, the patient should receive intramuscular injections of 100 µg of cyanocobalamin and 1 to 5 mg of folic acid. For the next 1 to 2 weeks the patient should receive daily intramuscular injections of 100 µg of cyanocobalamin, together with a daily oral supplement of 1 to 2 mg of folic acid.

The therapeutic response may be monitored by study of the hematopoietic system. Within 48 hours of the initiation of appropriate therapy, megaloblastic erythropoiesis disappears, and as efficient erythropoiesis begins, the concentration of iron in plasma falls to normal or below normal values. The reticulocyte count begins to rise on the second or third day and reaches a peak by the fifth to seventh days; the reticulocyte index reflects the proliferative state of the marrow. Finally, the hematocrit begins to rise during the second week. Patients with complicating iron deficiency, an infection or other inflammatory state, or renal disease may be unable to correct their anemia. Therefore, it is important to monitor the reticulocyte index over the first several weeks. If it does not continue at elevated levels while the hematocrit is less than 35%, plasma concentrations of iron and folic acid should again be determined and the patient reevaluated for an illness that could inhibit the response of the marrow.

The degree and rate of improvement of neurological signs and symptoms depend on the severity and the duration of the abnormalities. Those that have been present for only a few months usually disappear relatively rapidly. When a defect has been present for many months or years, full return to normal function may never occur.

Once begun, vitamin B_{12} therapy must be maintained for life. This fact must be impressed on the patient and family, and a system must be established to guarantee continued monthly injections of cyanocobalamin. Intramuscular injection of 100 µg of cyanocobalamin every 4 weeks is sufficient to maintain a normal concentration of vitamin B_{12} in plasma and an adequate supply for tissues. Patients with severe neurological symptoms and signs may be treated with larger doses of vitamin B_{12} in the period immediately after the diagnosis. Doses of 100 µg/d or several times per week may be given for several months with the hope of encouraging faster and more complete recovery. It is important to monitor vitamin B_{12} concentrations in plasma and to obtain peripheral blood counts at intervals of 3 to 6 months to confirm the adequacy of therapy. Because refractoriness to therapy can develop at any time, evaluation must continue throughout the patient's life.

> **GENERAL PRINCIPLES OF FOLIC ACID THERAPY (Cont.)**
>
> by dihydrofolate reductase to $H_4PteGlu$; this circumvents the methylfolate "trap." Folate therapy does not prevent or alleviate the neurological defects of vitamin B_{12} deficiency, and these may progress and become irreversible.

SECTION IV   Inflammation, Immunomodulation, and Hematopoiesis

KEY CONCEPTS

➥ Recombinant erythropoietin is used routinely for patients with the anemia of renal insufficiency, inflammation, and anemia associated with cancer or the therapy of cancer.

➥ Myeloid growth factors (eg, GM-CSF and G-CSF) are used to hasten the recovery of granulocytes after myelosuppressive therapy, to help mobilize hematopoietic stem cells into the peripheral blood to allow their harvest for transplantation, and to augment the number of mature leukocytes in the peripheral blood so that they can be used in patients with overwhelming infection.

➥ IL-11 and small molecules that activate the thrombopoietin receptor are used to treat acquired and hereditary thrombocytopenias.

➥ Iron deficiency is the most common nutritional disorder and can result from a variety of causes, including conditions with increased iron requirements such as pregnancy, infancy, menstruation, and blood loss.

➥ Deficiency of vitamin B_{12} and folic acid result in a characteristic megaloblastic anemia, but vitamin B_{12} deficiency can also lead to serious neurological lesions.

➥ The megaloblastic anemia that results from folate deficiency cannot be distinguished from that caused by vitamin B_{12} deficiency; thus it is important to consider both deficiencies when initiating treatment and monitoring therapy to avoid irreversible neurologic damage.

SUMMARY QUIZ

QUESTION 25-1 Used prophylactically in pregnant women to prevent neural tube defects in the fetus:

a. Riboflavin
b. Pyridoxine
c. Iron
d. Vitamin B_{12}
e. Folic acid

QUESTION 25-2 Indicated for use in patients suffering from cyclic neutropenia to stimulate neutrophil production:

a. Epoetin alfa
b. Filgrastim
c. Darbepoetin alfa
d. Romiplostim
e. Oprelvekin

QUESTION 25-3 Therapy with folinic acid is used to treat anemia associated with the

a. antituberculosis drugs isoniazid and pyrazinamide.
b. antiparkinson drug levodopa.
c. antibiotic chloramphenicol.
d. anticancer agent carboplatin.
e. anticancer agent methotrexate.

QUESTION 25-4 Deficiency in folic acid is characterized by

a. microcytic, hypochromic anemia.
b. sideroblastic anemia.
c. neutropenia.

(Continued)

d. red-cell aplasia.

e. megaloblastic anemia.

QUESTION 25-5 Which of the following agents activates the thrombopoietin receptor on megakaryocytes?

a. Epoetin alfa

b. Filgrastim

c. Darbepoetin alfa

d. Romiplostim

e. Oprelvekin

SUMMARY QUIZ ANSWER KEY

QUESTION 25-1 Answer is **e**. Folate deficiency has been implicated in the incidence of neural tube defects, including spina bifida, encephaloceles, and anencephaly. This is true even in the absence of folate-deficient anemia or alcoholism. The daily ingestion of a multivitamin preparation containing 400 to 500 µg of folic acid has become standard practice before and during pregnancy to reduce the incidence of neural tube defects and for as long as a woman is breast-feeding. In women with a history of a pregnancy complicated by a neural tube defect, an even larger dose of 4 mg/d has been recommended.

QUESTION 25-2 Answer is **b**. Filgrastim is a recombinant form of G-CSF that is administered by subcutaneous injection or slow intravenous infusion. Unlike natural G-CSF, it is not glycosylated and carries an extra N-terminal methionine. The principal action of filgrastim is the stimulation of CFU-G to increase neutrophil production (see Figure 25-1). It also enhances the phagocytic and cytotoxic functions of neutrophils. Its primary indication is in the treatment of severe neutropenia after autologous hematopoietic stem cell transplantation and high-dose cancer chemotherapy. Cyclic neutropenia is a congenital neutropenia that is characterized by a neutropenia that recurs every 14 to 35 days, with most patients exhibiting a cycle of 21 days. In patients with cyclic neutropenia, G-CSF therapy will increase the level of neutrophils and shorten the length of the cycle sufficiently to prevent recurrent bacterial infections.

QUESTION 25-3 Answer is **e**. Folinic acid (leucovorin calcium, citrovorum factor) is the 5-formyl derivative of tetrahydrofolic acid. The principal therapeutic uses of folinic acid are to circumvent the inhibition of dihydrofolate reductase as a part of high-dose methotrexate therapy and to potentiate fluorouracil in the treatment of colorectal cancer (see Chapter 45). It also has been used as an antidote to counteract the toxicity of folate antagonists such as pyrimethamine or trimethoprim.

Anemias can be a side effect of other drug therapies and the vitamin pyridoxine can correct some of these. Oral therapy with pyridoxine is of proven benefit in correcting the sideroblastic anemias associated with the antituberculosis drugs isoniazid and pyrazinamide, which act as vitamin B_6 antagonists. A daily dose of 50 mg of pyridoxine completely corrects the defect without interfering with treatment, and routine supplementation of pyridoxine often is recommended (see Chapter 42). In contrast, if pyridoxine is given to counteract the sideroblastic abnormality associated with administration of levodopa, the effectiveness of levodopa in controlling Parkinson disease is decreased. Pyridoxine therapy does not correct the sideroblastic abnormalities produced by chloramphenicol or lead.

QUESTION 25-4 Answer is **e**. An early sign of folic acid or vitamin B_{12} deficiency is megaloblastic anemia. Abnormal macrocytic red blood cells are produced, and the patient becomes severely anemic. This pattern of abnormal hematopoiesis is also termed *pernicious anemia*. The characteristic abnormality in red blood cell morphology is important for diagnosis and as a therapeutic guide following administration of the vitamins.

SECTION IV Inflammation, Immunomodulation, and Hematopoiesis

The anemia characteristic of severe iron deficiency is microcytic, hypochromic anemia. Copper deficiency also results in microcytic anemia because of the effects of copper deficiency on iron metabolism and heme production. Pyridoxine deficiency results in a characteristic sideroblastic anemia.

QUESTION 25-5 Answer is **d.** Romiplostim contains 4 copies of a small peptide grafted onto an immunoglobulin scaffold that binds with high affinity and activates the thrombopoietin receptor on megakaryocytes. It is approved for use in patients with immune (idiopathic) thrombocytopenic purpura (ITP) who have failed to respond to more conventional treatments. Romiplostim was found safe and efficacious in 2 randomized controlled studies in patients with ITP. Overall, ~84% of patients responded to the drug with substantial increases in platelet levels, of which approximately half were durable (platelets >50,000/μL for 6 of the last 8 weeks of study). The drug is administered weekly by subcutaneous injection, starting with a dose of 1 μg/kg, titrated to a maximum of 10 μg/kg, until platelet count increases above 50,000/μL.

Oprelvekin is recombinant IL-11 that increases peripheral platelet counts through its effects on the IL-11 receptor (see Figure 25-1 and Table 25-1). IL-11 acts synergistically with thrombopoietin.

SUMMARY: HEMATOPOIETIC AGENTS

CLASS AND SUBCLASSES	NAMES	CLINICAL USES	TOXICITIES COMMON	UNIQUE; CLINICALLY IMPORTANT
Erythropoiesis-Stimulating Agents (ESAs)	Epoetin alfa Darbepoetin alfa	Treatment of anemia, especially in patients with chronic renal failure, but also anemia associated with surgery, AIDS, cancer chemotherapy, prematurity, and certain chronic inflammatory diseases	Aggravation of hypertension (20-30% of patients) Iron deficiency (absolute or functional); virtually all patients will require supplemental iron	Thromboembolism Increased risk of cancer recurrence in patients with cancer- or chemotherapy-induced anemia Seizures with epoetin alfa in ~2.5% of patients on dialysis during first 90 d of therapy
Myeloid Growth Factors	GM-CSF (sargramostim)	Stimulate myelopoiesis in patients undergoing autologous bone marrow transplant, and in patients receiving intensive cancer chemotherapy, and some patients with cyclic neutropenia, myelodysplasia, aplastic anemia, or AIDS-associated neutropenia	Higher doses are associated with bone pain, malaise, flulike symptoms, fever, diarrhea, dyspnea, and rash	An acute reaction to first dose in sensitive patients includes flushing, hypotension, nausea, vomiting, dyspnea, fall in arterial PO_2 Capillary leak syndrome with prolonged administration in some patients Transient supraventricular arrhythmia, dyspnea, elevation of serum creatinine, bilirubin, and liver enzymes
	G-CSF (filgrastim) Pegylated recombinant G-CSF (pegfilgrastim)	Stimulation of neutrophil production (and phagocytic and cytotoxic functions of neutrophils) in patients with severe neutropenia after autologous stem cell transplantation, high-dose cancer chemotherapy, severe congenital neutropenia, and other neutropenia Used in peripheral blood stem cell (PBSC) collection to promote release of CD34+ progenitor cells	Mild to moderate bone pain with high doses over long periods Local skin reactions at site of subcutaneous injection Marked granulocytosis in patients receiving drug over prolonged periods, but not associated with increased morbidity or mortality Mild to moderate splenomegaly with long-term therapy	Rare cutaneous necrotizing vasculitis Patients with hypersensitivity to proteins produced in *Escherichia coli* should not receive the drug

Hematopoietic Agents — CHAPTER 25

CLASS AND SUBCLASSES	NAMES	CLINICAL USES	TOXICITIES COMMON	UNIQUE; CLINICALLY IMPORTANT
Thrombopoietic Growth Factors	IL-11 (oprelvekin)	Used in patients with chemotherapy-induced thrombocytopenia to increase platelet production	Fluid retention and associated cardiac symptoms, such as tachycardia, palpitation, edema, and shortness of breath; in elderly patients it often requires concomitant therapy with diuretics Blurred vision, injection-site rash or erythema, and paresthesia	
	Romiplostim Eltrombopag	Approved for use in patients with immune thrombocytopenic purpura (ITP) who have failed to respond to more conventional treatments		
Iron Supplements—Oral	Ferrous sulfate Ferrous fumarate Ferrous succinate, aspartate, and other ferrous salts Ferrous gluconate Polysaccharide-ferrihydrite complex	Treatment of iron deficiency anemia due to dietary iron deficiency, blood loss, and as an adjunct in patients treated with erythropoietin Prophylactic use of oral iron should be reserved for patients at high risk, including pregnant women, women with excessive menstrual blood loss, and infants	Heartburn, nausea, upper gastric discomfort, and diarrhea or constipation	Severe iron poisoning via accidental ingestion by children can be fatal; symptoms include abdominal pain, diarrhea, or vomiting of brown or bloody stomach contents containing pills; of particular concern are pallor or cyanosis, lassitude, drowsiness, hyperventilation due to acidosis, and cardiovascular collapse
Iron Supplements—Parenteral	Iron dextran Sodium ferric gluconate Ferumoxytol Iron sucrose	Used when oral iron therapy fails Common indications are iron malabsorption (eg, sprue, short bowel syndrome), severe oral iron intolerance, as a routine supplement to total parenteral nutrition, and in patients who are receiving erythropoietin, especially in hemodialysis patients	Reactions to intravenous iron include headache, malaise, fever, generalized lymphadenopathy, arthralgia, urticaria, and exacerbation of rheumatoid arthritis in some patients	Parenteral iron therapy should be used only when clearly indicated because acute hypersensitivity, including anaphylactic and anaphylactoid reactions, can occur in 0.2-3% of patients
Copper Supplement	Cupric sulfate	Supplementation (beginning with a therapeutic trial) in patients when a low plasma copper concentration is determined in the presence of leukopenia and anemia		
Vitamins—Pyridoxine	Pyridoxine Riboflavin	Pyridoxine is used to improve hematopoiesis in patients with either hereditary or acquired sideroblastic anemia (ie, sideroblastic anemia associated with the antituberculosis drugs isoniazid and pyrazinamide) Riboflavin used in the nutritional management of patients with gross, generalized malnutrition to treat or prevent red cell aplasia		

SECTION IV — Inflammation, Immunomodulation, and Hematopoiesis

CLASS AND SUBCLASSES	NAMES	CLINICAL USES	TOXICITIES — COMMON	TOXICITIES — UNIQUE; CLINICALLY IMPORTANT
Vitamins—Vitamin B_{12}	Cyanocobalamin (vitamin B_{12}) Hydroxocobalamin (vitamin B_{12})	Treatment of vitamin B_{12} deficiency; deficiency can manifest as severe megaloblastic anemia with neurological symptoms including paresthesia of the hands and feet, decreased vibration and position senses with resultant unsteadiness, decreased deep tendon reflexes, and in the later stages, confusion, moodiness, loss of memory, loss of central vision, hallucinations, and overt psychosis (see Side Bars CAUSES OF VITAMIN B_{12} DEFICIENCY and GENERAL PRNCIPLES OF VITAMIN B_{12} THERAPY)	Once begun, vitamin B_{12} therapy must be maintained for life; it is important to monitor vitamin B_{12} concentrations in plasma and to obtain peripheral blood counts at intervals of 3-6 mo to confirm the adequacy of therapy and monitor development of refractoriness to therapy	Cyanocobalamin should never be given intravenously due to rare reports of transitory exanthema and anaphylaxis after injection; if a patient reports a previous sensitivity to injections of vitamin B_{12}, an intradermal skin test should be performed before the full dose is administered
Vitamins—Folic Acid and Derivatives	Folic acid (pteroylglutamic acid [PteGlu], L-methylfolate) Folinic acid (leucovorin calcium, citrovorum factor)	Treatment or prevention of folate deficiency which can cause folate-deficient megaloblastic erythropoiesis and elevated plasma homocysteine Prevention of neural tube defects (folate supplements may be required early in pregnancy) Folinic acid is used to circumvent the inhibition of dihydrofolate reductase as a part of high-dose methotrexate therapy and to potentiate fluorouracil in the treatment of colorectal cancer and as an antidote to counteract the toxicity of folate antagonists such as pyrimethamine or trimethoprim (see Side Bars COMMON CAUSES OF FOLATE DEFICIENCY and GENERAL PRINCIPLES OF FOLIC ACID THERAPY)	The megaloblastic anemia that results from folate deficiency cannot be distinguished from that caused by vitamin B_{12} deficiency (see Figure 25-3); however, folate deficiency is rarely, if ever, associated with neurological abnormalities; thus the observation of characteristic abnormalities in vibratory and position sense and in motor and sensory pathways is incompatible with an isolated deficiency of folic acid Folic acid and leucovorin should never be used for the treatment of pernicious anemia or other megaloblastic anemia secondary to a deficiency of vitamin B_{12} because their use can result in an apparent response of the hematopoietic system, but neurological damage may occur or progress if already present	Rare reports of reactions to parenteral injections of folic acid and leucovorin; caution should be exercised in patients with a history of a reaction Folic acid in large amounts may counteract the antiepileptic effect of phenobarbital, phenytoin, and primidone, and increase the frequency of seizures in susceptible children

Hormones and Hormone Antagonists

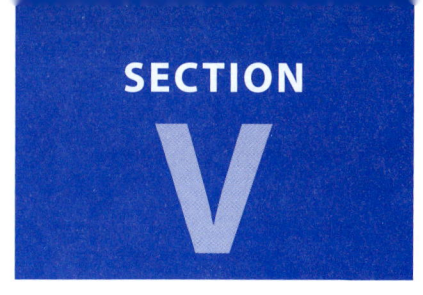

SECTION V

26. Introduction to Endocrinology: The Hypothalamic–Pituitary Axis 422
27. Thyroid and Antithyroid Drugs 431
28. Estrogens, Progestins, Contraception, and Androgens 441
29. ACTH, Adrenal Steroids, and Pharmacology of the Adrenal Cortex 459
30. Endocrine Pancreas and Pharmacotherapy of Diabetes Mellitus and Hypoglycemia 470
31. Drug Therapy of Mineral Ion Homeostasis and Bone Turnover Disorders 480

CHAPTER 26

Introduction to Endocrinology: The Hypothalamic–Pituitary Axis

DRUGS INCLUDED IN THIS CHAPTER

Bromocriptine (PARLODEL, CYLOSERT, others)
Cabergoline (CABERLIN, DOSTINEX, CABASER)
Cetrorelix (CETROTIDE)
Choriogonadotropin alfa (OVIDREL)
Follitropin α (GONAL-F)
Follitropin β (FOLLISTIM, PUREGON)
Ganirelix (ANTAGON)
Gonadorelin (FACTREL, LUTREPULSE)
Goserelin (ZOLADEX)
Histrelin (VANTAS, SUPPRELIN LA)
Lanreotide (SOMATULINE LA, SOMATULINE DEPOT)
Leuprolide (LUPRON, ELIGARD)
Lutropin alfa (LUVERIS, LHADI)
Mecasermin (INCRELEX)
Menotropins (REPRONEX)
Nafarelin (SYNAREL)
Octreotide (SANDOSTATIN, SANDOSTATIN-LAR DEPOT)
Oxytocin
Pegvisomant (SOMAVERT)
Pergolide (PERMAX)
Quinagolide (NORPROLAC)
Recombinant human growth hormon-eGH (ACCRETRTROPIN, GENOTROPIN, HUMATROPE, NORDITROPIN, NUTROPIN, OMNITROPE, SAIZEN, SERPSTIM, TEV-TROPIN, ZORBTIVE, NUTROPINE DEPOT)
Triptorelin (TRELSTAR DEPOT LA)
Urine-derived human chorionic gonadotropin (hCG; NOVAREL, PREGNYL, PROFASI)
Urofollitropin (uFSH; BRAVELLE, MENOPUR)

This chapter will be most useful after having a basic understanding of the material in Chapter 38, Introduction to Endocrinology: The Hypothalamic Pituitary Axis in *Goodman & Gilman's The Pharmacological Basis of Therapeutics*, 12th Edition. In addition to the material presented here, the 12th Edition includes:

- A detailed discussion of the hypothalamic-pituitary-endocrine axis
- A description of the pituitary hormones and their releasing factors
- A discussion of the therapy of growth hormone (GH) deficiency
- A discussion of the glycoprotein hormones: thyroid stimulating hormone (TSH) and gonadotropins
- A discussion of the posterior pituitary hormones: oxytocin and vasopressin

LEARNING OBJECTIVES

☑ Understand the functioning of the hypothalamic-pituitary axis.
☑ Describe the pharmacotherapy of GH excess and GH deficiency.
☑ Develop knowledge of the clinical uses of gonadotropin-releasing hormone (GnRH) and its analogs.

MECHANISMS OF ACTION OF DRUGS THAT ACT ON THE HYPOTHALAMIC-PITUITARY AXIS

DRUG CLASS	DRUG	MECHANISM OF ACTION
Somatostatin (SST) Analogs	Octreotide	SST analog that inhibits the release of GH from the pituitary (see Figures 26-1 and 26-2)
	Lanreotide	SST analog that inhibits the release of GH from the pituitary (see Figures 26-1 and 26-2)
Growth Hormone (GH) Antagonist	Pegvisomant	GH receptor antagonist (see Figure 26-3)
Dopamine (DA) Receptor Agonists	Quinagolide	DA receptor agonist; inhibits release of prolactin (see Figure 26-4)
	Bromocriptine	DA receptor agonist; inhibits release of prolactin (see Figure 26-4)
	Cabergoline	DA receptor agonist; inhibits release of prolactin (see Figure 26-4)
Recombinant GH	Recombinant GH	Binds to GH receptor (see Figure 26-3)
Insulin-like Growth Factor-1 (IGF-1)	Mecasermin	Mimics effects of GH (see Figure 26-2)
Gonadotropin-Releasing Hormone (GnRH) Agonists	GnRH	Signals through a specific GPCR on gonadotropic cells in the anterior pituitary to release follicle-stimulating hormone (FSH) and luteinizing hormone (LH) (see Figure 26-5)
	Goserelin	GnRH agonist
	Naferelin	GnRH agonist
	Triptorelin	GnRH agonist

(Continued)

Introduction to Endocrinology: The Hypothalamic–Pituitary Axis

CHAPTER 26

DRUG CLASS	DRUG	MECHANISM OF ACTION
	Histrelin	GnRH agonist
	Leuprolide	GnRH agonist
GnRH Antagonists	Cetrorelix	Antagonizes the effect of GnRH on gonadotropic cells
	Ganirelix	Antagonizes the effect of GnRH on gonadotropic cells
Follicle-Stimulating Hormone (FSH)	Menotropin	FSH preparation that acts on the FSH receptor
	Urofollitropin (uFSH)	FSH preparation that acts the FSH receptor
	Follitropin α	Recombinant FSH that acts on the FSH receptor
	Follitropin β	Recombinant FSH that acts on the FSH receptor
Human Chorionic Gonadotropin (hCG)	Choriogonadotropin alfa	Recombinant hCG that acts on the LH receptor
LuteinizingHormone (LH)	Lutropin alfa	Recombinant LH that acts on the LH receptor
Posterior Pituitary Hormones	Oxytocin	Acts via specific GPCR to enhance voltage-sensitive Ca^{2+} channels
	Arginine vasopressin	See Chapter 15

CASE 26-1

A 43-year-old man of normal height has been diagnosed with acromegaly.

a. **What is acromegaly and why is this patient's height normal?**

Acromegaly is the result of excess secretion of GH from an anterior pituitary adenoma. The organization of the posterior and anterior pituitary glands is shown in Figure 26-1. In adults, the signs and symptoms of acromegaly are arthropathy, carpal tunnel syndrome, visceromegaly, macroglossia, hypertension, glucose intolerance, headache, lethargy, excess perspiration, and sleep apnea. If the epiphyses are unclosed (presumably the epiphyses are closed in this patient), the GH excess results in increased longitudinal growth and gigantism.

b. **How is GH secretion regulated?**

Growth hormone–releasing hormone (GHRH) and somatostatin (SST), released from the hypothalamus, stimulate or inhibit the release of GH from the pituitary, respectively (see Figure 26-2). Insulin-like growth factor (IGF-1), a product of GH action on peripheral tissues, causes negative feedback inhibition of GH release at the level of the hypothalamus and the pituitary.

c. **How does GH cause its myriad of effects on various tissues?**

GH and prolactin act on specific receptors in target tissues. The GH receptor is a widely distributed cell surface receptor that consists of an extracellular hormone-binding domain, a single membrane-spanning region, and an intracellular domain that mediates signal transduction (see Figure 26-3).

d. **What are the options for treatment of acromegaly in this patient?**

Treatment options include transphenoidal surgery, radiation, and drugs that inhibit GH secretion. Increased attention has been given to pharmacological treatment of acromegaly either as primary treatment or for the treatment of persistent GH

(Continued)

SECTION V — Hormones and Hormone Antagonists

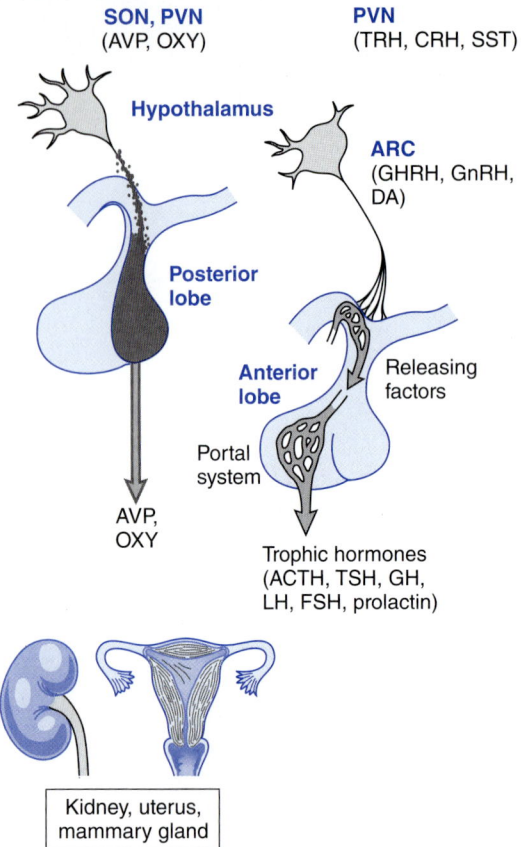

FIGURE 26-1 Organization of the anterior and posterior pituitary gland. Hypothalamic neurons in the supraoptic (SON) and paraventricular (PVN) nuclei synthesize arginine vasopressin (AVP) or oxytocin (OXY). Most of their axons project directly to the posterior pituitary, from which AVP and OXY are secreted into the systemic circulation to regulate their target tissues. Neurons that regulate the anterior lobe cluster in the mediobasal hypothalamus, including the PVN and the arcuate (ARC) nuclei. They secrete hypothalamic-releasing hormones, which reach the anterior pituitary via the hypothalamic-adenohypophyseal portal system and stimulate distinct populations of pituitary cells. These cells, in turn, secrete the trophic (signal) hormones, which regulate endocrine organs and other tissues. ACTH, Adrenocorticotrophic hormone; CRH, corticotropin-releasing hormone; DA, dopamine; FSH, follicle-stimulating hormone; GH, growth hormone; GHRH, growth hormone-releasing hormone; GnRH, gonadotropin-releasing hormone; LH, luteinizing hormone; TRH, thyrotropin-releasing hormone; TSH, thyroid-stimulating hormone.

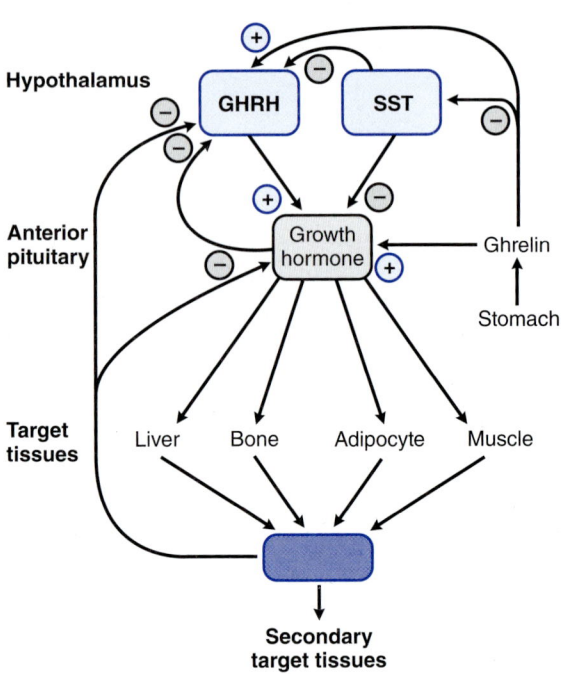

FIGURE 26-2 Growth hormone secretion and actions. Two hypothalamic factors, growth hormone–releasing hormone (GHRH) and somatostatin (SST) stimulate or inhibit the release of growth hormone (GH) from the pituitary, respectively. Insulin-like growth factor-1 (IGF-1), a product of GH action on peripheral tissues, causes negative feedback inhibition of GH release by acting at the hypothalamus and the pituitary. The actions of GH can be direct or indirect (mediated by IGF-1). Inhibition, −; stimulation, +.

excess after transphenoidal surgery. Octreotide and lanreotide are 2 SST analogs that are used widely to treat acromegaly. Both are available as long-acting formulations that require an intramuscular injection once every 4 weeks.

Pegvisomant is a GH receptor antagonist (see Figure 26-3) that is approved for the treatment of acromegaly. Pegvisomant binds to the GH receptor, but does not initiate signaling or stimulate IGF-1 secretion.

e. What adverse effects should this patient be warned about as a result of this treatment?

Diarrhea, nausea, and abdominal pain are common with octreotide and lanreotide but may diminish over time. Patients receiving these drugs may develop gallbladder sludge or gallstones. Inhibitory effects on thyroid-stimulating hormone (TSH) secretion may lead to hypothyroidism and thyroid function tests should be monitored periodically.

Pegvisomant should not be used in patients with elevated hepatic transaminases and hepatic function should be assessed in all patients. Loss of negative feedback of GH and IGF-1 may increase growth of GH-secreting adenomas.

Introduction to Endocrinology: The Hypothalamic–Pituitary Axis

CHAPTER 26

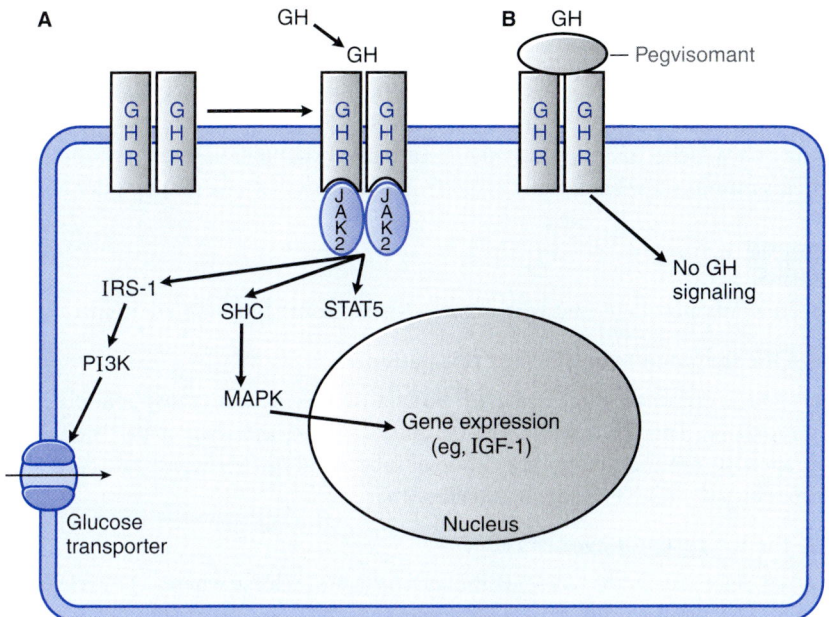

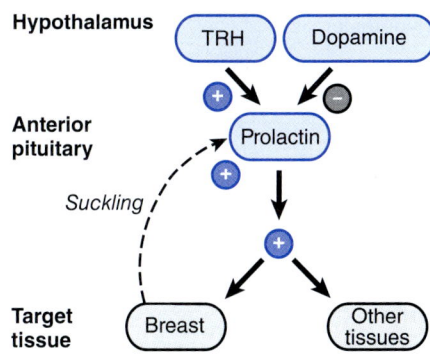

FIGURE 26-3 Mechanisms of growth hormone and prolactin action and of GH receptor antagonism. **Left (A):** The binding of GH to a homodimer of the GH receptor (GHR) induces autophosphorylation of JAK2. JAK2 then phosphorylates cytoplasmic proteins that activate downstream signaling pathways, including STAT5 and mediators upstream of MAPK, which ultimately modulate gene expression. The structurally related prolactin receptor also is a ligand-activated homodimer that recruits the JAK-STAT signaling pathway. The GHR also activates IRS-1, which may mediate the increased expression of glucose transporters on the plasma membrane. The diagram does not reflect the localization of the intracellular molecules, which presumably exist in multicomponent signaling complexes. JAK2, janus kinase 2; IRS-1, insulin receptor substrate-1; PI3K, phosphatidyl inositol-3 kinase; STAT, signal transducer and activator of transcription; MAPK, mitogen-activated protein kinase; SHC, Src homology containing. **Right (B):** Pegvisomant, a recombinant pegylated variant of human GH, contains amino acid substitutions that increase the affinity for 1 site of the GHR but do not activate its downstream signaling cascade. It thus interferes with GH signaling in target tissues.

FIGURE 26-4 Prolactin secretion and actions. Prolactin is the only anterior pituitary hormone for which a unique stimulatory releasing factor has not been identified. Thyrotropin-releasing hormone (TRH), however, can stimulate prolactin release and dopamine can inhibit it. Suckling induces prolactin secretion, and prolactin affects lactation and reproductive functions but also has varied effects on many other tissues. Prolactin is not under feedback control by peripheral hormones.

CASE 26-2

A 56-year-old man with advanced prostate cancer is being treated with leuprolide.

a. What is leuprolide and why is it used to treat prostate cancer?

Leuprolide is a synthetic gonadotropin-releasing hormone (GnRH) agonist that has greater receptor affinity, reduced enzymatic degradation, and is more potent than the naturally occurring GnRH. Endogenous GnRH is released from the hypothalamus and acts on the pituitary to release luteinizing hormone (LH) and follicle-stimulating hormone (FSH). LH acts on the testes to promote the secretion of androgens (see Figures 26-1 and 26-5).

Androgens stimulate the growth of normal and cancerous prostate cells (see Chapter 46). Standard therapy for advanced prostate cancer is surgical or pharmacological androgen deprivation therapy (see Chapter 46).

b. How does a GnRH agonist suppress androgen secretion?

The GnRH agonists bind to GnRH receptors on pituitary gonadotropin-producing cells, causing an initial release of LH and FSH and a subsequent increase in testosterone production from testicular Leydig cells. After approximately 1 week of therapy, GnRH receptors are downregulated on the gonadotropin-producing cells, causing a decline in the pituitary response and a subsequent decline in testosterone production.

(Continued)

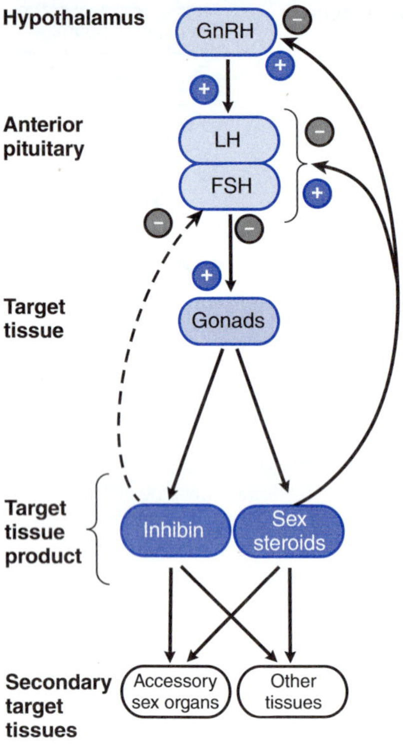

SECTION V

Hormones and Hormone Antagonists

FIGURE 26-5 The hypothalamic-pituitary-gonadal axis. A single hypothalamic-releasing factor, gonadotropin-releasing hormone (GnRH), controls the synthesis and release of both gonadotropins (LH and FSH) in males and females. Gonadal steroid hormones (androgens, estrogens, and progesterone) exert feedback inhibition at the level of the pituitary and the hypothalamus. The preovulatory surge of estrogen also can exert a stimulatory effect at the level of the pituitary and the hypothalamus. Inhibins, a family of polypeptide hormones produced by the gonads, specifically inhibit FSH secretion by the pituitary.

c. **What untoward effects might this patient expect as a result of the leuprolide therapy?**

He should be told to expect hot flashes, possible decreased bone density, and erectile dysfunction. There is an apparent increase in the incidence of pituitary apoplexy, a syndrome of headache, neurological manifestations, and impaired pituitary function; these effects mimic ones that usually result from an infarction of a pituitary adenoma.

CASE 26-3

A 32-year-old woman is diagnosed with a prolactin-secreting pituitary adenoma.

a. **What are the therapeutic options for this patient?**

The therapeutic options for patients with prolactinomas include transphenoidal surgery, radiation, and treatment with dopamine (DA) receptor agonists. The DA receptor agonists are the treatment of choice since the surgical success rate is 75% for microadenomas and 33% for macroadenomas.

b. **Why are the DA receptor agonists effective?**

Thyrotropin-releasing factor (TRH) stimulates prolactin release whereas DA released from the hypothalamus inhibits prolactin release (see Figure 26-4). The DA receptor agonists decrease both prolactin secretion and the size of the adenoma, thereby improving the endocrine abnormalities and the neurological symptoms (including visual field defects).

c. **What DA receptor agonists are used to treat hyperprolactinemia?**

The drugs in this class include bromocriptine, cabergoline, and quinagolide. Bromocriptine normalizes serum prolactin concentrations in 70% to 80% of patients and decreases tumor size in more than 50% of patients. Typically, hyperprolactinemia and tumor growth recur upon cessation of therapy.

Cabergoline has a higher affinity and greater selectivity for the D_2 receptor than bromocriptine. It is becoming the preferred drug in this setting. Cabergoline may induce remission in a significant number of patients with prolactinomas.

Quinagolide is not approved by the FDA but has been used extensively in Europe and Canada.

d. **What adverse effects might be expected from therapy with bromocriptine or cabergoline?**

Bromocriptine frequently causes nausea, vomiting, headache, and postural hypotension, particularly on initial use. Less frequently, bromocriptine may cause nasal congestion, digital vasospasm, and CNS effects such as psychoses, hallucinations, nightmares, or insomnia.

Cabergoline causes much less nausea than bromocriptine, but may still cause dizziness and hypotension. Cabergoline has been linked to valvular heart disease and echocardiographic assessment is appropriate for patients receiving chronic therapy.

KEY CONCEPTS

➡ The peptide hormones of the anterior pituitary are essential for the regulation of growth and development, reproduction, response to stress, and intermediary metabolism.

➡ The synthesis and secretion of the pituitary hormones are controlled by hypothalamic hormones and by hormones from the peripheral endocrine organs (see Figure 26-1).

➡ The most striking physiological effect of GH is the stimulation of the longitudinal growth of bones (see Figure 26-2).

(Continued)

Introduction to Endocrinology: The Hypothalamic–Pituitary Axis

CHAPTER 26

➡ GH excess is treated with the SST analogs octreotide and lanreotide.
➡ GH deficiency is treated with recombinant human GH.
➡ Analogs of GnRH are used predominantly to treat advanced prostate cancer (see Chapter 46).

SUMMARY QUIZ

QUESTION 26-1 A 78-year-old woman has received GH injections from an antiaging clinic. She is likely to experience which of the following effects?

a. Growth of the long bones in her legs
b. Carpal tunnel syndrome
c. Blurred vision
d. Decreased hearing
e. A metallic taste

QUESTION 26-2 A 6-year-old boy is diagnosed with central or GnRH-dependent precocious puberty. He is being treated with nafarelin, a GnRH analog, as a nasal spray. GnRH analogs are effective in precocious puberty because they

a. downregulate GnRh receptors on pituitary gonadotropes.
b. block the action of testosterone on muscle cells.
c. stimulate testicular estrogen synthesis.
d. antagonize the effect of luteinizing hormone (LH).
e. antagonize the effect of GnRH release from the hypothalamus.

QUESTION 26-3 A 20-year-old male cyclist is suspected of using performance-enhancing drugs. Although his urine testosterone concentration is elevated, his testosterone/epitestosterone (T/E) (a measure of exogenous testosterone administration) ratio is normal. He has achieved this state by the use of which of the following?

a. Estrogen
b. Progestin
c. Human chorionic gonadotropin (hCG)
d. Low dose testosterone
e. Growth hormone (GH)

QUESTION 26-4 A 4-year-old boy with short stature is diagnosed with growth hormone (GH) deficiency. His GH replacement therapy should be continued until

a. he is in the 90th percentile on growth charts.
b. he is in the 60th percentile on growth charts.
c. his epiphyses are fused.
d. he begins to develop secondary sex characteristics.
e. he has permanent teeth.

QUESTION 26-5 A 22-year-old man is determined to have impaired fertility secondary to gonadotropin deficiency. He is being treated with recombinant FSH. The most common side effect with gonadotropin therapy is

a. hirsutism.
b. alopecia.
c. erectile dysfunction.
d. dry skin.
e. gynecomastia.

SECTION V — Hormones and Hormone Antagonists

SUMMARY QUIZ ANSWER KEY

QUESTION 26-1 Answer is **b**. Side effects associated with the initiation of GH therapy in adults include peripheral edema, carpal tunnel syndrome, arthralgia, or myalgia, which occur most frequently in patients who are older or obese.

QUESTION 26-2 Answer is **a**. The intermittent release of GnRH is crucial for the proper synthesis and release of the gonadotropins; the continuous administration of GnRH leads to desensitization and downregulation of GnRH receptors on pituitary gonadotropes and forms the basis for the clinical use of long-acting GnRH agonists to suppress gonadotropin secretion.

QUESTION 26-3 Answer is **c**. The administration of hCG can stimulate testosterone secretion in males with normal Leydig cell function. Epitestosterone is an inactive epimer of testosterone secreted from the testes. The normal T/E ratio is approximately one. A ratio much larger than this would suggest the exogenous administration of testosterone. hCG administration would stimulate endogenous testosterone secretion and thus the T/E ratio would be close to one.

QUESTION 26-4 Answer is **c**. Although the most pronounced increase in growth occurs during the first 2 years of therapy, GH is continued until the epiphyses are fused and may be extended into the transition period from childhood to adulthood.

QUESTION 26-5 Answer is **e**. The most common side effect of gonadotropin therapy in males is gynecomastia, which occurs in up to a third of patients and presumably reflects increased production of estrogens due to the induction of aromatase.

SUMMARY: DRUGS THAT ACT ON HYPOTHALAMIC–PITUITARY AXIS

CLASS AND SUBCLASSES	NAMES	CLINICAL USES	TOXICITIES COMMON	TOXICITIES UNIQUE; CLINICALLY IMPORTANT
Somatostatin (SST) Analogs	Octreotide	Treatment of acromegaly	Diarrhea, nausea, abdominal pain	Gallbladder sludge; Hypothyroidism because of inhibition of TSH secretion
	Lanreotide	Treatment of acromegaly	Diarrhea, nausea, abdominal pain	Gallbladder sludge; Hypothyroidism because of inhibition of TSH secretion
Growth Hormone (GH) Antagonist	Pegvisomant	Treatment of acromegaly	Lipohypertrophy at injection site	Should not be used in patients with elevated hepatic transaminases
Dopamine (DA) Receptor Agonists	Quinagolide	Treatment of hyperprolactinemia (Not approved by FDA, but available in Europe and Canada)		
	Bromocriptine	Treatment of hyperprolactinemia	Nausea, vomiting, headache	Postural hypotension
	Cabergoline	Treatment of hyperprolactinemia	Less nausea than bromocriptine	Postural hypotension; Linked with valvular heart disease
Recombinant GH	Recombinant GH	Treatment of GH deficiency	Peripheral edema, carpal tunnel syndrome, arthralgia, myalgia	Should not be used in patients with neoplasia, proliferative retinopathy, or acute respiratory failure
Insulin-like Growth Factor-1 (IGF-1)	Mecasermin	Treatment of impaired growth due to mutations in GH receptor or postreceptor pathway	Hypoglycemia, lipohypertrophy	Should not be used in patients with closed epiphyses or in patients with neoplasia

(Continued)

Introduction to Endocrinology: The Hypothalamic–Pituitary Axis — CHAPTER 26

CLASS AND SUBCLASSES	NAMES	CLINICAL USES	TOXICITIES COMMON	UNIQUE; CLINICALLY IMPORTANT
Gonadotropin-Releasing Hormone (GnRH) Agonist	GnRH	Problems with availability have limited its use		
	Goserelin	Approved for use in endometriosis, prostate and breast cancer	Hot flashes; Decreased bone density in both sexes; Vaginal dryness and atrophy in women, erectile dysfunction in men	Syndrome mimicking pituitary adenoma infarction, including headache, impaired pituitary function and neurological manifestation; Contraindicated in pregnant women
	Naferelin	Approved for use in endometriosis and central precocious puberty	Hot flashes; Decreased bone density in both sexes; Vaginal dryness and atrophy in women, erectile dysfunction in men	Syndrome mimicking pituitary adenoma infarction including headache, impaired pituitary function and neurological manifestation; Contraindicated in pregnant women
	Triptorelin	Approved for advanced prostate cancer	Hot flashes; Decreased bone density in both sexes; Vaginal dryness and atrophy in women, erectile dysfunction in men	Syndrome mimicking pituitary adenoma infarction, including headache, impaired pituitary function and neurological manifestation; Contraindicated in pregnant women
	Histrelin	Approved for advanced prostate cancer and central precocious puberty	Hot flashes; Decreased bone density in both sexes; Vaginal dryness and atrophy in women, erectile dysfunction in men	Syndrome mimicking pituitary adenoma infarction, including headache, impaired pituitary function and neurological manifestation; Contraindicated in pregnant women
	Leuprolide	Approved for use in endometriosis, uterine fibroids, prostate cancer, and central precocious puberty	Hot flashes; Decreased bone density in both sexes; Vaginal dryness and atrophy in women, erectile dysfunction in men	Syndrome mimicking pituitary adenoma infarction, including headache, impaired pituitary function and neurological manifestation; Contraindicated in pregnant women
GnRH Antagonists	Cetrorelix	Prevention of LH surge and premature ovulation in ovarian-stimulation protocols (see Chapter 28)		Hypersensitivity reactions, including anaphylaxis; Contraindicated in pregnant women
	Ganirelix	Prevention of LH surge and premature ovulation in ovarian-stimulation protocols (see Chapter 28)		Hyper-sensitivity reactions, including anaphylaxis; Contraindicated in pregnant women
Follicle-Stimulating Hormone (FSH)	Menotropin	Ovarian stimulation or in vitro fertilization; Development of tests for the diagnosis of reproductive disorders		
	Urofollitropin	Ovarian stimulation or in vitro fertilization; Development of tests for the diagnosis of reproductive disorders		

(Continued)

SECTION V — Hormones and Hormone Antagonists

CLASS AND SUBCLASSES	NAMES	CLINICAL USES	TOXICITIES COMMON	TOXICITIES UNIQUE; CLINICALLY IMPORTANT
	Follitropin α	Ovarian stimulation or in vitro fertilization. Development of tests for the diagnosis of reproductive disorders		
	Follitropin β	Ovarian stimulation or in vitro fertilization. Development of tests for the diagnosis of reproductive disorders		
Human Chorionic Gonadotropin (hCG)	Choriogonadotropin alfa	Treatment of male infertility and cryptorchidism	Gynecomastia	
Luteinizing Hormone	Lutropin alfa	Development of tests of LH surge to determine ovulation. Diagnosis of reproductive disorders		
Posterior Pituitary Hormones	Oxytocin	Used to induce or augment labor or to prevent post-partum hemorrhage (see Chapter 28)		

Thyroid and Antithyroid Drugs

CHAPTER 27

This chapter will be most useful after having a basic understanding of the material in Chapter 39, Thyroid and Antithyroid Drugs in *Goodman & Gilman's The Pharmacological Basis of Therapeutics*, 12th Edition. In addition to the material presented here, the 12th Edition contains:

- A discussion of the chemistry and biosynthesis of the thyroid hormones.
- Figure 39-1 Thyronine, thyroid hormones, and precursors, shows the chemical structures of the thyroid hormones
- A detailed discussion of thyroid hormone metabolism and the conversion of thyroxine to triiodothyronine in peripheral tissues
- A discussion of the actions of thyroid hormone including the non-genomic effects of thyroid hormones, the effects of thyroid hormone metabolites, the effects of thyroid hormones on growth and development, and the thermogenic, cardiovascular, and metabolic effects of thyroid hormones
- Table 39-5 Selected Pharmacokinetic Features of Anti-Thyroid Drugs, shows selected pharmacokinetic features of propylthiouracil and methimazole

DRUGS INCLUDED IN THIS CHAPTER

- Carbimazole (NEO-MERCAZOLE)
- Desiccated thyroid (ARMOR THYROID, others)
- Iodide
- Levothyroxine (L-T_4, LEVOTHROID, LEVOXYL, SYNTHROID, UNITHROID, others)
- Liotrix (a thyroxine/triiodothyronine 4:1 mixture; THYROLAR)
- Methimazole (TAPAZOLE, others)
- Propylthiouracil
- Sodium iodine (IODOPEN)
- Sodium iodine ^{131}I (HICON, others)
- Triiodothyroxine (CYTOMEL, TRIOSTAT, others)

LEARNING OBJECTIVES

- ☑ Understand the principles of thyroid hormone regulation.
- ☑ Describe the diagnosis and treatment of hypothyroidism and hyperthyroidism, including during pregnancy.
- ☑ Describe the treatment options for well-differentiated thyroid cancer.

MECHANISMS OF ACTION OF THYROID AND ANTITHYROID DRUGS

DRUG CLASS	DRUG	MECHANISM OF ACTION
Thyroid Hormone	Levothyroxine Triiodothyroxine Liotrix Desiccated thyroid	Binding of 3,5,3'-triiodothyronine T_3 to thyroid hormone receptors (members of the nuclear receptor superfamily of transcription factors) on target tissues
Antithyroid Drugs	Propylthiouracil Methimazole Carbimazole	Interferes with the incorporation of iodine into tyrosyl residues to form iodothyronine (see Figure 27-1)
Ionic Thyroid Inhibitors	Iodide Sodium iodine	At high concentrations, iodide inhibits the synthesis of iodotyrosines and iodothyronines; high concentrations also inhibit the release of thyroid hormones
Radioactive Iodine	Sodium iodine ^{131}I	Incorporated into iodoamines and deposited into the colloid of thyroid follicles where the destructive β particles are released

THYROID FUNCTION TESTS

TSH (Thyroid-stimulating hormone)	Elevated in hypothyroidism; decreased in hyperthyroidism
T_4 (Thyroxine)	Elevated levels suggest hyperthyroidism; decreased levels suggest hypothyroidism
T_3 (Triiodothyronine)	Elevated levels suggest hyperthyroidism; decreased levels suggest hypothyroidism

SECTION V

Hormones and Hormone Antagonists

SYMPTOMS OF THYROID DISEASE

HYPOFUNCTION	HYPERFUNCTION
Fatigue	Exophthalmus—Graves disease
Lethargy	Excessive production of heat
Cold intolerance	Increased motor activity
Mental slowness	Increased sensitivity to catecholamines
Depression	Flushed skin
Dry skin	Warm moist skin
Constipation	Weak muscles
Mild weight gain	Tremulousness
Fluid retention	Rapid, forced heart rate
Muscle aches	Increased appetite
Irregular menses	Weight loss if intake is inadequate
Infertility	Heat intolerance
	Increased frequency of bowel movements

CASE 27-1

A 69-year-old man goes to his family doctor because he has been feeling fatigued and lethargic. His doctor does a complete evaluation. This patient had a myocardial infarction and has a recurrent ventricular arrhythmia. The patient's TSH is elevated and his T_4 is slightly decreased. The doctor suspects hypothyroidism and begins replacement therapy with levothyroxine.

a. Why is the TSH elevated in this patient?

The regulation of thyroid function is shown in Figure 27-2. Thyrotropin-releasing hormone (TRH) is released from the hypothalamus when circulating concentrations of thyroid hormone (T_4 and T_3) are low. TRH stimulates the release of preformed TSH granules from the pituitary. The released TSH binds to a GPCR receptor on the plasma membrane of thyroid cells and eventually all phases of thyroid hormone synthesis and release are stimulated (see Figure 27-2). When thyroid hormone levels are low, the negative feedback inhibition on the hypothalamic TRH release is removed and TSH secretion is increased.

b. What factors might affect the levothyroxine dose in this patient?

Table 27-1 lists some of the factors that may influence the dose of levothyroxine. This patient has had a myocardial infarction and is being treated for a ventricular arrhythmia with amiodarone (see Chapter 18). Amiodarone is an iodine-containing drug which may impair the conversion of T_4 to T_3.

c. What commonly prescribed drugs are associated with iodine-induced hypothyroidism?

Table 27-2 lists the iodine content of commonly prescribed drugs.

d. What is the goal of levothyroxine replacement therapy?

Levothyroxine is the hormone of choice for thyroid hormone replacement therapy. With this therapy one relies on the type 1 and 2 deiodinases to convert T_4 to T_3 to maintain a steady serum concentration of T_3 (see Figure 27-1). The goal of therapy is to normalize the serum TSH (in primary hypothyroidism) or free T_4 (in secondary hypothyroidism) and to relieve the symptoms of hypothyroidism.

(Continued)

Thyroid and Antithyroid Drugs CHAPTER 27

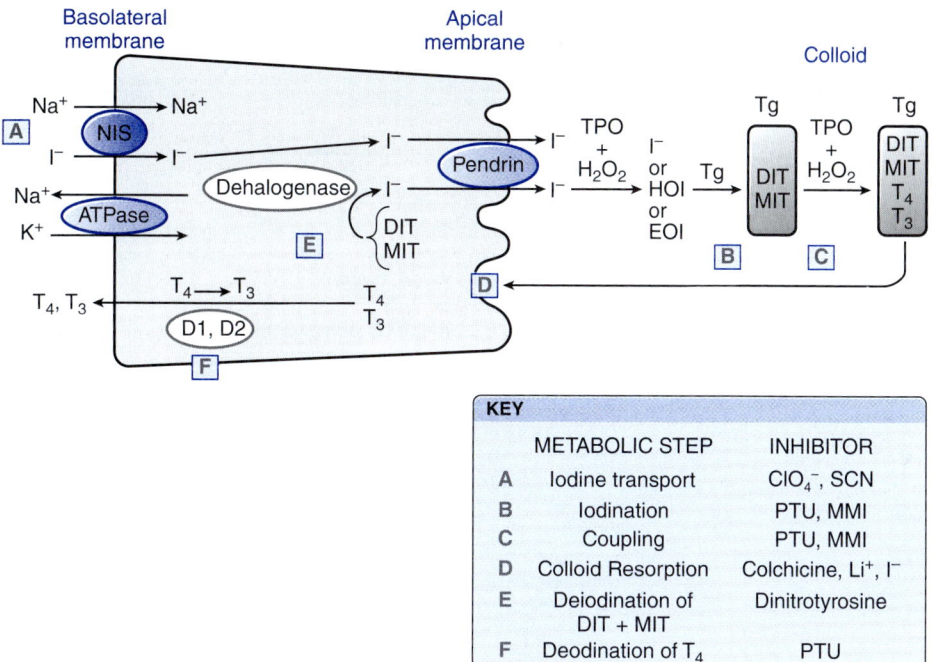

FIGURE 27-1 Major pathways of thyroid hormone biosynthesis and release. D1 and D2, deiodinases; DIT, diiodotyrosine; EOI, enzyme-linked species; HOI, hypoiodous acid; MMI, methimazole; MIT, monoiodotyrosine; PTU, propylthiouracil; Tg, thyroglobulin; TPO, thyroid peroxidase.

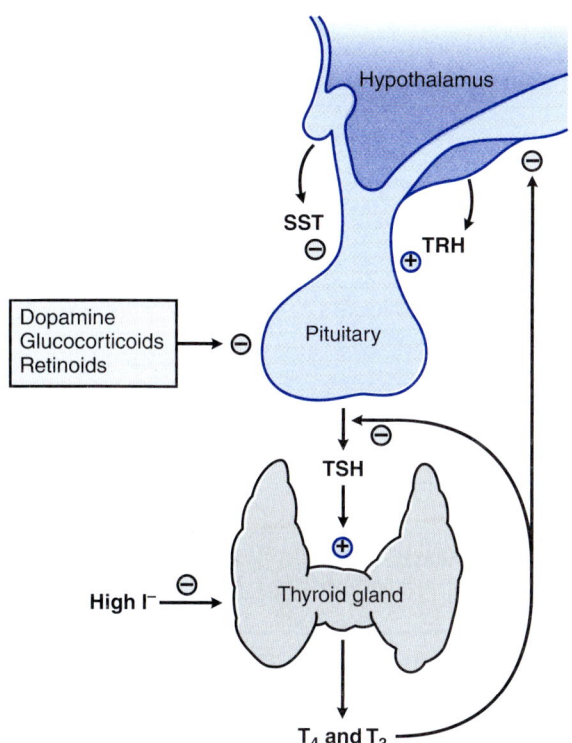

FIGURE 27-2 Regulation of thyroid hormone secretion. Myriad neural inputs influence hypothalamic secretion of thyrotropin-releasing hormone (TRH). TRH stimulates release of thyrotropin (TSH, thyroid-stimulating hormone) from the anterior pituitary; TSH stimulates the synthesis and release of the thyroid hormones T_3 and T_4. T_3 and T_4 feed back to inhibit the synthesis and release of TRH and TSH. Somatostatin (SST) can inhibit TRH action, as can dopamine and high concentrations of glucocorticoids. Low levels of I^- are required for thyroxine synthesis, but high levels inhibit thyroxin synthesis and release.

(Continued)

SECTION V — Hormones and Hormone Antagonists

TABLE 27-1 Factors Influencing Oral Levothyroxine Therapy

Drugs and other factors that may increase levothyroxine dosage requirements

Impaired levothyroxine absorption
- Aluminum-containing antacids
- Bile acid sequestrants (cholestyramine, colestipol, colesevelam)
- Calcium carbonate (effect generally small)
- Chromium picolinate
- Food
- Iron salts
- Lactose intolerance (single case report)
- Phosphate binders (lanthanum carbonate, sevelamer)
- Proton pump inhibitors
- Raloxifene
- Soy products (effect generally very small)
- Sucralfate

Increased thyroxine metabolism, CYP3A4 induction of hepatic
- Bexarotene
- Carbamapzepine
- Phenytoin
- Rifampin
- Sertraline

Impaired $T_4 \rightarrow T_3$ conversion
- Amiodarone

Mechanisms uncertain or multifactorial
- Estrogen pregnancy
- Ethionamide
- Tyrosine kinase inhibitors (imatinib, sunitinib)
- Lovastatin, simvastatin

Drugs and other factors that may decrease levothyroxine dosage requirements
- Advancing age (>65 years)
- Androgen therapy in women

Drugs that may decrease TSH without changing free T_4 in levothyroxine-treated patients
- Metformin

TABLE 27-2 Commonly Used Iodine-Containing Drugs

DRUGS	IODINE CONTENT
Oral or local	
Amiodarone	75 mg/tablet
Calcium iodide syrup	26 mg/mL
Iodoquinol (diiodohydroxyquin)	134-416 mg/tablet
Echothiophate iodide ophthalmic solution	5-41 µg/drop
Hydriodic acid syrup	13-15 mg/mL
Iodochlorhydroxyquin	104 mg/tablet
Iodine-containing vitamins	0.15 mg/tablet
Idoxuridine ophthalmic solution	18 µg/drop
Kelp/seaweed	0.15 mg/tablet
Lugol's solution	6.3 mg/drop
PONARIS nasal emollient	5 mg/0.8 mL
KI, saturated solution (KISS)	38 mg/drop
Topical antiseptics	
Iodoquinol cream (diiodohydroxyquin)	6 mg/g
Iodine tincture	40 mg/mL
Iodochlorhydroxyquin cream	12 mg/g
Iodoform gauze	4.8 mg/100 mg gauze
Povidone–iodine	10 mg/mL
Radiology contrast agents	
Diatrizoate meglumine sodium	370 mg/mL
Propyliodone	340 mg/mL
Iopanoic acid	333 mg/tablet
Ipodate	308 mg/capsule
Iothalamate	480 mg/mL
Metrizamide (undiluted)	483 mg/mL
Iohexol	463 mg/mL

Adapted from Roti E, Cozani R, Braverman LE. Adverse effects of iodine on the thyroid. *Endocrinologist*, 1997, 7:245-254. With permission. Copyright © Lippincott Williams & Wilkins. http://lww.com.

e. **What are the adverse effects of levothyroxine therapy?**

Adverse effects of thyroid hormone would generally occur only upon overtreatment and would be similar to the consequences of hyperthyroidism. An excess of thyroid hormone can increase the risk of atrial fibrillation, especially in the elderly, and can increase the risk of osteoporosis, especially in postmenopausal women.

Thyroid and Antithyroid Drugs — CHAPTER 27

CASE 27-2

A 26-year-old first trimester pregnant woman is diagnosed with hyperthyroidism.

a. What are the treatment options for this woman?

Thyrotoxicosis occurs in approximately 0.2% of pregnancies and is caused by Graves disease. Graves disease is an autoimmune disorder characterized by increased thyroid hormone production, diffuse goiter, and immunoglobulin (Ig)G antibodies that bind and activate the TSH receptor. The characteristic exophthalmos associated with Graves disease is an infiltrative opthalmopathy. Antithyroid drugs are the treatment of choice; radioactive iodine is clearly contraindicated. Both propylthiouracil and methimazole cross the placenta equally and both may be used safely although concern for liver failure in pregnancy may favor the use of methimazole. Methimazole is rarely associated with congenital gut anomalies and should be used after organogenesis in the first trimester. Graves disease often improves during the course of pregnancy and it is not uncommon for patients either to be on very low doses or off antithyroid drugs completely by the end of pregnancy.

b. What is the mechanism of action of methimazole?

Antithyroid drugs inhibit the formation of thyroid hormones by interfering with the incorporation of iodine into tyrosyl residues of thyroglobulin; they also inhibit the coupling of these iodotyrosyl residues to form iodothyronines (see Figure 27-1).

c. What other compounds (other than the typical antithyroid drugs) are inhibitors of thyroid function?

Table 27-3 is a list of compounds that inhibit thyroid function and the process that is affected.

(Continued)

TABLE 27-3 Anti-thyroid Compounds

PROCESS AFFECTED	EXAMPLES OF INHIBITORS
Active transport of iodide	Complex anions: perchlorate, fluoborate, pertechnetate, thiocyanate
Iodination of thyroglobulin	Thionamides: propylthiouracil, methimazole, carbimazole Thiocyanate Aniline derivatives; sulfonamides Iodide
Coupling reaction	Thionamides Sulfonamides ?All other inhibitors of iodination
Hormone release	Lithium salts Iodide
Iodotyrosine deiodination	Nitrotyrosines
Peripheral iodothyronine deiodination	Thiouracil derivatives
	Oral cholecystographic agents
	Amiodarone
Hormone excretion/inactivation	Inducers of hepatic drug-metabolizing enzymes: phenobarbital, rifampin, carbamazepine, phenytoin
Hormone action	Thyroxine analogs Amiodarone ?Phenytoin Binding in gut: cholestyramine

Data adapted from Meier C.A., Burger A.C. Effects of drugs and other substances on thyroid hormone synthesis and metabolism. In: *Werner and Ingbar's The Thyroid*, 9th ed. (Braverman L.E. and Utiger R.D. eds.) Lippincott Williams & Wilkins, Philadelphia, 2005.

d. What adverse effects of methimazole therapy should this patient be cautioned about?

The most common adverse reaction is a purpuric, urticarial, papular rash which often subsides spontaneously. More serious is agranulocytosis although it is rare. A baseline white blood cell count and differential should be obtained before starting therapy with antithyroid drugs. Patients should be cautioned to immediately report the development of a sore throat or fever, which are often signs of the presence of leukopenia. Agranulocytosis is reversible upon discontinuation of the offending drug.

CASE 27-3

A 58-year-old woman has been diagnosed with well-differentiated papillary thyroid cancer.

a. What are the treatment options with this patient?

The mainstays of therapy for well-differentiated thyroid cancer (papillary, follicular) are surgical thyroidectomy, radioiodine, and levothyroxine to suppress TSH. The rationale for TSH suppression is that TSH is a growth factor for these cancers.

b. What is the standard course of treatment for this patient if metastatic disease is suspected?

Because most well-differentiated thyroid carcinomas accumulate very little iodine, stimulation of iodine uptake with TSH is required to treat metastases effectively. Currently, endogenous TSH stimulation is evoked by withdrawal of thyroid hormone replacement therapy (or by the administration of recombinant human TSH) in patients previously treated with near-total thyroidectomy. Total body ^{131}I scanning and measurement of thyroglobulin when the patient is hypothyroid (TSH >35 mU/L) help to identify metastatic disease or residual thyroid bed tissue. Depending on the residual uptake or the presence of metastatic disease, an ablative dose of ^{131}I is administered, with a repeat total body scan 1 week later.

TSH-suppressive therapy with levothyroxine is indicated in all patients after treatment for thyroid cancer.

Anaplastic cancer is the exception: it is highly malignant with survival usually less than 1 year. Medullary thyroid carcinomas do not accumulate iodine and cannot be treated with ^{131}I.

KEY CONCEPTS

- Replacement therapy for hypothyroidism typically uses oral thyroxine given once daily.
- The goals of therapy for hypothyroidism are to restore serum TSH concentration to the normal range, and to relieve the signs and symptoms of hypothyroidism.
- In pregnancy, the standard replacement dose of thyroid hormone is usually increased.
- Options available for treating hyperthyroid patients include antithyroid drugs (eg, propylthiouracil and methimazole), radioactive iodine, and surgery.
- Radioactive iodine may aggravate ophthalmopathy.
- Medical therapy with antithyroid drugs to reduce the concentration of thyroid hormone is the preferred approach in younger patients with hyperthyroidism.
- In older patients or those with cardiac disease, radioactive iodine is usually recommended after the patient has been rendered euthyroid with antithyroid medication.

(Continued)

Thyroid and Antithyroid Drugs — CHAPTER 27

> The initial treatment of thyroid cancer is surgical. Radioactive iodine is given to ablate remnant thyroid tissue.

> Following resection of well-differentiated thyroid carcinoma, the goal of thyroxine therapy is to suppress TSH to below normal concentrations, thereby removing the potential effect of TSH to stimulate the proliferation of the cancer cells.

SUMMARY QUIZ

QUESTION 27-1 A 34-year-old woman is being prepared for thyroidectomy. As part of the preparation, she is given a solution containing high iodide concentration. She wonders why she is being treated with something that is added to food (salt). The explanation is that

a. iodide in food is poorly absorbed.
b. iodide in food is rapidly taken up by skeletal muscle.
c. low concentrations of iodide are required for thyroxine synthesis, but high concentrations inhibit thyroxine synthesis and release.
d. iodide in food is not utilized by the thyroid gland.
e. high concentrations of iodide block the TRH receptor on the pituitary gland.

QUESTION 27-2 A 38-year-old South American woman has a large protrusion on her neck but is otherwise asymptomatic. Her condition is caused by a dietary deficiency of

a. iron.
b. magnesium.
c. potassium.
d. sodium.
e. iodine.

QUESTION 27-3 A 22-year-old woman has signs of hyperthyroidism. Her doctor orders blood tests to determine the pituitary regulation of thyroid function. Which of the following tests will be most helpful?

a. Iodine
b. T_4—thyroxine
c. T_3—triiodothyronine
d. TSH—thyroid-stimulating hormone
e. TRH—thyroid-releasing hormone

QUESTION 27-4 A 68-year-old woman has increasing lethargy, slight weight gain, and the onset of cognitive impairment. A serum TSH is slightly elevated and a T_4 is within normal limits. She is a candidate for

a. TRH.
b. levothyroxine.
c. methimazole.
d. iodide.
e. radioactive iodine.

QUESTION 27-5 A 25-year-old woman has been treated with thyroxine for hypothyroidism. She has become pregnant. She complains now of being constantly fatigued. The proper course of action would be to

a. do nothing, fatigue is normal during pregnancy.
b. increase the iodine in her diet.
c. measure her serum TSH during the first trimester and adjust her thyroxine dose based on the result.

(Continued)

d. double her dose of thyroxine.

e. decrease the dose of thyroxine as the need for thyroid replacement therapy decreases during pregnancy.

QUESTION 27-6 A 48-year-old woman with Graves disease with severe hyperthyroidism is being treated with radioactive iodine. She is also being treated with methimazole because of

a. the long period of time before hyperthyroidism is controlled by radioactive iodine.

b. the expectation that radioactive iodine will be ineffective.

c. methimazole is better absorbed than radioactive iodine.

d. methimazole will counteract the side effects of radioactive iodine.

e. radioactive iodine is not active unless administered with methimazole.

QUESTION 27-7 A 73-year-old man with a history of surgery for a benign thyroid nodule when he was 50 years old is now euthyroid but has developed a cardiac arrhythmia. Which of the antiarrhythmic drugs listed below might cause him to develop iodine-induced hypothyroidism?

a. Quinidine

b. Amiodarone

c. Diltiazam

d. Propranolol

e. Digoxin

QUESTION 27-8 A 53-year-old woman with the diagnosis of Graves disease is being treated with radioactive iodine. She should be warned of the high likelihood of

a. hyperthyroidism.

b. iodism.

c. hypothyroidism.

d. thyroid nodules.

e. thyroid cancer.

SUMMARY QUIZ ANSWER KEY

QUESTION 27-1 Answer is **c**. Low levels of iodine are required for thyroid synthesis, but high levels of iodine inhibit thyroid synthesis and release.

QUESTION 27-2 Answer is **e**. In some areas of the world, simple or nontoxic goiter is prevalent because of insufficient dietary iodine. Normal thyroid function obviously requires an adequate intake of iodine; without it, normal amounts of thyroid hormone cannot be made, TSH is secreted in excess (see Figures 27-1 and 27-2), and the thyroid becomes hyperplastic and hypertrophic. The enlarged and stimulated thyroid becomes remarkably efficient at extracting residual traces of iodine from the blood and usually succeeds in producing sufficient thyroid hormones. In more severe iodine deficiency, adult hypothyroidism and cretinism may occur.

QUESTION 27-3 Answer is **d**. In patients with normal pituitary function, serum measurement of TSH is the thyroid function test of choice because pituitary secretion of TSH is sensitively regulated in response to circulating concentrations of thyroid hormone.

QUESTION 27-4 Answer is **b**. Subclinical hypothyroidism is the presence of a mildly elevated serum TSH concentration and a normal T_4 without obvious symptoms. An elevated TSH is especially common among elderly patients. Patients with subclinical hypothyroidism who may benefit from levothyroxine to normalize the TSH include those with goiter, autoimmune thyroid disease, hypercholesterolemia, cognitive dysfunction,

(Continued)

Thyroid and Antithyroid Drugs   CHAPTER 27

or pregnancy, and those patients who have nonspecific symptoms that could be due to hypothyroidism. The decision to use levothyroxine therapy in these patients must be on an individual basis because treatment may not be appropriate for all patients.

QUESTION 27-5 Answer is **c**. The dose of levothyroxine in the hypothyroid patient who becomes pregnant usually needs to be increased, perhaps due to the increased serum concentration of thyroid-binding globulin (TBG) induced by estrogen. Most physicians measure a serum TSH during the first trimester and then adjust the dose of thyroxine based on the result. The increased dosage requirement plateaus at about gestation week 16 to 20, and dosage needs to fall back to prepregnancy levels immediately after delivery.

QUESTION 27-6 Answer is **a**. A disadvantage of radioactive iodine therapy is the long period of time that is sometimes required before the hyperthyroidism is controlled. Methimazole is an antithyroid drug that is the drug of choice in conjunction with radioactive iodine to hasten recovery while awaiting the effects of radiation.

QUESTION 27-7 Answer is **b**. Amiodarone contains 75 mg in each tablet (see Table 27-2). A euthyroid patient with a history of a wide variety of underlying thyroid disorders may develop iodine-induced hypothyroidism when exposed to large amounts of iodine present in many commonly prescribed drugs. Among the disorders that predispose patients to iodine-induced hypothyroidism are treated Graves disease, Hashimoto thyroiditis, postpartum lymphocytic thyroiditis, subacute painful thyroiditis, and lobectomy for benign nodules. (See the answer to question 27-1.)

QUESTION 27-8 Answer is **c**. The chief consequence of the use of radioactive iodine is the high incidence of hypothyroidism which will require lifelong treatment and monitoring. Even when elaborate procedures are used to estimate iodine uptake and gland size, most patients become hypothyroid.

SUMMARY: THYROID AND ANTITHYROID DRUGS

CLASS AND SUBCLASSES	NAMES	CLINICAL USES	TOXICITIES COMMON	UNIQUE; CLINICALLY IMPORTANT
Thyroid Hormones	Levothyroxine	Thyroid replacement therapy in patients with hypothyroidism; suppression of TSH in patients with thyroid cancer	Signs of overtreatment would be the same as for hyperthyroidism	Excess thyroxine can increase the risk of atrial fibrillation, especially in the elderly. Risk of osteoporosis in postmenopausal women
	Triiodothyroxine	Used when more rapid onset of action is needed such as myxedema coma or for more rapid termination of action such as in preparing a cancer patient for ^{131}I therapy	Same as for levothyroxine	Same as for levothyroxine
	Liotrix	Mixture of thyroxine and triiodothyroxine	Same as for levothyroxine	Same as for levothyroxine
	Desiccated thyroid	Mixture of thyroxine and triiodothyroxine	Same as for levothyroxine	Same as for levothyroxine
Antithyroid Drugs	Propylthiouracil	Used in treatment of hyperthyroidism in the following ways: definitive treatment; to hasten recovery while awaiting effects of radioactive iodine; preparation for surgical treatment	Purpuric urticarial popular rash. Pain, stiffness of joints, paresthesia, headache, nausea, skin pigmentation, loss of hair	Agranulocytosis. Hepatic failure; frequent monitoring of liver function is recommended

(Continued)

SECTION V — Hormones and Hormone Antagonists

CLASS AND SUBCLASSES	NAMES	CLINICAL USES	TOXICITIES COMMON	UNIQUE; CLINICALLY IMPORTANT
	Methimazole	Used in treatment of hyperthyroidism in the following ways: definitive treatment; to hasten recovery while awaiting effects of radioactive iodine; preparation for surgical treatment	Same as propylthiouracil	Agranulocytosis
	Carbimazole	Same as propylthiouracil; available in Europe, not available in the United States	Same as propylthiouracil	
Ionic Thyroid Inhibitors	Iodide Sodium iodine	Treatment of hyperthyroidism in preoperative period Used in conjunction with antithyroid drugs and propranolol in the treatment of thyrotoxic crisis		Allergy to iodine with anaphylactic reaction
Radioactive Iodine	Sodium iodine ^{131}I	Treatment of hyperthyroidism Diagnosis of disorders of thyroid function Treatment of thyroid cancer after stimulation of iodine uptake with TSH Medullary thyroid cancers do not accumulate I⁻ and cannot be treated with ^{131}I Treatment of toxic nodular goiter		Contraindicated in pregnancy High incidence of delayed hypothyroidism

CHAPTER 28

Estrogens, Progestins, Androgens, and Contraception

This chapter will be most useful after having a basic understanding of the material in Chapter 40, Estrogens and Progestins, Chapter 41, Androgens, and Chapter 66, Contraception and Pharmacotherapy of Obstetrical and Gynecological Disorders in *Goodman & Gilman's The Pharmacological Basis of Therapeutics*, 12th Edition. In addition to the material presented here, these chapters in the 12th Edition contain:

- The biosynthesis and physiological and pharmacological actions of the estrogens, progestins, and androgens
- A detailed discussion of gonadotropin and gonadal steroid concentrations during the menstrual cycle, the effects of cyclical gonadal steroids on the reproductive tract, and the metabolic effects of estrogens, progestins, and androgens
- A detailed discussion of fertility induction and the general principles of drug therapy of pregnant women, and the prevention or arrest of preterm labor
- A detailed discussion of the secretion and transport of testosterone, the physiological and pharmacologic effects of androgens, and the effects of androgens at different stages of life

LEARNING OBJECTIVES

☑ Describe the mechanisms of action of estrogens, progestins, and androgens.
☑ Understand the therapeutic use and side effects of postmenopausal hormone replacement therapy.
☑ Understand the therapeutic uses and side effects of contraceptive therapy.
☑ Describe the therapeutic use of selective estrogen receptor modulators, antiestrogens, and aromatase inhibitors.
☑ Describe the use of testosterone in the treatment of male hypogonadism.
☑ Describe the use of androgen receptor antagonists and 5α-reductase inhibitors to treat metastatic prostate cancer and benign prostatic hypertrophy, respectively.
☑ Understand the side effects of the 17α-alkylated androgens used by athletes to enhance performance.

DRUGS INCLUDED IN THIS CHAPTER

Anabolic steroids (various 17α-alkylated androgens)
Anastrozole (ARIMIDEX)
Bicalutamide (CASODEX, others)
Clomiphene (CLOMID, SERPPHENE, others)
Conjugated equine estrogens (PREMARIN)
Conjugated estrogens + medroxyprogesterone acetate (PREMPRO, PREMPHASE)
Dutasteride (AVODART)
Estradiol + drospirenone (ANGELO)
Estradiol + norethindrone (PREFEST)
Estradiol cypionate (DEPO-ESTRADIOL, others)
Estradiol micronized (ESTRACE, others)
Estradiol nonmicronized (FEMTRACE)
Estradiol topical gel (ESTROGEL)
Estradiol transdermal (ALORA, CLIMERA, ESTRADERM, VIVELLE, others)
Estradiol vaginal ring (ESTRING)
Estradiol vaginal tablets (VAGIFEM)
Estradiol valerate (DELESTROGEN, others)
Estrogen esterified esters (MENEST)
Estropipate (ORTHO-EST, OGEN, others)
Ethinyl estradiol + norethindrone (FEMHRT)
Exemestane (AROMASIN)
Finasteride (PROSCAR)
Flutamide (EULEXIN)
Formestane
Fulvestrant (FASLODEX)
Letrozole (FEMARA)
Medroxyprogesterone acetate (MPA; PROVERA, DEPO-PROVERA)
Megestrol acetate (MEGACE, others)
Mifepristone (RU 38486; MIFEPREX)
Nilutamide (NILADRON)
Progesterone micronized (PROMETRIUM)
Progesterone slow-release intrauterine device (PROGESTASERT)
Progesterone vaginal gel (CRINONE, PROCHIEVE)

(continues)

MECHANISMS OF ACTION OF ESTROGENS, PROGESTINS, AND ANDROGENS

DRUG CLASS	DRUG	MECHANISM OF ACTION
Estrogen	Estradiol nonmicronized Estradiol micronized Conjugated equine estrogens Estrogen esterified esters Synthetic conjugated estrogens Estropipate Estradiol transdermal Estradiol topical gel Estradiol vaginal ring Estradiol vaginal tablets Estradiol valerate Estradiol cypionate Conjugated estrogens + medroxyprogesterone acetate (MPA) Ethinyl estradiol + norethindrone Estradiol + norethindrone Estradiol + drospirenone	The biosynthetic pathway for the estrogens is shown in Figure 28-1 and the neuroendocrine control of gonadotropin secretion in females is shown in Figure 28-2. Estrogens exert their effects by interaction with receptors that are members of the superfamily of nuclear receptors; estrogen receptors are ligand-activated transcription factors that increase or decrease the transcription of target genes (see Figure 28-3)

(Continued)

441

SECTION V Hormones and Hormone Antagonists

DRUGS INCLUDED IN THIS CHAPTER (Cont.)

Progesterone vaginal insert (ENDOMETRIN)
Raloxifene (EVISTA)
See Table 28-1 for brand names and formulations of oral contraceptives
See Table 28-2 for brand names and formulations of agents used for hormone replacement therapy
Synthetic conjugated estrogens (CENESTIN; ENJUVIA)
Tamoxifen
Testosterone (HISTERONE, others)
Testosterone buccal tablet (STRIANT)
Testosterone cypionate (DEPO-TESTOSTERONE, others)
Testosterone enanthate (DELATESTRYL, others)
Testosterone gel (ANDROGEL, TESTIM)
Testosterone patch (ANDRODERM)
Testosterone undecanoate (ANDRIOL)
Toremifene (FARESTON)
Ulipristal (ELLA, ELLAONE)

DRUG CLASS	DRUG	MECHANISM OF ACTION
Selective Estrogen Receptor Modulators	Tamoxifen Raloxifene Toremifene	Compounds with estrogenic agonist, antagonist, or mixed activity depending on the species and targeted gene measured (see Chapter 46)
Estrogen Antagonists	Clomiphene Fulvestrant	Bind to estrogen receptors and block estradiol binding Clomiphene increases gonadotropin secretion and stimulates ovulation
Estrogen Synthesis Inhibitors	Formestane Exemestane Anastrozole Letrozole	Formestane and exemestane act to irreversibly inactivate aromatase (see Figure 28-1) Anastrozole and letrozole act to reversibly inhibit aromatase
Progestin	Progesterone micronized Progesterone vaginal gel Progesterone slow-release intrauterine device Progesterone vaginal insert Medroxyprogesterone acetate (MPA) Megestrol acetate	Interact with progesterone receptors in target tissues
Progesterone Antagonist	Mifepristone	Progesterone receptor antagonist
Selective Progesterone Receptor Modulator	Ulipristal	Partial agonist at progesterone receptors; antiproliferative effects in the uterus and inhibits ovulation
Oral Contraceptive	See Table 28-1	Supresses luteinizing hormone (LH) surge and prevents ovulation
Androgen	Testosterone Testosterone enanthate Testosterone cypionate Testosterone undecanoate Testosterone patch Testosterone gel Testosterone buccal tablet Anabolic steroids (various 17α-alkylated androgens)	The biological effects of testosterone are mediated either directly, by binding to the androgen receptor, or indirectly by conversion to dihydrotestosterone Testosterone can act as an estrogen by conversion to estradiol (see Figures 28-1, 28-4, 28-5, and 28-6)
Androgen Receptor Antagonist	Flutamide Bicalutamide Nilutamide	Act as antagonists at the androgen receptor (see Chapter 46)
5α-Reductase Inhibitors	Finasteride Dutasteride	Inhibit 5α-reductase and block the conversion of testosterone to dihydrotestosterone (see Figure 28-5 and Chapter 46)

TABLE 28-1 Brand Names and Formulations of Oral Contraceptives

PRODUCT	BRAND NAME[a]		
Combination[b] monophasic		Estrogen (µg)	Progestin (mg)
Ethinyl estradiol/desogestrel	DESOGEN	30	0.15
	ORTHO-CEPT	30	0.15
Ethinyl estradiol/drospirenone	YASMIN	30	3
Ethinyl estradiol/ethynodiol	DEMULEN 1/35	35	1
	DEMULEN 1/50	50	1
Ethinyl estradiol/levonorgestrel	ALESSE	20	0.1
	LEVLITE	20	0.1
	LYBREL	20	0.09
	NORDETTE	30	0.15
Ethinyl estradiol/norgestrel	LO/OVRAL	30	0.3
	OVRAL	50	0.5
Ethinyl estradiol/norethindrone	BREVICON	35	0.5
	FEMCON	35	0.4
	LOESTRIN 1/20	20	1
	LOESTRIN 1.5/30	30	1.5
	NORINYL 1+35	35	1
	ORTHO-NOVUM 1/35	35	1
	OVCON 35	35	0.4
	OVCON 50	50	1
Ethinyl estradiol/norgestimate	ORTHO-CYCLEN	35	0.25
Mestranol/norethindrone	NORINYL 1+50	50	1
	ORTHO-NOVUM 1/50	50	1
Combination biphasic		Estrogen (µg)	Progestin (mg)
Ethinyl estradiol/desogestrel	MIRCETTE	20	0.15 (21 tabs)
		10	— (5 tabs)
Ethinyl estradiol/norethindrone	ORTHO-NOVUM 10/11	35	0.5 (10 tabs)
		35	1 (11 tabs)
Combination triphasic		Estrogen (µg)	Progestin (mg)
Ethinyl estradiol/desogestrel	CYCLESSA	25	0.1 (7 tabs)
		25	0.125 (7 tabs)
		25	0.15 (7 tabs)
Ethinyl estradiol/levonorgestrel	TRI-LEVLEN	30	0.05 (6 tabs)
		40	0.075 (5 tabs)
		30	0.125 (10 tabs)

(*Continued*)

SECTION V — Hormones and Hormone Antagonists

PRODUCT	BRAND NAME[a]	Estrogen (μg)	Progestin (mg)
	TRIPHASIL	30	0.05 (6 tabs)
		40	0.075 (5 tabs)
		30	0.125 (10 tabs)
Ethinyl estradiol/norethindrone	ORTHO-NOVUM 7/7/7	35	0.5 (7 tabs)
		35	0.75 (7 tabs)
		35	1 (7 tabs)
	TRI-NORINYL	35	0.5 (7 tabs)
		35	1 (9 tabs)
		35	0.5 (5 tabs)
Ethinyl estradiol/norgestimate	ORTHO TRI-CYCLEN	35	0.18 (7 tabs)
		35	0.215 (7 tabs)
		35	0.25 (7 tabs)
	ORTHO TRI-CYCLEN LO	25	0.18 (7 tabs)
		25	0.215 (7 tabs)
		25	0.25 (7 tabs)
Combination estrophasic		**Estrogen (μg)**	**Progestin (mg)**
Ethinyl estradiol/norethindrone	ESTROSTEP	20	1 (5 tabs)
		30	1 (7 tabs)
		35	1 (9 tabs)
Combination extended cycle		**Estrogen (μg)**	**Progestin (mg)**
Ethinyl estradiol/drospirenone	YAZ	20	3 (24 tabs)
Ethinyl estradiol/levonorgesterol	LYBREL	20	0.09 (28 tabs)
	SEASONALE	30	0.15 (84 tabs)
	SEASONIQUE	30	0.15 (84 tabs)
		10	— (7 tabs)
Ethinyl estradiol/norethindrone	LOESTRIN 24	20	1 (24 tabs)
Progestin only		**Estrogen (μg)**	**Progestin (mg)**
Norethindrone	MICRONOR	—	0.35[c]
	NOR-QD	—	0.35[c]
Norgestrel	OVRETTE	—	0.075[c]
Emergency contraception			
Levonorgestrel	PLAN B	—	0.75 × 2 doses
Ulipristal (progesterone partial agonist)	ella; ellaOne	—	30 mg × 1 dose

Unless otherwise indicated, the products are packaged with 21 active (hormone-containing) pills and 7 placebo tablets. For formulations that differ from this standard (eg, multiphasic pills, extended-cycle formulations), the numbers of tablets of each pill strength are indicated.

[a]Some formulations also contain iron to diminish the risk of Fe-deficiency anemia; these are not listed separately here.
[b]Combination formulations contain both an estrogen and a progestin.
[c]Denotes continuous administration of active pills.

TABLE 28-2 Brand Names and Formulations of Agents Used for Hormone Replacement Therapy

PREPARATION	BRAND	DOSE (mg)	FREQUENCY
Oral estrogen (tablets)			
Conjugated estrogens	CENESTIN	0.3, 0.45, 0.625, 0.9, 1.25	1/day
	ENJUVIA		
	PREMARIN		
Estropipate	OGEN	0.625, 1.25, 1.5	1/day
	ORTHO-EST	0.75, 1.5	
Micronized estrogen	ESTRACE	0.5, 1, 2	1/day
Estradiol	FEMTRACE	0.45, 0.9, 1.8	1/day
Esterified estrogens	MENEST	0.3, 0.625, 1.25, 2.5	1/day
Transdermal estradiol			
Patch	ALORA	0.025, 0.05, 0.075, 0.1	2/week
	CLIMARA	0.025, 0.0375, 0.05, 0.06, 0.075, 0.1	1/week
	ESCLIM	0.025, 0.0375, 0.05, 0.075, 0.1	2/week
	ESTRADERM	0.05, 0.1	2/week
	MENOSTAR	0.014	1/week
	VIVELLE	0.05, 0.1	2/week
	VIVELLE-DOT	0.025, 0.0375, 0.05, 0.075, 0.1	2/week
Gel	DIVIGEL	0.25, 0.5, 1 g/packet	1/day
	ELESTRIN	0.87 g/pump	1/day
	ESTROGEL	1.25 g/pump	1/day
Emulsion	ESTRASORB	1.74 g/pouch	2/day
Spray	EVAMIST	1.53 mg/spray	1-3 sprays/day
Vaginal estrogen			
Estradiol	ESTRACE (cream)	0.1 mg/g	1/day, then 1-3/week
	ESTRING (ring)	7.5 µg/24 hr	1/90 days
	FEMRING (ring)	0.05, 0.1 mg/day	1/3 months
	VAGIFEM (tabs)	25 µg	1/day for 2 weeks, then 2/week
Conjugated estrogens	PREMARIN (cream)	0.625 mg/g	1/day
Oral progestin			
Norethindrone	AYGESTIN	5 mg	1/day
Progesterone (micronized)	PROMETRIUM	100, 200 mg	
Medroxyprogesterone	PROVERA	2.5, 5, 10 mg	

(*Continued*)

SECTION V — Hormones and Hormone Antagonists

PREPARATION	BRAND	DOSE (mg)		FREQUENCY
		Estrogen (mg)	Progesterone (mg)	
Oral estrogen plus progesterone				
Estradiol/norethindrone	ACTIVELLA	1	0.5	1/day
Estradiol/drospirenone	ANGELIQ	1	0.5	
Ethinyl estradiol/norethindrone	FEMHRT	0.5	2.5 µg	
		1	5 µg	
Transdermal estrogen plus progesterone				
Estradiol/levonorgestrel	CLIMARA PRO	0.045 mg/day	0.015 mg/day	1/week
Estradiol/norethindrone	COMBIPATCH	0.05 mg/day	0.14 mg/day	2/week
		0.05 mg/day	0.25 mg/day	2/week

CASE 28-1

A 49-year-old woman has been 6 months without menstruation. She is now experiencing severe "hot flashes" that are impacting her daily life. She would like some therapy that would make her more comfortable.

a. What hormone replacement therapy is available for her?

Table 28-2 lists the brand names and formulations used for hormone replacement therapy. Regardless of the specific agent or regimen, menopausal hormone therapy with estrogens should use the lowest dose and shortest duration necessary to achieve an appropriate therapeutic goal.

(Continued)

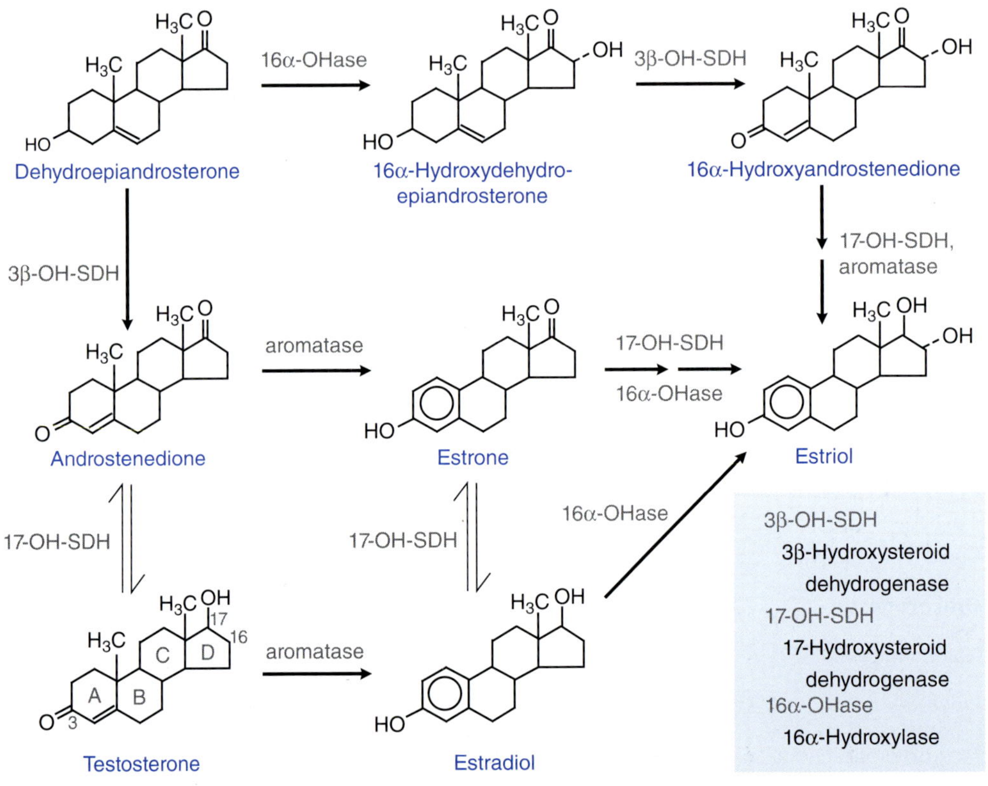

FIGURE 28-1 The biosynthetic pathway for the estrogens.

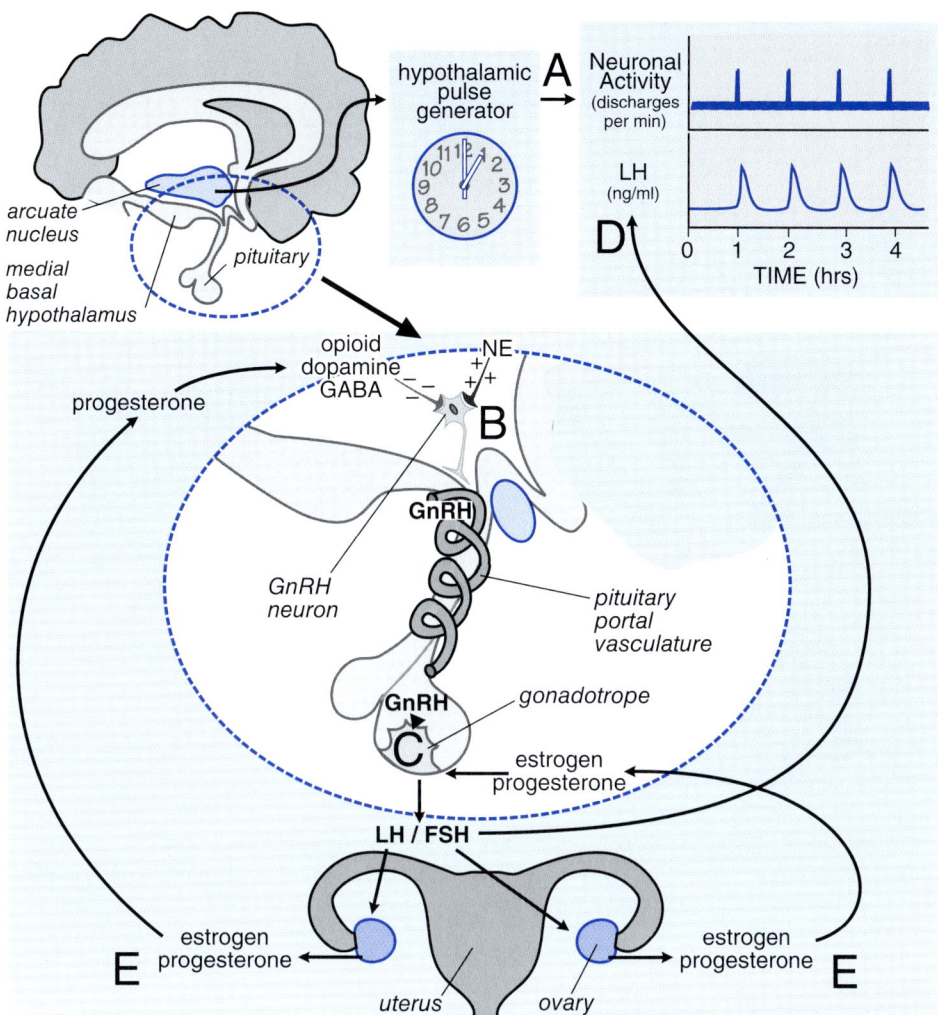

FIGURE 28-2 Neuroendocrine control of gonadotropin secretion in females. The hypothalamic pulse generator located in the arcuate nucleus of the hypothalamus functions as a neuronal "clock" that fires at regular hourly intervals. **A.** This results in the periodic release of gonadotropin-releasing hormone (GnRH) from GnRH-containing neurons into the hypothalamic-pituitary portal vasculature **B.** GnRH neurons receive inhibitory input from opioid, dopamine, and GABA neurons and stimulatory input from noradrenergic neurons (NE, norepinephrine). The pulses of GnRH trigger the intermittent release of luteinizing hormone (LH) and follicle-stimulating hormone (FSH) from pituitary gonadotropes **C,** resulting in the pulsatile plasma profile **D.** FSH and LH regulate ovarian production of estrogen and progesterone, which exert feedback controls **E.**

b. **She is being treated with a combination estrogen/progesterone product (ethinyl estradiol/norethindrone, FEMHRT). Why is the progesterone added to the estrogen?**

The use of unopposed estrogen for hormone treatment in postmenopausal women increases the risk of endometrial carcinoma by 5- to 15-fold. This increased risk can be prevented if a progestin is coadministered with the estrogen.

c. **What are the mechanisms of action estrogen and progesterone?**

Figure 28-3 describes the mechanism of action of a nuclear estrogen receptor. Estrogen and progesterone receptors are ligand-activated transcription factors that increase or decrease the transcription of target genes.

d. **What are the risks of hormone replacement therapy that should be discussed with the patient?**

Oral estrogens (and estrogen-progestin combinations) have a small but significant risk of thromboembolic disease in healthy women and in women with preexisting cardiovascular disease.

(Continued)

SECTION V   Hormones and Hormone Antagonists

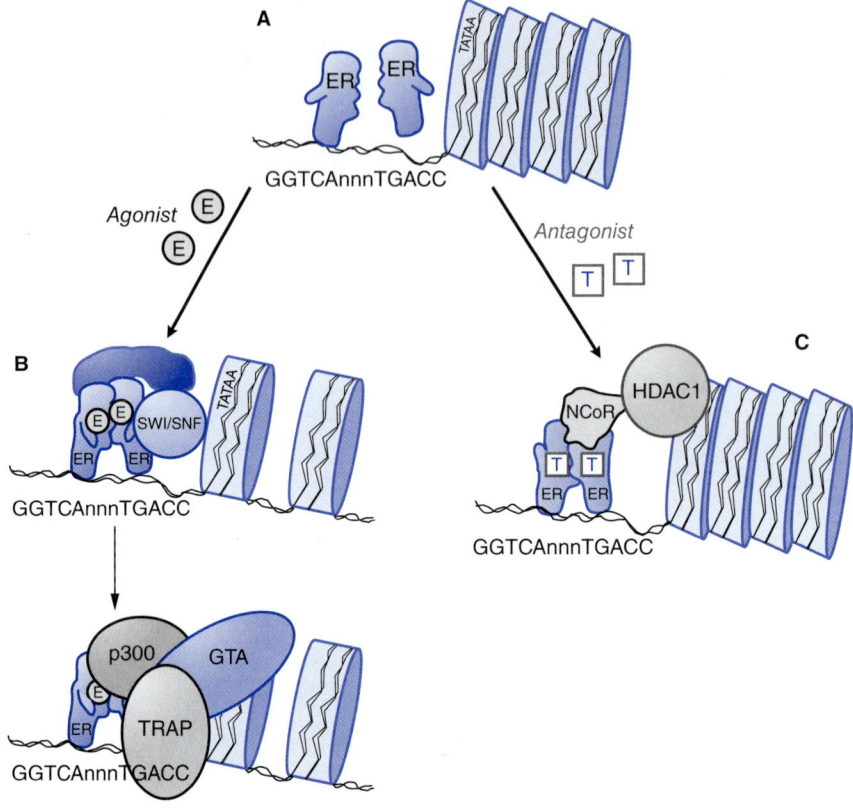

FIGURE 28-3 Molecular mechanism of action of nuclear estrogen receptor. **A.** Unliganded estrogen receptor (ER) exists as a monomer within the nucleus. **B.** Agonists such as 17β-estradiol bind to the ER and cause a ligand-directed change in conformation that facilitates dimerization and interaction with specific estrogen response element (ERE) sequences in DNA. The ER-DNA complex recruits coactivators such as SWI/SNF that modify chromatin structure, and coactivators such as steroid-receptor coactivator-1 (SRC-1) that has histone acetyltransferase (HAT) activity and that further alters chromatin structure. This remodeling facilitates the exchange of the recruited proteins such that other coactivators (eg, p300 and the TRAP complex) associate on the target gene promoter and proteins that comprise the general transcription apparatus (GTA) are recruited, with subsequent synthesis of mRNA. **C.** Antagonists such as tamoxifen (T) also bind to the ER but produce a different receptor conformation. The antagonist-induced conformation also facilitates dimerization and interaction with DNA, but a different set of proteins called corepressors, such as nuclear-hormone receptor corepressor (NcoR), are recruited to the complex. NcoR further recruits proteins such as histone deacetylase I (HDAC1) that act on histone proteins to stabilize nucleosome structure and prevent interaction with the GTA.

The progestin component in combined hormone-replacement therapy plays a major role in the increased risk of breast cancer. The available data suggest that the excess risk of breast cancer associated with menopausal use appears to abate 5 years after discontinuing therapy. Thus, hormone replacement therapy for less than or equal to 5 years is often prescribed to mitigate hot flashes and likely has a minimal effect on the risk of breast cancer.

CASE 28-2

A 22-year-old woman is asking for an oral contraceptive.

a. What are the options available for her?

Table 28-1 lists the brand names and formulations of oral contraceptives. The majority of available products contain estrogen and progestin in a constant amount of the estrogen and progestin (monophasic) that are packaged with 21 pills containing active hormone and 7 placebo tablets. In an effort to maximize the antiovulatory effects and

(Continued)

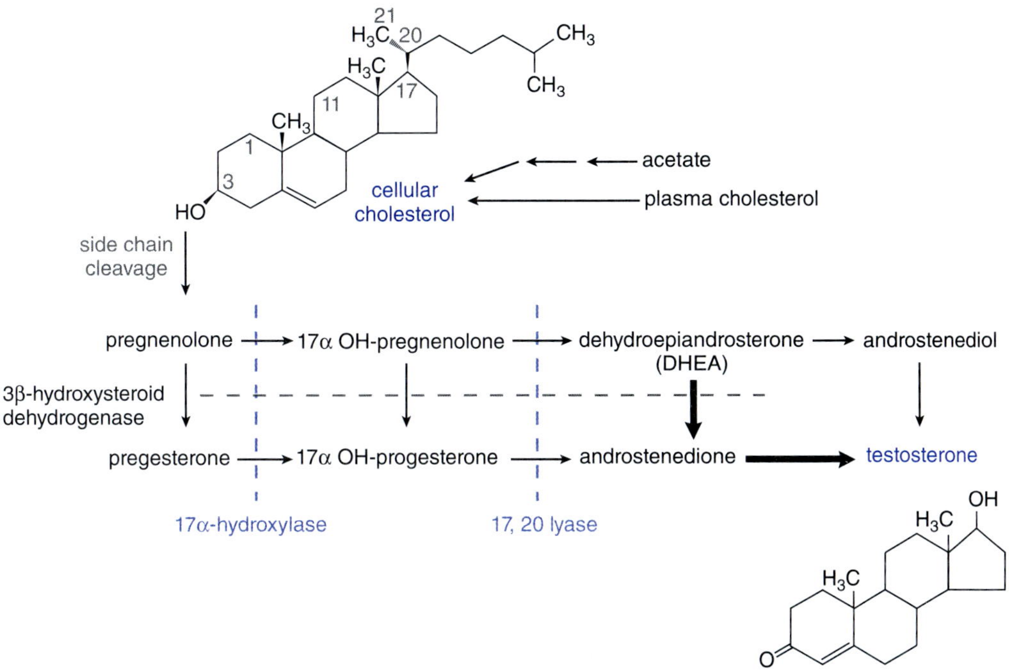

Estrogens, Progestins, Androgens, and Contraception   CHAPTER 28

FIGURE 28-4 Pathway of synthesis of testosterone in the Leydig cells of the testes. In Leydig cells, the 11 and 21 hydroxylases (present in adrenal cortex) are absent but CYP17 (17 α-hydroxylase) is present. Thus androgens and estrogens are synthesized; corticosterone and cortisol are not formed. Bold arrows indicate favored pathways.

prevent breakthrough bleeding while minimizing total exposure to the hormones, some formulations provide active pills with two (biphasic) or three (triphasic) different amounts of one or both hormone to be used sequentially during each cycle.

Formulations called extended-cycle contraceptives extend the number of active pills per cycle and thus decrease the duration of menstrual bleeding.

(*Continued*)

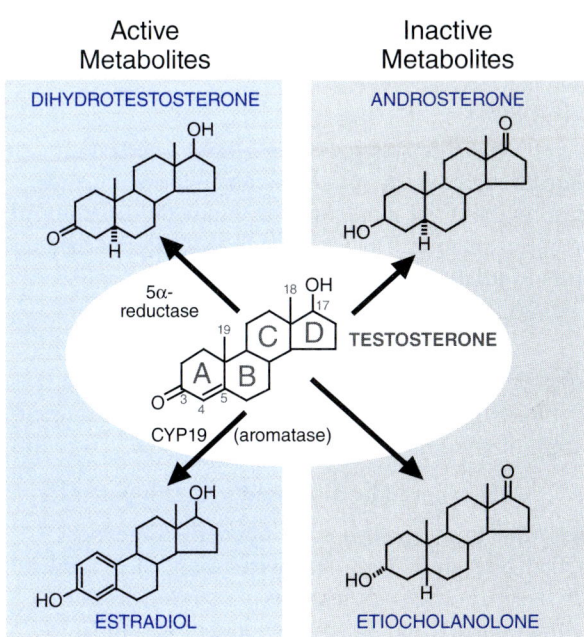

FIGURE 28-5 Metabolism of testosterone to its major active and inactive metabolites.

449

SECTION V

Hormones and Hormone Antagonists

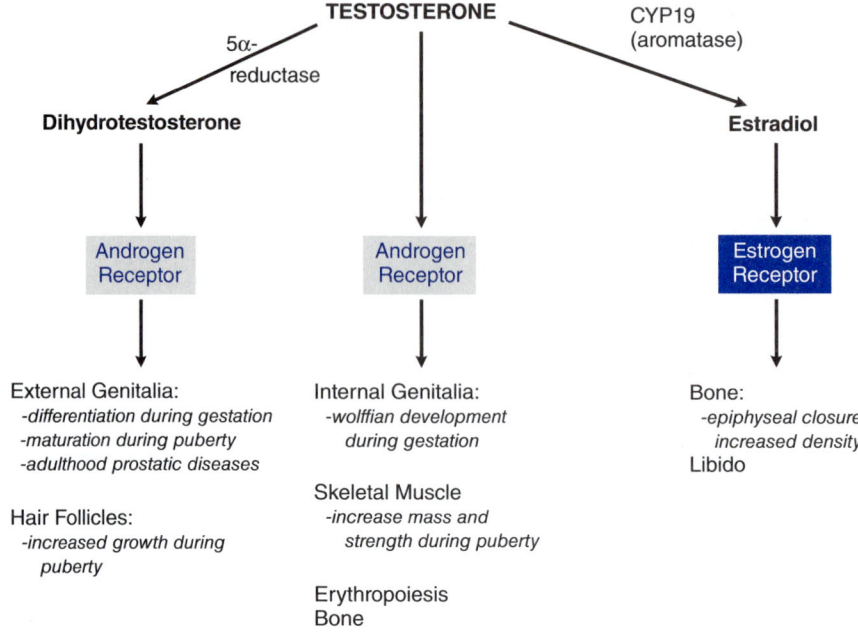

FIGURE 28-6 Direct effects of testosterone and effects mediated indirectly via dihydrotestosterone or estradiol.

A weekly transdermal patch (ORTHO EVRA) releases ethinyl estradiol and norelgestromin. Pharmacokinetic data suggests that it provides higher estrogen exposure than the low-dose oral contraceptives and the FDA has required a warning that this product may have increased risk of venous thromboembolism.

A vaginal ring (NUVARING) also is available that releases ethinyl estradiol and etonogestrel.

b. Why do some products contain a progesterone?

The structural features of the various progestins are shown in Figure 28-7. The major functions of the estrogen components are to sensitize the hypothalamus and pituitary gonadotropes (see Figure 28-2) to the feedback inhibitory effects of the progestin and to minimize breakthrough bleeding. The progestin exerts negative feedback, which suppresses the LH surge and thereby prevents ovulation and protects against uterine cancer by opposing the proliferative effects of the estrogen on the uterine endometrium.

c. What are progestin-only contraceptives?

The progestin-only contraceptives contain derivatives of 17α-alkyl-19-nortestosterone but do not contain an estrogen. Although they do inhibit ovulation to some degree, their efficacy also reflects changes in the cervical mucosa that inhibit fertilization and endometrial changes that inhibit implantation. They are slightly less effective than the combination estrogen/progestin formulations, particularly when doses are missed, but provide an alternative in settings when estrogen-containing formulations are contraindicated.

Progestins are also used for long-acting contraception. A depot formulation of medroxyprogesterone (DEPO-PROVERA) injected subcutaneously or intramuscularly provides effective contraception for 3 months.

d. What are the risks and side effects that should be discussed with this patient?

Thromboembolic disease, largely due to the estrogenic component, is the most common serious side effect. Other side effects include hypertension, edema, gallbladder disease, and elevations in serum triglycerides. Pills containing drospirenone, which antagonizes the mineralocorticoid receptor, should be accompanied

(Continued)

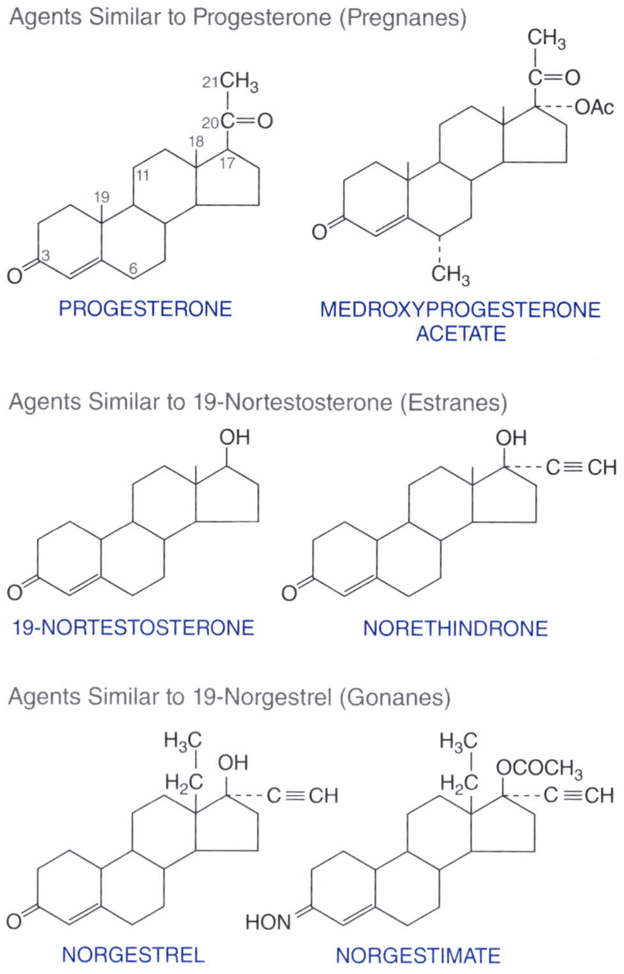

Estrogens, Progestins, Androgens, and Contraception CHAPTER 28

FIGURE 28-7 Structural features of various progestins.

with careful monitoring of the serum K^+. The long-acting progestin-only formulations (DEPO-PROVERA) are associated with decreased bone mineral density. Teenagers and younger women who have not achieved maximal bone density may be particularly at risk.

CASE 28-3

A 53-year-old woman is diagnosed with breast cancer. The "lump" is removed and lymph nodes are negative for signs of cancer. She is started on tamoxifen, a selective estrogen receptor modulator (SERM).

a. What are SERMs?

Selective estrogen receptor modulators, or SERMs, are compounds with tissue-selective actions. The pharmacological goals of these drugs are to produce beneficial estrogenic actions in certain tissues (eg, bone, brain, and liver) during postmenopausal hormone therapy but antagonist activity in tissues such as breast and endometrium, where estrogenic actions (eg, carcinogenesis) might be deleterious. Tamoxifen is highly efficacious in the treatment of breast cancer (see Chapter 46).

b. What are the untoward effects and risk of tamoxifen therapy?

Tamoxifen treatment causes a 2- to 3-fold increase in the relative risk of deep vein thrombosis and pulmonary embolism and a roughly 2-fold increase in endometrial carcinoma. The most common side effect is hot flashes.

SECTION V   Hormones and Hormone Antagonists

CASE 28-4

A 24-year-old woman with polycystic ovary syndrome is being treated with clomiphene for infertility.

a. What kind of drug is clomiphene and what is its mechanism of action?

Clomiphene is an antiestrogen and is a pure estrogen antagonist in all tissues studied. Clomiphene binds to estrogen receptors (see Figure 28-3), increases gonadotropin secretion and stimulates ovulation. It increases the amplitude of LH and FSH pulses (see Figure 28-2) without changing pulse frequency by acting largely at the pituitary level to block inhibitory actions of estrogen on gonadotropin release and/or somehow causing the hypothalamus to release larger amounts of GnRH per pulse.

b. What are the untoward effects of clomiphene?

Clomiphene should not be administered to pregnant women due to reports of teratogenicity in animals. Its untoward effects include ovarian hyperstimulation, increased incidence of multiple births, ovarian cysts, hot flashes, headaches, and blurred vision. Prolonged use may increase the risk of ovarian cancer.

CASE 28-5

A 23-year-old woman comes into the clinic requesting emergency contraception following unprotected sexual intercourse 12 hours earlier. She is given ulipristal.

a. What kind of drug is ulipristal and what is its mechanism of action?

Ulipristal functions as a selective progesterone receptor modulator (SPRM), acting as a partial agonist at progesterone receptors. It has antiproliferative effects in the uterus; however, its most relevant actions to date involve its capacity to inhibit ovulation. Ulipristal's antiovulatory actions likely occur due to progesterone regulation at many levels, including inhibition of LH release through the hypothalamus and pituitary, and inhibition of LH-induced follicular rupture within the ovary. It is effective up to 120 hours (5 days) after intercourse.

b. What other treatment options are available for this patient?

Plan B (see Table 28-1) contains 2 tablets of the progestin levonorgestrel and may be obtained in the United States without prescription by women who are 18 years of age or older. Other options for postcoital contraception include mifepristone that is not FDA approved for this use but is highly effective, and copper intrauterine devices when inserted within 4 days of unprotected intercourse.

c. What side effects might be expected following ulipristal administration?

The most severe side effect in clinical trials using ulipristal has been a self-limited headache and abdominal pain.

CASE 28-6

A 46-year-old man is diagnosed with hypogonadism and low serum testosterone.

a. What options are available for his testosterone replacement?

Figure 28-8 shows the androgens that are available for therapeutic use. Even though ingested testosterone is readily absorbed into the hepatic circulation, the rapid hepatic catabolism ensures that hypogonadal men generally cannot ingest it in sufficient amounts and with sufficient frequency to maintain a normal serum testosterone concentration. Most pharmaceutical preparations of androgens, therefore, are designed to bypass hepatic catabolism of testosterone.

Esterifying a fatty acid to the 17α hydroxyl group of testosterone creates a compound that is even more lipophilic than testosterone itself. When an ester such as testosterone enthanthate or cypionate is dissolved in oil and administered

(Continued)

Estrogens, Progestins, Androgens, and Contraception

CHAPTER 28

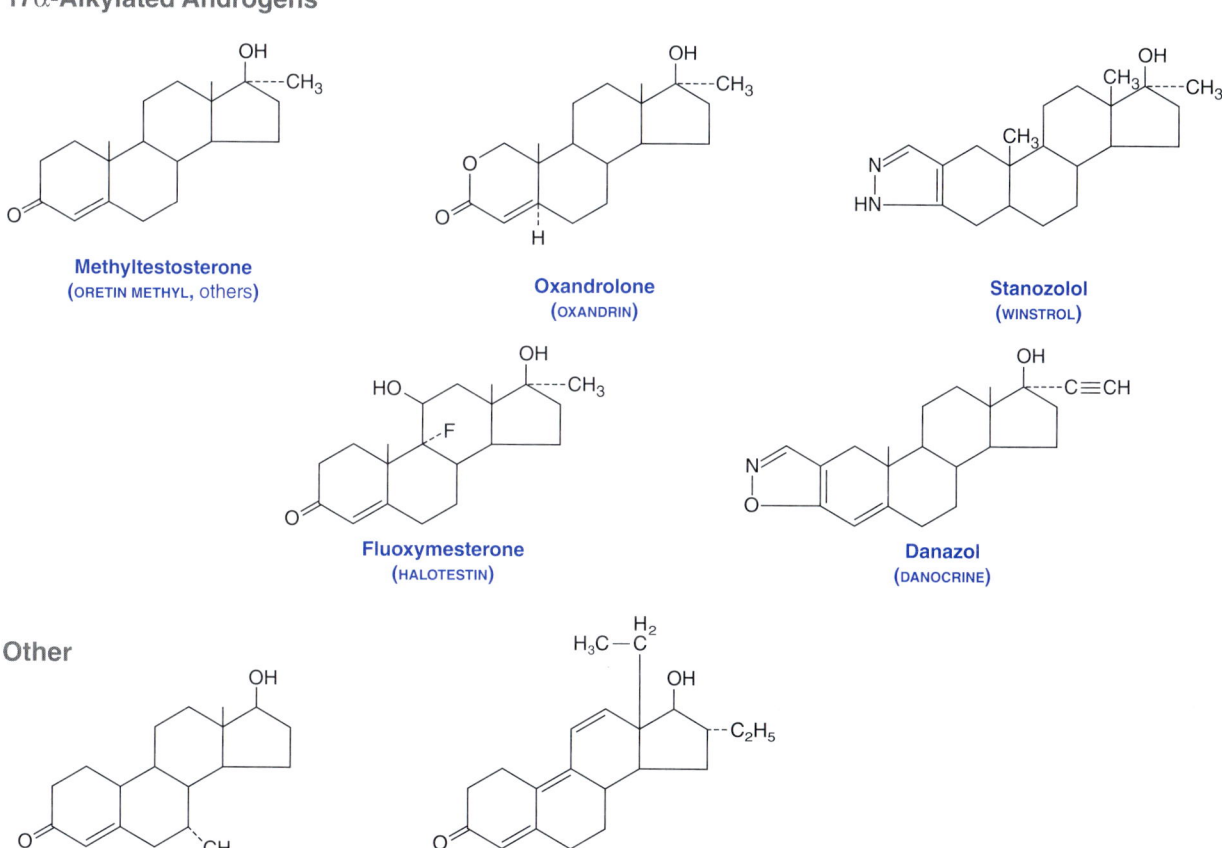

FIGURE 28-8 Structures of androgens available for therapeutic use.

intramuscularly every 2 to 4 weeks the resulting testosterone concentrations range from higher than normal in the first few days after injection to low normal just before the next injection. The undecanoate ester of testosterone, when dissolved in oil and ingested orally, is absorbed into the lymphatic circulation, thus bypassing initial hepatic catabolism.

(Continued)

A testosterone gel, a testosterone patch, and a testosterone buccal tablet are also available.

The 17α-alkylated androgens also are less prone to hepatic catabolism; however, they are less androgenic than testosterone and can cause hepatotoxicity.

b. What are the risks and untoward effects of testosterone therapy that should be discussed with this patient?

The major side effects of testosterone administration are acne, gynecomastia, and aggressive sexual behavior. Prolonged administration may be associated with benign prostatic hypertrophy and prostate cancer. The 17α-alkylated androgens are the only androgens that cause hepatotoxicity.

CASE 28-7

A 29-year-old male cyclist has been taking testosterone on the advice of his trainer. His trainer has rationalized that since testosterone is an endogenous substance, it will be difficult to detect.

a. What side effects might this athlete expect to experience?

The pathways of synthesis of testosterone are shown in Figure 28-4. All androgens suppress gonadotropin secretion when taken in high doses and thereby suppress endogenous testicular function. Thus, there is decreased endogenous testosterone and sperm production with resultant diminished fertility. Chronic administration may result in reduced testicular size. Androgens in high doses can be converted to estrogens, which may cause gynecomastia. The 17α-alkylated androgens can cause hepatotoxicity, including cholestasis and peliosis hepatis, blood-filled cysts.

b. Is it sound rationale that testosterone will be difficult to detect?

Endogenous testosterone can be detected by 1 of 2 methods. One is T/E ratio, the ratio of testosterone glucuronide to its endogenous epimer, epitestosterone glucuronide in urine. Administration of exogenous testosterone suppresses secretion of both endogenous testosterone and epitestosterone and replaces them with only the exogenous testosterone, so the T/E ratio is higher than normal. Both testosterone and epitestosterone are measured in urine by gas chromatography-mass spectrometry.

A second method for detecting the administration of exogenous testosterone employs gas chromatography-combustion isotope ratio mass spectrometry to detect the presence of ^{13}C and ^{12}C compounds. Urinary steroids with a low $^{13}C/^{12}C$ ratio are likely to have originated from pharmaceutical sources as opposed to endogenous physiological sources.

CASE 28-8

A 56-year-old man with metastatic prostate cancer is being treated with flutamide.

a. What is flutamide and what are its mechanisms of actions?

Flutamide is an androgen receptor antagonist that is used in the treatment of metastatic prostate cancer (see Chapter 46). When used alone flutamide causes an increased secretion of LH, which in turn increases serum testosterone concentrations. Androgen receptor antagonists are used primarily in conjunction with a GnRH agonist which during chronic therapy downregulates GnRH receptors causing a decline in the pituitary response. The fall in LH results in decreased serum testosterone concentrations. In this setting, flutamide blocks the actions of adrenal androgens, which are not inhibited by GnRH agonists.

b. What are the untoward effects of flutamide?

Common side effects of flutamide are diarrhea, breast tenderness, and nipple tenderness. Less commonly nausea, vomiting, and hepatotoxicity occur.

Estrogens, Progestins, Androgens, and Contraception

CHAPTER 28

KEY CONCEPTS

- In postmenopausal woman, hormone replacement therapy is most commonly used to treat vasomotor disturbances ("hot flashes").
- In postmenopausal women with an intact uterus, a progestin is included in the hormone replacement therapy to prevent endometrial cancer.
- Regardless of the specific drug(s), hormone replacement therapy should use the minimum dose and duration for the desired therapeutic end point.
- Estrogens and progestins are widely used as combination contraceptives and are 99% effective in preventing ovulation.
- Tamoxifen is a selective estrogen receptor modulator widely used for the adjuvant treatment of breast cancer and for prophylaxis in high-risk women, but treatment should be limited to 5 years.
- Fulvestrant, a pure estrogen antagonist, is used to treat breast cancer.
- Clomiphene is an estrogen antagonist used to treat infertility.
- Progestin-only contraceptives are available when estrogen-containing products are contraindicated.
- A levonorgestrel-only product and ulipristal are available for emergency contraception within 72 hours or 120 hours of unprotected intercourse, respectively.
- Mifepristone, administered with a prostaglandin, is used as an antiprogestin for medical abortion.
- Testosterone delivery systems are designed to avoid hepatic catabolism that occurs when testosterone is ingested orally.
- Androgen receptor antagonists such as flutamide are used to treat metastatic prostate cancer.
- Finasteride, a 5α-reductase inhibitor, is used to treat benign prostatic hypertrophy.
- The 17α-alkylated androgens are the only androgens that cause hepatotoxicity.

SUMMARY QUIZ

QUESTION 28-1 A 30-year-old woman is being started on birth control pills for the first time. She has a history of migraine headaches with aura. Therapy with which one of the following contraceptive formulations is contraindicated in this patient?

a. Levonorgestrel
b. Mifepristone
c. Norethindrone
d. Ethinyl estradiol/norethindrone
e. Ulipristal

QUESTION 28-2 A 56-year-old woman with an intact uterus is being treated with hormone replacement therapy with a product that contains an estrogen/progestin combination (estradiol/norethindrone). The progestin is added to

a. decrease the risk of endometrial cancer.
b. decrease the incidence of breast cancer.
c. increase the effectiveness in treating vasomotor symptoms.
d. decrease the risk of coronary heart disease.
e. decrease the risk of cognitive impairment.

QUESTION 28-3 A 25-year-old woman is being treated with clomiphene for fertility. Clomiphene acts by

a. blocking estrogen effects on the uterus.
b. increasing FSH concentrations.

(Continued)

c. blocking progesterone effects on the ovary.

d. decreasing LH concentrations.

e. increasing progesterone secretion by the ovary.

QUESTION 28-4 A 51-year-old woman is beginning menopause. Hormone replacement therapy should be considered for therapy of her hot flashes as well as to decrease the risk of

a. coronary heart disease.

b. dementia.

c. thromboembolic disease.

d. bone fractures.

e. liver impairment.

QUESTION 28-5 A 62-year-old man is being treated with testosterone for hypogonadism of old age. A likely side effect would be

a. hepatotoxicity.

b. dementia.

c. gynecomastia.

d. optic neuritis.

e. peripheral neuropathy.

QUESTION 28-6 A 68-year-old man is being treated with flutamide for advanced prostate cancer. In this setting flutamide should be administered with a GnRH agonist because flutamide, when used alone, causes an

a. increased LH secretion.

b. increased estrogen secretion.

c. increased TSH secretion.

d. increased progesterone secretion.

e. decreased testosterone secretion.

QUESTION 28-7 A 55-year-old man with benign prostatic hypertrophy is being treated with finasteride. Finasteride acts by blocking the conversion of

a. testosterone to estradiol.

b. testosterone to dihydrotestosterone.

c. cortisol to cortisone.

d. cholesterol to pregnenolone.

e. progesterone to androstenedione.

QUESTION 28-8 A 53-year-old woman with breast cancer is being treated with tamoxifen. Tamoxifen is a(n)

a. progesterone antagonist.

b. androgen agonist.

c. inhibitor of 5α-reductase.

d. inhibitor of aromatase.

e. selective estrogen receptor modulator.

SUMMARY QUIZ ANSWER KEY

QUESTION 28-1 Answer is **d**. The combination (estrogen/progestin) contraceptives are contraindicated in women with a history of thromboembolic disease, cerebrovascular disease, migraine headaches with aura, estrogen-dependent cancer, impaired hepatic function or active liver disease, undiagnosed uterine bleeding, and suspected pregnancy. Levonorgestrel and ulipristal are used as emergency contraception and

Estrogens, Progestins, Androgens, and Contraception

CHAPTER 28

mifepristone is used to terminate pregnancy. Norethindrone is a progestin-only oral contraceptive. While slightly less effective than the combination estrogen/progestin formulations, norethindrone provides an alternative in settings where estrogen-containing formulations are contraindicated.

QUESTION 28-2 Answer is **a.** In postmenopausal women with an intact uterus, a progestin is included in hormone replacement therapy to prevent endometrial cancer. The structural features of various progestins are shown in Figure 28-7.

QUESTION 28-3 Answer is **b.** Clomiphene is a potent antiestrogen that primarily is used for treatment of anovulation in the setting of an intact hypothalamic-pituitary axis and adequate estrogen production. Clomiphene acts by inhibiting the negative feedback effects of estrogen at hypothalamic-pituitary levels, increasing follicular-stimulating hormone (FSH) concentrations and thereby enhancing follicular maturation (see Figure 28-2).

QUESTION 28-4 Answer is **d.** In the Women's Health Initiative (WHI), treatment of postmenopausal women with conjugated estrogen plus medroxyprogesterone (in women with a uterus) or with conjugated estrogen alone (in women without a uterus), there was improved bone density and a decreased risk of bone fractures.

QUESTION 28-5 Answer is **c.** When administered in high doses, androgens, such as testosterone can be converted to estrogens, causing gynecomastia (see Figures 28-1 and 28-5). The 17α-alkylated androgens are the only androgens that cause hepatotoxicity.

QUESTION 28-6 Answer is **a.** Flutamide is a potent androgen receptor antagonist and has limited efficacy when used alone because it increases LH secretion that stimulates higher serum testosterone concentrations. It is used primarily in conjunction with a GnRH agonist in the treatment of metastatic prostate cancer (see Chapter 46).

QUESTION 28-7 Answer is **b.** Finasteride is an antagonist of 5α-reductase that blocks the conversion of testosterone to dihydrotestosterone, especially in male external genitalia (see Figure 28-5).

QUESTION 28-8 Answer is **e.** Tamoxifen is a selective estrogen receptor modulator with tissue-selective actions. The pharmacological goal of tamoxifen therapy is to produce beneficial estrogenic actions in certain tissues (eg, bone, brain, and liver), but antagonistic estrogen activity in tissues such as breast and endometrium where estrogenic actions (eg, carcinogenesis) might be deleterious (see Chapter 46).

SUMMARY: ESTROGENS, PROGESTINS, CONTRACEPTIVES, AND ANDROGENS

CLASS AND SUBCLASSES	NAMES	CLINICAL USES	TOXICITIES COMMON	TOXICITIES UNIQUE; CLINICALLY IMPORTANT
Estrogen	Estradiol nonmicronized Estradiol micronized Conjugated equine estrogens Estrogen esterified esters Synthetic conjugated estrogens Estropipate Estradiol transdermal Estradiol topical gel Estradiol vaginal ring Estradiol vaginal tablets Estradiol valerate Estradiol cypionate Conjugated estrogens + medroxyprogesterone acetate (MPA) Ethinyl estradiol + norethindrone Estradiol + norethindrone Estradiol + drospirenone	Menopausal hormone therapy Combination in oral contraceptives (see Table 28-1)		Unopposed use for hormone treatment increases the risk of endometrial carcinoma; this risk is prevented if progestin added to therapy Increased risk of thromboembolic disease May cause migraine in some women May reactivate or exacerbate endometriosis Drosperinone antagonizes the mineralocorticoid receptor and may cause serum K⁺ to rise particularly in patients on potassium-sparing diuretics

(Continued)

SECTION V — Hormones and Hormone Antagonists

CLASS AND SUBCLASSES	NAMES	CLINICAL USES	TOXICITIES COMMON	TOXICITIES UNIQUE; CLINICALLY IMPORTANT
Selective Estrogen Receptor Modulators	Tamoxifen Raloxifene Toremifene	Treatment of breast cancer (see Chapter 46) Raloxifene used to treat osteoporosis		Increased risk of endometrial cancer and thromboembolic disease
Estrogen Antagonists	Clomiphene Fulvestrant	Used to treat infertility due to anovulation		Ovarian hyper-stimulation, increased incidence of multiple births, ovarian cysts, hot flashes, and blurred vision
Estrogen Synthesis Inhibitors	Formestane Exemestane Anastrozole Letrozole	Used to treat breast cancer (see Chapter 46)	Hot flashes	Do not increase the risk of uterine cancer or thromboembolic disease
Progestin	Progesterone micronized Progesterone vaginal gel Progesterone slow-release intrauterine device Progesterone vaginal insert Medroxyprogesterone acetate (MPA) Megestrol acetate Levonorgestrel	Used in combination with estrogen as menopausal hormone therapy (see Table 28-2) Used either alone or in combination with estrogen as oral contraceptives (see Table 28-1) Levonorgestrel is used as emergency contraception after intercourse		
Progesterone Antagonist	Mifepristone	Used in combination with misoprostol (see Chapter 32) or other prostaglandin for the termination of early pregnancy	Nausea, vomiting, and diarrhea	Vaginal bleeding, abdominal pain, uterine cramps
Selective Progesterone Receptor Modulator	Ulipristal	Used as emergency contraception	Abdominal pain and self-limited headache	
Oral Contraceptive	See Table 28-1	Oral contraception	Nausea, edema, and headache	Thromboembolic disease
Androgen	Testosterone Testosterone enanthate Testosterone cypionate Testosterone undecanoate Testosterone patch Testosterone gel Testosterone buccal tablet Anabolic steroids (see Figure 28-8)	Therapeutic androgen replacement Treatment of AIDS-related muscle wasting in men		Diminished fertility Gynecomastia in high doses 17α-alkylated androgens are associated with hepatotoxicity
Androgen Receptor Antagonist	Flutamide Bicalutamide Nilutamide	Treatment of metastatic prostate cancer (see Chapter 46)		
5α-Reductase Inhibitors	Finasteride Dutasteride	Used to treat benign prostatic hyperplasia		Impotence is an infrequent side effect Gynecomastia has been reported

ACTH, Adrenal Steroids, and Pharmacology of the Adrenal Cortex

CHAPTER 29

This chapter will be most useful after having a basic understanding of the material in Chapter 42, ACTH, Adrenal Steroids, and the Pharmacology of the Adrenal Cortex in *Goodman & Gilman's The Pharmacological Basis of Therapeutics*, 12th Edition. In addition to the material presented here, the 12th Edition contains:

- A detailed discussion of the chemistry, actions, and regulation of the secretion of adrenocorticotropic hormone (ACTH)
- A description of the physiological functions of the adrenocorticosteroids
- A detailed description of the pharmacological effects of the adrenocorticosteroids
- A depiction of the chemical structures of the adrenocorticosteroids and their synthetic derivatives
- A discussion of inhibitors of the biosynthesis and action of the adrenocorticosteroids

LEARNING OBJECTIVES

- ☑ Understand the mechanisms of action and the physiological effects of the adrenocorticosteroids.
- ☑ Describe the differences in the anti-inflammatory and sodium-retaining potencies of the glucocorticoids.
- ☑ Describe the side effects of prolonged therapy with glucocorticoids.
- ☑ Understand the effect of abrupt cessation of glucocorticoid therapy.

DRUGS INCLUDED IN THIS CHAPTER

- Aminoglutethimide (CYTADREN)
- Corticorelin (ACTHREL)
- Cosyntropin (COSTROSYN, SYNACTHEN)
- Etomidate (AMIDATE)
- Human corticotropin-releasing hormone (CRH)
- Ketoconazole (NIZORAL; see also Chapter 43)
- Metyrapone (METOPIRONE)
- Mifepristone (MIFUPREX, RU-486; see also Chapter 28)
- Mitotane (LYSODREN)

Table 29-1 lists available preparations of adrenocortical steroids and their synthetic analogs

MECHANISMS OF ACTION OF ACTH, ADRENOCORTICOSTEROIDS, AND INHIBITORS OF THE SYNTHESIS OF ADRENOCORTICOSTEROIDS

DRUG CLASS	DRUGS	MECHANISM OF ACTION
Adrenocorticotropic Hormone (ACTH) Analog	Cosyntropin	Corresponds to residues 1-24 of ACTH; it stimulates the synthesis and release of adrenocortical hormones (see Figures 29-1 and 29-2)
Corticotropin-Releasing Hormone (CRH)	Corticorelin	Binds to specific membrane receptors on corticotropes in the anterior pituitary (see Figure 29-2)
Adrenocortical Steroids	See Table 29-1 for specific drugs	Binds to specific receptor proteins in target tissues to regulate the expression of corticosteroid-responsive genes, thereby changing the levels and array of proteins synthesized by the various target tissues (see Figure 29-3)
Inhibitors of the Biosynthesis of Adrenocortical Steroids	Ketoconazole	In doses higher than those employed in antifungal therapy, it is an effective inhibitor of adrenal and gonadal steroidogenesis, primarily because of its inhibition of the activity of CYP17 (17α-hydroxylase)
	Metyrapone	Inhibitor of CYP11B1 (11β-hydroxylase), which converts 11-deoxycortisol to cortisol
	Etomidate	Inhibitor of CYP11B1 (11β-hydroxylase), which converts 11-deoxycortisol to cortisol
	Aminoglutethimide	Inhibits CYP11A1, which catalyzes the initial and rate-limiting step in the biosynthesis of all steroids; also inhibits CYP11B1 and CYP19 (aromatase)
Adrenocorticolytic Agent	Mitotane	Cytolytic action is due to its metabolic conversion to a reactive acyl chloride by adrenal mitochondria and subsequent reaction with cellular proteins
Antiglucocorticoids	Mifepristone	At high doses, it inhibits the glucocorticoid receptor

SECTION V Hormones and Hormone Antagonists

TABLE 29-1 Available Preparations of Adrenocortical Steroids and Their Synthetic Analogs

NONPROPRIETARY NAME	TRADE NAME	TYPE OF PREPARATION
Alclometasone dipropionate	ACLOVATE	Topical
Amcinonide		Topical
Betamethasone acetate and sodium phosphate	CELESTONE SOLUSPAN	Injectable
Beclomethasone dipropionate	BECONASE AQ, QVAR40, QVAR80	Inhaled
	DIPROLENE, DIPROLINE AF	Topical
Betamethasone sodium phosphate	CELESTONE	Oral
Betamethasone valerate	BETA-VAL, DERMABET, LUXIQ	Topical
Budesonide	ENTOCORT EC	Oral
	PULMICORT	Inhaled
	RHINOCORT	Nasal
Ciclesonide	ALVESCO, OMNARIS	Inhaled
Clobetasol propionate	CLOBEX, CORMAX EMBELINE, OLUX, TEMOVATE	Topical
Clocortolone pivalate	CLODERM	Topical
Desonide	DESONATE, DESOWEN, VERDESO	Topical
Desoximetasone	TOPICORT	Topical
Dexamethasone		Oral
Dexamethasone sodium phosphate	MAXIDEX	Ophthalmic
Diflorasone diacetate	PSORCON	Topical
Fludrocortisone acetate*		Oral
Flunisolide	AEROBID, AEROSPAN HFA	Inhaled
	NASAREL	Nasal
Fluocinolone acetonide	DERMA-SMOOTHE/FS, FS, SYNALAR	Topical
	RETISERT	Intravitreal implant
Fluocinonide	LIDEX, LIDEX-E, VANOS	Topical
Fluorometholone	FML, FML FORTE	Ophthalmic
Fluorometholone acetate	FLAREX	Ophthalmic
Flurandrenolide	CORDRAN CORDRAN SP	Topical
Halcinonide	HALOG	Topical
Hydrocortisone	ALA-CORT, HYTONE, NUTRACORT, STIE-CORT, SYNACORT, TEXACORT	Topical
	CORTEF	Oral
Hydroxycortisone acetate	MICORT-HC	Topical
	CORTIFOAM	Rectal
Hydroxycortisone butyrate	LOCOID	Topical
Hydrocortisone cypionate	CORTEF	Oral
Hydrocortisone sodium succinate	A-HYDROCORT, SOLU-CORTEF	Injectable
Hydrocortisone valerate	WESTCORT	Topical
Methylprednisolone acetate	MEDROL	Oral
	DEPO-MEDROL	Injectable

(Continued)

ACTH, Adrenal Steroids, and Pharmacology of the Adrenal Cortex — CHAPTER 29

NONPROPRIETARY NAME	TRADE NAME	TYPE OF PREPARATION
Methylprednisolone sodium succinate	A-METHAPRED, SOLU-MEDROL	Injectable
Mometasone furoate	ASMANEX	Inhaled
	NASONEX	Nasal
	ELOCON	Topical
Prednisolone		Oral
Prednisolone acetate	FLO-PRED	Oral
	OMNIPRED, PRED FORT, PRED MILD	Ophthalmic
Prednisolone sodium phosphate	ORAPRED, ORAPRED ODT, PEDIAPRED	Oral
Prednisone		Oral
Triamcinolone acetonide	AZMACORT	Inhaled
	NASACORT AQ	Nasal
	KENOLOG	Topical
	KENOLOG-10, KENALOG-40, TRIESENCE, TRIVARIS	Injectable
Triamcinolone hexacetonide	ARISTOSPAN	Injectable
	AZMACORT	Inhaled

*Fludrocortisone acetate is intended for use as a mineralocorticoid.

Note: *Topical* preparations include agents for application to skin or mucous membranes in creams, solutions, ointments, gels, pastes (for oral lesions), and aerosols; *ophthalmic* preparations include solutions, suspensions, and ointments; *inhalation* preparations include agents for nasal or oral inhalation.

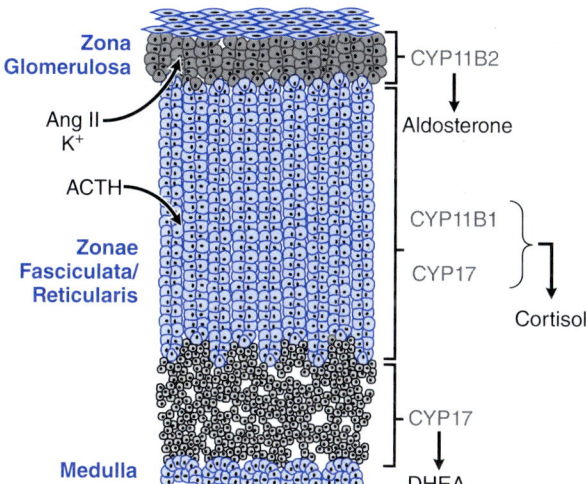

FIGURE 29-1 The adrenal cortex contains 3 anatomically and functionally distinct compartments. The major functional compartments of the adrenal cortex are shown, along with the steroidogenic enzymes that determine the unique profiles of corticosteroid products. Also shown are the predominant physiological regulators of steroid production: angiotensin II (Ang II) and K^+ for the zona glomerulosa and ACTH for the zona fasciculata. The physiological regulator(s) of dehydroepiandrosterone (DHEA) production by the zona reticularis are not known, although ACTH acutely increases DHEA biosynthesis.

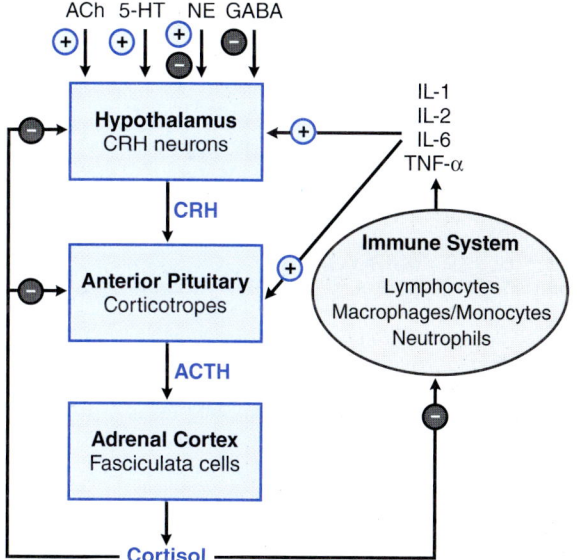

FIGURE 29-2 Overview of the hypothalamic-pituitary-adrenal (HPA) axis and the immune inflammatory network. Also shown are inputs from higher neuronal centers that regulate corticotropin-releasing hormone (CRH) secretion. + indicates a positive regulator, − indicates a negative regulator, + and − indicates a mixed effect, as for NE (norepinephrine). In addition, arginine vasopressin stimulates release of ACTH from corticotropes.

SECTION V: Hormones and Hormone Antagonists

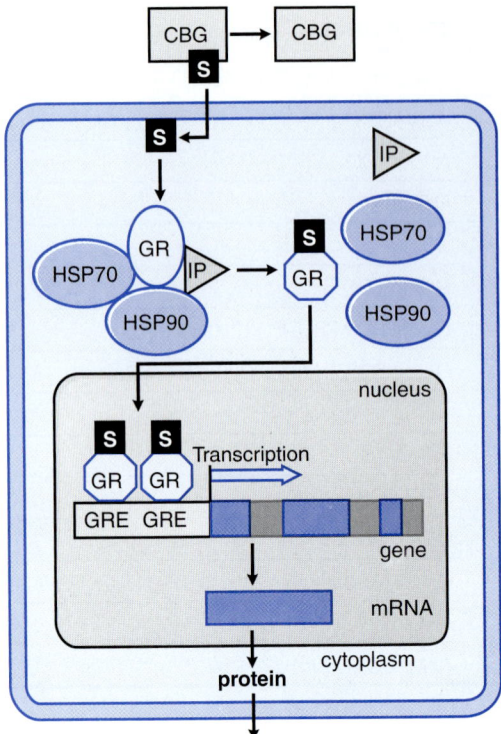

FIGURE 29-3 Intracellular mechanism of action of the glucocorticoid receptor. The figure shows the molecular pathway by which cortisol (labeled S) enters cells and interacts with the glucocorticoid receptor (GR) to change GR conformation (indicated by the change in shape of the GR), induce GR nuclear translocation, and activate transcription of target genes. The example shown is one in which glucocorticoids activate expression of target genes; the expression of certain genes, including proopiomelanocortin (POMC) expression by corticotropes, is inhibited by glucocorticoid treatment. CBG, corticosteroid-binding globulin; GR, glucocorticoid receptor; GRE, glucocorticoid-response elements in the DNA that are bound by GR, thus providing specificity to induction of gene transcription by glucocorticoids; HSP70, the 70-Kd heat-shock protein; IP, the 56-Kd immunophilin; HSP90, the 90-Kd heat-shock protein; S, steroid hormone. Within the gene are introns (gray) and exons (blue); transcription and mRNA processing leads to splicing and removal of introns and assembly of exons into mRNA.

PHYSIOLOGIC FUNCTIONS AND PHARMACOLOGIC EFFECTS OF ADRENOCORTICAL STEROIDS

PHYSIOLOGIC FUNCTION OR ORGAN AFFECTED	MECHANISM
Carbohydrate and Protein Metabolism	Stimulates the liver to form glucose from amino acids and glycerol and to store glucose as glycogen Decreases glucose utilization in periphery; increases protein breakdown
Lipid Metabolism	Redistributes body fat; increased fat in the back of neck, face, and supraclavicular area with loss of fat in the extremities Permissive facilitation of the lipolytic effect of growth hormone and β adrenergic agonists resulting in an increase in free fatty acids
Electrolyte and Water Balance	Mineralocorticoids act on the distal tubules and collecting ducts to enhance reabsorption of Na^+, and to enhance urinary excretion of K^+ and H^+ Decreases total body Ca^{2+} stores by lowering Ca^{2+} uptake from the gut and increasing Ca^{2+} excretion by the kidney
Cardiovascular System	Mineralocorticoid-induced changes in renal Na^+ exacerbate congestive heart failure Enhanced vascular reactivity of other vasoactive substances such as norepinephrine and angiotensin II and exacerbation of hypertension
Skeletal Muscle	Corticosteroids are required for the normal function of skeletal muscle; adrenocortical insufficiency results in muscle weakness; in aldosteronism, muscle weakness results from hypokalemia; glucocorticoid excess results in muscle wasting termed "steroid myopathy"

(Continued)

ACTH, Adrenal Steroids, and Pharmacology of the Adrenal Cortex

CHAPTER 29

PHYSIOLOGIC FUNCTION OR ORGAN AFFECTED	MECHANISM
Central Nervous System	Adrenocortical steroids exert direct effects on the CNS such as effects on mood, behavior, and brain excitability; frank psychosis has also been noted
Formed Elements of Blood	Corticosteroids exert effects on erythrocytes and produce a decrease in circulating lymphocytes, monocytes, basophils, and eosinophiles; certain lymphoid malignancies are destroyed by glucocorticoid treatment
Anti-Inflammatory and Immunosuppressive Actions	Glucocorticoids profoundly alter the immune response of lymphocytes and suppress inflammation; they are useful in managing the inflammatory response to diseases of humoral immunity such as urticarial as well as diseases of cellular immunity such as transplantation rejection (see Side Bar THE THERAPEUTIC USES OF ADRENOCORTICAL STEROIDS)

CASE 29-1

A 53-year-old woman with rheumatoid arthritis involving the joints of both hands and both hips has developed an exacerbation of her disease in the past two weeks. Fifteen years ago she responded well to a short course of prednisone. For the past 3 months, she has been receiving methotrexate. She is started back on prednisone now for relief of her symptoms.

a. Why was prednisone chosen?

Table 29-2 shows the relative potencies and equivalent doses of representative corticosteroids. Prednisone is a more potent anti-inflammatory agent than cortisol, but not as potent as dexamethasone. Prednisone has much less sodium-retaining potency than fludrocortisone, which has predominant mineralocorticoid activity. Prednisone is considered to be intermediate in its duration of action compared to cortisol and dexamethasone, which are short- and long-acting, respectively.

To facilitate drug tapering and/or conversion to alternate-day therapy, the intermediate-acting glucocorticoid such as prednisone is preferred to the longer-acting dexamethasone.

(Continued)

THERAPEUTIC USES OF ADRENOCORTICAL STEROIDS

- Replacement therapy
  - Acute adrenal Insufficiency
  - Chronic adrenal insufficiency
  - Congenital adrenal hyperplasia
- Nonendocrine diseases
  - Rheumatic disorders
  - Renal disease
  - Allergic disease
  - Bronchial asthma and other pulmonary conditions
  - Infectious diseases
  - Ocular diseases
  - Skin diseases
  - Gastrointestinal diseases
  - Hepatic diseases
  - Malignancies
  - Cerebral edema
  - Sarcoidosis
  - Thrombocytopenia
  - Autoimmune destruction of erythrocytes
  - Organ transplantation
  - Spinal cord injury

TABLE 29-2 Relative Potencies and Equivalent Doses of Representative Corticosteroids

COMPOUND	ANTI-INFLAMMATORY POTENCY	Na⁺-RETAINING POTENCY	DURATION OF ACTION[a]	EQUIVALENT DOSE (mg)[b]
Cortisol	1	1	S	20
Cortisone	0.8	0.8	S	25
Fludrocortisone	10	125	I	[c]
Prednisone	4	0.8	I	5
Prednisolone	4	0.8	I	5
6α-Methylprednisolone	5	0.5	I	4
Triamcinolone	5	0	I	4
Betamethasone	25	0	L	0.75
Dexamethasone	25	0	L	0.75

[a] S, short (ie, 8-12 hour biological $t_{1/2}$); I, intermediate (ie, 12-36 hour biological $t_{1/2}$); L, long (ie, 36-72 hour biological $t_{1/2}$).
[b] These dose relationships apply only to oral or intravenous administration, as glucocorticoid potencies may differ greatly following intramuscular or intraarticular administration.
[c] This agent is not used for glucocorticoid effects.

SECTION V

Hormones and Hormone Antagonists

GENERAL PRINCIPLES FOR THE USE OF GLUCOCORTICOIDS

- The decision to institute therapy requires careful consideration of the relative risks and benefits in each patient.
- For any disease and any patient, the appropriate dose to achieve a given therapeutic effect must be determined by trial and error and must be reevaluated periodically.
- A single dose of a glucocorticoid, even a large one, is virtually without harmful effects and a short course of up to 1 week, in the absence of specific contraindications, is unlikely to be harmful.
- As the duration of glucocorticoid therapy extends beyond 1 week, there are time and dose-related increases in the incidence of disabling and potential lethal effects.
- Except in the setting of replacement therapy the glucocorticoids are neither specific nor curative.
- Abrupt cessation of glucocorticoids after prolonged therapy is associated with the risk of adrenal insufficiency, which may be fatal.

The use of glucocorticoids in a disease such as rheumatoid arthritis is largely empirical and the use of glucocorticoids should follow the principles in the Side Bar GENERAL PRINCIPLES FOR THE USE OF GLUCOCORTICOIDS.

b. What is the mechanism of action of adrenocortical steroids?

The glucocorticoids interact with receptors in the various target tissues that are members of the nuclear receptor family of transcription factors (see Figure 29-3). In the target tissues, proteins are expressed that alter cellular functions resulting in the physiologic functions and pharmacologic effects shown in the Table PHYSIOLOGICAL FUNCTIONS AND PHARMACOLOGICAL EFFECTS OF THE ADRENOCORTICAL STEROIDS.

CASE 29-2

A 43-year-man has been diagnosed with primary adrenal insufficiency (Addison's disease). He requires replacement therapy with adrenocortical steroids.

a. What is the difference between primary and secondary adrenal insufficiency?

Adrenal insufficiency can result from structural or functional lesions of the adrenal cortex (primary adrenal insufficiency or Addison's disease) or from functional or structural lesions of the anterior pituitary or hypothalamus (secondary adrenal insufficiency). See Figures 29-1 and 29-2 for the anatomical and functional structure of the adrenal gland and for the regulation of corticosteroids from the anterior pituitary, respectively.

b. Why is hydrocortisone chosen to treat this patient?

Hydrocortisone is the active form of cortisone (see Figure 29-4). Although some patients with primary adrenal insufficiency can be maintained on hydrocortisone and liberal salt intake, most also require a mineralocorticoid such as fludrocortisone acetate to maintain water and electrolyte balance.

c. What are the major considerations in maintaining the proper dose of hydrocortisone in this patient?

Glucocorticoid doses often must be adjusted upward in patients who are also taking drugs that increase the plasma clearance of glucocorticoids (eg, phenytoin, rifampin, or barbiturates). The stress of concurrent illness may also necessitate a dose adjustment. During minor illnesses, the glucocorticoid dose should be doubled. If nausea or vomiting precludes the retention of oral medications, the patient's physician should be notified, and family members should be trained to administer parenteral dexamethasone and then seek medical attention immediately.

TOXICITIES OF ADRENOCORTICAL STEROIDS

- Adrenal insufficiency with abrupt withdrawal of therapy
- Fluid and electrolyte abnormalities (hypertension)
- Metabolic changes (hyperglycemia)
- Immune response (susceptibility to infection)
- Risk of peptic ulcers
- Myopathy
- Behavioral changes
- Cataracts
- Osteoporosis
- Osteonecrosis (aseptic necrosis of femoral head)
- Growth retardation in children

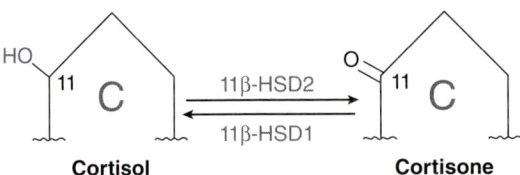

FIGURE 29-4 Receptor-independent mechanism by which 11β-hydroxysteroid dehydrogenase confers specificity of corticosteroid action. Type 2 11β-hydroxysteroid dehydrogenase (11β-HSD2) converts cortisol, which binds to both the mineralocorticoid receptor (MR) and the glucocorticoid receptor (GR), to cortisone, which binds to neither MR nor GR, thereby protecting the MR from the high circulating concentrations of cortisol. This inactivation allows specific responses to aldosterone in sites such as the distal nephron. The type 1 isozyme of 11β-HSD (11β-HSD1) catalyzes the reverse reaction, which converts inactive cortisone to active cortisol in such tissues as liver and fat. Only ring C of the corticosteroid is depicted.

ACTH, Adrenal Steroids, and Pharmacology of the Adrenal Cortex

CHAPTER 29

CASE 29-3

The patient in Case 29-1 was treated with 40 mg of prednisone daily for 2 weeks and then the dose was lowered to 20 mg daily. Attempts to further lower the dose have resulted in a flare-up of her disease. After 2 months of prednisone therapy, she became uncomfortable with her increased weight and the development of roundness in her face. Despite warnings not to do so, she stopped the use of her prednisone.

a. **What side effects is she likely to experience?**

The most severe complication of steroid cessation is the life-threatening condition of acute adrenal insufficiency characterized by nausea, vomiting, abdominal pain, hyponatremia, hyperkalemia, weakness, lethargy, and hypotension.

b. **How could this situation possibly have been avoided?**

Patients who are taking chronic glucocorticoid therapy should be cautioned against discontinuing the therapy without a significant tapering of the dose. There is significant variation among patients with respect to the degree and duration of adrenal suppression after glucocorticoid therapy. Patients who have received supraphysiological doses of glucocorticoids for a period of 2 to 4 weeks should be considered to have some hypothalamic-pituitary-adrenal (HPA) suppression. A gradual reduction in their glucocorticoid dose is required. Many patients recover from glucocorticoid-induced HPA suppression within several weeks to months; however, in some patients the time to recovery can be a year or longer.

CASE 29-4

A 22-year-old woman with the diagnosis of Crohn's disease has been successfully treated with sulfasalazine (see Chapter 33). A recent exacerbation of her disease has necessitated the addition of prednisone to her therapeutic regimen. She has noted, since starting the prednisone that she has been nervous and has had difficulty sleeping.

a. **What are the potential toxicities of adrenocortical steroids to warn the patient about?**

The toxicities of glucocorticoid therapy are listed in the Side Bar TOXICITIES OF ADRENOCORTICAL STEROIDS. Behavioral changes are particularly common. These might include nervousness, insomnia, changes in mood, and even overt psychosis. Suicidal tendencies are not uncommon.

b. **What are other treatment options available to this patient?**

Budesonide, (see Chapter 33) a potent glucocorticoid that is inactivated by first-pass hepatic metabolism, has diminished systemic side effects commonly associated with glucocorticoids. The drug can be administered by a delayed-release capsule that delivers steroid to the ileum and ascending colon, or as a retention enema for the treatment of ulcerative colitis.

CASE 29-5

A 36-year-old woman is suspected of having Cushing's syndrome. It is recommended that she have a dexamethasone suppression test.

a. **What is a dexamethasone suppression test and how is it interpreted?**

To determine if patients with clinical manifestations of hypercortisolism have biochemical evidence of increased cortisol biosynthesis, an overnight dexamethasone suppression test has been devised in which patients are given 1 mg of dexamethasone orally at 11 PM, and plasma cortisol is measured at 8 AM the following morning. Suppression of plasma cortisol to less than 1.8 µg/dL suggests that the patient does not have Cushing's syndrome.

(Continued)

SECTION V — Hormones and Hormone Antagonists

In a more formal dexamethasone suppression test, baseline plasma cortisol concentrations are measured for 48 hours and then dexamethasone is administered 0.5 mg every 6 hours for 48 hours. This dose markedly suppresses plasma cortisol in normal patients, but does not suppress cortisol concentrations in patients with Cushing's syndrome.

CASE 29-6

A 68-year-old man is diagnosed with bacterial conjunctivitis. He is prescribed a combination eye drop that contains dexamethasone and an antibiotic.

a. Why use an adrenocorticoal steroid in an eye infection?

Glucocorticoids can dramatically decrease inflammation in the conjunctiva when administered topically into the conjunctival sac (see Chapter 47).

b. What are the concerns with the use of this combination product?

Topical glucocorticoid therapy frequently increases intraocular pressure in normal eyes and exacerbates intraocular hypertension in patients with antecedent glaucoma. The glaucoma is not always reversible on cessation of the glucocorticoid therapy. Intraocular pressure should be monitored when glucocorticoids are applied to the eye for more than 2 weeks.

CASE 29-7

A 28-year-old woman is diagnosed with Cushing's syndrome from an ectopic ACTH-producing tumor. She is being treated with metyrapone.

a. What is metyrapone and how does it act?

Metyrapone is a relatively selective inhibitor of CYP11B (11β-hydroxylase), which converts 11-deoxycortisol to cortisol in the terminal reaction in the glucocorticoid biosynthetic pathway. Thus, the biosynthesis of cortisol is markedly impaired.

b. What are the untoward effects of long-term metyrapone therapy?

Chronic administration of metyrapone can cause hirsutism, which results from increased synthesis of androgens upstream from the enzymatic block. Metyrapone can also cause hypertension, which results from increased concentrations of 11-deoxycortisol. Other side effects include nausea, headache, sedation, and rash.

KEY CONCEPTS

- The rate of glucocorticoid secretion is determined by fluctuations in the release of ACTH by the pituitary corticotropes (see Figure 29-2).
- Adrenocortical steroids act by activating glucocorticoid receptors or mineralocorticoid receptors in various tissues (see Figure 29-3).
- Glucocorticoids are administered in many formulations (oral, parenteral, and topical) for disorders that share an inflammatory or immunological basis (see Table 29-1).
- Except for replacement therapy for adrenal insufficiency, glucocorticoids are neither specific nor curative.
- Corticosteroid preparations vary widely in their anti-inflammatory effects and duration of action. Some corticosteroids possess mineralocorticoid activity while others do not (see Table 29-2).
- Glucocorticoids have several potentially serious side effects (see Side Bar TOXICITIES OF ADRENOCORTICAL STEROIDS), which necessitates:
  - Limiting the dose to the minimal needed to achieve a therapeutic effect.
  - Periodic reevaluation.

(Continued)

ACTH, Adrenal Steroids, and Pharmacology of the Adrenal Cortex

CHAPTER 29

➡ A single dose of a glucocorticoid is virtually without long-term harmful effects.

➡ As the duration of glucocorticoid therapy increases beyond 1 week, adverse effects increase in a time- and dose-related manor.

➡ Abrupt cessation of glucocorticoids after prolonged therapy is associated with the risk of adrenal insufficiency.

SUMMARY QUIZ

QUESTION 29-1 A 34-year-old man is diagnosed with secondary adrenal insufficiency. He does not require the administration of a mineralocorticoid because

a. the adrenal medulla is intact.
b. the zona glomerulosa is intact.
c. the zona reticularis is intact.
d. the zona fasciculata is intact.
e. 11β-hydroxylase is not inhibited.

QUESTION 29-2 A 54-year-old man has been diagnosed with hypertension caused by his excessive consumption of licorice. Licorice is a known inhibitor of 11β-hydroxysteroid dehydrogenase that is involved in the inactivation of

a. cortisol.
b. aldosterone.
c. ACTH.
d. dehydroepiandrosterone.
e. progesterone.

QUESTION 29-3 A 34-year-old woman with Crohn's disease has been taking prednisone daily for 1 year. She has been experiencing a thickness in the back of her neck. This is likely due to a(n)

a. edema.
b. increase in muscle growth.
c. redistribution of lipid.
d. protein deposition.
e. ectopic thyroid tissue.

QUESTION 29-4 A 63-year-old man with type 2 diabetes and osteoarthritis in his left knee is given an intra-articular injection of a glucocorticoid to decrease pain in his knee. An elevation in his blood sugar for the next 3 days is likely due to an effect of the glucocorticoid on

a. diminished peripheral glucose utilization.
b. increased protein breakdown.
c. activation of lipolysis.
d. increased glucose synthesis in the liver.
e. all of the above.

QUESTION 29-5 A 48-year-old woman with a chronic pulmonary disease is being treated with an inhaled glucocorticoid product. She is likely to experience which of the following side effects?

a. Buffalo hump
b. Acute adrenal insufficiency
c. Hyperglycemia
d. Oral candidiasis
e. Hepatitis

SECTION V — Hormones and Hormone Antagonists

SUMMARY QUIZ ANSWER KEY

QUESTION 29-1 Answer is **b**. The zona glomerulosa is the site of aldosterone synthesis and secretion (see Figure 29-1). In secondary adrenal insufficiency, which usually involves pituitary or hypothalamic dysfunction, mineralocorticoid biosynthesis is preserved.

QUESTION 29-2 Answer is **a**. 11β-Hydroxysteroid dehydrogenase catalyzes the conversion of cortisol (active) to cortisone (inactive) (see Figure 29-4). Aldosterone is resistant to the enzyme's actions. The inhibition of the enzyme by licorice results in a state of mineralocorticoid excess resulting in hypertension.

QUESTION 29-3 Answer is **c**. A significant untoward effect of the pharmacological use of glucocorticoids is the dramatic redistribution of body fat. There is increased fat in the back of the neck ("buffalo hump"), face ("moon face"), and the supraclavicular area, coupled with a loss of fat in the extremities. One hypothesis for this effect is that truncal adipocytes are more sensitive than peripheral adipocytes to the elevated insulin concentrations that result from glucocorticoid-induced hyperglycemia.

QUESTION 29-4 Answer is **e**. Corticosteroids profoundly affect carbohydrate and protein metabolism, which can be viewed as protecting glucose-dependent tissues such as the heart and brain. They stimulate the liver to form glucose from amino acids and glycerol, and to store glucose as liver glycogen. In the periphery, glucocorticoids diminish glucose utilization, increase protein breakdown, increase the synthesis of glutamine, and activate lipolysis, thereby providing amino acids and glycerol for gluconeogenesis. The net result is to increase blood glucose concentrations.

QUESTION 29-5 Answer is **d**. In many patients, inhaled steroids can either reduce the need for oral corticosteroids or replace them altogether. The oral bioavailability of inhaled steroids vary considerably and those with low bioavailability will have less steroid-induced side effects. However, the deposition of steroid in the oral cavity may cause the growth of *Candida*. The incidence of this effect can be reduced by using a product such as ciclesonide or beclomethasone which are inactive prodrugs that are activated at their site of action by lung esterases. Therefore, they are less likely to adversely affect the oral cavity.

SUMMARY: ACTH, ADRENAL STEROIDS, AND PHARMACOLOGY OF THE ADRENAL CORTEX

CLASS AND SUBCLASSES	NAMES	CLINICAL USES	TOXICITIES COMMON	TOXICITIES UNIQUE; CLINICALLY IMPORTANT
Adrenocorticotropic Hormone (ACTH) Analog	Cosyntropin	Testing the integrity of the hypothalamic-pituitary axis		
Corticotropin-Releasing Hormone (CRH)	Corticorelin	Diagnostic testing of hypothalamic-pituitary axis	Flushing if drug is administered as an intravenous bolus	
Adrenocortical Steroids	See Table 29-1 for specific drugs	See Side Bar THERAPEUTIC USES OF ADRENOCORTICAL STEROIDS for the therapeutic use of adrenocortical steroids for selected specific examples, and the Side Bar GENERAL PRINCIPLES FOR THE USE OF GLUCOCORTICOIDS for principles related to the use of adrenocortical steroids		Acute adrenal insufficiency if withdrawal of chronic therapy is not tapered. Pseudotumor cerebri rarely associated with withdrawal of therapy. See Side Bar TOXICITIES OF ADRENOCORTICAL STEROIDS for side effects of adrenocortical steroid therapy

(Continued)

ACTH, Adrenal Steroids, and Pharmacology of the Adrenal Cortex — CHAPTER 29

CLASS AND SUBCLASSES	NAMES	CLINICAL USES	TOXICITIES COMMON	UNIQUE; CLINICALLY IMPORTANT
Inhibitors of the Biosynthesis of Adrenocortical Steroids	Ketoconazole	Antifungal agent used to inhibit steroid biosynthesis in patients with hypercortisolism		Hepatic dysfunction Inhibition of CYPs may lead to serious drug interactions
	Metyrapone	Used to impair the biosynthesis of cortisol in patients with adrenal neoplasms or tumors producing ACTH ectopically	Nausea, headache, sedation, rash	Precipitation of acute adrenal insufficiency Chronic administration may cause hirsutism
	Etomidate	Used to treat hypercortisolism by intravenous administration in patients who cannot take oral medication		Sedation
	Aminoglutethimide	Inhibits biosynthesis of cortisol; recently withdrawn from the market by the manufacturer		
Adrenocorticolytic Agent	Mitotane	Used to treat inoperable adrenocortical carcinoma		Severe GI disturbances and ataxia
Antiglucocorticoids	Mifepristone	Investigational use in high doses to treat patients with inoperable causes of cortisol excess (see Chapter 28)		See Chapter 28

Endocrine Pancreas and Pharmacotherapy of Diabetes Mellitus and Hypoglycemia

This chapter will be most useful after having a basic understanding of the material in Chapter 43, Endocrine Pancreas and Pharmacotherapy of Diabetes Mellitus and Hypoglycemia in *Goodman & Gilman's The Pharmacological Basis of Therapeutics*, 12th Edition. In addition to the material presented here, the 12th Edition includes:

- A detailed discussion of the regulation of blood glucose
- A description of pancreatic islet cell physiology and the synthesis and processing of insulin
- A discussion of the signaling pathway that is activated by insulin resulting in its effects on target cells
- A description of the pathogenesis of type 1 and type 2 diabetes
- Drugs that are in development for type 2 diabetes
- Table 43-5 Properties of Insulin Preparations

LEARNING OBJECTIVES

☑ Understand the mechanisms of action of insulin and the oral antidiabetic drugs.
☑ Describe the components for management of the diabetic patient including the goals of therapy.
☑ Describe the pharmacotherapeutic options for the treatment of patients with type 1 or type 2 diabetes.
☑ Learn about the adverse effects of insulin and the oral antidiabetic drugs.
☑ Understand the treatment of hypoglycemia.

DRUGS INCLUDED IN THIS CHAPTER

Acarbose (PRECOSE, others)
Alogliptin (NESINA)
Bromocriptine (CYCLOSET, not yet available in the United States for treatment of diabetes)
Colesevelam (WELCHOL)
Diazoxide (PROGLYCEM)
Exenatide (BYETTA)
Gliclazide (DIAMICRON, others, unavailable in the United States)
Glimepiride (AMARYL)
Glipizide (GLUCOTROL, others)
Glucagon
Glyburide (Glibenclamide; MICRONASE, DIABETA, others)
Insulin aspart (NOVOLOG)
Insulin determir (LEVEMIR)
Insulin glargine (LANTUS)
Insulin glulisine (APIDRA)
Insulin lispro (HUMALOG)
Insulin protamine hagedorn (NPH, insulin isophane)
Liraglutide (VICTOZA)
Metformin (GLUCOPHAGE, others)
Miglitol (GLYSET)
Nateglinide (STARLIX)
Pioglitazone (ACTOS)
Pramlintide (SYMLIN)
Repaglinide (PRANDIN)
Rosiglitazone (AVANDIA)
Saxagliptin (ONGLYZA)
Sitagliptin (JANIVIA)
Vidagliptin (GALVUS, ZOMELIS, JAIRA, not available in the United States)
Voglibose (VOGLIB, not available in the United States)

MECHANISMS OF ACTION INSULIN AND ORAL ANTIDIABETIC DRUGS

DRUG CLASS	DRUGS	MECHANISM OF ACTION
Insulin	Insulin	Insulin binds to a plasma membrane receptor that initiates a cascade of signaling events, which results in glucose utilization and glycogen synthesis (see Figure 30-1)
Biguanides	Metformin	Increases the activity of AMP-dependent protein kinase (AMPK); activated AMPK stimulates fatty acid oxidation, glucose uptake, and nonoxidative metabolism, and it reduces lipogenesis and gluconeogenesis; the net result is increased glycogen storage in skeletal muscle, lower rates of hepatic glucose production, increased insulin sensitivity, and lower blood glucose concentrations
Insulin Secretagogues—Sulfonylureas	Glyburide Glipizide Gliclazide Glimepiride	Stimulate insulin release by binding to a specific site on the β cell K_{ATP} channel complex and inhibiting its activity (see Figure 30-2)
Insulin Secretagogues—Nonsulfonylureas	Repaglinide Nateglinide	Stimulates insulin release by closing K_{ATP} channels in pancreatic β cells (see Figure 30-2)
Thiazolidinediones	Rosiglitazone Pioglitazone	Ligands for the peroxisome proliferation activating receptor γ ($PPAR_\gamma$) that are involved in the regulation of genes related to glucose and lipid metabolism

(Continued)

Endocrine Pancreas and Pharmacotherapy

CHAPTER 30

DRUG CLASS	DRUGS	MECHANISM OF ACTION
GLP-1 Agonists	Exenatide, Liraglutide	Glucagon-like peptide 1 (GLP-1) agonists that activate the GLP-1 receptor, activate the cAMP-PKA pathway, and initiate signals through PKC and P13K (see Figure 30-2)
Dipeptidyl Peptidase-4 (DPP-4) Inhibitors	Sitagliptin, Saxagliptin, Vidagliptin, Alogliptin	Inhibit the DPP-4 enzyme that is critical for the inactivation of GLP-1 and GIP (glucose-dependent insulinotropic polypeptide); thus the AUC of GLP-1 and GIP is increased when their secretion is stimulated by a meal (see Figure 30-3)
α-Glucosidase Inhibitors	Acarbose, Miglitol, Voglibose	Reduces intestinal absorption of carbohydrates from the GI tract and blunts the rate of rise of postprandial glucose by inhibiting α-glucosidase in the intestinal brush border
Amylin Agonists	Pramlintide	Synthetic form of amylin; it acts through the amylin receptor in the brain causing reduction in glucagon release, delayed gastric emptying, and satiety
Bile Acid Sequestrants	Colesevelam	Mechanism by which bile acid binding and removal from the enterohepatic circulation lowers blood glucose has not been established
Agents Used to Treat Hypoglycemia	Glucagon	Interacts with GPCR receptor on target cells; the effects of glucagon on the liver are mediated by cAMP
	Diazoxide	Hyperglycemia results from inhibition of insulin secretion (see Figure 30-2)

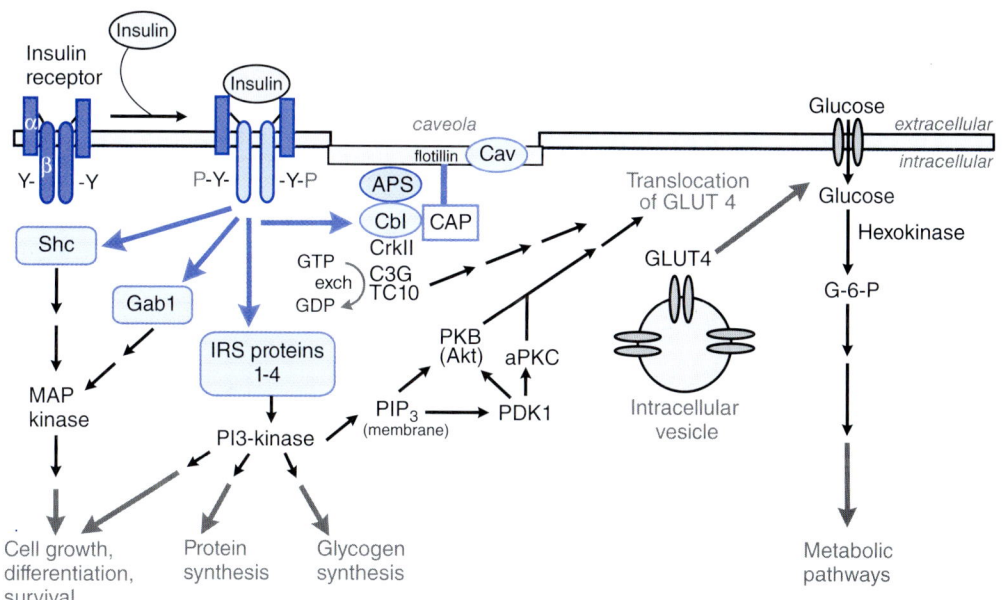

FIGURE 30-1 Pathways of insulin signaling. The binding of insulin to its plasma membrane receptor activates a cascade of downstream signaling events. Insulin binding activates the intrinsic tyrosine kinase activity of the receptor dimer, resulting in the tyrosine phosphorylation (Y-P) of the receptor's β subunits and a small number of specific substrates (light blue shapes): the insulin receptor substrate (IRS) proteins, Gab-1 and SHC; within the membrane, a caveolar pool of insulin receptor phosphorylates caveolin (Cav), APS, and Cbl. These tyrosine-phosphorylated proteins interact with signaling cascades via SH2 and SH3 domains to mediate the effects of insulin, with specific effects resulting from each pathway. In target tissues such as skeletal muscle and adipocytes, a key event is the translocation of the Glut4 glucose transporter from intracellular vesicles to the plasma membrane; this translocation is stimulated by both the caveolar and noncaveolar pathways. In the noncaveolar pathway, the activation of PI3K is crucial, and PKB/Akt (anchored at the membrane by PIP3) and/or an atypical form of PKC is involved. In the caveolar pathway, caveolar protein flotillin localizes the signaling complex to the caveola; the signaling pathway involves a series of SH2 domain interactions that add the adaptor protein CrkII, the guanine nucleotide exchange protein C3G, and small GTP-binding protein, TC10. The pathways are inactivated by specific phosphoprotein phosphatases (eg, PTB1B). In addition to the actions shown, insulin also stimulates the plasma membrane Na^+,K^+-ATPase by a mechanism that is still being elucidated; the result is an increase in pump activity and a net accumulation of K^+ in the cell. Abbreviations: aPKC, atypical isoform of protein kinase C; APS, adaptor protein with PH and SH2 domains; CAP, Cbl associated protein; CrkII, chicken tumor virus regulator of kinase II; GLUT4, glucose transporter 4; Gab-1, Grb-2 associated binder; MAP kinase, mitogen-activated protein kinase; PDK, phosphoinositide-dependent kinase; PI3 kinase, phosphatidylinositol-3-kinase; PIP3, phosphatidylinositol trisphosphate; PKB, protein kinase B (also called Akt); Y, tyrosine residue; Y-P, phosphorylated tyrosine residue.

SECTION V Hormones and Hormone Antagonists

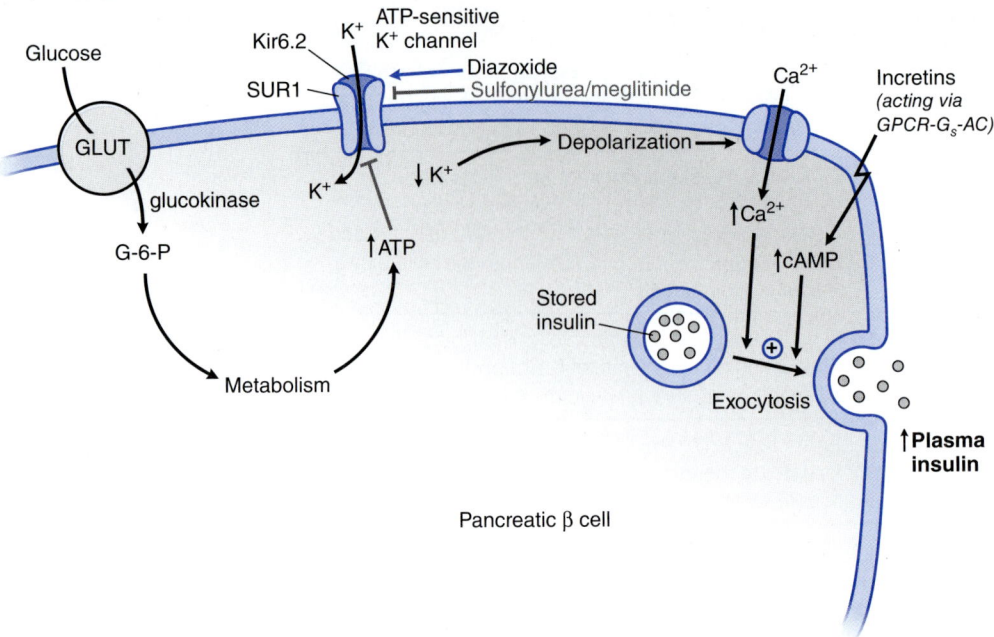

FIGURE 30-2 Regulation of insulin secretion from a pancreatic β cell. The pancreatic β cell in a resting state (fasting blood glucose) is hyperpolarized. Glucose, entering via GLUT transporters (primarily GLUT1 in humans, GLUT2 in rodents), is metabolized and elevates cellular ATP, which inhibits K+ entry through the K_{ATP} channel; the decreased K+ conductance results in depolarization, leading to Ca^{2+}-dependent exocytosis of stored insulin. The K_{ATP} channel, actually a hetero-octamer composed of SUR1 and Kir 6.2 subunits, is the site of action of several classes of drugs: ATP binds to and inhibits Kir6.2; sulfonylureas and meglitinides bind to and inhibit SUR1; all 3 agents thereby promote insulin secretion. Diazoxide and ADP-Mg^{2+} (low ATP) bind to and activate SUR1, thereby inhibiting insulin secretion. Incretins enhance insulin secretion.

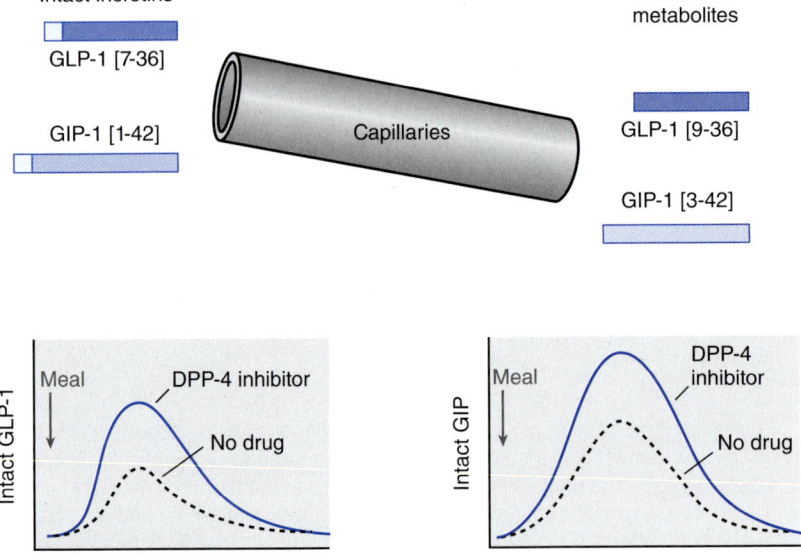

FIGURE 30-3 Pharmacological effects of DDP-4 inhibition. DPP-4, an ectoenzyme located on the luminal side of capillary endothelial cells metabolizes the incretins, glucagon-like peptide 1 (GLP-1), and glucose-dependent insulinotropic polypeptide (GIP), by removing the 2 N-terminal amino acids. The target for DPP-4 cleavage is a proline or alanine residue in the second position of the primary peptide sequence. The truncated metabolites GLP-1 [9-36] and GIP [3-42] are the major forms of the incretins in plasma and are inactive as insulin secretagogues. Treatment with a DPP-4 inhibitor increases the concentrations of intact GLP-1 and GIP.

Endocrine Pancreas and Pharmacotherapy

CHAPTER 30

TABLE 30-1 Criteria for the Diagnosis of Diabetes

- Symptoms of diabetes plus random blood glucose concentration ≥11.1 mM (200 mg/dL)[a] or
- Fasting plasma glucose ≥7.0 mM (126 mg/dL)[b] or
- Two-hour plasma glucose ≥11.1 mM (200 mg/dL) during an oral glucose tolerance test[c]
- HbA_{1c} ≥6.5%

[a]Random is defined as without regard to time since the last meal.
[b]Fasting is defined as no caloric intake for at least 8 h.
[c]The test should be performed using a glucose load containing the equivalent of 75 g anhydrous glucose dissolved in water; this test is not recommended for routine clinical use.

Note: In the absence of unequivocal hyperglycemia and acute metabolic decompensation, these criteria should be confirmed by repeat testing on a different day.

Data adapted from Diabetes Care, 2010; 33:S62–S69.

CASE 30-1

A 10-year-old girl is diagnosed with type 1 diabetes. She will start on insulin therapy.

a. How is the diagnosis of type 1 diabetes made?

The diagnosis of diabetes mellitus is currently based on the correlation of diabetes-specific complications with a particular level of glycemia, that is, the level of glycemia at which a diabetes-specific complication like retinopathy begins to appear. The criterion for the diagnosis of diabetes is shown in Table 30-1.

b. How should diabetes in this patient be managed? What are the goals of therapy?

Therapy of diabetes has to be individualized for each patient. Figure 30-4 shows the components of sound diabetes management. Table 30-2 lists the indexes of therapy and the goals for diabetic patients in general.

c. What is hemoglobin A_{1c} (A1C) and how does it differ from fasting blood glucose?

Exposure of proteins to an elevated glucose concentration produces nonenzymatic glycation of proteins including hemoglobin (Hb). Thus, the level of HbA_{1c} (A1C) represents the average glucose concentration to which the Hb has been exposed over the past 2 to 3 months.

d. What is the mechanism of action of insulin?

The pancreatic β cell is a highly specialized cell that quickly senses and responds to the external glucose concentration. The transport of glucose into the pancreatic β cell via a facilitative transporter (see Figure 30-2) results in increased intracellular calcium which, in turn, results in exocytotic release of insulin from storage vesicles.

Once in the circulation, insulin binds, in various tissues, to its plasma membrane receptor (see Figure 30-1) that activates a cascade of downstream intracellular signaling events. The tissues that are considered critical for the regulation of blood glucose are liver, skeletal muscle, and fat.

(Continued)

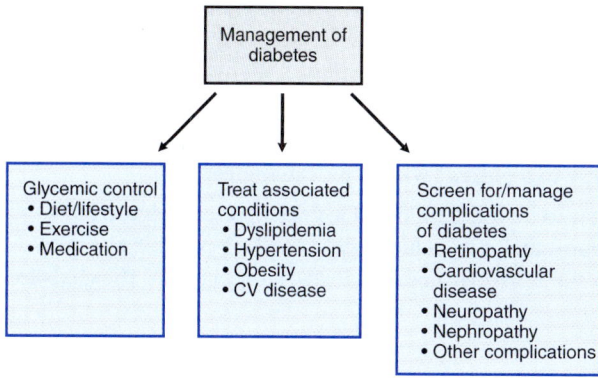

FIGURE 30-4 Components of comprehensive diabetes care.

SECTION V Hormones and Hormone Antagonists

TABLE 30-2 Goals of Therapy in Diabetes

INDEX	GOAL[a]
Glycemic control[b]	
A1C	<7.0%[c]
Preprandial capillary plasma glucose	3.9-7.2 mmol/L (70-130 mg/dL)
Peak postprandial capillary plasma glucose	10.0 mmol/L (<180 mg/dL)[d]
Blood pressure	<130/80
Lipids[e]	
Low-density lipoprotein	<2.6 mmol/L (<100 mg/dL)[f]
High-density lipoprotein	>1.1 mmol/L (>40 mg/dL)[g]
Triglycerides	<1.7 mmol/L (<150 mg/dL)

[a]As recommended by the ADA, goals should be individualized for each patient. Goals may be different for certain patient populations.
[b]A1C is primary goal.
[c]While the ADA recommends an A1C <7.0% in general, in the individual patient it recommends an appropriate goal for the individual patient be based on age, duration of diabetes, life expectancy, other medical conditions, and cardiovascular disease.
[d]One to two hours after beginning of a meal.
[e]In decreasing order of priority.
[f]In individuals with coronary artery disease, an LDL <1.8 mmol (70 mg/dL) is the goal.
[g]For women, some suggest a goal that is 0.25 mmol/L (10 mg/dL) or higher.
Data adapted from *Diabetes Care* 33:S11, 2010.

e. **What are the options with insulin therapy with this patient?**

Insulin preparations are classified according to their duration of action into short-acting and long-acting (see Table 45-3 in *Goodman and Gilman's The Pharmacological Basis of Therapeutics*, 12th Edition). In most patients, insulin-replacement therapy includes long-acting insulin (basal) and short-acting insulin to provide postprandial needs. Most insulin is injected subcutaneously. Short-acting insulins are the only form of the hormone used in subcutaneous infusion pumps.

CASE 30-2

A 53-year-old man is diagnosed with type 2 diabetes. His doctor follows the treatment algorithm for the management of type 2 diabetes as shown in Figure 30-5. The patient's initial A1C is 8.1%. After attempts at weight reduction, increased physical activity, and metformin pharmacotherapy his A1C is 7.8%.

a. **How is the diagnosis of type 2 diabetes made?**

The diagnosis of type 2 diabetes is made using the same criteria as shown in Table 30-1.

b. **What are the goals of therapy in a patient with type 2 diabetes?**

Therapy of type 2 diabetes has to be individualized for each patient. Figure 30-4 shows the components of sound diabetes management and is applicable to type 1 and type 2 diabetes patients. Table 30-2 lists the indexes of therapy and the goals for diabetic patients in general.

(Continued)

Endocrine Pancreas and Pharmacotherapy

CHAPTER 30

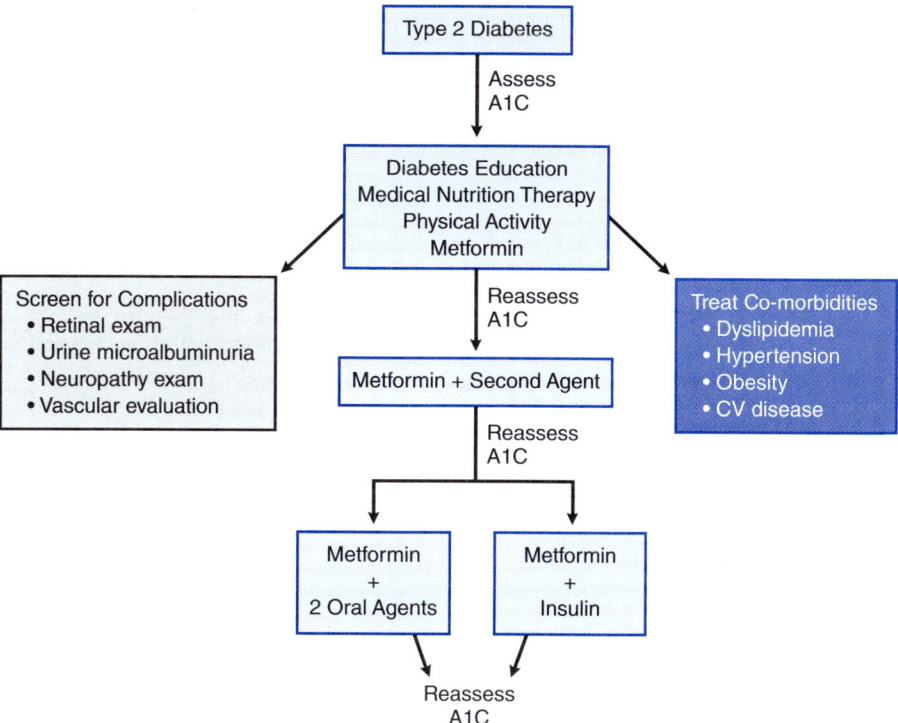

FIGURE 30-5 Treatment algorithm for management of type 2 diabetes mellitus. Patients diagnosed with type 2 diabetes, either by fasting glucose, oral glucose tolerance testing, or A1C, should have diabetes education that includes instruction on medical nutrition therapy and physical activity. Most patients newly diagnosed with type 2 diabetes have had subclinical or undiagnosed diabetes for many years previously and should be evaluated for diabetic complications (retinal examination, test for excess protein or albumin excretion in the urine, and clinical evaluation for peripheral neuropathy and vascular insufficiency); common comorbidities (hypertension and dyslipidemia) should be treated. Metformin is the consensus first line of therapy and should be started at the time of diagnosis. Failure to reach the glycemic target, generally an A1C ≤7% within 3-4 months, should prompt the addition of a second oral agent. Reinforce lifestyle interventions at every visit and check A1C every 3 months. Treatment may escalate to metformin plus 2 oral agents or metformin plus insulin, if necessary.

c. **What are the options to lower his A1C in addition to lifestyle modifications?**

One option that is commonly followed is to add a sulfonylurea drug. Other options include the insulin secretagogues that are nonsulfonylureas or the thiazolidinediones.

d. **What are the untoward effects of sulfonylurea drugs?**

The most severe untoward effect of the sulfonylurea drugs is hypoglycemia. Weight gain is also a common side effect of this class of drugs. Less common effects include nausea, vomiting, cholestatic jaundice, blood dyscrasias, and dermatological reactions.

CASE 30-3

The patient in Case 30-2 has an A1C that is 7.5% after pharmacotherapy with metformin plus a sulfonylurea.

a. **What are the options with this patient?**

The progressive insulin deficiency in type 2 diabetes often makes it increasingly difficult to achieve tight glycemic control solely with oral antihyperglycemic agents (see Figure 30-5). One option would be the addition of a thiazolidinedione drug such as rosiglitazone or pioglitazone. If this does not achieve the desired goal then the addition of insulin is another option.

(Continued)

SECTION V — Hormones and Hormone Antagonists

b. What are the untoward effects of the thiazolidinediones?

The most common side effect of the thiazolidinediones is weight gain and edema. Of greatest concern are the increased incidence of congestive heart failure and the risk of cardiovascular events (myocardial infarction or stroke). Treatment with thiazolidinediones may increase the risk of bone fracture in women.

If this patient already has a risk of cardiovascular disease, a better choice might be to add insulin to his diabetic regimen.

c. What type of insulin should be used?

The different types of insulin are shown in Table 43-5 in *Goodman and Gilman's The Pharmacological Basis of Therapeutics*, 12th Edition. Patients with type 2 diabetes are usually best treated with long-acting insulin such as glargine. Glargine has a sustained peakless absorption profile and provides better once-daily insulin coverage than NPH insulin. Glargine also has a lower risk of hypoglycemia, particularly overnight, compared to NPH insulin.

d. What other agents can be added?

If the addition of basal insulin still does not reach the target A1C, the addition of a glucagon-like peptide-1 (GLP-1) receptor agonist may be beneficial. A GLP-1 agonist such as exenatide or liraglutide stimulates insulin secretion, inhibits glucagon release, delays gastric emptying, reduces food intake, and normalizes fasting and postprandial insulin secretion. An alternative is a dipeptidyl peptidase-4 (DPP-4) inhibitor which results in a rise in the endogenous GLP-1 concentration by inhibiting its plasma clearance.

CASE 30-4

A 49-year-old woman without diabetes is diagnosed with recurring hypoglycemia. This is particularly troublesome because she awakes every morning with a headache.

a. What are the options for treating hypoglycemia?

Two agents are available for the treatment of hypoglycemia: glucagon and diazoxide.

b. What is the mechanism of action of glucagon?

Glucagon is used to treat severe hypoglycemia, particularly in diabetic patients when the patient cannot safely consume oral glucose and intravenous glucose is not available. Glucagon interacts with a GPCR on the plasma membrane of target cells.

c. What is the mechanism of action of diazoxide?

Diazoxide is an antihypertensive with potent hyperglycemic actions when given orally. The hyperglycemic action of diazoxide is primarily through the inhibition of insulin secretion (see Figure 30-2).

KEY CONCEPTS

- Insulin is the primary treatment of type 1 diabetes.
- There are many different types of insulin (see Table 45-3 in *Goodman and Gilman's The Pharmacological Basis of Therapeutics*, 12th Edition), including subcutaneous insulin pumps.
- Short-acting insulin is the only form of the hormone used in insulin pumps.
- Some drugs may promote hyperglycemia or hypoglycemia (see Table 30-3).
- Type 2 diabetes is a complex disease that requires multiple forms of treatment (see Figure 30-5) including diet, exercise, and medications.
- The goals of therapy for type 1 and type 2 diabetes are shown in Table 30-2.
- Insulin is the cornerstone of treatment of hyperglycemia in hospitalized patients.

(Continued)

TABLE 30-3 Some Drugs That May Promote Hyperglycemia or Hypoglycemia

HYPERGLYCEMIA	HYPOGLYCEMIA
Glucocorticoids	β Adrenergic antagonists
Antipsychotics (atypical, others)	Ethanol
Protease inhibitors	Salicylates
β Adrenergic agonists	Non-steroidal anti-inflammatory drugs
Diuretics (thiazide, loop)	Pentamidine
Hydantoins (phenytoin, others)	ACE inhibitors
Opioids (fentanyl, morphine, others)	Lithium chloride
Diazoxide	Theophylline
Nicotinic Acid	Bromocriptine
Pentamidine	Mebendazole
Epinephrine	
Interferons	
Amphotericin B	
Asparaginase	
Acamprosate	
Basiliximab	
Thyroid hormones	

➡ Metformin is the consensus first line of therapy for type 2 diabetes and should be started at the time of diagnosis.

➡ The most common and serious adverse effect of diabetes therapy is hypoglycemia. The more vigorous the attempt to achieve euglycemia, the more frequent are episodes of hypoglycemia.

SUMMARY QUIZ

QUESTION 30-1 A 45-year-old woman with type 2 diabetes is noticing an increase in her basal insulin dose needed to achieve the same effect. This is likely because of

a. increased insulin secretion.
b. insulin resistance in target tissues.
c. improper formulation of her insulin.
d. increased glucagon secretion.
e. increased consumption of carbohydrates.

QUESTION 30-2 A 69-year-old man with type 2 diabetes is hospitalized because of a knee replacement. His blood sugar postsurgery is 215 mg/dL. His hyperglycemia is best managed in the hospital by

a. increasing his metformin dose.
b. increasing his sulfonylurea dose.
c. adding a GLP-1 agent.
d. decreasing his food intake.
e. subcutaneous or intravenous insulin.

QUESTION 30-3 A 56-year-old woman with type 2 diabetes is being treated with metformin and glimepiride. These two drugs act synergistically because glimepiride

a. decreases the clearance of metformin.
b. acts to increase glycogen stores in the liver.
c. stimulates insulin release by binding to a specific site on β cells.
d. increases the activity of AMP-dependent protein kinase (AMPK).
e. decreases glucose reabsorption in the kidney.

SECTION V
Hormones and Hormone Antagonists

QUESTION 30-4 In the patient in Question 30-3, the metformin and glimepiride act synergistically because metformin

a. decreases the clearance of glimepiride.
b. acts to decrease glycogen stores in the liver.
c. stimulates insulin release by binding to a specific site on β cells.
d. increases the activity of AMP-dependent protein kinase (AMPK).
e. decreases glucose reabsorption in the kidney.

QUESTION 30-5 A 48-year-old man with type 2 diabetes is treated with glargine insulin once daily and lispro insulin with each meal. The main clinical difference in these 2 types of insulin is in their

a. effective duration of action.
b. the way they are administered.
c. storage.
d. metabolism by the liver.
e. penetration into the central nervous system.

QUESTION 30-6 The patient in Question 30-3 has developed onychomycosis and she is now being treated with fluconazole. She is at increased risk of hypoglycemia because fluconazole can

a. decrease the hepatic metabolism of metformin.
b. decrease the hepatic metabolism of glimepiride.
c. increase glucose uptake by skeletal muscle.
d. inhibit insulin secretion.
e. inhibit the action of glucagon.

SUMMARY QUIZ ANSWER KEY

QUESTION 30-1 Answer is **b**. Insulin sensitivity is a quantifiable parameter that is measured as the amount of glucose cleared from the blood in response to a dose of insulin. The failure of normal amounts of insulin to elicit the expected response is referred to as insulin resistance. The major insulin-responsive tissues are skeletal muscle, fat, and liver. Insulin resistance in muscle and fat is generally marked by a decrease in the transport of glucose from the circulation.

QUESTION 30-2 Answer is **e**. Insulin is the cornerstone of treatment of hyperglycemia in hospitalized patients. Intravenous insulin is the treatment of choice, but in patients who are more stable, subcutaneous insulin regimens using a combination of basal and prandial insulin is the standard.

QUESTION 30-3 Answer is **c**. Sulfonylureas such as glimepiride stimulate insulin release by binding to a specific site on the β cell K_{ATP} channel complex (the sulfonylurea receptor, SUR) and inhibiting its activity (see Figure 30-2).

QUESTION 30-4 Answer is **d**. Metformin increases the activity of the AMP-dependent protein kinase (AMPK). Activated AMPK stimulates fatty acid oxidation, glucose uptake and nonoxidative metabolism, and reduced lipogenesis and gluconeogenesis. The net result is increased glycogen storage in skeletal muscle, lower rates of hepatic glucose production, increased insulin sensitivity, and lower blood glucose concentrations.

QUESTION 30-5 Answer is **a**. See Table 45-3 in *Goodman and Gilman's The Pharmacological Basis of Therapeutics*, 12th Edition. The major clinical difference between glargine and lispro insulin is in their effective duration of action.

Endocrine Pancreas and Pharmacotherapy — CHAPTER 30

QUESTION 30-6 Answer is **b**. Hypoglycemia may be more frequent in patients taking a sulfonylurea and also taking an azole antifungal agent. Glimepiride is metabolized by CYP2C9, which is inhibited by fluconazole.

SUMMARY: DRUGS USED TO TREAT DIABETES MELLITUS AND HYPOGLYCEMIA

CLASS AND SUBCLASSES	NAMES	CLINICAL USES	TOXICITIES COMMON	TOXICITIES UNIQUE; CLINICALLY IMPORTANT
Insulin	Insulin	Treatment of type 1 and type 2 diabetes		Hypoglycemia Atrophy of subcutaneous fat Lipohypertrophy
Biguanides	Metformin	First-line treatment of type 2 diabetes	Nausea, diarrhea, indigestion, and abdominal pain	Lower blood concentrations of vitamin B_{12} Lactic acidosis
Insulin Secretagogues—Sulfonylureas	Glyburide Glipizide Gliclazide Glimepiride	Treatment of type 2 diabetes	Weight gain Nausea and vomiting	Hypoglycemia, cholestatic jaundice, agranulocytosis, aplastic anemia, hemolytic anemia, generalized hypersensitivity reactions, and dermatological reactions Ethanol may enhance the action of sulfonylureas and cause hypoglycemia Drug interactions with many drugs including azole antifungal agents and histamine H_2 antagonists
Insulin Secretagogues—Nonsulfonylureas	Repaglinide Nateglinide	Treatment of type 2 diabetes		Hypoglycemia Metabolized by liver and should be used cautiously in patients with hepatic insufficiency
Thiazolidinediones	Rosiglitazone Pioglitazone	Treatment of type 2 diabetes	Weight gain and edema	Increased incidence of congestive heart failure Rosiglitazone, but not pioglitazone may increase the risk of myocardial infarction and stroke Thiazolidinediones increase the risk of bone fracture in women
GLP-1 Agonists	Exenatide Liraglutide	Treatment of type 2 diabetes	Nausea and vomiting	Hypoglycemia is rare
Dipeptidyl Peptidase-4 (DPP-4) Inhibitors	Sitagliptin Saxagliptin Vidagliptin Alogliptin	Treatment of type 2 diabetes		Saxagliptin is metabolized by CYP3A4 and dose should be adjusted when coadministered with drugs that inhibit this enzyme
α-Glucosidase Inhibitors	Acarbose Miglitol Voglibose	Adjuncts to diet and exercise in type 2 diabetic patients not reaching glycemic targets	Malabsorption, flatulence, diarrhea, and abdominal bloating	Hypoglycemia when added to insulin or an insulin secretagogue Acarbose can decrease absorption of digoxin Miglitol can decrease the absorption of propranolol and ranitidine
Amylin Antagonists	Pramlintide	Used as an adjunct in patients with type 1 or type 2 diabetes who take insulin with meals	Nausea	Hypoglycemia Pregnancy category C May alter the pharmacokinetics of drugs that require GI absorption because of delayed gastric emptying
Bile Acid Sequestrants	Colesevelam	Treatment of hypercholesterolemia (see Chapter 20); may be used as an adjunct to diet and exercise to treat patients with type 2 diabetes	Constipation, dyspepsia, abdominal pain, and nausea	Interferes with the absorption of many commonly used drugs; most medications should be given 4 hours before colesevelam
Agents Used to Treat Hypoglycemia	Glucagon	Used to treat severe hypoglycemia		
	Diazoxide	Antihypertensive drug used to treat patients with chronic or recurring hypoglycemia		Sodium retention, edema, hyperuricemia, hypertrichosis, thrombocytopenia, and leukopenia

CHAPTER 31

Drug Therapy of Mineral Ion Homeostasis and Bone Turnover Disorders

DRUGS INCLUDED IN THIS CHAPTER

- 1α-hydroxycholecalciferol (1-OHD, alphacalcidol, ONE-ALPHA)
- 22-Oxacalcitrol (1,25-dihydroxy-22-oxavitamin D_3, OCT, maxacalcitol, OXAROL)
- Alendronate (FOSAMAX)
- Calcipotriene (DOVONEX, others)
- Calcitonin (CALCIMAR, MIACALCIN)
- Calcitriol (1,25-dihydroxycholecalciferol; CALCIJEX, ROCALTROL)
- Calcium salts
- Cinacalcet (SENSIPAR)
- Denosumab (investigational)
- Dihydrotachysterol (DHT, ROXANE)
- Doxercalciferol (1α-hydroxyvitamin D_2, HECTOROL)
- Ergocalciferol (calciferol, DRISDOL)
- Etidronate sodium (DIDRONEL)
- Ibandronate (BONIVA)
- Lanthanum carbonate (FOSRENOL)
- Pamidronate (AREDIA)
- Paricalcitol (1,25-dihydroxy-19-norvitamin D_2, ZEMPLAR)
- Plicamycin (MITHRACIN)
- Risedronate (ACTONEL)
- Sevelamer hydrochloride (RENAGEL)
- Teriparatide (FORTEO)
- Tiludronate (SKELID)
- Zoledronate (ZOMETA)

This chapter will be most useful after having a basic understanding of the material in Chapter 44, Agents Affecting Mineral Ion Homeostasis and Bone Turnover in *Goodman & Gilman's The Pharmacological Basis of Therapeutics*, 12th Edition. In addition to the material presented here, the 12th Edition contains:

- A detailed discussion of the physiology of mineral ion homeostasis
- A description of the hormonal regulation of calcium and phosphorous homeostasis
- A discussion of bone physiology
- A detailed discussion of the pharmacological treatment of disorders of mineral ion homeostasis and bone metabolism, including the therapeutic uses of vitamin D, calcitonin, bisphosphonates, parathyroid hormone (PTH), and calcium sensor mimetics
- A description of an integrated approach to the prevention and treatment of osteoporosis

LEARNING OBJECTIVES

- ☑ Understand calcium and phosphorous homeostasis.
- ☑ Describe the roles of PTH, calcitonin, and vitamin D in calcium homeostasis.
- ☑ Understand the concept of bone resorption and bone formation.
- ☑ Describe the mechanism of action and untoward effects of bisphosphonates.
- ☑ Describe the role of bisphosphonates in the prevention and treatment of osteoporosis.
- ☑ Describe the pharmacological management of hypocalcemia and hypercalcemia.

MECHANISMS OF ACTION OF DRUGS USED IN MINERAL HOMEOSTASIS AND BONE TURNOVER DISORDERS

DRUG CLASS	DRUGS	MECHANISM OF ACTION
Hormones	Calcitonin Teriparatide	Calcitonin actions are mediated by the calcitonin receptor (CTR), which is a member of the parathyroid PTH/secretin subfamily of GPCRs; the hypocalcemic and hypophosphatemic effects of calcitonin are caused by direct inhibition of osteoclastic bone resorption Teriparatide is a synthetic PTH fragment (1-34); intermittant exposure to PTH promotes anabolic actions on bone and is the basis for teriparatide's use in treating severe osteoporosis

(Continued)

Drug Therapy of Mineral Ion Homeostasis and Bone Turnover Disorders

CHAPTER 31

DRUG CLASS	DRUGS	MECHANISM OF ACTION
Vitamin D and Vitamin D Analogs	Calcitriol (biologically active metabolite of Vitamin D); (see Figure 31-1) Doxercalciferol Dihydrotachysterol 1α-Hydroxycholecalciferol Ergocalciferol Calcipotriene Paricalcitol 22-Oxacalcitrol	Actions of vitamin D and analogs are mediated by the vitamin D receptor (VDR), a nuclear receptor; calcitriol and other drugs in this class act to maintain normal calcium and phosphate in plasma by facilitating their absorption in the small intestine, by interacting with PTH to enhance their mobilization from bone, and by decreasing their renal excretion
Phosphate Binders	Sevelamer hydrochloride Lanthanum carbonate	Sevelamer is a nonabsorbable phosphate-binding polymer Lanthanum is a poorly permeable trivalent cation that binds phosphate
Bisphosphonates	Etidronate sodium Pamidronate Tiludronate Alendronate Risedronate Zoledronate Ibandronate	The bisphosphonates directly inhibit bone resorption by either osteoclast apoptosis (etidronate, pamidronate, tiludronate, risedronate, and zoledronate) or by inhibition of components of the cholesterol biosynthetic pathway that activate proteins important for osteoclast function (alendronate and ibandronate)
Calcium Sensor Mimetic ("calcimimetic")	Cinacalcet	Mimic the stimulatory effect of calcium on the calcium-sensing receptor (CaSR) to inhibit PTH secretion by the parathyroid glands; by enhancing the sensitivity of the CaSR to extracellular calcium, calcimimetics lower the concentration of calcium at which PTH secretion is suppressed
Monoclonal Antibody	Denosumab (investigational)	Blocks osteoclast formation and activation by binding with high affinity to RANKL and thereby reducing the binding of RANKL to RANK; see Figures 31-2 and 31-3 for details
Miscellaneous	Plicamycin (no longer available)	Plicamycin is a cytotoxic antibiotic that also decreases plasma Ca^{++} concentrations by inhibiting bone resorption

THERAPEUTIC USES OF VITAMIN D

- Prophylaxis and cure of nutritional rickets
- Treatment of metabolic rickets and osteomalacia, particularly in the setting of chronic renal failure
- Treatment of hypoparathyroidism
- Prevention and treatment of osteoporosis

SECTION V   Hormones and Hormone Antagonists

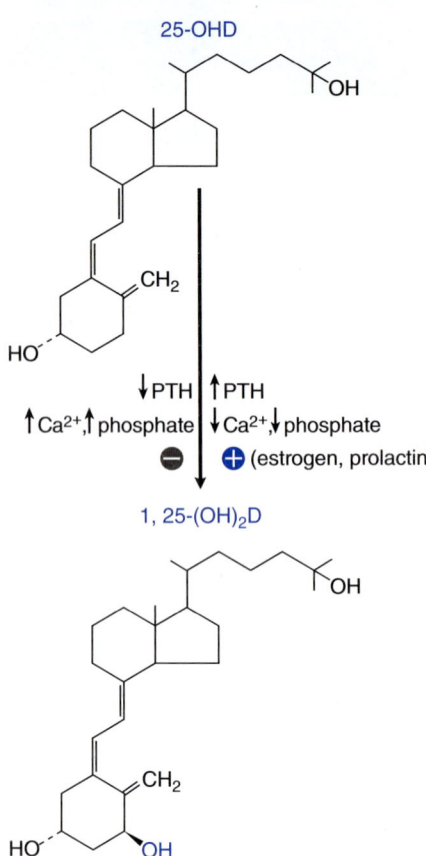

FIGURE 31-1 Regulation of 1α-hydroxylase activity. Changes in the plasma levels of PTH, Ca^{2+}, and phosphate modulate the hydroxylation of 25-OH vitamin D to the active form, 1,25-dihydroxyvitamin D. 25-OHD, 25-hydroxycholecalciferol; 1,25-$(OH)_2$-D, calcitriol; PTH, parathyroid hormone.

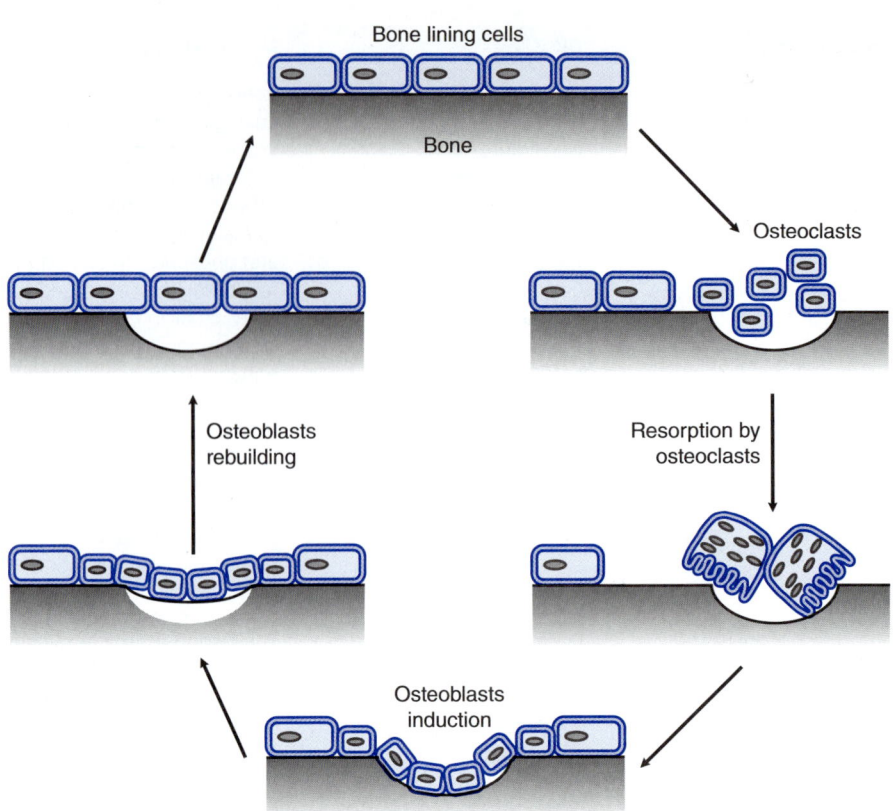

FIGURE 31-2 The bone remodeling cycle. Osteoclast precursors fuse and are activated to resorb a lacuna in a previously quiescent surface. These cells are replaced by osteoblasts that deposit new bone to restore the integrity of the tissue. *(Adapted with permission from Skerry TM, Gowen M. Bone cells and bone in remodelling in rheumatoid arthritis. In: Henderson B, Edwards JCW, Pettipher ER, eds. Mechanisms and Models in Rheumatoid Arthritis. London: Academic Press; 1995, pp 205-220.)*

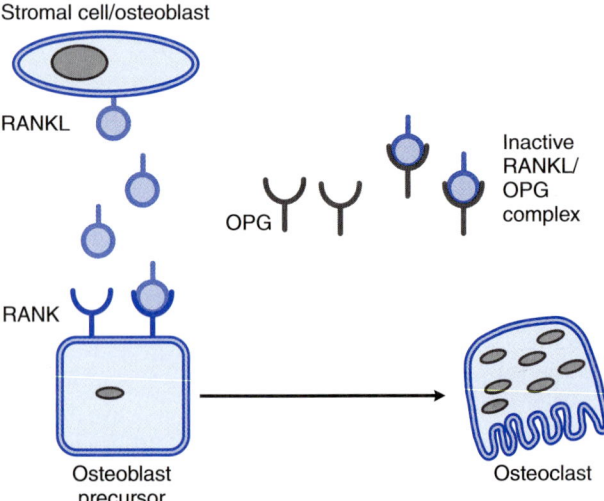

FIGURE 31-3 Receptor for activating NF-κB ligand (RANKL) and osteoclast formation. RANKL, acting on RANK, promotes osteoclast formation and subsequent resorption of bone matrix. Osteoprotegerin (OPG) binds to RANKL, reducing its binding to RANK and thereby inhibiting osteoclast differentiation.

Drug Therapy of Mineral Ion Homeostasis and Bone Turnover Disorders

CHAPTER 31

CASE 31-1

A 56-year-old man with a diagnosis of lung cancer is hospitalized because of lethargy, weakness, and polyuria. His serum calcium is 13 mg/dL.

a. Why is his serum calcium elevated?

Newly diagnosed hypercalcemia in hospitalized patients is most often caused by systemic malignancy, either with or without bone metastasis. PTH-related protein (PTHrP) is a primitive, highly conserved protein that may be abnormally expressed in malignant tissue, particularly in squamous cell and other epithelial cancers. Other tumors release cytokines or prostaglandins that stimulate bone resorption.

b. How does PTH cause hypercalcemia?

The primary function of PTH is to maintain a constant concentration of calcium and phosphorous in the extracellular fluid. The principal processes regulated are renal calcium and phosphorous absorption and mobilization of bone calcium (Figure 31-4). The actions of PTH on target tissues are mediated by at least 2 receptors: the PTH_1 receptor which binds both PTH and PTHrP; and the PTH_2 receptor found in vascular tissue, brain, pancreas, and placenta which binds only PTH.

c. What are the treatment options for this patient?

Calcitonin may be useful in managing hypercalcemia. Reduction in serum calcium can be rapid, although "escape" from the hormone commonly occurs within several days.

Intravenous bisphosphonates (pamidronate and zoledronate) have proven very effective in the management of hypercalcemia. They act by inhibiting bone resorption (see Case 31-3).

(Continued)

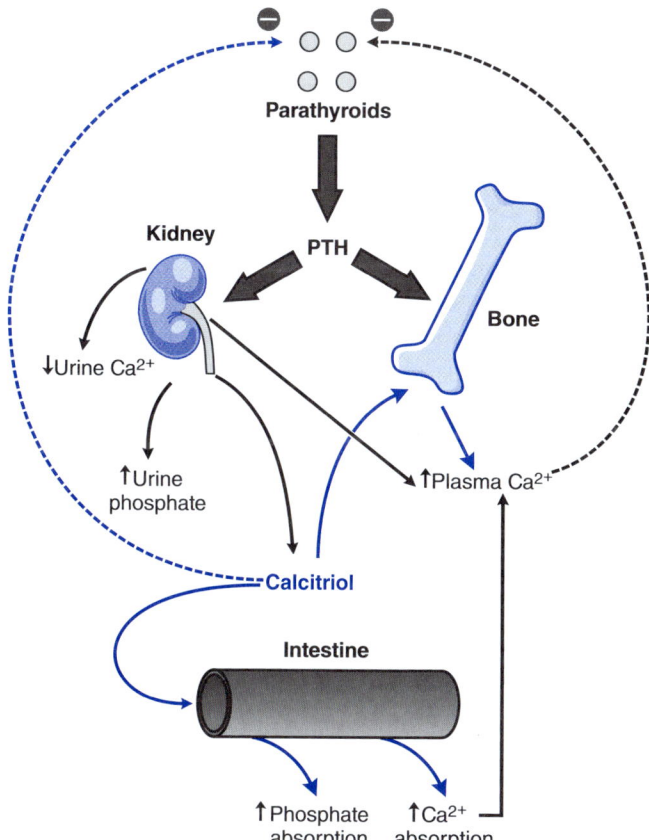

FIGURE 31-4 Calcium homeostasis and its regulation by parathyroid hormone (PTH) and 1,25-dihydroxyvitamin D. PTH has stimulatory effects on bone and kidney, including the stimulation of 1α-hydroxylase activity in kidney mitochondria leading to the increased production of 1,25-dihydroxyvitamin D (calcitriol) from 25-hydroxycholecalciferol, the monohydroxylated vitamin D metabolite. Calcitriol is the biologically active metabolite of vitamin D.

d. What is the mechanism of action of calcitonin?

Calcitonin actions are mediated by the calcitonin receptor (CTR). The hypocalcemic and hypophosphatemic effects of calcitonin are caused predominantly by direct inhibition of osteoclastic bone resorption.

CASE 31-2

A 42-year-old man with chronic renal disease is showing signs of decreased bone density. This was first diagnosed as osteomalacia, but later the diagnosis was changed to renal osteodystrophy.

a. What are osteomalacia and renal osteodystrophy?

Patients with chronic renal disease are at risk for developing osteomalacia (under-mineralization of bone matrix), which occurs commonly during sustained phosphate depletion. Patients with chronic renal disease are also at risk for developing a complex bone disease called renal osteodystrophy. In this setting, bone metabolism is stimulated by an increase in PTH and by a delay in bone mineralization that is due to decreased renal synthesis of calcitriol. In renal osteodystrophy, low bone mineral density (BMD) may accompany high-turnover bone lesions typically seen in patients with uncontrolled hyperparathyroidism. In another form of the disease, low mineral density is accompanied by low bone remodeling activity seen in patients with adynamic bone disease.

b. What is the role of phosphate binders in managing renal osteodystrophy?

The therapeutic approach to the patient with renal osteodystrophy of the high-turnover disease with deficient mineralization is dietary phosphate restriction, generally in combination with a phosphate binder. Highly effective phosphate binders have been developed. Sevelamer is a nonabsorbable phosphate-binding polymer that effectively lowers the serum phosphate concentration, with a corresponding reduction in the calcium × phosphate product. Lanthanum carbonate is a poorly permeable trivalent cation that is useful in treating the hyperphosphatemia associated with renal osteodystrophy.

c. What is the role of vitamin D in the management of renal osteodystrophy?

Renal osteodystrophy associated with low bone turnover is increasingly common and may be due to oversuppression of PTH with aggressive use of either calcitriol or other vitamin D analog. Current guidelines suggest that treatment with an active vitamin D preparation (see Figure 31-1) is indicated if serum 25-hydroxy vitamin D (25-OHD) levels are less than 30 ng/mL and serum calcium is less than 9.5 mg/dL. However, if 25-OHD and serum calcium levels are elevated, vitamin D supplementation should be discontinued. If the serum calcium is less than 9.5 mg/dL, treatment with a vitamin D analog is warranted irrespective of the 25-OHD level.

CASE 31-3

A 55-year-old woman is concerned because her mother and sister developed fractures in their legs and vertebra after menopause. She wants to know what osteoporosis is and if she is susceptible when she has never had a broken bone. She is also asking for a medication and other advice that will prevent osteoporosis. She wants to know if taking only a calcium supplement will prevent her from having fractures.

a. How is bone physiology involved in the development of osteoporosis?

Osteoporosis is a condition of low bone mass and microarchitectural disruption that results in fractures with minimal trauma. Osteoporosis can be categorized as primary or secondary. Primary osteoporosis represents 2 fundamentally different conditions: type I osteoporosis is characterized by loss of trabecular bone owing to estrogen lack at menopause, and type II osteoporosis is characterized by loss of cortical and trabecular bone in men and women due to long-term remodeling inefficiency, dietary inadequacy, and activation of the parathyroid axis with age. Secondary osteoporosis is due to systemic illness or medications such as glucocorticoids.

(Continued)

Drug Therapy of Mineral Ion Homeostasis and Bone Turnover Disorders

CHAPTER 31

Growth and development of endochondral bone are driven by a process called modeling. Once new bone is laid down, it is subjected to a continuous process of breakdown and renewal called remodeling by which bone mass is adjusted throughout adult life (see Figures 31-2 and 31-3). In women, loss of estrogen at menopause accelerates the rate of bone loss. Primary regulators of adult bone mass include physical activity, reproductive endocrine status, and calcium intake. Optimal maintenance of BMD requires sufficiency in all 3 areas, and deficiency of one is not compensated by excessive attention to another. Thus, taking only a calcium supplement is not sufficient to maintain BMD.

b. **This patient is started on ibandronate, a bisphosphonate. What are bisphosphonates and how are they used in the prevention and treatment of osteoporosis?**

Pharmacological treatment for the prevention and treatment of osteoporosis is aimed at restoring bone strength and preventing fractures. Bisphosphonates are the most frequently used drugs for the prevention and treatment of osteoporosis. Bisphosphonates concentrate at sites of active bone remodeling. Because they are highly charged, bisphosphonates are membrane impermeable but are incorporated into the bone matrix by fluid-phase endocytosis. The antiresorptive activity involves 2 primary mechanisms: (1) osteoclast apoptosis and (2) inhibition of components of the cholesterol biosynthetic pathway. The first-generation bisphosphonates, medronate, etidronate, clodronate, and tiludronate act by the first mechanism, whereas the second-generation bisphosphonates, pamidrone, alendronate, ibandronate, risedronate, and zoledronate act by the latter mechanism.

c. **What are the untoward effects of bisphosphonates?**

Oral bisphosphonates can cause heartburn, esophageal irritation, or esophagitis. These symptoms often abate when patients take the medication after an overnight fast, with tap water, and remain upright.

Serious osteonecrosis of the jaw is associated with the use of bisphosphonates.

Zoledronate has a profound effect on calcium and is capable of causing hypocalcemia. It has also been associated with decreased renal function. Patients should have laboratory tests for renal function prior to its use and renal function should be monitored periodically after treatment.

d. **What are other options for this patient?**

Teriparatide, a PTH fragment, is available to use in treating severe osteoporosis. In postmenopausal women with osteoporosis, teriparatide increases BMD and reduces the risk of vertebral and nonvertebral fractures. Candidates for teriparatide treatment include women who have a history of osteoporotic fracture, who have multiple risk factors for fracture, or who failed or are intolerant of previous osteoporosis therapy.

In animal studies, teriparatide has been associated with the development of osteosarcoma.

KEY CONCEPTS

➡ The steady-state content of calcium in bone reflects the net effect of bone resorption and bone formation.

➡ PTH is a polypeptide hormone that helps regulate plasma calcium by affecting bone resorption/formation, renal calcium excretion/reabsorption, and calcitriol synthesis (thus GI calcium absorption).

➡ The primary active metabolite of vitamin D is 1,25-hydroxyvitamin D. The enzyme system responsible for the 1α-hydroxylation of 25-hydroxyvitamin D (25-OHD) is located in the proximal tubules of the kidney.

➡ Calcitonin is a hypocalcemic hormone produced and secreted by the thyroid parafollicular C cells. The actions of calcitonin generally oppose those of PTH.

(Continued)

SECTION V — Hormones and Hormone Antagonists

- In women, loss of estrogen at menopause accelerates the rate of bone loss (see Figures 31-2 and 31-3).
- Patients with chronic renal disease are at risk for developing osteomalacia or a complex bone disease called renal osteodystrophy.
- Osteoporosis is a condition of low bone mass and microarchitectural disruption that results in fractures with minimal trauma.
- Bisphosphonates are the most frequently used drugs for the prevention and treatment of osteoporosis.
- Bisphosphonates are associated with severe untoward effects such as esophageal distress and osteonecrosis of the jaw.
- Teriparatide is a PTH fragment used for the treatment of severe osteoporosis.

SUMMARY QUIZ

QUESTION 31-1 A 43-year-old man with intestinal bypass surgery is at risk of developing a deficiency of

a. vitamin D.
b. calcium.
c. phosphorous.
d. vitamin C.
e. parathyroid hormone.

QUESTION 31-2 25-hydroxyvitamin D (25-OHD) is converted to its active form 1,25-OHD by the enzyme 1α-hydroxylase in the proximal renal tubules. 1α-hydroxylase is activated by a dietary deficiency of

a. potassium.
b. iron.
c. calcium.
d. zinc.
e. sodium.

QUESTION 31-3 Calcitonin is a hormone produced and secreted from the thyroid parafollicular C cells and is regulated by the serum concentration of

a. potassium.
b. calcium.
c. zinc.
d. iron.
e. sodium.

QUESTION 31-4 A 42-year-old man with lung cancer had a serum calcium measurement 1 month ago that was 9.0 mg/dL. He is hospitalized now with severe muscle weakness, fatigue, anorexia, and constipation. His serum calcium is 13.5 mg/dL. The severity of his symptoms is due to the

a. rate of rise in his serum calcium.
b. decrease in the intestinal excretion of calcium.
c. malabsorption of vitamin D.
d. formation of a parathyroid adenoma.
e. ingestion of large quantities of calcium.

Drug Therapy of Mineral Ion Homeostasis and Bone Turnover Disorders

CHAPTER 31

QUESTION 31-5 A 35-year-old woman with a parathyroid adenoma is being treated with cinacalcet, a calcium sensor mimetic. The principal adverse event with this drug is

a. hyperphosphatemia.
b. hypercalcemia.
c. hypervitaminosis D.
d. decreased vitamin D absorption.
e. hypocalcemia.

QUESTION 31-6 A 55-year-old woman is treated with a bisphosphonate drug to prevent osteoporosis during postmenopause. She should be cautioned about which of the following adverse events?

a. Congestive heart failure.
b. Tinnitus.
c. Macular degeneration.
d. Esophagitis.
e. Peripheral neuropathy.

SUMMARY QUIZ ANSWER KEY

QUESTION 31-1 Answer is **a.** Bile is essential for the absorption of vitamin D. Patients who have intestinal bypass surgery or otherwise have severe shortening or inflammation of the small intestine may fail to absorb vitamin D sufficiently to maintain normal levels.

QUESTION 31-2 Answer is **c.** See Figure 31-1. Vitamin D 1α-hydroxylase is subject to tight regulatory control that results in changes in calcitriol formation appropriate for optimal calcium homeostasis. Dietary deficiency of vitamin D, calcium, or phosphate enhances enzyme activity. Conversely high calcium, phosphate, or vitamin D intake suppresses enzyme activity.

QUESTION 31-3 Answer is **b.** The biosynthesis and secretion of calcitonin are regulated by the serum calcium concentration. Calcitonin secretion increases when serum calcium is high and decreases when serum calcium is low.

QUESTION 31-4 Answer is **a.** The degree of hypercalcemia and the rate of rise in serum calcium concentration largely dictate the extent of symptoms. Chronic elevation of serum calcium to 12 to 14 mg/dL generally causes few manifestations, whereas an acute rise to the same levels may cause marked neuromuscular manifestations owing to an increased threshold for excitation of nerve and muscle. The ingestion of large quantities of calcium by itself generally does not cause hypercalcemia; an exception is the hyperthyroid patient who absorbs calcium with increased efficiency.

QUESTION 31-5 Answer is **e.** Calcimimetics are drugs that mimic the stimulatory effect of calcium on the calcium-sensing receptor (CaSR) to inhibit PTH secretion by the parathyroid glands. The principal adverse event with calcimimetics is hypocalcemia.

QUESTION 31-6 Answer is **d.** Oral bisphosphonates can cause heartburn, esophageal irritation, or esophagitis (see Case 31-3). For patients in whom oral bisphosphonates cause severe esophageal distress despite counter measures, intravenous zoledronate or ibandronate offers skeletal protection without causing adverse GI effects.

SECTION V

Hormones and Hormone Antagonists

SUMMARY: DRUGS USED IN MINERAL HOMEOSTASIS AND BONE TURNOVER DISORDERS

CLASS AND SUBCLASSES	NAMES	CLINICAL USES	TOXICITIES — COMMON	TOXICITIES — UNIQUE; CLINICALLY IMPORTANT
Hormones	Calcitonin Teriparatide	Calcitonin is useful in managing hypercalcemia; it is also effective in patients with Paget disease and in some patients with osteoporosis Teriparatide is used to treat severe osteoporosis	Side effects of calcitonin are nausea, hand swelling, urticaria, and rarely intestinal cramping	Calcitonin is effective for the initial 6 hours but due to receptor downregulation, patients become refractory after a few days Teriparatide has been associated with osteosarcoma in animals Use of teriparatide should be limited to 2 years
Vitamin D and Vitamin D Analogs	Calcitriol Doxercalciferol Dihydrotachysterol 1α-Hydroxycholecalciferol Ergocalciferol Calcipotriene Paricalcitol 22-Oxacalcitrol	Therapeutic uses of vitamin D are shown in the Side Bar THERAPEUTIC USES OF VITAMIN D Calcipotriene is used as a topical preparation to treat psoriasis		Hypercalcemia with or without hyperphosphatemia Paricalcitol, and 22-oxacalcitrol reduce serum PTH but have less or negligible hypercalcemic activity
Phosphate Binders	Sevelamer hydrochloride Lanthanum carbonate	Sevelamer is useful in treating hyperphosphatemia in hemodialysis patients Lanthanum is useful in treating hyperphosphatemia in patients with renal osteodystrophy	Side effects of sevelamer include nausea, vomiting, diarrhea, and dyspepsia	
Bisphosphonates	Etidronate sodium Pamidronate Tiludronate Alendronate Risedronate Zoledronate Ibandronate	Treatment of Paget disease Ibandronate is approved for the prevention and treatment of postmenopausal osteoporosis Pamidronate and zoledronate are useful in treating hypercalcemia associated with malignancy	Heartburn, esophageal irritation esophagitis, abdominal pain, and diarrhea	Osteonecrosis of the jaw Parenteral infusion of pamidronate may cause flushing, flu-like symptoms, nausea and vomiting Zoledronate is capable of causing severe hypocalcemia
Calcium Sensor Mimetic ("calcimimetic")	Cinacalcet	Approved for the treatment of secondary hyperparathyroidism due to chronic renal disease		Hypocalcemia Metabolized by CYP3A4, 2D6, and 1A2; coadministration of inhibitors of these enzymes should be cautioned
Monoclonal Antibody	Denosumab (investigational)	Proposed to treat osteoporosis		

Drugs Affecting Gastrointestinal Function

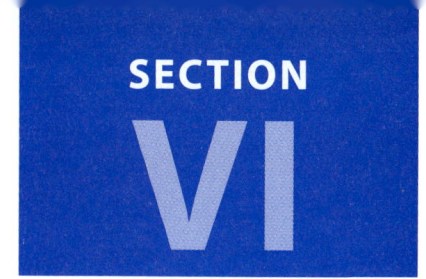

32. Pharmacotherapy of Gastric Acidity, Peptic Ulcers, and Gastroesophageal Reflux Disease 490

33. Drugs Used for the Treatment of Bowel Disorders 497

CHAPTER 32
Pharmacotherapy of Gastric Acidity, Peptic Ulcers, and Gastroesophageal Reflux Disease

DRUGS INCLUDED IN THIS CHAPTER
Cimetidine (TAGAMET, others)
Dexlansoprazole (KAPIDEX)
Esomeprazole (NEXIUM)
Famotidine (PEPSID, others)
Lansoprazole (PREVACID)
Misoprostol (CYTOTEC)
Nizatidine (AXID, others)
Omeprazole (PRILOSEC, others)
Pantoprazole (PROTONIX)
Rabeprazole (ACIPHEX)
Ranitidine (ZANTEC, others)
Sucralfate (CARAFATE, others)

This chapter will be most useful after having a basic understanding of the material in Chapter 45, Pharmacotherapy of Gastric Acidity, Peptic Ulcers, and Gastroesophageal Reflux Disease in *Goodman & Gilman's The Pharmacological Basis of Therapeutics*, 12th Edition. In addition to the material presented here, the 12th Edition contains:

- A description of the physiology of gastric secretion
- Therapeutic strategies for the treatment of specific acid-peptic disorders
- Table 45-2 which shows the composition and acid neutralizing capacities of popular antacid preparations

LEARNING OBJECTIVES

- ☑ Identify the sites in the gastric parietal cell where drugs act to suppress acid secretion.
- ☑ Describe the mechanism of action of proton pump inhibitors, H_2 receptor antagonists, and prostaglandin analogs to suppress gastric acid secretion.
- ☑ Describe the limitations to the use of H_2 receptor antagonists in chronic acid suppression.
- ☑ Identify potential drug interactions with proton pump inhibitors and H_2 receptor antagonists.
- ☑ Describe the mechanism of action of drugs that enhance gastric cytoprotection.
- ☑ Describe the recommendations for therapy of gastroesophageal reflux disease (GERD) and peptic ulcer disease.
- ☑ Understand the role of *Helicobacter pylori* infection in peptic ulcer disease and the therapeutic principles for its eradication.
- ☑ Describe appropriate therapy for NSAID-induced ulcers.

MECHANISMS OF ACTION OF DRUGS USED TO TREAT GASTRIC ACID DISEASES

DRUG CLASS	DRUGS	MECHANISM OF ACTION
H_2 Receptor Antagonists	Cimetidine Ranitidine Famotidine Nizatidine	Competes with histamine for binding to H_2 receptors on the basolateral membrane of parietal cells (see Figure 32-1)
Proton Pump Inhibitors	Lansoprazole Pantoprazole Omeprazole Esomeprazole Dexlansoprazole Rabeprazole	The activated form binds covalently with sulfhydryl groups on cysteine in the H^+,K^+-ATPase located on the luminal membrane of the parietal cell to suppress acid secretion (see Figure 32-1)
Prostaglandin Analog	Misoprostol	Binds to the EP_3 receptor on parietal cells decreasing cyclic AMP and gastric acid secretion (see Figure 32-1)
Cytoprotective Agent	Sucralfate	Forms a viscous, sticky polymer that adheres to epithelial cells and ulcer craters and is cytoprotective
Antacids	Various over-the-counter (OTC) products	Neutralize gastric acid
Bismuth	Various OTC products	Binds to the base of ulcers and promotes mucin and bicarbonate production

Pharmacotherapy of Gastric Acidity

CHAPTER 32

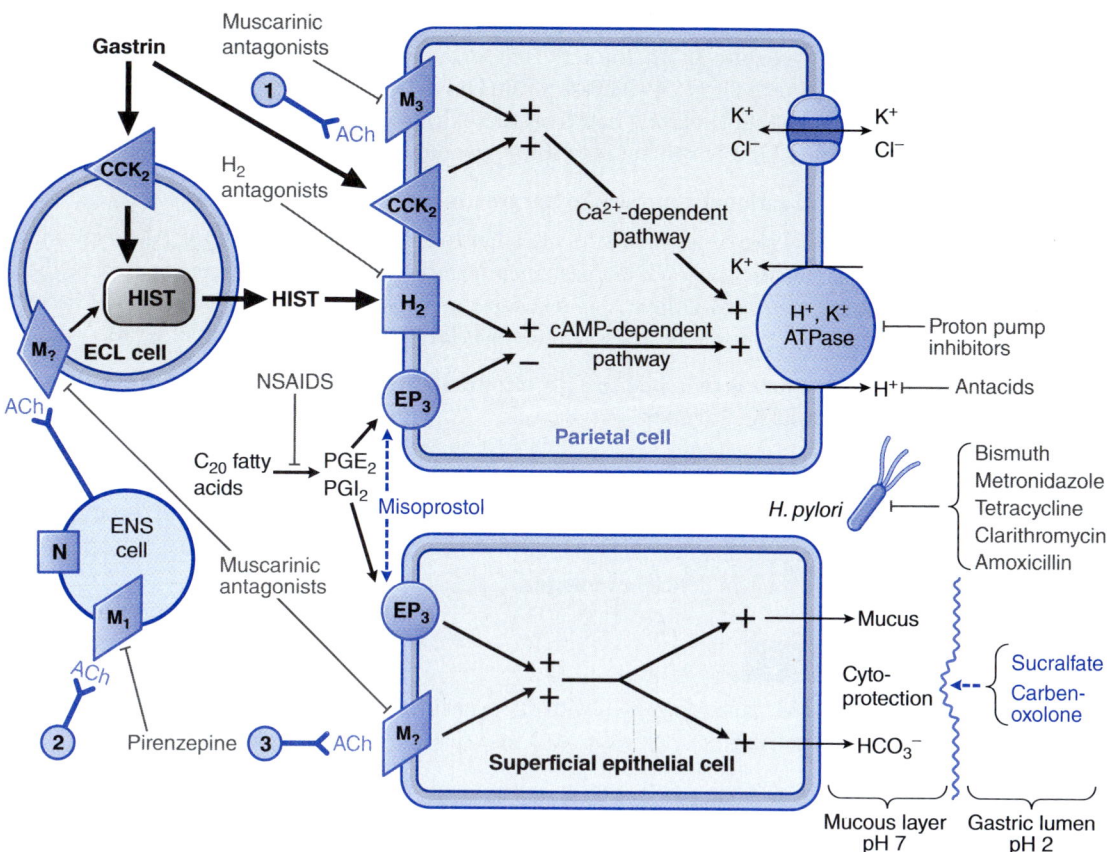

FIGURE 32-1 Physiological and pharmacological regulation of gastric secretion: the basis for therapy of acid-peptic disorders. Shown are the interactions among an enterochromaffin-like (ECL) cell that secretes histamine, a ganglion cell of the enteric nervous system (ENS), a parietal cell that secretes acid, and a superficial epithelial cell that secretes mucus and bicarbonate. Physiological pathways, shown in solid black, may be stimulatory (+) or inhibitory (–). *1* and *3* indicate possible inputs from postganglionic cholinergic fibers; *2* shows neural input from the vagus nerve. Physiological agonists and their respective membrane receptors include acetylcholine (ACh), muscarinic (M), and nicotinic (N) receptors; gastrin, cholecystokinin receptor 2 (CCK_2); histamine (HIST), H_2 receptor; and prostaglandin E_2 (PGE_2), EP_3 receptor. A gray ⟶ indicates targets of pharmacological antagonism. A blue dashed arrow indicates a drug action that mimics or enhances a physiological pathway. Shown in gray are drugs used to treat acid-peptic disorders. NSAIDs are nonsteroidal anti-inflammatory drugs, which can induce ulcers via inhibition of cyclooxygenase (see Chapter 22).

CASE 32-1

A 42-year-old woman is seen because of worsening heartburn during the past week. She was first diagnosed with GERD 1 month ago and treatment was begun with cimetidine 400 mg once daily. Two weeks later the cimetidine dosage was increased to 400 mg twice daily.

a. What is the reason for the worsening of her GERD symptoms?

Cimetidine is an H_2 receptor antagonist and tolerance to acid suppressing effects of these drugs has been shown to develop as early as 2 to 5 days after beginning treatment. One mechanism for this phenomenon is secondary to the hypergastrinemia that stimulates histamine release and overcomes the H_2 receptor blockade.

b. What are the mechanisms of action of H_2 receptor blockers and proton pump inhibitors?

The mechanisms of action of these drugs is shown in Figure 32-1. The H_2 receptor blockers suppress gastric acid secretion by competing with histamine for binding to H_2 receptors on the basolateral membrane of parietal cells. The structural similarity of the H_2 receptor antagonists and histamine is shown in Figure 32-2.

(Continued)

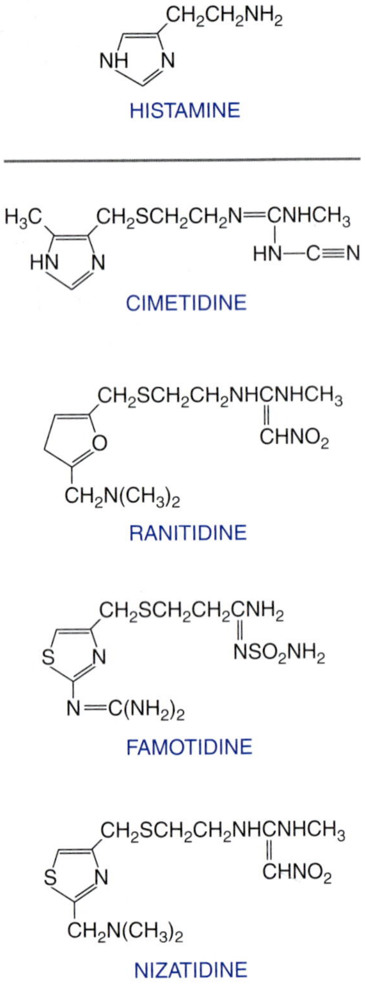

SECTION VI
Drugs Affecting Gastrointestinal Function

HISTAMINE

CIMETIDINE

RANITIDINE

FAMOTIDINE

NIZATIDINE

FIGURE 32-2 Histamine and H_2 receptor antagonists.

The proton pump inhibitors are prodrugs that require activation in an acid environment (see Figure 32-3). The activated form binds covalently with sulfhydryl groups on cysteine in the H^+,K^+-ATPase located on the luminal membrane of the parietal cell. Despite the short plasma half-lives (0.5-2 h) of the parent drug, acid suppression continues for 24 to 48 hours or until new pump molecules are synthesized.

c. What is a rational approach to her treatment?

A rational choice would be to switch her to a proton pump inhibitor. Although these drugs can also cause a hypergastrinemia, it does not result in tolerance because the inhibition occurs at the H^+,K^+-ATPase which is the final step in gastric acid secretion. Figure 32-4 shows the general guidelines for medical management of GERD.

d. If the patient is switched to a proton pump inhibitor, of what adverse effects should she be warned?

Proton pump inhibitors are metabolized by hepatic CYPs and they may interfere with the elimination of other drugs cleared by this route. Chronic treatment with proton pump inhibitors decreases the absorption of vitamin B_{12}. The loss of gastric acidity may affect the bioavailability of drugs, most notably iron salts. This may result in an iron deficiency anemia.

CASE 32-2

A 56-year-old man is diagnosed with duodenal ulcer complicated by *H. pylori* infection. He has been treated with amoxicillin for 2 weeks, but his symptoms of stomach pain persist.

a. Why has his therapeutic regimen not been effective? What problems might be the result of this therapeutic regimen?

H. pylori, a gram negative rod, has been associated with gastritis and subsequent development of gastric and duodenal ulcers, gastric adenoma, and gastric B-cell lymphoma. Single antibiotic therapy for *H. pylori* infection is not effective for eradication and may result in bacterial resistance that is more difficult to treat than the initial infection.

b. What would you recommend for the treatment of his condition?

A common therapeutic approach would be to use a proton pump inhibitor plus clarithromycin plus either metronidazole or amoxicillin for 14 days. Another common approach would be to use a proton pump inhibitor plus metronidazole plus bismuth plus tetracycline. These regimens are shown in Table 32-1.

c. What is the most common problem observed with your recommended regimen?

The most common problem observed with these therapeutic regimens is poor patient compliance due to the number of medications that must be taken each day and to medication-related side effects.

CASE 32-3

A 64-year-old man is referred because of stomach pain. He has been diagnosed with osteoarthritis and has been taking a COX-1 inhibitor for the past 3 months. Workup shows that he has a duodenal ulcer that you suspect is a result of his NSAID use.

a. Describe the pathogenesis of NSAID-induced ulcers.

NSAIDs diminish prostaglandin formation by inhibiting cyclooxygenase. This effect can result in enhanced gastric acid secretion (prostaglandins may lower gastric acid secretion). In addition, prostaglandins stimulate gastric mucin production that provides a cytoprotective effect to the gastric mucosa which is diminished by NSAIDs.

b. What are your therapeutic options?

One option is to change this patient to an NSAID that is a selective inhibitor of COX-2, although this may not completely eliminate the risk of ulcer formation.

(Continued)

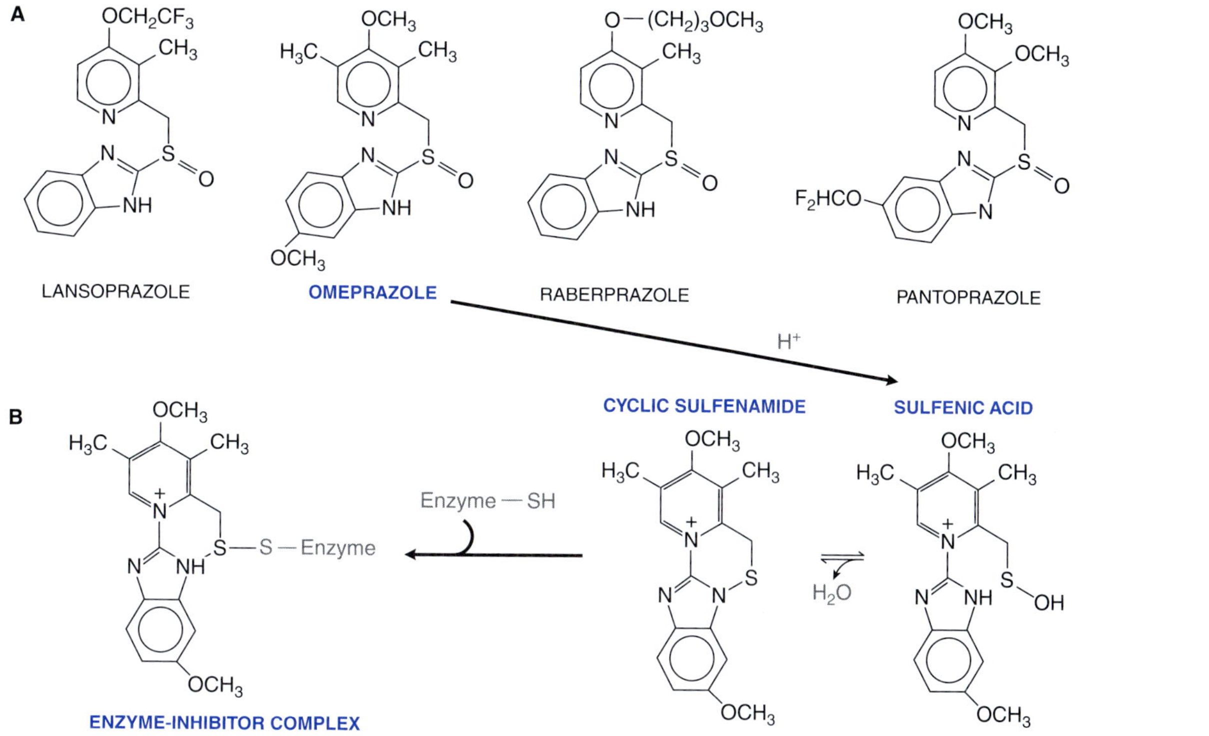

FIGURE 32-3 Proton pump inhibitors. **A.** Inhibitors of gastric H^+,K^+-ATPase (proton pump). **B.** Conversion of omeprazole to a sulfenamide in the acidic secretory canaliculi of the parietal cell. The sulfenamide interacts covalently with sulfhydryl groups in the proton pump, thereby irreversibly inhibiting its activity. The other 3 proton pump inhibitors undergo analogous conversions.

Another option is to try misoprostol although it has numerous gastrointestinal side effects and 4-times-daily dosing is inconvenient. Finally, NSAID-induced ulcers can be managed with acid suppression using either an H_2 receptor antagonist or proton pump inhibitor. Proton pump inhibitors can effectively heal active ulcers and prevent recurrence in the setting of continued NSAID administration.

Severity of GERD	Medical Management
Stage I Sporadic uncomplicated heartburn, often in setting of known precipitating factor. Often not the chief complaint. Less than 2-3 episodes per week. No additional symptoms.	Lifestyle modification, including diet, positional changes, weight loss, *etc*. Antacids and/or histamine H_2 receptor antagonists as needed.
Stage II Frequent symptoms, with or without esophagitis. Greater than 2-3 episodes per week.	Proton pump inhibitors more effective than histamine H_2 receptor antagonists.
Stage III Chronic, unrelenting symptoms; immediate relapse off therapy. Esophageal complications (*eg.*, stricture, Barrett's metaplasia).	Proton pump inhibitor either once or twice daily.

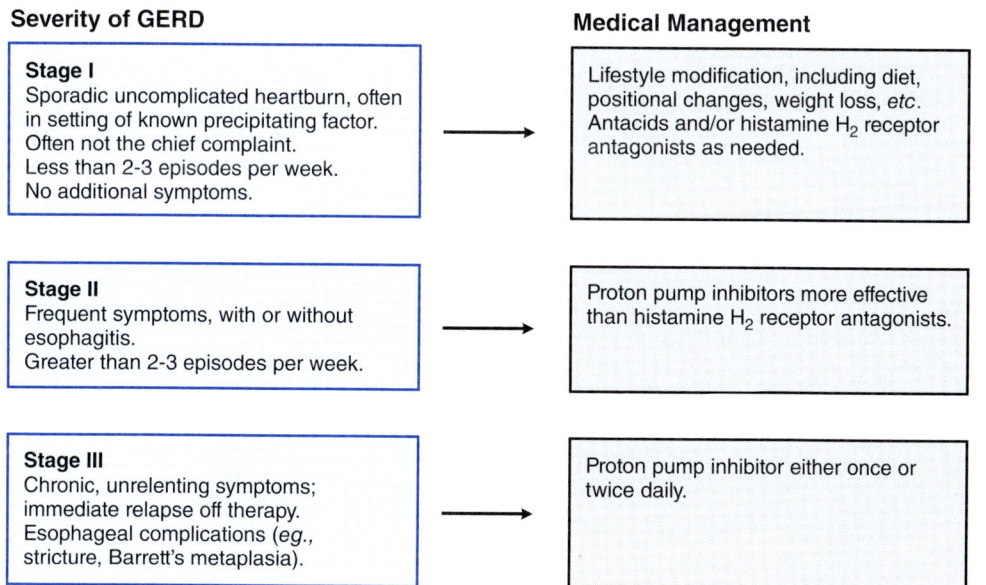

FIGURE 32-4 General guidelines for the medical management of gastroesophageal reflux disease (GERD). Only medications that suppress acid production or that neutralize acid are shown. *(Adapted with permission from Wolfe MM, Sachs G. Acid suppression. Gastroenterology, 2000;118:S24. Copyright © Elsevier.)*

SECTION VI   Drugs Affecting Gastrointestinal Function

TABLE 32-1 Therapy of *Helicobacter pylori* Infection

Triple therapy × 14 days: Proton pump inhibitor + clarithromycin 500 mg plus metronidazole 500 mg or amoxicillin 1 g twice a day (tetracycline 500 mg can be substituted for amoxicillin or metronidazole)

Quadruple therapy × 14 days: Proton pump inhibitor twice a day + metronidazole 500 mg three times daily plus bismuth subsalicylate 525 mg + tetracycline 500 mg four times daily

or

H_2 receptor antagonist twice a day plus bismuth subsalicylate 525 mg + metronidazole 250 mg + tetracycline 500 mg four times daily

Dosages:

Proton pump inhibitors:

   Omeprazole: 20 mg

   Lansoprazole: 30 mg

   Rabeprazole: 20 mg

   Pantoprazole: 40 mg

   Esomeprazole: 40 mg

H_2 receptor antagonists:

   Cimetidine: 400 mg

   Famotidine: 20 mg

   Nizatidine: 150 mg

   Ranitidine: 150 mg

KEY CONCEPTS

➥ Proton pump inhibitors are superior to H_2 receptor antagonists for acid suppression in patients with GERD and peptic ulcers.

➥ Tolerance to the acid-suppressing effects of the H_2 receptor antagonists is commonly observed and limits their continuous use.

➥ *H. pylori* is effectively eradicated with a combination of acid-suppressing drugs and multiple antibiotics administered for 10 to 14 days.

➥ NSAID-induced ulcers can be effectively treated with a proton pump inhibitor even during continued NSAID administration.

SUMMARY QUIZ

QUESTION 32-1 A 24-year-old woman presents with symptoms of esophageal reflux. She is 6 months pregnant. Which of the following drugs is contraindicated in this patient?

a. Ranitidine

b. Lansoprazole

c. Misoprostol

d. Sucralfate

e. Aluminum hydroxide antacid

QUESTION 32-2 A 48-year-old man with a duodenal ulcer disease is treated with cimetidine. After 6 weeks of treatment, he complains that his stomach pain is returning and wonders if the dose of cimetidine should be increased. The most likely reason for the decreased effectiveness of cimetidine in this patient is

a. tolerance.

b. diminished GI absorption.

c. enhanced plasma protein binding.

d. increased hepatic metabolism.

e. poor patient compliance.

Pharmacotherapy of Gastric Acidity

CHAPTER 32

QUESTION 32-3 Esomeprazole has a plasma half-life of a few hours yet suppresses acid secretion for 24 to 48 hours. The reason for this paradox is

a. acid suppression continues until new H^+,K^+-ATPase molecules are synthesized.
b. gastrin depletion occurs long after esomeprazole disappears from the plasma.
c. prostaglandin synthesis is enhanced by esomeprazole.
d. *H. pylori* is effectively suppressed by esomeprazole for 24 to 48 hours.
e. acid suppression continues until new H_2 receptors are synthesized.

QUESTION 32-4 A 48-year-old woman has been diagnosed with a duodenal ulcer that is complicated by *H. pylori* infection. A suitable therapeutic regimen for this patient would be

a. a single antibiotic.
b. a single antibiotic plus a proton pump inhibitor.
c. misoprostol plus a proton pump inhibitor.
d. an H_2 receptor antagonist.
e. 2 antibiotics plus a proton pump inhibitor.

QUESTION 32-5 A 60-year-old woman has had symptoms of heartburn for 6 months. She first treated herself with antacids but as the frequency and severity of the pain increased she switched to over-the-counter omeprazole which she has been taking daily for 3 months. She now comes to your office complaining of fatigue and lethargy. Her physical examination is unusual only in that her skin is remarkably pale. An analysis of her blood reveals hypochromic, microcytic red blood cells. The most likely explanation for this finding is

a. poor absorption of calcium.
b. poor absorption of vitamin B_{12}.
c. poor absorption of folic acid.
d. poor absorption of iron salts.
e. a direct effect of omeprazole on the bone marrow production of red blood cells.

SUMMARY QUIZ ANSWER KEY

QUESTION 32-1 Answer is **c**. Misoprostol is contraindicated in pregnancy because it can increase uterine contractility.

QUESTION 32-2 Answer is **a**. H_2 receptor antagonists are known to produce tolerance. One cause for this tolerance is the secondary increase in gastrin which stimulates histamine release and overcomes the H_2 receptor blockade.

QUESTION 32-3 Answer is **a**. Proton pump inhibitors irreversible bind to the H^+,K^+-ATPase and suppress acid secretion by the gastric parietal cell until new pump molecules are synthesized.

QUESTION 32-4 Answer is **e**. *H. pylori* infection is effectively eradicated with an acid-suppressing drug plus at least 2 antibiotics (see Table 32-1). A single antibiotic or acid-suppressing drug alone is not effective in eradicating *H. pylori*.

QUESTION 32-5 Answer is **d**. Proton pump inhibitors are so effective at the suppression of gastric acid secretion that the absorption of many substances that require an acidic environment is affected. One of these substances is iron salts and the resulting iron deficiency can be manifested by a hypochromic, microcytic anemia. The absorption of folic acid and vitamin B_{12} may also be decreased in the presence of acid-suppressing drugs but a deficiency in these would not result in a hypochromic, microcytic anemia (see AccessMedicine, *Harrison's Principles of Internal Medicine*, 18th Edition Online, Chapter 57, Anemia and Polycythemia).

SECTION VI: Drugs Affecting Gastrointestinal Function

SUMMARY: DRUGS USED TO TREAT GASTRIC ACIDITY, PEPTIC ULCERS, AND GASTROESOPHAGEAL REFLUX DISEASE

CLASS AND SUBCLASSES	NAMES	CLINICAL USES	TOXICITIES COMMON	TOXICITIES UNIQUE; CLINICALLY IMPORTANT
H_2 Receptor Antagonists	Cimetidine Ranitidine	Promote healing of gastric and duodenal ulcers, treatment of uncomplicated GERD, and to prevent occurrence of stress ulcers	Diarrhea, headache, drowsiness, fatigue, muscular pain, and constipation Tolerance occurs with long-term use	Inhibition of hepatic CYPs Delirium and confusion with IV use in elderly patients Gynecomastia in men Galactorrhea in women
	Famotidine	Same as cimetidine	Same as cimetidine	No inhibition of hepatic CYPs
	Nizatidine	Same as cimetidine	Same as cimetidine	No inhibition of hepatic CYPs
Proton Pump Inhibitors	Omeprazole Esomeprazole Lansoprazole Pantoprazole Rabeprazole	Treatment of gastric and duodenal ulcers and GERD	Nausea, flatulence, abdominal pain, constipation	Metabolized by hepatic CYPs and may affect other drugs that are metabolized by hepatic CYPs Decreased absorption of folic acid, vitamin B_{12}, and iron salts
Prostaglandin Analog	Misoprostol	Prevention of NSAID-induced mucosal injury	Diarrhea	Clinical exacerbation of inflammatory bowel disease Contraindicated in pregnancy
Cytoprotective Agents	Sucralfate	Treatment of peptic ulcer disease	Constipation	Avoid in patients with renal failure May inhibit the absorption of other drugs
Bismuth	OTC products	Treatment of peptic ulcer particularly in patients with *H. pylori* infection (see Table 32-1)	Black tongue and stools	Bismuth subsalicylate is associated with salicylate poisoning
Antacids	Various OTC products	OTC for heartburn and excess gastric acidity	See *Goodman and Gilman's Gilman's The Pharmacological Basis of Therapeutics*, 12th Edition, Chapter 45, for a discussion of the common adverse effects of the various antacids	Decreased drug absorption by increasing gastric pH

CHAPTER 33

Drugs Used for the Treatment of Bowel Disorders

The material in this chapter covers the material presented in Chapters 46 and 47 of *Goodman and Gilman's The Pharmacological Basis of Therapeutics*, 12th Edition; this chapter will be most useful after having a basic understanding of these chapters in the 12th Edition. In addition to the material presented here, Chapters 46 and 47 of the 12th Edition contain:

- A description of gastric motility (see Chapter 46)
- A description of the pathophysiology of constipation (see Chapter 46), including Table 46-3 that provides a classification and comparison of representative laxatives, and Table 46-4 that shows the properties of different dietary fibers
- The general principles and approaches to the treatment of diarrhea (see Chapter 46)
- A general description of irritable bowel syndrome (IBS) (see Chapter 46)
- A pharmacological approach to the management of nausea and vomiting (see Chapter 46), including Table 46-6 that shows the receptor specificity of antiemetic agents, and Table 46-7 that shows some antiemetic regimens used in cancer chemotherapy and their initial doses
- A description of the pharmacological management of chronic pancreatitis and steatorrhea (see Chapter 46)
- The pathogenesis of inflammatory bowel disease (IBD) (see Chapter 47), including Table 47-1 which details medications commonly used to treat IBD

LEARNING OBJECTIVES

- ☑ Describe the mechanisms of action of laxatives and cathartics, and understand their use.
- ☑ Describe the mechanisms of action of antidiarrheal agents and understand their use.
- ☑ Understand the pharmacotherapy of IBS.
- ☑ Identify drugs used to treat nausea and vomiting, and describe the mechanisms of action of these drugs.
- ☑ Identify the drugs used to treat IBD, their mechanisms of action, untoward effects, and understand how they are used to treat IBD.

DRUGS INCLUDED IN THIS CHAPTER

- Adalimumab (HUMIRA)
- Alosetron (LOTRONEX)
- Alvimopan (ENTEREG)
- Aprepitant (EMEND)
- Azathioprine (IMMURAN)
- Balsalazide (COLAZIDE)
- Bisacodyl (DULCOLAX, CORRECTOL, others)
- Bismuth (OTC PEPTO-BISMOL)
- Budesonide (ENTOCORT ER)
- Carboxymethylcellulose
- Certolizumab pegol (CIMZIA)
- Cholestyramine (QUESTRAN, others)
- Cisapride (PROPULSID) available only in a limited-access program
- Cyclosporine
- Dexpanthenol (ILOPAN, others)
- Dicyclomine (BENTYL, others)
- Difenoxin (MOTOFEN)
- Diphenoxylate (LOMOTIL)
- Docusate sodium (COLACE, DOXINATE, others)
- Domperidone (MOTILIUM)—not available in the United States
- Dronabinol (MARINOL)
- Glycopyrrolate (ROBINUL, others)
- Hyoscyamine (LEVSIN, others)
- Infliximab (REMIDCADE)
- Lactulose (CEPHULAC, others)
- Loperamide (IMODIUM, others)
- Lubiprostone (AMITIZA)
- Mesalamine (5-aminosalicylic acid, 5-ASA)
- Methotrexate
- Methscopolamine (PAMINE, others)
- Methylnaltrexone (RELISTOR)
- Metoclopramide (REGLAN, others)
- Nabilone (CESAMET)
- Natalizumab (TYSABRI)
- Octreotide (SANDOSTATIN)
- Olsalazine (DIPENTUM)

(continues)

MECHANISMS OF ACTION OF DRUGS USED TO TREAT BOWEL DISORDERS

DRUG CLASS	DRUGS	MECHANISM OF ACTION
Prokinetic Agents	Metoclopramide	D_2 receptor antagonist may also involve 5-HT_4 receptor agonism, vagal, and central 5-HT_3 antagonism
	Domperidone	D_2 receptor antagonist
	Cisapride Prucalopride	5-HT_4 receptor agonist
	Erythromycin	Mimics the effects of motilin, a peptide that contracts the upper GI tract
	Lubiprostone	Prostanoid activator of Cl^- channels

(Continued)

SECTION VI — Drugs Affecting Gastrointestinal Function

DRUGS INCLUDED IN THIS CHAPTER (Cont.)

- Ondansetron (ZOFRN, others)
- Polyethylene glycol (COLYTE, GOLYTELY, others)
- Prucalopride (RESELOR)—available in Europe for use in women with chronic constipation
- Saline laxatives
- Senna (SENOKOT, EX-LAX, others)
- Sulfasalazine (AZULFIDINE)

MECHANISMS OF ACTION OF LAXATIVES

- Enhanced retention of intraluminal fluid by hydrophilic or osmotic mechanisms
  - Bulk-forming agents (bran, psyllium, etc); hydrophilic colloids (methylcellulose, etc)
  - Osmotic agents (nonabsorbable inorganic salts or sugars)
  - Stool-wetting agents (surfactants) and emollients (docusate)
- Decreased net absorption of fluid by effects on small- and large-bowel fluid and electrolyte transport
  - Diphenylmethanes (bisacodyl)
  - Anthraquinones (senna and cascara)
  - Castor oil
- Altered motility by either inhibiting segmenting (nonpropulsive) contractions or stimulating propulsive contractions
  - 5-HT$_4$ receptor agonists
  - Dopamine receptor antagonists
  - Motilides (erythromycin)

DRUG CLASS	DRUGS	MECHANISM OF ACTION
	Methylnaltrexone, Alvimopan	Peripheral μ opioid receptor antagonist (see Chapter 10)
	Dexpanthenol	Enhances acetylcholine synthesis in the gut
Laxatives	Saline laxatives: Magnesium sulfate, hydroxide, citrate; Sodium phosphate	Osmotic increase in intraluminal fluid and increased motility
	Lactulose	Nondigestible sugar which causes an osmotic increase in intraluminal fluid and increased motility
	Polyethylene glycol	Nondigestible alcohol which causes an osmotic increase in intraluminal fluid and increased motility
	Docusate sodium	Anionic surfactant that lowers the surface tension of stool, softens stool, and permits easier defecation
	Bisacodyl	Stimulation of enterocytes, enteric neurons, and GI smooth muscle
Antidiarrheal Agents	Carboxymethylcellulose	Absorbs intestinal liquids
	Cholestyramine	Binds bile acids and some bacterial toxins
	Bismuth	Antisecretory, anti-inflammatory and antimicrobial effects
	Loperamide, Diphenoxylate, Difenoxin	μ opioid receptor agonist (see Chapter 10)
	Clonidine	α$_2$ receptor agonist
	Octreotide	Somatostatin analog
	Alosetron	5-HT$_3$ antagonist that produces a decrease in GI contractility and increased fluid absorption
Antispasmodics	Dicyclomine, Hyoscyamine, Glycopyrrolate, Methscopolamine	Anticholinergic (see Chapter 6)
Antinausea and Antiemetic Agents	Ondansetron	5-HT$_3$ antagonist
	Aprepitant	Substance P receptor antagonist
	Dronabinol, Nabilone	Stimulation of cannabinoid receptors
Agents to Treat Inflammatory Bowel Disease	Sulfasalazine, Olsalazine, Balsalazide, Mesalamine (5-ASA)	Intestinal anti-inflammatory effect (see Chapter 22)
	Budesonide	Enteric glucocorticoid with local anti-inflammatory effects (see Chapter 29)
	Azathioprine	Impairs purine synthesis and cell proliferation (see Chapter 23)

(Continued)

Drugs Used for the Treatment of Bowel Disorders

CHAPTER 33

DRUG CLASS	DRUGS	MECHANISM OF ACTION
	Cyclosporine	Calcineurin inhibitor (see Chapter 23)
	Methotrexate	Inhibition of dihydrofolate reductase (see Chapter 46)
	Infliximab Adalimumab Certolizumab pegol	Binds to and neutralizes TNF_α (see Chapter 23)
	Natalizumab	Binds α4 integrin (see Chapter 23)

CASE 33-1

A 56-year-old man returns to his orthopedic surgeon 2 weeks after repair of a torn anterior cruciate ligament. He has had a considerable amount of pain and has been taking oral hydrocodone on a regular basis daily. He complains today of constipation manifested by decreased stool frequency and difficulty with his bowel movements.

a. What is the likely cause of his constipation?

Figure 33-1 shows the volume and composition of fluid that traverses the small and large intestine daily. Opiate analgesics such as hydrocodone reduce propulsatile activity in the small and large intestine, and decrease intestinal secretions (see Chapter 10). These actions lead to increased water absorption, increasing viscosity of bowel contents and constipation.

b. What is a rational approach to this type of constipation?

Table 33-1 shows a classification of laxatives and Table 33-2 shows the effects of some laxatives on bowel function. In this case the constipation is specifically due to the use of an opioid narcotic for pain. Decreasing the use of the opiate narcotic should improve the situation. If this is not possible, increasing fiber in the diet as well as good hydration should be encouraged.

c. Is there an alternative if a high fiber diet is not effective?

Methylnaltrexone is a peripherally acting μ opioid receptor antagonist that specifically targets the underlying reason for the constipation, without limiting centrally produced analgesia.

CAUSES OF DIARRHEA

- Increased osmotic load within the intestine.
- Excessive secretion of electrolytes and water into the intestinal lumen.
- Exudation of protein and fluid from the intestinal mucosa.
- Altered intestinal motility resulting in rapid transit (and decreased fluid absorption).

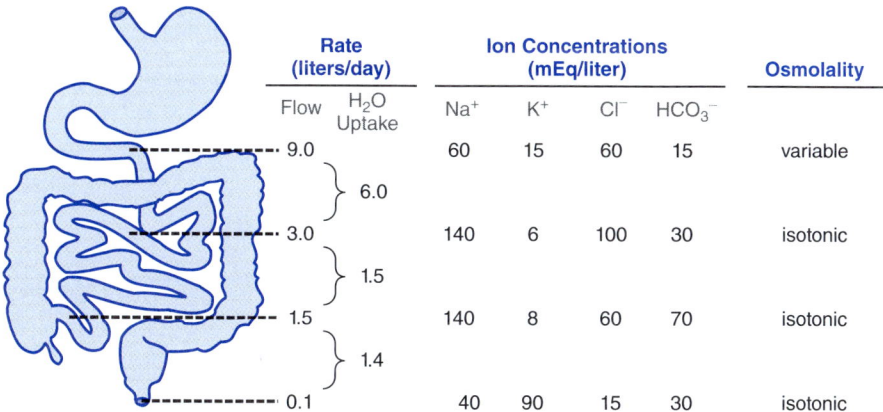

FIGURE 33-1 The approximate volume and composition of fluid that traverses the small and large intestines daily. Of the 9 L of fluid typically presented to the small intestine each day, 2 L are from the diet and 7 L are from secretions (salivary, gastric, pancreatic, and biliary). The absorptive capacity of the colon is 4 to 5 L per day.

SECTION VI
Drugs Affecting Gastrointestinal Function

TABLE 33-1 Classification of Laxatives

1. **Luminally active agents**
   Hydrophilic colloids; bulk-forming agents (bran, psyllium, etc)
   Osmotic agents (nonabsorbable inorganic salts or sugars)
   Stool-wetting agents (surfactants) and emollients (docusate, mineral oil)
2. **Nonspecific stimulants or irritants (with effects on fluid secretion and motility)**
   Diphenylmethanes (bisacodyl)
   Anthraquinones (senna and cascara)
   Castor oil
3. **Prokinetic agents (acting primarily on motility)**
   $5\text{-}HT_4$ receptor agonists
   Dopamine receptor antagonists
   Motilides (erythromycin)

CASE 33-2

A 36-year-old woman presents with a 2-day history of diarrhea and abdominal pain following a weekend camping trip. She appears acutely ill and is dehydrated.

a. What are the issues to address in this particular patient?

The presumptive diagnosis in this patient is giardiasis which has resulted from the ingestion of *Giardia intestinalis* in contaminated drinking water (see Chapter 36). The diagnosis is made by identification of cysts or trophozoites in fecal specimens or trophozoites in duodenal contents. While waiting on a definitive diagnosis, treatment with an antimicrobial such as metronidazole can be started, and her dehydration should be addressed.

b. What drugs might be used to treat her diarrhea?

An opioid that acts through peripheral opioid receptors such as loperamide or diphenoxylate/atropine should be effective in decreasing the diarrhea. Neither drug should be used for a prolonged period of time.

(Continued)

TABLE 33-2 Summary of Effects of Some Laxatives on Bowel Function

AGENT	SMALL BOWEL		COLON		
	TRANSIT TIME	MIXING CONTRACTIONS	PROPULSIVE CONTRACTIONS	MASS ACTIONS	STOOL WATER
Dietary fiber	↓	?	↑	?	↑
Magnesium	↓	—	↑	↑	↑↑
Lactulose	↓	?	?	?	↑↑
Metoclopramide	↓	?	↑	?	—
Cisapride	↓	?	↑	?	↑
Erythromycin	↓	?	?	?	?
Naloxone	↓	↓	—	—	↑
Anthraquinones	↓	↓	↑	↑	↑↑
Diphenylmethanes	↓	↓	↑	↑	↑↑
Docusates	—	?	?	?	—

Modified from Kreek, M.J. Constipation syndromes. In, A Pharmacological Approach to Gastrointestinal Disorders. (Lewis, J.H., ed.) Williams & Wilkins, Baltimore, 1994, pp. 179–208. With permission. http://lww.com.

Drugs Used for the Treatment of Bowel Disorders — CHAPTER 33

c. What untoward effects might this patient expect?

Loperamide lacks significant abuse potential and is more effective in treating diarrhea than diphenoxylate. Overdose can result in CNS depression (especially in children) and paralytic ileus. In patients with IBD loperamide should be used with caution to prevent the development of toxic megacolon.

CASE 33-3

A 57-year-old man comes to hospital for his first cycle of chemotherapy for small cell lung cancer.

a. What drug is a good choice for prophylactic antiemesis therapy for this patient?

Figure 33-2 shows the myriad of signaling pathways that are involved in the control of emesis and shows that cytotoxic drugs stimulate 5-HT$_3$ receptors in the GI system and chemoreceptor trigger zone. Table 33-3 is a general classification of antiemetic agents and shows drugs that are effective in treating cytotoxic drug-induced emesis. Ondansetron is one of the 5-HT$_3$ receptor antagonists that are effective in this setting. It should be administered intravenously 30 minutes before chemotherapy.

b. Is there any clinical situation in which the dose of ondansetron should be altered?

Ondansetron is extensively metabolized in the liver by CYP1A2, CYP2D6, and CYP3A4. Patients with hepatic dysfunction have reduced plasma clearance and some adjustment of the dosage is advisable.

(Continued)

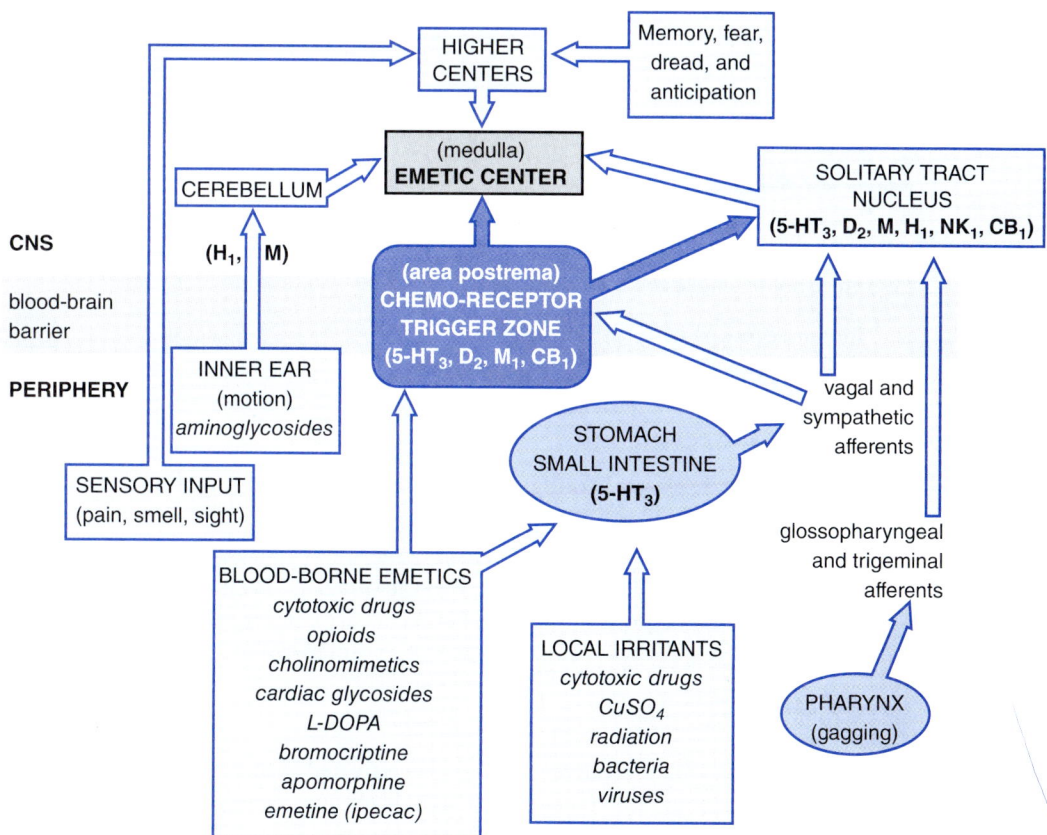

FIGURE 33-2 Pharmacologist's view of emetic stimuli. Myriad signaling pathways lead from the periphery to the emetic center. Stimulants of these pathways are noted in *italics*. These pathways involve specific neurotransmitters and their receptors (**bold** type). Receptors are shown for dopamine (D$_2$), acetylcholine (muscarinic, M), histamine (H$_1$), cannabinoids (CB$_1$), substance P (NK$_1$), and 5-hydroxytryptamine (5-HT$_3$). Some of these receptors also may mediate signaling in the emetic center.

SECTION VI Drugs Affecting Gastrointestinal Function

TABLE 33-3 General Classification of Anti-emetic Agents

ANTI-EMETIC CLASS	EXAMPLES	TYPE OF VOMITING MOST EFFECTIVE AGAINST
5-HT$_3$ receptor antagonists[a]	Ondansetron	Cytotoxic drug induced emesis
Centrally acting dopamine receptor antagonists	Metoclopramide[b] Promethazine[c]	Cytotoxic drug induced emesis
Histamine H$_1$ receptor antagonists	Cyclizine	Vestibular (motion sickness)
Muscarinic receptor antagonists	Hyoscine (scopolamine)	Motion sickness
Neurokinin receptor antagonists	Aprepitant	Cytotoxic drug induced emesis (delayed vomiting)
Cannabinoid receptor agonists	Dronabinol	Cytotoxic drug induced emesis

[a]The most effective agents for chemotherapy-induced nausea and vomiting are the 5-HT$_3$ antagonists and metoclopramide. In addition to their use as single agents, they are often combined with other drugs to improve efficacy as well as reduce the incidence of side effects.
[b]Also has some peripheral activity at 5-HT$_3$ receptors.
[c]Also has some antihistaminic and anticholinergic activity.

c. **If the ondansetron is not effective in this patient, is there an additional therapy that may be used?**

Dronabinol and nabilone are cannabinoids that react with the cannabinoid receptor (CB$_1$) and are useful prophylactic agents in patients receiving cancer chemotherapy when other antiemetic medications are not effective.

CASE 33-4

A 42-year-old man with ulcerative colitis is having a flare in symptoms with severe abdominal pain and bloody diarrhea for the past 24 hours. He is being treated with sulfasalazine but has not been compliant because of a persistent annoying rash.

a. **What are options with his therapy?**

The first option that should be considered is glucocorticoid therapy to rapidly alleviate his intestinal inflammation and curtail his diarrhea. If he is volume depleted, this should also be addressed.

b. **What are the side effects of sulfasalazine therapy and what might be done to increase this patient's compliance?**

Figure 33-3 shows the structures of sulfasalazine and related agents. Since the side effects of sulfasalazine are mostly related to the sulfapyridine moiety, an option in this patient would be to switch from sulfasalazine to a newer preparation such as olsalazine or balsalazide which does not contain sulfapyridine.

CASE 33-5

A 37-year-old man with ulcerative colitis has been treated in the past with azathioprine but after 6 months of therapy, there was no significant improvement in his symptoms.

a. **How is azathioprine metabolized?**

Figure 33-4 shows the metabolism of azathioprine. Azathioprine is a prodrug that is converted to mercaptopurine. Mercaptopurine is metabolized by thiopurine

(Continued)

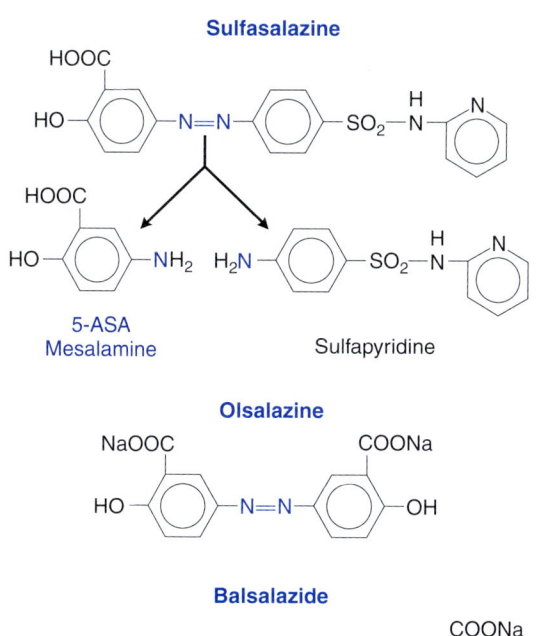

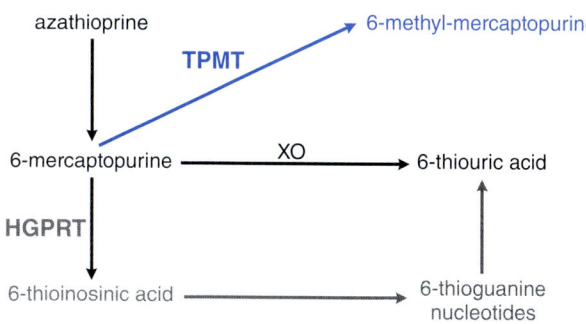

FIGURE 33-3 Structures of sulfasalazine and related agents. The blue N atoms indicate the diazo linkage that is cleaved to generate the active moiety.

FIGURE 33-4 Metabolism of azathioprine and 6-mercaptopurine. HGPRT, hypoxanthine–guanine phosphoribosyl transferase; TPMT, thiopurine methyltransferase; XO, xanthine oxidase. The activities of these enzymes vary among humans because genetic polymorphisms are expressed differentially, explaining responses and side effects when azathioprine–mercaptopurine therapy is employed.

methyltransferase (TPMT) to 6-methyl-mercaptopurine and by hypoxanthine-guanine phosphoribosyl transferase (HGPRT) to 6-thioguanine nucleotides.

b. How might polymorphisms in the metabolism of azathioprine lead to the lack of response to azathioprine in this patient?

Mercaptopurine has 3 metabolic fates: (1) conversion by xanthine oxidase to 6-thiouric acid, (2) metabolism by TPMT to 6-methyl-mercaptopurine (6-MMP), and (3) conversion to 6-thioguanine nucleotides by HGPRT (see Figure 33-4). Polymorphisms of TPMT in a given individual will determine the fate of mercaptopurine and the levels of 6-thioguanine and 6-MMP in each patient. Prior to initiating therapy patients may benefit from an evaluation of TPMT activity to establish the likelihood of an adverse effect such as suppression of bone marrow, or after the therapy has been started to measure the 6-thioguanine/6-MMP levels in individuals not responding to therapy.

CASE 33-6

A 32-year-old woman with the diagnosis of Crohn's disease initially had a good response to glucocorticoid therapy with a one-year remission. However, despite glucocorticoid therapy, she is now having frequent flares of abdominal pain and bloody diarrhea.

a. What options are available for her treatment of this relapse?

Patients who relapse frequently may be treated with immunosuppressive agents such as azathioprine-mercaptopurine. Infliximab is an immunoglobulin that neutralizes TNFα and is particularly useful in closing fistulas associated with Crohn's disease. The combination of infliximab and azathioprine is more effective than infliximab alone in induction of remission and mucosal healing in steroid-resistant patients.

(Continued)

b. How should this patient be monitored for the appearance of serious side effects?

The most serious idiosyncratic reaction to azathioprine is pancreatitis. The most serious dose-related adverse reaction to azathioprine is bone marrow suppression. Circulating blood counts should be monitored closely when azathioprine therapy is initiated and at 3-month intervals during maintenance therapy. Antibodies to infliximab can decrease its clinical efficacy. Infliximab is also associated with increased incidence of respiratory infections. Of particular concern is reactivation of tuberculosis or other granulomatous infections with subsequent dissemination.

KEY CONCEPTS

- Although many choices exist for treating constipation, most therapies are empirical and nonspecific.
- Most cases of constipation can be addressed by increasing fiber intake, avoiding constipating medications, and the judicious use of osmotic laxatives on an as-needed basis.
- Stimulant laxatives, although effective, should be avoided for long-term use.
- If no underlying cause can be determined, chronic diarrhea can be treated empirically with bulk-forming and hygroscopic agents followed by opiates such as loperamide.
- $5\text{-}HT_3$ receptor antagonists, such as ondansetron, are primary therapy for nausea and vomiting, especially in the postchemotherapy and postoperative settings.
- The cannabinoids, dronabinol or nabilone, may be effective for refractive cases of nausea and vomiting.
- Acute exacerbations of ulcerative colitis are treated with colonic-release preparations of mesalamine (5-ASA) and glucocorticoids.
- Maintenance therapy for patients with ulcerative colitis is with one of the 5-ASA compounds; in patients who relapse, azathioprine-mercaptopurine may be used.
- Monitoring the activity of TPMT and the metabolites of mercaptopurine may provide personalized therapy with this drug.
- Drugs used in mild to moderately active Crohn's disease include sulfasalazine, budesonide, and oral corticosteroids.
- Infliximab and other biological agents are useful in closing fistulas associated with Crohn's disease, but their use in maintaining patients in remission must be balanced against the risk of adverse effects.
- Antibiotics, particularly metronidazole, are used for the acute treatment of complications associated with Crohn's disease, but are not used as a routine therapy.

SUMMARY QUIZ

QUESTION 33-1 A 23-year-old woman with a history of type 1 diabetes since age 6 presents with nausea and vomiting associated with gastroparesis and delayed gastric emptying. Which of the following medications would be the most suitable treatment of the nausea and vomiting in this patient?

a. Dephenoxylate

b. Metoclopramide

c. Ondansetron

d. Dronabinol

e. Loperamide

(Continued)

Drugs Used for the Treatment of Bowel Disorders

CHAPTER 33

QUESTION 33-2 A 64-year-old woman is receiving ondansetron for the prophylactic treatment of emesis secondary to chemotherapy. Ondansetron's main mechanism of action is antagonism of

a. central μ opioid receptors.
b. peripheral H_2 receptors.
c. central dopamine receptors.
d. central 5-HT_3 receptors.
e. peripheral muscarinic receptors.

QUESTION 33-3 A 35-year-old woman has severe irritable bowel syndrome characterized by frequent and profuse diarrhea. She is being treated with alosetron because she has not responded to other forms of antidiarrheal therapy. The physician treating this patient must diligently monitor for

a. ischemic colitis.
b. congestive heart failure.
c. drug-induced hepatitis.
d. renal failure.
e. pulmonary fibrosis.

QUESTION 33-4 A 44-year-old man has been treated for chronic back pain with opioid narcotics. He has been plagued with constipation that he has managed to treat by increasing the fiber in his diet. This is no longer effective. Which of the following medications is likely to be of benefit in this patient?

a. Naltrexone
b. Metoclopramide
c. Methylnaltrexone
d. Bisacodyl
e. Lactulose

QUESTION 33-5 A 53-year-old man with a long history of alcohol abuse and hepatic cirrhosis is now developing hepatic encephalopathy. Which of the following agents may be most effective in reducing the signs and symptoms of this patient's hepatic encephalopathy?

a. Loperamide
b. Bisacodyl
c. Glycerin
d. Docusate sodium
e. Lactulose

QUESTION 33-6 A 27-year-old woman with ulcerative colitis is being treated with sulfasalazine. She should be closely monitored for which of the following common adverse effects with this drug?

a. Hearing loss
b. Skin rash
c. Blood in her urine
d. Heart arrhythmia
e. Onset of seizures

QUESTION 33-7 A 42-year-old woman with Crohn's disease has been treated with glucocorticoid therapy. During her initial high dose therapy, she responded well and the dose was tapered over 3 months. However, she relapsed with severe

(Continued)

symptoms during the last month of her taper. The reason for her relapse is most likely because

a. her taper was too rapid.
b. she is glucocorticoid-responsive.
c. she is glucocorticoid-unresponsive.
d. she was noncompliant with her steroid therapy.
e. she is glucocorticoid-dependent.

QUESTION 33-8 A 56-year-old man with ulcerative colitis is being treated with azathioprine. It is determined that his blood concentration ratio of 6-thioguanine/6-methylmercaptopurine is lower than normal. The most likely reason for this finding is that he has increased activity of which of following enzymes?

a. Xanthine oxidase
b. Hypoxanthine-guanine phosphoribosyl transferase (HGPRT)
c. Acetyl transferase
d. Thiopurine methyltransferase (TPMT)
e. Cytochrome P450 3A4

QUESTION 33-9 A 19-year-old woman with ulcerative colitis had to stop taking sulfasalazine because of a skin rash. She is now taking olsalazine which is also converted to 5-ASA but she has experienced no side effects. The most likely reason for the lack of side effects with olsalazine in this patient is because the olsalazine

a. is absorbed in the jejunum after oral use.
b. does not contain a sulfa moiety.
c. has a pH-sensitive release formulation.
d. is given intravenously.
e. is given by enema.

SUMMARY QUIZ ANSWER KEY

QUESTION 33-1 Answer is **b**. Metoclopramide is a dopamine (DA) receptor antagonist that is commonly used to treat the symptoms of delayed gastric emptying. Another drug that might be used is cisapride although it is available only through a limited use program because of its incidence of serious cardiovascular toxicities. Erythromycin is also a possible alternative.

QUESTION 33-2 Answer is **d**. Ondansetron is a central 5-HT$_3$ receptor antagonist. Table 33-3 shows a general classification of anti-emetic drugs.

QUESTION 33-3 Answer is **a**. Alosetron is a 5-HT$_3$ receptor antagonist that reduces GI contractility with decreased colonic transit and increased fluid absorption. The drug was withdrawn from the US market (then reapproved by the FDA) because of an unusually high incidence of ischemic colitis (up to 3 per 1000 patients). The cause is not fully established but may result from the drug's ability to suppress intestinal relaxation.

QUESTION 33-4 Answer is **c**. Methylnaltrexone is an antagonist of peripheral μ opioid receptors that is effective in increasing bowel movements in patients with opioid-induced constipation without limiting centrally produced analgesia.

QUESTION 33-5 Answer is **e**. Lactulose is a synthetic disaccharide of galactose and fructose that resists intestinal disaccharidase activity and osmotically draws water into the intestinal lumen. Patients with severe liver disease have an impaired capacity to detoxify ammonia coming from the colon, where it is produced by bacterial

(Continued)

metabolism of fecal urea. The drop in luminal pH that accompanies hydrolysis of lactulose to short-chain fatty acids in the colon results in "trapping" of ammonia by its conversion to the polar ammonium ion. Combined with the increases in colonic transit, lactulose therapy significantly lowers circulating ammonia levels.

QUESTION 33-6 Answer is **b.** Sulfapyridine, the sulfa moiety of sulfasalazine (see Figure 33-3), is responsible for most of its adverse reactions. Skin rash is a particularly common reaction with sulfa drugs and may be a harbinger of Stevens-Johnson syndrome.

QUESTION 33-7 Answer is **e.** Patients who are glucocorticoid-dependent respond initially to glucocorticoids but then experience a relapse of symptoms as the steroid dose is tapered. These patients are classified as glucocorticoid-dependent (see Chapter 29).

QUESTION 33-8 Answer is **d.** Patients who are rapid metabolizers with respect to TPMT shunt mercaptopurine metabolism away from 6-thioguanine nucleotides and toward 6-MMP (see Figure 33-4 and Case 33-5).

QUESTION 33-9 Answer is **b.** Olsalazine does not contain a sulfapyridine moiety (see Figure 33-3).

SUMMARY: DRUGS USED TO TREAT BOWEL DISORDERS

CLASS AND SUBCLASSES	NAMES	CLINICAL USES	TOXICITIES COMMON	UNIQUE; CLINICALLY IMPORTANT
Prokinetic Agents	Metoclopramide	Ameliorate the nausea and vomiting associated with GI dysmotility		Extrapyramidal effects, tardive dyskinesia
	Domperidone	Gastroparesis		
	Cisapride	Available only through a limited access program for GERD, gastroparesis, pseudoobstruction		Cardiac arrhythmia including ventricular tachycardia
	Prucalopride	Treatment of chronic constipation in women		
	Erythromycin	Diabetic gastroparesis		See Chapter 41
	Lubiprostone	Chronic constipation and irritable bowel syndrome with constipation	Nausea, headache, diarrhea, allergic reactions	
Opioid Antagonists	Methylnaltrexone Alvimopan	Opioid-induced constipation		
Enhancer of Acetylcholine Synthesis	Dexpanthenol	Treatment of postoperative ileus	Mild hypotension and local irritation	Shortness of breath
Laxative	Saline laxatives Magnesium sulfate, hydroxide, citrate Sodium phosphate	Treatment of constipation		Increased salt load Prolonged use associated with electrolyte imbalance
	Lactulose	Treatment of constipation Treatment of hepatic encephalopathy	Abdominal discomfort, flatulence	Prolonged use associated with electrolyte imbalance
	Polyethylene glycol	Treatment of constipation Bowel preparation for endoscopy and surgery		Prolonged use associated with electrolyte imbalance

(Continued)

SECTION VI Drugs Affecting Gastrointestinal Function

CLASS AND SUBCLASSES	NAMES	CLINICAL USES	TOXICITIES COMMON	UNIQUE; CLINICALLY IMPORTANT
	Docusate sodium	Stool softening and promotes ease of defecation		
	Bisacodyl	Treatment of constipation		Prolonged use associated with electrolyte imbalance and atonic colon
Antidiarrheal Agents	Carboxymethylcellulose	Treatment of diarrhea		
	Cholestyramine	Treatment of bile salt-induced diarrhea	See Chapter 20	
	Bismuth	Treatment of diarrhea		Danger of salicylate poisoning with bismuth subsalicylate
	Loperamide	Treatment of diarrhea		Used with caution in patients with inflammatory bowel disease to prevent toxic megacolon
	Diphenoxylate combined with atropine Difenoxin combined with atropine	Treatment of diarrhea	Combined with low dose of atropine to prevent abuse	High doses cause CNS depression and anticholinergic effects
	Clonidine	Treatment of chronic diarrhea in diabetics	See Chapter 7	See Chapter 7
	Octreotide	Treatment of hormone-secreting tumors of the pancreas and GI tract	Nausea and bloating	Long-term treatment can lead to gallstones and hypo- or hyperglycemia
	Alosetron	Treatment of diarrhea in women with irritable bowel syndrome (IBS)		Ischemic colitis in a small number of patients
Antispasmodics	Dicyclomine Hyoscyamine	Treatment of pain associated with IBS	Light-headedness, drowsiness, nervousness	
	Glycopyrrolate	Treatment of pain associated with IBS		
	Methscopolamine	Treatment of pain associated with IBS		
Antinauseants and Antiemetic Agents	Ondansetron	Treatment of nausea and chemotherapy-induced emesis	Constipation or diarrhea, headache, light-headedness	
	Aprepitant	Treatment of chemotherapy-induced nausea and emesis		Contraindicated in patients with life-threatening QT prolongation Interacts with other substrates of CYP3A4
	Dronabinol Nabilone	Treatment of chemotherapy-induced nausea and emesis	Palpitations, tachycardia, hypotension	Marijuana "highs" and abstinence syndrome upon withdrawal

(Continued)

Drugs Used for the Treatment of Bowel Disorders — CHAPTER 33

CLASS AND SUBCLASSES	NAMES	CLINICAL USES	TOXICITIES COMMON	UNIQUE; CLINICALLY IMPORTANT
Agents to Treat Inflammatory Bowel Disease (IBD)	Sulfasalazine	Treatment of IBD particularly ulcerative colitis	Headache, nausea, fatigue	Rash, bone marrow suppression, Stevens-Johnson syndrome, hepatitis, pneumonia: All due to sulfa moiety
	Mesalamine (5-ASA)	Treatment of IBD particularly ulcerative colitis	Headache, dyspepsia, skin rash	Has been associated with interstitial nephritis; renal function should be monitored in all patients
	Olsalazine	Treatment of IBD particularly ulcerative colitis	Headache, nausea, dyspepsia, diarrhea	
	Balsalazide	Treatment of IBD particularly ulcerative colitis	Headache, nausea, dyspepsia	
	Budesonide	Enteric release of synthetic steroid used for ileocecal Crohn's disease		
	Azathioprine	Treatment of IBD	Fever, rash, arthralgias, nausea, and vomiting	Idiosyncratic pancreatitis Dose-related bone marrow suppression Rare cholestatic hepatitis
	Cyclosporine	Second-line treatment of IBD		See Chapter 23
	Methotrexate	Treatment of steroid-resistant IBD		See Chapter 48
	Infliximab	Treatment of IBD		Increased incidence of respiratory infections and potential reactivation of TB
	Adalimumab Certolizumab pegol Natalizumab	Treatment of IBD		Natalizumab reacts with other immune-modulating drugs to increase the risk of multifocal leukoencephalopathy

Chemotherapy of Microbial Diseases

SECTION VII

34. General Principles of Antimicrobial Therapy 512

35. Chemotherapy of Malaria 520

36. Chemotherapy of Protozoal Infections:
Amebiasis, Giardiasis, Trichomoniasis, Trypanosomiasis,
Leishmaniasis, and Other Protozoal Infections 530

37. Chemotherapy of Helminth Infections 536

38. Sulfonamides, Trimethoprim-Sulfamethoxazole,
Quinolones, and Agents for Urinary Tract Infections 542

39. Penicillins, Cephalosporins,
and Other β-Lactam Antibiotics 549

40. Aminoglycosides 559

41. Protein Synthesis Inhibitors and Miscellaneous
Antibacterial Agents 568

42. Chemotherapy of Tuberculosis, *Mycobacterium Avium*
Complex Disease, and Leprosy 578

43. Antifungal Agents 588

44. Antiviral Agents and Treatment of HIV Infection 600

CHAPTER 34

General Principles of Antimicrobial Therapy

CLASSIFICATION OF ANTIMICROBIAL AGENTS

- The first broad classification of antimicrobial agents is according to the microorganisms they are active against: antibacterial, antiviral, antifungal, antiparasitic.
- Further classification of an antibiotic is based on:
  - The class and spectrum of the microorganisms it kills
  - The biochemical pathway it interferes with
  - The chemical structure of its pharmacophore (the chemical moiety of the drug that binds to a microbial receptor)

This chapter will be most useful after having a basic understanding of the material in Chapter 48, General Principles of Antimicrobial Therapy in *Goodman & Gilman's The Pharmacological Basis of Therapeutics*, 12th Edition. Neither Mechanisms of Action nor Clinical Summary Tables are included in this chapter because this information is provided in subsequent chapters.

In addition to the material presented here, Chapter 48 of the 12th Edition contains:
- A detailed discussion of the pharmacokinetic basis for antimicrobial therapy
- A thorough discussion of the types and goals of antimicrobial therapy

LEARNING OBJECTIVES

- ☑ Describe the pharmacokinetic basis of antimicrobial therapy.
- ☑ Identify the importance of susceptibility testing of antimicrobial agents.
- ☑ Identify the factors that form the basis for selection of an antimicrobial dose and dosing schedule.
- ☑ Describe the types and goals of antimicrobial therapy.
- ☑ Identify the mechanisms of resistance to antimicrobial agents.

DRUGS INCLUDED IN THIS CHAPTER

The pharmacology of specific drugs is not included in this chapter. The drugs presented in the cases are used as examples to illustrate various aspects of antimicrobial therapy; the specific pharmacology of these drugs is presented in the subsequent chapters of this section.

FACTORS THAT AFFECT THE PENETRATION OF A DRUG INTO AN ANATOMICAL COMPARTMENT

- Physical barriers (eg, blood–brain barrier)
- Chemical properties of the drug (eg, octanol-water partition coefficient)
- Membrane transporters (eg, p-glycoprotein)

CASE 34-1

A 34-year-old woman has a diagnosis of pneumococcal meningitis. The pathogen is determined to be sensitive to penicillin and she is being treated with high-dose penicillin.

a. **How does the chemical nature of a drug affect its penetration into various anatomic compartments such as the brain?**

An important factor is the drug's lipid solubility or its octanol:water partition coefficient. The higher the octanol:water partition coefficient, the more likely it is to penetrate physical barriers erected by layers of cells. The more charged a drug molecule, and the larger it is, the poorer its penetration across physical barriers.

b. **What is unique about the brain in terms of drug penetration?**

The central nervous system (CNS) is guarded by the blood–brain barrier. The movement of antibiotics across the blood–brain barrier is restricted by tight junctions that connect endothelial cells of cerebral microvessels to one another in the brain parenchyma, as well as by protein transporters. Antimicrobial agents that are polar at physiological pH, such as penicillin G, generally penetrate poorly. Some drugs, such as penicillin G, are actively transported out of the cerebrospinal fluid. However, the integrity of the blood–brain barrier is diminished during active bacterial infection, such as pneumococcal meningitis, leading to an opening of the tight junctions and the penetration of even polar drugs.

(Continued)

General Principles of Antimicrobial Therapy

CHAPTER 34

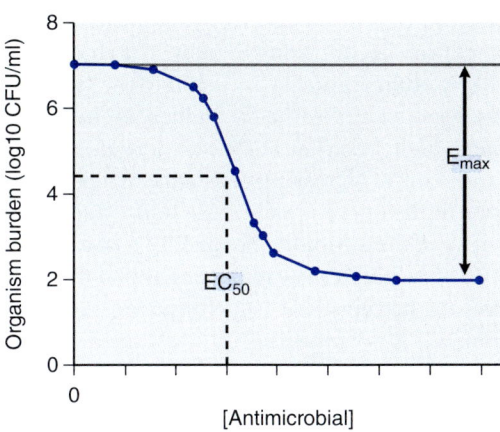

FIGURE 34-1 Inhibitory sigmoid E_{max} curve. CFU, colony forming units.

c. **What other anatomical compartments require special attention for antimicrobial therapy?**

The ocular cavity, pulmonary epithelial linings, endocardial vegetations, and prosthetic devices such as artificial heart valves, long-dwelling catheters, artificial hips, and devices for internal fixation of bone fractures are compartments in which antibiotic penetration is poor.

d. **How should the drug and its antimicrobial target be viewed?**

Antimicrobial molecules should be viewed as ligands whose receptors are microbial proteins and the relationship between drug concentration and effect on a population of organisms is modeled using the standard Hill-type curve for receptor and agonist (see Figure 34-1). The inhibitory concentration 50 or IC_{50} (also termed EC_{50} or effective concentration 50) is a measure of the antimicrobial agent's potency; the E_{max} is the antimicrobial agent's maximum effect.

CASE 34-2

A 62-year-old man with chronic obstructive pulmonary disease develops a pumonary infection that rapidly becomes a systemic bacteremia requiring antibiotic therapy. The microorganism has been isolated and susceptibility testing has been completed. The minimum inhibitor concentration (MIC) is 0.5 mg/L and the serum $t_{½}$ of the antibiotic is 3 hours.

a. **In choosing a drug and dose regimen that will be most effecitve in this patient what must be considered?**

The microbiology laboratory plays a central role in the decision to choose a particular antimicrobial agent over others. Their first function is the identification and isolation of the pathogenic organism. Once this is accomplished, the rational choice of the class of antibiotics to administer to the patient can be made. Then the laboratory performs susceptibility testing to narrow down the list of possible antimicrobials that could be used. Susceptibility testing for bacteria employs antibiotics in serially diluted concentrations of solid agar or in broth medium that contains a culture of the test microorganism. The lowest concentration of the agent that prevents visible growth after 18 to 24 hours of incubation is known as the MIC.

In choosing a dose regimen, the first consideration is to index drug exposure to the MIC. Second, dose itself is a poor measure of drug exposure, given between-patient and within-patient pharmacokinetic variability. The optimal dose of the antibiotic for a patient is the dose that achieves inhibitory concentration (IC) of IC_{80} to IC_{90} exposures at the site of infection. A third consideration is that optimal microbial kill by the antibiotic may be best achieved by optimizing certain shapes

(Continued)

of the concentration-time curve (see answer to Case 34-2b below). Last, changes in susceptibility to drug (ie, drug-resistance) can occur during therapy. The change in drug susceptibility of an organism is depicted in Figure 34-2. A shift to the right of the antimicrobial concentration versus response curve, that is, an increase in the IC_{50} (see Figure 34-2A), means that much higher concentrations are now needed to show a specific response to the drug and reflects increasing resistance to a particular antibiotic. A second possible change in the curve is a decrease in E_{max} (see Figure 34-2B), such that increasing the dose of the antibiotic beyond a certain point will achieve no further effect. This occurs because the available microbial target proteins have been reduced or the microbe has developed an alternative pathway to overcome the biochemical inhibition.

b. How does the dose administration schedule (once daily or 3 divided doses) affect the drug concentration-time profile?

Figure 34-3A depicts the concentration-time curve of an antibiotic in which the peak concentration (C_{Pmax}), area under the curve (AUC), and the fraction of the dosing interval (T) for which the drug concentration remains above the MIC (T > MIC) are shown. Figure 34-3B shows concentration-time curves when the same dose of the antibiotic is given as 3 equal doses administered at 0, 8, and 16 hours. The AUC_{0-24} will be similar whether the dose was given once a day or 3 times a day. Thus, for the same pathogen, the change in dose schedule does not change the AUC_{0-24}/MIC. However, the C_{Pmax} will decrease by a third when the total dose is split into 3 doses and administered more frequently (see Figure 34-3B). In addition, the time that the drug concentration persists above MIC (T > MIC) is slightly increased with the more frequent dosing schedule.

(Continued)

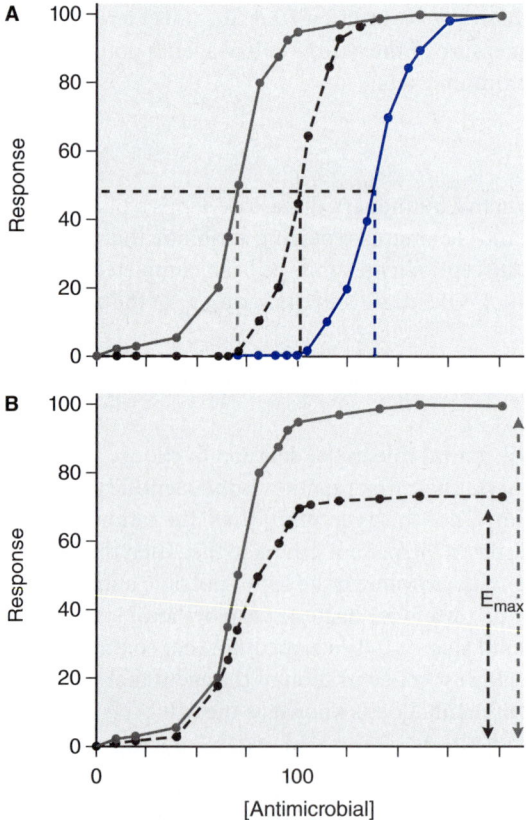

FIGURE 34-2 Changes in sigmoid E_{max} model with increases in drug resistance. Increase in resistance may show changes in IC_{50} (**panel A:** the IC_{50} increases from 70 [gray line] to 100 [black line], to 140 [blue line]) or decrease in E_{max} (**panel B:** efficacy decreases from full response [gray line] to 70% [black line]).

General Principles of Antimicrobial Therapy

CHAPTER 34

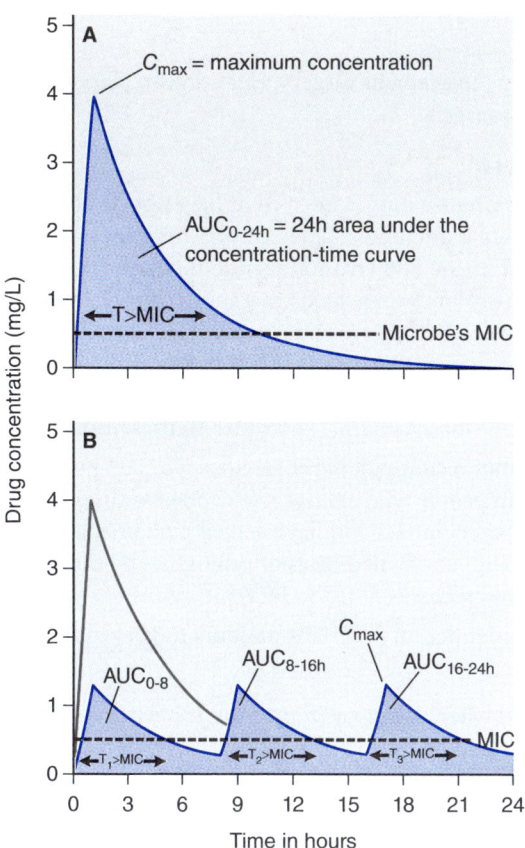

FIGURE 34-3 Effect of different dose schedules on shape of concentration-time curve. The total AUC for the fractionated dose in **curve B** is determined by adding AUC_{0-8h}, AUC_{8-16h}, and AUC_{16-24h}, which adds up to the same AUC_{0-24h} in **curve A**. The time concentration exceeds MIC is also determined by adding up $T_1>MIC$, $T_2>MIC$, and $T_3>MIC$, which results in a fraction greater than that for curve A.

c. **Which indices, AUC/MIC, or C_{Pmax}/MIC or T > MIC is the most important to determine the microbial kill?**

This depends on the antimicrobial. Some antibiotics (β-lactam antibiotics, eg, penicillin) kill best when drug concentration persists above MIC for longer durations of the dosing interval. A drug optimized by T > MIC should be dosed more frequently. Indeed the effectiveness of penicillin is enhanced when it is given as a continuous infusion.

The peak concentration is what matters for some antimicrobial agents. Aminoglycosides are a good example of this class as they previously were given three times a day but experience has shown that aminoglycosides are highly effective when given once a day (see Chapter 40).

There is a third group of antimicrobial agents for which the dosing schedule has no effect on efficacy, but it is the cummulative effect that matters. Daptomycin is an example of this group of drugs. These drugs also have a long postantibiotic effect (PAE). Their effect continues long after antibiotic concentrations decline below the MIC.

d. **How does the dosing schedule relate to resistance suppression?**

In many instances, the drug exposure required for resistance suppression is much higher than for optimal kill. Unfortunately, this higher exposure is also associated with drug toxicity when doses are increased. Although the relationship between microbial kill and exposure is based on the inhibitory sigmoid E_{max} model, this model does not apply to resistance suppression.

PATIENTS AT RISK FOR INFECTIVE ENDOCARDITIS FOR WHICH PROPHYLACTIC THERAPY IS RECOMMENDED

- Those with prosthetic material used for heart valve repair or replacement
- Those who have had previous infective endocarditis
- Those with congenital heart disease such as unrepaired cyanotic heart disease, or within 6 months of repair of the heart disease with prosthetic material, or those with residual defects adjacent to the prosthetic material
- Postcardiac transplant patients with heart valve defects

MECHANISMS OF ANTIMICROBIAL RESISTANCE

- Reduced entry of antibiotic into pathogen
- Enhanced export of antibiotic by pathogen efflux pumps (see Side Bar MAJOR SYSTEMS OF EFFLUX PUMPS THAT ARE RELEVANT TO ANTIMICROBIAL AGENTS)
- Release of microbial enzymes that destroy the antibiotic
- Alterations of microbial enzymes that are required to transform prodrugs to the effective moieties
- Alteration of target proteins
- Development of alternative biochemical pathways to those inhibited by the antibiotic

SECTION VII — Chemotherapy of Microbial Diseases

MAJOR SYSTEMS OF EFFLUX PUMPS THAT ARE RELEVANT TO ANTIMICROBIAL AGENTS

- Multidrug and toxic compound extruder (MATE)
- Major facilitator superfamily (MFS) transporters
- Small multidrug resistance (SMR) system
- Resistance nodulation division (RND) exporters
- ATP-binding cassette (ABC) transporters

CHEMOPROPHYLAXIS USED TO PREVENT WOUND INFECTIONS SHOULD FOLLOW THESE PRINCIPLES

- Antimicrobial activity must be present at the time of wound closure
- Antimicrobial therapy must be active against the most likely contaminating microorganisms for that type of surgery
- In clean surgical procedures, the expected incidence of wound infection is less than 5%, and antibiotics should not be used routinely

CASE 34-3

A 54-year-old woman is undergoing hip replacement surgery. Her surgeon placed her on a broad-spectrum antibiotic prior to surgery.

a. What is the goal of this antibiotic use?

Prophylaxis involves treating patients who are not yet infected or have not yet developed disease (see Figure 34-4). It is used in immunosuppressed patients such as those with HIV-AIDS, or are post-transplantation and on antirejection medications (see Chapter 23). In these patients, antimicrobial prophylactic therapy is administered based on the well-defined pattern of pathogens that are major causes of morbidity during immunosuppression. Infections for which prophylaxis is commonly given include *Pneumocystis jirovecii*, *Mycobacterium avium*-intracellulare, *Toxoplasma gondii*, *Candida* species, *Aspergillus* species, *Cytomegalovirus*, and other Herpesviridae.

Postexposure prophylaxis is sometimes recommended as in rifampin therapy to prevent meningococcal meningitis in people who are in close contact with a case, prevention of gonorrhea or syphilis after contact with an infected person, macrolide antibiotic therapy after contact with confirmed cases of pertussis, and those patients or health care workers inadvertently exposed to HIV infection.

Prophylactic therapy is also recommended in pregnant patients to prevent transmission of HIV and syphilis.

b. What principles should be followed when using antibiotics to prevent wound infections?

These guidelines are listed in the Side Bar CHEMOPROPHYLAXIS USED TO PREVENT WOUND INFECTIONS SHOULD FOLLOW THESE PRINCIPLES. The surgeon has followed the first guideline by placing the patient on the antibiotic prior to the surgery so there is sufficient antimicrobial activity at the time of wound closure.

c. This patient has had a previous episode of infective endocarditis. Does this make her a stronger candidate for prophylactic therapy?

This definitely changes the situation with regard to prophylactic antibiotic therapy. The situations in which prophylactic therapy is recommended for patients at risk of infective endocarditis are shown in the Side Bar PATIENTS AT RISK FOR INFECTIVE ENDOCARDITIS FOR WHICH PROPHYLACTIC THERAPY IS RECOMMENDED.

CASE 34-4

A 59-year-old transient man comes to the emergency department with fever and difficulty breathing. He is diagnosed with pneumonia and after blood and sputum cultures are obtained he is started on a β-lactam antibiotic. The next day his cultures show that the pathogen is resistant to the β-lactam antibiotic and he is switched to a combination of a fluoroquinolone and an aminoglycoside.

(Continued)

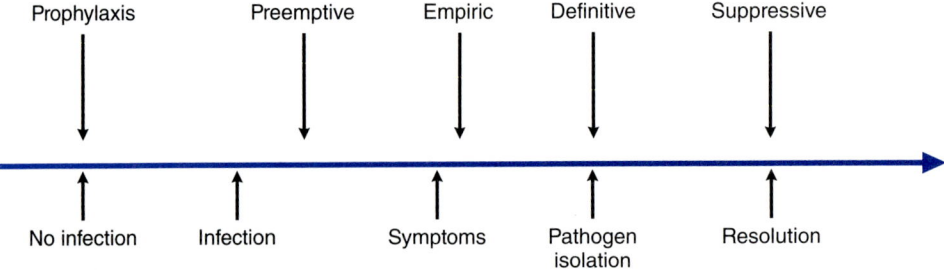

FIGURE 34-4 Antimicrobial therapy-disease progression timeline. Stages of disease progression are below the horizontal arrow; categories of antimicrobial therapy are above the arrow.

General Principles of Antimicrobial Therapy

CHAPTER 34

a. **Has the β-lactam antibiotic caused the pathogen to be resistant?**

Mutation and antibiotic selection of the resistant mutant are the molecular basis for resistance for many bacteria, viruses, and fungi. Mutations are not caused by drug exposure per se. They are random events that confer a survival advantage when drug is present. Drug resistance may be acquired by mutation and selection with passage of the trait vertically to daughter cells. Drug resistance more commonly is acquired by horizontal transfer of resistance determinants from a donor cell, often from another bacterial species, by transduction, transformation, or conjugation. Resistance acquired by horizontal transfer disseminates rapidly and widely either by clonal spread of the resistant strain or by subsequent transfers to other susceptible recipient strains.

b. **What are the mechanisms of resistance to antimicrobial agents?**

Nowadays, every major antimicrobial class is associated with the emergence of significant resistance. The mechanisms of microbial resistance are shown in the Side Bar MECHANISMS OF ANTIMICROBIAL RESISTANCE. The emergence of antibiotic resistance is associated with 2 factors: evolution and clinical/environmental practices. Microorganisms develop 1 of the mechanisms of resistance by acquiring genetic elements that code for the resistance mechanism, by mutating under antimicrobial pressure, or by constitutive induction of a resistance mechanism.

Small polar molecules, including many antibiotics, enter the pathogen cell through protein channels called porins. Absence of, mutation in, or loss of a favored porin channel can slow the rate of drug entry or prevent entry altogether. Or, if the target is intracellular and the drug requires active transport across the cell membrane, a mutation or phenotypic change that slows or abolishes this transport mechanism can confer resistance.

c. **How are efflux pumps in microbial membranes responsible for resistance?**

Efflux pumps (see Side Bar MAJOR SYSTEMS OF EFFLUX PUMPS THAT ARE RELEVANT TO ANTIMICROBIAL AGENTS) are also a prominent mechanism of resistance for parasites, bacteria, and fungi. Drug resistance to most antimalarial drugs (see Chapter 35), but specifically to chloroquine is mediated by an ABC transporter encoded by *Plasmodium falciparum* multidrug resistance gene 1 (*Pfmdr1*). Point mutations in the *Pfmdr1* gene lead to drug resistance and failure of chemotherapy.

d. **Give some other examples of mechanisms of antimicrobial resistance.**

Another mechanism of drug resistance is for the bacteria to enzymatically inactivate the drug. Bacterial resistance to β-lactam antibiotics (eg, penicillin, see Chapter 39) is due to production of a β-lactamase enzyme which destroys the antibiotic.

A common mechanism for antimicrobial resistance is either single point or multiple point mutations that result in a change in amino acid sequence and conformation of a target protein. This change leads to a reduced affinity of drug for its target (eg, methicillin-resistant *Staphylococcus aureus* [MRSA] caused by production of a low-affinity penicillin-binding protein).

Rarely an organism not only becomes resistant to an antimicrobial agent but subsequently starts requiring it for growth (eg, enterococcus, which develops vancomycin resistance, can, after prolonged exposure, develop vancomycin-requiring strains).

Nucleoside reverse transcriptase inhibitors such as zidovudine (see Chapter 44) are incorporated into the viral DNA chain and cause chain termination. Resistance emerges when mutations occur at a variety of points in the reverse transcriptase gene, and phosphorolytic excision of the incorporated chain-terminating nucleoside analog is enhanced.

SPECIAL CIRCUMSTANCES THAT FAVOR COMBINATION ANTIMICROBIAL THERAPY

- Preventing resistance to monotherapy
- Accelerating the rapidity of microbial kill
- Enhancing therapeutic efficacy by use of synergistic antibiotic interactions
- Paradoxically, reducing toxicity (ie, when full efficacy of a standard antibacterial agent can only be achieved at doses that are toxic to the patient)

SECTION VII: Chemotherapy of Microbial Diseases

CASE 34-5

A 35-year-old patient with HIV infection is started on 3 drugs in combination.

a. What are the problems of using combination therapy?

Using multiple antimicrobial agents where only one is required leads to increased toxicity and unnecessary damage to the patient's otherwise protective fungal and bacterial flora.

b. Why is this patient started on 3 drugs?

There are special circumstances where evidence is unequivocal in favor of combination therapy. These are listed in the Side Bar SPECIAL CIRCUMSTANCES THAT FAVOR COMBINATION ANTIMICROBIAL THERAPY. Clinical situations for which combination therapy is used are discussed in the relevant chapters but include antiretroviral therapy for AIDS (see Chapter 44), antiviral therapy for hepatitis B and C (see Chapter 44), and the treatment of tuberculosis (see Chapter 42).

KEY CONCEPTS

- Antimicrobial agents should be viewed as ligands whose receptors are microbial proteins.
- Knowledge of an antibiotic's pharmacokinetic variability (due to such factors as genetics, age, weight, disease status) leads to better dose adjustments.
- Proper interpretation of microbial susceptibility testing (minimum inhibitory concentration, MIC) is the first step in the selection of an antibiotic dose and dosing schedule.
- Maximizing the antibiotic concentration-time curve by selection of the proper dosing schedule is critical to obtaining optimal microbial kill.
- Monotherapy of antibiotics is preferred in order to limit the risk of toxicity and the emergence of resistance; however, there are circumstances that favor combination antibiotic therapy.
- Resistance to antibiotics develops when there is acquisition of genetic elements that code for one of several resistance mechanisms, or when mutations develop under antibiotic pressure, or under constitutive induction.
- Mutations that result in drug resistance are not caused by drug exposure per se, rather they are random events that confer a survival advantage when drug is present.

SUMMARY QUIZ

QUESTION 34-1 A 43-year-old man is neutropenic and has developed a fever. After obtaining the appropriate cultures, you decide to start him on a broad-spectrum antibacterial and antifungal therapy. Your decision fits which of the following goals of antimicrobial therapy?

a. Prophylaxis
b. Definitive
c. Empirical
d. Preemptive
e. Post-treatment suppression

General Principles of Antimicrobial Therapy CHAPTER 34

QUESTION 34-2 Typically the time when the antibiotic concentration is greater than the MIC is less with once-daily dosing than if the antibiotic were administered in 3 equally divided doses. However, aminoglycoside antibiotics are commonly administered once daily. The efficacy of once-daily dosing of aminoglycosides is due to

a. decreased toxicity.
b. increased renal excretion at higher doses.
c. less bacterial resistance to the antibiotic.
d. postantibiotic effect.
e. the rate of increase in the initial plasma concentration.

QUESTION 34-3 Bacterial resistance to β-lactam antibiotics (eg, penicillin) is usually due to the bacterial production of β-lactamase. This results in

a. destruction of the antibiotic.
b. reduced affinity to a bacterial protein.
c. enhanced efflux of the antibiotic from the bacteria.
d. decreased entry of the antibiotic into the bacteria.
e. development of an alternative mechanism of bacterial survival in the presence of antibiotic.

QUESTION 34-4 A 35-year-old patient with HIV infection is being started on 3 drugs in combination. The primary reason he is started on 3 drugs rather than 1 is

a. the drugs only come in combinations of 3.
b. the potential for reducing toxicity.
c. preventing resistance to monotherapy.
d. enhanced antiviral effect of each drug.
e. a decrease in urinary excretion of each drug.

SUMMARY QUIZ ANSWER KEY

QUESTION 34-1 Answer is **c**. This is termed empiric therapy (see Figure 34-4). Neutropenic patients with fever have a high risk of mortality, and when febrile, they are presumed to have either a bacterial or fungal infection. Once the pathogen is identified and susceptibility determined the broad-spectrum therapy can be switched to a specific antimicrobial agent.

QUESTION 34-2 Answer is **d**. The peak antibiotic plasma concentration is what matters for some antimicrobial agents, such as aminoglycosides, and the persistence above MIC has less relevance. These drugs can be administered less frequently due to their long duration of postantibiotic effect. That is, their antibacterial effect continues long after antibiotic concentrations decline below the MIC.

QUESTION 34-3 Answer is **a**. β-lactamase is an enzyme that destroys antibiotics that contain a β-lactam in their chemical structure (see Chapter 39).

QUESTION 34-4 Answer is **c**. It is standard of care to start patients with HIV infection on a regimen of 3 drugs primarily to prevent the development of resistant virus (see Chapter 44).

CHAPTER 35

Chemotherapy of Malaria

DRUGS INCLUDED IN THIS CHAPTER

- Artemisinin and Artemisinin—combination therapies
- Atovaquone/Proguanil (MALARONE)
- Chloroquine (ARALEN)
- Doxycycline—see Chapter 41
- Hydroxychloroquine (PLAQUENIL)
- Mefloquine (LARIUM)
- Primaquine
- Pyrimethamine (DARAPRIM)
- Quinine/Quinidine
- Sulfadoxine/Pyrimethamine (FANSIDAR)

This chapter will be most useful after having a basic understanding of the material in Chapter 49, Chemotherapy of Malaria in *Goodman & Gilman's The Pharmacological Basis of Therapeutics*, 12th Edition. In addition to the material presented here, Chapter 49 in the 12th Edition contains:

- Tables 49-2, 49-3, and 49-4 which provide information about appropriate regimens, including adult and pediatric dosages, for the prevention, treatment, and presumptive self-treatment of malaria
- Figure 49-4 which is an algorithm approach to the treatment of malaria

LEARNING OBJECTIVES

- ☑ Know the stages of the malaria parasite in the human body.
- ☑ Classify antimalarial drugs into those that are effective against only the blood stages of the parasite, those that are effective against both the blood and liver stages, and those that are effective against only the liver stages of the parasite.
- ☑ Understand the use of antimalarial drugs in clinical context, particularly with regard to their mechanism of action, therapeutic uses, and toxicities.
- ☑ Describe the principles and guidelines for the chemoprophylaxis and treatment of malaria.

CRITERIA FOR THE DIAGNOSIS OF MALARIA

- Signs and symptoms consistent with malaria, including fever, chills, malaise, myalgia, headache, ± severe malaria criteria (see Table CRITERIA FOR DIAGNOSIS OF SEVERE MALARIA), plus
- Demonstration of the malaria parasite:
  - Light microscope examination of stained thin or thick smear
  - Rapid diagnostic test
  - Molecular or biophysical-based testing

CRITERIA FOR DIAGNOSIS OF SEVERE MALARIA

Prostration	Jaundice
Impaired consciousness/coma	Severe anemia
Respiratory distress	Acute renal failure
Multiple convulsions	Disseminated intravascular coagulation
Circulatory shock	Acidosis
Pulmonary edema	Hemoglobinuria
Acute respiratory distress syndrome	Parasitemia >5%
Abnormal bleeding	

ANTIMALARIAL DRUG MECHANISMS OF ACTION AND RESISTANCE

DRUG	MECHANISM OF ACTION	MECHANISM OF RESISTANCE
Artemisinin and Derivatives	Production of toxic heme-adducts	Not known at this time
Atovaquone	Inhibits mitochondrial electron transport in the cytochrome bc_1 complex	Nucleotide polymorphisms in the cytochrome b gene
Proguanil	Inhibits dihydrofolate reductase-thymidylate synthase	Mutations in the amino acid sequence near the dihydrofolate-reductase binding site

(Continued)

Chemotherapy of Malaria

CHAPTER 35

DRUG	MECHANISM OF ACTION	MECHANISM OF RESISTANCE
Pyrimethamine	Inhibits *Plasmodium* dihydrofolate-reductase	Mutations in dihydrofolate-reductase binding site
Sulfadoxine	Inhibition of *Plasmodium* dihydropteroate synthase	Mutations in dihydropteroate synthase gene
Chloroquine/ Hydroxychloroquine	Production of toxic heme adducts	Production of a chloroquine efflux transporter
Quinine/Quinidine	Production of toxic heme adducts	Production of an efflux transporter; amplification of *pfmdr 1* gene
Mefloquine	Production of toxic heme adducts. There is also a cytosolic mode of action	Amplification of *pfmdr 1* gene that accumulates drug in digestive vacuole away from cytosolic site of action
Primaquine	Production of reactive oxygen species	Not known at this time

CURRENT ARTEMISININ COMBINATION THERAPY (ACT) REGIMENS

Artemether-lumefantrine*

Artesunate-mefloquine

Artesunate-amodiaquine

Artesunate-sulfoxadine-pyrimethamine

Dihydroartemisinin-piperaquine

*Lumefantrine shares structural similarities with mefloquine and is only formulated with artemether (COARTEM)

CASE 35-1

A 43-year-old woman develops the signs and symptoms of uncomplicated malaria caused by *Plasmodium falciparum*. Her symptoms include fever, chills, malaise, and headache. A microscopic examination of a blood smear confirms the diagnosis. She is treated with the combination therapy artemether-lumefantrine.

a. Why is she treated with the combination product rather than either artemether or lumefantrine alone?

Artemether-lumefantrine is one of several artemisinin-based combination therapies (ACTs). The artemisinins are very potent and fast-acting antimalarials. However, the emergence of *P. falciparum* isolates with an increased tolerance to artemisinins has recently been found. The primary goal of these combination products is to increase treatment efficacy and reduce selection pressure for the emergence of drug resistance. The short $t_{1/2}$ of the artemisinins results in substantial treatment failure rates when artemisinins are used as monotherapy. Combining an artemisinin with a longer-lasting partner drug assures sustained antimalarial activity.

b. What are the pharmacokinetic properties of lumefantrine that make it a good choice in combination with artemether?

Artemisinins rapidly achieve peak serum concentrations; intramuscular artemether peaks at 2 to 6 hours, due to a depot effect at the injection site. Lumefantrine has a large apparent volume of distribution and a terminal elimination $t_{1/2}$ of 4 to 5 days. Administration with a high-fat meal is recommended because it significantly increases lumefantrine absorption. The advantages and disadvantages of the other combination drugs are discussed in detail in Chapter 49 in *Goodman and Gilman's The Pharmacological Basis of Therapeutics*, 12th Edition.

CASE 35-2

A 23-year-old female college student is planning a trip to an area of Africa that is endemic for chloroquine-resistant *P. falciparum*. She has been advised to take atovaquone-proguanil for chemoprophylaxis.

a. When should the drug be started?

Chemoprophylaxis for malaria should begin before exposure and preferably before the traveler leaves home. This is to establish therapeutic blood concentrations and to detect early signs or symptoms of intolerance so that the regimen can be

(Continued)

modified before departing. The regimen should be taken daily while in the malarious area and for 7 days after leaving the area. (see Table 35-1 below and Table 49-2 in *Goodman and Gilman's The Pharmacological Basis of Therapeutics*, 12th Edition for detailed chemoprophylactic regimens.)

b. **What side effects might this patient expect?**

This combination is generally considered safe with no serious side effects. The most common side effects are nausea, vomiting, diarrhea, and headache.

c. **Why is the combination atovaquone-proguanil used rather than either drug alone?**

Resistance to atovaquone when used alone occurs easily. The addition of proguanil markedly reduces the frequency of atovaquone resistance. However, once atovaquone resistance is present the effect of adding the proguanil diminishes.

d. **How do the mechanisms of atovaquone and proguanil work synergistically?**

Atovaquone acts selectively on the mitochondrial cytochrome bc_1 complex to inhibit electron transport and collapse the mitochondrial membrane potential. The antimalarial activity of proguanil is ascribed to cycloguanil (structurally similar to pyrimethamine), a selective inhibitor of the bifunctional plasmodial dihydrofolate reductase-thymidylate synthetase that is crucial for parasite purine and pyrimidine synthesis. Inhibition of this enzyme causes inhibition of DNA synthesis and depletion of folate cofactors. The synergy between proguanil and atovaquone results from the ability of proguanil to enhance the mitochondrial toxicity of atovaquone.

TABLE 35-1 Regimens for the Prevention of Malaria in Nonimmune Individuals (For complete details see Table 49-2 in *Goodman & Gilman's The Pharmacological Basis of Therapeutics*, 12th Edition, Chapter 49)

DRUG	USAGE	COMMENTS
Atovaquone/Proguanil	Prophylaxis in all areas	Begin 1-2 days before travel to malarious areas; take daily at the same time each day while in the malarious area and for 7 days after leaving such area
Chloroquine Phosphate	Prophylaxis only in areas with chloroquine-sensitive malaria	Begin 1-2 weeks before travel to malarious areas; take weekly on the same day of the week while in the malarious area and for 4 weeks after leaving such area
Doxycycline	Prophylaxis in all areas	Begin 1-2 days before travel to malarious areas; take daily at the same time each day while in the malarious area and for 4 weeks after leaving such area
Hydroxychloroquine Sulfate	Alternative to chloroquine for prophylaxis only in areas with chloroquine-sensitive malaria	Begin 1-2 weeks before travel to malarious areas; take weekly on the same day of the week while in the malarious area and for 4 weeks after leaving such area
Mefloquine	Prophylaxis in areas with mefloquine-sensitive malaria	Begin 1-2 weeks before travel to malarious areas; take weekly on the same day of the week while in the malarious area and for 4 weeks after leaving such area
Primaquine	Prophylaxis for short duration travel to areas principally with *Plasmodium vivax*	Begin 1-2 days before travel to malarious areas; take daily at the same time each day while in the malarious area and for 7 days after leaving such area
	For presumptive antirelapse therapy (terminal prophylaxis) to decrease the risk of relapse (*P. vivax, Plasmodium ovale*)	Indicated for persons with prolonged exposure to *P. vivax* and *P. ovale* or both

Source: From the United States Centers for Disease Control and Prevention, Health Information for International Travel 2010 (Yellow Book). http://wwwnc.cdc.gov/travel/content/yellowbook/home-2010.aspx. Accessed January 12, 2010.

Chemotherapy of Malaria　　CHAPTER 35

CASE 35-3

A 28-year-old female university student in Turkey contracts uncomplicated malaria with symptoms of fever, chills, malaise, myalgia, and headache. The director of the clinic in which you work wants to treat her with chloroquine.

a. Is chloroquine an appropriate drug to treat uncomplicated malaria in the country of Turkey?

Chloroquine is highly effective against the erythrocytic forms of *Plasmodium ovale*, *Plasmodium vivax*, *Plasmodium malariae*, *Plasmodium knowlesi*, and chloroquine-sensitive strains of *Plasmodium falciparum*. Turkey is a country in which

(Continued)

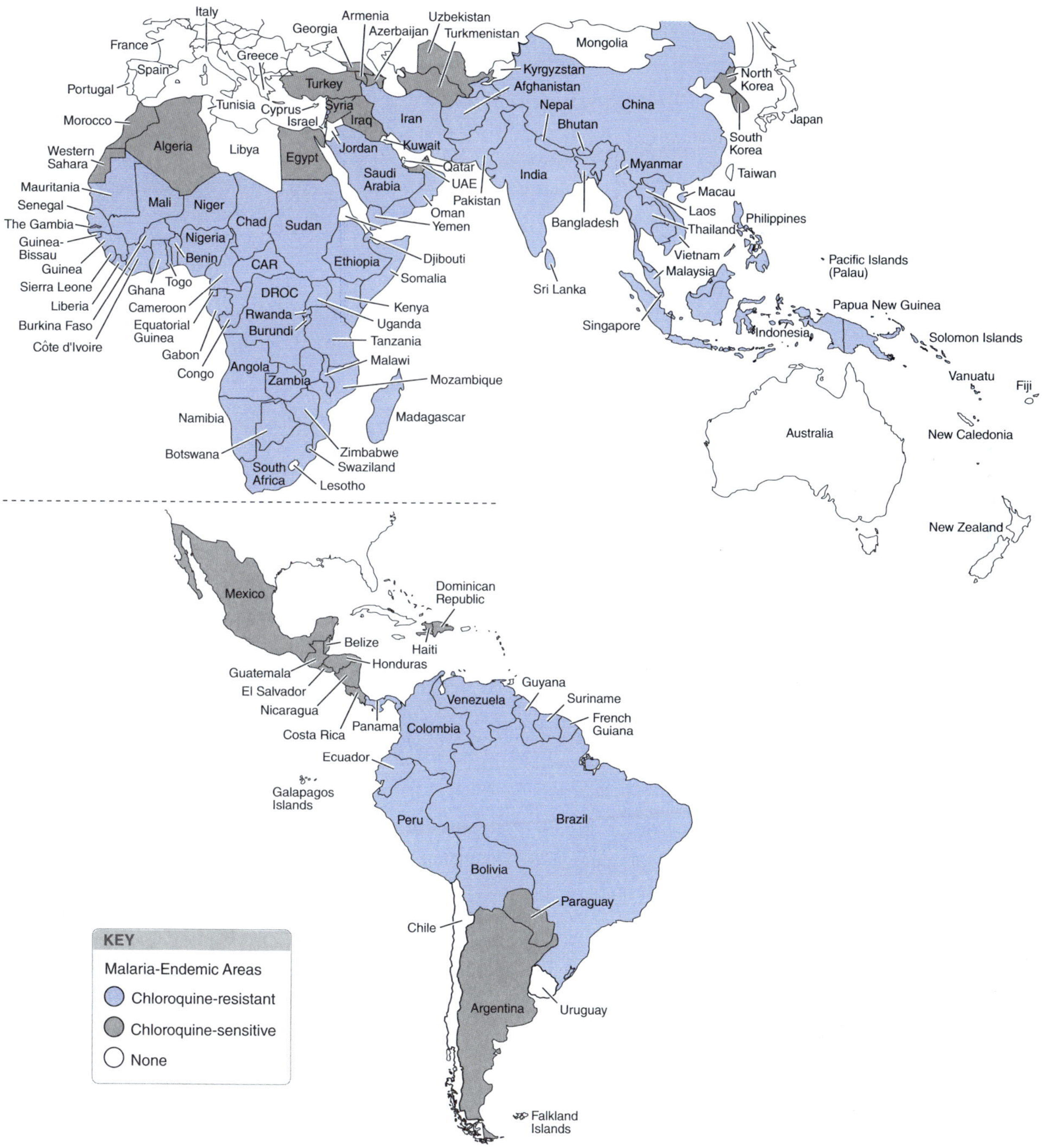

FIGURE 35-1 Malaria-endemic countries in the Americas (bottom) and in Africa, the Middle East, Asia, and the South Pacific (top), 2007. CAR, Central African Republic; DCOR, Democratic Republic of the Congo; UAE, United Arab Emirates. *(Reproduced with permission from Anthony S. Fauci, Eugene Braunwald, Dennis L Kasper, et al, Eds. Harrison's Principles of Internal Medicine, 17 ed. McGraw-Hill, Inc., New York, 2008. Figure 203-2, p. 1282.)*

523

SECTION VII — Chemotherapy of Microbial Diseases

P. falciparum is still chloroquine-sensitive (see Figure 35-1). Although inexpensive and safe, chloroquine has, because of the spread of chloroquine-resistant strains of *P. falciparum* across most malaria-endemic regions of the world (see Figure 35-1), been largely replaced by artemisinin-based combination therapies.

b. **Describe the mechanism of chloroquine's antimalarial activity and the mechanism that *P. falciparum* use to become resistance to its use.**

Malarial parasites digest hemoglobin in the host erythrocytes and sequester the heme as an insoluble, chemically inert pigment called hemozoin. It is thought that chloroquine interferes with this heme detoxification.

A parasite-encoded efflux mechanism may explain the reduced concentrations of chloroquine in the digestive vacuoles of chloroquine-resistant parasites. The polymorphic gene (*pfcrt*, for *P. falciparum* chloroquine resistance transporter) encodes a putative chloroquine transporter that resides in the membrane of the parasite digestive vacuole at the site of hemoglobin degradation and chloroquine action.

c. **What chloroquine toxicities should this student be cautioned about?**

Chloroquine is not recommended for treating patients with epilepsy or myasthenia gravis, and it can cause hemolytic anemia in patients with G6PD deficiency. It should be used cautiously in patients with advanced liver disease. Chloroquine inhibits CYP2D6 and interacts with drugs metabolized by this enzyme.

CASE 35-4

A 34-year-old man has developed uncomplicated malaria in an area that is known to have chloroquine-resistant *P. falciparum* (see Figure 35-1) and is being treated with quinine plus doxycycline.

a. **What are the common toxicities of quinine that should be watched for in this patient?**

Quinine has a triad of dose-related toxicities: cinchonism, hypoglycemia, and hypotension. Cinchonism consists of tinnitus, high-tone deafness, visual disturbances, headache, dysphoria, nausea, vomiting, and postural hypotension. These effects disappear soon after the drug is withdrawn. Hypoglycemia is also common and can be life-threatening if not treated promptly with intravenous glucose.

b. **What are the more severe and rare toxicities and precautions of quinine use?**

Quinine rarely causes cardiac complications (ie, arrhythmias) unless therapeutic plasma concentrations are exceeded. Severe hemolysis can result from hypersensitivity to quinine and therapy should be discontinued immediately if evidence of hemolysis appears. Quinine should be avoided in patients with tinnitus or optic neuritis and in patients with cardiac arrhythmias, the same precautions as for quinidine (see Chapter 29 in *Goodman and Gilman's The Pharmacological Basis of Therapeutics*, 12th Edition).

c. **What are other therapeutic options?**

Other possible choices for treatment of *P. falciparum* malaria in a chloroquine-resistant area are artemether-lumefantrine, atovaquone-proguanil, clindamycin (used in combination with quinine or quinidine), or mefloquine (except in Southeast Asia).

CASE 35-5

A 34-year-old-man in Cambodia has been treated with mefloquine for severe malaria. He returns to the clinic because his symptoms have not subsided.

a. **What is a major limitation to the use of mefloquine in Southeast Asia?**

Mefloquine is reserved for the prevention and treatment of drug-resistant *P. falciparum* and *P. vivax*, but is no longer considered first-line treatment. In areas where malaria is due to multiple drug-resistant strains of *P. falciparum*, such as Southeast Asia, mefloquine is used in combination with an artemisinin compound.

(Continued)

b. What is the mechanism of action of mefloquine?

Mefloquine binds to intraerythrocytic hemozoin similar to chloroquine. It appears that *pfmdr1* gene amplification is a major determinant of mefloquine treatment failure and in vitro mefloquine resistance.

c. Describe the major limitations to the use of mefloquine.

Mefloquine is not recommended for use during pregnancy and pregnancy should be avoided for 3 months after stopping mefloquine because of its prolonged elimination. Mefloquine is associated with neuropsychiatric signs and symptoms, including dizziness, confusion, and headache in 10% (or greater) of patients. Vivid dreams are common. Severe neurotoxicity such as psychosis or seizures is rare.

CASE 35-6

A 46-year-old man with a primary hepatic stage of *P. falciparum* is treated with primaquine.

a. Why was primaquine chosen and what are its major therapeutic uses?

Figure 35-2 shows the life cycle of malaria parasites and Table 35-2 shows the malarial parasite developmental stages targeted by antimalarial drugs. Primaquine acts against primary and latent hepatic stages of *Plasmodium* spp. and prevents relapses in *P. vivax* and *P. ovale* infections. Primaquine is used primarily for the

(Continued)

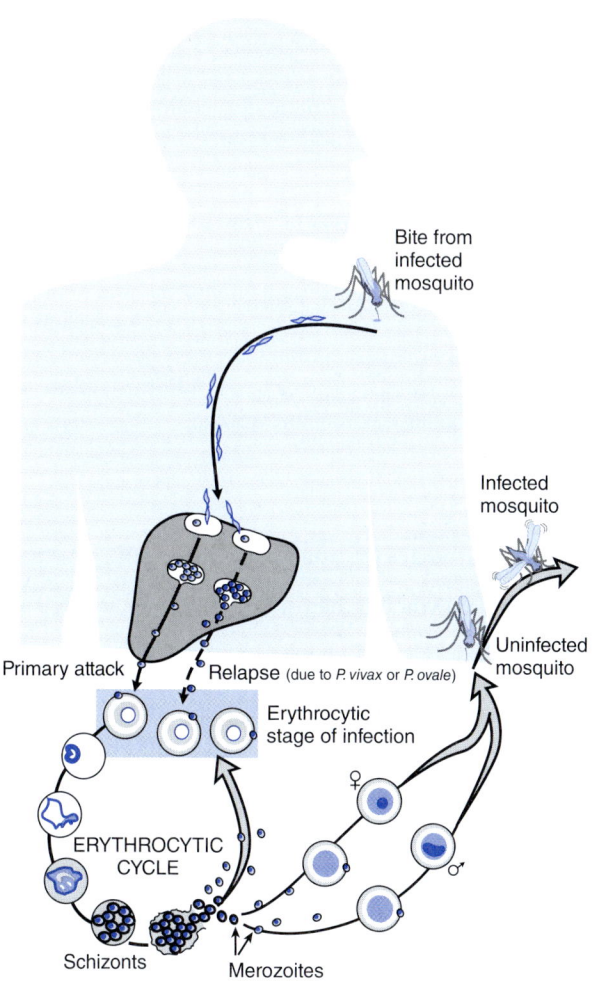

FIGURE 35-2 Life cycle of malaria parasites.

SECTION VII — Chemotherapy of Microbial Diseases

TABLE 35-2 Malarial Parasite Developmental Stages Targeted by Antimalarial Drugs

		EFFECT OF DRUG ON PARASITE VIABILITY				
			LIVER STAGES		BLOOD STAGES	
GROUP	DRUGS	SPOROZOITE	PRIMARY	HYPNOZOITE	ASEXUAL	GAMETOCYTE
1	Artemisinins	–	–	–	+	+
	Chloroquine	–	–	–	+	+/–
	Mefloquine	–	–	–	+	–
	Quinine/Quinidine	–	–	–	+	+/–
	Pyrimethamine	–	–	–	+	–
	Sulfadoxine	–	–	–	+	–
	Tetracycline	–	–	–	+	–
2	Atovaquone/Proguanil	–	+	–	+	+/–
3	Primaquine	–	+	+	–	+

–, no activity; +/–, low to moderate activity; +, important activity.

terminal chemoprophylaxis (shortly before or immediately after a patient leaves an endemic area), and for radical cure of *P. vivax* and *P. ovale* infections because of its high activity against the latent tissue forms of these *Plasmodium* species. Primaquine is often given together with a blood schizonticide, usually chloroquine, to eradicate erythrocytic stages of these *Plasmodia* and to reduce the possibility of emerging drug resistance.

b. **What toxicity is of major concern with primaquine and what precautions are necessary with primaquine?**

Therapeutic or higher doses of primaquine may cause acute hemolysis and hemolytic anemia in patients with G6PD deficiency. About 11% of African-Americans have the A variant of G6PD, and are therefore susceptible to hemolysis caused by primaquine. G6PD deficiency should be ruled out prior to the administration of primaquine. Primaquine should not be given to pregnant women.

CASE 35-7

The student in Case 35-3 asks your general advice regarding malaria therapy.

a. **What is your advice to her (beside what you told her in Case 35-3) regarding chemoprophylaxis for malaria?**

Regimens for malaria chemoprophylaxis include primarily 3 drugs: atovaquone-proguanil and doxycycline that can both be used in all areas, and mefloquine that can be used in areas with mefloquine-sensitive malaria. Other options include chloroquine or hydroxychloroquine in the few areas with chloroquine-sensitive malaria, and primaquine for short duration travel to areas with principally *P. vivax*.

b. **She also asks for advice about treatment should she contract malaria.**

For uncomplicated malaria, chloroquine is the drug of choice for *P. ovale*, *P. knowlesi*, *P. malariae*, and chloroquine-sensitive strains of *P. vivax* and *P. falciparum*. Primaquine

(Continued)

must not be given to patients with G6PD deficiency. For uncomplicated malaria caused by chloroquine-resistant *P. falciparum*, 4 treatment options are available:

- Artemether-lumefantrine
- Atovaquone-proguanil
- Oral quinine with other effective but slower-acting blood schizonticides such as doxycycline or clindamycin
- Mefloquine

For the treatment of severe malaria, no matter the region where the infection was acquired, the recommended treatments are based on intravenous artesunate or quinidine plus a second drug.

c. She is also concerned about getting pregnant during her stay in Turkey and asks if there is a recommended treatment for malaria in pregnant patients?

Chemoprophylaxis during pregnancy is complex, and women should evaluate with expert medical staff the benefits and risks of different strategies. Severe malaria during pregnancy should be treated with intravenous antimalarial treatment according to the general guidelines, taking into account the drugs that should be avoided during pregnancy such as primaquine, mefloquine, and tetracycline.

KEY CONCEPTS

- *P. falciparum* has become progressively more resistant to antimalarial drugs.
- Effective chemoprophylaxis regimens include atovaquone-proguanil, doxycycline, or mefloquine.
- Chemoprophylaxis should be started before exposure, ideally before the traveler leaves home, and continued after returning from a malarious region.
- First-line therapy for uncomplicated malaria is artemether-lumefantrine.
- First-line therapy for severe malaria is IV artesunate followed by atovaquone-proguanil, doxycycline, or mefloquine.
- Primaquine and mefloquine should not be used in pregnant women and primaquine should not be used in patients with G6PD deficiency.

SUMMARY QUIZ

QUESTION 35-1 A physician is planning to treat a 27-year-old woman with primaquine for a documented *P. vivax* infection. Prior to beginning treatment the physician must test the patient for

a. elevated serum amylase.
b. glucose-6-phosphate dehydrogenase deficiency.
c. iron deficiency.
d. elevated serum calcium.
e. vitamin B_{12} deficiency.

QUESTION 35-2 A 35-year-old man will be traveling to an area that is endemic for malaria. His physician starts him on an oral artemisinin derivative prior to his trip. This drug is likely to be ineffective as chemoprophylactic therapy because

a. it is effective against only the blood stages of *P. falciparum*.
b. its side effects are so severe that compliance is unlikely.
c. it is likely to have cross-resistance with chloroquine.
d. its active metabolite dihydroartemisinin has a short plasma $t_{1/2}$.
e. its effectiveness after oral administration is poor.

SECTION VII

Chemotherapy of Microbial Diseases

QUESTION 35-3 A 42-year-old man is being treated with atovaquone-proguanil for uncomplicated *P. falciparum* malaria. This combination product is preferred to the use of atovaquone alone because

a. there is a reduced risk of resistance.
b. proguanil improves the absorption of atovaquone.
c. proguanil decreases the clearance of atovaquone.
d. proguanil decreases the side effects of atovaquone.
e. atovaquone improves the absorption of proguanil.

QUESTION 35-4 Chloroquine-resistance is now common in most parts of the world. The cause of chloroquine-resistance is

a. enhanced metabolism by the *P. falciparum* parasite.
b. poor absorption in the human GI tract.
c. induced metabolism by the human liver after repeat dosing.
d. sequestration of the drug in fat stores.
e. enhanced efflux of drug from the digestive vacuoles of drug-resistant parasites.

QUESTION 35-5 A 19-year-old woman will be traveling to an area that is endemic for mefloquine-sensitive *P. falciparum*. She is to be treated with mefloquine chemoprophylactically. She should be warned about which of the following common side effect?

a. Nosebleeds
b. Tinnitus
c. Vivid dreams
d. Blurred vision
e. A metallic taste

SUMMARY QUIZ ANSWER KEY

QUESTION 35-1 Answer is **b**. Primaquine may cause acute hemolysis and hemolytic anemia in humans with G6PD deficiency. More than 400 genetic variants of G6PD deficiency produce a variable response to oxidative stress. About 11% of African-Americans have a variant of G6PD deficiency; primaquine-induced hemolysis can be even more severe in white ethnic groups, including Sardinians, Sephardic Jews, Greeks, and Iranians as these populations have a G6PD variant in which 2 amino acid substitutions impair both enzyme stability and activity.

QUESTION 35-2 Answer is **d**. Artemisinins have a relatively short plasma $t_{1/2}$ that makes them unsuitable for prophylactic therapy.

QUESTION 35-3 Answer is **a**. Resistance to atovaquone alone in *P. falciparum* develops easily and it is conferred by a nucleotide polymorphisms in the cytochrome b gene located in the parasite's mitochondrial genome. These polymorphyisms appear to affect atovaquone binding. The addition of proguanil markedly reduces the frequency of appearance of atovaquone-resistance.

QUESTION 35-4 Answer is **e**. Chloroquine acts by interfering with heme detoxification in parasite digestive vacuoles. A parasite-encoded efflux mechanism reduces the concentration of chloroquine in the digestive vacuoles of chloroquine-resistant parasites.

QUESTION 35-5 Answer is **c**. Vivid dreams are common with mefloquine. Other toxicities, including disturbed sleep, dysphoria, headache, GI disturbances, and dizziness, can all occur at chemoprophylactic doses. Severe CNS toxicity with mefloquine treatment is not common but can be as high as 0.5% and include seizures, confusion, acute psychosis, and disabling vertigo.

Chemotherapy of Malaria — CHAPTER 35

SUMMARY: ANTIMALARIAL DRUGS

CLASS AND SUBCLASSES	NAMES	CLINICAL USES	RESISTANCE	TOXICITIES COMMON	TOXICITIES UNIQUE; CLINICALLY IMPORTANT
Artemisinins	Dehydroartemisinin Artemether Artesunate Artemether/Lumefantrine	Severe malaria Uncomplicated malaria	No significant cross-resistance to other drugs	Allergic reaction in 1:3000 patients	Reversible decreases in reticulocyte and neutrophil count and increases in transaminases
Atovaquone	MEPRONE	Rarely used by itself	Resistance if used alone	Nausea, vomiting, diarrhea, and headache	May compete with other drugs for plasma protein binding Rifampin and tetracycline reduce plasma concentrations
Proguanil		Rarely used by itself	Resistance develops if used alone	Nausea and diarrhea	Polymorphism in CYP2C family may alter metabolism
Atovaquone-Proguanil	MALARONE	Prophylaxis and treatment of drug-resistant strains of P. falciparum or P. vivax	Resistance to the combination is uncommon unless strain is initially resistant to atovaquone	Nausea, vomiting, abdominal pain, mild reversible elevations in liver transaminases	Not indicated for use in pregnant women due to limited data
Pyrimethamine	Pyrimethamine-sulfadoxine	No longer recommended for the treatment of uncomplicated malaria	Resistance is extensive	Well tolerated in therapeutic doses	Megaloblastic anemia resembling folate deficiency Skin rashes from the sulfa moiety
Chloroquine	ARALEN	Used to treat P. ovale, P. vivax, P. malariae, P. knowlesi, and chloroquine-sensitive P. falciparum	Resistance of P. falciparum is extensive	Well tolerated in therapeutic doses	Not to be used in patients with epilepsy or myasthenia gravis Hemolysis in patients with G6PD deficiency
Quinine/Quinidine		Not used for chemoprophylaxis Treatment of P. falciparum from chloroquine-resistant areas IV quinidine used to treat severe malaria	Resistance is increasing	Cinchonism, Hypoglycemia Hypotension	Should not be used in patients with tinnitus or optic neuritis Use with caution in patients with cardiac arrhythmias Severe hemolysis may occur
Mefloquine	LARIUM	Used for treatment and chemoprophylaxis	Used in combination with an artemisinin compound in area with high drug resistance	Vivid dreams, nausea, vomiting, and vertigo	Contraindicated in patients with seizures or other neuropsychiatric disorders Not recommended in patients with cardiac disorders
Primaquine		Terminal chemoprophylaxis of P. vivax and P. ovale	Partial resistance to P. vivax is reported	Well tolerated in therapeutic doses Nausea and vomiting	Contraindicated in patients with G6PD deficiency and pregnant women

CHAPTER 36

Chemotherapy of Protozoal Infections: Amebiasis, Giardiasis, Trichomoniasis, Trypanosomiasis, Leishmaniasis, and Other Protozoal Infections

DRUGS INCLUDED IN THIS CHAPTER

- Amphotericin B (see Chapter 43)
- Eflornithine (ORNIDYL)
- Fumagillin (FUMIDIL)
- 8-Hydroxyquinolines (iodoquinol; YODOXIN)
- Melarsoprol
- Metronidazole (FLAGYL)
- Miltefosine (IMPAVIDO)
- Nitazoxanide (ALINA)
- Nifurtimox (LAMPIT)
- Benznidazole (ROCHAGAN)
- Paromomycin
- Pentamidine
- Sodium stibogluconate
- Suramin

PROTOZOAL INFECTIONS DISCUSSED IN THIS CHAPTER

- Amebiasis
- Giardiasis
- Cryptosporidiosis

This chapter will be most useful after having a basic understanding of the material in Chapter 50, Chemotherapy of Protozoal Infections in *Goodman & Gilman's The Pharmacological Basis of Therapeutics*, 12th Edition. In addition to the material presented here, the 12th Edition contains:

- A detailed discussion of protozoal infections, including amebiasis, giardiasis, toxoplasmosis, trichomoniasis, cryptosporidiosis, trypanosomiasis, leishmaniasis, babesiosis, balantidiasis, *Isospora belli*, and microsporidia

LEARNING OBJECTIVES

☑ Understand the most common protozoal infections, the clinical symptoms, and the mainstays of therapy.
☑ Describe the mechanisms of action of antiprotozoal drugs.
☑ Understand the treatment of giardiasis, amebiasis, and cryptosporidiosis.
☑ Identify the therapeutic uses of antiprotozoal drugs.
☑ Describe the toxicities and precautions to the use of antiprotozoal drugs.

MECHANISMS OF ACTION AND RESISTANCE OF ANTI-PROTOZOAL DRUGS

DRUG	MECHANISM OF ACTION	MECHANISM OF RESISTANCE
Amphotericin	Binds ergosterol in protozoal membranes to form pores and increase membrane permeability	No significant protozoal resistance
Eflornithine	Inhibition of ornithine decarboxylase	Mutations in ornithine decarboxylase
Fumagillin	Inhibition of methionine-aminopeptidase-2	
Melarsoprol	Inhibition of many enzymes	Mutations in drug transporters
Metronidazole	Forms highly reactive nitro radical anion that targets DNA and other vital biomolecules. Interferes with the pyruvate:ferredoxin oxidoreductase (PFOR) enzyme-dependent electron-transfer reaction, which is essential to anaerobic metabolism in protozoan and bacterial species	Impaired O_2 scavenging capabilities leading to higher local O_2 concentrations and decreased activation of metronidazole. Also mutations in nitroreductase
Miltefosine	Not completely known	Point mutations in transporter which leads to decreased drug uptake
Nitazoxanide	Nitazoxanide (like metronidazole) interferes with the pyruvate:ferredoxin oxidoreductase (PFOR) enzyme-dependent electron-transfer reaction, which is essential to anaerobic metabolism in protozoan and bacterial species	Resistance to nitazoxanide has been induced in *Giardia* in vitro, but resistant clinical isolates have not been reported

(Continued)

Chemotherapy of Protozoal Infections   CHAPTER 36

DRUG	MECHANISM OF ACTION	MECHANISM OF RESISTANCE
Nifurtimox	Nifurtimox is activated by an NADH-dependent mitochondrial nitroreductase, leading to the intracellular generation of nitro radical anions that are thought to account for trypanocidal effects; these radicals form covalent attachments to macromolecules leading to cellular damage that kills the parasites	Reduced nitroreductase expression
Benznidazole	Same as nifurtimox	Same as nifurtimox
Paromomycin	Paromomycin binds to the 30S ribosomal subunit similar to neomycin and kanamycin (see Chapter 40) and shares their spectrum of antibacterial activity	
Pentamidine	In *Trypanosoma brucei* pentamidine is concentrated via an energy-dependent high-affinity uptake system in cells where it is thought to react with a variety of negatively charged intracellular targets	Although failure to concentrate pentamidine is the usual cause of resistance, other mechanisms also may be involved
Sodium Stibogluconate	Pentavalent antimonials act as prodrugs being reduced to the Sb^{3+} species; Sb^{3+} induces a rapid efflux of trypanothione and glutathione from the cells, and also inhibits trypanothione reductase, thereby causing a significant loss of thiol reduction potential in the treated cells	Resistance appears to result from overexpression of glutathione and polyamine biosynthetic enzymes, leading to increased trypanothione levels, which conjugate to the drug
Suramin	Suramin is a slow-acting trypanocide with an unknown mechanism of action; parasites take up the drug by receptor-mediated endocytosis of the protein-bound drug; once in the cell, suramin reacts reversibly with a variety of biomolecules inhibiting many trypanosomal and mammalian enzymes	No significant field resistance

CASE 36-1

A 35-year-old woman comes into your office complaining of diarrhea and abdominal pain for the past 3 days. She has recently returned from a white-water rafting trip. On the trip she fell out of the boat and although she had a life preserver on, she believes that she swallowed considerable amounts of river water.

a. You suspect giardiasis and want to begin treatment after obtaining appropriate specimens. What is giardiasis?

Giardiasis is caused by the protozoan *Giardia intestinalis*, is prevalent worldwide, and is the most common intestinal protozoal infection in the United States. *Giardia* is a zoonosis and cysts shed in the feces of animals and humans can contaminate recreational and drinking water supplies. Infection with *Giardia* results in an asymptomatic carrier state, acute self-limited diarrhea, or chronic diarrhea.

b. How is the diagnosis of giardiasis made?

The diagnosis of giardiasis is made by identification of cysts or trophozoites in fecal specimens or of trophozoites in duodenal contents.

(Continued)

SECTION VII Chemotherapy of Microbial Diseases

COMMON ROUTES OF TOXOPLASMOSIS INFECTION IN HUMANS

- Ingestion of undercooked meat containing cysts
- Ingestion of vegetables contaminated with soil containing cysts
- Direct oral contact with feces of cats shedding cysts
- Transplacental fetal infection with *tachyzoites* from acutely infected mothers

---

c. **After instructing your patient in how to collect fecal specimens, what is the most appropriate therapy to limit the acute diarrhea, to prevent the development of chronic diarrhea, and to prevent the development of a "carrier state"?**

Chemotherapy with a 5-day course of metronidazole or a single dose of tinidazole is usually successful. Paromomycin has been used to treat pregnant women to avoid any possible mutagenic effects of the other drugs.

d. **What are the potential side effects of metronidazole therapy which this patient should be informed about?**

The most common side effects of metronidazole are headache, nausea, dry mouth, vomiting, and diarrhea, and are rarely severe enough to discontinue therapy. More severe neuropathies may include dizziness, vertigo, and rarely encephalopathy, seizures, incoordination, ataxia, and numbness or paresthesias of the extremities; these neuropathies warrant discontinuation of metronidazole.

Metronidazole has a well-documented disulfiram-like effect (see Chapter 9) and patients should be warned not to drink alcoholic beverages during or within 3 days of therapy.

CASE 36-2

A 10-year-old boy is brought into the emergency department with a 2-day history of severe diarrhea. The child is otherwise well with no chronic diseases but appears dehydrated and lethargic. It is summer and the child has been swimming in the public pool every day for the past week.

a. **What organism is most likely causing this child's diarrhea?**

Cryptosporidia protozoa cause diarrhea in a number of animal species including humans. *Cryptosporidium parvum* and *Cryptosporidium hominis* account for almost all infections in humans. Oocysts in feces may be spread by direct human-to-human contact or by contaminated water supplies.

b. **Are there special populations that are vulnerable to cryptosporidiosis?**

Those at risk include travelers, children in day-care facilities, male homosexuals, animal handlers, and health care personnel. Immunocompromised individuals are especially vulnerable.

c. **Are there specific treatments for cryptosporidiosis?**

In most individuals, the infection is self-limited. However, immunocompromised individuals may require hospitalization and supportive care. The most effective therapy for cryptosporidiosis in AIDS patients is the restoration of their immune function. Nitazoxanide is currently the only drug approved for the treatment of cryptosporidiosis in the United States.

CASE 36-3

A 56-year-old woman is diagnosed with amebic colitis. She is started on metronidazole but an infectious disease consultant recommends adding paromomycin to her therapeutic regimen.

a. **Why add the paromomycin when *Entamoeba histolytica* is usually susceptible to metronidazole?**

The cornerstone of therapy for amebiasis is metronidazole which is the drug of choice for the treatment of amebic colitis, amebic liver abscess, and any other extraintestinal form of amebiasis. Because metronidazole is so well absorbed in the gut, concentrations may not be therapeutic in the colonic lumen such that the drug is less effective

(Continued)

Chemotherapy of Protozoal Infections — CHAPTER 36

against cysts. Patients with amebic colitis or amebic liver abscess also should receive a luminal agent such as paromomycin or the 8-hydroxyquinoline compound, iodoquinol. Nitazoxanide, a drug approved for the treatment of cryptosporidiosis and giardiasis, is also active against *E. histolytica*.

b. What is paromomycin and what toxicities and side effects should this patient be warned of?

Paromomycin (aminosidine) is an aminoglycoside used as an oral agent to treat *E. histolytica* infection. Adverse effects after oral administration are rare but include abdominal pain and cramping, epigastric pain, nausea, vomiting, steatorrhea, and diarrhea.

Parenteral administration carries the same risks of nephrotoxicity and ototoxicity as with other aminoglycosides (see Chapter 40).

KEY CONCEPTS

- Amebiasis, giardiasis, trichomoniasis, toxoplasmosis, cryptosporidiosis, trypanosomiasis, and leishmaniasis are common protozoal infections seen worldwide.
- Protozoa multiply rapidly in their hosts and effective vaccines are unavailable.
- Therapy of protozoal infections often requires multiple drugs.
- Antiprotozoal drugs have severe toxicities that require careful monitoring.
- Giardiasis, prevalent worldwide, is the most commonly reported protozoal infection in the United States.
- Trichomoniasis is a sexually transmitted disease common in the United States.
- Treatment of patients with giardiasis or trichomoniasis using either metronidazole or tinidazole is usually successful.

SUMMARY QUIZ

QUESTION 36-1 A 36-year-old woman with the diagnosis of *Trichomonas vaginalis* returns to your office one day after receiving a 2 g oral dose of metronidazole with complaints of flushing, headache, vomiting, and abdominal pain. She states that her symptoms began after she and her husband celebrated their 10th wedding anniversary at a restaurant. The most likely cause of her symptoms is

a. chocolate.
b. red wine.
c. cabbage.
d. pork.
e. coffee.

QUESTION 36-2 A 24-year-old man with the diagnosis of late stage trypanosomiasis caused by *T. brucei gambiense* is being treated with eflornithine. Eflornithine is an inhibitor of ornithine decarboxylase. The parasite and human enzyme are equally susceptible to inhibition by eflornithine. The selective toxicity of eflornithine in parasites is because the

a. human enzyme is protected within vacuoles.
b. parasite accumulates the drug in high concentrations.
c. human enzyme is turned over more rapidly than the parasitic enzyme.
d. human enzyme contains a different molecular site of binding of eflornithine.
e. product of the enzyme in parasites is putrescine.

SECTION VII

Chemotherapy of Microbial Diseases

QUESTION 36-3 Miltefosine is the first orally active drug for the treatment of visceral leishmaniasis. However, because of its teratogenic potential, miltefosine is contraindicated in pregnant women. A suitable alternative in a pregnant woman might be

a. metronidazole.
b. fumagillin.
c. melarsoprol.
d. sodium stibogluconate.
e. pentamidine.

QUESTION 36-4 Amphotericin B is a highly effective drug for the treatment of visceral leishmaniasis. Amphotericin B works in leishmania by

a. inhibiting protein synthesis.
b. binding with and depleting calcium.
c. competing for enzymes that are responsible for folic acid synthesis.
d. inhibiting DNA synthesis.
e. binding with ergosterol precursors in the cell membrane.

QUESTION 36-5 Melarsoprol is the only drug effective for the treatment of

a. late (CNS) stages of *Trypanosoma brucei rhodesiense*.
b. late (CNS) stages of *Trypanosoma brucei gambiense*.
c. early stages of *Trypanosoma brucei rhodesiense*.
d. early stages of *Trypanosoma brucei gambiense*.
e. *Toxoplasma gondii*.

SUMMARY QUIZ ANSWER KEY

QUESTION 36-1 Answer is **b**. Patients taking metronidazole may have a disulfiram-like reaction (see Chapter 9) if they drink alcohol. The symptoms often include flushing, headache, vomiting, and abdominal pain.

QUESTION 36-2 Answer is **c**. The molecular mechanism of eflornithine clearly is inhibition of ornithine decarboxylase. Eflornithine irreversibly inhibits both mammalian and trypanosomal ornithine decarboxylases, thereby preventing the synthesis of putrescine, a precursor of polyamines needed for cell division. Eflornithine inactivates the enzyme through covalent binding of an active-site cysteine residue. The mammalian enzyme is turned over rapidly, whereas the parasite enzyme is stable, and this difference likely plays a role in the drug's selective toxicity. In addition, mammalian cells may be able to replenish polyamine pools through uptake of extracellular polyamines. The parasite lacks efficient polyamine transport mechanisms.

QUESTION 36-3 Answer is **d**. The classic therapy for all species of *Leishmania* is pentavalent antimony (sodium stibogluconate). Though widely used, resistance to this compound has led to widespread failure of this drug in India. Other alternatives might be amphotericin B and paromomycin. Pentamidine is useful for the treatment of cutaneous leishmaniasis.

QUESTION 36-4 Answer is **e**. The mechanism of action of amphotericin B against leishmania is similar to the basis for the drug's antifungal activity (see Chapter 43). Amphotericin complexes with ergosterol precursors in the cell membrane, forming pores that allow ions to enter the cell. Leishmania have a membrane sterol composition similar to fungal pathogens, and the drug binds to these sterols preferentially over the host membrane cholesterol.

QUESTION 36-5 Answer is **a**. Despite the fact that it causes an often fatal encephalopathy in 2 to 10% of patients, melarsoprol has remained the only drug for the treatment of late (CNS) stages of East African trypanosomiasis (sleeping sickness) caused by *Trypanosoma brucei rhodesiense*. This disease is 100% fatal if untreated.

Chemotherapy of Protozoal Infections — CHAPTER 36

SUMMARY: ANTIPROTOZOAL DRUGS

CLASS AND SUBCLASSES	NAMES	CLINICAL USES	RESISTANCE	TOXICITIES COMMON	TOXICITIES UNIQUE; CLINICALLY IMPORTANT
Amphotericin B	AMBISOME	Visceral leishmaniasis (This is an antifungal agent discussed in Chapter 43)	Not of clinical importance	See Chapter 43	See Chapter 43
Eflornithine	DFMO, ORNIDYL	Trypanosomiasis caused by *T. brucei gambiense*	Ineffective against East African trypanosomiasis	Abdominal pain and headache	Pneumonia, fever, seizures, diarrhea
Fumagillin	FUMIDIL B	Keratoconjunctivitis caused by *Encephalitozoon hellem*			
8-Hydroxyquinolines	Iodoquinol and clioquinol	Intestinal colonization with *E. histolytica* (Preferred luminal agent is paromomycin to treat amebiasis)	Not of clinical importance		Peripheral neuropathy and myelo-optic neuropathy
Melarsoprol	MEL B; ARSOBAL	Only drug for treatment of late (CNS) stage of East African trypanosomiasis			Fatal encephalopathy in 2-10% of patients, peripheral neuropathy, hypertension, myocardial damage
Metronidazole	FLAGYL Tinidazole Secnidazole Ornidazole Benznidazole	Trichomoniasis, amebiasis, and giardiasis	Clinical resistance to *T. vaginalis*, anaerobic bacteria, *Helicobacter pylori*	Headache, nausea, dry mouth, vomiting, diarrhea	Dizziness, vertigo, seizures, ataxia, paresthesias
Miltefosine	IMPAVIDO	Leishmaniasis		Vomiting and diarrhea	Contraindicated in pregnant women
Nifurtimox	LAMPIT	American trypanosomiasis		Nausea and vomiting	Psychic disturbance, polyneuritis, CNS excitability
Benznidazole	ROCHAGAN	American trypanosomiasis		Nausea and vomiting	
Nitazoxanide	ALINA	Cryptosporidiosis and giardiasis		Abdominal pain, diarrhea, vomiting, headache	
Paromomycin	HUMATIN	Amebiasis, used in combination with metronidazole to treat amebic colitis and amebic liver abscess		Abdominal pain, nausea, vomiting, diarrhea	Risk of nephrotoxicity and ototoxicity with parenteral use
Pentamidine	PENTAM 300	Early stage *T. brucei gambiense* Used as an aerosol (NEBUPENT) to treat *Pneumocystis carinii*			Intravenous use associated with hypotension, tachycardia, headache, hypoglycemia
Sodium Stibogluconate	PENTOSTAM	Leishmaniasis	Clinical resistance is common	Pain at IM injection site, chemical pancreatitis, elevation of serum hepatic enzymes	Bone marrow suppression, ECG changes include T-wave flattening and prolongation of QT interval
Suramin	BAYER 205	African trypanosomiasis	Not effective against American trypanosomiasis	Nausea, vomiting, malaise, fatigue	Mazzotti reaction with concomitant onchocerciasis (see Chapter 37), renal toxicity, delayed neurotoxicity

CHAPTER 37

Chemotherapy of Helminth Infections

DRUGS INCLUDED IN THIS CHAPTER

- Albendazole (ALBENZA and ZENTEL)
- Diethylcarbamazine (DEC)
- Doxycycline
- Ivermectin (MECTIZAN, STROMECTOL)
- Mebendazole (VERMOX, others)
- Metrifonate (trichlorfon; BILARCIL)
- Niclosamide
- Oxamniquine
- Piperazine
- Praziquantel (BILTRICIDE, DISTOCIDE)
- Pyrantel Pamoate (PIN-X, others)

This chapter will be most useful after having a basic understanding of the material in Chapter 51, Chemotherapy of Helminth Infections in *Goodman & Gilman's The Pharmacological Basis of Therapeutics*, 12th Edition. In addition to the material presented here, the 12th Edition contains:

- A detailed discussion of helminth infections and their treatment including nematodes (roundworms), cestodes (flatworms), and trematodes (flukes)

LEARNING OBJECTIVES

- ☑ Understand the common helminth infections, the clinical symptoms, and the mainstays of therapy.
- ☑ Describe the therapeutic uses of antihelmintic drugs.
- ☑ Understand the mechanisms of actions of antihelmintic drugs.
- ☑ Identify the toxicities and contraindications of antihelmintic drugs.

CASE 37-1

A 3-year-old boy is brought into your office. His mother is complaining that her child is scratching between his legs which has caused irritation and redness.

a. Although you suspect a pinworm (*Enterobius vermicularis*) infection, how is the diagnosis made?

Often the worms or their eggs can be seen in the perianal area early in the morning. A "tape test" is used to diagnose pinworm. In the morning before bathing or using the toilet a piece of cellophane tape is pressed in the skin around the anus, and removed. The tape is then examined with a microscope to look for the worms or their eggs.

b. What is the appropriate treatment of this child?

The relative incidence of common helminthic infections in humans worldwide is illustrated in Figure 37-1. *Enterobius*, pinworm, is one of the most common helminth infections in temperate climates, including the United States. Although this parasite rarely causes serious complications, pruritus in the perianal region can be severe, and scratching may cause secondary infection. Salpingitis or even peritonitis is a rare complication in female patients.

Pyrantel pamoate, mebendazole, or albendazole as a single dose are highly effective in the treatment of *Enterobius* infection. A second dose is often recommended to be administered 2 weeks after the first. The infection easily spreads throughout members of a family, a school, or an institution, and may require treatment of all individuals in close contact with an infected person.

CASE 37-2

A 53-year-old man comes into your office with a 3-month history of weight loss, abdominal pain, and fatigue. His history is also significant for the consumption of partially cooked fish during a camping trip 6 months previously. A physical examination reveals a blood pressure of 140/60 mm Hg, pulse of 72 beats/min, and a respiratory rate of 16 breaths/min. The remainder of his physical examination is also normal with the exception of pale nail beds and skin. A complete blood count shows the presence of a megaloblastic anemia. An examination of a fresh stool specimen reveals the eggs and segments of a worm.

(Continued)

Chemotherapy of Helminth Infections
CHAPTER 37

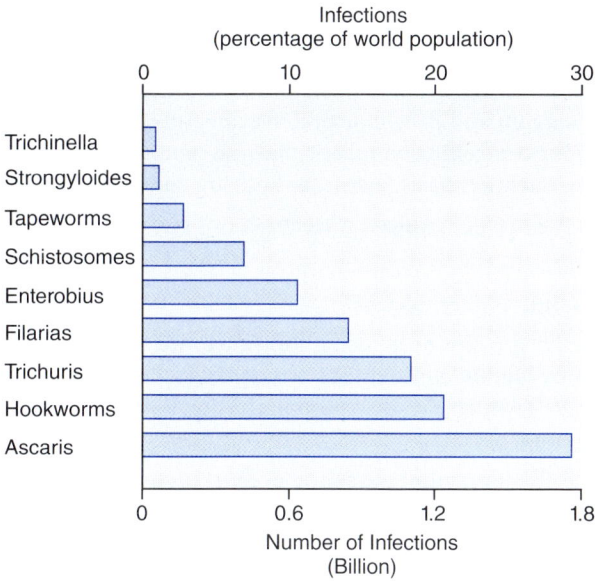

FIGURE 37-1 Relative incidence of helminth infections worldwide.

a. **What is the likely diagnosis?**

Diphyllobothrium latum, known as fish tapeworm, is found most commonly in rivers and lakes of the Northern Hemisphere. Eating inadequately cooked infected fish introduces the larvae into the human intestine. Although most infected individuals are asymptomatic, the most frequent manifestations include abdominal symptoms and weight loss.

b. **What is the cause of this patient's anemia?**

Megaloblastic anemia develops due to a deficiency of vitamin B_{12} (see Chapter 25), which is taken up by the parasite.

c. **What is an appropriate treatment for this patient?**

Praziquantel eliminates the worm and ensures hematological remission.

d. **What are the likely side effects of this treatment?**

Abdominal discomfort, particularly pain, nausea, and diarrhea, may occur shortly after taking praziquantel, and is transient and dose-related. Other adverse effects include headache, dizziness, and drowsiness, and patients should be warned not to drive or operate machinery after taking a dose. Praziquantel is contraindicated in ocular cysticercosis because the host response can irreversibly damage the eye.

CASE 37-3

As a medical missionary to sub-Saharan Africa you are involved with the administration of ivermectin to rural communities for the treatment of onchocerciasis caused by *Onchocerca volvulus*.

a. **What is onchocerciasis?**

Onchocerca volvulus is transmitted by blackflies near fast-flowing streams and rivers in sub-Saharan Africa. Inflammatory reactions, primarily to microfilariae rather than adult worms, affect the subcutaneous tissues, lymph nodes, and eyes. Onchocerciasis is a leading cause of infectious blindness worldwide and results from the cumulative destruction of microfilariae in the eyes that occurs over decades.

b. **What are the usual therapeutic uses of ivermectin?**

Ivermectin is the drug of choice for treatment of onchocerciasis, in adults and children 5 years or older. It is also given in mass drug administration programs in

(Continued)

the Americas and in sub-Saharan Africa. Ivermectin is not curative because it has little effect on adult *Onchocerca volvulus*.

A single annual dose of ivermectin is effective and safe for mass chemotherapy of infections with *Wuchereria bancrofti* and *Brugia malayi*. Ivermectin is as effective as diethylcarbamazine (DEC) for controlling lymphatic filariasis, and unlike DEC, it can be used in regions where onchocerciasis, loiasis, or both are endemic.

Ivermectin administration is the drug of choice for treatment of human strongyloidiasis.

c. Describe the mechanism of action of ivermectin?

Ivermectin immobilizes affected organisms by inducing a tonic paralysis of the musculature. This appears to occur by binding to glutamate-activated Cl^- channels found in nematode nerve or muscle cells, which causes hyperpolarization by increasing intracellular chloride concentration.

Ivermectin has no discernible effect on adult parasites, even in high doses, but affects developing larvae and blocks egress of microfilariae from the uterus of adult female worms.

d. How is ivermectin administered and how is it metabolized?

Peak concentrations of ivermectin in plasma are achieved within 4 to 5 hours after oral administration. The long terminal $t_{1/2}$ of approximately 57 hours reflects a low systemic clearance and a large apparent volume of distribution. Ivermectin is extensively metabolized by hepatic CYP3A4 to at least 10 metabolites.

A P-glycoprotein efflux pump drug transporter located in the endothelium of brain microvasculature appears to reduce ivermectin penetration into the CNS and may explain the paucity of CNS side effects in humans.

e. What are the common side effects associated with the use of ivermectin and what precautions should be considered in the treatment of onchocerciasis?

Ivermectin is well tolerated by uninfected humans. In filarial infections, ivermectin therapy frequently causes a Mazzotti-like reaction to dying microfilariae. The intensity of these reactions relates to the microfilarial burden.

Ivermectin is not approved for use in children younger than 5 years or pregnant women.

KEY CONCEPTS

- Worms pathogenic for humans are classified into roundworms (nematodes), flatworms and flukes (trematodes), and tapeworms (cestodes).
- Anthelmintics are drugs that act either locally within the GI tract to cause expulsion of worms, or systemically against helminthes residing outside the GI tract.
- Acquired resistance to anthelmintics in humans has yet to become a major clinical problem.
- Treatment of loiasis or onchocerciasis should proceed with caution in patients with large parasite burden due to tissue damage caused by destruction of the microfilariae (Mazzotti-like reaction).

SUMMARY QUIZ

QUESTION 37-1 A 32-year-old man is seen because of megaloblastic anemia of unknown origin. After considerable workup, he is discovered to have an intestinal fish tapeworm, *Diphyllobothrium latum*. Treatment with praziquantel eliminates the worm

(Continued)

and cures his anemia. The cause of the anemia in patients with *Diphyllobothrium latum* infection is

a. iron deficiency.
b. vitamin B_{12} deficiency.
c. folic acid deficiency.
d. vitamin E deficiency.
e. intestinal blood loss.

QUESTION 37-2 A 23-year-old woman returns from several years in sub-Saharan Africa. She has lymphadenitis and decreasing eyesight. She is diagnosed with onchocerciasis. Both ivermectin and diethylcarbamazine (DEC) are known to be effective against *Onchocerca volvulus*. Why is ivermectin chosen over DEC in the treatment of onchocerciasis?

a. DEC may worsen ocular lesions.
b. DEC is not absorbed from the GI tract.
c. Ivermectin may be given by intramuscular injection.
d. Resistance to DEC is common.
e. DEC is contraindicated in women.

QUESTION 37-3 A 4-year-old boy is brought into your office because of a possible pinworm infection. Examination of the anal area confirms the diagnosis of *Enterobius* (pinworm). Which of the following drugs would you recommend to treat this infection?

a. Ivermectin
b. DEC
c. Praziquantel
d. Pyrantel pamoate
e. Metrifonate

QUESTION 37-4 A 25-year-old woman immigrant from Guatemala is diagnosed with *Taenia solium* (pork tapeworm) upon examination of a stool specimen. Tests reveal that she has cysticercosis although a magnetic resonance image of the brain with a contrast agent shows no signs of neurocysticercosis. Which of the following drugs would be appropriate for her treatment?

a. Ivermectin
b. DEC
c. Pyrantel pamoate
d. Metrifonate
e. Albendazole

QUESTION 37-5 A 28-year-old man returns to the United States after living 2 years in Brazil. He complains of lethargy. Examination reveals mild liver dysfunction. He is diagnosed with *Schistosoma mansoni*. Which of the following drugs is most appropriate for treating this patient?

a. Praziquantel
b. Ivermectin
c. DEC
d. Albendazole
e. Metrifonate

SUMMARY QUIZ ANSWER KEY

QUESTION 37-1 Answer is **b.** The cause of anemia in *Diphyllobothrium latum* infections is a deficiency of vitamin B_{12}, which is taken up by the parasite.

(Continued)

SECTION VII — Chemotherapy of Microbial Diseases

QUESTION 37-2 Answer is **a.** DEC is contraindicated for the treatment of onchocerciasis because it causes severe reactions related to microfilarial destruction, including worsening ocular lesions. Such reactions are far less severe in response to ivermectin.

QUESTION 37-3 Answer is **d.** In the United States, pyrantel pamoate is sold as an over-the-counter pinworm treatment. High cure rates are achieved after a single oral dose, although it is wise to repeat the treatment after an interval of 2 weeks. If the child is in a day-care center, it may be prudent to recommend that other children in the center seek consultation with a physician and treatment if necessary. An alternate choice would be mebendazole.

QUESTION 37-4 Answer is **e.** Niclosamide is the preferred drug for treatment of intestinal infections with *T. solium*. However, niclosamide poses a risk to people infected with *T. solium* because ova released from drug-damaged gravid worms develop into larvae that can cause cysticercosis. Albendazole is the drug of choice for treating cysticercosis. Treatment of neurocysticercosis is controversial because anthelmintic treatment can shrink brain cysts but also can have adverse consequences leading to seizures and hydrocephalus. Pretreatment with glucocorticoids is advised. Chemotherapy for neurocysticercosis is appropriate only when it is directed at live cysticerci and not against dead or dying cysticerci (as evidenced by neuroimaging).

QUESTION 37-5 Answer is **a.** Praziquantel is the drug of choice for treatment of schistosomiasis. Metrifonate has been used with success in the treatment of *Schistosoma haematobium*, but it is not effective against *S. mansoni*.

SUMMARY: ANTHELMINTIC DRUGS

CLASS AND SUBCLASSES	NAMES	CLINICAL USES	RESISTANCE	TOXICITIES COMMON	TOXICITIES UNIQUE; CLINICALLY IMPORTANT
Benzimidazoles	Albendazole Mebendazole	GI nematodes, including enterobiasis Cystic hydatid disease due to *E. granulosus* Cysticercosis caused by *T. solium*	Resistance among human nematodes is confined to *T. trichiura*	Mild GI symptoms	Liver dysfunction in long-term use Albendazole should not be given to pregnant women
Diethylcarbamazine	DEC	Lymphatic filariasis	Not of clinical significance	Anorexia, nausea, headache	Contraindicated for treatment of onchocerciasis because of Mazzotti reaction
Doxycycline		Treatment of bacterial symbionts of the genus *Wolbachia*		See Chapter 41	See Chapter 41
Ivermectin	MECTIZAN STROMECTOL	Onchocerciasis Lymphatic filariasis Strongyloidiasis	Not of clinical significance Resistance has been observed in livestock and is of concern in mass treatment programs		Mazzotti-like reaction in filarial infections Not approved in children <5 years or in pregnant women
Praziquantel	BILTRICIDE DISTOCIDE	Most cestodes and trematodes that infect humans Schistosomiasis and liver fluke infections	Not of clinical significance	GI symptoms, headache, dizziness	In neurocysticercosis, inflammatory reactions may produce meningismus and seizures

(Continued)

Chemotherapy of Helminth Infections — CHAPTER 37

CLASS AND SUBCLASSES	NAMES	CLINICAL USES	RESISTANCE	TOXICITIES COMMON	UNIQUE; CLINICALLY IMPORTANT
Metrifonate	Trichlorfon	*Schistosoma haematobium*	Not of clinical significance		
Oxamniquine		Second-line drug after praziquantel for *S. mansoni* infection			
Niclosamide		Second-line drug after praziquantel for *T. saginata*, *D. latum*; no longer approved for use in the United States	Not of clinical significance		Poses a risk of causing cysticercosis in patients with *T. solium*
Piperazine		Highly effective against *Ascaris lumbricoides* and *Enterobius vermicularis*, but is superseded by the better tolerated benzimidazoles	Not of clinical significance		
Pyrantel pamoate	PIN-X, others	Pinworm, roundworm, and hookworm infections	Not of clinical significance	Mild GI symptoms, headache, dizziness	Not recommended in pregnant women or children <2 years

CHAPTER 38

Sulfonamides, Trimethoprim-Sulfamethoxazole, Quinolones, and Agents for Urinary Tract Infections

DRUGS INCLUDED IN THIS CHAPTER

- Mafenide (SULFAMYLON) Methenamine
- Nitrofurantoin (FURADANTIN, MICROBID, others)
- Phenazopyridine (PYRIDIUM, others)
- Quinolones (norfloxacin [NOROXIN, others], ofloxacin, [FLOXIN, others], ciprofloxacin [CIPRO, others], moxifloxacin [AVELOX])
- Silver sulfadiazine (SILVADENE, others)
- Sulfacetamide
- Sulfadiazine
- Sulfadoxine (FANSIDAR)
- Sulfamethoxazole
- Sulfasalazine (AZULFADINE, others)
- Sulfisoxazole
- Trimethoprim-sulfamethoxazole (BACTRIM, SEPTRA, others)

BACTERIAL RESISTANCE TO SULFONAMIDES

Resistance to sulfonamides is the consequence of altered enzymatic constitution of the bacterial cell characterized by:

- A lower affinity of dihydropteroate synthesis enzymes.
- Decreased bacterial permeability or active efflux of the drug.
- An alternative metabolic pathway for synthesis of an essential metabolite.
- Increased production of an essential metabolite or drug antagonist.

BACTERIAL RESISTANCE TO QUINOLINES

Resistance to quinolines may develop during therapy via mutations in the bacterial chromosomal genes encoding DNA gyrase or topoisomerase IV (see Figure 38-3), or by active transport of the drug out of the bacteria.

This chapter will be most useful after having a basic understanding of the material in Chapter 52, Sulfonamides, Trimethoprim-Sulfamethoxazole, Quinolones, and Agents for Urinary Tract Infections in *Goodman & Gilman's The Pharmacological Basis of Therapeutics*, 12th Edition. In addition to the material presented here, the 12th Edition contains:

- Structural formulas for each of the drugs in this chapter, in addition to the figures reproduced here
- Table 52-2 which is a compilation of the structural formulas for selected quinolones and fluoroquinolones

LEARNING OBJECTIVES

☑ Understand the mechanism of action of sulfonamide drugs.

☑ Identify the various sulfonamide drugs and categorize them according to their absorption from the gastrointestinal (GI) tract.

☑ Identify the therapeutic uses and untoward effects of sulfonamide drugs including trimethoprim-sulfamethoxazole.

☑ Describe the therapeutic uses, mechanisms of action, and toxicities of quinolone antibiotic drugs.

☑ Identify the uses and limitations of antiseptic and analgesic drugs for the treatment of urinary tract infections.

The mechanism of action of sulfonamides is shown in Figure 38-2 and the resistance to sulfonamides is described in the side bar BACTERIAL RESISTANCE TO SULFONAMIDES

The mechanism of action of quinolines is shown in Figure 38-3 and the resistance to quinolines is described in the side bar BACTERIAL RESISTANCE TO QUINOLINES.

CASE 38-1

A 56-year-old woman presents with symptoms of her second urinary tract infection within 2 months. She has no fever and her white blood cell count is not elevated. A previous culture showed *Escherichia coli*, and she responded well to the combination of trimethoprim-sulfamethoxazole. After obtaining the appropriate cultures and sensitivities you decide to treat her again with this combination.

a. **What is unique about the mechanism of action of this combination that makes it effective in treating bacterial infections?**

The sulfonamides can be classified on the basis of the rapidity with which they are absorbed and excreted (see Table 38-1). The structural formulas of selected members of this class are shown in Figure 38-1.

The antimicrobial activity of the combination of trimethoprim and sulfamethoxazole results from its actions on 2 steps of the enzymatic pathway for the synthesis of tetrahydrofolic acid (see Figure 38-2). Mammalian cells use preformed folates from the diet and do not synthesize the compound. Trimethoprim is a highly selective inhibitor of dihydrofolate reductase of lower organisms. This relative selectivity is vital because dihydrofolate reductase function is essential to all species.

b. **The culture of the urine shows again *Escherichia coli* sensitive to the combination of trimethoprim-sulfamethoxazole. Why is this step necessary in this patient with a previous urinary tract infection?**

(Continued)

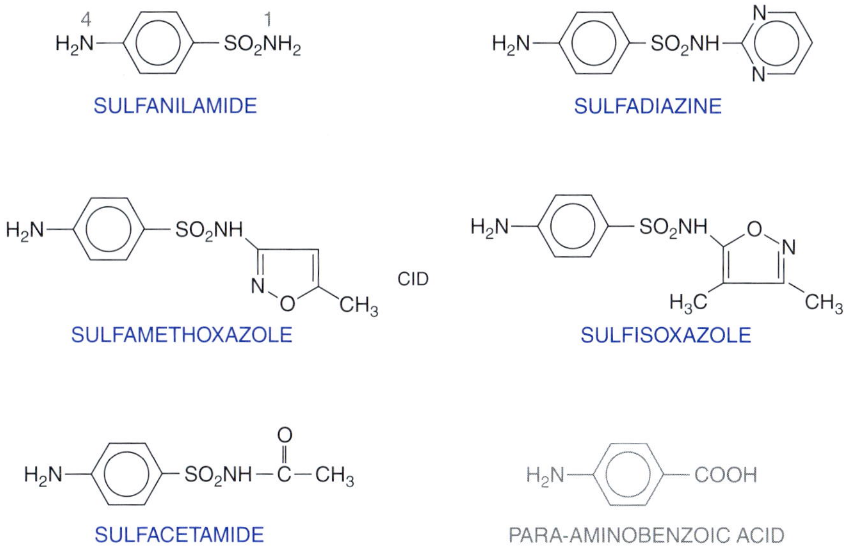

Sulfonamides, Trimethoprim-Sulfamethoxazole, Quinolones, and Agents

CHAPTER 38

FIGURE 38-1 Structural formulas of selected sulfonamides and para-aminobenzoic acid. The N of the para-NH_2 group is designated as N4; that of the amide NH_2, as N1.

Treatment of uncomplicated lower urinary tract infection (UTI) with trimethoprim-sulfamethoxazole often is highly effective for sensitive bacteria. The combination appears to have special efficacy in chronic and recurrent infections of the urinary tract.

Bacterial resistance to trimethoprim-sulfamethoxazole is an increasing problem, although resistance is lower than it is to either agent alone. Resistance is often due to the acquisition of a plasmid that codes for an altered dihydrofolate reductase.

c. Since the combination trimethoprim-sulfamethoxazole affects folate synthesis, does it induce folate deficiency in humans? Of what untoward effects should this patient be warned?

Trimethoprim-sulfamethoxazole, in recommended dosage, does not induce folate deficiency in normal persons. The margin between toxicity for bacteria and that for humans may be relatively narrow when the cells of the patient are deficient in folate. In such cases, trimethoprim-sulfamethoxazole may cause or precipitate megaloblastosis, leucopenia, or thrombocytopenia.

About 75% of the untoward effects involve the skin and are due to the sulfa moiety in sulfamethoxazole. Exfoliative dermatitis, Stevens-Johnson syndrome, and epidermal necrolysis are rare, occurring primarily in older individuals. Glossitis and stomatitis are relatively common.

TABLE 38-1 Classification of Sulfonamides According to Absorption and Elimination Kinetics

CLASS	SULFONAMIDE	SERUM $t_{1/2}$ (hours)
Absorbed and eliminated rapidly	Sulfisoxazole Sulfamethoxazole Sulfadiazine	5-6 11 10
Poorly absorbed, active in bowel	Sulfasalazine	–
Used topically	Sulfacetamide Silver sulfadiazine	– –
Long-acting (absorbed rapidly but eliminated slowly)	Sulfadoxine	100-230

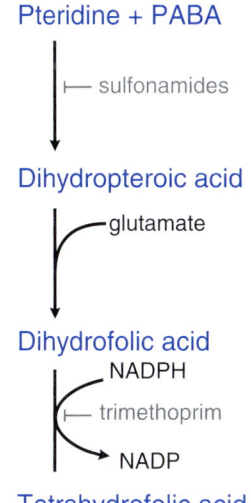

FIGURE 38-2 Steps in folate metabolism blocked by sulfonamides and trimethoprim. PABA, para-amino benzoic acid

SECTION VI Chemotherapy of Microbial Diseases

CASE 38-2

A 42-year-old man has been treated with ciprofloxacin for a known *Hemophilus influenza* infection of the respiratory tract for 2 weeks without improvement of symptoms. Although an initial culture showed sensitivity of the organism to ciprofloxacin, a repeat culture shows that the organism is now resistant.

a. How does resistance develop to the quinolones?

Resistance to the quinolone drugs may develop during therapy via mutations in the bacterial chromosomal genes encoding DNA gyrase or topoisomerase IV, or by active transport of the drug out of the bacteria (see Side Bar BACTERIAL RESISTANCE TO QUINOLINES). Resistance has increased after the introduction of the fluoroquinolones, especially in *Pseudomonas* and *Staphylococci*. Increasing resistance is being observed in *C. jejuni*, *Salmonella*, *N. gonorrhoeae*, and *S. pneumoniae*.

b. How can the manner in which quinolones are administered affect the development of resistance?

As mentioned in Chapter 34, the pharmacokinetic and pharmacodynamic parameters of antimicrobial agents are important in preventing the selection and spread of resistant strains and have led to the concept of the mutation-prevention concentration, which is the lowest concentration of antimicrobial that prevents selection of resistant bacteria from high bacterial inocula. β-Lactams are time-dependent agents without significant post-antibiotic effects, resulting in bacterial eradication when unbound serum concentrations exceed MICs of these agents against infecting pathogens for more than 40 to 50% of the dosing interval. By contrast, fluoroquinolones are concentration- and time-dependent agents, resulting in bacterial eradication when unbound serum area-under-the-curve-to-MIC ratios exceed 25 to 30. An extended release formulation of ciprofloxacin exemplifies this principle.

c. What is the mechanism of action of the quinolones?

The quinolone antibiotics target bacterial DNA gyrase and topoisomerase IV (see Figure 38-3). For many gram-positive bacteria (such as *S. aureus*), topoisomerase IV is the primary activity inhibited by the quinolones. In contrast, DNA gyrase is the primary quinolone target in many gram-negative microbes (such as *E. coli*).

The quinolones inhibit gyrase-mediated DNA supercoiling at concentrations that correlate well with those required to inhibit bacterial growth. Mutations of the gene that encodes the gyrase A subunit polypeptide can confer resistance to these drugs.

Topoisomerase IV separates interlinked (catenated) daughter DNA molecules that are the product of DNA replication. Eukaryotic cells do not contain DNA gyrase, but they do contain a conceptually and mechanistically similar type II DNA topoisomerase that removes positive supercoils from DNA to prevent its tangling during replication. Quinolones inhibit eukaryotic type II topoisomerase only at concentrations much higher than those that inhibit bacterial DNA gyrase.

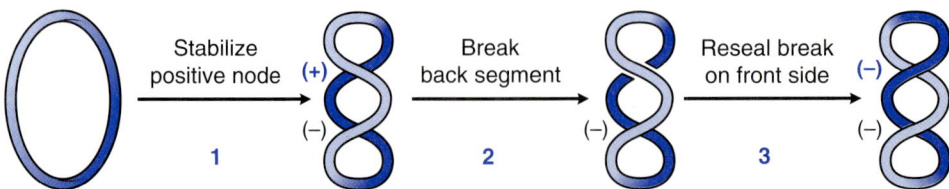

FIGURE 38-3 Model of the formation of negative DNA supercoils by DNA gyrase. The enzyme binds to 2 segments of DNA (1), creating a node of positive (+) superhelix. The enzyme then introduces a double-strand break in the DNA and passes the front segment through the break (2). The break is then resealed (3), creating a negative (−) supercoil. Quinolones inhibit the nicking and closing activity of the gyrase and, at higher concentrations, block the decatenating activity of topoisomerase IV. (*From Cozzarelli NR. DNA gyrase and the supercoiling of DNA. Science, 1980, 207:953-960. Reprinted with permission from AAAS.*)

Sulfonamides, Trimethoprim-Sulfamethoxazole, Quinolones, and Agents

CHAPTER 38

CASE 38-3

A 48-year-old man has had chronic urinary tract infections due to loss of bladder control following a spinal cord injury. He is now being treated with nitrofurantoin chronically to suppress *E. coli* which has been the organism most commonly cultured from his urinary tract.

a. What kind of a drug is nitrofurantoin and what is its mechanism of action?

Nitrofurantoin is used for the prevention and treatment of infections of the urinary tract. Enzymes capable of reducing nitrofurantoin result in the formation of reactive intermediates that damage DNA. The selective antimicrobial activity is due to the fact that bacteria reduce nitrofurantoin more rapidly than do mammalian cells. The antibacterial activity is higher in an acidic urine. Nitrofurantoin is approved only for the treatment of urinary tract infections caused by microorganisms known to be susceptible to the drug. Resistance to nitrofurantoin occurs more frequently than resistance to fluoroquinolones or trimethoprim-sulfamethoxazole, making nitrofurantoin a second-line agent for treatment of urinary tract infections.

b. Should this patient develop a systemic infection, would nitrofurantoin be effective?

Nitrofurantoin is absorbed rapidly and completely from the GI tract, but antibacterial concentrations are not achieved in plasma because the drug is eliminated rapidly. Forty percent of nitrofurantoin is excreted unchanged into the urine.

c. What are the common untoward effects of nitrofurantoin?

The most common untoward effects of nitrofurantoin are nausea, vomiting, and diarrhea. Hypersensitivity reactions include chills, fever, leucopenia, granulocytopenia, hemolytic anemia (associated with glucose-6-phosphate dehydrogenase [G6PD] deficiency), cholestatic jaundice, and hepatocellular damage. Chronic active hepatitis is an uncommon but serious side effect. Interstitial pulmonary fibrosis can occur in patients taking the drug chronically. Nitrofurantoin colors the urine brown.

KEY CONCEPTS

- Sulfonamides inhibit the incorporation of para-amino-benzoic acid (PABA) into tetrahydrofolic acid (see Figure 38-2).
- Trimethoprim prevents the reduction of dihydrofolate to tetrahydrofolate (see Figure 38-2).
- The combination of sulfamethoxazole and trimethoprim inhibits 2 sequential steps in the bacterial synthesis of tetrahydrofolate, thus increasing its antibacterial activity and reducing the development of resistance.
- Sulfonamide drugs (see Table 38-1) can be divided into:
    - Those that are well-absorbed and rapidly excreted
    - Those that are poorly absorbed and are effective in bowel lumen or used topically
    - Those that are long-acting
- Sulfonamides have activity against gram-positive and gram-negative organisms.
- Resistant strains have become common.
- Adverse reactions to sulfonamides frequently involve the skin and some are serious.
- Hypersensitivity reactions to repeated use of sulfonamides are common.
- Quinolones are effective orally for a wide variety of microorganisms and are commonly used to treat urinary tract infections, traveler's diarrhea, and respiratory tract infections.
- Urinary antiseptics are commonly used to prevent or suppress urinary tract infections in susceptible patients.
- Phenazopyridine, a urinary analgesic, is used to treat the symptoms of dysuria and frequency.

SECTION VI
Chemotherapy of Microbial Diseases

SUMMARY QUIZ

QUESTION 38-1 Sulfonamide drugs are selective for sensitive bacteria as compared to mammalian cells because

a. mammalian cells have the ability to extrude sulfonamide drugs.
b. mammalian cells do not take up sulfonamide drugs.
c. mammalian cells require preformed folic acid.
d. bacterial cells accumulate sulfonamide drugs more than mammalian cells.
e. sulfonamide drugs interfere with the synthesis of vitamin B_{12} in bacterial cells but not mammalian cells.

QUESTION 38-2 Mafenide is a sulfonamide drug that is used topically in burn patients. If the burn area is extensive and mafenide is sufficiently absorbed, a metabolic acidosis may occur because the mafenide

a. inhibits carbonic anhydrase.
b. is an acid.
c. inhibits folic acid excretion.
d. depresses respiration and causes the accumulation of carbon dioxide.
e. causes an accumulation of dihydropteroic acid.

QUESTION 38-3 In the combination drug trimethoprim-sulfamethoxazole, the trimethoprim moiety is selective for bacterial cells compared to mammalian cells because the trimethoprim

a. is accumulated in bacterial cells.
b. is a selective inhibitor of dihydrofolate reductase in lower organisms.
c. destroys bacterial cell walls.
d. inhibits the incorporation of PABA into dihydropteroic acid.
e. inhibits bacterial protein synthesis.

QUESTION 38-4 A 23-year-old pregnant woman presents with the signs and symptoms of a urinary tract infection. She is 3 months pregnant. The choice of a trimethoprim-sulfisoxazole drug over a fluoroquinolone drug might be recommended because

a. the likely bacteria involved in a UTI during pregnancy are not sensitive to fluoroquinolones.
b. in pregnancy, the fluoroquinolone drugs are not absorbed after oral administration.
c. the fluoroquinolones are contraindicated in pregnancy.
d. trimethoprim-sulfisoxazole achieves much higher plasma concentrations than fluoroquinolone drugs in pregnancy.
e. trimethoprim-sulfamethoxazole also has urinary analgesic effects.

QUESTION 38-5 A 46-year-old woman has a urinary tract infection which has become a systemic infection with fever and lethargy. Nitrofurantoin, an effective urinary antiseptic, would not be recommend for her treatment because

a. the bacterial organism is likely not sensitive to nitrofurantoin.
b. nitrofurantoin is bacteriostatic.
c. effective concentrations of nitrofurantoin are not achieved in the kidney or bladder.
d. effective concentrations of nitrofurantoin are not achieved in the plasma.
e. bacterial resistance to nitrofurantoin is common.

Sulfonamides, Trimethoprim-Sulfamethoxazole, Quinolones, and Agents

CHAPTER 38

SUMMARY QUIZ ANSWER KEY

QUESTION 38-1 Answer is **c**. In sensitive bacteria, sulfonamide drugs inhibit the enzyme responsible for the incorporation of PABA into dihydropteroic acid, the immediate precursor of folic acid (see Figure 38-2). Mammalian cells require preformed folic acid, cannot synthesize it, and are insensitive to drugs that act by inhibiting the synthesis of folic acid.

QUESTION 38-2 Answer is **a**. Mafenide and its metabolite inhibit carbonic anhydrase, and the urine becomes alkaline. Metabolic acidosis with compensatory tachypnea and hyperventilation may ensue.

QUESTION 38-3 Answer is **b**. Trimethoprim is a highly selective inhibitor of dihydrolate reductase in bacteria; approximately 100,000 times more drug is required to inhibit human reductase than the bacterial enzyme. This relative selectivity is vital because this enzymatic function is essential to all species.

QUESTION 38-4 Answer is **c**. The fluoroquinolones are contraindicated in pregnancy.

QUESTION 38-5 Answer is **d**. Antibacterial concentrations of nitrofurantoin are not achieved in plasma following oral administration of recommended doses because the drug is eliminated rapidly.

SUMMARY: SULFONAMIDES, TRIMETHOPRIM-SULFAMETHOXAZOLE, QUINOLONES, AND AGENTS FOR URINARY TRACT INFECTIONS

CLASS AND SUBCLASSES	NAMES	CLINICAL USES	RESISTANCE	TOXICITIES COMMON	TOXICITIES UNIQUE; CLINICALLY IMPORTANT
	Sulfisoxazole	Rapidly absorbed and eliminated. Used in combination with erythromycin for otitis media		Because of high solubility, it infrequently causes hematuria or crystalluria	Use with caution in patients with impaired renal function. Hypersensitivity reactions
	Sulfamethoxazole Fixed-dose combinations with trimethoprim	Urinary tract infections. Slightly slower absorption than sulfisoxazole			Insoluble acetylated form in the urine may cause crystalluria
	Sulfadiazine	Absorbed rapidly and acetylated form is excreted slowly			Insoluble acetylated form may cause crystalluria
	Sulfasalazine (see Chapter 33)	Poorly absorbed and is used for ulcerative colitis and regional enteritis		Side effects and toxicities are due to the sulfapyridine moiety	Infertility in males. Should not be used in patients with known sulfa drug hypersensitivity
	Sulfacetamide	Used primarily for ophthalmic infections			Should not be used in patients sensitive to sulfa drugs
	Silver sulfadiazine	Used topically to reduce the incidence of infections from burns	Resistance is known to occur	Burning, itching, and rash	Should not be used in patients with known hypersensitivity to sulfa drugs

SECTION VI: Chemotherapy of Microbial Diseases

CLASS AND SUBCLASSES	NAMES	CLINICAL USES	RESISTANCE	TOXICITIES COMMON	TOXICITIES UNIQUE; CLINICALLY IMPORTANT
	Mafenide	Used topically to prevent colonization of burns		Intense pain at site of application	Superinfection with *Candida* may be a problem. Due to inhibition of carbonic anhydrase metabolic acidosis may occur
	Sulfadoxine	Prophylaxis and treatment of malaria (see Chapter 35)			Severe skin reactions, eg, Stevens-Johnson syndrome
	Trimethoprim—Sulfamethoxazole	Urinary tract infections. Treatment of *Pneumocystis jirovecii* in AIDS patients	The emergence of resistant bacteria may limit its usefulness	Skin rashes and other dermatologic reactions. Glossitis and stomatitis are common	Should not be used in patients with known hypersensitivity to sulfa drugs
Quinolones	Ciprofloxacin, Ofloxacin, Norfloxacin, Levofloxacin, Moxifloxacin	Urinary tract infections, prostatitis, sexually transmitted diseases, traveler's diarrhea, respiratory infections, bone, joint, and soft tissue infections	Resistance may develop during therapy	Nausea, vomiting, abdominal discomfort	Headache and dizziness. Photosensitivity. Achilles tendon rupture in patients >60 years of age. Should be used with caution in patients taking antiarrhythmic agents that prolong QT interval
Urinary Antiseptics	Methenamine	Chronic suppressive therapy of urinary tract infections			Combines with sulfa drugs causing mutual antagonism. Mandelate moiety causes crystalluria
	Nitrofurantoin	Urinary tract infections; cannot be used for systemic infections	Resistance is more common than to fluoroquinolones	Nausea, vomiting, diarrhea	Colors urine brown. Hypersensitivity reactions. Interstitial pulmonary fibrosis. Should not be used in pregnant women or patients with impaired renal function
Urinary Analgesics	Phenazopyridine	Urinary analgesia to alleviate symptoms of dysuria			Colors urine orange or red

Penicillins, Cephalosporins, and Other β-Lactam Antibiotics

CHAPTER 39

This chapter will be most useful after having a basic understanding of the material in Chapter 53, Penicillins, Cephalosporins, and Other β-Lactam Antibiotics in *Goodman & Gilman's The Pharmacological Basis of Therapeutics*, 12th Edition. In addition to the material presented here, the 12th Edition contains:

- A detailed discussion of the mechanisms of action and resistance of the penicillins and cephalosporins
- A detailed discussion of each of the penicillins and cephalosporins, including their pharmacokinetics and therapeutic uses in specific infections
- Figure 53-3 which shows a comparison of the structure and composition of gram-positive and gram-negative bacterial cell walls
- Table 53-1 which shows the chemical structures and major properties of the various penicillins
- Table 53-2 which shows the chemical structures and dosage forms of selected cephalosporins and related compounds
- Table 53-3 which shows the cephalosporin generations and the useful spectrum of each generation

LEARNING OBJECTIVES

- ☑ Understand the mechanisms of action of the penicillins, cephalosporins, and other β-lactam antibiotics.
- ☑ Understand the mechanisms of resistance of the penicillins, cephalosporins, and other β-lactam antibiotics.
- ☑ Describe the therapeutic effects of the penicillins, cephalosporins, and other β-lactam antibiotics.
- ☑ Describe the untoward effects and contraindications of the penicillins, cephalosporins, and other β-lactam antibiotics.

DRUGS INCLUDED IN THIS CHAPTER

Penicillins
- Penicillin G
- Penicillin V
- Methicillin
- Oxacillin (BACTOCILL)
- Nafcillin
- Ampicillin
- Amoxicillin
- Carbenicillin
- Ticarcillin
- Mezlocillin
- Piperacillin

Cephalosporins
- Cephazolin (ANCEF, KEFZOL, others)
- Cephalexin (KEFLEX, others)
- Cefadroxil (DURACEF)
- Cephradine (VELOCEF)
- Cefuroxime (ZANACEF)
- Cefuroxime axetil (CEFTIN)
- Cefprozil (CEFZIL)
- Cefmetazole (ZEFAZONE)
- Loracarbef (LORABID)
- Cefotaxime (CLAFORAN)
- Ceftriaxone (ROCEPHIN)
- Cefdinir (OMNICEF)
- Cefditoren pivoxil (SPECTRACEF)
- Ceftibuten (CEDAX)
- Cefpodoxime proxetil (VANTIN)
- Ceftizoxime (CEFIZOX)
- Cefoperazone (CEFOBID)
- Ceftazidime (FORTAZ, others)
- Cefepime (MAXIPINE)

Other β-Lactam Antibiotics
- Imipenem (PRIMAXIN)
- Meropenem (MERREM)
- Doripenem (DORIBAX)
- Ertapenem (INVANZ)
- Aztreonam (AZACTAM)

(continues)

MECHANISMS OF ACTION AND RESISTANCE OF PENICILLINS, CEPHALOSPORINS, AND β-LACTAMASE INHIBITORS

DRUGS	MECHANISM OF ACTION	MECHANISM OF RESISTANCE
Penicillins	Inhibition of cell wall peptidoglycan synthesis (see Figure 39-1) Binding to penicillin-binding proteins (see Figure 53-3 Goodman and Gilman's The Pharmacological Basis of Therapeutics, 12th Edition)	Inactivated by β-lactamases (see Figure 39-2) Antibiotic efflux pumps of gram-negative bacteria (see Figure 39-3)
Cephalosporins	Same as for penicillins	Same as for penicillins
Carbapenems	Same as for penicillins	Resistant to hydrolysis by β-lactamases (see individual drugs
β-Lactamase Inhibitors	Inactivate certain β-lactamases	Not appropriate

SECTION VII

Chemotherapy of Microbial Diseases

DRUGS INCLUDED IN THIS CHAPTER (Cont.)

β-Lactamase Inhibitors

- Clavulanic acid (AUGMENTUM, combination with amoxicillin; TIMENTIN, combination with ticarcillin)
- Sulbactam (UNASYN, combination with ampicillin)
- Tazobactam (ZOSYN, combination with piperacillin)

MECHANISMS OF BACTERIAL RESISTANCE TO PENICILLINS AND CHEPHALOSPORINS

- Structural differences in penicillin-binding proteins (PBPs)
- Decreased affinity for PBPs
- Inability of antibiotic to penetrate to site of action
- Efflux pumps that extrude antibiotic (see Figure 39-3)
- Enzymatic (β-lactamase) destruction of antibiotic (see Figure 39-2)

CLASSES OF β-LACTAMASE ENZYMES

- Class A—includes the extended-spectrum β-lactamases (ESBLs) that degrade penicillins, some cephalosporins, and, in some instances, carbapenems.
- Class B—are Zn^{2+}-dependent enzymes that destroy all β-lactams except aztreonam.
- Class C—active against cephalosporins.
- Class D—includes cloxacillin-degrading enzymes.

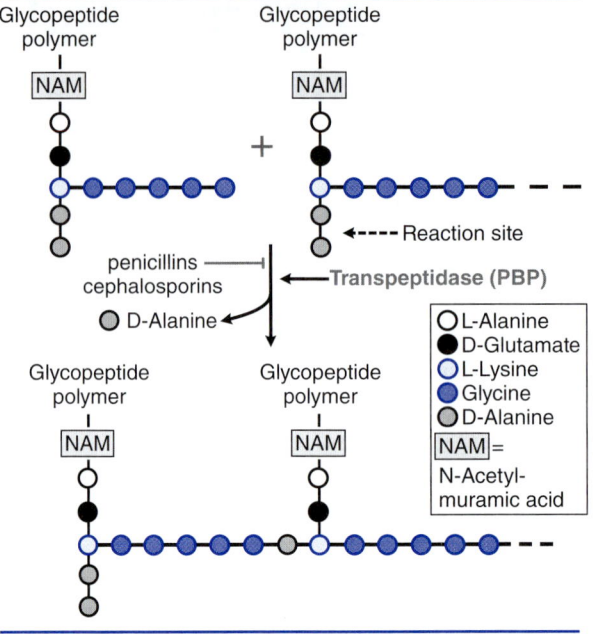

FIGURE 39-1 Action of β-lactam antibiotics in *Staphylococcus aureus*. The bacterial cell wall consists of glycopeptide polymers (a NAM-NAG amino-hexose backbone) linked via bridges between amino acid side chains. In *S. aureus,* the bridge is $(Gly)_5$-D-Ala between lysines. The cross-linking is catalyzed by a transpeptidase, the enzyme that penicillins and cephalosporins inhibit. NAM, *N*-acetyl-muramic acid; NAG, *N*-acetyl-glucosamine.

CASE 39-1

A 56-year-old man is brought to hospital with a productive cough and temperature of 103°F. A chest X-ray reveals pneumonia in the left lower lobe. After obtaining sputum and blood cultures he is started on an intramuscular injection of penicillin G. His symptoms do not improve over the next 24 hours and the cultures return showing *S. pneumoniae* not sensitive to penicillin.

a. What is the mechanism of action of penicillin to sensitive bacteria?

The cell walls of bacteria are essential for their normal growth and development. Peptidoglycan is a heteropolymeric compound of the cell wall that provides rigid mechanical stability by virtue of its highly cross-linked latticework structure (see Figure 39-1). Figure 53-3 in *Goodman and Gilman's The Pharmacological Basis of Therapeutics*, 12th Edition shows a comparison of the structure and composition of

(Continued)

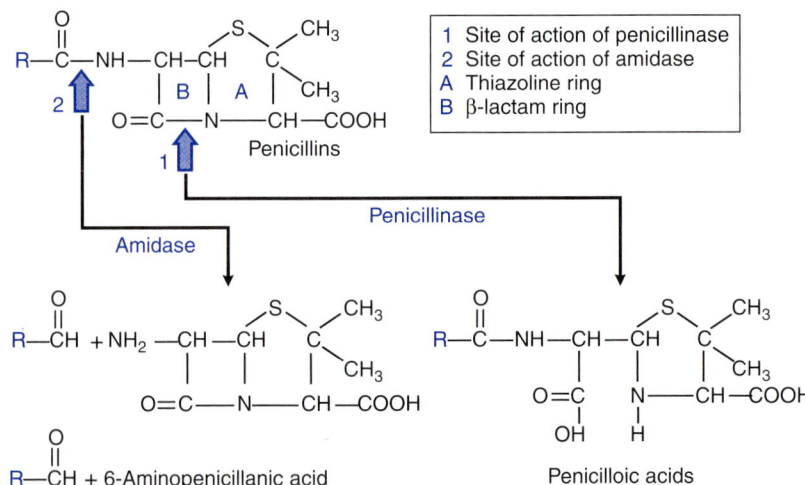

FIGURE 39-2 Structure of penicillins and products of their enzymatic hydrolysis.

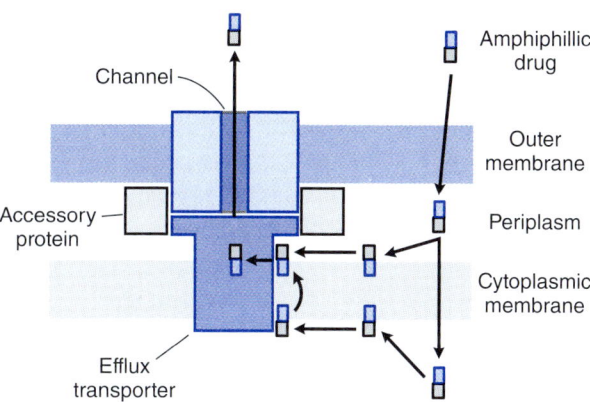

FIGURE 39-3 Antibiotic efflux pumps of gram-negative bacteria. Multidrug efflux pumps traverse both the inner and outer membranes of gram-negative bacteria. The pumps are composed of a minimum of 3 proteins and are energized by the proton motive force. Increased expression of these pumps is an important cause of antibiotic resistance. (*Reprinted with permission from Oxford University Press. Nikaido H. Antibiotic resistance caused by gram-negative multidrug efflux pumps.* Clin Infect Dis, *1998, 27[suppl I]:S32-S41. © 1998 by the Infectious Diseases Society of America. All rights reserved.*)

gram-positive and gram-negative cells. In the synthesis of the bacterial cell wall, the terminal glycine residue of the pentaglycine bridge is linked to the fourth residue of the pentapeptide (D-alanine), releasing the fifth residue (also D-alanine). It is this step in peptidoglycan synthesis that is inhibited by the β-lactam antibiotics and glycopeptide antibiotics such as vancomycin (see Chapter 41). There are additional targets for the actions of penicillins and cephalosporins that are collectively termed penicillin-binding proteins (PBP). The PBPs vary in their affinities for different β-lactam antibiotics, although the interactions eventually become covalent.

b. What is the mechanism of bacterial resistance to the penicillins?

β-Lactam antibiotics are capable of being inactivated by β-lactamases that are present in large quantities (see Figure 39-2). The β-lactamases are grouped into 4 classes (see Side Bar CLASSES OF β-LACTAMASE ENZYMES). Some Class A and D enzymes are inhibited by β-lactamase inhibitors such as clavulanate and tazobactam. Bacterial resistance to the β-lactam antibiotics may also develop by mechanisms other than destruction by β-lactamases (see Side Bar MECHANISMS OF BACTERIAL RESISTANCE TO PENICILLINS AND CHEPHALOSPORINS).

CASE 39-2

A 68-year-old woman has contracted an *S. epidermidis* infection that is not methicillin-resistant. An infectious disease consultant recommends the use of a penicillinase-resistant penicillin.

a. What are the penicillinase-resistant penicillins?

The penicillinase-resistant penicillins (oxacillin, dicloxacillin, and cloxacillin) are resistant to hydrolysis by staphylococcal penicillinase (see Table 39-1). Nafcillin is a semisynthetic penicillin that is highly resistant to penicillinase and has proven effective against infections caused by penicillinase-producing strains of *S. aureus*.

b. What are their therapeutic uses?

The role of these penicillins as the agents of choice for most staphylococcal disease is changing with the increasing incidence of isolates of methicillin-resistant (MRSA) microorganisms. This term denotes resistance of these bacteria to all the penicillinase-resistant penicillins and cephalosporins. Hospital-acquired strains usually are resistant to the aminoglycosides, tetracyclines, erythromycin, and clindamycin as well. Vancomycin (see Chapter 41) is considered the drug of choice for hospital-acquired resistant strains, although resistance to vancomycin is also emerging.

SECTION VII   Chemotherapy of Microbial Diseases

TABLE 39-1 Classification of The Penicillins and Summary of Their Pharmacological Properties

DRUG	ACTIVITY	SPECIAL CIRCUMSTANCES
Penicillin G and V	Sensitive strains of gram-positive cocci	Hydrolyzed by penicillinase. Ineffective against most strains of *S. aureus*
Penicillinase-Resistant: Methicillin (discontinued in the United States), Nafcillin, Oxacillin, Cloxacillin (not in the United States), Dicloxacillin	Less sensitive than penicillin G and V	Agents of first choice for penicillinase-producing *S. aureus* and *S. epidermidis* that are not methicillin-resistant
Ampicillin, Amoxicillin, and Others	Activity extended to gram-negative organisms such as *H. influenzae, E. coli,* and *Proteus mirabilis*	Frequently administered with β-lactamase inhibitors to prevent hydrolysis by Class A β-lactamases
Carbenicillin (discontinued in the United States) and Ticarcillin	Activity extended to include *Pseudomonas, Enterobacter,* and *Proteus* spp.	Inferior to ampicillin against gram-positive cocci and less active than piperacillin against *Pseudomonas*
Mezlocillin, Azlocillin (both discontinued in the United States), and Piperacillin	Excellent activity against *Pseudomonas, Klebsiella,* and certain other gram-negative organisms	Utility is threatened by the emergence of broad-spectrum β-lactamases. Piperacillin retains the activity of ampicillin against gram-positive cocci

CASE 39-3

A 7-year-old girl is treated with amoxicillin for an otitis media of 3 days duration. After the first dose, the girl's mother notices swelling of the child's lips and mild difficulty breathing. The girl is seen in the emergency room where the diagnosis of penicillin allergy is made, and the amoxicillin is discontinued.

a. **The mother does not recall her daughter ever taking penicillin. Is this possible?**

Hypersensitivity reactions are by far the most common adverse effects noted with the penicillins, which probably are the most common cause of drug allergy. Hypersensitivity reactions may occur with any dosage form of penicillin; allergy to 1 penicillin exposes the patient to a greater risk of reaction if another penicillin is given. Hypersensitivity reactions may appear in the absence of a previous known exposure to the drug. A detailed discussion of hypersensitivity reactions and the management of the patient potentially allergic to penicillin can be found in Chapter 53 of the 12th Edition of *Goodman and Gilman's The Pharmacological Basis of Therapeutics*.

b. **What is the cause of penicillin allergy?**

Penicillins and their breakdown products act as haptens after covalent reaction to proteins. The most abundant breakdown product is the penicilloyl moiety (major determinant moiety, MDM), which is formed when the β-lactam ring is opened (see Figure 39-2). A large percentage of immunoglobulin (Ig)E-mediated reactions are to the MDM, but at least 25% of reactions are to other breakdown products (minor determinants). These products are formed in vivo and also can be found in solutions of penicillin prepared for administration. Anaphylactic reactions to penicillin usually are mediated by IgE antibodies against the minor determinants.

c. **Is there a means of detecting penicillin allergy prior to giving a dose of penicillin?**

Evaluation of the patient's history is the most practical way to avoid the use of penicillin in patients who are at the greatest risk of adverse reaction. Most patients who give a history of allergy to penicillin should be treated with another antibiotic. Unfortunately, there is no totally reliable means to confirm a history of allergy to penicillin.

Penicillins, Cephalosporins, and Other β-Lactam Antibiotics

CHAPTER 39

CASE 39-4

A 43-year-old man is treated with the third-generation cephalosporin, ceftazidime, for an infection with *Pseudomonas*.

a. What is the therapeutic distinction in the different generations of cephalosporin antibiotics?

See Table 53-3 in *Goodman & Gilman's The Pharmacological Basis of Therapeutics*, 12th Edition and the Summary Table at the end of this chapter for individual drugs. The first-generation cephalosporin antibiotics have good activity against gram-positive bacteria and modest activity against gram-negative microorganisms. The second-generation cephalosporins have somewhat increased activity against the gram-negative microorganisms, but are much less active than the third-generation agents. The third-generation cephalosporins generally are less active against gram-positive cocci; these agents are much more active against *Enterobacteriacae*, though resistance is dramatically increasing due to β-lactamase-producing strains. Fourth-generation cephalosporins have an extended spectrum of activity compared to the third-generation agents and have increased stability from hydrolysis by plasmid and chromosomally mediated β-lactamases.

b. Why was this man treated with ceftazidime?

Ceftazidime has activity against the *Enterobacteriaceae* very similar to cefotaxime, but its distinguishing feature is its excellent activity against *Pseudomonas* and other gram-negative bacteria.

CASE 39-5

A 43-year-old man is being treated with aztreonam for a gram-negative bacterial infection.

a. How is aztreonam different from the penicillins or cephalosporins?

Aztreonam belongs to the subclass of β-lactam drugs called carbapenems. But even within this subclass, aztreonam is unique. Carbapenems have a broader spectrum of activity than most other β-lactam antibiotics. Aztreonam has activity only against gram-negative bacteria; it has no activity against gram-positive bacteria and anaerobic organisms. However, activity against *Enterobacteriaceae* and *P. aeruginosa* is excellent. It is also highly active in vitro against *H. influenzae* and gonococci.

b. How is aztreonam administered and what precautions should be followed?

Aztreonam is administered either intramuscularly or intravenously and most of the drug is recovered unaltered in the urine. The usual dose of aztreonam should be reduced in patients with renal insufficiency.

CASE 39-6

A 64-year-old woman with type 2 diabetes develops a severe sore throat. She has been caring for her 3-year-old grandchild who has similar symptoms. She is treated with a combination of amoxicillin and clavulanic acid because of a concern that the organism may be resistant to amoxicillin alone.

a. What are β-lactamase inhibitors and how are they used to prevent bacterial resistance to the penicillins?

β-Lactamase inhibitors (clavulanic acid, sulbactam, and tazobactam) prevent the destruction of β-lactam antibiotics by β-lactamase. They are most active against plasmid-encoded β-lactamases; they are inactive at clinically achievable concentrations against the type I chromosomal β-lactamase.

b. What other antibiotics are combined with β-lactamase inhibitors?

Sulbactam is combined with ampicillin. Tazobactam is combined with piperacillin.

MECHANISM OF BACTERIAL RESISTANCE TO THE CEPHALOSPORINS

- Inability of antibiotic to reach site of action
- Alterations in penicillin-binding proteins (PBPs)
- β-Lactamases that hydrolyze the β-lactam ring

SECTION VII: Chemotherapy of Microbial Diseases

KEY CONCEPTS

- Penicillins and cephalosporins act by inhibiting bacterial cell wall synthesis.
- Bacterial resistance to the penicillins and cephalosporins is a serious clinical problem.
- Penicillinase-resistant penicillins (nafcillin, oxacillin, dicloxacillin, and cloxacillin) are less active against microorganisms sensitive to penicillin but are the agents of first choice for the treatment of penicillinase-producing *S. aureus* and *S. epidermidis* that are not methicillin resistant.
- The cephalosporins can be divided into first-, second-, third-, and fourth-generation agents, with each generation having a different spectrum of activity.
- The carbapenems (imipenem, meropenem, doripenem, ertapenem, and aztreonam) are β-lactam antibiotics with a broader spectrum of activity than most other β-lactam antibiotics.
- β-Lactamase inhibitors are added to some β-lactam antibiotics to extend their activity against strains of bacteria that produce β-lactamase.

SUMMARY QUIZ

QUESTION 39-1 A 23-year-old woman develops a rash following her first dose of penicillin V. The most likely cause of the rash is an allergy to penicillin. What component of penicillin is the most frequent cause of an allergic reaction?

a. The intact penicillin molecule
b. The penicilloic acid moiety (major determinant moiety)
c. The 6-aminopenicillanic acid moiety
d. Other breakdown products (minor determinant moiety)
e. The side chain attached to the β-lactam ring through the amide linkage

QUESTION 39-2 A 48-year-old woman has an infection that cultures a *S. aureus* known to elaborate penicillinase. It is appropriate that she be treated with nafcillin because

a. blood concentrations of nafcillin are sufficiently high to kill all *S. aureus*.
b. nafcillin is more potent against *S. aureus* than penicillin G.
c. nafcillin is resistant to penicillinase.
d. nafcillin is active against methicillin-resistant microorganisms (MRSA).
e. nafcillin is a naturally occurring penicillin.

QUESTION 39-3 A 62-year-old man is being treated for gonorrhea with a third-generation cephalosporin, ceftriaxone. Ceftriaxone is the drug of choice for gonorrhea rather than a first- or second-generation cephalosporin because

a. this third-generation cephalosporin has a shorter plasma half-life than the first- or second-generation cephalosporins.
b. ceftriaxone has a half-life of about 8 hours making it effective as a single dose.
c. it has a much lower incidence of adverse reactions compared to other cephalosporins.
d. it is active against methicillin-resistant bacteria.
e. ceftriaxone is well absorbed after oral administration.

QUESTION 39-4 A 37-year-old woman is being treated with the combination drug, imipenem and cilastatin. Cilastatin is added to imipenem because the cilastatin

a. inhibits the destruction of imipenem by a renal tubular dipeptidase.
b. inhibits β-lactamase.
c. increases the oral absorption of imipenem.

(Continued)

Penicillins, Cephalosporins, and Other β-Lactam Antibiotics

CHAPTER 39

d. decreases the incidence of nausea and vomiting caused by imipenem.

e. inhibits the possibility of allergic reactions in patients who have had allergic reactions to other β-lactam antibiotics.

QUESTION 39-5 A 16-year-old boy is treated for an infection with a strain of staphylococci known to produce β-lactamase with a combination of amoxicillin and clavulanic acid. Clavulanic acid is added to amoxicillin because it

a. increases the oral absorption of amoxicillin.

b. decreases the renal excretion of amoxicillin.

c. decreases the protein binding of amoxicillin.

d. enhances the binding of amoxicillin to penicillin-binding proteins.

e. inhibits β-lactamase.

SUMMARY QUIZ ANSWER KEY

QUESTION 39-1 Answer is **b**. A large percentage of immunoglobulin E-mediated reactions are to the major determinant moiety, but at least 25% of reactions are to other breakdown products which can be found in solutions of penicillin for administration.

QUESTION 39-2 Answer is **c**. Nafcillin is a semisynthetic penicillin that is highly resistant to penicillinase and has proven effective against infections caused by penicillinase-producing strains of *S. aureus*. There is an increasing incidence of isolates of methicillin-resistant microorganisms (eg, MRSA) that are resistant to all penicillinase-resistant penicillins including nafcillin.

QUESTION 39-3 Answer is **b**. A single dose of ceftriaxone is effective in the treatment of urethral, cervical, rectal, or pharyngeal gonorrhea. A single dose is effective because of its $t_{1/2}$ of ~8 hours allows it to be administered intramuscularly as a single dose.

QUESTION 39-4 Answer is **a**. Imipenem, which is not absorbed orally, is marketed in combination with cilastatin, a drug that inhibits the degradation of imipenem by a renal tubular dipeptidase. Patients who are allergic to other β-lactam antibiotics may have hypersensitivity reactions to imipenem.

QUESTION 39-5 Answer is **e**. Clavulanic acid is a suicide inhibitor that irreversibly binds β-lactamases produced by a wide range of gram-positive and gram-negative microorganisms. It has been combined with amoxicillin as an oral preparation and with ticarcillin as a parenteral preparation.

SUMMARY: PENICILLINS, CEPHALOSPORINS, CARBAPENEMS, AND OTHER β-LACTAM ANTIBIOTICS

CLASS AND SUBCLASSES	NAMES	CLINICAL USES	RESISTANCE	TOXICITIES COMMON	UNIQUE; CLINICALLY IMPORTANT
Penicillins	Penicillin G and Penicillin V	Sensitive strains of gram-positive cocci	Strains of bacteria that produce β-lactamases and MRSA		Allergic reactions
	Oxacillin	Sensitive strains of staphylococci that elaborate penicillinase	Methicillin-resistant *S. aureus* (MRSA)		Allergic reactions
	Cloxacillin Dicloxacillin Nafcillin	Same as oxacillin	Same as oxacillin		Allergic reactions
	Amoxicillin Ampicillin	Bacteriocidal for gram-positive and gram-negative bacteria	Sensitive to penicillinase and MRSA		Allergic reactions Dose reduced in patients with renal failure

(Continued)

SECTION VII — Chemotherapy of Microbial Diseases

CLASS AND SUBCLASSES	NAMES	CLINICAL USES	RESISTANCE	TOXICITIES COMMON	TOXICITIES UNIQUE; CLINICALLY IMPORTANT
	Carbenicillin	*P. aeruginosa* and some *Proteus* strains that are resistant to ampicillin	Sensitive to penicillinase and MRSA		Allergic reactions May cause heart failure due to administration of excessive Na^+ May interfere with platelet function
	Ticarcillin	More active against *P. aeruginosa* than carbenicillins	Sensitive to penicillinase and MRSA		Allergic reactions
	Mezlocillin	More active against *Klebsiella* than carbenicillin; discontinued in the United States	Sensitive to penicillinase and MRSA		Allergic reactions
	Piperacillin	Activity against *P. aeruginosa*, Enterobacteriaceae, many *Bacteroides* spp., and *E. faecalis*	Sensitive to penicillinase and MRSA		Allergic reactions
Cephalosporins-First Generation	Cephazolin Cephalexin Cefadroxil Cephradine	Sensitive strains of streptococci and *Staphylococci aureus*	Resistant to bacteria that produce β-lactamases and MRSA		Allergic reactions
Cephalosporins-Second Generation	Cefuroxime	Similar to cefaclor with broader gram-negative activity	Resistant to bacteria that produce β-lactamases and MRSA		Allergic reactions
	Cefoxitin	Treatment of certain anaerobic and mixed aerobic-anaerobic infections such as pelvic inflammatory disease and lung abscess	Resistant to destruction by some β-lactamases		Allergic reactions
	Cefaclor	Used orally Activity is similar to cephalexin More active against *H. influenzae* and *Moraxella catarrhalis*	Some β-lactamase–producing organisms are resistant		Allergic reactions
	Cefotetan	Activity against *B. fragilis*	Resistant to bacteria that produce β-lactamases and MRSA		Allergic reactions
	Cefuroxime axetil	Prodrug of cefuroxime	Resistant to bacteria that produce β-lactamases and MRSA		Allergic reactions
	Cefprozil	Orally administered More active than first-generation agents against penicillin-sensitive streptococci, *E. coli*, *P. mirabilis*, *Klebsiella* spp. and *Citrobacter* spp.	Resistant to bacteria that produce β-lactamases and MRSA		Allergic reactions

(Continued)

Penicillins, Cephalosporins, and Other β-Lactam Antibiotics — CHAPTER 39

CLASS AND SUBCLASSES	NAMES	CLINICAL USES	RESISTANCE	TOXICITIES COMMON	UNIQUE; CLINICALLY IMPORTANT
	Cefmetazole	Activity against *B. fragilis*; discontinued in the United States			Allergic reactions
	Loracarbef	Similar to cefaclor	More stable against some β-lactamases		Allergic reactions
Cephalosporins-Third Generation	Cefotaxime	Gram-positive and gram-negative aerobic bacteria	Resistant to many β-lactamases		Allergic reactions
	Ceftriaxone	Similar to cefotaxime Single dose used to treat gonorrhea; $t_{1/2}$ is 8 hours	Resistant to bacteria that produce β-lactamases and MRSA		Allergic reactions
	Cefdinir	Gram-positive and gram-negative infections Indicated for treatment of otitis media, soft tissue, and respiratory infections Inactive against *Pseudomonas* and *Enterobacter* spp.	Resistant to bacteria that produce β-lactamases and MRSA		Allergic reactions
	Cefixime	Treatment of otitis media caused by *H. influenzae* and *S. pyogenes*	Resistant to bacteria that produce β-lactamases and MRSA		Allergic reactions
	Cefditoren pivoxil	Indicated for the treatment of pharyngitis, tonsillitis, uncomplicated skin infections and acute exacerbations of chronic bronchitis	Resistant to bacteria that produce β-lactamases and MRSA		Allergic reactions
	Ceftibuten	Administered orally Activity limited *to S. pneumoniae, S. pyogenes, H. influenzae*, and *M. catarrhalis*	Resistant to bacteria that produce β-lactamases and MRSA		Allergic reactions
	Cefpodoxime proxetil	Administered orally Similar activity to cefepime except it is more active against *Enterobacter* and *Pseudomonas* spp	Resistant to bacteria that produce β-lactamases and MRSA		Allergic reactions
	Ceftizoxime	Similar to cefotaxime except it is less active against *S. pneumoniae*	Resistant to bacteria that produce β-lactamases and MRSA		Allergic reactions
	Cefoperazone	Effective against *Pseudomonas*	Resistant to bacteria that produce β-lactamases and MRSA		Allergic reactions May cause a clotting disorder May cause a disulfiram-like reaction with alcohol ingestion
	Ceftazidime	Excellent activity against *Pseudomonas* and other gram-negative bacteria	Resistant to bacteria that produce β-lactamases and MRSA		Allergic reactions

(Continued)

SECTION VII — Chemotherapy of Microbial Diseases

CLASS AND SUBCLASSES	NAMES	CLINICAL USES	RESISTANCE	TOXICITIES COMMON	UNIQUE; CLINICALLY IMPORTANT
Cephalosporins–Fourth Generation	Cefepime	Comparable to second- and third-generation agents	Stable to hydrolysis by many β-lactamases		Allergic reactions Dose reduced in patients with renal insufficiency
Other β-Lactam Antibiotics	Imipenem	Broader spectrum of activity than most other β-lactam agents	Resistant to hydrolysis by most β-lactamases, but not *Klebsiella pneumoniae* carbapenemase (KPC)-producing strains		Seizures in 1.5% of patients Allergic reactions Dose reduced in patients with renal insufficiency
	Meropenem	Broader spectrum of activity than most other β-lactam agents	Resistant to hydrolysis by most β-lactamases, but not KPC-producing strains		Less risk of seizures than imipenem Allergic reactions Dose reduced in patients with renal insufficiency
	Doripenem	Broader spectrum of activity than most other β-lactam agents	Resistant to hydrolysis by most β-lactamases, but not KPC-producing strains		Allergic reactions Dose reduced in patients with renal insufficiency
	Ertapenem	Broader spectrum of activity than most other β-lactam agents	Resistant to hydrolysis by most β-lactamases, but not KPC-producing strains		Allergic reactions
	Aztreonam	Activity only against gram-negative bacteria; active against *Enterobacteriaceae*, *P. aeruginosa*, and *H. influenzae*	Resistant to hydrolysis by most β-lactamases, but not KPC-producing strains		Dose reduced in patients with renal insufficiency Allergic reactions
β-Lactamase Inhibitors	Clavulanic acid	Combined with amoxicillin and with ticarcillin			
	Sulbactam	Combined with ampicillin			
	Tazobactam	Combined with piperacillin			

CHAPTER 40

Aminoglycosides

This chapter will be most useful after having a basic understanding of the material in Chapter 54, Aminoglycosides in *Goodman & Gilman's The Pharmacological Basis of Therapeutics*, 12th Edition. In addition to the material presented here, the 12th Edition contains:

- Figure 54-1 which shows the sites of activity of various plasmid-mediated enzymes capable of inactivating aminoglycosides
- Table 54-1 which provides the minimal inhibitory concentrations of aminoglycosides that will inhibit 90% (MIC_{90}) of clinical isolates for several bacterial species
- Table 54-2 which provides an algorithm for dose reduction of aminoglycosides based on creatinine clearance

LEARNING OBJECTIVES

☑ Understand aminoglycoside mechanisms of action and resistance.

☑ Describe the advantages and disadvantages of multiple daily dosing versus once daily extended-interval dosing regimens for aminoglycosides.

☑ Describe the rationale and the methods of plasma concentration monitoring of aminoglycoside therapy.

☑ Describe the causes and clinical signs of aminoglycoside ototoxicity and nephrotoxicity and the best means of monitoring therapy to avoid these serious toxicities.

☑ Understand the unique clinical differences among the aminoglycosides.

The mechanisms of action and resistance of the aminoglycosides are shown in the side bars MECHANISMS OF ACTION OF AMINOGLYCOSIDE and MECHANISMS OF AMINOGLYCOSIDE RESISTANCE, respectively.

CASE 40-1

A 56-year-old woman is in hospital for the treatment of pneumonia. Her case is complicated because she acquired the pneumonia in another hospital while undergoing post-surgical rehabilitation for a hysterectomy. She was being treated with a cephalosporin at the other hospital, but gentamicin is now added.

a. Why was the aminoglycoside added to her therapeutic regimen?

An aminoglycoside in combination with a β-lactam antibiotic is recommended as standard therapy for hospital-acquired pneumonia in which a multiple-drug resistant gram-negative aerobe is a likely causative agent. If it is established that the β-lactam is active against the causative agent, there is generally no need to continue the aminoglycoside.

b. Why is the combination of a β-lactam antibiotic and an aminoglycoside effective?

These 2 antibiotic classes have distinctly different mechanisms of action and their effectiveness should be complementary. β-Lactam antibiotics inhibit cell wall synthesis (see Chapter 39). Aminoglycosides act at the 30S ribosomal subunit to disrupt the normal cycle of ribosomal function by interfering with the initiation of protein synthesis, also by leading to accumulation of abnormal initiation complexes and premature termination, and by causing misreading of the mRNA template and incorporation of incorrect amino acids into the growing polypeptide chains (see Figure 40-1).

CASE 40-2

A 23-year-old woman is being treated with gentamicin for an enterococci infection. Twenty-four hours after beginning treatment it is learned that the organism is resistant to gentamicin.

(Continued)

DRUGS INCLUDED IN THIS CHAPTER

- Amikacin
- Gentamicin (GARAMYCIN, others)
- Kanamycin
- Neomycin
- Netilmicin (NETROMYCIN)
- Streptomycin
- Tobramycin (TOBREX, others)

MECHANISMS OF ACTION OF AMINOGLYCOSIDES

- The aminoglycosides are rapidly bactericidal and their bacterial killing is concentration-dependent
- Aminoglycosides exhibit a postantibiotic effect, that is, the bactericidal activity persists after serum concentration falls below the MIC
- Duration of postantibiotic effect is also concentration-dependent
- Inside the bacterial cell, the aminoglycosides bind to polysomes and interfere with protein synthesis by causing misreading and premature termination of mRNA translation (see Figure 40-1)

MECHANISMS OF AMINOGLYCOSIDE RESISTANCE

- Failure of the aminoglycoside to penetrate the bacteria cell
- Inactivation of the aminoglycoside by microbial enzymes
- Low affinity of the aminoglycoside for the bacterial ribosome

SECTION VII Chemotherapy of Microbial Diseases

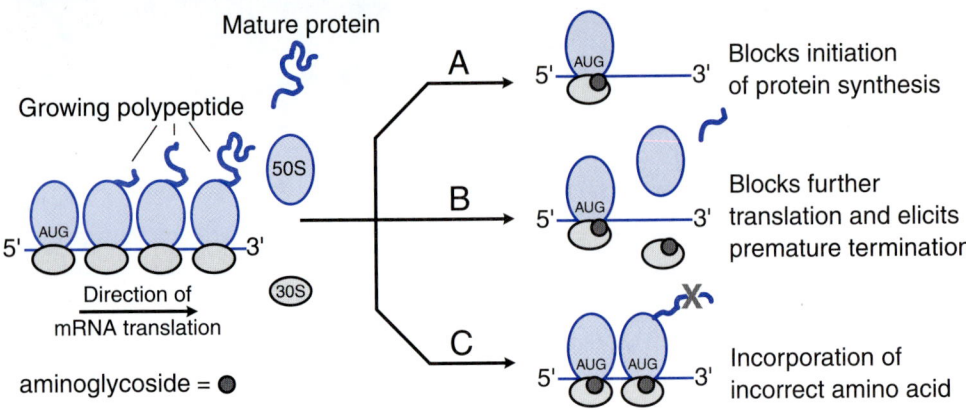

FIGURE 40-1 Effects of aminoglycosides on protein synthesis. **A.** Aminoglycoside (represented by dark grey circles) binds to the 30S ribosomal subunit and interferes with initiation of protein synthesis by fixing the 30S to 50S ribosomal complex at the start codon (AUG) of mRNA. As 30S to 50S complexes downstream complete translation of mRNA and detach, the abnormal initiation complexes, the so-called streptomycin monosomes, accumulate, blocking further translation of the message. Aminoglycoside binding to the 30S subunit also causes misreading of mRNA, leading to **B**, premature termination of translation with detachment of the ribosomal complex and incompletely synthesized protein or **C**, incorporation of incorrect amino acids (indicated by the grey X), resulting in the production of abnormal or nonfunctional proteins.

a. **Does resistance to gentamicin mean resistance to other aminoglycosides?**

Resistance to gentamicin indicates cross-resistance to tobramycin, amikacin, kanamycin, and netilmicin because the inactivating enzyme is bifunctional and can modify all these aminoglycosides. The chemical structure of streptomycin is sufficiently different from gentamicin that this inactivating enzyme does not modify streptomycin; consequently gentamicin-resistant strains of enterococci may be susceptible to streptomycin.

Amikacin is a suitable substrate for only a few of the inactivating enzymes that confer gentamicin-resistance; thus, strains that are resistant to multiple other aminoglycosides tend to be susceptible to amikacin.

A significant percentage of clinical isolates of *Enterococcus faecalis* and *E. faecium* are highly resistant to all aminoglycosides.

b. **What are the likely mechanisms of aminoglycoside resistance?**

See Side Bar MECHANISMS OF AMINOGLYCOSIDE RESISTANCE. Clinically, drug inactivation is the most common mechanism for acquired microbial resistance to aminoglycosides. The genes encoding aminoglycoside-modifying enzymes are acquired primarily by conjugation and transfer of resistance plasmids. These enzymes phosphorylate, adenylate, or acetylate specific hydroxyl or amino groups.

Other mechanisms of aminoglycoside resistance include the inability of the aminoglycoside to penetrate bacterial intracellular space and a reduced affinity of the aminoglycoside for the bacterial ribosome.

CASE 40-3

A 65-year-old man is in hospital for the treatment of community-acquired pneumonia that is sensitive to an aminoglycoside. He is being treated with 5.1 mg/kg of gentamicin as a single dose once every 24 hours.

a. **Based on a half-life of 2 to 3 hours, aminoglycosides have been historically administered in 3 equally divided doses over a 24-hour period. Is this patient's single dose expected to be effective?**

Numerous studies and meta-analyses demonstrate that administration of the total dose of aminoglycoside once daily is just as effective as multiple-dose regimens. In addition, extended-interval administration costs less, is administered more easily, and is associated with less nephrotoxicity.

(Continued)

A comparison of high-dose, extended-interval dosing to traditional divided-dose methods is illustrated in Figure 40-2. Because of the postantibiotic effect of aminoglycosides, good therapeutic response can be attained even when the concentrations of aminoglycosides fall below bacterial inhibitory concentrations for a substantial period of the dosing interval.

b. How does the once-daily dosing affect aminoglycoside toxicity?

The high-dose, extended-interval dosing methods for aminoglycosides reduce the characteristic oto- and nephrotoxicity of these drugs. High-dose, extended-interval dosing regimens, despite higher peak concentrations, provide a longer period when concentrations fall below the threshold for toxicity than does a multiple-dose regimen (12 hours vs less than 3 hours total in the example shown in Figure 40-2), potentially accounting for the lower toxicity of this approach. This diminished toxicity is probably due to a threshold effect from accumulation of drug in the inner ear or in the kidney (see Cases 40-5 and 40-6).

c. Is this once-a-day dosing of aminoglycosides suitable for all patients?

One key exception to the use of extended-interval dosing is for aminoglycoside use as a combination therapy with a cell wall-active agent in the treatment of gram-positive infections, such as endocarditis.

Although schemes exist for adjusting the dosages of aminoglycosides dosed by extended-interval methods in patients with renal dysfunction, some clinicians prefer to use the traditional multiple-dose regimens in such patients.

d. After administration of an aminoglycoside, how should the plasma concentration be monitored?

For multiple-daily-dosing regimens, both peak and trough plasma concentrations are determined. The trough sample is obtained just before a dose, and the peak sample is obtained 60 minutes after an intramuscular injection or 30 minutes after an intravenous infusion given over 30 minutes. The peak concentration documents that the dose produces therapeutic concentrations, generally accepted to be 4 to 10 µg/mL for gentamicin, netilmicin, and tobramycin, and 15 to 30 µg/mL for amikacin and streptomycin. The trough concentration is used to avoid toxicity by monitoring for accumulation of the drug. Trough concentrations should be less than 1 to 2 µg/mL for gentamicin, netilmicin, and tobramycin and less than 10 µg/mL for amikacin and streptomycin.

Monitoring of aminoglycoside plasma concentrations also is important when using an extended-interval dosing regimen, although peak concentrations are not

(*Continued*)

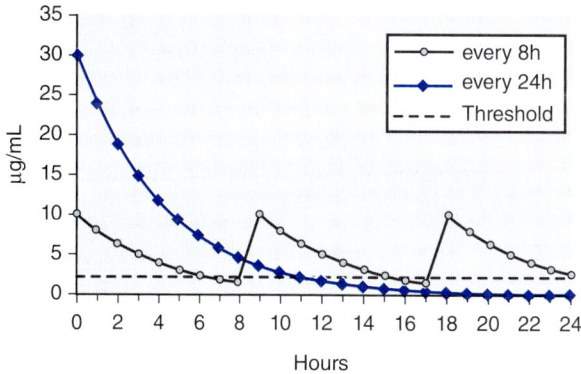

FIGURE 40-2 Plasma concentrations (µg/mL) after administration of 5.1 mg/kg of gentamicin intravenously to a hypothetical patient either as a single dose (every 24 hours) or as 3 divided doses (every 8 hours). The threshold for toxicity has been chosen to correspond to a plasma concentration of 2 µg/mL, the maximum recommended. The high-dose, extended-interval (once-daily) regimen produces a 3-fold higher plasma concentration, which enhances efficacy that otherwise might be compromised due to prolonged sub-MIC concentrations later in the dosing interval compared with the every-8-hours regimen. The once-daily regimen provides a 12-hour period during which plasma concentrations are below the threshold for toxicity, thereby minimizing the toxicity that otherwise might result from the high plasma concentrations early on. The every-8-hours regimen, in contrast, provides only a brief period during which plasma concentrations are below the threshold for toxicity.

determined routinely (these will be 3-4 times higher than the peak achieved with a multiple-daily-dosing regimen).

The most accurate method for monitoring plasma concentrations for dose adjustment during an extended-interval dosing regimen is to measure the concentration of 2 plasma samples drawn several hours apart (eg, at 2 and 12 hours after a dose). The clearance can then be calculated and the dose adjusted to achieve the desired target range.

CASE 40-4

A 46-year-old man with chronic renal insufficiency is brought into the emergency department suffering from an elevated temperature of 104 °F. His medical chart is not available. It is decided to treat him with gentamicin, but his last creatinine clearance is not known.

a. The dose of aminoglycoside should be decreased in patients with poor renal function. Since this patient's creatinine clearance is unknown, what initial dose should he be started on?

The concentration of aminoglycoside in plasma produced by the initial dose depends only on the volume of distribution of the drug. Thus (assuming his volume of distribution is normal), this patient can be treated initially with a standard dose of gentamicin, for example, 5 mg/kg given over 30 to 60 minutes. The next dose (24 hours later) can be adjusted for his reduced renal function which should then be known.

b. Why is it important to reduce the dose of aminoglycosides in patients with decreased renal function?

The elimination of aminoglycosides depends almost entirely on the kidney and a linear relationship exists between the concentration of creatinine in the plasma and the $t_{1/2}$ of all aminoglycosides in patients with moderately compromised renal function. In anephric patients, the $t_{1/2}$ varies from 20 to 40 times that of normal individuals. Because the incidence of nephrotoxicity and ototoxicity is likely related to the overall drug exposure to aminoglycosides, it is critical to reduce the maintenance dosage of these drugs in patients with impaired renal function.

c. How is a maintenance dose determined?

For patients with impaired renal function, it is common to rely upon algorithms such as the one shown in Table 54-2 in the 12th Edition of *The Pharmacological Basis of Therapeutics* or those published in other medical texts and reference books. It should be understood that such algorithms are only a guideline and that plasma concentrations must be monitored as discussed in Case 40-3 above and in Appendix II of the *The Pharmacological Basis of Therapeutics*, 12th Edition. Determination of the concentration of drug in plasma is an essential guide to the proper administration of aminoglycosides. In patients with life-threatening systemic infections, aminoglycoside concentrations should be determined several times per week (more frequently if renal function is changing) and should be determined within 24 to 48 hours of any change in dosage.

CASE 40-5

During a course of gentamicin therapy, a 76-year-old man develops ringing in his ears.

a. What are the clinical symptoms of ototoxicity with aminoglycosides?

A high-pitched tinnitus often is the first sign of cochlear toxicity. If the drug is not stopped, auditory impairment may develop after a few days. The affected individual is not always aware of the difficulty, and it will not be detected except by careful auditory examination.

Moderately intense headache lasting 1 to 2 days may precede the onset of vestibular toxicity. This is followed immediately by nausea and vomiting. Difficulty with equilibrium may develop and persist for 1 to 2 weeks. Prominent symptoms of

(Continued)

vestibular toxicity include vertigo in the upright position, inability to perceive termination of movement, and difficulty in sitting or standing without visual clues.

b. **What are the risk factors for producing ototoxicity?**

It is generally thought the ototoxicity seen with aminoglycosides is more likely to occur in patients with persistently elevated concentration of drug in plasma.

Ototoxicity is largely irreversible and results from progressive destruction of vestibular or cochlear sensory cells. Accumulation within the perilymph and endolymph occurs predominantly when aminoglycoside concentrations in plasma are high. Diffusion back into the bloodstream is slow; the half-lives of the aminoglycosides are 5 to 6 times longer in otic fluids than in plasma. Back diffusion is concentration-dependent and facilitated at the trough concentration of the drug in plasma. However, studies have not consistently shown an association between ototoxicity and risk factors such as aminoglycoside plasma concentrations, total dose, duration of exposure, and renal dysfunction.

c. **How should aminoglycosides be monitored to avoid ototoxicity?**

If it is anticipated that the patient will be treated with an aminoglycoside for more than 3 to 4 days then plasma concentrations should be monitored to avoid drug accumulation. See the answer to Case 40-3d for a description of a rational approach to aminoglycoside plasma concentration monitoring.

CASE 40-6

A 63-year-old woman has been treated with gentamicin for 7 days. During these 7 days, her serum creatinine has risen from 1.0 mg/dL to 2.2 mg/dL and there is concern for the development of nephrotoxicity. She is scheduled for another 3 days of gentamicin therapy.

a. **What variables are important for the development of aminoglycoside nephrotoxicity?**

Approximately 8 to 26% of patients who receive an aminoglycoside for several days develop mild renal impairment that is almost always reversible. The toxicity correlates with the total amount of drug administered and consequently with longer courses of therapy. Advanced age, liver disease, diabetes, and septic shock have been suggested as risk factors for the development of aminoglycoside nephrotoxicity. The nephrotoxic potential varies among individual aminoglycosides. Neomycin concentrates to the greatest degree in the renal cortex, is highly nephrotoxic, and should not be administered systemically. Streptomycin does not concentrate in the renal cortex and is the least nephrotoxic. The difference in the nephrotoxicity of gentamicin and tobramycin is slight. Other drugs such as amphotericin B, cyclosporin, vancomycin, angiotensin-converting enzyme inhibitors, and cisplatin may potentiate the nephrotoxicity of the aminoglycosides. Clinical studies have not proven conclusively that furosemide potentiates aminoglycoside nephrotoxicity, but the volume depletion and K^+ wasting that accompany the use of furosemide may predispose to aminoglycoside toxicity.

b. **What are the mechanisms of aminoglycoside nephrotoxicity?**

Aminoglycoside nephrotoxicity results from the accumulation and retention of the aminoglycoside in the renal proximal tubular cells. The biochemical events leading to tubular cell damage and glomerular dysfunction probably involve perturbations of the structure of cellular membranes. The initial manifestation of damage is excretion of enzymes of the renal tubular brush border. After several days, there is a defect in the renal concentrating ability, mild proteinuria, and the appearance of hyaline and granular casts. The glomerular filtration rate is reduced after several additional days. Aminoglycoside renal impairment is almost always reversible because the proximal tubular cells have the capacity to regenerate.

(Continued)

SECTION VII

Chemotherapy of Microbial Diseases

c. **What methods are available for monitoring aminoglycoside therapy to avoid or manage nephrotoxicity?**

Monitoring plasma trough concentrations, as described in Case 40-3, are used to avoid toxicity by measuring drug accumulation. Trough concentrations should be less than 1 to 2 μg/mL for gentamicin, netilmicin, and tobramycin and less than 10 μg/mL for amikacin and streptomycin.

KEY CONCEPTS

- Aminoglycosides are bactericidal by disrupting the normal cycle of ribosomal functioning thereby interfering with bacterial protein synthesis.
- Resistance to aminoglycosides is most commonly caused by drug-inactivating enzymes produced by bacteria.
- Aminoglycosides are characterized by a postantibiotic effect, that is, residual bactericidal activity persisting after the serum concentration has fallen below the minimum inhibitory concentration (MIC).
- High-dose, extended-interval dosing regimens are effective in most instances and may reduce the characteristic oto- and nephrotoxicity of aminoglycosides.
- Plasma concentration monitoring of aminoglycosides is an essential guide to the proper administration of aminoglycosides.
- All aminoglycosides have the potential to produce irreversible cochlear and vestibular toxicity.
- All aminoglycosides have the potential to produce nephrotoxicity that is almost always reversible.

SUMMARY QUIZ

QUESTION 40-1 A 36-year-old woman is being treated with gentamicin in hospital for a gram-negative infection. Her trough blood concentrations are below the known minimum inhibitory concentration (MIC) of the bacteria. An infectious disease consultant is not concerned about this because

a. the MIC for most bacteria are notoriously too high.
b. gentamicin plasma concentrations are not an effective way to monitor therapy.
c. gentamicin has residual bacteriocidal activity which persists after the plasma concentration has fallen below the MIC.
d. gentamicin is bacteriostatic.
e. the mechanism of action of gentamicin is inhibition of cell wall synthesis.

QUESTION 40-2 A 64-year-old man is suffering from a gas gangrene infection of his right foot due to a mid-calf arterial clot. The bacteria involved is *Clostridium perfringens*. An aminoglycoside is not a good choice for antibiotic therapy because aminoglycosides are

a. bacteriostatic.
b. not active against anaerobic bacteria.
c. more toxic under anaerobic conditions.
d. only effective if they are injected directly into anaerobic tissue.
e. metabolized more rapidly under anaerobic conditions.

QUESTION 40-3 A 26-year-old woman has the diagnosis of bacterial meningitis. The organism cultured is a gram-negative *Pseudomonas* susceptible to gentamicin. There is concern about treatment of this patient with gentamicin because

a. aminoglycosides are not generally active against gram-negative bacteria.
b. aminoglycosides can cause seizures at therapeutic concentrations.

(Continued)

c. patients with meningitis have a tendency to be more susceptible to the nephrotoxic effects of the aminoglycosides.
d. aminoglycosides are polar and do not penetrate the central nervous system.
e. aminoglycosides are rapidly metabolized in the brain and do not reach therapeutic concentrations.

QUESTION 40-4 A 40-year-old woman is being treated with intravenous gentamicin 3 times daily. Her therapy was begun 3 days ago and is expected to continue for an additional 10 days. What is the recommended monitoring of plasma gentamicin concentrations?

a. No plasma concentration monitoring is necessary.
b. Measure peak and trough concentrations several times per week.
c. Measure only peak plasma concentrations.
d. Measure only trough concentration once after 3 days of therapy.
e. Monitor peak and trough plasma concentrations only if renal dysfunction is apparent.

QUESTION 40-5 A 43-year-old man is being treated with gentamicin and penicillin mixed in the same IV solution for a serious pulmonary infection that is sensitive to gentamicin. After 3 days of therapy, his temperature remains elevated and his pulmonary congestion is worsening. A possible cause is that the

a. gentamicin is inactivated by the penicillin in the IV mixture in vitro.
b. penicillin enhances the elimination of gentamicin.
c. gentamicin causes a destruction of penicillin in vivo.
d. penicillin inhibits the entry of gentamicin into the bacterial cell.
e. penicillin prevents the ribosomal binding of gentamicin.

QUESTION 40-6 A 23-year-old woman has developed a pulmonary infection of unknown cause. Patients in the same hospital have recently developed infections with organisms shown to be resistant to gentamicin and tobramycin. An infectious disease consultant recommends initially starting the patient on amikacin along with another antibiotic that is known to inhibit cell wall synthesis. The choice of amikacin is made because it is

a. less expensive than gentamicin or tobramycin.
b. less nephrotoxic than gentamicin or tobramycin.
c. less ototoxic than gentamicin or tobramycin.
d. more concentrated in pulmonary tissue than gentamicin or tobramycin.
e. resistant to many of the aminoglycoside-inactivating enzymes.

SUMMARY QUIZ ANSWER KEY

QUESTION 40-1 Answer is **c**. A postantibiotic effect, that is, residual bactericidal activity persisting after the serum concentration has fallen below the MIC, is characteristic of the aminoglycoside antibiotics; the duration of this effect is concentration-dependent.

QUESTION 40-2 Answer is **b**. Aminoglycosides must penetrate intracellularly to be effective. Transport of aminoglycosides across the cytoplasmic membrane is an oxygen-dependent active process. Thus, anaerobic bacteria are resistant to the aminoglycosides because they lack the necessary transport system.

QUESTION 40-3 Answer is **d**. Because of their polar nature, the aminoglycosides do not penetrate into most cells, the CNS, or the eye. Concentrations of aminoglycosides achieved in the CSF with parenteral administration usually are subtherapeutic. If CNS therapy with an aminoglycoside is necessary, a preservative-free formulation of an

(Continued)

aminoglycoside is administered directly intrathecally or intraventricularly once daily. Such treatment may cause local inflammation and can result in radiculitis and other complications.

QUESTION 40-4 Answer is **b**. Determination of the concentration of gentamicin in plasma is an essential guide to its proper administration. In patients with life-threatening infections for which gentamicin may be administered more than for a few days, it is recommended that plasma concentrations be determined several times per week or more frequently if renal function is changing. Plasma aminoglycoside concentrations should be determined within 24 to 48 hours of a change in dosage.

Peak plasma concentrations of aminoglycosides are used to determine that the dose produces a therapeutic concentration; trough plasma concentrations are used to monitor drug accumulation. Peak concentrations are not routinely measured during an extended-interval dosing regimen.

QUESTION 40-5 Answer is **a**. Aminoglycosides can be inactivated by various penicillins in vitro and thus should not be admixed in solution.

QUESTION 40-6 Answer is **e**. Amikacin is resistant to many of the aminoglycoside-inactivating enzymes. It is the preferred agent for the initial therapy of serious nosocomial gram-negative infections in hospitals where resistance to gentamicin and tobramycin has become a significant problem.

SUMMARY: AMINOGLYCOSIDES

CLASS AND SUBCLASSES	NAME	CLINICAL USES	RESISTANCE	TOXICITY COMMON	TOXICITY UNIQUE; CLINICALLY IMPORTANT
Aminoglycosides	Gentamicin	Urinary tract infection: not indicated for routine use Pneumonia: in combination with a β-lactam antibiotic for the treatment of hospital-acquired pneumonia in which a multiple drug-resistant gram-negative aerobe is a likely causative agent Bacterial endocarditis: low-dose gentamicin (3 mg/kg/d in divided doses) in combination with penicillin or vancomycin for treatment due to gram-positive organisms; in cases of enterococcal endocarditis, the administration of penicillin and gentamicin for 4-6 weeks is recommended because of the unacceptably high relapse rate with penicillin alone Sepsis: inclusion of an aminoglycoside is recommended for the febrile patient with granulocytopenia and when *P. aeruginosa* is a potential pathogen	Clinical bacterial resistance is increasingly common Aminoglycosides have little activity against anaerobic bacteria or facultative bacteria under aerobic conditions Aminoglycoside activity against most gram-positive bacteria is limited and they should not be used as a single agent in the treatment of infections caused by gram-positive bacteria		Nephrotoxicity (reversible), irreversible ototoxicity When applied topically to large areas of denuded skin, plasma concentrations may reach the toxic range
	Tobramycin	Similar to gentamicin	Similar to gentamicin		Similar to gentamicin

(Continued)

Aminoglycosides — CHAPTER 40

CLASS AND SUBCLASSES	NAME	CLINICAL USES	RESISTANCE	TOXICITY COMMON	TOXICITY UNIQUE; CLINICALLY IMPORTANT
	Amikacin	Broader spectrum than gentamicin. Amikacin is less active than gentamicin against enterococci and should not be used for this organism. Amikacin is active against *M. tuberculosis*, including streptomycin-resistant strains and atypical mycobacteria	Because of its resistance to many of the aminoglycoside-inactivating enzymes, it is recommended for the initial treatment of nosocomial gram-negative infections in hospitals where resistance to gentamicin and tobramycin has become a significant problem		Similar to gentamicin
	Netilmicin	Its antibacterial activity is broad against aerobic gram-negative bacilli	It is not metabolized by most of the aminoglycoside-inactivating enzymes and may be active against certain bacteria that are resistant to gentamicin		Similar to gentamicin
	Streptomycin	Rarely used because it is less active against gram-negative aerobes than other aminoglycosides. Streptomycin (or gentamicin) is the drug of choice for the treatment of tularemia	Gentamicin-resistant strains of enterococci may be susceptible to streptomycin		Ototoxicity of streptomycin is primarily vestibular and irreversible
	Kanamycin	Its spectrum of activity is limited compared with other aminoglycosides; the use of kanamycin has become obsolete			Similar to gentamicin
	Neomycin	Available for topical administration in combination with polymyxin, bacitracin, other antibiotics and corticosteroids. Neomycin and polymyxin B have been used for irrigation of the urinary bladder		Hypersensitivity reactions are reported and involve primarily skin rashes when the drug is applied topically	Similar to gentamicin

CHAPTER 41

Protein Synthesis Inhibitors and Miscellaneous Antibacterial Agents

DRUGS INCLUDED IN THIS CHAPTER

- Azithromycin (ZITHROMAX)
- Bacitracin
- Chloramphenicol
- Clarithromycin (BIAXIN, others)
- Clindamycin (CLEOCIN PHOSPHATE, others)
- Daptomycin (CUBICIN)
- Doxycycline
- Erythromycin
- Linezolid (ZYVOX)
- Mupirocin (BACTROBAN)
- Polymyxin
- Quinupristin/dalfopristin (SYNERCID)
- Spectinomycin
- Teicoplanin
- Telithromycin (KETEX)
- Tetracycline
- Tigecycline
- Vancomycin (VANCOCIN)

This chapter will be most useful after having a basic understanding of the material in Chapter 55, Protein Synthesis Inhibitors and Miscellaneous Antibacterial Agents in *Goodman & Gilman's The Pharmacological Basis of Therapeutics*, 12th Edition. In addition to the material presented here Chapter 55 contains:

- Table 55-2 which provides information about the activity of most of the antibacterial agents covered in this chapter against key gram-positive pathogens

LEARNING OBJECTIVES

- ☑ Understand the mechanisms of action and resistance of tetracyclines, macrolides, vancomycin, linezolid, daptomycin, and quinupristin/dalfopristin
- ☑ Describe the unique toxicities of antibiotics that are inhibitors of bacterial protein synthesis
- ☑ Describe the uses and untoward reactions of vancomycin
- ☑ Identify the drug–drug interactions that occur with some of these antibiotics
- ☑ Understand how linezolid, daptomycin, and quinupristin/dalfopristin are used to treat methicillin-resistant and vancomycin-resistant organisms

MECHANISMS OF ACTION AND RESISTANCE OF PROTEIN SYNTHESIS INHIBITORS

DRUGS	MECHANISM OF ACTION	MECHANISM OF RESISTANCE
Tetracycline, Doxycycline, Tigecycline	Inhibition of protein synthesis by binding to the 30S bacterial ribosome subunit (see Figure 41-1)	Decreased bacterial cell accumulation of tetracycline Bacterial production of a ribosomal protection protein that displaces drug from its target Enzymatic destruction of drug
Chloramphenicol	Inhibition of protein synthesis by binding to the 50S bacterial ribosome subunit (see Figure 41-2)	Bacterial production of acetyltransferase that inactivates the drug
Erythromycin, Clarithromycin, Telithromycin, Azithromycin	Inhibition of protein synthesis by binding to the 50S bacterial ribosome subunit (see Figure 41-3)	Enhanced efflux from bacterial cell Ribosomal protection by production of methylase enzymes Hydrolysis by esterases Mutation of 50S ribosomal protein
Clindamycin	Inhibition of protein synthesis by binding to the 50S bacterial ribosome subunit	Ribosomal protection by constitutively produced methylase enzyme Altered metabolism
Quinupristin/Dalfopristin	Inhibition of protein synthesis by binding to the 50S bacterial ribosome subunit	Production of methylase enzyme that prevents binding to target Production of acetyltransferase that inactivates the drug Enhanced efflux from bacterial cell

Protein Synthesis Inhibitors and Miscellaneous Antibacterial Agents — CHAPTER 41

DRUGS	MECHANISM OF ACTION	MECHANISM OF RESISTANCE
Linezolid	Inhibition of protein synthesis by binding to the 50S bacterial ribosome subunit to prevent formation of larger ribosomal complex	Point mutations in rRNA
Spectinomycin	Inhibition of protein synthesis by binding to the 30S bacterial ribosome subunit	Mutations in rRNA; Modifications of the drug by adenyltransferase
Polymyxin	As surface-active agents, polymyxins interact with phospholipids and disrupt bacterial cell wall	Resistance is rare
Vancomycin, Teicoplanin	Inhibit cell wall synthesis by binding to D-alanyl-D-alanine terminus of cell wall precursor units (see Figure 41-4)	Bacterial alteration of drug target
Daptomycin	Binds to bacterial membranes resulting in depolarization, loss of membrane potential and cell death	Not fully characterized
Bacitracin	Inhibits synthesis of bacterial cell wall	*Pseudomonas*, *Candida* spp. and *Nocardia* are resistant but mechanism is not known
Mupirocin	Inhibition of protein synthesis by binding to isoleucyl transfer-RNA synthetase	Production of a "bypass" synthetase that binds mupirocin poorly

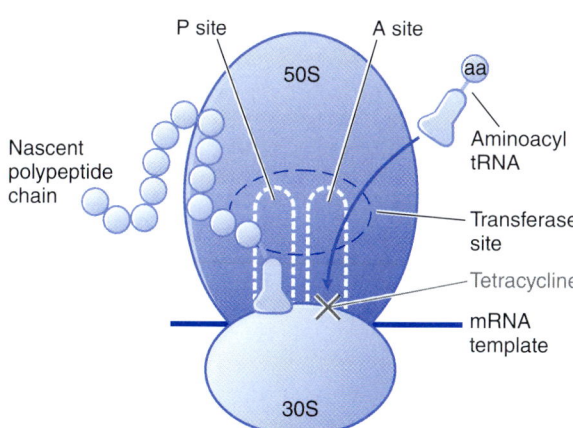

FIGURE 41-1 Inhibition of bacterial protein synthesis by tetracyclines. Messenger RNA (mRNA) attaches to the 30S subunit of bacterial ribosomal RNA. The P (peptidyl) site of the 50S ribosomal RNA subunit contains the nascent polypeptide chain; normally, the aminoacyl tRNA charged with the next amino acid (aa) to be added to the chain moves into the A (acceptor) site, with complementary base pairing between the anticodon sequence of tRNA and the codon sequence of mRNA. Tetracyclines inhibit bacterial protein synthesis by binding to the 30S subunit and blocking tRNA binding to the A site.

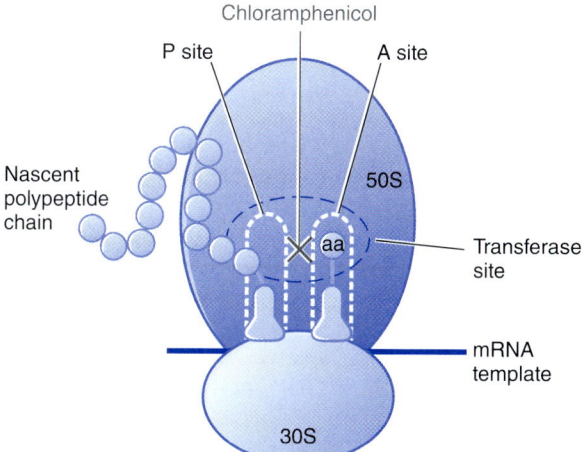

FIGURE 41-2 Inhibition of bacterial protein synthesis by chloramphenicol. Chloramphenicol binds to the 50S ribosomal subunit at the peptidyltransferase site and inhibits the transpeptidation reaction. Chloramphenicol binds to the 50S ribosomal subunit near the site of action of clindamycin and the macrolide antibiotics. These agents interfere with the binding of chloramphenicol and thus may interfere with each other's actions if given concurrently. See Figure 41-1 and its legend for additional information.

SECTION VII
Chemotherapy of Microbial Diseases

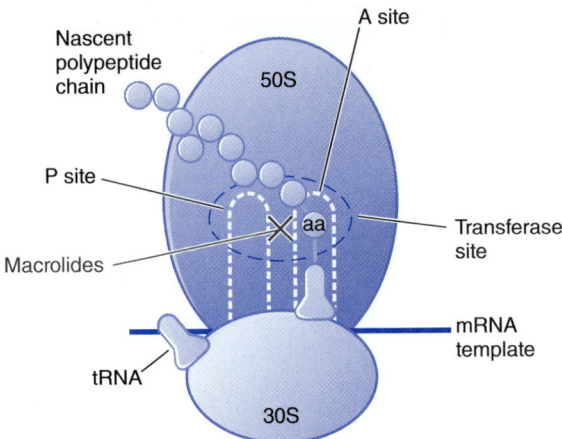

FIGURE 41-3 Inhibition of bacterial protein synthesis by the macrolide antibiotics erythromycin, clarithromycin, and azithromycin. Macrolide antibiotics are bacteriostatic agents that inhibit protein synthesis by binding reversibly to the 50S ribosomal subunits of sensitive organisms. Erythromycin appears to inhibit the translocation step such that the nascent peptide chain temporarily residing at the A site of the transferase reaction fails to move to the P, or donor, site. Alternatively, macrolides may bind and cause a conformational change that terminates protein synthesis by indirectly interfering with transpeptidation and translocation. See Figure 41-1 and its legend for additional information.

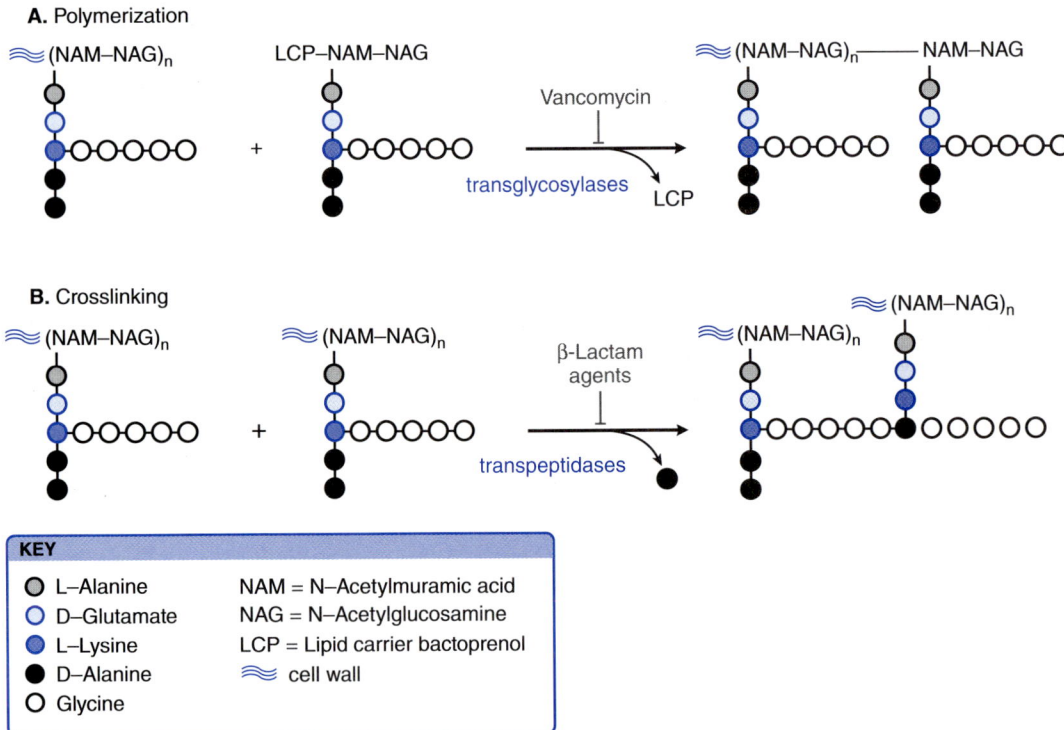

FIGURE 41-4 Inhibition of bacterial cell wall synthesis: vancomycin and β-lactam agents. Vancomycin inhibits the polymerization or transglycosylase reaction (**A**) by binding to the D-alanyl-D-alanine terminus of the cell wall precursor unit attached to its lipid carrier and blocks linkage to the glycopeptide polymer (indicated by the subscript n). These (NAM–NAG)$_n$ peptidoglycan polymers are located within the cell wall. Van A-type resistance is due to expression of enzymes that modify cell wall precursor by substituting a terminal D-lactate for D-alanine, reducing vancomycin binding affinity by 1000 times. β-Lactam antibiotics inhibit the cross-linking or transpeptidase reaction (**B**) that links glycopeptide polymer chains by formation of a cross-bridge with the stem peptide (the 5 glycines in this example) of 1 chain, displacing the terminal D-alanine of an adjacent chain. See also Figure 39-1.

Protein Synthesis Inhibitors and Miscellaneous Antibacterial Agents CHAPTER 41

CASE 41-1

A 56-year-old man has developed a community-acquired skin infection that is shown to be methicillin-resistant *S. aureus*. An infectious disease consultant recommends initial treatment with doxycycline.

a. **Why doxycycline?**

Tetracyclines, doxycycline, and minocycline have generally retained excellent levels of activity against staphylococci, including methicillin-resistant *Staphylococcus aureus* (MRSA). Community-acquired strains of MRSA often are susceptible to tetracycline, doxycycline, or minocycline.

b. **What is the mechanism of action of doxycycline?**

Tetracyclines and glycylcyclines inhibit bacterial protein synthesis by binding to the 30S bacterial ribosome and preventing access of aminoacyl tRNA to the acceptor site on the mRNA-ribosome complex (see Figure 41-1).

c. **Another consultant has recommended chloramphenicol. Is this a good choice?**

Chloramphenicol use should be limited to infections for which the benefits of the drug outweigh the risks of the potential toxicities. In this case, the benefits do not outweigh the risks.

Chloramphenicol is potentially toxic to the bone marrow in two ways: (1) a dose-related toxicity that presents as anemia, leukopenia, or thrombocytopenia, and (2) an idiosyncratic response manifested by aplastic anemia. This latter response may be fatal if the bone marrow aplasia is complete. The risk of aplastic anemia does not contraindicate the use of chloramphenicol in situations in which it may be lifesaving. However, the drug should never be used in undefined situations or in diseases that are readily, safely, and effectively treated with other less toxic antibiotics.

CASE 41-2

A 23-year-old woman college student is given a prescription for clarithromycin for a *Haemophilus influenzae* infection.

a. **What is the mechanism of action of clarithromycin and how does it differ from that of tetracycline and chloramphenicol?**

Clarithromycin acts by binding to the bacterial 50S ribosome (see Figure 41-3) to inhibit bacterial protein synthesis. This is the same site of action for chloramphenicol and clindamycin and these agents (macrolides, clindamycin, and chloramphenicol) may interfere with each other's actions if given concurrently. Tetracycline binds to the 30S subunit of the bacterial ribosome.

b. **What atypical infectious disease is commonly treated with clarithromycin?**

Clarithromycin is used in combination with omeprazole (or other proton pump inhibitor) and amoxicillin for the treatment of peptic ulcer disease caused by *H. pylori* (see Chapter 32).

c. **What toxicities should this patient be warned against?**

Macrolides commonly cause GI upset which may include nausea, vomiting, and abdominal pain. Erythromycin, clarithromycin, and telithromycin have been reported to cause cardiac arrhythmias, including QT prolongation and ventricular tachycardia. Most patients who experience cardiac toxicity have underlying risk factors, such as hereditary long QT syndrome, hypokalemia or hypomagnesemia, profound bradycardia, or are receiving certain antiarrhythmic drugs (eg, quinidine, procainamide, amiodarone) or other agents that prolong QTc (see Chapter 18).

(Continued)

d. **What serious drug-interactions should this patient be advised of?**

Macrolide antibiotics inhibit CYP3A4 and are associated with significant drug interactions such as potentiation of the effects of drugs metabolized by the same pathway. Inducers of CYP3A4 such as rifampin may decrease the serum concentration of the macrolide antibiotics. Inhibitors of CYP3A4, such as itraconazole, may increase the serum concentrations of the macrolide antibiotics. Azithromycin appears to be free of these drug interactions, but caution should be used when using azithromycin in conjunction with drugs known to interact with other macrolide antibiotics.

CASE 41-3

A 34-year-old woman in hospital has developed an *E. faecium* infection that is resistant to vancomycin. An infectious disease consultant has recommended she be treated with quinupristin/dalfopristin.

a. **Why is quinupristin given in combination with dalfopristin?**

Quinupristin binds at the same site (on the 50S bacterial ribosome) as the macrolides and has a similar effect. Dalfopristin binds at a site nearby, resulting in a conformational change in the 50S ribosome, synergistically enhancing the binding of quinupristin at its target site.

b. **What are the hazards of using this combination?**

Quinupristin/dalfopristin inhibits CYP3A4. The concomitant administration of other CYP3A4 substrates may result in significant toxicity. Appropriate caution and monitoring are recommended for drugs in which the toxic/therapeutic window is narrow or for drugs that prolong the QTc interval.

c. **Linezolid is another drug that might be useful in treating this patient. Why might this drug be an effective alternative?**

Linezolid is FDA approved for the treatment of infections caused by vancomycin-resistant *E. faecium*. However, this agent is associated with some significant adverse effects.

d. **What are the hazards of linezolid therapy?**

Patients receiving long-term therapy with linezolid have developed peripheral neuropathy, optic neuritis, and lactic acidosis. These effects are not always reversible.

Linezolid is a weak nonspecific inhibitor of monoamine oxidase and patients receiving concomitant therapy with an SSRI may develop serotonin syndrome.

CASE 41-4

A 62-year-old man has developed a soft tissue infection following an auto accident. Cultures are pending.

a. **Is empirical treatment with vancomycin warranted?**

Vancomycin is frequently used in the empirical and definitive treatment of skin/soft-tissue and bone/joint infections, where gram-positive organisms including MRSA are the leading pathogens. Vancomycin and teicoplanin have been used to treat a wide variety of infections, including osteomyelitis and endocarditis, caused by methicillin-resistant and methicillin-susceptible staphylococci, streptococci, and enterococci.

b. **What is the mechanism of action of vancomycin**

Vancomycin inhibits the polymerization or transglycosylase reaction by binding to the D-alanyl-D-alanine terminus of the cell wall precursor unit attached to its lipid carrier thus blocking linkage to the glycoprotein polymer (see Figure 41-4).

(Continued)

Protein Synthesis Inhibitors and Miscellaneous Antibacterial Agents — CHAPTER 41

c. **What are the concerns about starting vancomycin empirically?**

A major concern for using vancomycin empirically is the development of resistance. Glycopeptide-resistant strains of enterococci have emerged as major nosocomial pathogens in hospitals in the United States. Resistance to vancomycin is due to the expression of enzymes that modify cell wall precursors by substituting a terminal D-lactate for D-alanine reducing vancomycin binding by 1000 times.

d. **What are the hazards of intravenous vancomycin?**

Rapid intravenous infusion of vancomycin may cause erythematous or urticarial reactions, flushing, tachycardia, and hypotension. Extreme flushing is referred to as "red man" syndrome. This effect is due to direct toxic effect of vancomycin on mast cells, causing them to release histamine.

CASE 41-5

Cultures from the patient in Case 41-4 are methicillin-resistant *S. aureus* that is also resistant to vancomycin. The decision has been made to switch the patient to daptomycin.

a. **Why daptomycin?**

Daptomycin may be active against vancomycin-resistant strains, although minimum inhibitory concentrations (MICs) tend to be higher for these organisms than for their vancomycin-susceptible counterparts.

b. **What is the mechanism of action of daptomycin?**

Daptomycin is an ionophore that binds to bacterial membranes resulting in depolarization, loss of membrane potential, and cell death.

CASE 41-6

A 6-year-old boy has fallen and scraped his knee. His mother goes to the pharmacy to obtain an antibiotic ointment. The pharmacist recommends an over-the-counter preparation containing polymyxin, bacitracin, and neosporin.

a. **Why is this combination of drugs available over-the-counter?**

Polymyxin and bacitracin are available for the topical treatment of minor skin infections. Neosporin is an aminoglycoside that is also available in topical preparations. Products that contain these antibiotics for otic or ophthalmic use are not available over-the-counter.

b. **What are the mechanisms of actions of the miscellaneous antibiotic agents bacitracin, polymyxin, and mupirocin?**

Polymyxins are surface-active amphipathic agents that interact with phospholipids and disrupt the structure of cell membranes. Bacitracin is an inhibitor of bacterial cell wall synthesis. Mupirocin inhibits bacterial protein synthesis by reversibly binding and inhibiting isoleucyl transfer-RNA synthetase.

KEY CONCEPTS

- Doxycycline is a drug of choice for sexually transmitted diseases, rickettsial infections, plague, brucellosis, tularemia, and spirochetal infections.
- Macrolide antibiotics are effective for treatment of respiratory tract infections caused by the common pathogens of community-acquired pneumonia, including *S. pneumoniae*, *Haemophilus* spp., *Chlamydia*, mycoplasma, and *Legionella*.

(Continued)

SECTION VII — Chemotherapy of Microbial Diseases

- Macrolides, except azithromycin, have important drug interactions because they inhibit hepatic CYPs.
- Chloramphenicol is rarely indicated because it can cause irreversible bone marrow toxicity.
- Vancomycin, daptomycin, quinupristin/dalfopristin, and linezolid are indicated for the treatment of gram-positive infections caused by drug-resistant organisms.
- Quinupristin/dalfopristin and linezolid are indicated for the treatment of vancomycin-resistant *E. faecium* infections.
- Quinupristin/dalfopristin, linezolid, and daptomycin are active against vancomycin-resistant strains of *S. aureus*.
- Polymyxin, bacitracin, and mupirocin are effective for the topical treatment of minor skin infections.

SUMMARY QUIZ

QUESTION 41-1 A-47-year-old man is receiving intravenous vancomycin. He develops flushing, tachycardia, and hypotension. The flushing, caused by the rapid infusion of vancomycin (referred to as "red man" syndrome), is caused by

a. testosterone released by sertoli cells.
b. glucagon released by hepatic cells.
c. histamine released by mast cells.
d. dopamine released by endothelial cells.
e. growth hormone released by pituitary cells.

QUESTION 41-2 A 25-year-old woman is receiving tetracycline for the treatment of acne. She should be warned against the concurrent ingestion of

a. milk.
b. caffeine.
c. chocolate.
d. green leafy vegetables.
e. water.

QUESTION 41-3 The patient in Question 41-2 should also be warned of

a. discoloration of her hair.
b. discoloration of her urine.
c. an excessive growth of finger and toe nails.
d. night blindness.
e. photosensitivity.

QUESTION 41-4 A 41-year-old woman is being treated with clindamycin for an infection in the skin of her leg that resulted from a bicycle accident. She should be warned about what serious side effect?

a. Discoloration around the infection site
b. Watery diarrhea
c. Constipation
d. Painful urination
e. A change in her hearing

Protein Synthesis Inhibitors and Miscellaneous Antibacterial Agents — CHAPTER 41

QUESTION 41-5 A 63-year-old woman has developed a vancomycin-resistant *E. faecium* infection. It is recommended that she be treated with quinupristin/dalfopristin. Which of this patient's medications should be discontinued or at least be monitored closely while she is on quinupristin/dalfopristin therapy?

a. Hydrochlorthiazide

b. Acetaminophen

c. Aspirin

d. Fluoxetine

e. None of the above

QUESTION 41-6 The patient in Question 41-5 is switched to daptomycin. Which of this patient's medications should be discontinued or at least monitored closely while she is on daptomycin therapy?

a. Hydrochlorthiazide

b. Acetaminophen

c. Aspirin

d. Fluoxetine

e. None of the above

SUMMARY QUIZ ANSWER KEY

QUESTION 41-1 Answer is **c**. Rapid intravenous infusion of vancomycin may cause a flushing reaction referred to as "red man" syndrome. This is not an allergic reaction but a direct toxic effect of vancomycin on mast cells, causing them to release histamine. This reaction is generally not observed with teicoplanin.

QUESTION 41-2 Answer is **a**. Oral absorption of most tetracyclines is incomplete. Absorption is further impaired by the concurrent ingestion of dairy products, antacids, aluminum hydroxide gels, calcium, magnesium, iron or zinc salts, and bismuth subsalicylate (PEPTO BISMOL). The cations in these products result in chelation with the tetracycline and decreased absorption.

QUESTION 41-3 Answer is **e**. Tetracyclines may produce mild to severe photosensitivity reactions in the skin of treated individuals exposed to sunlight.

QUESTION 41-4 Answer is **b**. The reported incidence of diarrhea associated with the administration of clindamycin ranges from 2 to 20%. A number of patients (up to 10%) have developed pseudomembranous colitis caused by the toxin from the organism *C. difficile*. This colitis is characterized by watery diarrhea, fever, and elevated peripheral white blood cell counts. This syndrome may be fatal. Treatment with metronidazole or oral vancomycin is usually curative, although relapses may occur.

QUESTION 41-5 Answer is **d**. Quinupristin/dalfopristin inhibits CYP3A4. The concomitant administration of other CYP3A4 substrates, such as fluoxetine, should be used with caution or monitored carefully.

QUESTION 41-6 Answer is **e**. Daptomycin neither inhibits nor induces CYPs, and there are no significant drug–drug interactions.

SECTION VII: Chemotherapy of Microbial Diseases

SUMMARY: PROTEIN SYNTHESIS INHIBITORS AND MISCELLANEOUS ANTIBIOTICS

CLASS AND SUBCLASSES	NAME	CLINICAL USES	RESISTANCE (SEE SIDE BAR MECHANISMS OF ACTION AND RESISTANCE OF PROTEIN SYNTHESIS INHIBITORS)	TOXICITY COMMON	TOXICITY UNIQUE; CLINICALLY IMPORTANT
Tetracyclines	Tetracycline, Doxycycline, Tigecycline	First-line therapy of infections caused by rickettsia, mycoplasmas, and Chlamydia	Resistance has limited the use of these agents for the common bacterial infections	GI irritation	Photosensitivity; Hepatic toxicity in doses >2 g/d; Aggravation of azotemia; Fanconi syndrome with outdated products; Brown discoloration of teeth in children or infants; Depressed bone growth in premature infants
Chloramphenicol	Chloramphenicol	Limited to use in infections for which the benefits outweigh the potential toxicities	Resistance is reported	Hypersensitivity	Bone marrow toxicity resulting in aplastic anemia; "Gray baby syndrome" in neonates
Macrolides and Ketolides	Erythromycin, Clarithromycin, Telithromycin, Azithromycin	Respiratory tract infections caused by Streptococcus pneumonia and H. influenzae; Alternatives for treatment of erysipelas and cellulitis; Chlamydial infections; Pertussis and Campylobacter infections; Helicobacter pylori (clarithromycin); Disseminated mycobacterial infections (clarithromycin)	Resistance is common	GI distress	Cardiac arrhythmias in patients with risk factors such as prolonged QT syndrome; Inhibition of CYP3A4, associated with drug interactions with other drugs metabolized by this CYP
Lincosamides	Clindamycin	Similar to erythromycin, but more active against anaerobic bacteria especially B. fragilis	Similar to erythromycin, but clindamycin is not a substrate for macrolide efflux pumps	Nausea, vomiting, and diarrhea	Pseudomembranous colitis caused by C. difficle
Streptogramins	Quinupristin/Dalfopristin	Bacteriocidal against streptococci and many strains of staphylococci but bacteriostatic against E. faecium	Similar to macrolides	Pain and phlebitis at infusion site	Inhibition of CYP3A4 which may cause toxicity of other drugs metabolized by this enzyme
Oxazolidinones	Linezolid	Treatment of infections caused by vancomycin-resistant E. faecium; nosocomial pneumonia, caused by methicillin-susceptible and resistant strains of S. aureus; community-acquired pneumonia	Should be reserved as an alternative agent for treatment of infections caused by multiple drug-resistant strains	GI distress	Hematologic toxicity including myelosuppression
Aminocyclitols	Spectinomycin	Treatment of gonorrhea resistant to first-line drugs			
Polymyxins	Polymyxin B, Polymyxin E	Not absorbed orally; available for ophthalmic, otic, and topical use in combination with other agents	Emergence of resistance while on therapy is documented	None, probably due to poor systemic absorption	

(Continued)

Protein Synthesis Inhibitors and Miscellaneous Antibacterial Agents — CHAPTER 41

CLASS AND SUBCLASSES	NAME	CLINICAL USES	RESISTANCE (SEE SIDE BAR MECHANISMS OF ACTION AND RESISTANCE OF PROTEIN SYNTHESIS INHIBITORS)	TOXICITY COMMON	TOXICITY UNIQUE; CLINICALLY IMPORTANT
Glycopeptides	Vancomycin, Teicoplanin	Used to treat infections caused by methicillin-sensitive and methicillin-resistant strains of staphylococci, streptococci, and enterococci	Resistant strains of enterococci have emerged as major nosocomial pathogens	Hypersensitivity reactions	"Red man" syndrome from rapid IV infusion. Auditory impairment
Lipopeptides	Daptomycin	Treatment of complicated skin and soft tissue infections and complicated bacteremia	Not well-characterized		Musculoskeletal toxicity including rhabdomyolysis in rare cases
Bacitracin	Bacitracin	Use restricted to topical application including ophthalmic and skin ointments	Not a major clinical problem		Hypersensitivity reactions are rare
Mupirocin	Mupirocin	Available for topical use for treatment of traumatic skin lesions and impetigo secondarily infected with S. aureus or S. pyogenes. Nasal ointment is approved for the eradication of S. aureus nasal carriage	No cross-resistance with other classes of antibiotics	Irritation and sensitization at the site of application	Polyethylene glycol in the ointment can be absorbed from damaged skin

CHAPTER 42

Chemotherapy of Tuberculosis, *Mycobacterium Avium* Complex Disease, and Leprosy

DRUGS INCLUDED IN THIS CHAPTER

- Aminoglycosides (streptomycin, amikacin, kanamycin) (See Chapter 40)
- Capreomycin (CAPASTAT)
- Clofazimine (LAMPRENE)
- Cycloserine (SEROMYCIN)
- Dapsone
- Ethambutol (MYAMBUTOL)
- Ethionamide (TRECATOR)
- Fluoroquinolones (ofloxacin, ciprofloxacin, moxifloxacin) (See Chapter 38)
- Isoniazid (NYDRAZID)
- PA-824
- Pyrazinamide
- Rifamycins: Rifampin (RIFADIN, RIMAC-TANE, others), Rifapentine (PRIFTIN), Rifabutin (MYCOBUTIN)
- TMC-207

This chapter will be most useful after having a basic understanding of the material in Chapter 56, Chemotherapy of Tuberculosis, Mycobacterium Avium Complex Disease, and Leprosy in *Goodman & Gilman's The Pharmacological Basis of Therapeutics*, 12th Edition. In addition to the material presented here, the 12th Edition contains:

- Table 56-1 Pathogenic Mycobacterial Rapid and Slow Growers (Runyon Classification)
- Table 56-2 Population Pharmacokinetic Parameter Estimates for Antimycobacteial Drugs in Adult Patients
- Table 56-3 Pharmacokinetic Parameters of Rifampin, Rifabutin, and Rifapentine
- Table 56-5 Drugs Used in the Treatment of Mycobacteria Other Than for Tuberculosis, Leprosy, or MAC (*Mycobacterium Avium* Complex)
- Figure 56-4 Multimodal distribution of isoniazide (INH) clearance due to NAT2 polymorphisms

LEARNING OBJECTIVES

- ☑ Understand the rationale for combination drug therapy in the treatment of tuberculosis (TB).
- ☑ Know the mechanisms of action and resistance for drugs used to treat TB and leprosy.
- ☑ Describe the adverse effects and drug interactions commonly associated with anti-TB drugs.
- ☑ Know the principles of anti-TB chemotherapy.
- ☑ Understand the principles of therapy of *Mycobacterium Avium* Complex (MAC) disease.
- ☑ Understand the principles of antileprosy therapy.

MECHANISMS OF ACTION AND RESISTANCE OF DRUGS USED TO TREAT TUBERCULOSIS AND LEPROSY

DRUG	MECHANISM OF ACTION (see Figure 42-1)	MECHANISM OF RESISTANCE (see Figure 42-2)
Rifamycins	Binds to the β subunit of DNA-dependent RNA polymerase to form a stable drug-enzyme complex thus suppressing chain formation in RNA synthesis	Mutations causing an alteration in the drug target
Pyrazinamide	In *Mycobacterium tuberculosis* pyrazinamidase deaminates pyrazinamide to pyrazinoic acid (POA) which is protonated in an acidic environment to POAH which is responsible for microbial killing (see Side Bar PROPOSED MECHANISMS FOR MICROBIAL KILLING BY PYRAZINAMIDE)	Pyrazinamidases with reduced affinity for pyrazinamide
Isoniazid	Activated in bacilli by catalase-peroxidase (KatG) to an isonicotinoyl radical that reacts with mycobacterial NAD and NADP to form protein adducts; adduct formation inhibits the formation of mycolic acid and mycobacterial dihydrofolate reductase, thereby interfering with nucleic acid synthesis (see Figure 42-3)	Preexistent resistance can be expected in pulmonary TB cavities of untreated patients; these resistant mycobacteria are selected and amplified by isoniazid monotherapy; resistance is associated with mutation or deletion of KatG, also by enhancement of efflux pump activity
Ethambutol	Inhibition of arabinosyl transferase III with disruption of mycobacterial cell wall	Mutations in the *embB* gene and possibly by enhanced efflux pump activity

(Continued)

Chemotherapy of TB, MAC Disease, and Leprosy

CHAPTER 42

DRUG	MECHANISM OF ACTION (see Figure 42-1)	MECHANISM OF RESISTANCE (see Figure 42-2)
Clofazimine	Possible mechanisms of action include: • membrane disruption • inhibition of phospholipase A_2 • inhibition of K^+ transport • interference with electron transport	Unknown
Ethionamide	Mycobacteria convert ethionamide to a sulfoxide and another toxic intermediate; this results in inhibition of mycolic acid biosynthesis and impairment of cell wall synthesis	Resistance occurs via changes in the enzyme that activates ethionamide
TMC-207	Targets subunit c of ATP synthase resulting in inhibition of proton pump and interference of energy metabolism	Mutation of ATP synthase c subunit
PA-824	Inhibition of mycolic acid and protein synthesis	Mutation in target protein
Cycloserine	Inhibition of alanine racemase and stopping reactions in which D-alanine is incorporated into cell wall synthesis	Resistance in clinical isolates has been demonstrated although mechanism is unknown
Capreomycin	Inhibition of protein synthesis similar to aminoglycosides	Resistance develops when given alone; there is cross-resistance with kanamycin and neomycin
Dapsone	Structural analog of *para*-aminobenzoic acid (PABA) and inhibitor of dihydropteroate synthase in folate pathway (see Figure 42-4)	Mutations in genes encoding dihydropteroate synthase

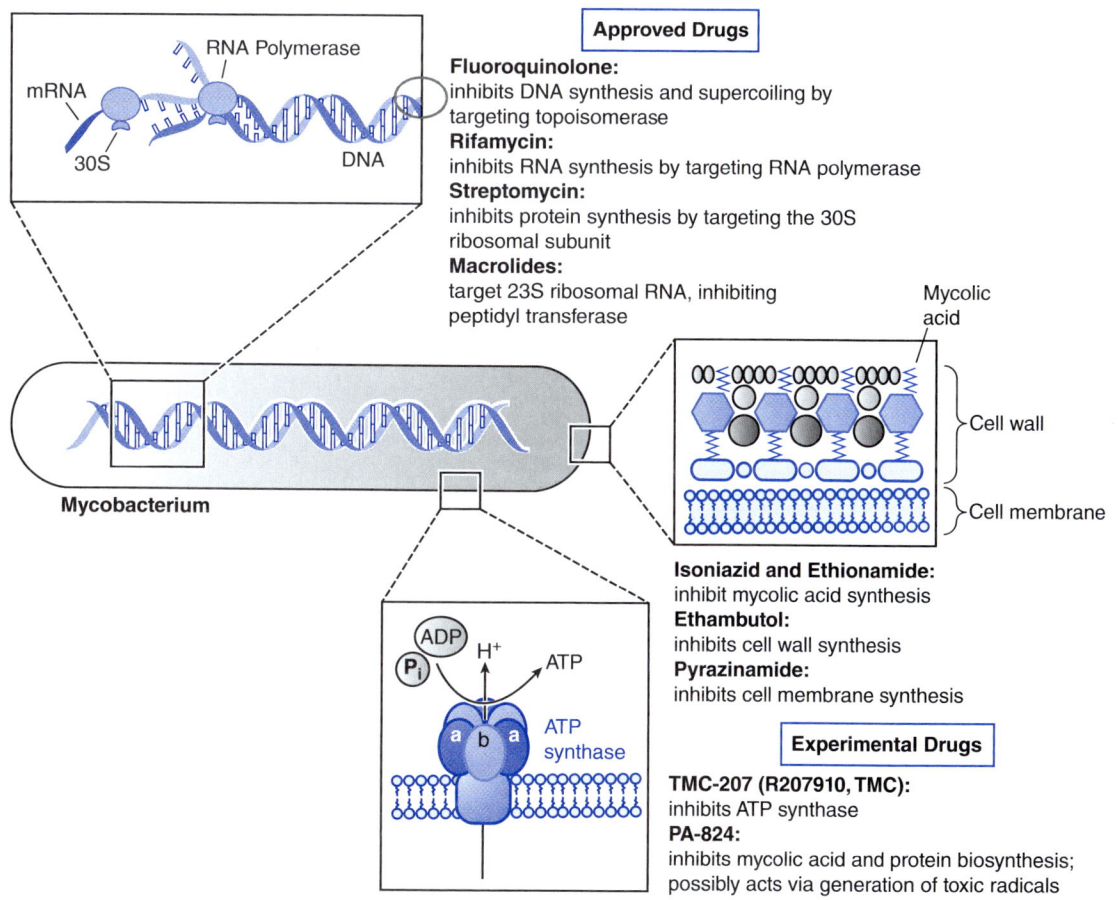

FIGURE 42-1 Mechanisms of action of established and experimental drugs used for the chemotherapy of mycobacterial infections. Shown at the top are the sites of action of approved drugs for the chemotherapy of mycobacterial diseases. Rifamycin is used as a generic term for several drugs, of which rifampin is used most frequently. Also included are 2 experimental drugs now under investigation: TMC-207 and PA-824. Clofazimine, whose mode of action is not understood, is omitted.

SECTION VII Chemotherapy of Microbial Diseases

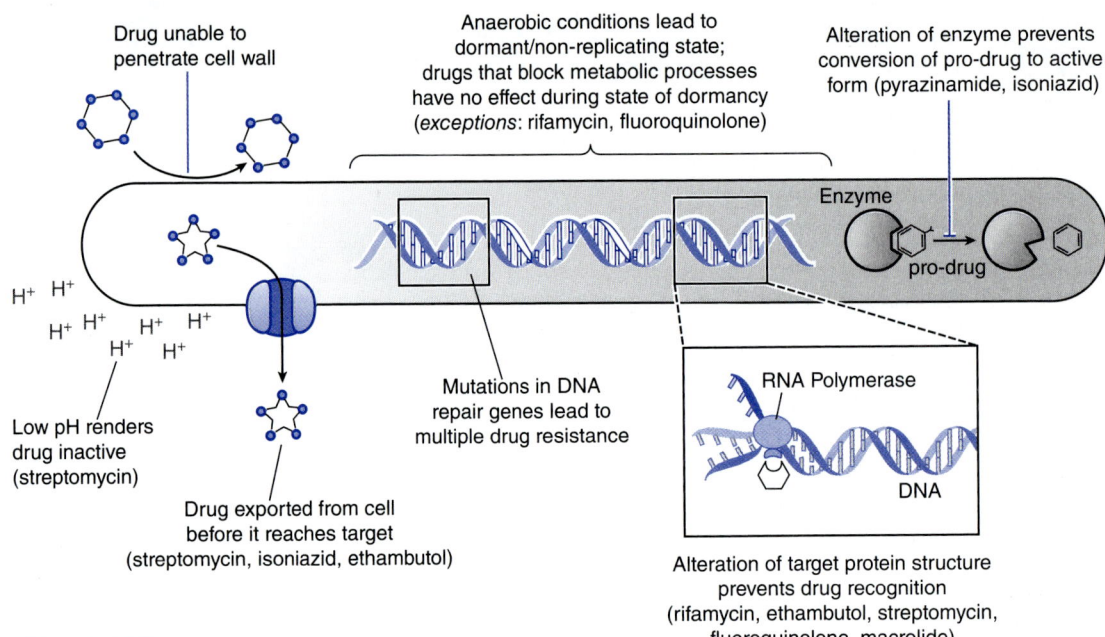

FIGURE 42-2 Mechanisms of resistance of *Mycobacteria* to different chemotherapeutic drugs. Shown are the various mechanisms by which mycobacteria resist antibacterial effects of the currently approved chemotherapeutic agents.

PROPOSED MECHANISMS FOR MICROBIAL KILLING BY PYRAZINAMIDE

- Inhibition of fatty acid synthesis type I leading to interference with mycolic acid synthesis
- Reduction of intracellular pH
- Disruption of membrane transport by protonated pyrazinoic acid (POAH)

CRITERION FOR PROPHYLACTIC ANTITUBERCULOSIS THERAPY

Mantoux reaction is more than or equal to 5 mm and those who meet one of following criteria:

- Recently exposed to TB
- HIV co-infection
- Fibrotic changes on chest radiograms
- Immunosuppressed

Mantoux reaction is more than or equal to 10 mm and those who meet one of the following criteria:

- Recent (≤5 years) immigrants from area of high TB prevalence
- Children younger than 4 years
- Children exposed to adults with TB
- Intravenous (IV) drug users
- Residents and employees in high-risk settings

Anyone with a Mantoux reaction more than 15 mm

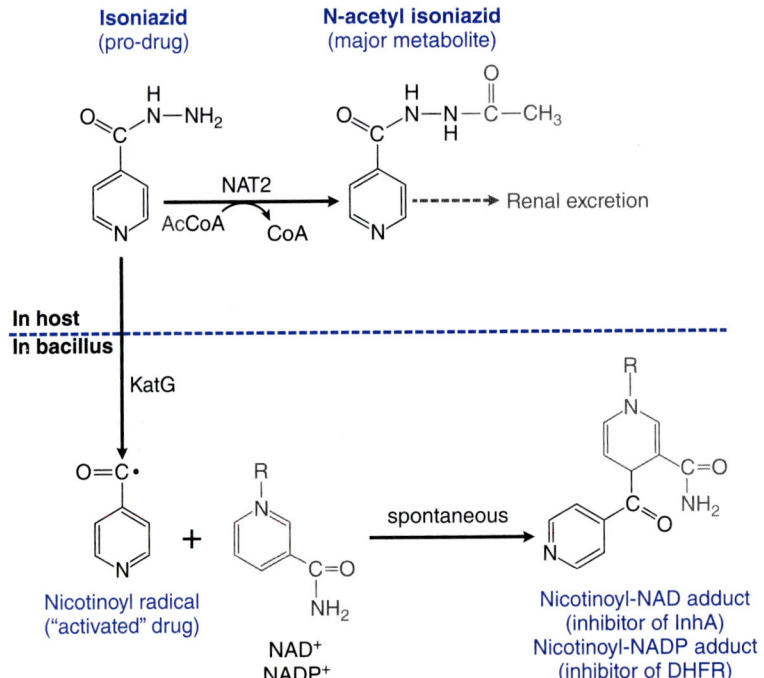

FIGURE 42-3 Metabolism and activation of isoniazid. The prodrug isoniazid is metabolized in humans by NAT2 isoforms to its principal metabolite, N-acetyl isoniazid, which is excreted by the kidney. Isoniazid diffuses into mycoplasma where it is "activated" by KatG (oxidase/peroxidase) to the nicotinoyl radical, which reacts spontaneously with NAD^+ or $NADP^+$ to produce adducts that inhibit important enzymes in cell wall and nucleic acid synthesis. DHFR, dihydrofolate reductase.

Chemotherapy of TB, MAC Disease, and Leprosy

CHAPTER 42

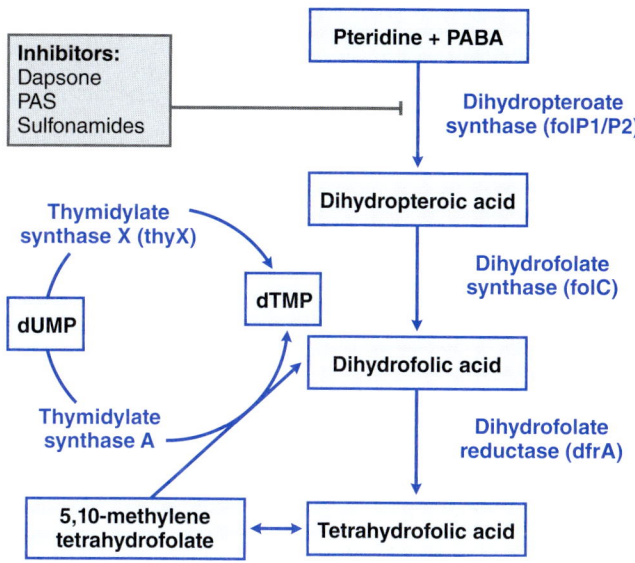

FIGURE 42-4 Effects of antimicrobials on folate metabolism and deoxynucleotide synthesis.

DEFINITIVE ANTITUBERCULOSIS THERAPY

All active TB cases should be confirmed by culture with antimicrobial susceptibility determined.

For the first 2 months:
- Isoniazid (5 mg/kg, maximum 300 mg/d), pyridoxine (10 to 50 mg/d)
- Rifampin (10 mg/kg, maximum 600 mg/d)
- Pyrazinamide (15 to 30 mg/kg, maximum 2 g/d)

Follow-up therapy, 2 or 3 times per week, for next 4 months:
- Isoniazid (15 mg/kg), pyridoxine (10 to 50 mg/d)
- Rifampin (10 mg/kg)

CASE 42-1

On a recent trip to India, a 45-year-old man contracted tuberculosis that was confirmed by culture. Antimicrobial susceptibility was performed and the patient was started on isoniazid, rifampin, and pyrazinamide as definitive therapy for tuberculosis.

a. Why did this patient receive three drugs?

Only combination anti-TB therapy is currently recommended for treatment of TB. When anti-TB drug monotherapy was administered to TB patients, resistance emergence terminated the effectiveness of these drugs. The mutation rates to first-line TB drugs are between 10^{-7} and 10^{-10} so that the likelihood of resistance is high to any single anti-TB drug in patients with cavitary TB who have $\sim 10^9$ CFU (colony forming units) of bacilli in a 3-cm pulmonary lesion. However, the likelihood that bacilli would develop mutations to 2 or more different drugs is the product of 2 mutation rates which makes the probability of resistance emergence to more than 2 drugs acceptably small. Multidrug therapy has also led to a reduction in length of therapy.

b. What is the mechanism of action of rifampin?

Rifampin enters bacilli in a concentration-dependent manner where it binds to the β subunit of DNA-dependent RNA polymerase to form a stable drug-enzyme complex. Drug binding suppresses chain formation in RNA synthesis (see Figure 42-1).

c. How should rifampin therapy be optimized?

Rifampin's bactericidal activity is best optimized by a regimen to achieve a high AUC/MIC (area under the curve/minimal inhibitory concentration) ratio, but resistance suppression and rifampin's enduring postantibiotic effect are best optimized by high C_{Pmax}/MIC therapy (see Chapter 34). Therefore, the duration of time that the rifampin concentration persists above the MIC is of less importance than reaching a high C_{Pmax}. The $t_{1/2}$ of rifampin is less of an issue in optimizing therapy, and if patients could tolerate it, higher doses would lead to higher bactericidal activities while suppressing resistance.

d. For what clinical diseases, other than TB, might rifampin be useful?

Rifampin is also useful for the prophylaxis of meningococcal disease and *Haemophilus influenza* meningitis. Combined with a β-lactam antibiotic or vancomycin, rifampin may be useful for therapy in selected cases of staphylococcal endocarditis

(Continued)

or osteomyelitis, especially those caused by staphylococci "tolerant" to penicillin. Rifampin may also be used for the eradication of staphylococcal nasal carrier state.

e. What adverse effects should this patient be warned of with the use of rifampin?

Rifampin is generally well tolerated, but patients should be warned that it will cause an orange-tan discoloration of skin, urine, feces, saliva, tears, and contact lenses.

CASE 42-2

A 35-year-old woman hospital employee has a routine tuberculin skin test reaction of 18 mm. She is started on prophylactic isoniazid therapy of 300 mg daily. She is also started on pyridoxine (vitamin B_6).

a. What is the mechanism of action of isoniazid?

Isoniazid is activated within the *bacillus* to an isonicotinoyl radical by KatG, a multifunctional catalase-peroxidase (see Figure 42-3). This radical interacts with mycobacterial NAD and NAPD to form adducts that inhibit the activities of enzymes responsible for the synthesis of mycolic acid, an essential component of the mycobacterial cell wall. The adducts also inhibit mycobacterial dihydrofolate reductase and interfere with nucleic acid synthesis.

b. How is isoniazid metabolized?

Isoniazid is metabolized by hepatic arylamine *N*-acetyltransferase type 2 (see Figure 42-3). Isoniazid clearance in patients can be classified into 2 phenotypic groups: slow and fast acetylators as seen in Figure 56-4 of *Goodman and Gilman's The Pharmacological Basis of Therapeutics*, 12th Edition. Recently the phenotypic groups have been expanded to fast, intermediate, and slow acetylators. The number of *NAT2*4* alleles accounts for 88% of the variability of isoniazid clearance. Slow acetylators may be a greater risk for adverse effects from isoniazid, sulfonamides, and procainamide. Fast acetylators may have diminished responses to standard doses of these agents but a greater risk from bioactivation by NAT2 of arylamine/hydrazine carcinogens.

CASE 42-3

In the patient in Case 42-2:

a. What are the potential side effects of isoniazid therapy in this otherwise healthy woman?

Isoniazid is converted to acetylisoniazid which can be converted to acetylhydrazine and hepatotoxic metabolites by CYP2E1. Rapid acetylators will form diacetylhydrazine which is nontoxic, while slow acetylators or CYP2E1 induction will lead to more hepatotoxic metabolites. Rifampin, a potent inducer of CYP2E1, potentiates isoniazid hepatotoxicity.

Isoniazid also can cause a peripheral neuritis (see answer to Case 42-3c below).

b. What drug interactions should she be warned of?

Isoniazid is a potent inhibitor of CYP2C19, CYP3A, and a weak inhibitor of CYP2D6. Isoniazide induces CYP2E1. Drugs metabolized by these enzymes will potentially be affected. Table 42-1 lists the potential drug interactions that might occur with isoniazid and their adverse effects.

c. Why is she also given a vitamin?

As mentioned above in the answer to question a of this case, isoniazid causes a peripheral neuritis (most commonly paresthesias of the feet and hands). This neuropathy is more frequent in slow acetylators and in individuals with diabetes mellitus, poor nutrition, or anemia. The prophylactic administration of pyridoxine (vitamin B_6) prevents the development of peripheral neuritis even when therapy lasts as long as 2 years.

Chemotherapy of TB, MAC Disease, and Leprosy

CHAPTER 42

TABLE 42-1 Isoniazid-Drug Interactions via Inhibition and Induction of CYPs

CO-ADMINISTERED DRUG	CYP ISOFORM	ADVERSE EFFECTS
Acetaminophen	CYP2E1 inhibition-induction	Hepatotoxicity
Carbamazepine	CYP3A inhibition	Neurological toxicity
Diazepam	CYP3A and CYP2C19 inhibition	Sedation and respiratory depression
Ethosuximide	CYP3A inhibition	Psychotic behavior
Isoflurane and enflurane	CYP2E1 induction	Decreased effectiveness
Phenytoin	CYP2C19 inhibition	Neurological toxicity
Theophylline	CYP3A inhibition	Seizures, palpitation, nausea
Vincristine	CYP3A inhibition	Limb weakness and tingling
Warfarin	CYP2C9 inhibition	Possibility of increased bleeding (single case reported)

CASE 42-4

A 25-year-old medical resident has developed active TB after being exposed in the hospital. It is known that the patient she was exposed to had a strain of *M. tuberculosis* that was resistant to isoniazid. She is started on rifampin, pyrazinamide, and ethambutol.

a. What is the mechanism of action of ethambutol?

Ethambutol inhibits arabinosyl transferase III which disrupts the assembly of the mycobacterial cell wall.

b. If this patient's *M. tuberculosis* is resistant to isoniazid, might it also be resistant to ethambutol?

Mycobacterial resistance to ethambutol develops via mutations in the *embB* gene. However, enhanced efflux pump activity may induce resistance to both isoniazid and ethambutol. Thus, resistance to isoniazid does not necessarily predict resistance to ethambutol.

c. What serious side effect of ethambutol should this patient be warned about?

About 1% of patients receiving ethambutol experience diminished visual acuity. Approximately 15% of patients receiving a dose of ethambutol of 50 mg/kg/d will develop optic neuritis resulting in decreased visual acuity and an inability to distinguish red from green. The incidence of this reaction is proportional to the dose of ethambutol with approximately 1% of patients who receive a dose of 15 mg/kg/d experiencing this effect.

CASE 42-5

A 36-year-old man in Central Africa has developed leprosy. He is being treated with rifampin, clofazimine, and dapsone.

a. Why 3 drugs?

The reasons for using combination therapy in the treatment of leprosy include reduction in the development of resistance, the need for adequate therapy when primary resistance already exists, and reduction in the duration of therapy. Rifampin is the most bactericidal drug in the regimen. Clofazimine is only bacteriostatic against *Mycobacterium leprae*; however, it also has anti-inflammatory effects.

(Continued)

SECTION VII

Chemotherapy of Microbial Diseases

TREATMENT OF DRUG-RESISTANT TUBERCULOSIS

Therapy should be based on evidence of susceptibility and should include the following:

- At least 3 drugs to which the pathogen is susceptible, one of them injectable
- Use of 4 to 6 medications for MDR-TB (multiple drug resistant-TB)
- 18 months of therapy

PRINCIPLES OF THERAPY OF *MYCOBACTERIUM AVIUM* COMPLEX (MAC)

- MAC is made up of 2 species: *M. intracellulare* and *M. avium*.
- After isolating MAC from pulmonary specimens, first determine whether disease is present or if the organism is merely part of environmental contamination.
- Criteria for therapy:
  - Positive cultures from 2 sputum specimens, or 1 positive culture from bronchoalveolar lavage, or pulmonary biopsy with positive culture or histopathological features
  - Clinical evidence of infection
  - Radiological evidence of infection
- For newly diagnosed patients with MAC pneumonia, therapy should include rifamycin, ethambutol, and macrolide (clarithromycin or azithromycin).
- Therapy should continue for 12 months after last negative culture.

PRINCIPLE OF ANTILEPROSY THERAPY

Therapy for leprosy is based on multidrug regimens using the following:

- Rifampin
- Clofazimine
- Dapsone

---

b. What is the mechanism of action of dapsone?

Dapsone is a competitive inhibitor of dihydropteroate synthase in the folate pathway (see Figure 42-4). Dapsone also has anti-inflammatory effects by inhibiting tissue damage caused by neutrophils.

c. What enzyme deficiency should this patient be tested for before starting dapsone therapy?

Dapsone, an oxidant, causes severe hemolysis in patients with glucose-6-phosphate dehydrogenase (G6PD) deficiency. Thus, G6PD deficiency testing should be performed prior to the use of dapsone wherever possible.

CASE 42-6

A 58-year-old man develops active TB confirmed by positive culture. An infectious disease consultant recommends therapy with isoniazid, rifampin, and pyrazinamide. Susceptibility testing reveals that the *M. tuberculosis* cultured from this patient is resistant to isoniazid and rifampin.

a. What are the considerations in treating this patient?

Multidrug-resistant tuberculosis (MDR-TB) is present if an isolate is resistant simultaneously to isoniazid and rifampin. In documented drug resistance, therapy should be based on evidence of susceptibility and should include the principles shown in the Side Bar TREATMENT OF DRUG-RESISTANT TUBERCULOSIS.

CASE 42-7

Following a liver transplant, a 38-year-old man develops a sputum culture that is positive for *Mycobacterium intracellulare*.

a. What is the first course of action?

M. intracellulare is 1 of the species that make up MAC, *Mycobacterium avium* is the other species. These bacteria are ubiquitous in the environment and can be encountered in food, water, and soil. *M. intracellulare* often infects immunocompromised patients. The first decision after isolating MAC from pulmonary specimens is to determine whether disease is actually present or if the organism is merely part of environmental contamination (see Side Bar PRINCIPLES OF THERAPY OF *MYCOBACTERIUM AVIUM* COMPLEX).

b. If the diagnosis is confirmed, what is the recommended therapy?

In newly diagnosed patients with MAC pneumonia, therapy with rifampin, ethambutol, and a macrolide antibiotic—either clarithromycin or azithromycin—is recommended. Therapy should be continued for 12 months after the last negative culture.

KEY CONCEPTS

- Combination therapy is the desirable approach for mycobacterial disease to ensure effective eradication and to prevent the emergence of resistance.
- Isoniazid, rifamycins, ethambutol, streptomycin, and pyrazinamide are first-line agents for the treatment of tuberculosis.
- Antimicrobial agents with excellent activity against MAC include rifabutin, clarithromycin, azithromycin, and fluoroquinolones.
- Clinical monitoring of patients with mycobacterial infections is important because drug interactions and adverse drug reactions are common with the multiple-drug regimens used.
- Considerable progress has been achieved in eliminating leprosy through the use of multiple-drug chemotherapy, including dapsone, rifampin, and clofazimine.

Chemotherapy of TB, MAC Disease, and Leprosy — CHAPTER 42

SUMMARY QUIZ

QUESTION 42-1 A 35-year-old man has developed a tuberculin skin reaction that is 20 mm in size. He is being treated with a triple-drug regimen of isoniazid, rifampin, and pyrazinamide but is concerned because of the number of medications he must take every day. He is a slow acetylator of isoniazid. He asks why other antibiotics like penicillin are not effective in treating tuberculosis. Your answer is that the tuberculosis bacteria

a. have developed a resistance to penicillin.
b. have a rigid cell wall that does not allow penicillin to get inside the cell.
c. destroy the penicillin.
d. multiply too rapidly for the penicillin to be effective.
e. are anaerobic.

QUESTION 42-2 The patient in Case 42-1 should be instructed to take his rifampin on an empty stomach because

a. food decreases the peak plasma concentration of rifampin by one-third.
b. rifampin may affect the taste of food.
c. food increases the absorption of rifampin and may cause toxicity.
d. food increases gastric transit.
e. food increases gastric acid secretion which may destroy the rifampin.

QUESTION 42-3 The plasma concentration of rifampin in the patient in Case 42-1 is only above the MIC approximately 25% of the dosing interval. This is of little concern because the rifampin

a. $t_{1/2}$ in this patient is prolonged.
b. bactericidal activity is optimized by a high AUC/MIC.
c. volume of distribution is very small.
d. pharmacokinetics are best described by a two-compartment model.
e. induces CYP3A4.

QUESTION 42-4 After 1 month of treatment, the patient in case 42-1 is complaining of numbness and tingling in his feet. The likely problem is

a. tight shoes.
b. a blood clot in the femoral artery.
c. undiagnosed diabetes mellitus.
d. heart failure.
e. isoniazid-induced peripheral neuritis.

QUESTION 42-5 The patient in Case 42-1 is taking other medications for medical problems unrelated to tuberculosis. Which of the following drugs should be monitored closely after starting isoniazid therapy?

a. Aspirin
b. Dexamethasone
c. Phenytoin
d. Metformin
e. Nitroglycerine

QUESTION 42-6 A 63-year-old woman has developed leprosy and is being treated with a combination of rifampin, clofazimine, and dapsone. A deficiency of which of the following enzymes is of specific concern with dapsone therapy?

a. *N*-acetyltransferase
b. DNA gyrase

(Continued)

SECTION VII Chemotherapy of Microbial Diseases

c. Pyrazinamidase
d. Glucose-6-phosphate dehydrogenase
e. Glutathione transferase

SUMMARY QUIZ ANSWER KEY

QUESTION 42-1 Answer is **b**. The name *Mycobacterium* refers to their waxy appearance due to the composition of their cell walls. More than 60% of their cell wall is lipid, mainly mycolic acids. This extraordinary shield prevents many pharmacological compounds, such as penicillin, from getting into the bacterial cell wall or inside the cell.

QUESTION 42-2 Answer is **a**. After oral administration, the rifamycins are absorbed to variable extents. Food decreases the rifampin C_{Pmax} by one-third. A high-fat meal increases the area under the curve (AUC) of rifapentine by 50%.

QUESTION 42-3 Answer is **b**. Rifampin's bactericidal activity is best optimized by a high AUC/MIC ratio. However, the resistance suppression and rifampin's postantibiotic effect are best optimized by high C_{Pmax}/MIC. Therefore, the duration of time that the rifampin concentration persists above the MIC is of less importance.

QUESTION 42-4 Answer is **e**. Paresthesia of the feet and hands (peripheral neuritis) is encountered in about 2% of patients receiving isoniazid 5 mg/kg daily. Neuropathy is more frequent in slow acetylators of isoniazid. The prophylactic administration of pyridoxine (vitamin B_6) prevents the development of the peripheral neuritis as well as other nervous system disorders.

QUESTION 42-5 Answer is **c**. Isoniazid is a potent inhibitor of CYP2C19, CYP3A, and a weak inhibitor of CYP2D6. Drugs that are metabolized by these enzymes will potentially be affected. Phenytoin metabolism by CYP2C19 is inhibited by isoniazid with potential neurotoxicity resulting.

QUESTION 42-6 Answer is **d**. Glucose-6-phosphate dehydrogenase (G6PD) protects red blood cells against oxidative damage. Dapsone, an oxidant, causes severe hemolysis in patients with G6PD deficiency. G6PD deficiency occurs in nearly half a billion people worldwide. Thus, G6PD deficiency testing should be performed prior to the use of dapsone wherever possible.

SUMMARY: DRUGS USED IN THE TREATMENT OF TUBERCULOSIS, MAC, AND LEPROSY

CLASS AND SUBCLASSES	NAME	CLINICAL USES	RESISTANCE	TOXICITY COMMON	TOXICITY UNIQUE; CLINICALLY IMPORTANT
Rifamycins	Rifampin, rifapentine, rifabutin	Available for the treatment of TB either alone, or in fixed dose combinations with isoniazid or isoniazid plus pyrazinamide Also useful for prophylaxis of meningococcal disease and *H. influenzae* meningitis	The prevalence of rifampin-resistant isolates are 1 in every 10^7 to 10^8 bacilli	Rash, nausea, and vomiting	Rarely hepatitis Skin and body fluid discoloration
Pyrazinamide		Coadministration with isoniazid or rifampin has led to a one-third reduction in the duration of TB therapy and a two-thirds reduction in TB relapse	Pyrazinamide-resistant *M. tuberculosis* have pyrazinamidases with reduced affinity for pyrazinamide	Elevated blood uric acid levels	Hepatic injury Gout

(Continued)

Chemotherapy of TB, MAC Disease, and Leprosy — CHAPTER 42

CLASS AND SUBCLASSES	NAME	CLINICAL USES	RESISTANCE	TOXICITY COMMON	TOXICITY UNIQUE; CLINICALLY IMPORTANT
Isoniazid	NYDRAZID	Available to treat TB either alone, or in combination with rifampin or pyrazinamide	Prevalence of resistance is about 1 in 10^6 bacilli; preexisting resistance can be expected in pulmonary TB cavities of untreated patients		Hepatic injury due to the formation of hepatotoxic metabolites; Peripheral neuropathy that is prevented by the prophylactic administration of pyridoxine
Ethambutol	MYAMBUTOL	Oral administration for the treatment of TB, disseminated MAC, and *Mycobacterium kansaii* infection	30-70% of clinical isolates are resistant to ethambutol	Lowered visual acuity, rash, drug fever	Optic neuritis with loss of visual acuity
Clofazimine	LAMPRENE	Part of multiple drug therapy with rifampin and dapsone for the treatment of leprosy		Abdominal pain, diarrhea, nausea, and vomiting	Body fluid discoloration
TMC-207		Good activity against *M. tuberculosis*, MAC, *M. leprae*, *Mycobacterium bovis*, *Mycobacterium marinum*, *M. kansaii*, *Mycobacterium ulcerans*, *Mycobacterium fortuitum*, *Mycobacterium szulgai*, and *Mycobacterium abscessus*		Nausea and diarrhea	Full side-effect profile is not clear at this time
PA-824		In vitro it kills non-replicating *M. tuberculosis* under aerobic conditions and replicating bacilli in ambient air		Not known at this time	Not known at this time
Ethionamide	TRECATOR	Second-line drug for the treatment of TB	Resistance occurs via mutations in the enzyme that activates ethionamide	GI upset	Severe postural hypotension; Mental depression, drowsiness, blurred vision, diplopia, dizziness, paresthesias; neurologic symptoms are relieved by pyridoxine (vitamin B_6)
Cycloserine	SEROMYCIN	Second-line drug for the treatment of TB; inhibits *M. tuberculosis* at concentrations of 5-20 mg/L; Good activity against MAC, *Escherichia coli*, *Staphylococcus aureus*, *Nocardia*, and *Chlamydia*	Resistance in clinical isolates of *M. tuberculosis* has been detected		Neuropsychiatric symptoms are common in 50% of patients; Contraindicated in patients with a history of epilepsy
Capreomycin	CAPASTA	Second-line drug for the treatment of TB; Antimicrobial activity is similar to aminoglycosides	Resistance develops when given alone	Hearing loss, tinnitus, proteinuria	Should not be administered with other drugs that damage cranial nerve VIII
Dapsone		Bacteriostatic against *M. leprae*; Highly effective against *Plasmodium falciparum*	Resistance occurs from mutations in genes encoding dihydropteroate synthase	Skin rashes	Hemolysis in patients with G6PD deficiency treated with 200-300 mg/d; Rarely psychosis

CHAPTER 43

Antifungal Agents

DRUGS INCLUDED IN THIS CHAPTER

- Amphotericin B (FUNGIZONE); colloidal dispersion (AMPHOTEC, AMPHOCIL); liposomal formulation (AMBISOME); lipid complex (ABELCET)
- Anidulafungin (ERAXIS)
- Butenafine (MENTAX, LOTRIMIN ULTRA)
- Butoconazole (FEMSTAT 3, others)
- Caspofungin (CANCIDAS)
- Ciclopirox olamine (LOPROX, others)
- Clotrimazole (LOTRIMIN, MYCELEX, GYNE-LOTRIMIN, others)
- Fluconazole (DIFLUCAN, others)
- Flucytosine (ANCOBON)
- Griseofulvin (GRIFULVIN and GRIS-PEG)
- Haloprogin (HALOTEX)
- Isavuconazole (BAL 8557) (investigational)
- Itraconazole (SPORANOX, others)
- Ketoconazole (NIZORAL, others)
- Micafungin (MYCAMINE)
- Miconazole (MICATIN, ZEASORB-AF, MONISTAT 7, MONISTAT 3, MONISTAT 1, others)
- Naftifine (NAFTIN)
- Nystatin (MYCOSTATIN, NILSTAT, NYOTRAN, others)
- Oxiconazole (OXISTAT)
- Posaconazole (NOXAFIL)
- Sertaconazole (ERTACZO)
- Sulconazole (EXELDERM, SULCOSYN)
- Terbinafine (LAMISIL, others)
- Terconazole (TERAZOL, others)
- Tioconazole (VAGISTAT 1, others)
- Tolnaftate (AFTATE, TINACTIN, others)
- Undecylenic acid (DESENEX, others); Calcium undecylenate (CALDESENE, CRUEX)
- Voriconazole (VFEND)
- Whitfield's Ointment

This chapter will be most useful after having a basic understanding of the material in Chapter 57, Antifungal Agents in *Goodman & Gilman's The Pharmacological Basis of Therapeutics*, 12th Edition. In addition to the material presented here, the 12th Edition contains:

- Structural formulas for each of the antifungal agents in addition to the figures reproduced here
- Table 57-1 Pharmacotherapy of Mycoses which lists the drugs used for different mycoses
- Table 57-7 Pharmacokinetics of Echinocandins in Humans which shows the pharmacokinetic differences among caspofungin, micafungin, and anidulafungin

LEARNING OBJECTIVES

☑ Understand the mechanisms of action and resistance of antifungal agents.
☑ Describe the therapeutic uses of antifungal agents in the context of treatment for fungal diseases.
☑ Develop knowledge of the common and unique toxicities of antifungal agents.
☑ Understand the drug–drug interactions that can occur with the use of azole antifungal agents.
☑ Know the differences in treating invasive fungal infections with systemic drugs versus superficial infections with topical antifungal agents.

MECHANISMS OF ACTION AND RESISTANCE OF ANTIFUNGAL DRUGS

DRUG	MECHANISM OF ACTION (see Figure 43-1)	MECHANISM OF RESISTANCE
Amphotericin B	Binds to ergosterol in fungi membranes to form pores and increase membrane permeability	Resistance is rare, but may be caused by replacement of ergosterol with precursor sterols
Flucytosine	Converted in fungi to 5-fluorouracil (5-FU), which is incorporated into RNA and inhibits nucleic acid synthesis (see Figure 43-2)	Resistance is due to a loss of the fungal permease necessary for cytosine transport or a decrease in fungal cytosine deaminase activity
Imidazoles and Triazoles	Impaired ergosterol synthesis due to inhibition of 14-α-sterol demethylase	Mutation in *ERG11*, the gene coding for the 14-α-sterol demethylase
Echinocandins	Inhibition of 1,3-β-D-glucan synthesis in fungal cell wall resulting in loss of structural integrity, osmotic instability, and cell death	Mutations in glucan synthase complex genes
Griseofulvin	Inhibition of microtubule function and inhibition of fungal mitosis	Deficient energy-dependent transport system used to get antifungal agent to microtubules
Terbinafine	Inhibition of fungal squalene epoxidase, blocking ergosterol biosynthesis, and disruption of fungal cell membrane	Mutations in squalene epoxidase

Antifungal Agents CHAPTER 43

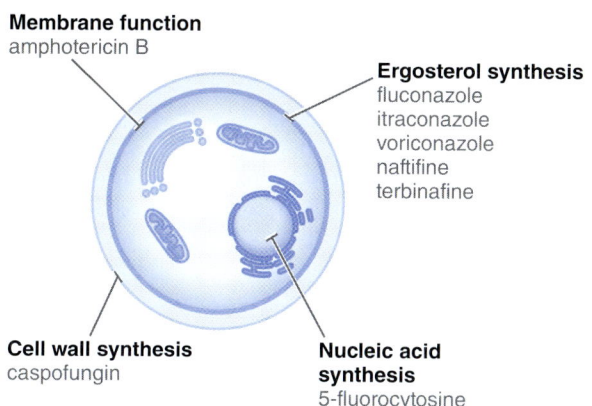

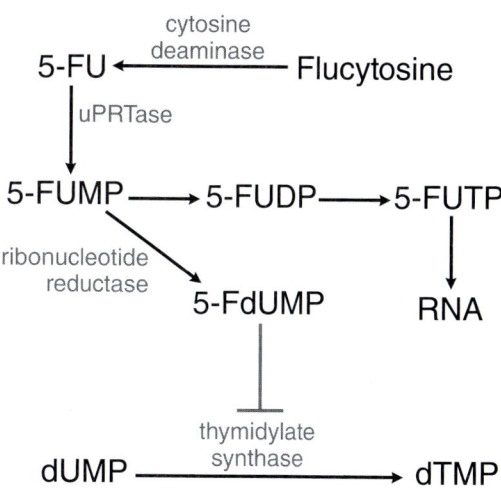

FIGURE 43-1 Sites of action of antifungal drugs. Amphotericin B and other polyenes, such as nystatin, bind to ergosterol in fungal cell membranes and increase membrane permeability. The imidazoles and triazoles, such as itraconazole and fluconazole, inhibit 14-α-sterol demethylase, prevent ergosterol synthesis, and lead to the accumulation of 14-α-methylsterols. The allylamines, such as naftifine and terbinafine, inhibit squalene epoxidase and prevent ergosterol synthesis. The echinocandins, such as caspofungin, inhibit the formation of glucans in the fungal cell wall.

FIGURE 43-2 Action of flucytosine in fungi. Flucytosine is transported by cytosine permease into the fungal cell, where it is deaminated to 5-fluorouracil (5-FU). The 5-FU is then converted to 5-fluorouracil-ribose monophosphate (5-FUMP) and then is either converted to 5-fluorouridine triphosphate (5-FUTP) and incorporated into RNA or converted by ribonucleotide reductase to 5-fluoro-2′-deoxyuridine-5′-monophosphate (5-FdUMP), which is a potent inhibitor of thymidylate synthase. 5-FUDP, 5-fluorouridine-5′-diphosphate; dUMP, deoxyuridine-5′-monophosphate; dTMP, deoxythymidine-5′-monophosphate.

CASE 43-1

A 56-year-old woman is diagnosed with mucormycoses involving the maxillary sinuses. An infectious disease consultant recommends that she be treated with amphotericin B.

a. What different formulations of amphotericin B are available for her treatment?

There are currently 4 formulations of amphotericin B commercially available: conventional amphotericin B (C-AMB), liposomal amphotericin B (L-AMB), amphotericin B lipid complex (ABLC), and amphotericin B colloidal dispersion (ABCD). Table 43-1 summarizes the pharmacokinetic properties of these different preparations.

b. What are the major differences in these formulations?

C-AMB is insoluble in water, but is formulated for intravenous use by complexing it with the bile salt, deoxycholate. ABCD forms a colloidal solution when dispersed in water and provides much lower blood concentrations than C-AMB.

(Continued)

TABLE 43-1 Pharmocokinetic Parameters for Amphotericin B Formulations after Multiple Administrations in Humans

PRODUCT	DOSE (mg/kg)	C_{MAX} (µg/mL)	$AUC_{(1-24hr)}$ (µg·hr/mL)	V (L/kg)	Cl (mL/hr/kg)
AmBisome (L-AMB)	5	83±35.2	555±311	0.11±0.08	11±6
Amphotec (ABCD)	5	3.1	43	4.3	117
Ablecet (ABLC)	5	1.7±0.8	14±7	131±7.7	426±188.5
Fungizone (C-AMB)	0.6	1.1±0.2	17.1±5	5±2.8	38±15

For details, see Boswell et al. (1998). From Boswell GW, Buell D, Bekersky I. AmBisome (Liposomal Amphotericin B): A comparative review. *J Clin Pharmacol*, 1998, 38:583-592. © 1998 The American College of Clinical Pharmacology. Reprinted by permission of SAGE Publications.

Infusion reactions of chills and fever are more common with ABCD than with C-AMB. L-AMB is supplied as a lyophilized powder and has equivalent blood concentrations as C-AMB. L-AMB is approved for empirical therapy of fever in the neutropenic host not responding to appropriate antibacterial agents, as well as for salvage therapy of aspirgillosis and candidiasis. ABLC provides blood concentrations of amphotericin B that are much lower than with the same dose of C-AMB. ABLC is approved for salvage therapy of deep mycoses.

The lipid formulations appear to reduce the risk of nephrotoxicity during therapy. The cost of the lipid formulations of amphotericin B greatly exceeds that of C-AMB.

c. **What is the mechanism of action of amphotericin?**

The anitifungal activity of amphotericin B depends principally on its binding to a sterol moiety, primarily ergosterol, in the membrane of sensitive fungi. By virtue of their interaction with these sterols, polyenes, appear to form pores or channels that increase the permeability of the membrane, allowing the outward leakage of a variety of small molecules (see Figure 43-1).

d. **What untoward effects should be watched for in this patient?**

Major untoward effects of amphotericin B are infusion-related reactions such as fever and chills. These are most severe with ABCD, slightly less with C-AMB, even less with ABLC, and least with L-AMB.

Nephrotoxicity with amphotericin, a major concern, is dose-dependent, usually transient, and increased by concurrent therapy with other nephrotoxic agents such as aminoglycosides or cyclosporine. Permanent functional renal impairment is uncommon in adults with normal renal function prior to treatment.

Hypochromic, normocytic anemia commonly occurs during treatment with C-AMB.

CASE 43-2

A 19-year-old woman with coccidiodal meningitis is being treated with fluconazole.

a. **Why is fluconazole chosen instead of amphotericin B?**

Fluconazole is the drug of choice for the treatment of coccidioidal meningitis because of good penetration into the cerebrospinal fluid and much less morbidity than with intrathecal amphotericin B.

b. **What are the limitations to the use of fluconazole?**

Fluconazole is a Category C agent that should be avoided during pregnancy unless the potential benefit justifies the possible risk to the fetus.

Fluconazole is an inhibitor of CYP3A4 and CYP2C9, and drug–drug interactions (shown in Tables 43-2 to 43-5) are a limitation to the use of this drug.

TABLE 43-2 Interaction of Azole Antifungal Agents with Hepatic CYPs

FLUCONAZOLE	VORICONAZOLE	ITRACONAZOLE	POSACONAZOLE
CYP3A4 inhibitor	CYP2C9 inhibitor and substrate	CYP3A4 inhibitor	CYP3A4 inhibitor
CYP2C9 inhibitor	CYP3A4 inhibitor		
CYP2C19 inhibitor	CYP2C19 inhibitor		

Antifungal Agents CHAPTER 43

TABLE 43-3 Drugs Exhibiting Elevated Plasma Concentrations When Co-Administered with Azole Anti-Fungal Agents

Alfentanil	Eplerenone	Losartan	Saquinavir
Alprazolam	Ergot alkaloids	Lovastatin	Sildenafil
Astemizole	Erlotinib	Methadone	Sirolimus
Buspirone	Eszopiclone	Methylprednisolone	Solifenacin
Busulfan	Felodipine	Midazolam	Sunitinib
Carbamazepine	Fexofenadine	Nevirapine	Tacrolimus
Cisapride	Gefitinib	Omeprazole	Triazolam
Cyclosporine	Glimepiride	Phenytoin	Vardenafil
Digoxin	Glipizide	Pimozide	Vinca alkaloids
Docetaxel	Halofantrine	Quinidine	Warfarin
Dofetilide	Haloperidol	Ramelteon	Zidovudine
Efavirenz	Imatinib	Ranolazine	Zolpidem
Eletriptan	Irinotecan	Risperidone	

Mechanism of interaction presumably occurs largely at the level of hepatic CYPs, especially CYPs 3 A4, 2C9, and 2D6, but can also involve P-glycoprotein and other mechanisms. Not all drugs listed interact equally with all azoles.

TABLE 43-4 Some Drugs That Decrease Azole Concentration When Co-Administered

DRUG	FLUCONAZOLE	VORICONAZOLE	ITRACONAZOLE	POSACONAZOLE
Antacids (simultaneous)	–		+	–
Barbiturates		+	+[a]	
Carbamazepine	+	+	+	+
H$_2$ antagonists			+	+
Didanosine			+	
Efavirenz		+	+	
Nevirapine		+	+	
Proton pump inhibitors	–	–[b]	+	+
Phenytoin	–	+	+	+
Rifampin	+	+	+	+
Rifabutin		+	+	+
Ritonavir		+		

[a]Phenobarbital only.

[b]Omeprazole and voriconazole increase each other's concentrations in plasma; reduce omeprazole dose by 50% when initiating voriconazole therapy.

Reproduced with permission from Zonios DI, Bennett JE. Update on azole antifungals. *Sem Respir Crit Care Med*. 2008;29:192–210.

SECTION VII Chemotherapy of Microbial Diseases

TABLE 43-5 Some Additional Contraindicated Azole Drug Combinations

DRUG	FLUCONAZOLE	VORICONAZOLE	ITRACONAZOLE	POSACONAZOLE
Alfuzosin		X	X	X
Artemether	X	X		
Bepridil	X			
Clopidogrel	X			
Conivaptan	X	X	X	X
Dabigatran			X	
Darunavir		X		
Dronedarone	X	X	X	X
Everolimus	X	X	X	X
Lopinavir		X		
Lumefantrine	X	X		
Mesoridazine	X			
Nilotinib	X	X	X	X
Nisoldipine	use with caution	X	X	X
Quinine	X	X		
Rifapentine		X	use with caution	use with caution
Ritonavir		X	use with caution	
Rivaroxaban		X	X	
Salmeterol		X	X	X
Silodosin		X	X	X
Simvastatin	use with caution		X	
St. John's wort		X		
Tetrabenazine	X	X		
Thioridazine	X	X		
Tolvaptan	X	X		X
Tolvaptan	X		X	
Topotecan			X	
Ziprasidone	X	X		

CASE 43-3

A 26-year-old woman has developed esophageal candidiasis. She is being treated with oral voriconazole. She is also being treated for a seizure disorder and depression, and during the course of her antifungal therapy, she will be taking several other drugs.

a. What is the mechanism of action of voriconazole?

Voriconazole, a triazole, is an inhibitor of 14-α-sterol demethylase and impairs the biosynthesis of ergosterol required for the fungal cytoplasmic membrane and thereby inhibits growth of fungi (see Figure 43-1).

(Continued)

Antifungal Agents CHAPTER 43

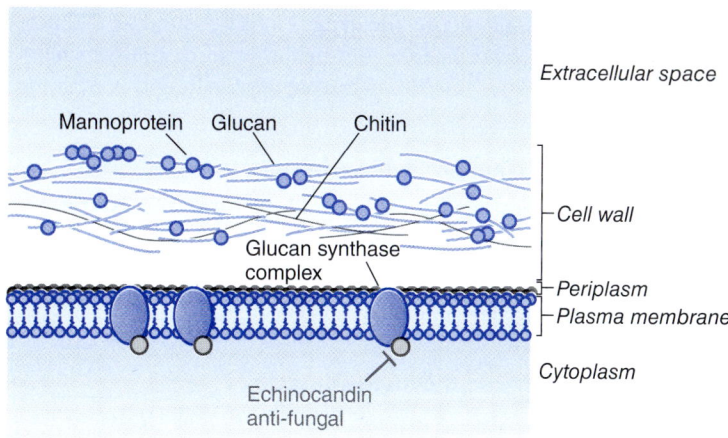

FIGURE 43-3 The fungal cell wall and membrane and the action of echinocandins. The strength of the fungal cell wall is maintained by fibrillar polysaccharides, largely β-1,3-glucan and chitin, which bind covalently to each other and to proteins. A glucan synthase complex in the plasma membrane catalyzes the synthesis of β-1,3-glucan; the glucan is extruded into the periplasm and incorporated into the cell wall. Echinocandins inhibit the activity of the glucan synthase complex, resulting in loss of the structural integrity of the cell wall. A subunit of glucan synthase designated Fks1p is thought to be the target of the echinocandin. Mutations in Fks1p, coded for by *FSK1*, cause resistance to echinocandins.

b. What drug interactions are of concern while this patient is taking voriconazole?

Voriconazole is metabolized by, and inhibits, CYPs 2C19, 2C9, and 3A4. Drug interactions with voriconazole are summarized in Tables 43-2, 43-3, 43-4, and 43-5.

c. What other untoward effects should this patient be warned of?

Voriconazole is contraindicated in pregnancy (Category D). Voriconazole also causes a prolongation of the QTc interval, which can become significant in patients with other risk factors for torsades de pointes.

CASE 43-4

An infectious disease consultant has suggested that the patient in Case 43-3 could be treated with caspofungin.

a. What is caspofungin and what is its role in the treatment of esophageal candidiasis?

Caspofungin belongs to the Echinocandin class of antifungal agents. Caspofungin is approved for initial therapy of deeply invasive candidiasis and as salvage therapy for patients with invasive aspergillosis who are failing or intolerant of approved drugs such as amphotericin B or voriconzaole. Caspofungin is approved for esophageal candidiasis.

b. What is the mechanism of action of the Echinocandin class of antifungal agents?

Echinocandins inhibit the activity of the glucan synthase complex, resulting in loss of the structural integrity of the fungal cell wall, osmotic instability, and cell death (see Figure 43-3).

CASE 43-5

A 47-year-old man has developed an irritated and itchy beard. The cause is diagnosed as tinea (*Trichophyton* spp.). He is being treated with griseofulvin orally.

a. What is the mechanism of action of griseofulvin and why is it effective in treating this patient?

Griseofulvin inhibits fungal microtubule function and thereby disrupts assembly of the mitotic spindle with inhibition of fungal mitosis. It is deposited in keratin

(Continued)

SECTION VII

Chemotherapy of Microbial Diseases

precursor cells; when these cells differentiate, the drug is tightly bound to, and persists in keratin, providing prolonged resistance to fungal infection. Thus, the new growth of hair or nails is the first to become free of disease. As the fungus-containing keratin is shed, it is replaced by normal tissue.

b. There are numerous antifungal creams available, why not use one of these?

Topical treatment is useful in many superficial fungal infections, that is, those confined to the stratum corneum, squamous mucosa, or cornea. Topical administration of antifungal agents usually is not successful for mycoses of the nails (onychomycosis) and hair (tinea capitis), and has no place in the treatment of subcutaneous mycoses, such as sporotrichosis and chromoblastomycosis.

c. What are the untoward effects of griseofulvin therapy?

The incidence of serious reactions due to griseofulvin is very low. Headache, which may be severe, usually disappears as therapy is continued. Hepatotoxicity has been reported. Leukopenia and neutropenia warrant the monitoring of weekly blood studies during the first month of therapy.

Griseofulvin induces hepatic CYPs and may increase the metabolism of warfarin and may reduce the efficacy of low-estrogen oral contraceptive agents.

CASE 43-6

A 36-year-old woman has developed vaginal candidiasis and is being treated with miconazole vaginal suppositories.

a. What are the advantages of using topical antifungal creams?

Vaginal creams, suppositories, and tablets, effective for the treatment of vaginal candidiasis, are all used once a day for 1 to 7 days, preferably at bedtime to facilitate retention. Approximately 3 to 10% of the vaginal dose is absorbed. The most common side effect is vaginal burning or itching. A male sexual partner may experience mild penile irritation.

KEY CONCEPTS

- Antifungal agents have 3 mechanisms of action: inhibit synthesis of cell wall components, inhibit synthesis of nucleic acids, or inhibit microtubule/mitotic spindle function.
- Amphotericin B comes in 4 formulations that have specific advantages and disadvantages.
- Imidazoles and triazoles are antifungal agents that share the same spectrum of activity and mechanism of action.
- The azoles interact with hepatic CYPs as substrates and inhibitors, and drug–drug interactions may limit their use in certain patients (see Tables 43-2, 43-3, 43-4, and 43-5).
- The echinocandins are well-tolerated antifungal agents, and are used mainly for invasive candidiasis and aspergillosis.
- Griseofulvin therapy is used for mycotic disease of the skin, hair, and nails due to *Microsporum*, *Trichophyton*, or *Epidermophyton*.
- Topical antifungal treatment is useful for superficial infections confined to the stratum corneum, squamous mucosa, or cornea.
- Antifungal agents are formulated in creams for vaginal use to treat vaginal candidiasis.

Antifungal Agents — CHAPTER 43

SUMMARY QUIZ

QUESTION 43-1 A 43-year-old man is being treated with amphotericin B for esophageal candidiasis. Which of the following serum laboratory tests should be monitored closely?

a. Bilirubin
b. Cholesterol
c. Glucose
d. Creatinine
e. Sodium

QUESTION 43-2 A 56-year-old man with cryptococcal meningitis is being treated with flucytosine and amphotericin B. Flucytosine is metabolized to 5-flurouracil by fungal cells which inhibits DNA synthesis. The selectivity of flucytosine is due to a lack of which enzyme in mammalian cells:

a. Cytosine deaminase
b. *N*-acetyltransferase
c. Fluorine oxidase
d. Uracil phosphoribosyl transferase
e. Thymidylate synthetase

QUESTION 43-3 A 48-year-old woman with a history of atrial fibrillation is being treated with warfarin. She has recently developed coccidiodal meningitis and treatment with fluconazole is started. A potential drug–drug interaction that may result in elevated plasma warfarin concentration is likely because fluconazaole inhibits

a. CYP3A4.
b. CYP2D6.
c. CYP2C9.
d. CYP2C19.
e. CYP4.

QUESTION 43-4 A 38-year-old man is being treated with voriconazole for invasive aspergillosis. His dose should be adjusted if it is determined that he has this disease:

a. Renal failure
b. Hepatic cirrhosis
c. Rheumatoid arthritis
d. Type 2 diabetes mellitus
e. Colon cancer

QUESTION 43-5 A 69-year-old man with onychomycosis is being treated with griseofulvin. His treatment has been going on for 1 month and he has been told that it may last for 1 year. Although he has had no serious side effects, his compliance is waning. Treatment of onchomycosis with griseofulvin is prolonged because it is

a. absorbed slowly.
b. metabolized rapidly.
c. metabolized completely and the metabolites are inactive.
d. excreted rapidly in the urine.
e. bound to keratin and requires shedding of fungal-containing keratin.

SECTION VII Chemotherapy of Microbial Diseases

QUESTION 43-6 What is an alternative therapy for the patient in question 43-5?

a. Amphotericin B
b. Flucytosine
c. Tolnaftate cream
d. Terbinafine
e. Undecylenic acid

SUMMARY QUIZ ANSWER KEY

QUESTION 43-1. Answer is **d.** Azotemia occurs in 80% of patients who receive C-AMB for deep mycoses. Lipid formulations are less nephrotoxic. Nephrotoxicity is dose-dependent, usually transient, and increased by concurrent therapy with other nephrotoxic agents.

QUESTION 43-2. Answer is **a.** The selective action of flucytosine is due to the lack of cytosine deaminase in mammalian cells, which prevents the metabolism to 5-flurouracil.

QUESTION 43-3. Answer is **c.** Fluconazole is an inhibitor of CYP3A4, CYP2C9, and CYP2C19 (see Table 43-3). Warfarin is metabolized by CYP2C9 (see Chapter 19). The inhibition of CYP2C9 would cause an increase in warfarin plasma concentrations unless the warfarin dose is adjusted accordingly.

QUESTION 43-4. Answer is **b.** Voriconazole is metabolized primarily by CYP2C19 and to a lesser extent CYP2C9 and CYP3A4. Patients with mild-to-moderate cirrhosis should receive the same loading dose of voriconazole but half of the maintenance dose. There are no data to guide dosing in patients with severe hepatic insufficiency.

QUESTION 43-5. Answer is **e.** Griseofulvin is deposited in keratin precursor cells; when these cells differentiate, the drug is tightly bound to, and persists in, keratin, providing prolonged resistance to fungal invasion. For this reason, the new growth of the hair or nails is the first to become free of disease. As the fungus-containing keratin is shed, it is replaced by normal tissue.

QUESTION 43-6. Answer is **d.** Terbinafine accumulates in skin, nails, and fat. It is somewhat more effective for onychomycosis than itraconazole. Duration of treatment varies with the site being treated but typically is 6 to 12 weeks. Efficacy in onychomycosis can be improved by the simultaneous use of amorofine 5% nail lacquer.

SUMMARY: ANTIFUNGAL DRUGS

CLASS AND SUBCLASSES	NAME	CLINICAL USES	RESISTANCE	TOXICITY COMMON	TOXICITY UNIQUE; CLINICALLY IMPORTANT
Amphotericin	Amphotericin B (C-AMB) Amphotericin B colloidal dispersion (ABCD) Amphotericin B liposomal (L-AMB) Amphotericin B lipid complex (ABLC)	Clinical activity against *Candida* spp., *Cryptococcus neoformans*, *Blastomyces dermatitidis*, *Histoplasma capsulatum*, *Sporothrix schenckii*, *Coccidiosis* spp., *Paracoccidioides braziliensis*, *Aspergillus* spp., *Penicillium marneffei*, and the agents of mucormycosis	Some *Candida* and *Aspergillus* spp. are resistant, but significant resistance is rare	Infusion-related fever and chills ABCD > C-AMB > ABLC > L-AMB	Dose-dependent renal toxicity; less with lipid formulations
Flucytosine	ANCOBON	Clinically useful against *Cryptococcus neoformans*, *Candida* spp., and the agents of chromoblastomycosis	Resistance during therapy (secondary resistance) is an important cause of therapeutic failure when flucytosine is used alone for cryptococcosis and candidiasis	Nausea, vomiting, diarrhea, and severe entero-colitis	Depression of bone marrow leading to leukopenia and throbocytopenia

(Continued)

Antifungal Agents — CHAPTER 43

CLASS AND SUBCLASSES	NAME	CLINICAL USES	RESISTANCE	TOXICITY COMMON	TOXICITY UNIQUE; CLINICALLY IMPORTANT
Imidazoles and triazoles	Itraconazole	Infections due to *B. dermatitides, H. capsulatum, P. braziliensis,* and *C. immitis*	Resistance emerges gradually during prolonged azole therapy	Drug interactions, see Tables 43-2, 43-3, 43-4, and 43-5	Doses of 300 mg twice daily have led to adrenal insufficiency and hypertension
	Fluconazole	Orophyarngeal candidiasis, uncomplicated vaginal candidiasis, cryptococcal meningitis, coccidiodal memingitis			Category C agent to be avoided in pregnancy unless benefit justifies risk
	Voriconazole	Invasive apergillosis, esophageal canididiasis, initial treatment of candidenia			Contraindicated in pregnancy (Category D) Hepatotoxicity has been reported and liver function should be monitored Prolongation of QTc interval in patients at risk for torsade de pointes
	Posaconazole	Similar to fluconazole, but fluconazole is the preferred drug due to safety, cost, and experience		Drug interactions, see Tables 43-2, 43-3, 43-4, and 43-5; GI distress	Not known to prolong QTc interval, but should not be administered with drugs that are CYP3A4 substrates and drugs that prolong QTc interval
Imidazoles and triazoles for topical use	Clotrimazole, cream, lotion, powder, aerosol solution, and solution; vaginal cream or tablets; troches	Cutaneous dermatophyte infections, including cutaneous and vulvovaginal candidiasis	Recurrences common in all infections	Local irritation, including vaginal burning; sexual partner may experience penile irritation	No serious systemic toxicities
	Econazole	Similar to miconazole		Local irritation	
	Miconazole cream, lotion, powder, aerosol solution, and aerosol powder; vaginal cream	Treatment of tinea pedis, tinea cruris, tinea versicolor, and vulvovaginal candidiasis		Vaginal irritation	
	Terconazole	Vaginal suppository and vaginal cream for treatment of vaginal candidiasis			
	Butoconazole	Vaginal cream similar to clotrimazole			Slower response in pregnancy requires a 6-day course in second or third trimester
	Tioconazole	Ointment used for treatment of vulvovaginal candidiasis			

(Continued)

SECTION VII — Chemotherapy of Microbial Diseases

CLASS AND SUBCLASSES	NAME	CLINICAL USES	RESISTANCE	TOXICITY COMMON	TOXICITY UNIQUE; CLINICALLY IMPORTANT
	Oxiconazole	Cream and lotion available for common dermatophytes			
	Sulconazole	Solution or cream available for common dermatophytes			
	Sertaconzole	Cream for treatment of tinea pedis			
	Ketoconazole	Cream, gel, foam, shampoo for common skin dermatophytes, tinea versicolor, and seborrheic dermatitis			
Echinocandins	Caspofungin	Deeply invasive candidiasis and as salvage therapy for aspergillosis; Esophogeal candidiasis	Resistance can be selected for *Candida albicans* during prolonged therapy	Phlebitis at infusion site	
	Micafungin	Deeply invasive candidiasis; Esophageal candidiasis	Resistance can be selected for *Candida albicans* during prolonged therapy		Mild inhibitor of CYP 3A4
	Andulafugin	Candidemia in non-neutropenic patients; Esophogeal candidiasis	Resistance can be selected for *Candida albicans* during prolonged therapy		
Griseofulvin	Micro-sized powder; Ultra-micro-sized powder	Mycotic diseases of the skin, hair, and nails due to *Microsporum, Trichophyton,* or *Epidermophyton*; itraconazole or terbinafine is more effective for onychomycosis		Headache usually disappears as therapy is stopped	Induction of CYP and increases the rate of metabolism of warfarin requiring an adjustment of warfarin dose
Terbinafine	LAMASIL, others	Onychomycosis, tinea capitus, ring worm; Cream or spray is used to treat tinea corporis, tinea cruris, and tinea pedis		Low incidence of GI distress, headache, or rash	Not recommended for treatment of patients with azotemia or hepatic failure; Pregnancy Category B
Ciclopirox olamine	PENLAC NAIL LACQUER, others	Available as a cream, gel, suspension, and lotion for treatment of cutaneous candidiasis, tinea corporis, cruris pedis, and versicolor; nail lacquer is available for onychomycosis		Hypersensitivity	No systemic accumulation
Haloprogin	HALOTEX *(Not available in the United States)*	Cream or solution is used to treat tinea pedis, cruris, tinea corporis, tinea manuum, and tinea versicolor			
Tolnaftate	AFTATE, TINACTIN	Cream, gel, powder, aerosol powder, topical solution, topical aerosol liquid are used for treatment of tinea pedis			No toxic or allergic reaction have been noted

(Continued)

Antifungal Agents — CHAPTER 43

CLASS AND SUBCLASSES	NAME	CLINICAL USES	RESISTANCE	TOXICITY COMMON	TOXICITY UNIQUE; CLINICALLY IMPORTANT
Naftifine	NAFTIN	Cream or gel effective for treatment of tinea cruris and tinea corporis		Local irritation and contact dermatitis	
Butenafine	MENTAX, LOTRAMIN ULTRA	Similar to naftifine			
Nystatin	MYCOSTATIN, NILSTAT, others	Available in preparations for treatment of cutaneous or vaginal candidiasis Suspension is available for treatment of oral candidiasis A liposomal formulation is in clinical trials for systemic candidemia		Bitter taste; adverse effects are uncommon	
Undecylenic acid	DESENEX, others Calcium undecylenate is available as a powder	Available as a cream, powder, spray powder, soap, and liquid for the treatment of various dermatomycoses, especially tinea pedis			
Whitfield's Ointment		An ointment that combines the fungistatic action of benzoic acid and the keratolytic action of salicylic acid; used to treat tinea capitis		Mild local irritation	

CHAPTER 44

Antiviral Agents and Treatment of HIV Infection

This chapter is a composite of Chapters 58 and 59 in *Goodman and Gilman's The Pharmacological Basis of Therapeutics*, 12th Edition. The material presented here will be more useful after having a basic understanding of the material presented in these chapters. This chapter does not contain detailed information about all antiviral or antiretroviral agents. For the details of agents not discussed here, see Chapters 58 and 59 in the 12th Edition of *Goodman and Gilman's The Pharmacological Basis of Therapeutics*. In addition to the material presented here, the 12th Edition contains:

- Table 58-2 which provides the nomenclature of antiviral agents
- Figures 58-2, 58-4, 58-6, 59-2, 59-4, and 59-6 which show the chemical structures of each of the drugs discussed in this chapter
- At the beginning of Chapter 59 in *Goodman and Gilman's The Pharmacological Basis of Therapeutics*, 12th Edition, there is an excellent overview of human immunodeficiency disease (HIV) infection and its treatment, the pathogenesis of HIV-related disease, and the principles of HIV chemotherapy
- Table 59-1 which is a list of antiretroviral agents approved in the United States
- Tables 59-2, 59-3, and 59-4 which provide detailed information on the pharmacokinetics of antiretroviral agents

LEARNING OBJECTIVES

- ☑ Understand the treatment of herpes virus infections and the use of antiherpes drugs.
- ☑ Know the treatment strategies for chronic hepatitis B and C infections.
- ☑ Understand the mechanisms of action and resistance, and the therapeutic use of the anti-influenza agents.
- ☑ Know the principles of HIV chemotherapy.
- ☑ Know the mechanisms of action and resistance, the untoward effects, and the therapeutic uses of the drugs used to treat HIV infections.

DRUGS INCLUDED IN THIS CHAPTER

GENERIC NAME	TRADE NAME	GENERIC NAME	TRADE NAME
Antiherpes Agents		**Antihepatitis Agents**	
Acyclovir	ZOVIRAX	Adefovir dipivoxil	HEPSERA
Cidofovir	VISTIDE	Entecavir	BARACLUDE
Penciclovir	FAMVIR, others; Famciclovir which is de-esterified to penciclovir	Interferon alfa-N1	WELLFERON[a]
Foscarnet	FOSCAVIR, others	Interferon alfa-N3	ALFERON N
Fomivirsen	VITRAVENE	Interferon alfacon-1	INFERGEN
Ganciclovir	CYTOVENE, VITRASERT, others	Interferon alfa-2B	INTRON A
Idoxuridine	HERPLEX, DENDRID	Interferon alfa-2A	ROFERON A
Docosanol		Lamivudine	EPIVIR, others

(Continued)

Antiviral Agents and Treatment of HIV Infection
CHAPTER 44

GENERIC NAME	TRADE NAME	GENERIC NAME	TRADE NAME
Trifluridine	VIROPTIC, others	Peginterferon alfa-2A	PEGASYS
Valacyclovir	VALTREX, others	Peginterferon alfa-2B	PEG-INTRON
Valganciclovir	VALCYTE, others		
Anti-influenza Agents		**Other Antiviral Agents**	
Amantadine	SYMMETREL, others	Ribavirin	VIRAZOLE, REBETROL, COPEGUS, others
Oseltamivir	TAMIFLU	Telbivudine	TYZEKA
Rimantadine	FLUMADINE, others		
Zanamivir	RELENZA	Imiquimod	ALDARA
Nucleoside Reverse Transcriptase Inhibitors (NRTIs)		**Protease Inhibitors**	
Zidovudine	RETROVIR, others[b]	Saquinavir	INVIRASE
Didanosine	VIDEX, VIDEC EC, others	Indinavir	CRIXIVAN
Stavudine	ZERIT	Ritonavir	NORVIR
Zalcitabine	HIVID[c]	Nelfinavir	VIRACEPT
Lamivudine	EPIVIR[b]	Amprenavir	AGENERASE, PROZEI[a]
Abacavir	ZIAGEN[b]	Lopinavir	KALETRA, ALUVIA[c]
Tenofovir disoproxil	VIREAD[b]	Atazanavir	REYATAZ, ZRIVADA
Emtricitabine	EMTRIVA[b]	Fosamprenavir	LEXIVA, TELZIR
Non-nucleoside Reverse Transcriptase Inhibitors (NNRTIs)		Tipranavir	APTIVUS
Nevirapine	VERAMUNE	Darunavir	PREZISTA
Efavirenz	SUSTIVA, STORCRIN[b]	**Entry Inhibitors**	
Delavirdine	RESCRIPTOR	Enfuvirtide	FUZEON
Etravirine	INTELENCE	Maraviroc	SELZENTRY, CELSENTRI
		Integrase Inhibitor	
		Raltegravir	ISENTRESS

[a]Not currently approved in the United States.
[b]A number of fixed-dose combinations are available: zidovudine + lamivudine (COMBIVIR); zidovudine + lamivudine + abacavir (TRIZIVIR); abacavir + lamivudine (EPZICOM); tenofovir + emtricitabine (TRUVADA); tenofovir + efavirenz + emtricitabine (ATRIPLA).
[c]Lopinavir is available only as a fixed-dose combination with ritonavir (KALETRA/ALUVIA).

MECHANISMS OF ACTION AND RESISTANCE OF ANTIVIRAL DRUGS

DRUG	MECHANISM OF ACTION	MECHANISM OF RESISTANCE
Acyclovir	See Figures 44-1 and 44-2; inhibition of DNA synthesis by interaction with HSV thymidine kinase and DNA polymerase	Impaired production of thymidine kinase, altered thymidine kinase substrate, or altered DNA polymerase
Cidofovir	Inhibits viral DNA synthesis by slowing and eventually terminating chain elongation; the diphosphate acts as a competitive inhibitor of deoxycytidine triphosphate (dCTP) and as alternative substrate for DNA polymerase	Resistance in cytomegalovirus (CMV) is due to mutations in DNA polymerase

SECTION VII   Chemotherapy of Microbial Diseases

DRUG	MECHANISM OF ACTION	MECHANISM OF RESISTANCE
Penciclovir	Inhibits viral DNA synthesis by competitive inhibition of viral DNA polymerase (see Figures 44-1 and 44-2)	Mutations in thymidine kinase or viral DNA polymerase
Foscarnet	Inhibits viral nucleic acid synthesis by interacting with herpes virus DNA polymerase or HIV reverse transcriptase (see Figure 44-1)	Mutations in herpes virus DNA polymerase
Fomivirsen	First approved antisense therapy for viral infections; inhibits CMV replication through sequence-specific and nonspecific mechanisms including virus binding to cells	
Ganciclovir	Competitive inhibitor of deoxyguanosine triphosphate incorporation into DNA and inhibition of viral DNA polymerase (see Figures 44-1 and 44-2)	CMV resistance is due to either mutations in viral phosphotransferase which reduces intracellular ganciclovir phosphorylation or mutations in viral DNA polymerase
Idoxuridine	The triphosphate inhibits viral DNA synthesis and is incorporated into viral DNA	
Trifluridine	The monophosphate inhibits thymidylate synthesis and the triphosphate inhibits thymidine triphosphate incorporation into DNA	Trifluridine-resistant HSV have altered thymidine substrate specificity
Ribavirin	Alteration of cellular nucleotide pool and inhibition of viral mRNA synthesis	Not documented, but cells that do not phosphorylate ribavirin to its active form have been reported
Adefovir dipivoxil	Competitive inhibition of viral DNA polymerase and reverse transcriptases	Point mutations in hepatitis B virus (HBV) polymerase
Entecavir	Inhibition of HBV polymerase (reverse transcriptase)	Mutation in HIV reverse transcriptase
Interferon	Activates JAK-STAT pathway that leads to synthesis of over 2 dozen proteins that contribute to antiviral activity at various stages of viral penetration (see Figure 44-3)	Block production or activity of interferon-inducible proteins
Lamivudine	Inhibitor of DNA polymerase/reverse transcriptase of HIV and HBV (see Figures 44-4 and 44-5)	Point mutations in HBV DNA polymerase
Amantadine	Inhibits viral replication by inhibition of viral uncoating (see Figure 44-1)	Mutation in the RNA sequence encoding for the M2 protein transmembrane domain
Oseltamivir	Selective inhibitor of viral neuraminidase which leads to virus aggregation at the cell surface and reduced virus spread (see Figure 44-1)	Mutations in viral hemagglutinin and/or neuraminidase
Rimantadine	Inhibits viral replication by inhibition of viral uncoating (see Figure 44-1)	Mutation in the RNA sequence encoding for the M2 protein transmembrane domain
Zanamivir	Inhibition of viral neuraminidase which leads to virus aggregation at the cell surface and reduced virus spread (see Figure 44-1)	Mutations in viral hemagglutinin and/or neuraminidase
Telbivudine	Inhibition of HBV DNA polymerase (reverse transcriptase) by competing with the natural substrate, thymidine 5'-triphosphate (see Figures 44-4 and 44-5)	Mutation of HBV DNA polymerase
Tenofovir disoproxil	Reverse transcriptase inhibitor of HIV and HBV (see Figures 44-4 and 44-5)	Mutations in reverse transcriptase
Imiquimod	Induces cytokines and chemokines with antiviral and immunomodulating effects	None known
Zidovudine	Inhibition of nucleoside reverse transcriptase (see Figures 44-4 and 44-5)	Mutations in reverse transcriptase

(Continued)

Antiviral Agents and Treatment of HIV Infection — CHAPTER 44

DRUG	MECHANISM OF ACTION	MECHANISM OF RESISTANCE
Didanoside	Reverse transcriptase inhibitor (see Figures 44-4 and 44-5)	Mutations in reverse transcriptase
Stavudine	Reverse transcriptase inhibitor (see Figures 44-4 and 44-5)	Mutations in reverse transcriptase
Abacavir	Reverse transcriptase inhibitor (see Figures 44-4 and 44-5)	Mutations in reverse transcriptase
Emtricitabine	Reverse transcriptase inhibitor (see Figures 44-4 and 44-5)	Mutations in reverse transcriptase
Saquinavir	HIV protease inhibitor (see Figures 44-5 and 44-6)	Accumulation of multiple resistance mutations
Indinavir	HIV protease inhibitor (see Figures 44-5 and 44-6)	Accumulation of multiple resistance mutations
Ritonavir	HIV protease inhibitor (see Figures 44-5 and 44-6)	Mostly used as a pharmacokinetic enhancer (CYP3A4 inhibitor) and at the low doses used is not known to induce resistance
Nelfinavir	Nonpeptidic protease inhibitor (see Figures 44-5 and 44-6)	Mutation in HIV protease
Amprenavir	HIV protease inhibitor (see Figures 44-5 and 44-6)	Mutation in HIV protease
Lopinavir	HIV protease inhibitor (see Figures 44-5 and 44-6)	Mutation in HIV protease
Atazanavir	HIV protease inhibitor (see Figures 44-5 and 44-6)	Mutation in HIV protease
Tipranavir	HIV protease inhibitor (see Figures 44-5 and 44-6)	Resistance requires accumulation of multiple mutations
Darunavir	HIV protease inhibitor (see Figures 44-5 and 44-6)	Resistance requires accumulation of multiple mutations
Nevirapine	Non-nucleoside reverse transcriptase inhibitor (see Figures 44-5 and 44-7)	Mutation in reverse transcriptase; cross-resistance extends to efavirenz and delavirdine
Efavirenz	Non-nucleoside reverse transcriptase inhibitor (see Figures 44-5 and 44-7)	Mutation in reverse transcriptase; cross-resistance extends to nevirapine and delavirdine
Delavirdine	Non-nucleoside reverse transcriptase inhibitor (see Figures 44-5 and 44-7)	Mutation in reverse transcriptase; cross-resistance extends to nevirapine and efavirenz
Etravirine	Non-nucleoside reverse transcriptase inhibitor (see Figures 44-5 and 44-7)	Mutation in reverse transcriptase; activity of etravirine is not affected by mutations that confer high-level resistance to efavirenz, delavirdine, and nevirapine
Enfuvirtide	Prevents formation of a complex critical for membrane fusion and viral entry into the host cell (see Figures 44-5 and 44-8)	Retains activity against viruses that have become resistant to antiviral agents of other classes
Maraviroc	A chemokine receptor antagonist that binds to host CCR5 receptor to block binding of viral gp120 (see Figures 44-5 and 44-8)	HIV that is predominantly CCR5-tropic shifts tropism to CXCR4; or there is a mutation in gp120 that allows virus binding in the presence of inhibitor
Raltegravir	Blocks the catalytic activity of HIV-encoded integrase, thus preventing the integration of virus DNA into the host chromosome (see Figures 44-5 and 44-9)	Mutations in the integrase gene

SECTION VII — Chemotherapy of Microbial Diseases

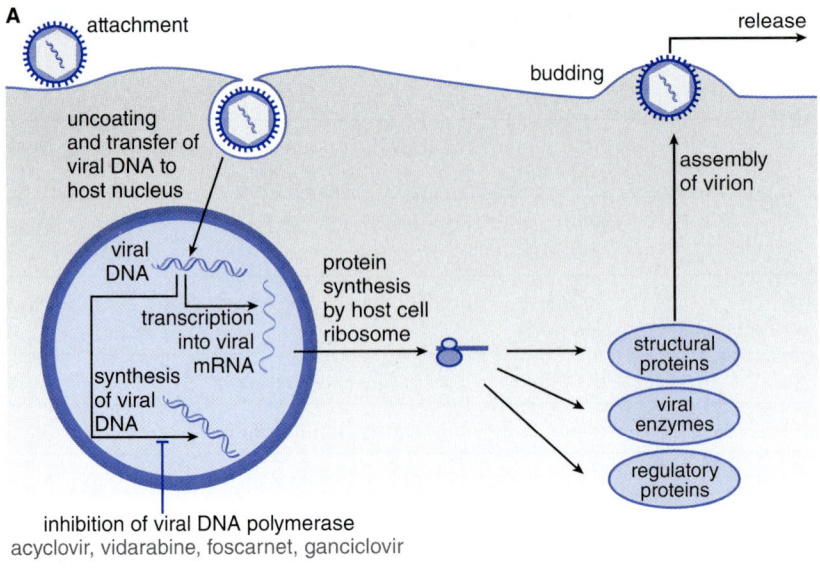

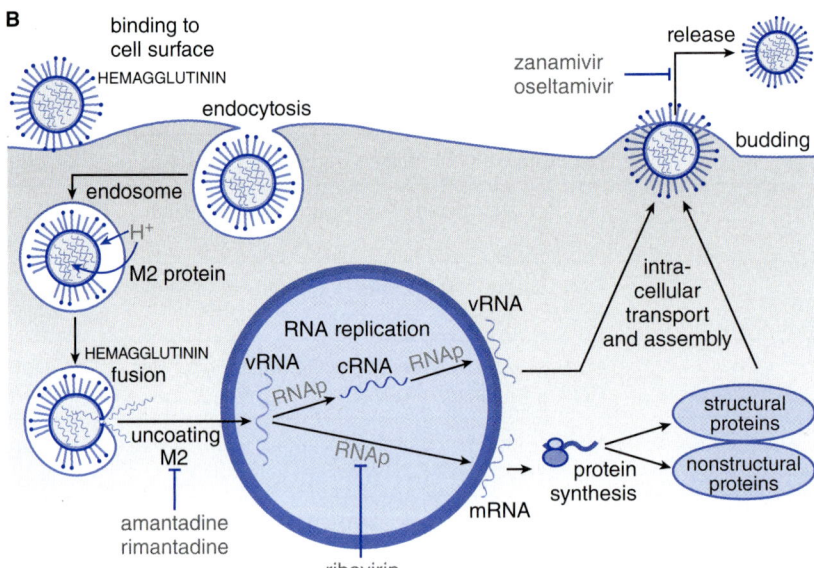

FIGURE 44-1 Replicative cycles of DNA (**A**) and RNA (**B**) viruses. The replicative cycles of herpesvirus (**A**) and influenza (**B**) are examples of DNA-encoded and RNA-encoded viruses, respectively. Sites of action of antiviral agents also are shown. cDNA, complementary DNA; cRNA, complementary RNA; DNAp, DNA polymerase; mRNA, messenger RNA; RNAp, RNA polymerase; vRNA, viral RNA. The symbol ("T-line") indicates a block to virus growth. **A.** Replicative cycles of herpes simplex virus, a DNA virus, and the probable sites of action of antiviral agents. Herpesvirus replication is a regulated multistep process. After infection, a small number of immediate-early genes are transcribed; these genes encode proteins that regulate their own synthesis and are responsible for synthesis of early genes involved in genome replication, such as thymidine kinases, DNA polymerases, etc. After DNA replication, the bulk of the herpesvirus genes (called late genes) are expressed and encode proteins that either are incorporated into or aid in the assembly of progeny virions. **B.** Replicative cycles of influenza, an RNA virus, and the loci for effects of antiviral agents. The mammalian cell shown is an airway epithelial cell. The M2 protein of influenza virus allows an influx of hydrogen ions into the virion interior, which in turn promotes dissociation of the RNP (ribonuclear protein) segments and release into the cytoplasm (uncoating). Influenza virus mRNA synthesis requires a primer cleared from cellular mRNA and used by the viral RNAp complex. The neuraminidase inhibitors zanamivir and oseltamivir specifically inhibit release of progeny virus. Small capitals indicate virus proteins.

Antiviral Agents and Treatment of HIV Infection

CHAPTER 44

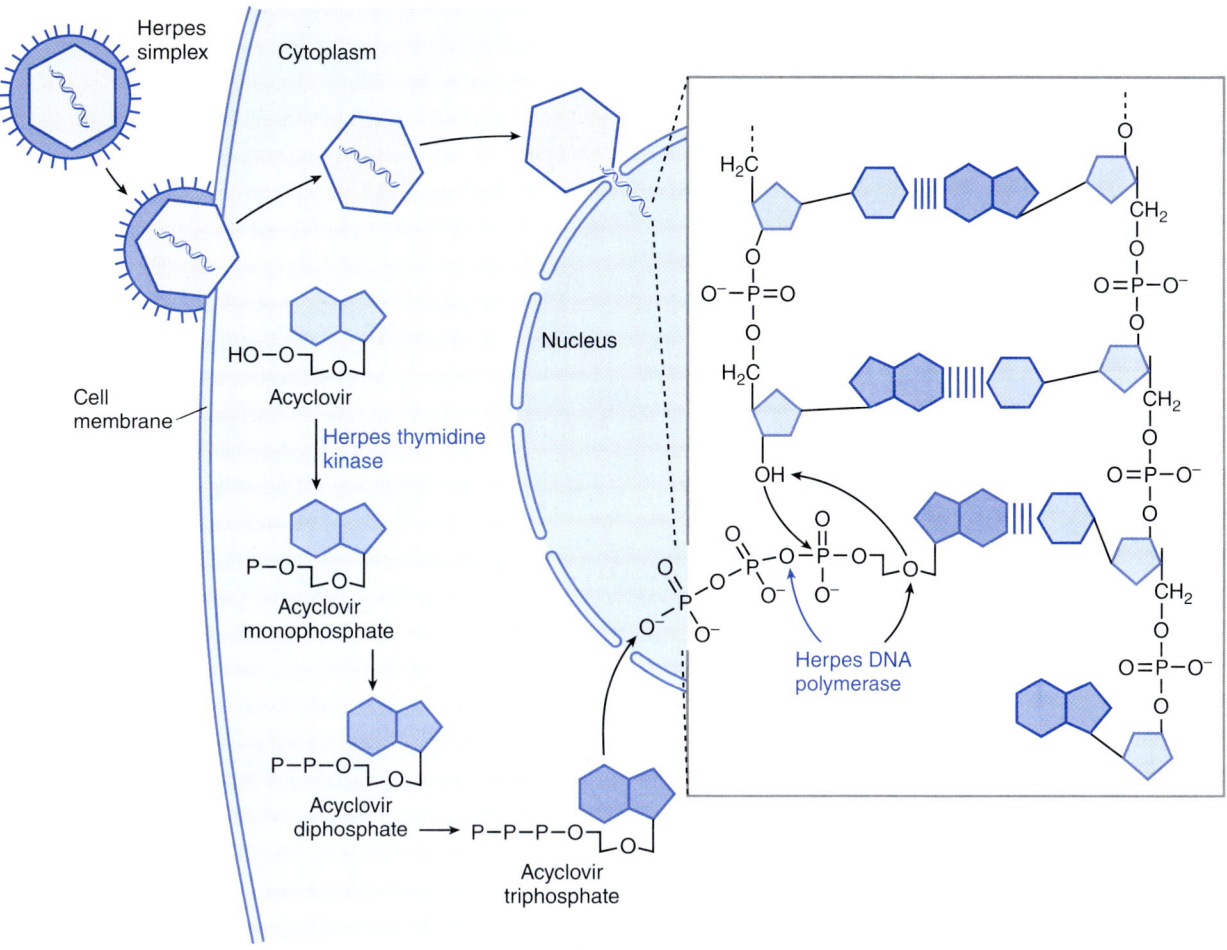

FIGURE 44-2 Mechanism of action of acyclovir in cells infected by herpes simplex virus. A herpes simplex virion is shown attaching to a susceptible host cell, fusing its envelope with the cell membrane, and releasing naked capsids that deliver viral DNA into the nucleus, where it initiates synthesis of viral DNA. Acyclovir molecules entering the cell are converted to acyclovir monophosphate by virus-induced thymidine kinase. Host-cell enzymes add 2 more phosphates to form acyclovir triphosphate, which is transported into the nucleus. After the herpes DNA polymerase cleaves pyrophosphate from acyclovir triphosphate (indicated by the blue arrow in the inset), viral DNA polymerase inserts acyclovir monophosphate rather than 2′-deoxyguanosine monophosphate into the viral DNA (indicated by black arrows in the inset). Further elongation of the chain is impossible because acyclovir monophosphate lacks the 3′ hydroxyl group necessary for the insertion of an additional nucleotide, and the exonuclease associated with the viral DNA polymerase cannot remove the acyclovir moiety. In contrast, ganciclovir and penciclovir have a 3′ hydroxyl group; therefore, further synthesis of viral DNA is possible in the presence of these drugs. Foscarnet acts at the pyrophosphate-binding site of viral DNA polymerase and prevents cleavage of the pyrophosphate from nucleoside triphosphates, thus stalling further primer template extension. The blue bands between the viral DNA strands in the inset indicate hydrogen bonding of the base pairs. (*Adapted from Balfour HH. Antiviral drugs. N Engl J Med. 1999, 340:1255–1268.*)

CASE 44-1

A 47-year-old man is immunocompromised because of the medications he is taking to prevent a heart transplant rejection. He develops a herpes simplex virus (HSV) infection of his lower lip.

a. What are his treatment options?

Infection with herpes simplex virus 1 (HSV-1) typically causes diseases of the mouth, face, skin, esophagus, or brain. Herpes simplex virus 2 (HSV-2) causes infections of the genitals, rectum, skin, hands, or meninges. Acyclovir and its ester prodrug, valacyclovir, are the prototypes of a class of drugs that are phosphorylated intracellularly to become inhibitors of viral DNA synthesis. Other drugs that use the same strategy include penciclovir, its prodrug famciclovir, and ganciclovir, and its prodrug valganciclovir. Cidofovir and foscarnet are available to treat acyclovir-resistant HSV infections. Idoxuridine is available for the topical (ophthalmic)

(Continued)

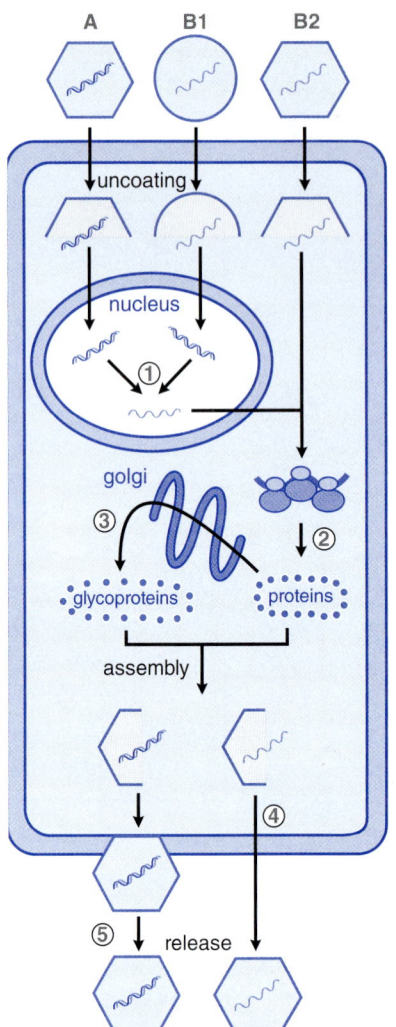

FIGURE 44-3 Interferon-mediated antiviral activity occurs via multiple mechanisms. The binding of interferon (IFN) to specific cell surface receptor molecules signals the cell to produce a series of antiviral proteins. The stages of viral replication that are inhibited by various IFN-induced antiviral proteins are shown. Most of these act to inhibit the translation of viral proteins (mechanism 2), but other steps in viral replication also are affected (mechanisms 1, 3, and 4). The roles of these mechanisms in the other actions of IFNs are under study. 2'5'A, 2'-5'-oligoadenylates; eIF-2α, protein synthesis initiation factor; IFN, interferon; mRNA, messenger RNA; Mx, IFN-induced cellular protein with antiviral activity; RNase L, latent cellular endoribonuclease; tRNA, transfer RNA. (*Modified from Baron, S., Coppenhaver, D.H., and Dianzani, F., et al. Introduction to the interferon system. In*, Interferons: Principles and Medical Applications. [*Baron, S., Dianzani, F., Stanton, G.J., et al., eds.*] University of Texas Medical Branch Dept. of Microbiology, Galveston, TX, 1992, pp. 1–15. With permission.)

treatment of HSV keratitis. Trifluridine is available for the topical treatment of keratoconjunctivitis and recurrent epithelial keratitis owing to HSV-1 and HSV-2. Topical trifluridine appears to be effective in some patients with acyclovir-resistant HSV cutaneous infections.

b. What is the mechanism of action of acyclovir?

The stages of viral replication and possible targets of action of antiviral agents are shown in Table 44-1. Acyclovir inhibits viral DNA synthesis via a mechanism outlined in Figure 44-2. Its selectivity of action depends on interaction with 2 viral proteins: HSV thymidine kinase and DNA polymerase.

c. What are the possible mechanisms of acyclovir resistance?

Acyclovir resistance in HSV has been linked to one of three mechanisms (see Table MECHANISMS OF ACTION AND RESISTANCE OF ANTIVIRAL DRUGS):

(Continued)

Antiviral Agents and Treatment of HIV Infection

CHAPTER 44

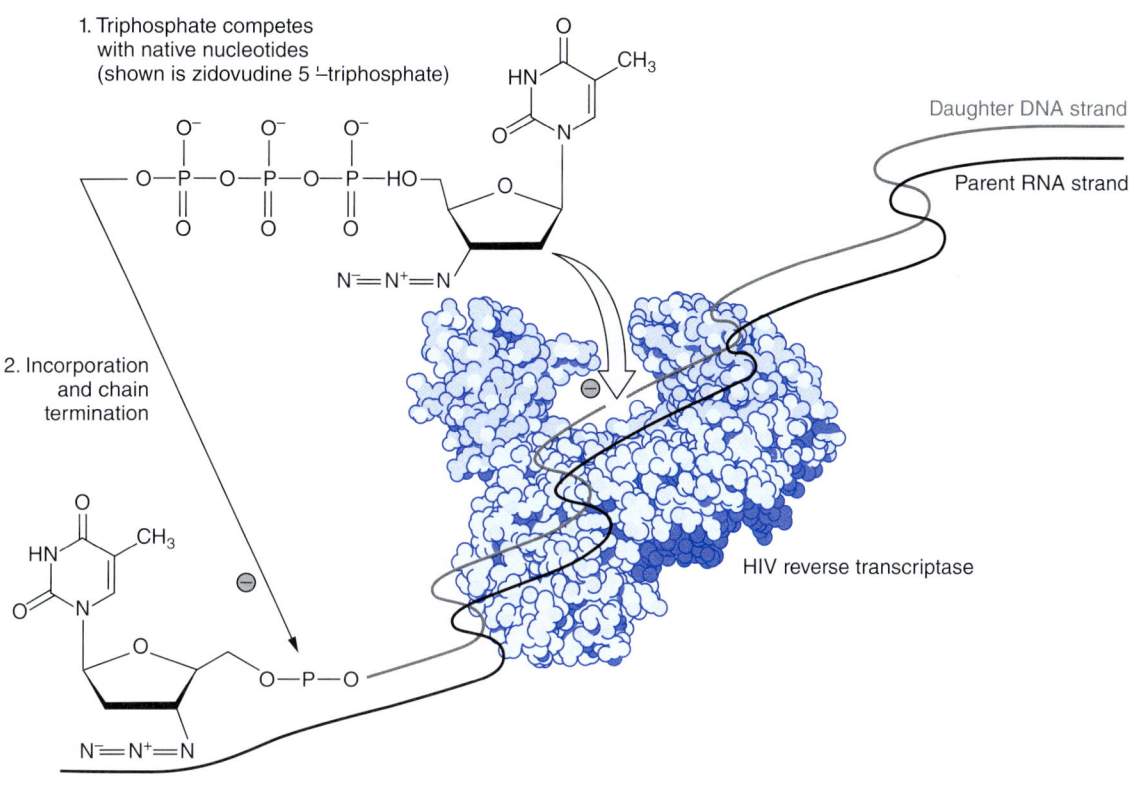

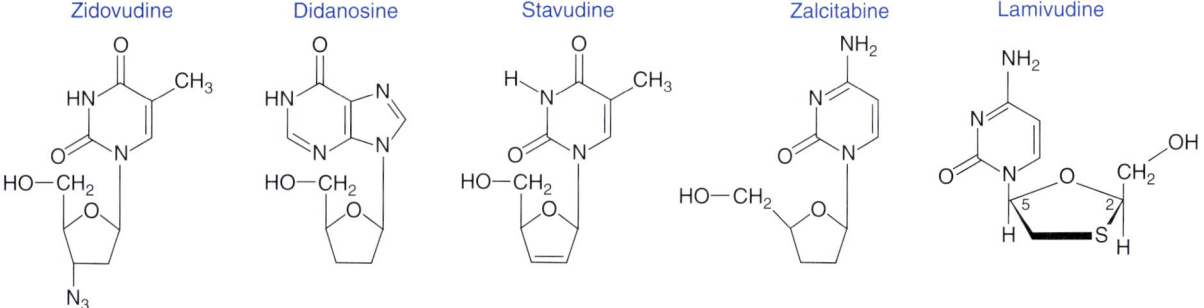

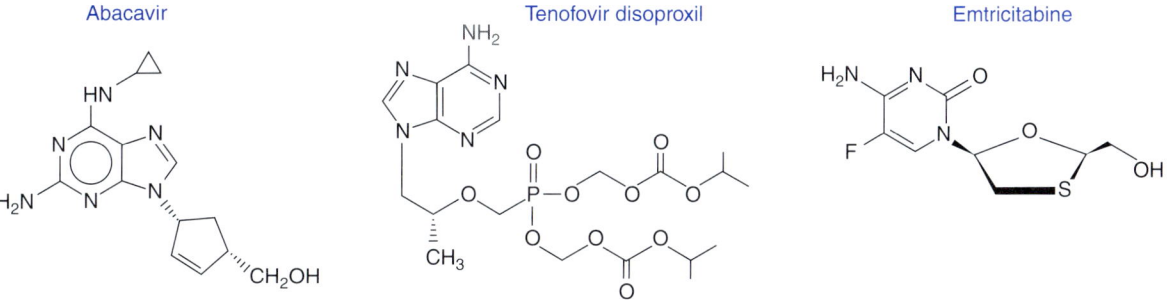

FIGURE 44-4 Structures and mechanism of nucleoside and nucleotide reverse transcriptase inhibitors.

impaired production of viral thymidine kinase, altered thymidine kinase substrate specificity (eg, phosphorylation of thymidine but not acyclovir), or altered viral DNA polymerase. The most common resistance mechanism in clinical HSV isolates is absent or deficient viral thymidine kinase activity.

(Continued)

SECTION VII
Chemotherapy of Microbial Diseases

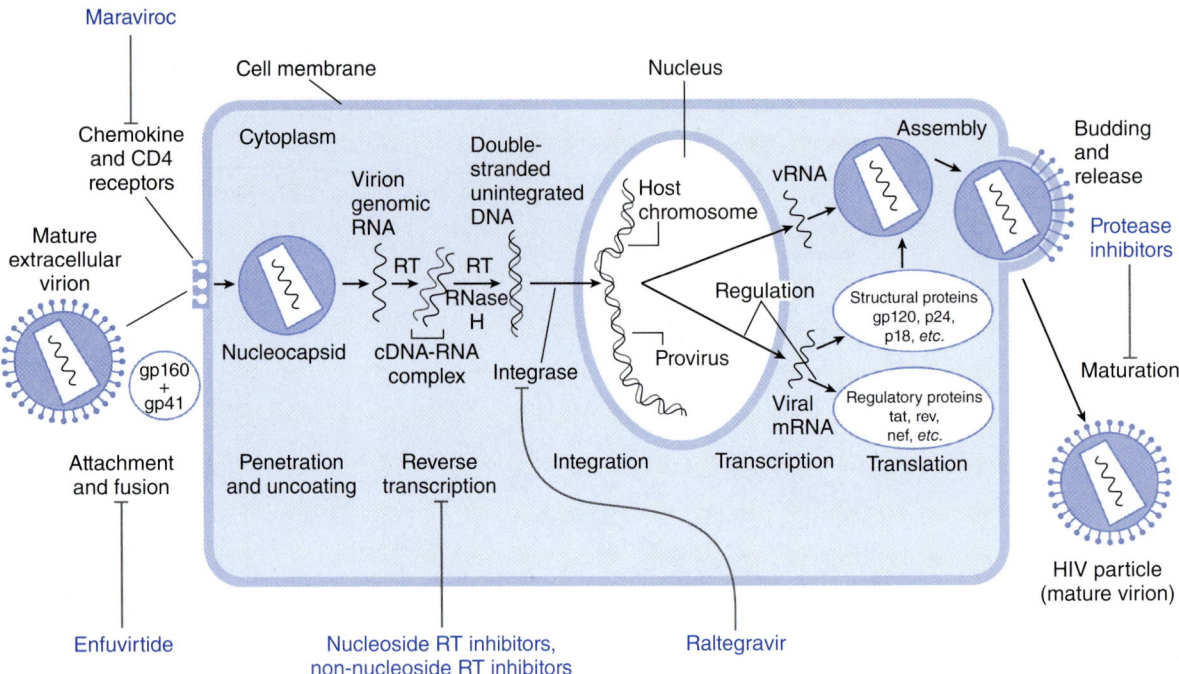

FIGURE 44-5 Replicative cycle of HIV-1 showing the sites of action of available antiretroviral agents. Available antiretroviral agents are shown in blue. cDNA, complementary DNA; gp120 + gp41, extracellular and intracellular domains, respectively, of envelope glycoprotein mRNA, messenger RNA; RNase H, ribonuclease H; RT, reverse transcriptase. (Adapted from Hirsch MS and D'Aquila RT. Therapy for human immunodeficiency virus infection. N Engl J Med. 1993, 328:1686–1695.)

d. If he is treated with acyclovir, what adverse events should this patient be warned about?

Oral acyclovir is associated with nausea, vomiting, diarrhea, rash, and headache. The principal dose-limiting toxicities of intravenous acyclovir are renal insufficiency and CNS side effects. The renal effects are due to high urine concentrations of the drug causing crystalline nephropathy. Neurotoxicity is manifested by altered sensorium, tremor, myoclonus, delirium, seizures, or extrapyramidal signs.

CASE 44-2

An otherwise healthy 76-year-old woman developed a rash on her side and back 5 days ago. She now describes considerable pain in the area. Her physician suspects varicella zoster virus (VZV) infection, commonly known as shingles.

a. What are the treatment options for this woman?

The 2 drugs most commonly used for VZV infections are acyclovir and penciclovir, or their prodrugs, valacyclovir, and famciclovir, respectively. Both drugs are effective if started within 24 hours of the rash.

b. Her physician elects to use famciclovir. Is it likely to be effective?

In immunocompetent adults with herpes zoster of less than or equal to 3 days' duration, famciclovir (500 mg 3 times a day for 10 days) is at least as effective as acyclovir (800 mg 5 times daily) in reducing healing time and zoster-associated pain, particularly in those more than or equal to 50 years of age. The fact that the rash started 5 days prior to the start of treatment makes it less likely that the treatment will be effective.

c. How is famciclovir absorbed and metabolized?

Famciclovir is well absorbed orally and is converted rapidly to penciclovir by deacetylation. The bioavailability of penciclovir is approximately 75% following oral administration of famciclovir.

Antiviral Agents and Treatment of HIV Infection

CHAPTER 44

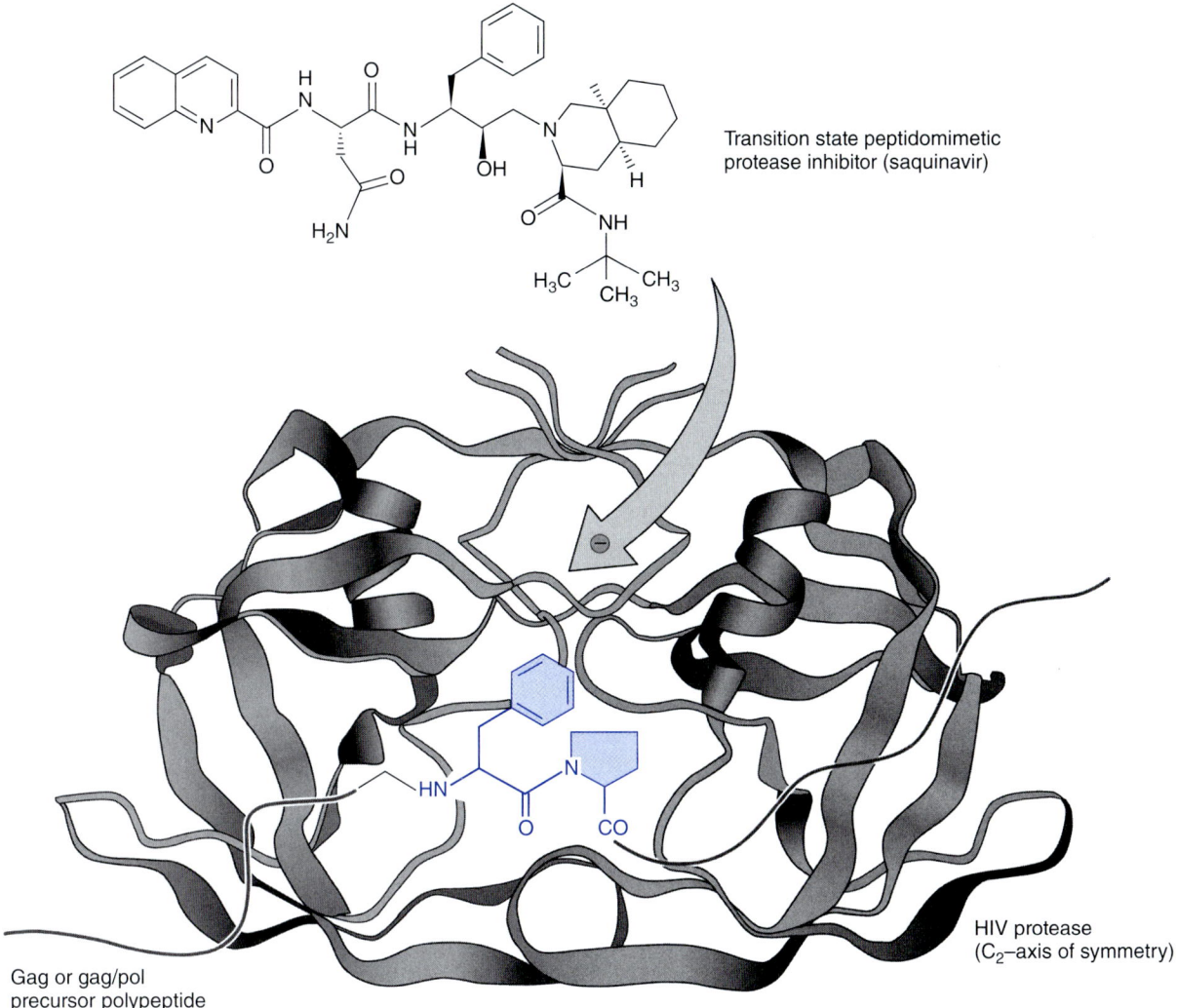

FIGURE 44-6 Mechanism of action of an HIV protease inhibitor. Shown here is a phenylalanine-proline target peptide sequence (in blue) for the protease enzyme (in black) with chemical structures of the native amino acids (in lower box) to emphasize homology of their structures to that of saquinavir (at top).

CASE 44-3

A 23-year-old man with AIDS has begun to develop blurred vision in the left eye. The diagnosis of cytomegalovirus (CMV) retinitis is made. He is started on intravenous foscarnet.

a. What treatment options, other than foscarnet, are available for the treatment of CMV retinitis?

Other than foscarnet, the treatment options for CMV retinitis include ganciclovir, fomivirsen, and cidofovir. Fomivirsen is given by intravitreal injection for patients intolerant of or unresponsive to other therapies.

(Continued)

SECTION VII Chemotherapy of Microbial Diseases

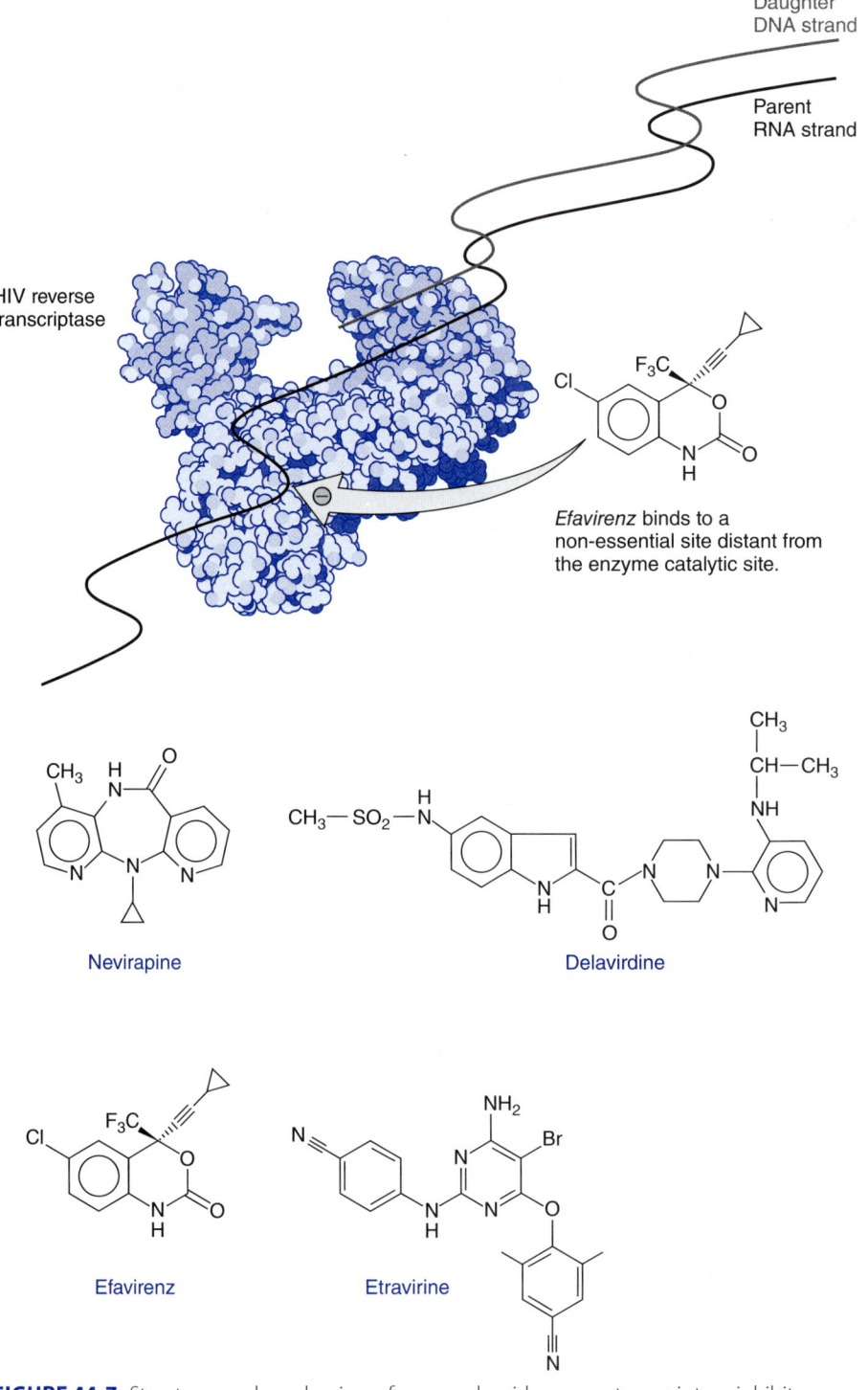

FIGURE 44-7 Structures and mechanism of non-nucleoside reverse transcriptase inhibitors.

b. What is the mechanism of action of foscarnet?

Foscarnet inhibits viral nucleic acid synthesis by interacting directly with herpesvirus DNA polymerase (see Figure 44-1). Foscarnet reversibly blocks the pyrophosphate binding site of the viral polymerase in a noncompetitive manner and inhibits cleavage of pyrophosphate from deoxynucleotide triphosphates.

c. Do patients develop resistance to foscarnet?

Resistant clinical isolates of herpesviruses have emerged during therapeutic use of foscarnet and may be associated with poor clinical response. Herpesviruses

(Continued)

Antiviral Agents and Treatment of HIV Infection

CHAPTER 44

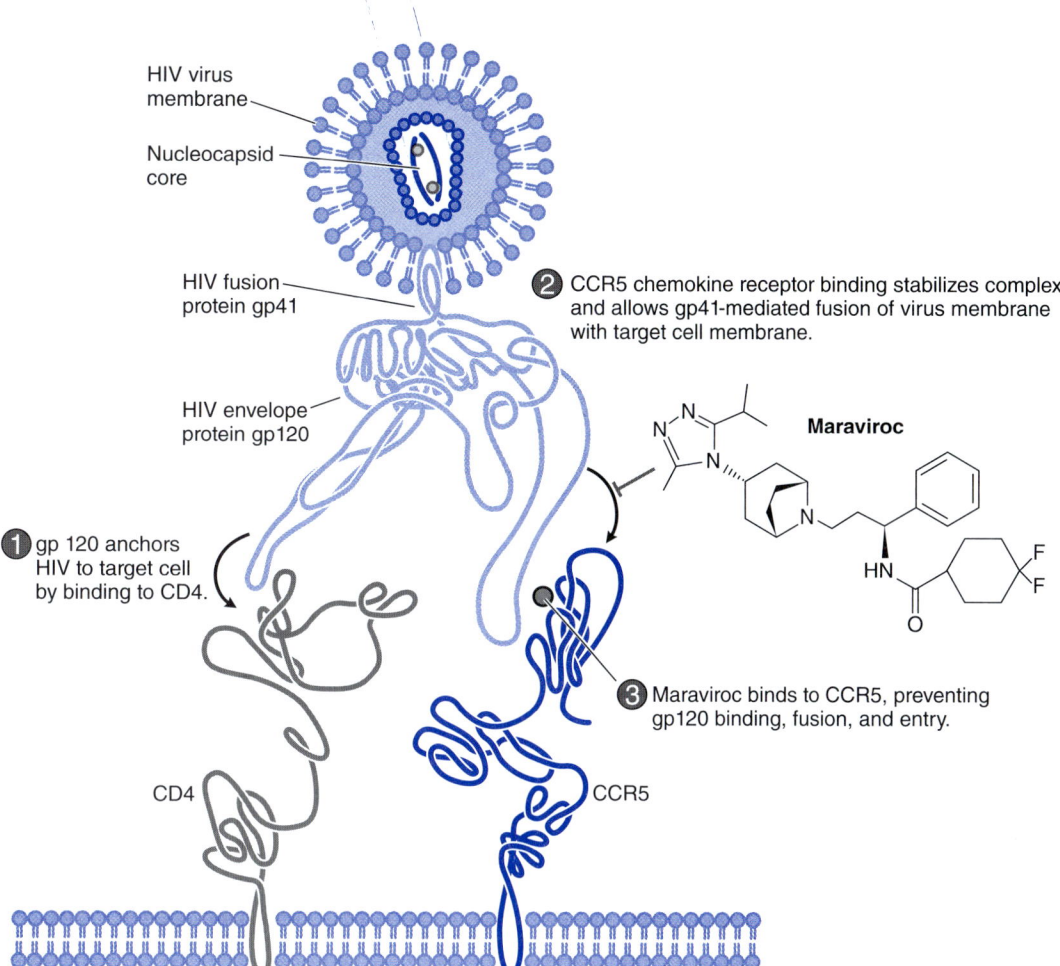

FIGURE 44-8 Mechanism of action of the HIV entry inhibitor maraviroc.

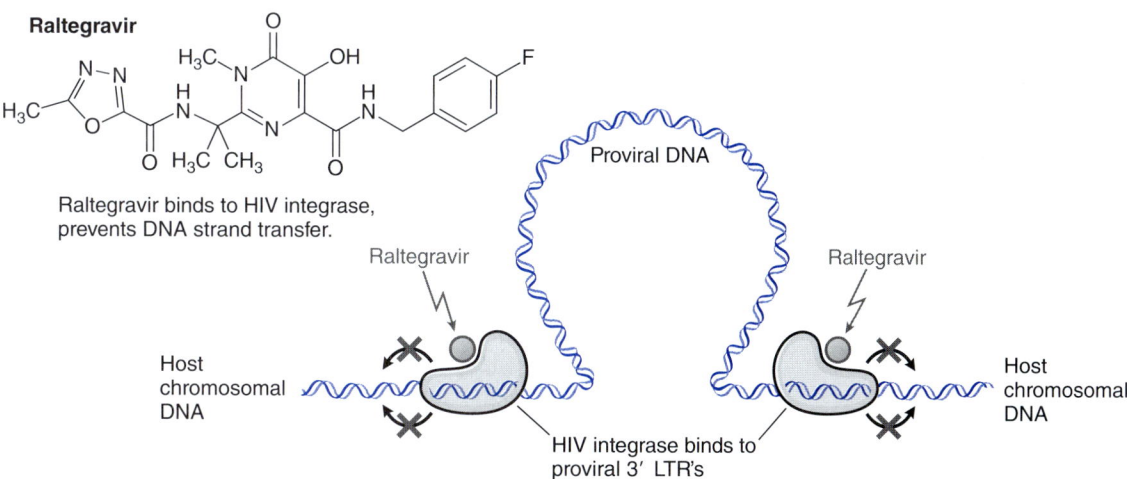

FIGURE 44-9 Mechanism of action of the HIV integrase inhibitor raltegravir.

SECTION VII   Chemotherapy of Microbial Diseases

TABLE 44-1 Stages of Virus Replication and Possible Targets of Action of Antiviral Agents

STAGE OF REPLICATION	CLASSES OF SELECTIVE INHIBITORS
Cell entry	
Attachment	Soluble receptor decoys, antireceptor antibodies, fusion protein inhibitors
Penetration	
Uncoating	Ion channel blockers, capsid stabilizers
Release of viral genome	
Transcription of viral genome[a]	Inhibitors of viral DNA polymerase, RNA polymerase, reverse transcriptase, helicase, primase, or integrase
Transcription of viral messenger RNA	
Replication of viral genome	
Translation of viral proteins	Interferons, antisense oligonucleotides, ribozymes
Regulatory proteins (early)	Inhibitors of regulatory proteins
Structural proteins (late)	
Post-translational modifications	
Proteolytic cleavage	Protease inhibitors
Myristoylation, glycosylation	
Assembly of virion components	Interferons, assembly protein inhibitors
Release	Neuraminidase inhibitors, antiviral antibodies, cytotoxic lymphocytes
Budding, cell lysis	

[a]Depends on specific replication strategy of virus, but virus-specified enzyme required for part of process.

resistant to foscarnet have point mutations in the viral DNA polymerase and are associated with 3- to 7-fold reductions in foscarnet activity in vitro.

d. This patient should be monitored for what major untoward effects?

Foscarnet's major dose-limiting toxicities are nephrotoxicity and symptomatic hypocalcemia. Acute tubular necrosis, crystalline glomerulopathy, nephrogenic diabetes insipidus, and interstitial nephritis have been described. Saline loading may reduce the risk of nephrotoxicity.

Foscarnet is highly ionized at physiological pH, and metabolic abnormalities are common. These include increases or decreases in calcium and phosphate, hypomagnesemia, and hypokalemia. Decreased serum ionized calcium may cause paresthesia, arrhythmias, tetany, seizures, and other CNS disturbances.

CASE 44-4

A 46-year-old woman is considered immunocompromised because of therapy for a bone marrow transplant. Influenza A is identified in the community in which she lives. Although she is asymptomatic, she is started on amantadine.

a. Why is she started on amantadine while she is asymptomatic?

Seasonal prophylaxis with amantadine is an alternative in high-risk patients if the influenza vaccine cannot be administered. Prophylaxis should be started as soon as influenza is identified in the community or region and should be continued throughout the period of risk because any protective effects are lost several days after cessation of therapy.

(Continued)

Antiviral Agents and Treatment of HIV Infection — CHAPTER 44

b. **What is the mechanism of action of amantadine?**

Amantadine and rimantadine have 2 mechanisms of action (see Figure 44-1). They inhibit an early step in viral replication, probably viral uncoating; for some strains they also have an effect on a late step in viral assembly, probably mediated through altering hemagglutinin processing. The primary locus of action is the influenza A virus M2 protein, an integral membrane protein that functions as an ion channel.

c. **Do patients treated with amantadine develop resistance to the drug?**

The utility of amantadine is limited by the development of resistance. Resistant variants appear to be pathogenic and can cause disabling influenza. Resistance to amantadine results from a mutation in the RNA sequence encoding for the M2 protein transmembrane domain. Resistant isolates typically appear in the treated patient within 2 to 3 days of starting therapy.

d. **What are the major limitations to the use of amantadine?**

The most common side effects of amantadine are dose-related CNS and gastrointestinal effects. These include nervousness, light-headedness, difficulty concentrating, insomnia, nausea, and loss of appetite. High plasma concentrations are associated with serious neurotoxic reactions including delirium, hallucinations, seizures, and coma.

CASE 44-5

A 37-year-old man with chronic hepatitis C virus (HCV) infection is being treated with interferon and ribavirin.

a. **What are this patient's therapeutic options?**

Current standard of care for treatment of HCV infection is a combination of peginterferon alpha and ribavirin, which produces a high cure rate in selected virus genotypes only. Recent advances in the development of highly effective oral agents include HCV protease inhibitors and polymerase inhibitors that are selective for this pathogen. It is likely that treatment recommendations will change radically in the near future.

b. **What interferon products are available and how do they differ?**

Interferons (IFNs) are potent cytokines that possess antiviral, immunomodulatory, and antiproliferative activities. Three classes of human interferons with significant antiviral activity currently are recognized: α, β, and γ. IFN-α and IFN-β may be produced in nearly all cells in response to viral infection. They exhibit antiviral and antiproliferative actions and stimulate the cytotoxic activity of lymphocytes, natural killer cells, and macrophages. Because IFNs induce long-lasting cellular effects, their activities are not easily predictable from the usual pharmacokinetic measures.

Attachment of IFN to large inert polyethylene glycol (PEG) molecules (pegylation) slows absorption, decreases clearance, and provides higher and more prolonged serum concentrations that enable once weekly dosing. The pegylated IFNs are generally better tolerated than standard IFNs.

c. **What is the mechanism of action of interferons?**

Following binding to specific cellular receptors, IFNs activate the JAK-STAT signal transduction pathway and lead to nuclear translocation of a cellular protein that binds to genes containing an IFN-specific response element. This in turn leads to synthesis of over 2 dozen proteins that contribute to viral resistance mediated at different stages of viral penetration (see Figure 44-3).

d. **What is ribavirin and why is it added to this patient's treatment regimen?**

Ribavirin is a purine nucleoside analog that inhibits the replication of RNA and DNA viruses. Oral ribavirin in combination with pegIFN alfa-2A or -2B has become the standard treatment for chronic HCV infection.

(Continued)

SECTION VII Chemotherapy of Microbial Diseases

e. **What untoward effects might be expected with this regimen?**

Injection of recombinant IFN usually is associated with an acute influenza-like syndrome beginning several hours after injection. The principal dose-limiting toxicities are depression, myelosuppression with granulocytopenia and thrombocytopenia, neurasthenia, and autoimmune disorders, including thyroiditis and hypothyroidism.

Systemic ribavirin causes dose-related reversible anemia owing to extravascular hemolysis and bone marrow suppression. Ribavirin is classified as FDA pregnancy category X.

CASE 44-6

A 42-year-old woman with recently diagnosed HIV infection is being started on medication to treat her disease.

a. **What clinical decisions are important for making treatment recommendations?**

Current treatment recommendations center on making 2 important clinical decisions: (1) When to start therapy in treatment-naïve individuals; and (2) when to change therapy in individuals that are failing their current regimen.

Several expert panels issue periodic recommendations for the use of antiretroviral drugs for treatment-naïve and treatment-experienced adults and children. In the United States, the Panel on Clinical Practices for treatment of HIV Infection issues updated guidelines approximately every 6 months; their most recent guidelines can be accessed at http://www.aidsinfo.nih.gov/Guidelines (Department of Health and Human Services).

b. **What principles drive treatment guidelines?**

In each clinical setting there is a complex algorithm of possible drug choices depending on patient and viral characteristics. The specific drugs recommended may change from year to year as new choices become available and clinical research data accumulate. However, it is likely that future treatment guidelines will continue to be driven by 3 principles: (1) Use of combination therapy to prevent the emergence of resistant virus; (2) Emphasis on regimen convenience, tolerability, and adherence to chronically suppress HIV replication; and (3) Realization of the need for lifelong treatment under most circumstances.

c. **What concerns about drug resistance should be considered in all patients?**

There is a high likelihood that all untreated infected individuals harbor viruses with single-amino acid mutations conferring some degree of resistance to every known antiretroviral drug because of the high mutation rate of HIV and the tremendous number of infectious virions. Drug therapy does not cause mutation but rather provides the necessary selective pressure to promote growth of drug-resistant viruses that arise naturally. A combination of active agents therefore is required to prevent drug resistance, analogous to strategies employed in the treatment of tuberculosis (see Chapter 42). The current standard of care is to use at least 3 drugs simultaneously for the entire duration of treatment.

CASE 44-7

A 45-year-old man with HIV infection is being treated with a combination of zidovudine, lamivudine, and abacavir.

a. **What are the mechanisms of action of these drugs?**

These drugs are nucleoside reverse transcriptase inhibitors (NRTIs). Their mechanism of action is summarized in Figures 44-1 and 44-5. The HIV-encoded, RNA-dependent DNA polymerase, also called reverse transcriptase, converts viral RNA into proviral DNA that is then incorporated into a host cell chromosome. Zidovudine, lamivudine, and abacavir are phosphorylated and their triphosphates

(Continued)

competitively inhibit incorporation of natural nucleotides by reverse transcriptase and also terminate the elongation of proviral DNA because they are incorporated into nascent DNA but lack a 3'-hydroxyl group.

b. Why is the combination therapy used?

The combination therapy is used to prevent drug resistance as described in Case 44-6.

c. What are the precautions and possible untoward effects of this combination?

Patients initiating zidovudine often complain of fatigue, malaise, myalgia, nausea, anorexia, headache, and insomnia.

Lamivudine is one of the least toxic antiretroviral drugs.

Abacavir is associated with a unique and potentially fatal hypersensitivity syndrome. This syndrome is characterized by fever, abdominal pain, and other GI complaints, a rash, and malaise or fatigue. The presence of a fever, abdominal pain, and rash within 6 weeks of starting abacavir is diagnostic and necessitates the discontinuation of the drug. Abacavir can never be restarted once discontinued for hypersensitivity because the reintroduction of the drug leads to rapid recurrence of severe symptoms and may lead to death.

CASE 44-8

A 25-year-old man with HIV infection is being treated with nevirapine as a single agent.

a. What is the mechanism of action of nevirapine?

Nevirapine is a non-nucleoside reverse transcriptase inhibitor (NNRTI) that binds to a hydrophobic pocket of the HIV reverse transcriptase where it induces a conformational change in the enzyme that greatly reduces its activity (see Figures 44-1 and 44-7). Unlike nucleoside reverse transcriptase inhibitors (NRTIs), the NNRTIs do not require intracellular phosphorylation to attain activity.

b. What is the problem in using this drug as a sole agent to treat HIV?

When nevirapine was used as monotherapy, there was a rapid fall in plasma HIV RNA concentrations that was followed by a return toward baseline within 8 weeks because of rapid emergence of resistance. Nevirapine should never be used as a single agent or as the sole addition to a failing regimen.

CASE 44-9

A 38-year-old woman with HIV infection is being treated with a combination product containing lopinavir and ritonavir.

a. What is the mechanism of action of these drugs?

Lopinavir and ritonavir are HIV protease inhibitors (see Figure 44-6). These drugs prevent the proteolytic cleavage of peptides and proteins that are essential structural and enzymatic components of HIV. Viral proteases are homodimers; human proteases (renin, pepsin, gastricsin, cathepsins) contain only 1 polypeptide chain and are not significantly inhibited by HIV protease inhibitors.

b. Why is the combination product used?

Ritonavir is one of the most potent known inhibitors of CYP3A4. Because lopinavir undergoes extensive hepatic oxidative metabolism by CYP3A4, ritonavir is used to inhibit the metabolism of lopinavir and increase its concentrations.

c. What precautions should be taken with the combination of lopinavir and ritonavir?

The most common adverse events with lopinavir/ritonavir are loose stools, diarrhea, nausea, and vomiting.

Because lopinavir is dependent on CYP3A4, the concomitant administration of agents that induce CYP3A4 such as rifampin and St. John's wort may lower plasma concentrations of lopinavir and loss of antiviral effectiveness.

(Continued)

SECTION VII Chemotherapy of Microbial Diseases

Ritonavir, beside being a potent inhibitor of CYP3A4, is also a moderate CYP inducer at the doses employed in the coformulation and can adversely decrease concentrations of some coadministered drugs such as oral contraceptives.

CASE 44-10

A 56-year-old man with HIV infection has been treated with 3 other antiretroviral agents. Despite this treatment, he has evidence of HIV replication. Treatment with enfuvirtide is recommended.

a. What is the mechanism of action of enfuvirtide?

Enfuvirtide is a synthetic peptide that prevents membrane fusion and viral entry into the host cell (see Figure 44-5). Enfuvirtide retains activity against viruses that have become resistant to antiretroviral agents of other classes because of its unique mechanism of action.

b. Why is enfuvirtide recommended only after treatment with other antiretroviral agents has failed?

Most patients develop local injection site reactions to the parenteral administration of enfuvirtide. Given the cost, inconvenience, and cutaneous toxicity of enfuvirtide, it is generally reserved for patients who have failed all other feasible antiretroviral agents. In fact, enfuvirtide is FDA approved for use only in treatment-experienced adults who have evidence of HIV replication despite ongoing antiretroviral therapy.

KEY CONCEPTS

- There are distinct stages of viral replication. The classes of antiviral agents that can act at each stage are shown in Table 44-1.
- Acyclovir is the prototype of a group of antiherpes viral agents that are phosphorylated intracellularly by a virus kinase and subsequently by host enzymes to become inhibitors of viral DNA synthesis.
- Amantadine and rimantadine are anti-influenza agents that inhibit viral replication by inhibiting viral uncoating; zanamivir and oseltamivir inhibit viral neuraminidase.
- The anti-influenza drugs are used for the prevention and treatment of influenza A, and some for influenza B.
- Drugs used to treat chronic hepatitis C virus infection are the interferons and ribavirin.
- Interferon and ribavirin can cure patients with chronic hepatitis B virus infection but are associated with a high rate of side effects, often leading to premature treatment discontinuation.
- Several antiretroviral nucleoside or nucleotide analog polymerase inhibitors, including lamivudine, telbivudine, and tenofovir, have potent anti-HBV activity and provide alternative therapy to interferon and ribavirin. Adefovir, dipivoxil, and entecavir also provide alternative therapy for chronic HBV infection.
- Three-drug combinations are the minimum standard of care for HIV infection. Starting therapy with only a single agent inevitably provokes the emergence of drug-resistant virus.
- Drugs used to treat HIV infection generally fall into 3 classes:
  - Nucleoside reverse transcriptase inhibitors (NRTIs).
  - Non-nucleoside reverse transcriptase inhibitors (NNRTIs).
  - Protease inhibitors.
- Ritonavir is a protease inhibitor that is a very potent inhibitor of CYP3A4. It is often added in combination with other drugs to enhance their pharmacokinetic profile.

(Continued)

Antiviral Agents and Treatment of HIV Infection

CHAPTER 44

➡ There are 2 drugs, maraviroc and enfuvirtide, that block the entry of HIV into host cells; raltegravir prevents the integration of virus DNA into the host chromosome.

➡ Prescribers of antiretroviral therapy must maintain a comprehensive and current fund of knowledge regarding the disease and its pharmacotherapy. The prescribing of antiretroviral agents to patients with HIV infection should be limited to those with specialized training.

SUMMARY QUIZ

QUESTION 44-1 A 48-year-old man with AIDS is diagnosed with CMV retinitis. He is being treated with intravenous foscarnet. A laboratory blood test for which of the following should be monitored closely?

a. Copper
b. Alanine aminotransferase
c. Calcium
d. Zinc
e. Bilirubin

QUESTION 44-2 Which of the following drugs is an option for the treatment of CMV retinitis in the patient in Question 44-1?

a. Acyclovir
b. Gancyclovir
c. Rimantadine
d. Oseltamivir
e. Ribavirin

QUESTION 44-3 A 36-year-old woman has been diagnosed with chronic hepatitis C. She is prescribed oral ribavirin in combination with which of the following agents for her treatment?

a. Tenofovir
b. Telbivudine
c. Enfuvirtide
d. PegINF alpha-2A
e. Cidofovir

QUESTION 44-4 A 27-year-old man with newly diagnosed HIV infection is started on zidovudine alone. This treatment regimen is unlikely to be therapeutically effective because

a. zidovudine is not active against HIV.
b. zidovudine is metabolized by hepatic CYPs.
c. the side effects of zidovudine do not warrant its use.
d. the use of zidovudine is limited by its absorption from the gastrointestinal tract.
e. resistance of the HIV is likely to develop from the use of a single agent.

QUESTION 44-5 A 43-year-old woman with HIV infection is treated with atazanavir and ritonavir. Ritonavir is added to the regiment because it

a. inhibits CYP3A4, decreases the metabolism of atazanavir, and raises its plasma concentrations.
b. prevents the renal excretion of atazanavir.
c. increases the oral absorption of atazanavir.

(Continued)

SECTION VII
Chemotherapy of Microbial Diseases

d. is a more potent inhibitor of HIV replication than atazanavir.

e. It decreases the neurotoxicity of atazanavir.

QUESTION 44-6 A 56-year-old man has been treated for HIV infection for 10 years. His HIV is now resistant to all previous antiretroviral drugs and there is evidence of HIV replication despite his treatment with 3 concomitant drugs. He is now being treated with enfuvirtide because it

a. is less expensive.

b. is less toxic.

c. is more effective against HIV.

d. has an unique mechanism of action.

e. can be administered orally.

QUESTION 44-7 A 35-year-old woman with HIV infection also has developed chronic hepatitis B. She is being treated with entecavir for her chronic HBV infection. Because she has recently developed symptoms of fatigue and nausea, she has stopped her entecavir therapy. She is at risk for developing

a. acute renal failure.

b. acute pancreatitis.

c. acute exacerbation of hepatitis B.

d. chronic hepatitis C.

e. acute neurotoxicity.

QUESTION 44-8 A 28-year-old man with HIV is being treated with lopinavir. He admits to using nutritional supplements bought over the Internet because it makes him feel in control of his therapy. This patient should be cautioned about the effect nutritional supplements may have on

a. HIV.

b. the metabolism of lopinavir.

c. the renal excretion of lopinavir.

d. the cardiac toxicity of lopinavir.

e. the skin toxicity of lopinavir.

SUMMARY QUIZ ANSWER KEY

QUESTION 44-1 Answer is **c**. Foscarnet is highly ionized at physiological pH, and metabolic abnormalities are common. These include increases or decreases in calcium and phosphate, hypomagnesemia, and hypokalemia. Decreased serum ionized calcium may cause paresthesia, arrhythmias, tetany, seizures, and other CNS disturbances. Concomitant intravenous pentamidine administration increases the risk of symptomatic hypocalcemia.

QUESTION 44-2 Answer is **b**. Acyclovir is ineffective therapeutically in established CMV infections, but gancyclovir is effective for treatment and chronic suppression of CMV retinitis in immunocompromised patients and for prevention of CMV in transplant patients.

QUESTION 44-3 Answer is **d**. Oral ribavirin in combination with injected pegINF alfa-2A or -2B has become standard treatment for chronic HCV infection.

QUESTION 44-4 Answer is **e**. Starting treatment with only a single antiretroviral drug inevitably provokes the emergence of drug-resistant virus. A combination of antiviral agents therefore is required to prevent drug resistance.

QUESTION 44-5 Answer is **a**. Atazanavir undergoes oxidative metabolism in the liver primarily by CYP3A4. Ritonavir is one of the most potent known inhibitors of

(Continued)

CYP3A4. Ritonavir inhibits the metabolism of all current HIV protease inhibitors and is frequently used in combination with most of these drugs, except nelfinavir, to enhance their pharmacokinetic profile and allow a reduction in dose and dosing frequency of the coadministered drug.

QUESTION 44-6 Answer is **d**. Enfuvirtide has a unique mechanism of antiretroviral action. It prevents viral entry into the host cell. Because of this unique mechanism of action, it retains activity against viruses that have become resistant to antiretroviral agents of other classes.

QUESTION 44-7 Answer is **c**. Severe acute exacerbations of hepatitis B have been reported in patients who have discontinued anti-HBV therapy. Hepatic function should be monitored closely with both clinical and laboratory follow-up for at least several months in patients who discontinue anti-HBV therapy.

QUESTION 44-8 Answer is **b**. Because lopinavir metabolism is highly dependent on CYP3A4, concomitant administration of agents that induce CYP3A4 may lower plasma lopinavir concentrations considerably. St. John's wort is a known inducer of CYP3A4, leading to lower concentrations of lopinavir and possible loss of antiviral effectiveness.

SUMMARY: ANTIVIRAL DRUGS

CLASS AND SUBCLASSES	NAME	CLINICAL USES	RESISTANCE	TOXICITY COMMON	TOXICITY UNIQUE; CLINICALLY IMPORTANT
Antiherpes Agents	Acyclovir	HSV infections	Impaired production of thymidine kinase, altered thymidine kinase substrate, or altered DNA polymerase	Nausea, diarrhea, rash, and headache	Renal insufficiency and CNS side effects, including altered sensorium, seizures, delirium, or extrapyramidal effects
	Cidofovir	Approved for treatment of CMV retinitis in HIV-infected patients	Resistance in CMV is due to mutations in DNA polymerase		Nephrotoxicity Use in pregnancy Category C
	Foscarnet	Useful for treatment of CMV retinitis and acyclovir-resistant HSV and VZV infections	Mutations in herpes virus DNA polymerase	Rash, fever, nausea	Nephrotoxicity and symptomatic hypocalcemia
	Fomivirsen	CMV retinitis			Iritis, vitritis, cataracts
	Ganciclovir	Chronic suppression of CMV retinitis and other CMV syndromes in AIDS patients	CMV resistance is due to either mutations in viral phosphotransferase which reduces intracellular ganciclovir phosphorylation or mutations in viral DNA polymerase	Rash, fever, nausea, vomiting Phlebitis	Neutropenia and thrombocytopenia CNS toxicity, including headache and seizures
	Idoxuridine	Topical treatment of HSV keratitis	Resistance develops readily in vitro and in viral isolates of idoxuridine-treated patients	Pruritus, inflammation and edema of eye or lids	
	Penciclovir	Treatment of HSV and varicella-zoster virus (VZV) infections	Mutations in thymidine kinase or viral DNA polymerase	Headache, diarrhea, nausea	
	Trifluridine	Treatment of HSV keratoconjunctivitis and recurrent epithelial keratitis	Trifluridine-resistant HSV have altered thymidine substrate specificity	Irritation and palpebral edema at injection site	

(Continued)

SECTION VII: Chemotherapy of Microbial Diseases

CLASS AND SUBCLASSES	NAME	CLINICAL USES	RESISTANCE	TOXICITY COMMON	TOXICITY UNIQUE; CLINICALLY IMPORTANT
Antihepatitis Agents	Adefovir dipivoxil	Treatment of chronic hepatitis B virus (HBV) infections	Point mutations in HBV polymerase	Headache, abdominal discomfort	Pregnancy Category C Dose-related nephrotoxicity
	Entecavir	Treatment of chronic hepatitis B virus (HBV) infections	Mutations in HIV reverse transcriptase	Headache, fatigue, dizziness, nausea	Severe exacerbations of hepatitis B in patients who have discontinued anti-HBV therapy
	Interferon	Treatment of condyloma acuminatum Chronic HCV infection Chronic HBV infection Kaposi's sarcoma in HIV-infected patients, other malignancies, and multiple sclerosis	Blocked production or activity of interferon-inducible proteins	Acute influenza-like syndrome several hours after injection	Granulocytopenia and thrombocytopenia Neurotoxicity manifested by somnolence, confusion, behavioral disturbance Debilitating neurasthenia and depression; thyroiditis and hypothyroidism
	Lamivudine	Treatment of chronic HBV hepatitis and HIV infection	Point mutations in HBV DNA polymerase		Generally well tolerated
Anti-influenza Agents	Amantadine	Prophylaxis against influenza A	Mutations in the RNA sequence encoding for the M2 protein trans-membrane domain	Nervousness light-headedness, insomnia, loss of appetite, and nausea	
	Oseltamivir	Treatment and prevention of influenza A and B virus infections	Mutations in viral hemagglutinin and/or neur aminidase	Nausea, vomiting	Pregnancy Category C
	Rimantadine	Prophylaxis against influenza A	Mutations in the RNA sequence encoding for the M2 protein trans-membrane domain		
	Zanamivir	Prevention and treatment of influenza A and B virus infections	Mutations in viral hemagglutinin and/or neuraminidase	Wheezing and bronchospasm	Not recommended for treatment of patients with underlying airway disease because of serious adverse events
Other Antiviral Agents	Ribavirin	Oral ribavirin in combination with pegIFN alfa-2A or -2B is standard treatment for chronic hepatitis C virus (HCV) infection Ribavirin aerosol is for treatment of RSV bronchiolitis and pneumonia in children	Resistance not documented, but cells that do not phosphorylate ribavirin to its active form have been reported	Conjunctival irritation, rash, transient wheezing	Pregnancy Category X Dose-related anemia due to extravascular hemolysis and bone marrow suppression
	Telbivudine	Treatment of chronic HBV infection	Mutations of HBV DNA polymerase	Increased creatine kinase, nausea, diarrhea, fatigue, myalgia, and myopathy	

(Continued)

Antiviral Agents and Treatment of HIV Infection — CHAPTER 44

CLASS AND SUBCLASSES	NAME	CLINICAL USES	RESISTANCE	TOXICITY COMMON	TOXICITY UNIQUE; CLINICALLY IMPORTANT
	Imiquimod	Topical treatment of condylomata acuminata		Local erythema, excoriation, itching, burning	
Nucleoside Reverse Transcriptase Inhibitors (NRTIs)	Zidovudine	Treatment of HIV infection in adults and children	Mutations in reverse transcriptase	Fatigue, nausea, malaise, myalgia, anorexia, insomnia	Bone marrow suppression with anemia
	Didanosine	Treatment of HIV infection in adults and children	Mutations in reverse transcriptase	Diarrhea	Peripheral neuropathy and pancreatitis
	Stavudine	Treatment of HIV infection in adults and children	Mutations in reverse transcriptase		Peripheral neuropathy Fat wasting and lipodystrophy Should not be used with either didanosine (increased peripheral neuropathy and fatal pancreatitis) or zidovudine (competition for intracellular phosphorylation)
	Zalcitabine	Treatment of advanced HIV			No longer marketed because of severe peripheral neuropathy
	Lamivudine	Treatment of chronic HBV hepatitis and HIV infection	Point mutations in DNA polymerase		Few significant adverse effects
	Abacavir	In combination with other antiretroviral agents for the treatment of HIV infection	Mutations in reverse transcriptase		Fatal hypersensitivity syndrome manifested by fever, abdominal pain, and rash; the adverse reaction is linked to the HLA-B*5701 genotype
	Tenofovir disoproxil	Treatment of chronic HBV infection and HIV infection	Mutations in reverse transcriptase; in HBV infection, resistance was not evident over 48 weeks of treatment	Flatulence	
	Emtricitabine	Treatment of HIV infection in adults	Mutations in reverse transcriptase	Prolonged exposure causes hyperpigmentation	Few significant adverse effects
Protease Inhibitors	Saquinavir	Treatment of HIV infection in adults Predominantly used in combination with ritonavir	Accumulation of multiple resistance mutations	Nausea, vomiting, diarrhea	Metabolized by intestinal and hepatic CYP3A4; substances that inhibit intestinal CYP3A4 increase AUC by 3 fold Long-term use associated with lipodystrophy
	Indinavir	No longer widely used because of nephrotoxicity	Accumulation of multiple resistance mutations		Nephrolithiasis and nephrotoxicity

(Continued)

SECTION VII — Chemotherapy of Microbial Diseases

CLASS AND SUBCLASSES	NAME	CLINICAL USES	RESISTANCE	TOXICITY COMMON	TOXICITY UNIQUE; CLINICALLY IMPORTANT
	Ritonavir	Used infrequently alone; ritonavir is a potent inhibitor of CYP3A4 and is used in combination to enhance the pharmacokinetic profile of other protease inhibitors	Mostly used as a pharmacokinetic enhancer (CYP3A4 inhibitor) and at the low doses use is not known to induce resistance	Nausea, vomiting, and diarrhea	Reduces the ethinyl estradiol AUC by 40%; alternative forms of contraception should be found
	Nelfinavir	Treatment of HIV infection in adults and children	Mutation in HIV protease	Diarrhea	Metabolized by CYP2C19 and CYP 3A4; concomitant administration of agents that induce these enzymes may be contraindicated
	Amprenavir	Treatment of HIV infection in adults and children, commonly in combination with ritonavir	Mutation in HIV protease	Diarrhea, nausea, vomiting	Amprenavir is both an inducer and inhibitor of CYP3A4 and drug interactions can occur and be unpredictable Substances that induce CYP3A4 may lower plasma amprenavir concentrations
	Lopinavir	Treatment of HIV infection in adults and children, commonly in combination with ritonavir	Mutation in HIV protease	Nausea, vomiting, diarrhea	Metabolized by CYP3A4; concomitant administration of substances that induce this enzyme may lower plasma concentration of lopinavir substantially
	Atazanavir	Used in combination with ritonavir to treat HIV-infected adults	Mutation in HIV protease	Unconjugated hyperbilirubinemia Diarrhea, nausea	Metabolized by CYP3A4; the concomitant administration of agents that induce this enzyme are contraindicated
	Tipranavir	Used in treatment-experienced adults and children whose HIV is resistant to other protease inhibitors	Resistance requires accumulation of multiple mutations	Rash	Associated with rare fatal hepatotoxicity Tipranavir is a substrate, inducer, and inhibitor of CYP enzymes
	Darunavir	Used in combination with ritonavir to treat HIV-infected adults	Resistance requires accumulation of multiple mutations	Rash, GI complaints	
Non-Nucleoside Reverse Transcriptase Inhibitors (NNRTIs)	Nevirapine	Treatment of HIV infection in adults and children	Mutations in reverse transcriptase; cross-resistance extends to efavirenz and delavirdine	Rash, fever, fatigue	Elevated hepatic transaminases

(Continued)

Antiviral Agents and Treatment of HIV Infection

CHAPTER 44

CLASS AND SUBCLASSES	NAME	CLINICAL USES	RESISTANCE	TOXICITY COMMON	TOXICITY UNIQUE; CLINICALLY IMPORTANT
	Efavirenz	Treatment of HIV infection in adults and children	Mutations in reverse transcriptase; cross-resistance extends to nevirapine and delavirdine	Headache and elevated hepatic trans-aminases	CNS symptoms including dizziness, impaired concentration, dysphoria, insomnia; frank psychosis Use should be avoided in women of childbearing potential unless 2 forms of birth control are used Metabolized by CYP2B6 and CYP 3A4; drugs that induced these enzymes should be avoided
	Delavirdine	Treatment of HIV infection in adults generally in combination with other nucleoside agents	Mutations in reverse transcriptase; cross-resistance extends to nevirapine and efavirenz	Rash	Substrate for and inhibitor of CYP3A4 and can alter metabolism of other CYP3A4 substrates
	Etravirine	Use in treatment-experienced HIV-infected adults		Rash	Inducer of CYP3A4 and glucuronosyl transferase Inhibitor of CYP2C9 and CYP 2C19 Should not be administered with tipranavir/ritonavir fosamprenavir/ritonavir or atazanavir/ritonavir Should not be combined with delavirdine, efavirenz, or nevirapine
EntryInhibitors	Enfuvirtide	Use in treatment-experienced adults who have evidence of HIV replication despite antiretroviral therapy		Injection site reactions	Not metabolized and no known drug interactions
	Maraviroc	Use in HIV-infected adults who have evidence of CCR5-tropic virus	HIV that is predominantly CCR5-tropic shifts tropism to CXCR4; or there is a mutation in gp120 that allows virus binding in the presence of inhibitor		Little significant toxicity CYP3A4 substrate; susceptible to drug interactions with drugs that are CYP3A4 inhibitors or inducers
Integrase Inhibitor	Raltegravir	Treatment of HIV-infected adults	Mutations in the integrase gene	Headache, nausea, fatigue	Little clinical toxicity

Chemotherapy of Neoplastic Diseases

SECTION VIII

45. Cancer Chemotherapy and Cytotoxic Agents.............................. 626

46. Targeted Anticancer Therapies 661

CHAPTER 45

Cancer Chemotherapy and Cytotoxic Agents

DRUGS INCLUDED IN THIS CHAPTER

- 2-Mercaptoethanesulfonate (mesna; MESNEX)—reacts with acrolein in urine and protects against severe hemorrhagic cystitis in high-dose cyclophosphamide regimens
- 5-Fluorouracil (5-FU)
- 6-Mercaptopurine (6-MP; PURINETHOL, others)
- 6-Thioguanine (6-TG)
- Altretamine (hexamethylmelamine; HEXALEN)
- Amifostine (WR-2721; ETHYOL, others)—thiophosphate cytoprotective agent (see cisplatin clinical toxicities)
- Arsenic trioxide (ATO; TRISENOX)
- Azacytidine (5-azacytidine)
- Bendamustine (TREANDA, others)
- Bleomycin (BLENOXANE, others)
- Busulfan (MYLERAN, BUSULFEX)
- Carmustine (BCNU; BICNU, GLIADEL)
- Capecitabine (XELODA)
- Carboplatin (CBDCA, JM-8; PARAPLATIN)
- Carboxypeptidase G2 (a methotrexate-cleaving enzyme used to reduce methotrexate in plasma)
- Chlorambucil (LEUKERAN)
- Cisplatin (PLATINOL, others)
- Cladribine (2-chlorodeoxyadenosine, 2-CdA; LEUSTATIN, others)
- Clofarabine (2-chloro-2′-fluoro-arabinosyladenine)
- Cyclophosphamide (LYOPHILIZED CYTOXAN, others)
- Cytarabine (1-β-D-arabinofuranosylcytosine, cytosine arabinoside, Ara-C; CYTOSAR-U, TARABINE PFS, DEPOCYT, others)
- Dacarbazine (DTIC; DTIC-DOME)
- Dactinomycin (actinomycin D; COSMEGEN)
- Daunorubicin (daunomycin, rubidomycin; CERUBIDINE, others)

(continues)

This chapter will be most useful after having a basic understanding of the material in Chapter 60 General Principles of Cancer Chemotherapy and Chapter 61 Cytotoxic Agents in *Goodman & Gilman's The Pharmacological Basis of Therapeutics*, 12th Edition. In addition to the material presented here, Chapters 60 and 61 of the 12th Edition contain:

- A description of the cell cycle, and cell cycle checkpoints and regulation
- The clinical pharmacology and toxicities of specific agents
- The molecular structures of cytotoxic agents used to treat cancer and other diseases such as immune disorders

LEARNING OBJECTIVES

☑ Understand the mechanisms of action of cytotoxic antineoplastic agents on tumor cells (see Figure 45-1).

☑ Understand the mechanisms of toxicity of cytotoxic antineoplastic agents on normal cells and strategies for reducing toxic effects.

☑ Understand the mechanisms of drug resistance to individual agents and strategies to avoid resistance.

☑ Know how pharmacogenetics can impact tumor sensitivity and toxicities of specific agents.

☑ Know the signs of acute toxicity and when chemotherapy should be altered or discontinued.

☑ Know the risk of long-term toxicities that can occur with individual chemotherapeutic agents.

☑ Know the therapeutic strategies that can reduce acute and chronic toxicities.

☑ Know which classes of agents are typically used in treating specific cancers.

☑ Know which drugs are used in combination to improve tumor cell killing and reduce the risk of resistance development.

CASE 45-1

A patient with a chronic lymphocytic leukemia is started on chemotherapy with cyclophosphamide.

a. What is the mechanism of action of cyclophosphamide?

Cyclophosphamide is a nitrogen mustard and is now the most widely used agent of this class of alkylating agents. Alkylating agents have in common the property of forming highly reactive carbonium ion intermediates. These reactive intermediates covalently link to sites of high electron density, such as phosphates, amines, sulfhydryl, and hydroxyl groups. Their chemotherapeutic and cytotoxic effects are directly related to the alkylation of reactive amine, oxygen, or phosphate groups on DNA (see Figure 45-1). The N7 atom of guanine is particularly susceptible to the formation of a covalent bond with bifunctional alkylating agents and may represent the key target that determines their biological effects (see Figure 45-2). Other atoms in the purine and pyrimidine bases of DNA, including N1 and N3 of the adenine ring, N3 of cytosine, and O6 of guanine, react with these agents, as do the amino and sulfhydryl groups of proteins and the sulfhydryl groups of glutathione.

(Continued)

Cancer Chemotherapy and Cytotoxic Agents

CHAPTER 45

MECHANISMS OF ACTION AND RESISTANCE OF ALKYLATING AGENTS AND PLATINUM COORDINATION COMPLEXES (SEE TABLE 45-1)

CLASSIFICATION	DRUG	MECHANISMS OF ACTION	MECHANISMS OF RESISTANCE
Nitrogen Mustards	Mechlorethamine HCl Cyclophosphamide Ifosfamide Melphalan Chlorambucil Bendamustine	Form highly reactive carbonium ion intermediates that alkylate reactive amines, oxygens, and phosphates on DNA (Figures 45-1 through 45-4) which leads to cell death	Overexpression of nucleotide excision repair (NER) pathway Mutations of p53 DNA repair by O^6-alkyl, methyl guanine methyltransferase (MGMT) Activated intermediates of cyclophosphamide can be degraded by aldehyde dehydrogenase, glutathione transferase, and other pathways (see Figure 45-4) See Side Bar MECHANISMS OF RESISTANCE TO ALKYLATING AGENTS
Ethyleneimines and Methylmelamines	Altretamine (hexamethylendiamine) Thiotepa	Cytotoxic mechanism of altretamine is unknown (it has no alkylating activity in vitro but is demethylated in liver microsomes to form formaldehyde) Thiotepa and its primary metabolite (TEPA) form DNA cross-links	Overexpression of NER pathway Mutations of p53 DNA repair by MGMT See Side Bar MECHANISMS OF RESISTANCE TO ALKYLATING AGENTS
Alkyl Sulfonates	Busulfan	Alkylate DNA through the release of methyl radicals (see Figures 45-1 and 45-3)	Overexpression of NER pathway Mutations of p53 DNA repair by MGMT See Side Bar MECHANISMS OF RESISTANCE TO ALKYLATING AGENTS
Nitrosoureas	Carmustine (BCNU) Lomustine (CCNU) Semustine (methyl-CCNU) Streptozocin (streptozotocin)	Exert their cytotoxicity through the spontaneous breakdown to an alkylating intermediate, the 2-chloroethyl diazonium ion, a strong electrophile, that can alkylate guanine, cytidine, and adenine bases, leading to interstrand or intrastrand cross-linking of DNA (see Figures 45-1, 45-3, and 45-5)	Overexpression of NER pathway Mutations of p53 DNA repair by MGMT See Side Bar MECHANISMS OF RESISTANCE TO ALKYLATING AGENTS

(Continued)

DRUGS INCLUDED IN THIS CHAPTER (Cont.)

- Decitabine (2'-deoxy-5-azacytidine)
- Docetaxel (TAXOTERE)
- Doxorubicin (ADRIAMYCIN)
- Epirubicin (ELLENCE, others)
- Estramustine (EMCYT)
- Etoposide (VP-16-213; VEPESID, others)
- Floxuridine (FUdR, fluorodeoxyuridine; FUDR, others)
- Fludarabine phosphate (FLUDARA, OFORTA)
- Gemcitabine (2',2'-difluorodeoxycytidine; dFdC, GEMZAR)
- High-dose methotrexate with leucovorin rescue (HDM-L)
- Hydroxyurea (HU; HYDREA, DROXIA, others)
- Idarubicin (IDAMYCIN PFS)
- Ifosfamide (IFEX, others)
- Irinotecan (CPT-11; CAMPTOSAR, others)
- Ixabepilone (IXEMPRA)
- L-asparaginase (L-ASP; ELSPAR)
- Leucovorin (folinic acid, citrovorum factor, 5-formyltetrahydrofolate, N^5-formyl FH_4)
- Lometrexol
- Lomustine (CCNU; CeeNU)
- Mechlorethamine HCl (MUSTARGEN)
- Melphalan (ALKERAN)
- Methotrexate (amethopterin; RHEUMATREX, TREXALL, others)
- Mitomycin (mitomycin-C; MUTAMYCIN, others)
- Mitotane (o,p'-DDD)
- Mitoxantrone (NOVANTRONE, others)
- Nab-paclitaxel (ABRAXANE)
- Nelarabine (6-methoxy-arabinosyl-guanine)
- Oxaliplatin (ELOXATIN)
- Paclitaxel (TAXOL, others)
- Pegaspargase (PEG-L-Asparaginase; ONCASPAR)
- Pemetrexed (MTA; ALIMTA)
- Pentostatin (2'-deoxycoformycin)
- Pralatrexate (FOLOTYN)
- Procarbazine (MATULANE)
- Raltitrexed (TOMUDEX)

(continues)

SECTION VIII
Chemotherapy of Neoplastic Diseases

DRUGS INCLUDED IN THIS CHAPTER (Cont.)

- Romidepsin (depsipeptide, FK228; ISTODAX)
- Semustine (methyl-CCNU)
- Streptozocin (streptozotocin; ZANOSAR)
- Temozolomide (TEMODAR)
- Teniposide (VM-26; VUMON)
- Thiotepa (triethylenethiophosphoramide; THIOPLEX, others)
- Topotecan (HYCAMTIN)
- Trabectedin (YONDELIS)—not currently approved in the United States
- Tretinoin (all-trans retinoic acid; ATRA)
- Trimetrexate (NEUTREXIN)
- Valrubicin (VALSTAR)
- Vinblastine sulfate ((VELBAN, others)
- Vincristine sulfate (VINCASAR PFS, others)
- Vinorelbine (NAVELBINE, others)
- Vorinostat (suberoylanilide hydroxamic acid, SAHA; ZOLINZA)

MECHANISMS OF CYTOTOXICITY

- Alkylating agents interfere with DNA integrity and function, and primarily induce cell death in rapidly proliferating tissues.
- Lethality of DNA alkylation depends on the following:
  - The recognition of the adduct by DNA repair systems.
  - The creation of DNA strand breaks by repair enzymes.
  - An intact apoptotic response.
- In nondividing cells, DNA damage activates a checkpoint that depends on the presence of a normal p53 gene.
  - Cells thus blocked in the G_1/S interface either repair DNA alkylation or undergo apoptosis.
  - Malignant cells with mutant or absent p53 fail to suspend cell-cycle progression, do not undergo apoptosis, and exhibit resistance to alkylating drugs.
- Bifunctional agents, in which cytotoxic effects predominate, cause DNA strand cross-linking.

(continues)

CLASSIFICATION	DRUG	MECHANISMS OF ACTION	MECHANISMS OF RESISTANCE
Triazenes	Dacarbazine (DTIC) Temozolomide	Spontaneous cleavage of the metabolite methyl-triazeno-imidazole-carboxamide (MTIC) yields a methyl diazonium ion that transfers methyl rather than ethyl groups to DNA (see Figures 45-1 and 45-3) Temozolomide is a monofunctional methylating agent	Overexpression of NER pathway Mutations of p53 DNA repair by MGMT See Side Bar MECHANISMS OF RESISTANCE TO ALKYLATING AGENTS Simple methylation can be bypassed by DNA polymerases
Methylhydrazines	Procarbazine	Converted by CYP-mediated oxidation to a highly reactive monofunctional methylating agent that can cause chromosomal damage, resulting in mutagenesis and carcinogenesis (see Figures 45-1 and 45-3)	Overexpression of NER pathway Mutations of p53 DNA repair by MGMT See Side Bar MECHANISMS OF RESISTANCE TO ALKYLATING AGENTS Simple methylation can be bypassed by DNA polymerases
Platinum Coordination Complexes	Cisplatin Carboplatin (CBDCA) Oxaliplatin	Platinum-coordinated ligands are replaced by water molecules in the cell yielding a highly reactive aquated molecule that reacts with nucleophilic sites on DNA and protein forming intrastrand and interstrand cross-links (see Figures 45-1 and 45-3)	Reduced uptake by Cu^{2+} transporter (CTR1) Increased efflux through Cu^{2+} efflux transporters ATP7A and ATP7B, and MRP 1 efflux transporters Intracellular sulfhydryls inactivate the drug Overexpression of NER pathway See Side Bar MECHANISMS OF RESISTANCE TO ALKYLATING AGENTS Resistance to cisplatin but not oxaliplatin is partly mediated by MMR system which recognizes platinum-DNA complexes and initiates apoptosis Oxaliplatin does not display cross-resistance to cisplatin and carboplatin in some tumors

Alkylation of the N7 of guanine in DNA exerts several biologically important effects. Guanine residues in DNA exist predominantly as the keto tautomer and readily make Watson-Crick base pairs by hydrogen bonding with cytosine residues. However, when the N7 of guanine is alkylated (to become a quaternary ammonium nitrogen), the guanine residue is more acidic and the enol tautomer is favored.

(Continued)

Cancer Chemotherapy and Cytotoxic Agents

CHAPTER 45

TABLE 45-1 Alkylating Agents

TYPE OF AGENT	NONPROPRIETARY NAMES	DISEASE
Nitrogen mustards	Mechlorethamine Cyclophosphamide Ifosfamide	Hodgkin's disease Acute and chronic lymphocytic leukemia; Hodgkin's disease; non-Hodgkin's lymphoma; multiple myeloma; neuroblastoma; breast, ovary, lung cancer; Wilms' tumor; cervix, testis cancer; soft-tissue sarcoma
	Melphalan Chlorambucil	Multiple myeloma Chronic lymphocytic leukemia; macroglobulinemia
Methylhydrazine derivative	Procarbazine (*N*-methylhydrazine, MIH)	Hodgkin's disease
Alkyl sulfonate	Busulfan	Chronic myelogenous leukemia, bone marrow transplantation
Nitrosoureas	Carmustine (BCNU) Streptozocin (streptozotocin) Bendamustine	Hodgkin's disease; non-Hodgkin's lymphoma; glioblastoma Malignant pancreatic insulinoma; malignant carcinoid Non-Hodgkin's lymphoma
Triazenes	Dacarbazine (DTIC; dimethyltriazenoi-midazole carboxamide), Temozolomide	Malignant melanoma; Hodgkin's disease; soft-tissue sarcomas; melanoma Malignant gliomas
Platinum coordination complexes	Cisplatin, carboplatin, oxaliplatin	Testicular, ovarian, bladder, esophageal, lung, head and neck, colon, breast cancer

The modified guanine can mispair with thymine residues during DNA synthesis, leading to the substitution of thymine for cytosine. Second, alkylation of the N7 creates lability in the imidazole ring, leading to opening of the ring and excision of the damaged guanine residue. Mispairing and imidazole ring opening can lead to attempts to repair the damaged stretch of DNA, causing strand breakage. Third, with bifunctional alkylating agents such as nitrogen mustards, the second 2-chloroethyl side chain can undergo a similar cyclization reaction and alkylate a second guanine residue or another nucleophilic moiety, resulting in the crosslinking of two nucleic acid chains or the linking of a nucleic acid to a protein, alterations that would cause a major disruption in nucleic acid function. Any of these effects could contribute to both the mutagenic and cytotoxic effects of alkylating agents. The extreme cytotoxicity of bifunctional alkylators correlates very closely with interstrand cross-linkage of DNA.

The capacity of alkylating agents to interfere with DNA integrity and function, and to induce cell death in rapidly proliferating tissues provides the basis for their therapeutic and toxic properties (see Side Bar MECHANISMS OF CYTOTOXICITY). Acute effects manifest primarily against rapidly proliferating tissues; however, certain alkylating agents may have damaging effects on tissues with normally low mitotic indices (eg, liver, kidney, and mature lymphocytes), which usually are affected in a delayed time frame.

(Continued)

MECHANISMS OF CYTOTOXICITY (Cont.)

- Monofunctional methylating agents (procarbazine, temozolomide) have greater capacity for mutagenesis and carcinogenesis:
  - Simple methylation may be bypassed by DNA polymerases, leading to mispairing reactions that permanently modify DNA sequence; these can be transmitted to subsequent generations leading to mutagenesis and carcinogenesis.

DNA REPAIR MECHANISMS

- Alkylation of a single strand of DNA (mono-adducts) is repaired by the nucleotide excision repair (NER) pathway.
- DNA strand cross-links require participation of nonhomologous end joining, an error-prone pathway, or the error-free homologous recombination pathway.
- The homologous recombination (end joining) pathway has multiple components:
  - Sensors of DNA integrity (such as p53)
  - Activation signals such as the ataxia-telangiectasia-mutated (ATM) and ataxia-telangiectasia and rad-related (ATR) proteins
  - Activated DNA repair complex composed of Fanconi anemia proteins and BRCA2, all of which localize at the site of DNA damage and initiate removal of the cross-linked segment of DNA
  - Homologous recombination, which allows re-synthesis of the damaged DNA sequence followed by religation of the repaired sequences
- The homologous recombination process depends on the presence and accurate functioning of multiple proteins; their absence or mutation, as in Fanconi anemia or ataxia telangiectasia, leads to extreme sensitivity to DNA cross-linking agents.
- Other repair enzymes are specific for removing methyl and ethyl adducts from the O^6 of guanine (MGMT), and for repair of alkylation of the N-3 of adenine and N-7 of guanine (3-methyladenine-DNA glycosylase).
- For the methylating drugs, nitrosoureas, cisplatin and carboplatin, and thiopurine analogs, the mismatch repair (MMR) pathway is essential for cytotoxicity, causing strand breaks at sites of adduct formation, creating mispairing of thymine residues, and triggering apoptosis.

SECTION VIII Chemotherapy of Neoplastic Diseases

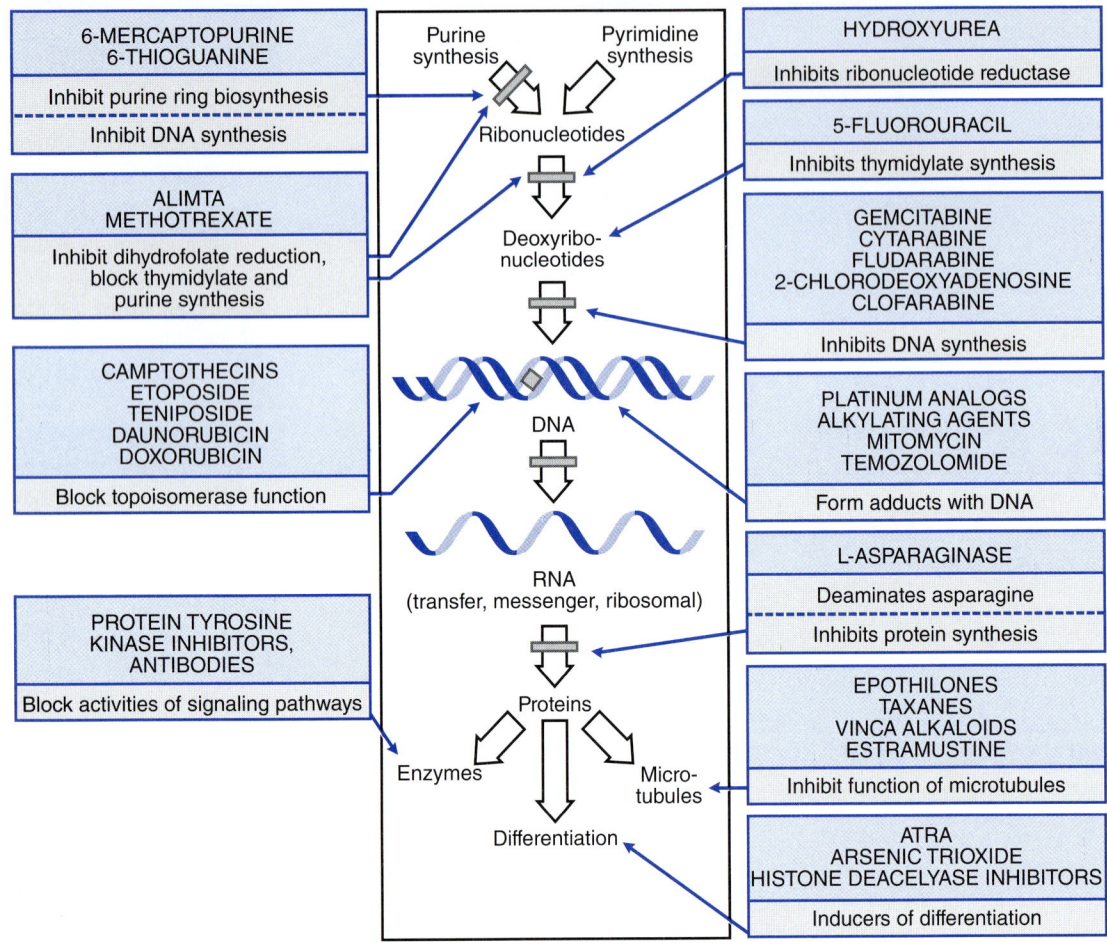

FIGURE 45-1 Summary of the mechanisms and sites of action of some chemotherapeutic agents useful in neoplastic disease.

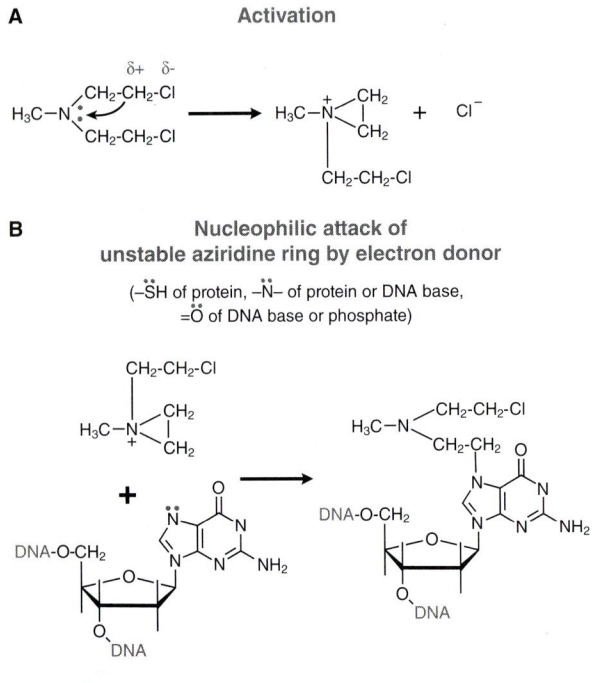

FIGURE 45-2 Mechanism of action of alkylating agents. **A.** Activation reaction. **B.** Alkylation of N7 of guanine.

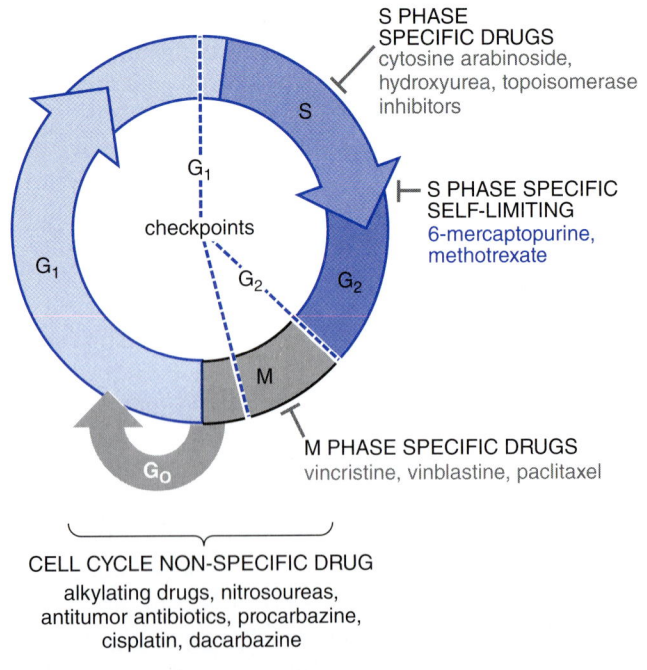

FIGURE 45-3 Cell cycle specificity of antineoplastic agents.

Cancer Chemotherapy and Cytotoxic Agents — CHAPTER 45

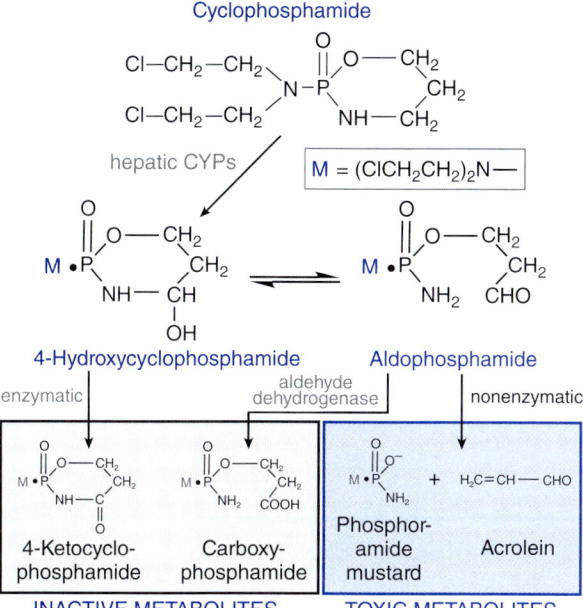

FIGURE 45-4 Metabolism of cyclophosphamide.

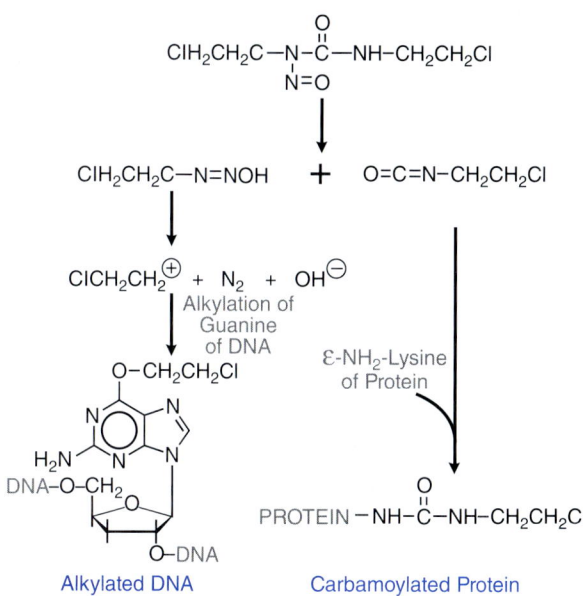

FIGURE 45-5 Degradation of carmustine (BCNU) with generation of alkylating and carbamylating intermediates.

b. How are the active alkylating species formed in vivo?

Cyclophosphamide is well absorbed orally and is activated to the 4-hydroxy intermediate in the liver by CYP2B (see Figure 45-4), with subsequent transport of the activated intermediate to sites of action. 4-Hydroxycyclophosphamide may be oxidized further by aldehyde oxidase, either in the liver or in tumor tissue, to inactive metabolites. 4-Hydroxycyclophosphamide and its tautomer, aldophosphamide, travel in the circulation to tumor cells where aldophosphamide cleaves spontaneously, generating stoichiometric amounts of phosphoramide mustard and acrolein. Phosphoramide mustard is responsible for antitumor effects, while acrolein is associated with significant toxicities.

c. What are the adverse effects of cyclophosphamide?

Alkylating agents are associated with a wide range of toxicities (see Side Bar TOXICITIES OF ALKYLATING DRUGS). Most alkylating agents (ie, melphalan, chlorambucil, cyclophosphamide, and ifosfamide) cause dose-limiting toxicity to bone marrow elements (myelosuppression) and, to a lesser extent, intestinal mucosa. Cyclophosphamide has lesser effects on peripheral blood platelet counts than do the other agents. Nausea and vomiting, which are due to neurotoxic effects, commonly follow agent administration of nitrogen mustard. High-dose therapy with cyclophosphamide can lead to organ damage, including GI ulceration, cystitis (see next paragraph), and, less commonly, pulmonary, renal, hepatic, and cardiac toxicities (a hemorrhagic myocardial necrosis). Dose-limiting major organ toxicities associated with alkylating agents are listed in Table 45-2.

Cyclophosphamide and ifosfamide release a nephrotoxic and urotoxic metabolite, acrolein (see Figure 45-4), which causes a severe hemorrhagic cystitis in high-dose regimens. This adverse effect can be prevented by coadministration of 2-mercaptoethanesulfonate (mesna), which conjugates acrolein in urine. Mesna does not negate the systemic antitumor activity of the drug. Patients should receive vigorous intravenous hydration during high-dose treatment. Brisk hematuria in a patient receiving daily oral therapy should lead to immediate drug discontinuation. Refractory bladder hemorrhage can become life threatening, and cystectomy may be necessary for control of bleeding. Inappropriate secretion of antidiuretic hormone

(Continued)

SECTION VIII — Chemotherapy of Neoplastic Diseases

MECHANISMS OF RESISTANCE TO ALKYLATING AGENTS

Specific biochemical changes implicated in the development of resistance to an alkylating agent when used as a single agent include the following:

- Decreased permeation of actively transported drugs (mechlorethamine and melphalan).
- Increased intracellular concentrations of nucleophilic substances, principally thiols such as glutathione, which can conjugate with and detoxify electrophilic intermediates.
- Increased activity of DNA repair pathways, which may differ for the various alkylating agents:
  - Increased activity of the complex NER pathway correlates with resistance to most chloroethyl and platinum adducts.
  - MGMT activity determines response to BCNU and to methylating drugs such as the triazenes, procarbazine, temozolomide, and busulfan.
- Increased rates of metabolic degradation of the activated forms of cyclophosphamide and ifosfamide to their inactive keto and carboxy metabolites by aldehyde dehydrogenase (see Figure 45-4), and detoxification of most alkylating intermediates by glutathione transferases.
- Loss of the ability to recognize adducts formed by nitrosoureas and methylating agents, as the result of defective MMR capability, confers resistance, as does defective checkpoint function for virtually all alkylating drugs.
- Impaired apoptotic pathways (eg, overexpression of bcl-2) confer resistance.

TOXICITIES OF ALKYLATING DRUGS (See Table 45-2)

- Most alkylating agents cause dose-limiting toxicity to bone marrow elements, with acute myelosuppression that peaks at 6-10 days and recovers in 14-21 days.
- Alkylating agents are highly toxic to dividing mucosal cells and to hair follicles, leading to oral mucosal ulceration, intestinal denudation, and alopecia.

TABLE 45-2 Dose-Limiting Extramedullary Toxicities of Single Alkylating Agents

DRUG	MTD,^{a} mg/m^2	FOLD INCREASE OVER STANDARD DOSE	MAJOR ORGAN TOXICITIES
Cyclophosphamide	7000	7	Cardiac, hepatic VOD
Ifosfamide	16,000	2.7	Renal, CNS, hepatic VOD
Thiotepa	1000	18	GI, CNS, hepatic VOD
Melphalan	180	5.6	GI, hepatic VOD
Busulfan	640	9	GI, hepatic VOD
Carmustine (BCNU)	1050	5.3	Lung, hepatic VOD
Cisplatin	200	2	PN, renal
Carboplatin	2000	5	Renal, PN, hepatic VOD

^{a}Maximum tolerated dose (MTD; cumulative) in treatment protocols.
CNS, central nervous system; GI, gastrointestinal; PN, peripheral neuropathy; VOD, veno-occlusive disease.

has been observed in patients receiving cyclophosphamide, usually at doses greater than 50 mg/kg. It is important to be aware of the possibility of water intoxication, because these patients usually are vigorously hydrated to prevent bladder toxicity.

All alkylating agents have toxic effects on the male and female reproductive systems, causing an often permanent amenorrhea, and an irreversible azoospermia in men.

Alkylating agents are highly leukemogenic. Acute nonlymphocytic leukemia peaks in incidence ~4 years after therapy and may affect up to 5% of patients treated on regimens containing alkylating drugs. Leukemia often is preceded by a period of neutropenia or anemia, and by bone marrow morphology consistent with myelodysplasia. Melphalan, the nitrosoureas, and the methylating agent procarbazine have the greatest propensity to cause leukemia, while it is less common after cyclophosphamide.

d. What are the mechanisms by which resistance to cyclophosphamide and other alkylating agents might develop?

The Side Bar MECHANISMS OF RESISTANCE TO ALKYLATING AGENTS describes mechanisms by which tumors can develop resistance to the alkylating agents. One mechanism of resistance is increased rates of metabolic degradation of the activated forms of cyclophosphamide to its inactive keto and carboxy metabolites by aldehyde dehydrogenase, as well as by inactivation by glutathione transferase and other enzymatic pathways (see Figure 45-4).

With all alkylating agents, lethality of DNA alkylation depends on the recognition of the DNA adduct, the creation of DNA strand breaks by repair enzymes, and an intact apoptotic response. The specific repair enzyme complex utilized will depend on two factors: the chemistry of the DNA adduct formed and the repair capacity of the cell involved. The process of recognizing and repairing DNA generally requires an intact NER complex. As described in the answer to Case 45-1a, the ability of the bifunctional nitrogen mustards to form interstrand DNA cross-links increases cytotoxicity over alkylation of single strands by monofunctional alkylating agents. Alkylation of a single strand of DNA (mono-adducts) is repaired by the NER pathway, while the less frequent DNA cross-links require participation of nonhomologous end joining, an error-prone pathway, or the error-free homologous recombination pathway (see Side Bar DNA REPAIR MECHANISMS).

(Continued)

Cancer Chemotherapy and Cytotoxic Agents

CHAPTER 45

Recognition of extensively damaged DNA by p53 can trigger apoptosis. In nondividing cells, DNA damage activates a checkpoint that depends on the presence of a normal p53 gene. Cells thus blocked in the G_1/S interface either repair DNA alkylation or undergo apoptosis. Malignant cells with mutant or absent p53 fail to suspend cell-cycle progression, do not undergo apoptosis, and exhibit resistance to alkylating drugs.

CASE 45-2

Carboplatin, cisplatin, and oxaliplatin are referred to as platinum coordination complexes, and are widely used cancer chemotherapy agents.

a. What is the mechanism of action of these agents?

The platinum coordination complexes have broad antineoplastic activity and have become the foundation for the treatment of many cancers (see Table 45-1). They covalently bind to nucleophilic sites on DNA and share many pharmacological attributes with alkylators (see Figure 45-1).

Cisplatin, carboplatin, and oxaliplatin enter cells by an active Cu^{2+} transporter, CTR1. Inside the cell, the chloride, cyclohexane, or oxalate ligands of the three analogs are displaced by water molecules, yielding a positively charged and highly reactive molecule. The aquated species of the drug can react with electron-rich molecules, such as sulfhydryls, and with various sites on DNA, forming both intrastrand and interstrand cross-links. The N-7 of guanine is a particularly reactive site, leading to platinum cross-links between adjacent guanines (GG intrastrand cross-links) on the same DNA strand; guanine–adenine cross-links also form and may contribute to cytotoxicity. Interstrand cross-links form less frequently. DNA-platinum adducts inhibit replication and transcription, lead to single- and double-stranded breaks and miscoding, and, if recognized by p53 and other checkpoint proteins, cause induction of apoptosis. For cisplatin and carboplatin, the mismatch repair (MMR) pathway is essential for cytotoxicity, causing strand breaks at sites of adduct formation, creating mispairing of thymine residues, and triggering apoptosis.

The analogs differ in the conformation of their adducts and the effects of adduct on DNA structure and function. The oxaliplatin adducts are bulkier and less readily repaired, create a different pattern of distortion of the DNA helix, and differ from cisplatin adducts in the pattern of hydrogen bonding to adjacent segments of DNA. Unlike the other platinum analogs, oxaliplatin exhibits a cytotoxicity that does not depend on an active MMR system, which may explain its greater activity in colorectal cancer. It also seems less dependent on the presence of high-mobility group (HMG) proteins that are required by the other platinum derivatives.

b. How does the mechanism of action of these agents differ from the alkylating agents?

Cisplatin and other platinum complexes do not form carbonium ion intermediates like other alkylating agents or formally alkylate DNA; however, they covalently bind to nucleophilic sites on DNA causing DNA strand cross-links, and thus share many pharmacological attributes with alkylators.

c. What are the common toxicities of these agents?

Many of the toxicities of these agents are similar to the alkylating agents (see Side Bar TOXICITIES OF ALKYLATING DRUGS; also see Table 45-2). The primary clinical toxicities differ somewhat among cisplatin, carboplatin, and oxaliplatin.

An important dose-limiting toxicity of cisplatin is renal toxicity. To prevent renal toxicity, it is important to establish a chloride diuresis by the infusion of 1-2 L of normal saline prior to treatment. The appropriate amount of cisplatin then is diluted in a solution containing dextrose, saline, and mannitol, and administered over 4-6 hours. Amifostine is a thiophosphate cytoprotective agent that reduces

(Continued)

TOXICITIES OF ALKYLATING DRUGS (See Table 45-2) (Cont.)

- Neurotoxic effects range from nausea and vomiting to more severe central and peripheral toxicities that include altered mental status, coma, generalized seizures, and cerebellar ataxia.
- Other organ toxicities may supervene after prolonged or high-dose use; these effects can appear after months or years and may be irreversible and even lethal:
  - Pulmonary fibrosis.
  - Vascular endothelial damage may precipitate veno-occlusive disease (VOD) of the liver, an often fatal side effect.
  - Nephrotoxic and urotoxic (ie, toxic metabolites in the urine that can damage the bladder and lower urinary tract) effects.
  - Unstable alkylating agents (particularly mechlorethamine and the nitrosoureas) have strong vesicant properties and cause damage to veins with repeated use and, if extravasated, produce ulceration.
  - Toxic effects on the male and female reproductive systems, causing an often permanent amenorrhea, particularly in perimenopausal women, and an irreversible azoospermia in men.
- Alkylating agents are highly leukemogenic.
  - Acute nonlymphocytic leukemia, often associated with partial or total deletions of chromosome 5 or 7, peaks in incidence ~4 years after therapy and may affect up to 5% of patients treated on regimens containing alkylating drugs.

renal toxicity associated with repeated administration of cisplatin, but is not commonly used.

Ototoxicity caused by cisplatin is unaffected by diuresis and is manifested by tinnitus and high-frequency hearing loss. The ototoxicity can be unilateral or bilateral, tends to be more frequent and severe with repeated doses, and may be more pronounced in children.

Marked nausea and vomiting occur in almost all patients receiving cisplatin and usually can be controlled with 5-HT$_3$ antagonists, NK1-receptor antagonists, and high-dose corticosteroids (see Chapter 33). At higher doses, or after multiple cycles of treatment, cisplatin causes a progressive peripheral motor and sensory neuropathy, which may worsen after discontinuation of the drug and may be aggravated by subsequent or simultaneous treatment with taxanes or other neurotoxic drugs. Cisplatin causes mild to moderate myelosuppression, with transient leukopenia and thrombocytopenia. Anemia may become prominent after multiple cycles of treatment. Electrolyte disturbances, including hypomagnesemia, hypocalcemia, hypokalemia, and hypophosphatemia, are common. Hypocalcemia and hypomagnesemia secondary to tubular damage and renal electrolyte wasting may produce tetany if untreated. Routine measurement of Mg^{2+} concentrations in plasma is recommended. Hyperuricemia, hemolytic anemia, and cardiac abnormalities are rare side effects. Anaphylactic-like reactions, characterized by facial edema, bronchoconstriction, tachycardia, and hypotension, may occur within minutes after administration and should be treated by intravenous injection of epinephrine and with corticosteroids or antihistamines.

Carboplatin is relatively well tolerated clinically, causing less nausea, neurotoxicity, ototoxicity, and nephrotoxicity than cisplatin. Instead, the dose-limiting toxicity is myelosuppression, primarily thrombocytopenia. It is more likely to cause a hypersensitivity reaction; in patients with a mild reaction, premedication, graded doses of drug, and more prolonged infusion lead to desensitization. Carboplatin is an effective alternative for responsive tumors in patients unable to tolerate cisplatin because of impaired renal function, refractory nausea, significant hearing impairment, or neuropathy, but doses must be adjusted for renal function.

The dose-limiting toxicity of oxaliplatin is a peripheral neuropathy. An acute form, often triggered by exposure to cold liquids, manifests as paresthesias and/or dysesthesias in the upper and lower extremities, mouth, and throat. It may be caused by rapid release of oxalate, with depletion of calcium and magnesium, and responds to infusion of these electrolytes. A second type of peripheral neuropathy is more closely related to cumulative dose and has features similar to cisplatin neuropathy: progressive sensory neurotoxicity, with dysesthesias, ataxia, and numbness of the extremities. Hematological toxicity is mild to moderate, except for rare immune-mediated cytopenias, and nausea is well controlled with 5-HT$_3$ receptor antagonists. Oxaliplatin may cause an acute allergic response with urticaria, hypotension, and bronchoconstriction.

All of the platinum analogs are mutagenic, teratogenic, and carcinogenic. Like other DNA adduct–forming drugs, these agents have been associated with pulmonary fibrosis and the development of leukemia, months to years after treatment.

d. What are the mechanisms for resistance and sensitivity to the platinum coordination complex agents?

Resistance to the platinum analogs likely is multifactorial (see Side Bar MECHANISMS OF RESISTANCE TO ALKYLATING AGENTS), and the compounds differ in their degree of cross-resistance. Carboplatin shares cross-resistance with cisplatin in most experimental tumors, while oxaliplatin does not.

Repair of platinum-DNA adducts requires participation of the NER pathway. Inhibition or loss of NER increases sensitivity to cisplatin in ovarian cancer patients, while overexpression of NER components is associated with poor

(Continued)

response to cisplatin or oxaliplatin-based therapy in lung, colon, and gastric cancer. Higher levels of expression of the NER component ERCC1, in tumor cells and peripheral white blood cells are associated with a lower response rate in patients with solid tumors.

Resistance to cisplatin, but not oxaliplatin, appears to be partly mediated through loss of function in the MMR proteins (hMLH1, hMLH2, or hMSH6), which recognize platinum-DNA adducts and initiate apoptosis.

In the absence of effective repair of DNA-platinum adducts, sensitive cells cannot replicate or transcribe affected portions of the DNA strand. However, it is clear that some DNA polymerases can bypass adducts, especially those created by cisplatin. Oxaliplatin adducts are less easily bypassed. It remains unproven whether these polymerases contribute to resistance.

Platinum coordination complex drugs enter cells by active transport and cisplatin resistance related to loss of active uptake has been demonstrated in vitro. The compounds are actively extruded from cells by ATP7A and ATP7B copper transporters and by multidrug resistance protein 1 (MRP1/ABCC1); variable expression of these transporters may contribute to clinical resistance. Overexpression of copper efflux transporters, ATP7A and ATP7B, correlates with poor survival after cisplatin-based therapy for ovarian cancer.

MECHANISMS OF ACTION AND RESISTANCE OF ANTIMETABOLITES (SEE TABLE 45-3)

CLASSIFICATION	DRUG	MECHANISMS OF ACTION	MECHANISMS OF RESISTANCE
Folic Acid Analogs (Antifolates)	Methotrexate (amethopterin) High-dose methotrexate with leucovorin rescue (HDM-L) Trimetrexate	Binds DHFR and prevents the formation of FH_4 (see Figure 45-6) and allows the accumulation of the toxic inhibitor substrate FH_2 polyglutamate, thus shutting down one-carbon transfer reactions needed for the de novo synthesis of purine nucleotides, thymidylate, and the synthesis of DNA and RNA (see Figures 45-1 and 45-3)	See Side Bar MECHANISMS OF RESISTANCE TO ANTIMETABOLITES
	Pemetrexed (MTA)	Inhibits DHFR, and is readily converted to polyglutamates, which more potently inhibit glycinamide ribonucleotide formyltransferase (GART) and thymidylate synthase (TS) (see Figures 45-1 and 45-6)	See Side Bar MECHANISMS OF RESISTANCE TO ANTIMETABOLITES
	Pralatrexate Raltitrexed	Exert their primary inhibitory effects on TS (see Figure 45-6)	See Side Bar MECHANISMS OF RESISTANCE TO ANTIMETABOLITES
	Lometrexol	Primary inhibitory effects are on GART to block early steps in purine biosynthesis (see Figure 45-6)	See Side Bar MECHANISMS OF RESISTANCE TO ANTIMETABOLITES
Pyrimidine Analogs	5-Fluorouracil (5-FU) Floxuridine (FUdR, fluorodeoxyuridine) Capecitabine	Enzymatically converted in cells to the nucleotide forms (see Figure 45-7); FUTP is incorporated into RNA, FdUTP is incorporated into DNA, and FdUMP inhibits TS (see Figures 45-1, 45-7, and 45-8)	See Side Bar MECHANISMS OF RESISTANCE TO ANTIMETABOLITES
	Cytarabine (cytosine arabinoside, Ara-C)	Enzymatically converted in cells to its active form, the 5′-monophosphate ribonucleotide (Ara-CMP), by deoxycytidine kinase (dCK); Ara-CMP is phosphorylated to form Ara-CDP and Ara-CTP, which inhibit DNA polymerase, thus blocking replication and repair synthesis, and elongation (see Figures 45-1 and 45-3)	See Side Bar MECHANISMS OF RESISTANCE TO ANTIMETABOLITES

(Continued)

SECTION VIII Chemotherapy of Neoplastic Diseases

CLASSIFICATION	DRUG	MECHANISMS OF ACTION	MECHANISMS OF RESISTANCE
	Azacytidine (5-azacytidine) Decitabine (2′-deoxy-5-azacytidine)	Incorporates into DNA and forms covalent adducts with DNA cytosine methyltransferase, leading to its depletion and global demethylation of DNA, and tumor cell differentiation and apoptosis Decitabine also induces double-strand DNA breaks	Sensitivity to the azanucleosides correlates with the presence of the influx carrier, human equilibrative nucleoside transporter 1 (hENT1)
	Gemcitabine (2′,2′-difluorodeoxyuridine)	Converted to difluorodeoxycytidine di- and triphosphates (dFdCDP and dFdCTP) which inhibit DNA synthesis by multiple mechanisms including incorporation of dFdCTP into DNA and subsequent DNA strand termination (see Figure 45-1)	See Side Bar MECHANISMS OF RESISTANCE TO ANTIMETABOLITES
Purine Analogs	6-Mercaptopurine (6-MP) 6-Thioguanine (6-TG)	Converted by hypoxanthine guanine phosphoribosyl transferase (HGPRT) into the corresponding ribonucleotides (6-MP to 6-thioGMP and 6-TG to T-IMP) T-IMP inhibits the synthesis of ribosyl-5-phosphate and is also converted to 6-thioGMP 6-thioGMP is incorporated into DNA causing strand breaks and base mispairing (see Figures 45-1 and 45-3)	See Side Bar MECHANISMS OF RESISTANCE TO ANTIMETABOLITES
	Fludarabine phosphate	Phosphorylated by dCK to the active triphosphate derivative, which inhibits DNA polymerase, DNA primase, DNA ligase, and ribonucleotide reductase (RNR), and becomes incorporated into DNA and RNA; chain termination occurs when incorporated into DNA (see Figure 45-1); incorporation into RNA inhibits RNA function, RNA processing, and mRNA translation	See Side Bar MECHANISMS OF RESISTANCE TO ANTIMETABOLITES
	Cladribine (2-chlorodeoxyadenosine, 2-CdA)	After phosphorylation by dCK to cladribine triphosphate, it is incorporated into DNA producing DNA strand breaks, depleting NAD and ATP, and leading to apoptosis (see Figure 45-1); it is a potent inhibitor of RNR	See Side Bar MECHANISMS OF RESISTANCE TO ANTIMETABOLITES
	Clofarabine (2-chloro-2′-fluoro-arabinosyladenine)	Phosphorylated by dCK to the active triphosphate derivative and is incorporated into DNA where it terminates DNA synthesis and leads to apoptosis; it inhibits RNR	
	Nelarabine (6-methoxy-arabinosyl-guanine)	Active metabolite is transported into tumor cells, where it is activated by dCK to Ara-G triphosphate (Ara-GTP), which is incorporated into DNA and terminates DNA synthesis	
	Pentostatin (2′-deoxycoformycin)	A transition-state analog of the intermediate in the adenosine deaminase (ADA) reaction that potently inhibits ADA, which leads to accumulation of intracellular adenosine and deoxyadenosine nucleotides, which can block DNA synthesis by inhibiting RNR; also inactivates S-adenosyl homocysteine hydrolase, can inhibit RNA synthesis and its triphosphate derivative is incorporated into DNA, resulting in strand breakage	

Cancer Chemotherapy and Cytotoxic Agents — CHAPTER 45

TABLE 45-3 Antimetabolites

TYPE OF AGENT	NONPROPRIETARY NAMES	DISEASE
Folic acid analogs	Methotrexate (amethopterin)	Acute lymphocytic leukemia; choriocarcinoma; breast, head, neck and lung cancers; osteogenic sarcoma; bladder cancer
	Pemetrexed	Mesothelioma, lung cancer
Pyrimidine analogs	Fluorouracil (5-fluorouracil; 5-FU), capecitabine	Breast, colon, esophageal, stomach, pancreas, head and neck; premalignant skin lesion (topical)
	Cytarabine (cytosine arabinoside)	Acute myelogenous and acute lymphocytic leukemia; non-Hodgkin's lymphoma
	Gemcitabine	Pancreatic, ovarian, lung cancer
	5-aza-cytidine	Myelodysplasia
	Deoxy-5-aza-cytidine	Myelodysplasia
Purine analogs and related inhibitors	Mercaptopurine (6-mercaptopurine; 6-MP)	Acute lymphocytic and myelogenous leukemia; small cell non-Hodgkin's lymphoma
	Pentostatin (2'-deoxycoformycin)	Hairy cell leukemia; chronic lymphocytic leukemia; small cell non-Hodgkin's lymphoma
	Fludarabine	Chronic lymphocytic leukemia
	Clofarabine	Acute myelogenous leukemia
	Nelarabine	T-cell leukemia, lymphoma

A   **Thymidylate synthesis**

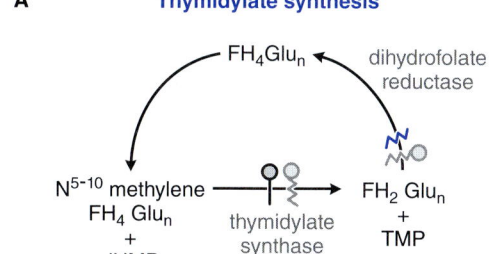

B   ***De novo* purine synthesis**

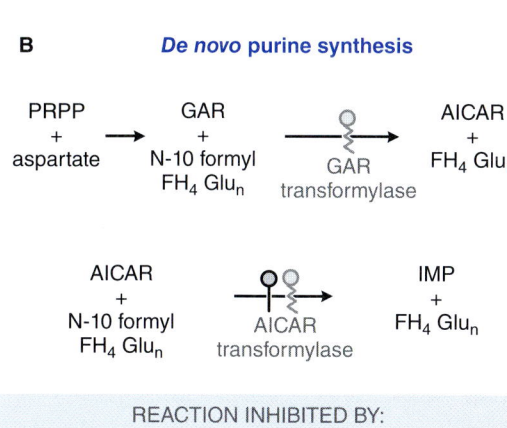

FIGURE 45-6 Sites of action of methotrexate and its polyglutamates. AICAR, aminoimidazole carboxamide; dUMP, deoxyuridine monophosphate; FH_2Glu_n, dihydrofolate polyglutamate; FH_4Glu_n, tetrahydrofolate polyglutamate; GAR, glycinamide ribonucleotide; IMP, inosine monophosphate; PRPP, 5-phosphoribosyl-1-pyrophosphate; TMP, thymidine monophosphate.

SECTION VIII Chemotherapy of Neoplastic Diseases

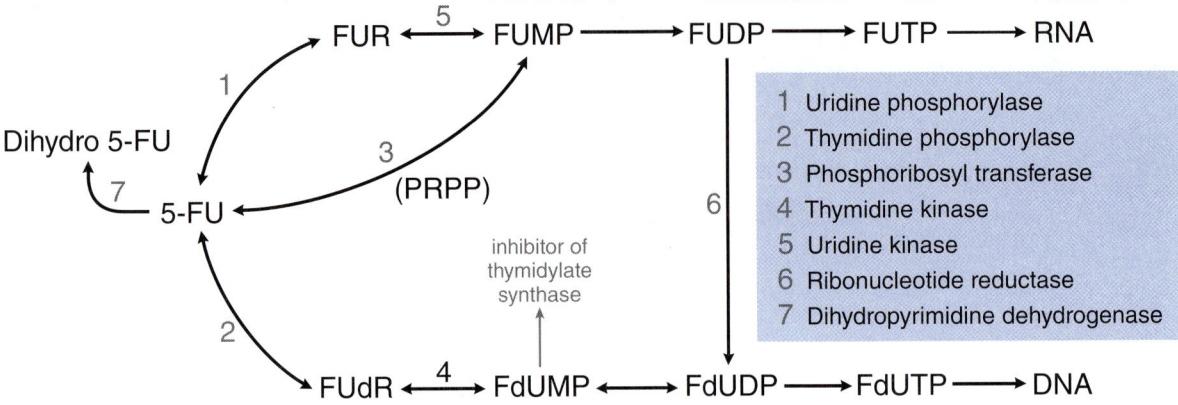

FIGURE 45-7 Activation pathways for 5-fluorouracil (5-FU) and 5-floxuridine (FUR). FdUDP, fluorodeoxyuridine diphosphate; FdUMP, fluorodeoxyuridine monophosphate; FdUTP, fluorodeoxyuridine triphosphate; FUDP, floxuridine diphosphate; FUdR, fluorodeoxyuridine; FUMP, floxuridine monophosphate; FUTP, floxuridine triphosphate; PRPP, 5-phosphoribosyl-1-pyrophosphate.

MECHANISMS OF RESISTANCE TO ANTIMETABOLITES

- Acquired resistance to methotrexate affects each known step in methotrexate action:
  - Impaired transport of methotrexate into cells
  - Production of altered forms of DHFR that have decreased affinity for the inhibitor
  - Increased concentrations of intracellular DHFR through gene amplification or altered gene regulation
  - Decreased ability to synthesize methotrexate polyglutamates
  - Increased expression of a drug efflux transporter of the MRP class (see Chapter 5 in *Goodman & Gilman's The Pharmacological Basis of Therapeutics*, 12th Edition for a comprehensive description of drug efflux transporters)
- Resistance to pemetrexed is incompletely understood but might arise from the following
  - Loss of influx transport
  - Thymidylate synthesis (TS) amplification
  - Changes in purine biosynthetic pathways
  - Loss of polyglutamation
- Resistance to the cytotoxic effects of 5-FU or FUdR has been ascribed to the following:
  - Loss or decreased activity of the enzymes necessary for activation of 5-FU
  - Amplification of TS
  - Mutation of TS to a form that is not inhibited by FdUMP

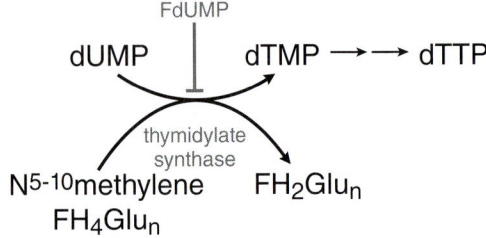

Other actions of 5-FU nucleotides:
- Inhibition of RNA processing
- Incorporation into DNA

FIGURE 45-8 Site of action of 5-fluoro-2′-deoxyuridine-5′-phosphate (5-FdUMP). 5-FU, 5-fluorouracil; dUMP, deoxyuridine monophosphate; FdUMP, fluorodeoxyuridine monophosphate; FH_2Glu_n, dihydrofolate polyglutamate; FH_4Glu_n, tetrahydrofolate polyglutamate; dTMP, deoxythymidine monophosphate; dTTP, deoxythymidine triphosphate.

CASE 45-3

A 6-year-old boy is being treated for acute lymphoblastic leukemia (ALL) using methotrexate with leucovorin rescue.

a. What is the mechanism of action of methotrexate?

Methotrexate is a folic acid analog, or antifolate, that interferes with folic acid metabolic pathways (see Figure 45-6). Folic acid is an essential dietary factor that is converted by enzymatic reduction to a series of tetrahydrofolate (FH_4) cofactors that provide methyl groups for the synthesis of precursors of DNA (thymidylate and purines) and RNA (purines). Interference with FH_4 metabolism reduces the cellular capacity for one-carbon transfer and the necessary methylation reactions in the synthesis of purine ribonucleotides and thymidine monophosphate (TMP), thereby inhibiting DNA replication (see Figure 45-1).

The primary target of methotrexate is the enzyme dihydrofolate reductase (DHFR; see Figure 45-6). Inhibition of DHFR leads to partial depletion of the FH_4 cofactors (N^{5-10} methylene tetrahydrofolic acid and N-10 formyl tetrahydrofolic acid). The absence of reduced folates shuts down the one-carbon transfer reactions crucial for the de novo synthesis of purine nucleotides and thymidylate, and interrupts the synthesis of DNA and RNA. In addition, methotrexate, like its physiological counterparts (the folates), undergoes conversion to a series of polyglutamates

(Continued)

Cancer Chemotherapy and Cytotoxic Agents

CHAPTER 45

(MTX-PGs) in both normal and tumor cells. These MTX-PGs constitute an intracellular storage form of folates and folate analogs, and dramatically increase inhibitory potency of the analog for additional sites, including thymidylate synthase (TS) and 2 early enzymes in the purine biosynthetic pathway (see Figure 45-6). Finally, the dihydrofolic acid polyglutamates that accumulate in cells behind the blocked DHFR reaction also act as inhibitors of TS and other enzymes (see Figure 45-6).

As with most antimetabolites, methotrexate is only partially selective for tumor cells and kills rapidly dividing normal cells, such as those of the intestinal epithelium and bone marrow. Folate antagonists kill cells during the S phase of the cell cycle (see Figure 45-3) and are most effective when cells are proliferating rapidly.

b. What is the rationale for the use of leucovorin?

To function as a cofactor in one-carbon transfer reactions, folate must first be reduced by DHFR to FH_4.

Introduction of high-dose methotrexate regimens with "rescue" of host toxicity by the reduced folate, leucovorin (folinic acid, citrovorum factor, 5-formyl tetrahydrofolate, N^5-formyl FH_4), extends the effectiveness of this drug to treat both systemic and CNS lymphomas, osteogenic sarcoma, and leukemias. The administration of leucovorin within 24 hours after high-dose infusions of methotrexate allows the use of regimens that produce cytotoxic concentrations of drug in the CSF and protects against leukemic meningitis. The toxic effects of methotrexate are rapidly terminated by administering leucovorin which repletes the intracellular pool of FH_4 cofactors.

c. How might pharmacogenetics affect the response of this patient to antifolate treatment?

The C677T substitution in methylenetetrahydrofolate reductase (MTHFR) reduces the activity of the enzyme that generates methylenetetrahydrofolate, the cofactor for TS (see Figure 45-6), and thereby increases methotrexate toxicity, especially GI toxicity (see Chapter 7 in *Goodman & Gilman's The Pharmacological Basis of Therapeutics*, 12th Edition for a more comprehensive description of the pharmacogenetics of methotrexate). The presence of this polymorphism in leukemic cells confers increased sensitivity to methotrexate and might also modulate the toxicity and therapeutic effect of pemetrexed, a predominant TS inhibitor. Likewise, polymorphisms in the promoter region of TS govern the translation efficiency of this message and, by governing the intracellular levels of TS in both normal and tumor cells, modulate the response and toxicity of both antifolates and fluoropyrimidines such as 5-fluorouracil. Other common polymorphisms that affect methotrexate pharmacotherapy include those in the genes that code for DHFR and proline transformylases (see Chapter 7 in *Goodman & Gilman's The Pharmacological Basis of Therapeutics*, 12th Edition).

d. How do other folate antagonists differ from methotrexate in their mechanism of action other important properties?

Pemetrexed and its polyglutamates have a somewhat different spectrum of biochemical actions. Like methotrexate, pemetrexed inhibits DHFR, but as a polyglutamate, it even more potently inhibits glycinamide ribonucleotide formyltransferase (GART) and thymidylate synthase (TS). Unlike methotrexate, it produces little change in the pool of reduced folates, indicating that the distal sites of inhibition (TS and GART) predominate. Its pattern of deoxynucleotide depletion, as studied in cell lines, also differs from methotrexate, as it causes a greater fall in thymidine triphosphate (TTP) than in other triphosphates. Like methotrexate, it induces p53 and cell-cycle arrest, but this effect does not seem to depend on downstream induction of p21. Pralatrexate is more effectively taken up and polyglutamated than methotrexate.

New folate antagonists that are better substrates for the reduced folate carrier have been identified. In efforts to bypass the obligatory membrane transport system and

(Continued)

MECHANISMS OF RESISTANCE TO ANTIMETABOLITES (*Cont.*)

- ▸ High levels of the degradative enzymes dihydrouracil dehydrogenase and thymidine phosphorylase
- ▸ Insufficient concentrations of 5, 10-methylenetetrahydrofolate, thus preventing formation of maximal levels of the inhibited ternary complex with TS
- Resistance to Ara-C has been attributed to the following:
  - ▸ Reduced influx through nucleoside carriers (eg, hENT1 transporter mutation)
  - ▸ Reduced activities of catabolic enzymes (deoxycytidine kinase [dCK] is the rate-limiting activating enzyme)
  - ▸ Increased activities of anabolic enzymes
    - ▸ Cytidine deaminase which converts Ara-C to nontoxic AraU
    - ▸ dCMP deaminase which converts Ara-CMP to inactive Ara-UMP
    - ▸ 5' nucleotidase which degrades Ara-CMP
- Gemcitabine resistance is found in tumors with low levels of dCK and high levels of cytidine deaminase.
- The most common mechanism of 6-MP resistance is deficiency or complete lack of the activating enzyme, HGPRT, or increased alkaline phosphate activity; other mechanisms for resistance include the following:
  - ▸ Decreased drug uptake
  - ▸ Increased efflux due to one of several active transporters
  - ▸ Alteration in allosteric inhibition of ribosylamine 5-phosphate synthase
  - ▸ Impaired recognition of DNA breaks and mismatches due to loss of a component (MSH6) of MMR
- Resistance to fludarabine is associated with the following:
  - ▸ Decreased activity of dCK (the enzyme that phosphorylates and thereby activates the drug)
  - ▸ Increased drug efflux
  - ▸ Increased ribonucleotide reductase (RNR) activity

(continues)

SECTION VIII

Chemotherapy of Neoplastic Diseases

MECHANISMS OF RESISTANCE TO ANTIMETABOLITES (Cont.)

- Resistance to cladribine is associated with the following:
  - Loss of the activating enzyme, dCK
  - Increased expression of RNR
  - Increased active efflux by ABCG2 or other members of the ABC cassette family of transporters

to facilitate penetration of the blood-brain barrier, lipid-soluble folate antagonists also have been synthesized. Trimetrexate, a lipid-soluble analog, has modest antitumor activity, primarily in combination with leucovorin rescue. However, it is beneficial in the treatment of *Pneumocystis jiroveci* (*Pneumocystis carinii*) pneumonia where leucovorin provides differential rescue of the host but not the parasite.

e. What are the mechanisms of acquired resistance to methotrexate and pemetrexed?

Resistance to the cytotoxic effects of folate analogs can develop by a number of mechanisms that affect drug transport into tumor cells, mutations in the enzymes involved in folic acid metabolism, changes in expression of these enzymes, and increased efflux of drug from tumor cells (see Side Bar MECHANISMS OF RESISTANCE TO ANTIMETABOLITES).

CASE 45-4

A 58-year-old man is prescribed topical 5-FU to treat precancerous skin lesions on his face and arms.

a. What is the mechanism of action of 5-FU?

5-FU is an analog of thymine. It is enzymatically converted in cells to a nucleotide, floxuridine monophosphate (FUMP), by one of several pathways (see Figure 45-7). FUMP can then follow several different pathways (see Figure 45-7). One pathway leads to the formation of the triphosphate FUTP, which is incorporated into RNA. 5-FU incorporation into RNA is one mechanism of cytotoxicity as the result of major effects on both the processing and functions of RNA.

In an alternative reaction sequence crucial for antineoplastic activity, FUMP is reduced to FUDP by RNR to the deoxynucleotide level and then to FdUMP, a potent inhibitor of thymidylate synthesis (TS; see Figures 45-7 and 45-8). TS is required for the physiological conversion of dUMP to dTMP, which is phosphorylated to dTTP and incorporated into DNA (see Figure 45-8). Thus, blocking TS prevents DNA synthesis (see Figure 45-1) and is another mechanism of cytotoxicity. In 5-FU–treated cells, both fluorodeoxyuridine triphosphate (FdUTP) and deoxyuridine triphosphate (dUTP) (the substrate that accumulates behind the blocked TS reaction) incorporate into DNA in place of the depleted physiological dTTP (see Figure 45-7). The significance of the incorporation of FdUTP and dUTP into DNA is unclear. Presumably, the incorporation of deoxyuridylate and/or fluorodeoxyuridylate into DNA would call into action the excision-repair process. This process may result in DNA strand breakage because DNA repair requires dTTP, but this substrate is lacking as a result of TS inhibition.

The folate cofactor, $N^{5,10}$ methylene tetrahydrofolate, and FdUMP form a covalently bound ternary complex with TS (see Figure 45-8). This inhibited complex resembles the transition state formed during the enzymatic conversion of dUMP to thymidylate. The physiological complex of TS-folate-dUMP progresses to the synthesis of thymidylate by transfer of the methylene group and 2 hydrogen atoms from folate to dUMP, but this reaction is blocked in the inhibited complex of TS-FdUMP-folate by the stability of the fluorine carbon bond on FdUMP; sustained inhibition of the enzyme results.

5-FU also may be converted by thymidine phosphorylase to the deoxyriboside fluorodeoxyuridine (FUdR) and then by thymidine kinase to FdUMP (see Figure 45-7). These complex metabolic pathways for the generation of FdUMP may be bypassed through administration of floxuridine (fluorodeoxyuridine; FUdR), which is converted directly to FdUMP by thymidine kinase (FUdR rarely is used in clinical practice).

b. When used to treat tumors, what are the mechanisms of resistance to the fluoropyrimidines?

Resistance to the cytotoxic effects of 5-FU or FUdR has been ascribed to loss or decreased activity of the enzymes necessary for activation of 5-FU, amplification of

(Continued)

Cancer Chemotherapy and Cytotoxic Agents

CHAPTER 45

TS, mutation of TS to a form that is not inhibited by FdUMP, and high levels of the degradative enzymes dihydrouracil dehydrogenase and thymidine phosphorylase.

TS levels are controlled by an autoregulatory feedback mechanism wherein the unbound enzyme interacts with and inhibits the translational efficiency of its own mRNA, which provides for the rapid TS modulation needed for cellular division. When TS is bound to FdUMP, inhibition of translation is relieved, and levels of free TS rise. This may be an important mechanism by which malignant cells become insensitive to the effects of 5-FU.

Some malignant cells appear to have insufficient concentrations of $N^{5,10}$ methylene tetrahydrofolate, and thus cannot form maximal levels of the inhibited ternary complex with TS. Addition of exogenous folate in the form of N^5-formyl FH_4 (leucovorin) increases formation of the complex and enhances responses to 5-FU in clinical trials.

c. What are the important toxicities when the fluoropyrimidines are used to treat tumors?

The earliest untoward symptoms during a course of therapy are anorexia and nausea, followed by stomatitis and diarrhea, which constitute reliable warning signs that a sufficient dose has been administered. Mucosal ulcerations occur throughout the GI tract and may lead to fulminant diarrhea, shock, and death, particularly in patients who are dihydropyrimidine dehydrogenase deficient.

5-FU is inactivated by reduction of the pyrimidine ring in a reaction carried out by dihydropyrimidine dehydrogenase (DPD), which is found in the liver, intestinal mucosa, tumor cells, and other tissues. Inherited deficiency of this enzyme leads to greatly increased sensitivity to the drug (see Figure 45-7). The rare individual who totally lacks this enzyme may experience profound drug toxicity following conventional doses of the drug. DPD deficiency can be detected either by enzymatic or molecular assays using peripheral white blood cells or by determining the plasma ratio of 5-FU to its metabolite, 5-fluoro-5,6-dihydrouracil.

Myelosuppression is also a major toxicity. Loss of hair, occasionally progressing to total alopecia, nail changes, dermatitis, and increased pigmentation and atrophy of the skin may be encountered. Hand-foot syndrome, a particularly prominent adverse effect of capecitabine (an orally administered prodrug of 5-FU), consists of erythema, desquamation, pain, and sensitivity to touch of the palms and soles. Acute chest pain with evidence of ischemia in the electrocardiogram may result from coronary artery vasospasms during or shortly after 5-FU infusion.

The significant risk of toxicity with fluoropyrimidines emphasizes the need for very skillful supervision by physicians familiar with the action and possible hazards.

CASE 45-5

A 32-year-old woman is being treated with 6-MP for her leukemia.

a. What is the mechanism of action of 6-mercaptopurine?

6-MP is a purine analog. 6-MP and a related 6-thiopurine, 6-thioguanine (6-TG), function as analogs of the natural purines, hypoxanthine and guanine. The substitution of sulfur for oxygen on C6 of the purine ring creates compounds that are readily transported into cells, including activated malignant cells. Nucleotides formed from 6-MP and 6-TG inhibit de novo purine synthesis and also become incorporated into nucleic acids (see Figure 45-1). Both 6-TG and 6-MP are excellent substrates for hypoxanthine guanine phosphoribosyl transferase (HGPRT) and are converted in a single step to the ribonucleotides 6-thioguanosine-5′-monophosphate (6-thioGMP) and 6-thioinosine-5′-monophosphate (T-IMP), respectively. Because T-IMP is a poor substrate for guanylyl kinase, the enzyme that converts guanosine monophosphate (GMP) to guanosine diphosphate (GDP), T-IMP accumulates intracellularly and in a second step is converted to 6-TGMP.

(Continued)

SECTION VIII
Chemotherapy of Neoplastic Diseases

T-IMP inhibits the new formation of ribosyl-5-phosphate, as well as conversion of inosine-5′-monophosphate (IMP) to adenine and guanine nucleotides. Of these, the most important point of attack seems to be the reaction of glutamine and PRPP to form ribosyl-5-phosphate, the first committed step in the de novo pathway. 6-thioguanine nucleotide is incorporated into DNA, where it induces strand breaks and base mispairing. Strand breaks depend on the presence of an intact MMR system, the absence of which leads to resistance.

b. What are the mechanisms of resistance to the thiopurine antimetabolites?

The most common mechanism of 6-MP resistance observed in vitro is deficiency or complete lack of the activating enzyme, HGPRT, or increased alkaline phosphate activity. Other mechanisms for resistance are listed in the Side Bar MECHANISMS OF RESISTANCE TO ANTIMETABOLITES.

c. What are the primary toxicities of 6-MP?

The principal toxicity of 6-MP is bone marrow depression, although in general, this side effect develops more gradually than with folic acid antagonists; accordingly, thrombocytopenia, granulocytopenia, or anemia may not become apparent for several weeks. When depression of normal bone marrow elements occurs, dose reduction usually results in prompt recovery, although myelosuppression may be severe and prolonged in patients with a polymorphism affecting thiopurine methyltransferase (TPMT), one of the enzymes responsible for the metabolic degradation of 6-MP.

TPMT catalyzes the methylation of the sulfhydryl group on 6-MP, which leads to subsequent oxidation. Enzymatic activity of TPMT reflects the inheritance of polymorphic alleles; up to 15% of the Caucasian population has decreased enzyme activity (see Chapter 7 in *Goodman & Gilman's The Pharmacological Basis of Therapeutics*, 12th Edition). Low levels of erythrocyte TPMT activity are associated with increased drug toxicity in individual patients and a lower risk of relapse after treatment with 6-MP. Testing for these TMPT polymorphisms prior to treatment is recommended.

Anorexia, nausea, or vomiting is seen in ~25% of adults, but stomatitis and diarrhea are rare; manifestations of GI effects are less frequent in children than in adults. Jaundice and hepatic enzyme elevations occur in up to one-third of adult patients treated with 6-MP and usually resolve upon discontinuation of therapy. Their appearance has been associated with bile stasis and hepatic necrosis on biopsy. 6-MP and its derivative, azathioprine, predispose to opportunistic infections such as reactivation of hepatitis B, fungal infection, and *Pneumocystis pneumonia*, and an increased incidence of squamous cell malignancies of the skin. 6-MP has teratogenic effects during the first trimester of pregnancy, and AML has been reported after prolonged 6-MP therapy for Crohn's disease.

MECHANISMS OF ACTION AND RESISTANCE OF CYTOTOXIC NAURAL PRODUCTS (SEE TABLE 45-4)

CLASSIFICATION	DRUG	MECHANISMS OF ACTION	MECHANISMS OF RESISTANCE
Microtubule-Damaging Agents—Vinca Alkaloids	Vinblastine sulfate Vinorelbine Vincristine sulfate	Bind to β tubulin blocking its polymerization with α tubulin into microtubules, thus preventing mitotic spindle formation which blocks cells in mitosis leading to apoptosis (see Figures 45-1 and 45-3)	See Side Bar MECHANISMS OF RESISTANCE TO CYTOTOXIC NATURAL PRODUCTS
Microtubule-Damaging Agents—Taxanes	Paclitaxel Nab-paclitaxel Docetaxel	Bind to β tubulin site (different than the vinca alkaloids) and promote rather than inhibit microtubule formation causing aberrant microtubule structures away from the centriole and arrest in mitosis (see Figures 45-1 and 45-3)	See Side Bar MECHANISMS OF RESISTANCE TO CYTOTOXIC NATURAL PRODUCTS

(Continued)

Cancer Chemotherapy and Cytotoxic Agents

CHAPTER 45

CLASSIFICATION	DRUG	MECHANISMS OF ACTION	MECHANISMS OF RESISTANCE
Microtubule-Damaging Agents—Estramustine	Estramustine	Bind to β tubulin and microtubule-associated proteins, causing microtubule disassembly and antimitotic actions (see Figure 45-1)	
Microtubule-Damaging Agents—Epothilones	Ixabepilone	Bind to β tubulin (at a site distinct from taxanes) and trigger microtubule nucleation at multiple sites away from the centriole (see Figure 45-1)	See Side Bar MECHANISMS OF RESISTANCE TO CYTOTOXIC NATURAL PRODUCTS
Topoisomerase inhibitors—Camptothecin Analogs	Topotecan Irinotecan (CPT-11)	Bind and stabilize the normally transient DNA-topoisomerase I cleavable complex, inhibiting religation and resulting in single-stranded DNA strand breaks (reversible) and double-stranded DNA strand breaks (irreversible) (see Figure 45-1)	See Side Bar MECHANISMS OF RESISTANCE TO CYTOTOXIC NATURAL PRODUCTS
Topoisomerase inhibitors—Epipodophyllotoxins	Etoposide (VP-16-213) Teniposide (VM-26)	Form a ternary complex with topoisomerase II and DNA that prevents resealing of the strand break; the enzyme remains bound to the free end of the broken DNA strand, leading to an accumulation of DNA breaks and cell death (see Figure 45-1)	See Side Bar MECHANISMS OF RESISTANCE TO CYTOTOXIC NATURAL PRODUCTS
Anticancer Antibiotics—Actinomycins	Dactinomycin (actinomycin D)	Bind double-stranded DNA, which prevents DNA-dependent RNA polymerase transcription; also causes single-strand breaks in DNA through a free-radical intermediate or as a result of the action of topoisomerase II (see Figure 45-2)	
Anticancer Antibiotics—Anthracyclines and Anthracenediones	Doxorubicin Daunorubicin (daunomycin, rubidomycin) Idarubicin Epirubicin Valrubicin Mitoxantrone	Intercalate with DNA, directly inhibiting transcription and replication Form a tripartite complex with topoisomerase II and DNA, which inhibits the religation of the broken DNA strands, leading to apoptosis (see Figures 45-1 and 45-2) Their quinone groups also generate free radicals which attack DNA and oxidize DNA bases	
Anticancer Antibiotics—Bleomycin	Bleomycin	Binds to DNA and the activated complex generates free radicals that cause oxidative damage to the deoxyribose of thymidylate and other nucleotides, leading to single- and double-stranded breaks in DNA; an excess of breaks results in apoptosis (see Figure 45-2)	
Anticancer Antibiotics—Mitomycin	Mitomycin (mitomycin-C)	Chemical reduction of the quinone and loss of the methoxy group converts mitomycin to a bifunctional or trifunctional alkylating agent that inhibits DNA synthesis and forms DNA cross-links; attempts to repair DNA lead to strand breaks (see Figures 45-1 and 45-2)	
Trabectedin	Trabectedin	Binds to the minor groove of DNA, allowing the alkylation of guanine and bending the helix toward the major groove; the bulky DNA adduct is recognized by the transcription-coupled nucleotide excision repair (NER) complex, which initiates attempts to repair the damaged strand, converting the adduct to a double-stranded break	
Enzymes	L-asparaginase (L-ASP) Pegaspargase (PEG-L-asparaginase)	Catalyzes the hydrolysis of circulating asparagine, thus depriving lymphocytic leukemias (which lack asparagine synthetase) of asparagine, leading to cell death (see Figure 45-1)	

SECTION VIII

Chemotherapy of Neoplastic Diseases

MECHANISMS OF RESISTANCE TO CYTOTOXIC NATURAL PRODUCTS

- The vinca alkaloids share cross-resistance to many tumors and their antitumor effects are blocked by:
  - Increased expression of the *mdr*-1 gene and its product, P-glycoprotein, a membrane efflux transporter
  - MRP and the closely related breast cancer resistance protein, may mediate multidrug resistance
  - Mutations in β tubulin or in the relative expression of isoforms of β tubulin; both changes prevent the inhibitors from effectively binding to their target
- The mechanism of resistance to taxanes clinically is not known, but several mechanisms are possible based on studies in vitro:
  - Increased expression of the *mdr*-1 gene and its product, P-glycoprotein
  - β Tubulin mutations (which may heighten sensitivity to vinca alkaloids)
  - An increase in survivin expression, an antiapoptotic factor
  - An increase in α aurora kinase expression, an enzyme that promotes completion of mitosis
  - Up-regulating the βIII isoform of tubulin (the tubulin subunit that taxanes bind preferentially)
  - Drugs that block cell-cycle progression prior to mitosis antagonize the toxic effects of taxanes
- Ixabepilone may be less susceptible to P-glycoprotein–mediated multidrug resistance when compared to taxanes, but resistance might result from the following:
  - Mutation of the β tubulin binding site
  - Up-regulation of isoforms of β tubulin
- A number of mechanisms of resistance to campothecins have been suggested based on in vitro studies (their relevance to clinical settings is still unclear) including the following:
  - Topotecan is a substrate for P-glycoprotein, but its efflux is much lower than other MDR substrates.
  - The MRP class of transporters have been associated with topotecan and irinotecan resistance.

(continues)

TABLE 45-4 Natural Products

TYPE OF AGENT	NONPROPRIETARY NAMES	DISEASE
Vinca alkaloids	Vinblastine Vinorelbine	Hodgkin's disease; non-Hodgkin's lymphoma; testis cancer; breast cancer; lung cancer
	Vincristine	Acute lymphocytic leukemia; neuroblastoma; Wilms' tumor; rhabdomyosarcoma; Hodgkin's disease; non-Hodgkin's lymphoma
Taxanes	Paclitaxel Docetaxel	Ovarian, breast, lung, prostate, bladder, head and neck cancer
Epipodophyllotoxins	Etoposide	Testis, small cell lung and other lung cancer; breast cancer; Hodgkin's disease; non-Hodgkin's lymphomas; acute myelogenous leukemia; Kaposi's sarcoma
	Teniposide	Acute lymphoblastic leukemia in children
Camptothecins	Topotecan irinotecan	Ovarian cancer; small cell lung cancer; colon cancer
Antibiotics	Dactinomycin (actinomycin D)	Choriocarcinoma; Wilms' tumor; rhabdomyosarcoma; testis cancer; Kaposi's sarcoma
	Daunorubicin (daunomycin, rubidomycin)	Acute myelogenous and acute lymphocytic leukemia
	Doxorubicin	Soft-tissue, osteogenic, and other sarcoma; Hodgkin's disease; non-Hodgkin's lymphoma; acute leukemia; breast, genitourinary, thyroid, lung, and stomach cancer; neuroblastoma and other childhood and adult sarcomas
Echinocandins	Yondelis	Soft-tissue sarcomas; ovarian cancer
Anthracenedione	Mitoxantrone	Acute myelogenous leukemia; breast and prostate cancer
	Bleomycin	Testis and cervical cancer; Hodgkin's disease; non-Hodgkin's lymphoma
	Mitomycin C	Stomach, anal, and lung cancer
Enzymes	L-Asparaginase	Acute lymphocytic leukemia

MECHANISMS OF ACTION AND RESISTANCE OF CYTOTOXIC AGENTS WITH DIVERSE MECHANISMS OF ACTION (SEE TABLE 45-5)

CLASSIFICATION	DRUG	MECHANISMS OF ACTION	MECHANISMS OF RESISTANCE
Adrenocortical Suppressants-Mitotane	Mitotane (o,p'-DDD)	Mechanism of action has not been elucidated Relatively selective cytotoxicity for adrenocortical cells, normal or neoplastic	

(Continued)

Cancer Chemotherapy and Cytotoxic Agents

CHAPTER 45

CLASSIFICATION	DRUG	MECHANISMS OF ACTION	MECHANISMS OF RESISTANCE
Substitutes Urea—Hydroxyurea (HU)	Hydroxyurea (HU)	Inhibits ribonucleoside diphosphate reductase (RNR), which catalyzes the reductive conversion of ribonucleotides to deoxyribonucleotides (a rate-limiting step in the biosynthesis of DNA), causing cells to arrest at or near the G_1–S interface through both p53-dependent and -independent mechanisms (see Figures 45-1 and 45-3)	Tumor cells become resistant to HU through increased synthesis of the hRRM2 subunit of ribonucleoside diphosphate reductase, thus restoring enzyme activity
Differentiating Agents—Retinoids	Tretinoin (all-transretinoic acid, ATRA)	The pharmacology of retinoids is described in Chapter 48 ATRA induces differentiation in acute promyelocytic leukemia (APL) cells by binding the oncogenic PML–RAR-α fusion gene (see Figure 45-1)	Resistance arises by further mutation of the fusion gene that abolishes ATRA binding; by induction of CYP26A1 in liver or leukemic cells; or by loss of expression of the PML–RAR-α fusion gene
Differentiating Agents—Arsenic Trioxide	Arsenic trioxide (ATO)	Mechanisms of antitumor action and differentiation induction are uncertain but may act by increasing reactive oxygen species (ROS) by inhibiting thioredoxin reductase and inactivating GSH (see Figure 45-1)	ATO's cytotoxic effects are antagonized by cell survival signals emanating from activation of the PI3 kinase cell survival pathway (Akt kinase, S6 kinase, and mammalian target of rapamycin [mTOR])
Differentiating Agents—HDAC Inhibitors	Vorinostat (suberoylanilide hydroxamic acid) Romidepsin (depsipeptide, FK228)	Antitumor action is unclear, but inhibits histone deacetylases (HDACs), increasing histone acetylation which enhances gene transcription of cell-cycle regulators, nuclear transcription factors, and pro-apoptotic genes (see Figure 45-1)	

MECHANISMS OF RESISTANCE TO CYTOTOXIC NATURAL PRODUCTS (Cont.)

- Irinotecan resistance may result from lack of carboxylesterase that converts the agent to its active metabolite, SN-38.
- Decreased expression or mutation of topoisomerase I.
- Enzyme phosphorylation or polyADP ribosylation may reduce the activity of topoisomerase I and its susceptibility to inhibition.
- Cells exposed to camptothecins up-regulate topoisomerase II, an alternative enzyme for DNA strand passage.
- Cellular repair processes may not readily recognize the stabilized drug-DNA-topoisomerase I complexes.
- Resistance to anthracyclines in tumor cells has been attributed to the following:
  - Overexpression of transcription-linked DNA repair
  - Multidrug resistance associated with expression of MRP transporters and by the breast cancer resistance protein
  - Increased glutathione peroxidase activity
  - Decreased activity or mutation of topoisomerase II
  - Enhanced ability to repair DNA strand breaks
- Tumor cells resistant to etoposide and teniposide demonstrate the following:
  - Amplification of the *mdr*-1 gene that encodes the P-glycoprotein drug efflux transporter
  - Mutation or decreased expression of topoisomerase II
  - Mutations of the p53 tumor suppressor gene, a required component of the apoptotic pathway
- Several mechanisms of bleomycin resistance have been described in resistant tumor cells:
  - High levels of hydrolase activity
  - A polymorphism of the hydrolase gene, SNP A1450G, that may be associated with increased hydrolase activity
  - Decreased uptake
  - Repair of strand breaks
  - Drug inactivation by thiols or thiol-rich proteins

(continues)

CASE 45-6

The standard curative regimen for Hodgkin's lymphoma is known as the ABVD regimen (doxorubicin [ADRIAMYCIN], bleomycin, vinblastine, and dacarbazine).

a. What is the mechanism of action of each agent in the ABVD regimen?

Doxorubicin (ADRIAMYCIN) is an anthracycline antibiotic derived from the fungus *Streptomyces peucetius* var. *caesius*. Cytotoxic agents of this class

(Continued)

SECTION VIII

Chemotherapy of Neoplastic Diseases

MECHANISMS OF RESISTANCE TO CYTOTOXIC NATURAL PRODUCTS (Cont.)

- Resistance to mitomycin has been ascribed to the following:
  - Deficient activation
  - Intracellular inactivation of the reduced quinone
  - P-glycoprotein–mediated drug efflux

TABLE 45-5 Miscellaneous Agents (some of these agents are covered in Chapter 46)

TYPE OF AGENT	NONPROPRIETARY NAMES	DISEASE
Substituted urea	Hydroxyurea	Chronic myelogenous leukemia; polycythemia vera; essential thrombocytosis
Differentiating agents	Tretinoin, arsenic trioxide	Acute promyelocytic leukemia
	Histone deacetylase inhibitor (vorinostat)	Cutaneous T-cell lymphoma
Protein tyrosine kinase inhibitors	Imatinib	Chronic myelogenous leukemia; GI stromal tumors (GIST); hypereosinophilia syndrome
	Dasatinib, nilotinib	Chronic myelogenous leukemia
	Gefitinib, erlotinib	EGFR inhibitors: non-small cell lung cancer
	Sorafenib	Hepatocellular cancer, renal cancer
	Sunitinib	GIST, renal cancer
	Lapatinib	Breast cancer
Proteasome inhibitor	Bortezomib	Multiple myeloma
Biological response modifiers	Interferon-alfa, interleukin-2	Hairy cell leukemia; Kaposi's sarcoma; melanoma; carcinoid; renal cell; non-Hodgkin's lymphoma; mycosis fungoides; chronic myelogenous leukemia
Immunomodulators	Thalidomide	Multiple myeloma
	Lenalidomide	Myelodysplasia (5q⁻ syndrome); multiple myeloma
mTOR Inhibitors	Temsirolimus, everolimus	Renal cancer
Monoclonal antibodies		(*see* Tables 46-1 and 46-2)

(the anthracyclines and anthracenediones: doxorubicin; daunorubicin; idarubicin; epirubicin; valrubicin; mitoxantrone) all have quinone and hydroquinone moieties on adjacent rings that permit the gain and loss of electrons. These compounds can intercalate with DNA, directly affecting transcription and replication. A more important action is the ability to form a tripartite complex with topoisomerase II and DNA. Topoisomerase II is an ATP-dependent enzyme that binds to DNA and produces double-strand breaks at the 3′-phosphate backbone, allowing strand passage and uncoiling of supercoiled DNA. Following strand passage, topoisomerase II religates the DNA strands. This enzymatic function is essential for DNA replication and repair. Formation of the tripartite complex with anthracyclines or with etoposide inhibits the religation of the broken DNA strands, leading to apoptosis. Anthracyclines, by virtue of their quinone groups, also generate free radicals in solution, and in both normal and malignant tissues. Anthracyclines can form semiquinone radical intermediates that can react with O_2 to produce superoxide anion

(*Continued*)

radicals. These can generate both hydrogen peroxide and hydroxyl radicals, which attack DNA and oxidize DNA bases.

Bleomycin is a member of unique group of DNA-cleaving antibiotics which are fermentation products of *Streptomyces verticillus*. Bleomycin's cytotoxicity results from its ability to cause oxidative damage to the deoxyribose of thymidylate and other nucleotides, leading to single- and double-stranded breaks in DNA. The bleomycin molecule is a glycopeptide that contains a metal-binding cage that is bound to either Fe^{2+} or Cu^{2+}. In the presence of O_2 and a reducing agent the metal–drug complex becomes activated and functions as a ferrous oxidase, transferring electrons from Fe^{2+} to molecular oxygen to produce oxygen radicals. Bleomycin binds to DNA, and the activated complex generates free radicals that are responsible for abstraction of a proton at the 3′ position of the deoxyribose backbone of the DNA chain, opening the deoxyribose ring and generating a strand break in DNA.

Vinblastine is a vinca alkaloid derived from the Madagascar periwinkle plant, *Catharanthus roseus*. Other vinca alkaloids with antitumor activity include vincristine, vindesine, and vinorelbine. The vincas bind specifically to β tubulin and block its polymerization with α tubulin into microtubules, thus preventing the formation of mitotic spindles. In the absence of an intact mitotic spindle, duplicated chromosomes cannot align along the division plate. They disperse throughout the cytoplasm (exploded mitosis) or may clump in unusual groupings, such as balls or stars. Cells are blocked in mitosis and undergo changes characteristic of apoptosis.

Dacarbazine (DTIC) is a triazene alkylating agent. It is metabolically activated by hepatic CYPs through an *N*-demethylation reaction. In the target cell, spontaneous cleavage of the metabolite, methyl-triazeno-imidazole-carboxamide (MTIC), yields an alkylating moiety, a methyl diazonium ion. This reactive species incorporates methyl groups into DNA. For a detailed description of DNA alkylation reactions, refer to Case 45-1a.

b. **What is the rationale for using combinations of cytotoxic drugs such as the ABVD regimen compared to single-agent therapies?**

Most cytotoxic drugs are used in combination with other cytotoxic agents with different mechanisms of action to enhance tumor cell killing and to avoid the development of resistance. Drugs in combination can negate the effects of a resistance mechanism specific for a single agent, and they may be synergistic because of their biochemical interactions. Ideally, drug combinations should not overlap in their major toxicities.

KEY CONCEPTS

- Cytotoxic antineoplastic agents are structurally and mechanistically diverse.
- The efficacy of many cytotoxic agents depends on intact cell cycle checkpoint regulation and apoptotic mechanisms.
- Rapidly dividing cells (including normal cells such as GI epithelial cells and bone marrow cells) are typically more sensitive to the effects of cytotoxic agents.
- Common acute toxicities of cytotoxic agents include GI damage and myelosuppression.
- Myelosuppression can lead to increased risk of opportunistic infections and bleeding disorders.
- DNA modifying agents are typically mutagenic and carcinogenic, resulting in increased risk of leukemias and other cancers months or years following treatment.
- Cytotoxic agents can cause chronic damage to critical organs, including the kidney, liver, and heart.
- Most cytotoxic chemotherapeutic agents are fetotoxic.

(Continued)

SECTION VIII
Chemotherapy of Neoplastic Diseases

- Resistance to the effectiveness of cytotoxic antineoplastic agents can develop through a variety of mechanisms, including changes in cellular influx and efflux, alterations in drug activation and inactivation, and mutations or changes in drug targets or cellular pathways needed for cytotoxicity.
- Antineoplastic agents are often used in combination or with radiation to minimize the development of resistance and enhance tumor cell killing.
- Individual patient tumor response and organ toxicity to cytotoxic chemotherapy can be affected by the patient's genetics, as well as many other factors such as renal and hepatic function.
- It is imperative to recognize toxicities early, to alter doses or discontinue offending medication to relieve symptoms and reduce risk, and to provide vigorous supportive care (platelet transfusions, antibiotics, and hematopoietic growth factors).

SUMMARY QUIZ

QUESTION 45-1 A nucleoside analog that is enzymatically converted by deoxycytidine kinase (dCK) to its active form, the 5′-monophosphate ribonucleotide is

a. leucovorin.
b. 5-fluorouracil (5-FU).
c. azacytidine.
d. gemcitabine.
e. cytarabine (Ara-C).

QUESTION 45-2 When administered prior to 5-FU, this agent enhances the activation of and antitumor activity by increasing pools of PRPP.

a. Leucovorin
b. Oxaliplatin
c. Methotrexate
d. Cytarabine (Ara-C)
e. Fluxuridine

QUESTION 45-3 An enzyme derived from *Escherichia coli* that deprives leukemia cells of a required amino acid is

a. pentostatin.
b. L-asparaginase (L-ASP).
c. deoxycytidine kinase (dCK).
d. trabectedin.
e. asparagine synthase.

QUESTION 45-4 Paclitaxel and the other taxanes have a central role in the therapy of ovarian, breast, lung, GI, genitourinary, and head and neck cancers. The cytotoxic effect of the taxanes in tumor cells is the result of

a. inhibition of microtubule formation.
b. inhibition of microtubule disassembly.
c. enhancement of microtubule disassembly.
d. inhibition of topoisomerase I.
e. inhibition of topoisomerase II.

Cancer Chemotherapy and Cytotoxic Agents

CHAPTER 45

QUESTION 45-5 The camptothecins, topotecan and irinotecan, are potent, cytotoxic neoplastic agents. They act by

a. intercalating DNA.
b. alkylating DNA.
c. stabilizing the DNA-topoisomerase I cleavable complex.
d. inhibiting DNA cleavage by topoisomerase I.
e. inhibiting topoisomerase I binding to DNA.

SUMMARY QUIZ ANSWER KEY

QUESTION 45-1 Answer is **e.** Cytarabine (1-β-D-arabinofuranosylcytosine; Ara-C) is the most important antimetabolite used in the therapy of acute myelocytic leukemia (AML). Ara-C is an analog of 2′-deoxycytidine with the 2′-hydroxyl in a position that hinders rotation of the pyrimidine base around the nucleoside bond and interferes with base pairing. The drug enters cells via a nucleoside transporter and is converted to its active form, the 5′-monophosphate ribonucleotide (Ara-CMP), by dCK. Polymorphisms of dCK may influence the rate of drug activation in individual patients.

Ara-CMP reacts with appropriate deoxynucleotide kinases to form diphosphate and triphosphates (Ara-CDP and Ara-CTP). Ara-CTP competes with the physiological substrate deoxycytidine 5′-triphosphate (dCTP) for incorporation into DNA by DNA polymerases. The incorporated Ara-CMP residue is a potent inhibitor of DNA polymerase, both in replication and repair synthesis, and blocks the further elongation of the nascent DNA molecule. The block in elongation activates checkpoint kinases (ATR and chk-1), which initiate attempts to remove the offending nucleotide. If DNA breaks are not repaired, apoptosis ensues.

QUESTION 45-2 Answer is **c.** A number of agents have been combined with 5-FU in attempts to enhance cytotoxic activity through biochemical modulation. Methotrexate, by inhibiting purine synthesis and increasing cellular pools of PRPP (see Figure 45-6), enhances the activation of 5-FU (see Figure 45-7), and increases antitumor activity of 5-FU when given prior to but not following 5-FU.

Some malignant cells appear to have insufficient concentrations of $N^{5,10}$ methylene tetrahydrofolate, and thus cannot form maximal levels of the inhibited ternary complex with TS. Addition of exogenous folate in the form of N^5-formyl FH_4 (leucovorin) increases formation of the complex and enhances responses to 5-FU (see Figure 45-8).

The combination of cisplatin and 5-FU has yielded impressive responses in tumors of the upper aerodigestive tract, but the molecular basis of their interaction is not well understood. Oxaliplatin, which downregulates TS expression, is commonly used with 5-FU.

Perhaps the most clinically important interaction is the enhancement of irradiation by fluoropyrimidines, the mechanistic basis for which is unclear. 5-FU with simultaneous irradiation cures anal cancer and enhances local tumor control in head and neck, cervical, rectal, gastroesophageal, and pancreatic cancers.

QUESTION 45-3 Answer is **b.** Most normal tissues are able to synthesize L-asparagine in amounts sufficient for protein synthesis, but lymphocytic leukemias lack adequate amounts of asparagine synthetase, and derive the required amino acid from plasma. L-ASP, by catalyzing the hydrolysis of circulating asparagine to aspartic acid and ammonia, deprives these malignant cells of asparagine, leading to cell death. The enzyme has become a standard agent for treating ALL. L-ASP is used in combination

SECTION VIII — Chemotherapy of Neoplastic Diseases

with other agents, including methotrexate, doxorubicin, vincristine, and prednisone for the treatment of ALL and for high-grade lymphomas. Resistance arises through induction of asparagine synthetase in tumor cells.

L-ASP toxicities result from its antigenicity as a foreign protein and its inhibition of protein synthesis. Hypersensitivity reactions, including urticaria and full-blown anaphylaxis, occur in 5-20% of patients and may be fatal. These reactions usually are heralded by the earlier appearance of circulating neutralizing antibody and accelerated enzyme clearance from plasma. In these patients, pegaspargase (a preparation in which the enzyme is conjugated to 5000-Da units of monomethoxy polyethylene glycol) is a safe and effective alternative. The so-called "silent" enzyme inactivation by antibodies occurs in a higher percentage of patients than overt hypersensitivity and may be associated with a negative clinical outcome, especially in high-risk ALL patients.

QUESTION 45-4 Answer is **b**. Paclitaxel and other taxanes (nab-paclitaxel and docetaxel) bind specifically to the β tubulin subunit of microtubules and antagonize the disassembly of this key cytoskeletal protein, with the result that bundles of microtubules and aberrant structures derived from microtubules appear in the mitotic phase of the cell cycle. Arrest in mitosis follows. Drugs that block cell cycle progression prior to mitosis antagonize the toxic effects of taxanes. Resistance to taxanes is associated in some cancer cells with increased expression of the *mdr-1* gene and its product, P-glycoprotein; other resistant cells have β tubulin mutations (these latter cells may display heightened sensitivity to vinca alkaloids). The taxanes preferentially bind to the βII tubulin subunit of microtubules; therefore, cells may become resistant by upregulating the βIII isoform of tubulin.

The vinca alkaloids and colchicine derivatives differ from the taxanes in that they bind to a different site on β tubulin site and inhibit microtubule formation rather than inhibit disassembly.

Estramustine binds to β tubulin and microtubule-associated proteins, causing microtubule disassembly and inhibition of mitosis.

Ixabepilone and other members of the epothilones class resemble taxanes in that they bind to β tubulin and trigger microtubule nucleation at multiple sites away from the centriole. This chaotic microtubule stabilization triggers cell cycle arrest at the G_2-M interface and apoptosis. Epothilones bind to a site distinct from that of taxanes. In vitro studies suggest that ixabepilone is less susceptible to P-glycoprotein-mediated multidrug resistance when compared to taxanes. Mechanisms implicated in epothilone resistance include mutation of the β tubulin binding site and up-regulation of isoforms of β tubulin.

QUESTION 45-5 Answer is **c**. The camptothecins bind to and stabilize the normally transient DNA-topoisomerase I cleavable complex.

The DNA topoisomerases are nuclear enzymes that reduce torsional stress in supercoiled DNA, allowing selected regions of DNA to become sufficiently untangled and relaxed to permit replication, repair, and transcription. Two classes of topoisomerase (I and II) mediate DNA strand breakage and resealing, and both have become the target of cancer chemotherapies. Camptothecin analogs inhibit the function of topoisomerase I, while a number of different chemical entities (eg, anthracyclines, epipodophyllotoxins, acridines) inhibit topoisomerase II. Topoisomerase I binds covalently to double-stranded DNA through a reversible transesterification reaction. This reaction yields an intermediate complex in which the tyrosine of the enzyme is bound to the 3′-phosphate end of the DNA strand, creating a single-strand DNA break. This "cleavable complex" allows for relaxation of the DNA torsional strain, either by passage of the intact single-strand through the nick or by free rotation of the DNA about the noncleaved strand. Once the DNA torsional strain has been relieved, the topoisomerase I reseals the cleavage and dissociates from the newly relaxed double helix.

(Continued)

Cancer Chemotherapy and Cytotoxic Agents

CHAPTER 45

The camptothecins do not affect the initial DNA cleavage action of topoisomerase I, but inhibit the DNA religation step, leading to the accumulation of single-stranded breaks in DNA. These lesions are reversible and are not by themselves toxic to the cell. However, the collision of a DNA replication fork with this cleaved strand of DNA causes an irreversible double-strand DNA break, ultimately leading to cell death. Camptothecins are therefore S phase-specific drugs (see Figure 45-3 for a representation of the cell cycle) because ongoing DNA synthesis is necessary for cytotoxicity. This has important clinical implications. S phase-specific cytotoxic agents generally require prolonged exposures of tumor cells to drug concentrations above a minimum threshold to optimize therapeutic efficacy. In fact, preclinical studies of low-dose, protracted administration of camptothecin analogs have less toxicity, and equal or greater antitumor activity, than shorter, more intense courses.

SUMMARY: CYTOTOXIC AGENTS USED IN THE TREATMENT OF CANCER

CLASS AND SUBCLASSES	NAMES	CLINICAL USES	TOXICITIES COMMON	TOXICITIES UNIQUE; CLINICALLY IMPORTANT
Nitrogen Mustards	Mechlorethamine HCl Cyclophosphamide Ifosfamide Melphalan Chlorambucil Bendamustine	See Table 45-1 and text of Chapter 61 of *Goodman & Gilman's The Pharmacological Basis of Therapeutics*, 12th Edition for uses of specific agents	See Side Bar TOXICITIES OF ALKYLATING DRUGS and Table 45-3 Major acute toxicities of mechlorethamine are nausea and vomiting, lacrimation, and myelosuppression	Acrolein is a toxic metabolite of cyclophosphamide (see Figure 45-4) and ifosfamide, and causes hemorrhagic cystitis which can be mitigated by coadministration of mesna; vigorous IV hydration should be given with high-dose therapy to prevent bladder toxicity
Ethyleneimines and Methylmelamines	Altretamine (hexamethylendiamine)	Palliative treatment for persistent or recurrent ovarian cancer following cisplatin-based combination therapy	See Side Bar TOXICITIES OF ALKYLATING DRUGS Main toxicities are myelosuppression and neurotoxicity Nausea and vomiting also are common side effects and may be dose-limiting Renal dysfunction may necessitate discontinuing the drug	Peripheral and central neurotoxicity (ataxia, depression, confusion, drowsiness, hallucinations, dizziness, and vertigo) Peripheral blood counts and a neurological examination should be performed prior to the initiation of each course of therapy Severe, life-threatening orthostatic hypotension may develop in patients who receive monoamine oxidase (MAO) inhibitors concurrently with altretamine
	Thiotepa	Primarily used for high-dose chemotherapy regimens	See Side Bar TOXICITIES OF ALKYLATING DRUGS	May cause neurotoxic symptoms, including coma and seizures in high-dose regimens
Alkyl Sulfonates	Busulfan	See Table 45-1	See Side Bar TOXICITIES OF ALKYLATING DRUGS Major toxic effects are related to myelosuppression Occasionally, patients experience nausea, vomiting, and diarrhea Long-term use leads to impotence, sterility, amenorrhea, and fetal malformation	Pulmonary fibrosis, GI mucosal damage, and hepatic veno-occlusive disease (VOD) are important toxicities with high-dose regimens VOD and hepatotoxicity is increased by coadministration with drugs that inhibit CYPs Anticonvulsants must be used concomitantly to protect against acute CNS toxicities, including tonic-clonic seizures, which may occur several hours after each dose

(Continued)

SECTION VIII Chemotherapy of Neoplastic Diseases

CLASS AND SUBCLASSES	NAMES	CLINICAL USES	TOXICITIES COMMON	UNIQUE; CLINICALLY IMPORTANT
Nitrosoureas	Carmustine (BCNU) Lomustine (CCNU) Semustine (methyl-CCNU) Streptozocin (streptozotocin)	See Table 45-1 and text of Chapter 61 of *Goodman & Gilman's The Pharmacological Basis of Therapeutics*, 12th Edition for uses of specific agents Carmustine, lomustine, and semustine are highly lipophilic, readily cross the blood-brain barrier and are used to treat brain tumors Streptozocin is used exclusively in the treatment of human pancreatic islet cell carcinoma and malignant carcinoid tumors	See Side Bar TOXICITIES OF ALKYLATING DRUGS With streptozocin, nausea is frequent and mild, reversible renal or hepatic toxicity occurs in approximately two-thirds of cases (renal toxicity may be cumulative), and hematological toxicity occurs in 20% of patients	With the exception of streptozocin, nitrosoureas cause profound and delayed myelosuppression with recovery 4-6 weeks after a single dose Renal failure with long-term treatment Highly carcinogenic and mutagenic BCNU in high doses with bone marrow rescue produces hepatic VOD, pulmonary fibrosis, renal failure, and secondary leukemia
Triazenes	Dacarbazine (DTIC) Temozolomide	See Table 45-1 and text of Chapter 61 of *Goodman & Gilman's The Pharmacological Basis of Therapeutics*, 12th Edition for uses of specific agents Primary indication for dacarbazine is in the combination chemotherapy of Hodgkin's disease; modestly effective against malignant melanoma and adult sarcomas Temozolomide is the standard agent in combination with radiation therapy for patients with malignant glioma and astrocytoma	See Side Bar TOXICITIES OF ALKYLATING DRUGS DTIC induces nausea and vomiting in >90% of patients Myelosuppression is mild and readily reversible within 1-2 weeks A flu-like syndrome consisting of chills, fever, malaise, and myalgias may occur Hepatotoxicity, alopecia, facial flushing, neurotoxicity, and dermatological reactions are less common	Temozolomide is administered cyclically, and hematological monitoring is necessary to guide dosing adjustments
Methylhydrazines	Procarbazine	See Table 45-1 and text of Chapter 61 of *Goodman & Gilman's The Pharmacological Basis of Therapeutics*, 12th Edition for uses of specific agents Currently employed for second-line therapy in malignant brain tumors; is rarely used in current practice	See Side Bar TOXICITIES OF ALKYLATING DRUGS Most common toxic effects include leukopenia and thrombocytopenia GI symptoms such as mild nausea and vomiting occur in most patients; diarrhea and rash are noted in 5-10% of cases	Augments sedative effects; concomitant use of CNS depressants should be avoided A weak MAO inhibitor Has disulfiram-like action, EtOH ingestion should be avoided Highly carcinogenic, mutagenic, and teratogenic, and is associated with a 5-10% risk of acute leukemia in combination with other agents or radiation Causes infertility, particularly in males

(Continued)

Cancer Chemotherapy and Cytotoxic Agents — CHAPTER 45

CLASS AND SUBCLASSES	NAMES	CLINICAL USES	TOXICITIES	
			COMMON	UNIQUE; CLINICALLY IMPORTANT
Platinum Coordination Complexes	Cisplatin Carboplatin (CBDCA) Oxaliplatin	See Table 45-1 and text of Chapter 61 of *Goodman & Gilman's The Pharmacological Basis of Therapeutics*, 12th Edition for uses of specific agents Oxaliplatin exhibits a range of antitumor activity (colorectal and gastric cancer) that differs from other platinum agents, perhaps due to its MMR- and HMG-independent effects	See Side Bar TOXICITIES OF ALKYLATING DRUGS Marked nausea and vomiting occur in almost all patients and usually can be controlled with 5-HT$_3$ antagonists, NK1-receptor antagonists, and high-dose corticosteroids Electrolyte disturbances, including hypomagnesemia, hypocalcemia, hypokalemia, and hypophosphatemia are common; routine monitoring of plasma Mg^{2+} recommended Ototoxicity Anaphylactic-like reactions Carboplatin is relatively well tolerated, causing less nausea, neurotoxicity, ototoxicity, and nephrotoxicity than cisplatin	Cisplatin-induced nephrotoxicity; to prevent renal toxicity with cisplatin, it is important to establish a chloride diuresis by the infusion of 1-2 L of normal saline prior to treatment Amifostine is a thiophosphate cytoprotective agent that reduces renal toxicity Ototoxicity Anaphylactic-like reactions Aluminum reacts with and inactivates cisplatin; the drug should not come in contact with needles or other infusion equipment that contain aluminum during its preparation or administration Dose-limiting toxicity of carboplatin is myelosuppression Dose-limiting toxicity of oxaliplatin is a peripheral neuropathy Platinum agents cause leukemia and pulmonary fibrosis months to years after administration
Folic Acid Analogs (Antifolates)	Methotrexate(amethopterin) High-dose methotrexate with leucovorin rescue (HDM-L) Trimetrexate Pemetrexed Pralatrexed Raltitrexed Lometrexol	See Table 45-3 and text of Chapter 61 of *Goodman & Gilman's The Pharmacological Basis of Therapeutics*, 12th Edition for uses of specific agents Methotrexate is also used to treat psoriasis and rheumatoid arthritis (see Chapter 23)	Primary toxicities of antifolates affect the bone marrow and the intestinal epithelium and usually resolve within 10-14 days Pemetrexed is also associated with a prominent erythematous and pruritic rash in 40% of patients which can be diminished with dexamethasone Additional toxicities include alopecia, dermatitis, an allergic interstitial pneumonitis, nephrotoxicity (after high-dose therapy), defective oogenesis or spermatogenesis, abortion, and teratogenesis	Myelosuppression can increase risk for spontaneous hemorrhage or life-threatening infection, and may require prophylactic transfusion of platelets and broad-spectrum antibiotics if febrile Prolonged myelosuppression may occur in patients with compromised renal function and requires dosage adjustment based on creatinine clearance

(Continued)

SECTION VIII Chemotherapy of Neoplastic Diseases

CLASS AND SUBCLASSES	NAMES	CLINICAL USES	TOXICITIES COMMON	UNIQUE; CLINICALLY IMPORTANT
Pyrimidine Analogs	5-Fluorouracil (5-FU) Floxuridine (FUdR, fluorodeoxyuridine) Capecitabine	See Table 45-3 and text of Chapter 61 of *Goodman & Gilman's The Pharmacological Basis of Therapeutics*, 12th Edition for uses of specific agents. 5-FU is rarely used as a single agent. 5-FU also is a potent radiation sensitizer. 5-FU is used topically for premalignant keratoses of the skin and multiple superficial basal cell carcinoma	Anorexia and nausea, followed by stomatitis and diarrhea constitute reliable warning signs that a sufficient dose has been administered. Alopecia, nail changes, dermatitis, and increased pigmentation and atrophy of the skin may occur	Mucosal ulcerations throughout the GI tract may lead to fulminant diarrhea, shock, and death, particularly in patients who are DPD deficient. Myelosuppression (more often with bolus regimens). Hand-foot syndrome (more often with infusional regimens). Coronary vasospasm with 5-FU infusion. The significant risk of toxicity with fluoropyrimidines emphasizes the need for very skillful supervision by physicians familiar with the action and possible hazards
	Cytarabine (cytosine arabinoside, Ara-C)	See Table 45-3 and text of Chapter 61 of *Goodman & Gilman's The Pharmacological Basis of Therapeutics*, 12th Edition for uses of specific agents	Acute, severe leukopenia, thrombocytopenia, and anemia with striking megaloblastic changes. GI disturbances, stomatitis, conjunctivitis, reversible hepatic enzyme elevations, noncardiogenic pulmonary edema, and dermatitis	After high-dose Ara-C (1-2 weeks) dyspnea, fever, and pulmonary infiltrates may occur, which may be fatal in 10-20% of patients. Intrathecal Ara-C (especially with systemic high-dose methotrexate) or high-dose systemic Ara-C may cause CNS toxicity including ataxia and slurred speech, seizures, delirium, myelopathy, or coma, especially in patients >40 years of age and/or patients with poor renal function
	Azacytidine (5-azacytidine) Decitabine (2′-deoxy-5-azacytidine)	See Table 45-3 and text of Chapter 61 of *Goodman & Gilman's The Pharmacological Basis of Therapeutics*, 12th Edition for uses of specific agents	Myelosuppression and mild GI symptoms	Severe nausea and vomiting when given intravenously in large doses
	Gemcitabine (2′,2′-difluorodeoxycytidine, dFdC)	See text of Chapter 61 of *Goodman & Gilman's The Pharmacological Basis of Therapeutics*, 12th Edition for uses of specific agents	Myelosuppression. Flu-like syndrome, asthenia, and rarely a posterior leukoencephalopathy syndrome. Mild elevation in liver transaminases may occur in ≥40% of patients and are reversible	Longer-duration infusions lead to greater myelosuppression and hepatic toxicity. Long-term regimens may lead to progressive hemolytic uremic syndrome, necessitating drug discontinuation. Gemcitabine is a very potent radiosensitizer and should not be used with radiotherapy

(Continued)

Cancer Chemotherapy and Cytotoxic Agents — CHAPTER 45

CLASS AND SUBCLASSES	NAMES	CLINICAL USES	TOXICITIES	
			COMMON	UNIQUE; CLINICALLY IMPORTANT
Purine Analogs	6-Mercaptopurine (6-MP) 6-Thioguanine (6-TG)	See Table 45-3 and text of Chapter 61 of Goodman & Gilman's The Pharmacological Basis of Therapeutics, 12th Edition for uses of specific agents The combination of methotrexate and 6-MP appears to be synergistic 6-MP is also used for Crohn's disease (see Chapter 23)	Myelosuppression (develops more gradually than with folic acid antagonists) Anorexia, nausea, or vomiting in ~25% of adults, but stomatitis and diarrhea are rare Jaundice and hepatic enzyme elevations occur in up to one-third of adult patients treated with 6-MP; usually resolves upon discontinuation of therapy	Myelosuppression may be severe and prolonged in patients with a polymorphism affecting TPMT Predisposes to opportunistic infection such as reactivation of hepatitis B, fungal infection, and *Pneumocystis* pneumonia and an increased incidence of squamous cell malignancies of the skin
	Fludarabine phosphate	See Table 45-3 and text of Chapter 61 of Goodman & Gilman's The Pharmacological Basis of Therapeutics, 12th Edition for uses of specific agents Also used as an immunosuppressant in nonmyeloablative allogeneic bone marrow transplantation, where it suppresses the host response and may encourage alloreactive donor T cells	Myelosuppression (World Health Organization grade 3 or 4) in about half of patients Nausea and vomiting in a minor fraction; infrequently chills and fever, malaise, anorexia, peripheral neuropathy, and weakness	Depletion of $CD4^+$ T cells Predisposes to opportunistic infections Tumor lysis syndrome (relatively infrequent) Altered mental status, seizures, optic neuritis, and coma at higher doses and in older patients Auto-immune events (acute hemolytic anemia or pure red cell aplasia, prolonged cytopenias) Myelodysplasia and acute leukemias may arise as late complications
	Cladribine (2-chlorodeoxyadenosine, 2-CdA)	See text of Chapter 61 of Goodman & Gilman's The Pharmacological Basis of Therapeutics, 12th Edition for uses of specific agents	Major toxicity is myelosuppression Cumulative thrombocytopenia with repeated doses Other toxic effects include nausea, high fever, headache, fatigue, skin rashes	Opportunistic infections are common Tumor lysis syndrome
	Clofarabine (2-chloro-2'-fluoro-arabinosyladenine)	See Table 45-3 and text of Chapter 61 of Goodman & Gilman's The Pharmacological Basis of Therapeutics, 12th Edition for uses of specific agents	Major toxicity is myelosuppression Elevated hepatic enzymes and increased bilirubin Nausea, vomiting, and diarrhea Hypokalemia and hypophosphatemia	Clinical syndrome of hypotension, tachyphemia, pulmonary edema, organ dysfunction, fever, are all suggestive of capillary leak syndrome and cytokine release; evidence of capillary leak should lead to immediate discontinuation of the drug
	Nelarabine (6-methoxy-arabinosyl-guanine)	See Table 45-3 and text of Chapter 61 of Goodman & Gilman's The Pharmacological Basis of Therapeutics, 12th Edition for uses of specific agents	Myelosuppression and liver function test abnormalities	Frequent, serious neurological sequelae such as seizures, delirium, somnolence, peripheral neuropathy, or Guillain-Barré syndrome; neurological side effects may not be reversible

(Continued)

SECTION VIII — Chemotherapy of Neoplastic Diseases

CLASS AND SUBCLASSES	NAMES	CLINICAL USES	TOXICITIES — COMMON	TOXICITIES — UNIQUE; CLINICALLY IMPORTANT
	Pentostatin (2′-deoxycoformycin)	See Table 45-3 and text of Chapter 61 of Goodman & Gilman's The Pharmacological Basis of Therapeutics, 12th Edition for uses of specific agents	Myelosuppression, GI symptoms, skin rashes, and abnormal liver function studies. Neutropenic fever and opportunistic infections may occur	Immunosuppression may persist for several years after discontinuation. Major renal and neurological complications are encountered with high doses. Severe or even fatal pulmonary toxicity may occur in combination with fludarabine phosphate
Microtubule-Damaging Agents—Vinca Alkaloids	Vinblastine sulfate, Vinorelbine, Vincristine sulfate	See Table 45-4 and text of Chapter 61 of Goodman & Gilman's The Pharmacological Basis of Therapeutics, 12th Edition for uses of specific agents	Mild myelosuppression and mild neurotoxicity. GI disturbances including nausea, vomiting, anorexia, and diarrhea may occur. Severe constipation with vincristine may be prevented by a prophylaxis with laxatives and bulk-forming agents. Alopecia occurs in ~20% of patients given vincristine, however, it is always reversible, frequently without cessation of therapy. Vinorelbine may cause allergic reactions and mild, reversible changes in liver enzymes	Syndrome of inappropriate secretion of antidiuretic hormone has been reported with vinblastine, less commonly with vincristine. Extravasation during injection may lead to cellulitis and phlebitis
Microtubule-Damaging Agents—Taxanes	Paclitaxel, Nab-paclitaxel, Docetaxel	See Table 45-4 and text of Chapter 61 of Goodman & Gilman's The Pharmacological Basis of Therapeutics, 12th Edition for uses of specific agents	Myelosuppression. Peripheral neuropathy with paclitaxel is dose-limiting; with high-dose schedules or prolonged use, a stocking-glove sensory neuropathy can be disabling. Hypersensitivity reactions in patients receiving paclitaxel infusions of short duration (1-6 h) are largely averted by pretreatment with dexamethasone, diphenhydramine, and histamine H_2 receptor antagonists. Higher rates of peripheral neuropathy with nab-paclitaxel compared to paclitaxel but rarely hypersensitivity reaction. Docetaxel causes greater neutropenia than paclitaxel but less peripheral neuropathy and less frequent hypersensitivity	After treatment with paclitaxel, myalgias for several days are common. Mucositis is common in 72- or 96-hour infusions and in the weekly schedule with paclitaxel. Asymptomatic bradycardia and occasional silent ventricular tachycardia can occur with paclitaxel. With multiple cycles of docetaxel therapy, progressive fluid retention can occur leading to peripheral edema, pleural and peritoneal fluid, and pulmonary edema in extreme cases; dexamethasone can prevent this

(Continued)

Cancer Chemotherapy and Cytotoxic Agents — CHAPTER 45

CLASS AND SUBCLASSES	NAMES	CLINICAL USES	TOXICITIES COMMON	TOXICITIES UNIQUE; CLINICALLY IMPORTANT
Microtubule-Damaging Agents—Estramustine	Estramustine	See text of Chapter 61 of *Goodman & Gilman's The Pharmacological Basis of Therapeutics*, 12th Edition for uses of specific agents	Myelosuppression	Possesses estrogenic side effects (gynecomastia, impotence, elevated risk of thrombosis, and fluid retention), hypercalcemia, acute attacks of porphyria, impaired glucose tolerance, and hypersensitivity reactions, including angioedema
Microtubule-Damaging Agents—Epothilones	Ixabepilone	See text of Chapter 61 of *Goodman & Gilman's The Pharmacological Basis of Therapeutics*, 12th Edition for uses of specific agents	Toxicities similar to those of the taxanes, namely neutropenia, peripheral sensory neuropathy, fatigue, diarrhea, and asthenia	
Topoisomerase inhibitors—Camptothecin Analogs	Topotecan Irinotecan (CPT-11)	See Table 45-4 and text of Chapter 61 of *Goodman & Gilman's The Pharmacological Basis of Therapeutics*, 12th Edition for uses of specific agents	Dose-limiting toxicity of topotecan with all dosing schedules is neutropenia, with or without thrombocytopenia, and GI side effects such as mucositis and diarrhea in some patients. Less common but mild topotecan-related toxicities include nausea and vomiting, elevated liver transaminases, fever, fatigue, and rash. Dose-limiting toxicity with irinotecan is delayed diarrhea which can be reduced by treatment with loperamide (see Chapter 33). Common but mild toxicities with irinotecan include nausea and vomiting, fatigue, vasodilation or skin flushing, mucositis, elevation in liver transaminases, and alopecia	Severe neutropenia and febrile neutropenia (which may be fatal with concomitant diarrhea). Inhibition of acetylcholinesterase activity by irinotecan may occur within the first 24 h causing a cholinergic syndrome (acute diarrhea, diaphoresis, hypersalivation, abdominal cramps, visual accommodation disturbances, lacrimation, rhinorrhea, asymptomatic bradycardia) which can be treated with atropine
Topoisomerase inhibitors—Epipodophyllotoxins	Etoposide (VP-16-213) Teniposide (VM-26)	See Table 45-4 and text of Chapter 61 of *Goodman & Gilman's The Pharmacological Basis of Therapeutics*, 12th Edition for uses of specific agents	Dose-limiting toxicity of etoposide is leukopenia; thrombocytopenia occurs less often and usually is not severe. Nausea, vomiting, stomatitis, and diarrhea occur with etoposide in ~15% of patients. Alopecia is common but reversible. Myelosuppression, nausea, and vomiting are teniposide's primary toxic effects	

(Continued)

SECTION VIII Chemotherapy of Neoplastic Diseases

CLASS AND SUBCLASSES	NAMES	CLINICAL USES	TOXICITIES COMMON	UNIQUE; CLINICALLY IMPORTANT
Anticancer Antibiotics—Actinomycins	Dactinomycin (actinomycin D)	See Table 45-4 and text of Chapter 61 of *Goodman & Gilman's The Pharmacological Basis of Therapeutics*, 12th Edition for uses of specific agents	Anorexia, nausea, and vomiting Hematopoietic suppression with pancytopenia Proctitis, diarrhea, glossitis, cheilitis, and ulcerations of the oral mucosa are common Dermatological manifestations (alopecia, erythema, desquamation, and increased inflammation and pigmentation) in areas previously or concomitantly subjected to X-ray radiation	Severe injury may occur as a result of local drug extravasation
Anticancer Antibiotics—Anthracyclines and Anthracenediones	Doxorubicin (ADRIAMYCIN) Daunorubicin (daunomycin, rubidomycin) Idarubicin Epirubicin Valrubicin Mitoxantrone	See Table 45-4 and text of Chapter 61 of *Goodman & Gilman's The Pharmacological Basis of Therapeutics*, 12th Edition for uses of specific agents	Myelosuppression, stomatitis, alopecia, GI disturbances, and rash are common toxicities Mitoxantrone causes less cardiac toxicity, nausea, vomiting, and alopecia than does doxorubicin Erythematous streaking near the site of infusion ("ADRIAMYCIN flare") is a benign local allergic reaction and should not be confused with extravasation	Cardiac toxicity (acute and chronic) characterized by tachycardia, arrhythmias, dyspnea, hypotension, pericardial effusion, and congestive heart failure poorly responsive to digitalis; chronic cardiomyopathy is cumulative dose-related and can occur years after treatment; concomitant administration of dexrazoxane may avert later cardiotoxicity
Anticancer Antibiotics—Bleomycin	Bleomycin	See Table 26-4 and text of Chapter 61 of *Goodman & Gilman's The Pharmacological Basis of Therapeutics*, 12th Edition for uses of specific agents	Skin toxicities, including hyperpigmentation, hyperkeratosis, erythema, ulceration, and rarely Raynaud's phenomenon Other toxicities include hyperthermia, headache, nausea and vomiting, and a peculiar acute fulminant reaction in ~1% patients with lymphomas or testicular cancer	Pulmonary toxicity (1-5% of patients), which begins with a dry cough, fine rales, and diffuse basilar infiltrates on X-ray and may progress to life-threatening pulmonary fibrosis (~1% die); risk of pulmonary toxicity is related to total dose
Anticancer Antibiotics—Mitomycin	Mitomycin (mitomycin-C)	See Table 45-4 and text of Chapter 61 of *Goodman & Gilman's The Pharmacological Basis of Therapeutics*, 12th Edition for uses of specific agents	Myelosuppression, characterized by marked leukopenia and thrombocytopenia	A hemolytic uremic syndrome (hemolysis, neurological abnormalities, interstitial pneumonia, and glomerular damage resulting in renal failure) believed to result from drug-induced endothelial damage; toxicity increases with dose (28% renal failure in total high dose); early recognition and immediate discontinuation of drug is needed to minimize toxicity Interstitial pulmonary fibrosis Heart failure, especially in combination with doxorubicin

(Continued)

Cancer Chemotherapy and Cytotoxic Agents — CHAPTER 45

CLASS AND SUBCLASSES	NAMES	CLINICAL USES	TOXICITIES — COMMON	TOXICITIES — UNIQUE; CLINICALLY IMPORTANT
Trabectedin	Trabectedin	Approved outside the United States for second-line treatment of soft tissue sarcomas and ovarian cancer in combination with doxorubicin	Mild myelosuppression	Significant hepatic enzyme elevations and fatigue in one-third of patients, but with dexamethasone pretreatment transaminase increases are less pronounced and rapidly reversed Rhabdomyolysis (rarely)
Enzymes	L-asparaginase (L-ASP Pegaspargase (PEG-L-asparaginase)	See Table 45-4 and text of Chapter 61 of Goodman & Gilman's The Pharmacological Basis of Therapeutics, 12th Edition for uses of specific agents	Toxicities resulting from inhibition of protein synthesis in normal tissues (eg, hyperglycemia due to insulin deficiency, clotting abnormalities due to deficient clotting factors, hypertriglyceridemia due to effects on lipoprotein production, hypoalbuminemia)	Hypersensitivity reactions to L-ASP, including urticaria and full-blown anaphylaxis, occur in 5-20% of patients and may be fatal; pegaspargase is a safe and effective alternative in patients who show hypersensitivity to L-ASP "Silent" enzyme inactivation by antibodies occurs in a higher percentage of patients than overt hypersensitivity and may be associated with a negative clinical outcome, especially in high-risk ALL patients Pancreatitis Dysregulated coagulation (thrombosis and hemorrhage)
Mitotane	Mitotane (*o,p'*-DDD)	Adrenal cortex cancer	Anorexia and nausea in most patients, somnolence and lethargy in ~34%, and dermatitis in 15-20%	Because of drug-induced adrenal cortex damage, adrenocorticosteroid replacement therapy is necessary
Hydroxyurea (HU)	Hydroxyurea (HU)	See Table 45-5 and text of Chapter 61 of Goodman & Gilman's The Pharmacological Basis of Therapeutics, 12th Edition for uses of specific agents	Myelosuppression, which is rapidly reversible with drug discontinuation Desquamative interstitial pneumonitis, GI disturbances, and dermatological reactions (including increased pigmentation and painful leg ulcers)	Potent teratogen; should not be used in women with childbearing potential
Differentiating Agents—Retinoids	Tretinoin (all-trans retinoic acid, ATRA)	See Table 45-5 and text of Chapter 61 of Goodman & Gilman's The Pharmacological Basis of Therapeutics, 12th Edition for uses of specific agents	Dry skin, cheilitis, reversible hepatic enzyme abnormalities, bone tenderness, pseudotumor cerebri, hypercalcemia, and hyperlipidemia	"Differentiation syndrome" or "retinoic acid syndrome" caused by an outpouring of cytokines and mature-appearing neutrophils of leukemic origin results in a syndrome of respiratory distress, fever, pulmonary infiltrates pleural and pericardial effusions, and mental status changes that affect 15-20% of patients and may have a fatal outcome; mitigated by dexamethasone pretreatment

(Continued)

SECTION VIII: Chemotherapy of Neoplastic Diseases

CLASS AND SUBCLASSES	NAMES	CLINICAL USES	TOXICITIES COMMON	TOXICITIES UNIQUE; CLINICALLY IMPORTANT
Differentiating Agents—Arsenic Trioxide	Arsenic trioxide (ATO)	See Table 45-5 and text of Chapter 61 of *Goodman & Gilman's The Pharmacological Basis of Therapeutics*, 12th Edition for uses of specific agents	Reversible side effects include hyperglycemia, hepatic enzyme elevations, fatigue, dysesthesias, and light-headedness	Differentiation syndrome similar to ATRA in 10% of patients which is reversed by oxygen, corticosteroids, and temporary discontinuation of ATO. Prolongation of QTc interval in 40% of patients (***torsades de pointes*** is rare); monitor serum electrolytes, treat hypokalemia, and avoid using ATO with other QT-prolonging drugs (see Chapter 18)
Differentiating Agents—HDAC Inhibitors	Vorinostat (suberoylanilide hydroxamic acid, SAHA) Romidepsin (depsipeptide)	See Table 45-5 and text of Chapter 61 of *Goodman & Gilman's The Pharmacological Basis of Therapeutics*, 12th Edition for uses of specific agents	Fatigue, nausea, diarrhea, and thrombocytopenia	Deep venous thrombosis and pulmonary embolism with vorinostat. Prolongation of QTc interval with vorinostat, requiring caution when used in patients with underlying cardiac disease, careful monitoring of the QTc interval, and correction of electrolyte (K^+, Mg^{++}) abnormalities, and avoidance of use with other QT-prolonging drugs (see Chapter 18)

CHAPTER 46

Targeted Anticancer Therapies

This chapter will be most useful after having a basic understanding of the material in Chapter 62 Targeted Therapies: Tyrosine Kinase Inhibitors, Monoclonal Antibodies, and Cytokines, and Chapter 63 Natural Products in Cancer Chemotherapy: Hormones, in *Goodman & Gilman's The Pharmacological Basis of Therapeutics*, 12th Edition. In addition to the material presented here, the 12th Edition contains:

- A discussion of the use of targeted anticancer therapies in combination with cytotoxic agents in Chapter 60 General Principles of Cancer Chemotherapy
- The molecular structures of small molecule drugs used in targeted anticancer therapies

LEARNING OBJECTIVES

- ☑ Understand the mechanisms of action and clinical uses of small molecule inhibitors of protein tyrosine kinases.
- ☑ Understand the mechanisms of action and clinical uses of monoclonal antibodies that target growth factor receptors and other tumor cell antigens.
- ☑ Understand the mechanisms of action and clinical uses of monoclonal antibodies that target the VEGF pathway.
- ☑ Understand the mechanism of action and clinical uses of anticancer drugs that target the mTOR pathway, and proteosome-mediated protein degradation.
- ☑ Understand the mechanism of action and clinical uses of anticancer drugs that target the IL-2 receptor.
- ☑ Understand the clinical uses of the immunomodulatory analogs (IMiDs) in treating multiple myeloma and myelodysplastic syndrome.
- ☑ Understand the mechanism of action and use of hormone therapy to treat hormone-dependent tumors.
- ☑ Know the common and important toxicities of targeted anticancer pharmacotherapies.
- ☑ Know mechanisms of acquired resistance to specific targeted anticancer therapies.

DRUGS INCLUDED IN THIS CHAPTER

- ^{131}I-Tositumomab (BEXXAR)
- ^{90}Y-Ibritumomab tiuxetan (ZEVALIN)
- Abarelix (PLENAXIS; withdrawn from market)
- Abiraterone (ZYTIGA)
- Aldesleukin (IL-2; PROLEUKIN)
- Alemtuzumab (CAMPATH)
- Anastrozole (ARIMIDEX)
- Bevacizumab (AVASTIN)
- Bicalutamide (CASODEX, others)
- Bortezomib (VELCADE)
- Buserelin (SUPREFACT)—not available in the United States
- Cetrorelix (CETROTIDE)
- Cetuximab (ERBITUX)
- Cyproterone—not available in the United States
- Dasatinib (BMS-354825; SPRYCEL)
- Degarelix (FIRMAGON)
- Denileukin diftitox (ONTAK)
- Deslorelin—not available in the United States
- Dexamethasone
- Erlotinib (TARCEVA)
- Everolimus (AFINITOR)
- Exemestane (AROMASIN)
- Flutamide (EULEXIN)
- Fulvestrant (FASLODEX)
- Ganirelix—not available in the United States
- Gefitinib (IRESSA)
- Gemtuzumab ozogamicin (MYLOTARG)— withdrawn from the US market in 2010
- GnRH (GONADORELIN)
- Goserelin (ZOLADEX)
- Histrelin (VANTAS)
- Imatinib mesylate (STI 571; GLEEVEC, GLIVEC)
- Ketoconazole (NIZORAL)
- Lapatinib (TYKERB)
- Lenalidomide (REVLIMID)

(continues)

MECHANISMS OF ACTION AND RESISTANCE OF TARGETED ANTICANCER DRUGS

DRUG CLASS	DRUG	MECHANISM OF ACTION	MECHANISM OF RESISTANCE
Protein Tyrosine Kinase Inhibitors— ATP Inhibitors	Imatinib mesylate Dasatinib Nilotinib Gefitinib Erlotinib Lapatinib Sunitinib Sorafenib	Inhibit disease-causing tyrosine kinase activity, usually by blocking ATP binding to the catalytic site VEGFR inhibitors (sunitinib and sorafenib) block angiogenesis	Point mutations in kinases that lower drug affinity and alter drug effects on kinase activity Amplification of kinase gene Drug efflux, activation of downstream pathways, and altered kinase trafficking are also possible

(Continued)

SECTION VIII

Chemotherapy of Neoplastic Diseases

DRUGS INCLUDED IN THIS CHAPTER (Cont.)

- Letrozole (FEMARA)
- Leuprolide (LUPRON, ELIGARD)
- Medroxyprogesterone (DEPO-PROVERA, others)
- Megestrol (MEGACE)
- Megestrol acetate (MEGACE, others)
- Nafarelin (SYNAREL)
- Nilotinib (AMN107; TASIGNA)
- Nilutamide (NILANDRON)
- Ofatumumab (ARZERRA)
- Panitumumab (VECTIBIX)
- Pazopanib (VOTRIENT)
- Prednisone
- Raloxifene (EVISTA)
- Ranibizumab (LUCENTIS)
- Rapamycin (sirolimus; RAPAMUNE)
- Rituximab (RITUXAN)
- Sorafenib (NEXAVAR)
- Sunitinib (SUTENT)
- Tamoxifen (NOLVADEX, others)
- Temsirolimus (TORISEL)
- Thalidomide (THALOMID)
- Toremifene (FARESTON)
- Trastuzumab (HERCEPTIN)
- Triptorelin (TRELSTAR, TRELSTARDEPOT)

DRUG CLASS	DRUG	MECHANISM OF ACTION	MECHANISM OF RESISTANCE
Monoclonal Antibodies—Growth Factor Receptors (EGFR, HER2/neu, VEGFRs, PDGFR) Antibodies	Cetuximab Panitumumab Trastuzumab	Binds the extracellular domain of the growth factor which prevents receptor activation and downstream signaling, downregulates receptor expression, and induces antibody-dependent cellular cytotoxicity (ADCC) (see Table 46-1)	
Monoclonal Antibodies—Growth Factor (VEGF) Antibodies	Bevacizumab Ranibizumab	Binds the ligand(s) of growth factor receptors, blocking interaction of the ligand with its cognate receptor (see Table 46-1)	
Monoclonal Antibodies—CD20 Antibodies	Rituximab ^{131}I-Tositumomab ^{90}Y-Ibritumomab tiuxetan Ofatumumab	Binds CD20 antigen on B-cell lymphoma and chronic lymphocytic leukemia (CLL) cells which inhibits CD20-mediated proliferation and differentiation (see Table 46-1) The radionuclide-conjugated antibodies target delivery of radiation to CD20-containing tumor cells (see Table 46-1) Ofatumumab causes B-cell lysis (both ADCC and complement-dependent cytotoxicity [CDC])	Downregulation of CD20 Genetic polymorphisms of target antigen Impaired antibody-dependent cellular cytotoxicity Decreased complement activation Limited effects on signaling and induction of apoptosis
Monoclonal Antibodies—CD52 Antibodies	Alemtuzumab	Binds CD52 antigen on B-cell CLL and T-cell lymphoma, causing tumor cell death through ADCC and CDC (see Table 46-1)	Genetic polymorphisms of target antigen
Monoclonal Antibodies—CD33 Antibodies	Gemtuzumab ozogamicin	Binds CD33 on acute myelocytic leukemia (AML) cells and other hemopoietic cells; following binding to CD33 and endocytosis, calicheamicin (the toxin) is cleaved from gemtuzumab ozogamicin, and the toxin enters the nucleus where it causes double-strand DNA breaks and cell death (see Table 46-1)	Genetic polymorphisms of target antigen

(Continued)

Targeted Anticancer Therapies — CHAPTER 46

DRUG CLASS	DRUG	MECHANISM OF ACTION	MECHANISM OF RESISTANCE
Thalidomide and Its Derivatives (Immunomodulatory analogs, IMiDs)	Thalidomide Lenalidomide	Multiple immunomodulatory mechanisms (see Figure 46-1)	
Proteasome Inhibitors	Bortezomib	Binds the 26S proteasome and Inhibits proteasome-mediated protein degradation, particularly IκB, thus preventing the transcriptional activity of NF-κB and downregulating survival responses Proteasome inhibition also disrupts degradation of other key cell cycle regulators leading cells to apoptosis	
mTOR Inhibitors	Rapamycin Temsirolimus Everolimus	Inhibits mTORC1 in the PI3 kinase pathway (Figure 46-2)	Resistance is incompletely understood but may arise through the action of a second mTOR complex, mTORC2, which is unaffected by rapamycins and which regulates Akt kinase (see Figure 46-2)
Interleukin-2 (IL-2) Receptor Agonists	Aldesleukin Denileukin diftitox	Binds the IL-2 receptor on immune effector cells which appears to enhance tumor cell killing by activated T cells, NK cells, and monocytes Denileukin diftitox is a recombinant immunotoxin consisting of IL-2 and the active fragment of diphtheria toxin which binds the high-affinity IL-2R receptor and introduces the toxin into cells causing cell death by inhibiting protein synthesis (see Table 46-1)	
Colony-Stimulating Factors	See Chapter 25	See Chapter 25	

(Continued)

SECTION VIII Chemotherapy of Neoplastic Diseases

DRUG CLASS	DRUG	MECHANISM OF ACTION	MECHANISM OF RESISTANCE
Glucocorticoids	Prednisone Dexamethasone	Binds to specific physiological receptors that translocate to the nucleus and induce antiproliferative and apoptotic responses in sensitive cells (see Chapter 29)	
Progestins	Medroxyprogesterone Megestrol acetate	See Chapter 28	
Estrogens and Androgens	See Chapter 28	See Chapter 28	
Antiestrogens—Selective Estrogen-Receptor Modulators (SERMs)	Tamoxifen Toremifene Raloxifene	Bind to the estrogen receptor (ER) and exert either estrogenic or antiestrogenic effects, depending on the specific organ (see Chapter 28)	Polymorphisms in CYP2D6 that reduce its activity (see Figure 46-3) Cross-talk between the ER and HER2/neu pathway Altered interactions between PAX2 and the ER co-activator AIB-1/SRC-3
Antiestrogens—Selective Estrogen-Receptor Downregulators (SERDs)	Fulvestrant	Similar to SERMs but devoid of any estrogen agonist effects Estradiol antagonist Reduce the number of ER molecules in target cells	
Anti-estrogens—Aromatase (CYP19) Inhibitors	Anastrozole Letrozole Exemestane	Block aromatase conversion of androgens to estrogens (see Figure 46-4) resulting in estrogen deprivation	
Gonadotropin-Releasing Hormone (GnRH) Agonists	GnRH Leuprolide Buserelin Nafarelin Deslorelin Histrelin Triptorelin Goserelin	Bind to GnRH receptors on pituitary gonadotropin-producing cells leading to GnRH receptor down-regulation, causing inhibition of testosterone production in Leydig cells	

(Continued)

DRUG CLASS	DRUG	MECHANISM OF ACTION	MECHANISM OF RESISTANCE
Gonadotropin-Releasing Hormone (GnRH) Antagonists	Cetrorelix Ganirelix Abarelix Degarelix	Antagonize GnRH receptors on pituitary gonadotropin-producing cells, causing inhibition of testosterone production in Leydig cells without causing the initial testosterone flare caused by GnRH agonists	
Antiandrogens—Steroidal	Cyproterone Megestrol	Bind to androgen receptors (ARs) inhibiting binding of testosterone and dihydrotestosterone	
Antiandrogens—Nonsteroidal	Flutamide Bicalutamide Nilutamide	Inhibit binding of testosterone and dihydrotestosterone and consequent AR translocation from the cytoplasm to the nucleus	
Estrogens	See Chapter 28	High estrogen levels reduce testosterone via negative feedback on the hypothalamic–pituitary axis. May exert a cytotoxic effect on prostate cancer cells by competing with androgens for steroid hormone receptors	
Inhibitors of Steroidogenesis	Ketoconazole Abiraterone	Ketoconazole inhibits both testicular and adrenal steroidogenesis by blocking CYPs, primarily CYP17 (17α-hydroxylase). Abiraterone is an irreversible inhibitor of both 17α-hydroxylase and C-17,20-lyase CYP17 activity (See Figure 46-4)	

CASE 46-1

A 34-year-old man is diagnosed with Philadelphia chromosome-positive (Ph⁺) chronic myelogenous leukemia (CML).

a. What is the molecular mechanism that causes this form of cancer?

A single molecular event, in this case the 9:22 chromosomal translocation which results in the Philadelphia chromosome (Ph⁺), leads to expression of the Abelson protooncogene kinase ABL fused to BCR (breakpoint cluster region), yielding a

(Continued)

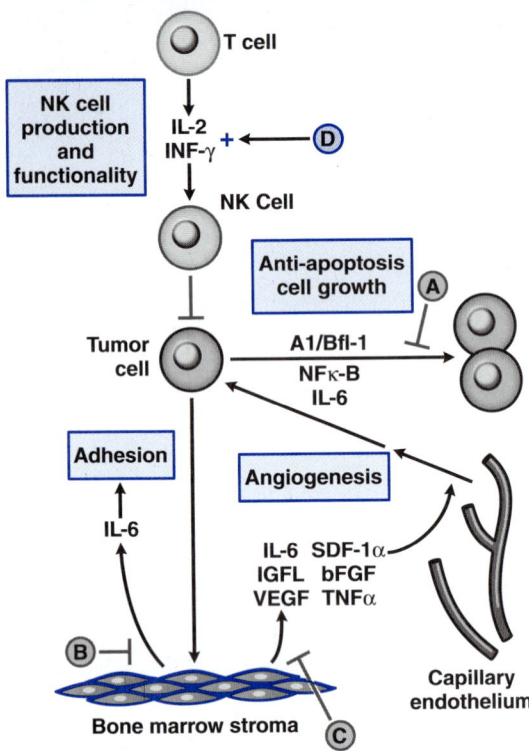

FIGURE 46-1 Schematic overview of proposed mechanisms of antimyeloma activity of thalidomide and its derivatives. Some biological hallmarks of the malignant phenotype are indicated in the boxes. The proposed sites of action for thalidomide (letters inside circles) are hypothesized to also be operative for thalidomide derivatives. **A.** Direct anti–multiple myeloma (MM) effect on tumor cells, including G1 growth arrest and/or apoptosis, even against MM cells resistant to conventional therapy. This is due to the disruption of the antiapoptotic effect of BCL-2 family members, blocking NF-κB signaling, and inhibition of the production of interleukin-6 (IL-6). **B.** Inhibition of MM-cell adhesion to bone marrow stromal cells partially due to the reduction of IL-6 release. **C.** Decreased angiogenesis due to the inhibition of cytokine and growth factor production and release. **D.** Enhanced T-cell production of cytokines, such as IL-2 and interferon-γ (IFN-γ), that increase the number and cytotoxic functionality of natural killer (NK) cells. VEGF, vascular endothelial growth factor.

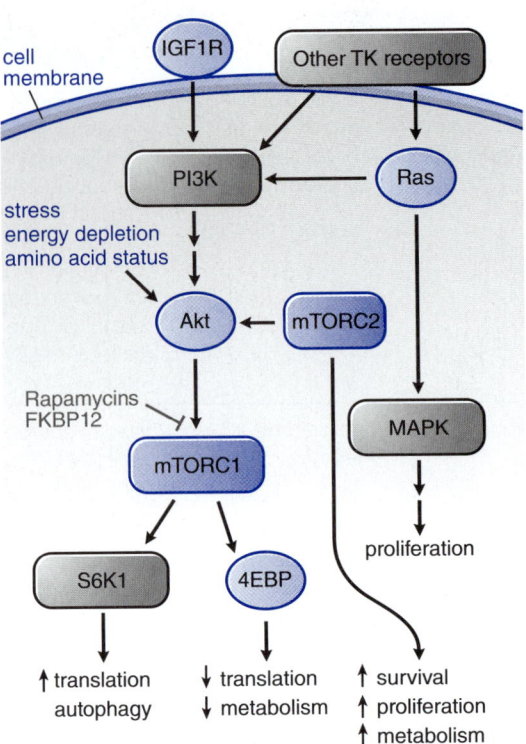

FIGURE 46-2 Insulin-like growth factor 1 receptor (IGF-1R) and other tyrosine kinase (TK) growth factor receptors signal through multiple pathways. A key pathway is regulated by phosphatidylinositol-3 kinase (PI3K) and its downstream partner, the mammalian target of rapamycin (mTOR). Rapamycins complex with FKBPP12 to inhibit the mTORC1 complex. mTORC2 remains unaffected and responds by upregulating Akt, driving signals through the inhibited mTORC1. The various downstream outputs of the 2 complexes are shown. Phosphorylation of 4EBP by mTOR inhibits the capacity of 4EBP to inhibit eif-4E and slow metabolism. 4EBP, eukaryotic initiation factor 4e (eif-4E) binding protein; FKBP12, the immunophilin target (binding protein) for tacrolimus (FK506); S6K1, S6 kinase 1.

constitutively activated protein tyrosine kinase, BCR-ABL, and then the malignant phenotype. This is the most common mechanism causing CML.

b. What is the first-line treatment for CML and what is the rationale for this pharmacotherapy?

Imatinib and the related compounds dasatinib and nilotinib induce clinical and molecular remissions in more than 90% of CML patients in the chronic phase of disease. These agents target the BCR-ABL tyrosine kinase and inhibit its activity.

c. What are the mechanisms of resistance to imatinib pharmacotherapy of CML?

Resistance to the tyrosine kinase inhibitors arises from point mutations in 3 separate segments of the BCR-ABL kinase domain. The contact points between imatinib and the enzyme become sites of mutations in drug-resistant leukemic cells; these mutations prevent tight binding of the drug and lock the enzyme in its open configuration, in which it has access to substrate. Most such mutations hold the enzyme in its open and enzymatically active confirmation. The most common resistance mutations affect amino acids 255 and 315, both of which serve as contact points

(Continued)

Targeted Anticancer Therapies

TABLE 46-1 Monoclonal Antibodies Approved for Hematopoietic and Solid Tumors

ANTIGEN AND TUMOR CELL TARGETS	ANTIGEN FUNCTION	NAKED ANTIBODIES	RADIOISOTOPE-BASED ANTIBODIES	TOXIN-BASED ANTIBODIES
Antigen: CD20				
Tumor type: B-cell lymphoma and CLL	Proliferation/differentiation	Rituximab (chimeric)	^{131}I-tositumomab; ^{90}Y-ibritumomab tiuxetan	None
Antigen: CD52				
Tumor type: B-cell CLL and T-cell lymphoma	Unknown	Alemtuzumab (humanized)	None	None
Antigen: CD33				
Tumor type: acute myelocytic leukemia	Unknown	Gemtuzumab (humanized)	None	Gemtuzumab ozogamicin
Antigen: HER2/neu (ErbB2)				
Tumor type: breast cancer	Tyrosine kinase	Trastuzumab (humanized)	None	None
Antigen: EGFR (ErbB1)				
Tumor type: colorectal, NSCLC, pancreatic, breast	Tyrosine kinase	Cetuximab (chimeric) Panitumumab (humanized)	None	None
Antigen: VEGF				
Tumor type: colorectal cancer	Angiogenesis	Bevacizumab (humanized)	None	None

CLL, chronic lymphocytic leukemia; EGFR, epidermal growth factor receptor; NSCLC, non-small cell lung cancer; VEGF, vascular endothelial growth factor.

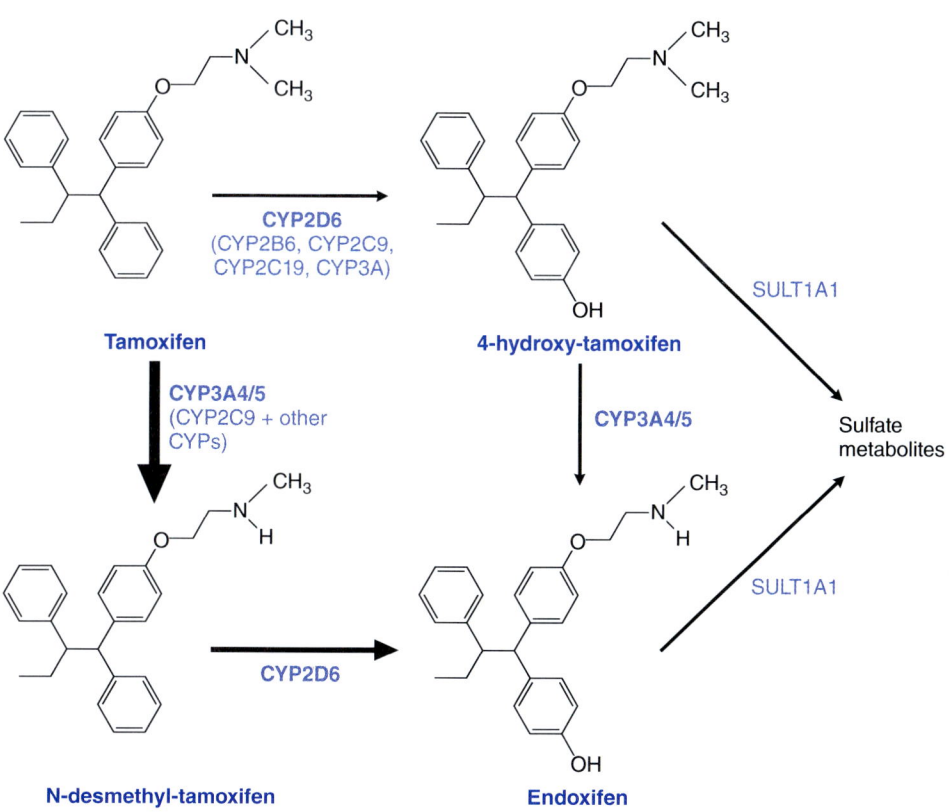

FIGURE 46-3 Tamoxifen and its metabolites.

SECTION VIII Chemotherapy of Neoplastic Diseases

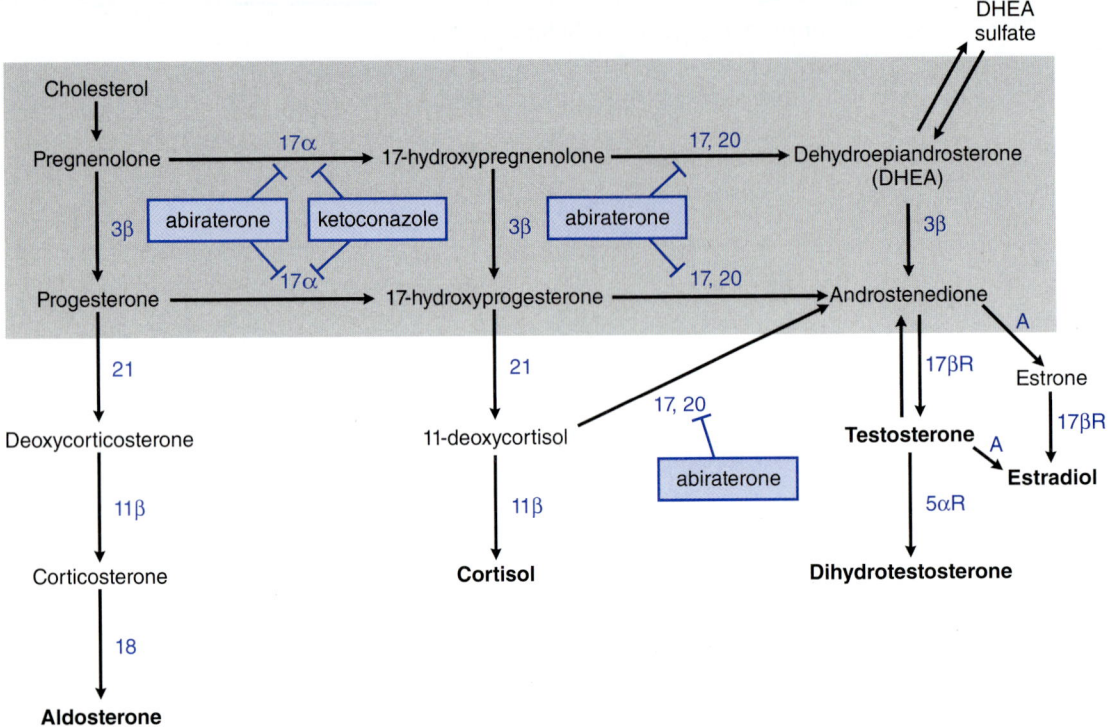

FIGURE 46-4 Steroid synthesis pathways. The enclosed shaded area contains the pathways used by the adrenal glands and gonads. Enzymes are shown next to their respective biochemical pathways, inhibitors are shown in boxes with T-shaped arrows pointing at the enzymes they inhibit. 11β, 11β-hydroxylase; 17,20, C-17,20-lyase (also CYP17); 17α, 17α-hydroxylase (CYP17); 17βR, 17β-reductase; 18, aldosterone synthase; 21, 21-hydroxylase; 3β, 3β-hydroxysteroid dehydrogenase; 5αR, 5α-reductase; A, aromatase.

for imatinib; these mutations confer high-level resistance to imatinib and nilotinib. Dasatinib is unaffected by mutation at 255 but is ineffective in the presence of mutation at 315. Nilotinib retains inhibitory activity in the presence of most point mutations (except at 315) that confer resistance to imatinib.

Other mutations affect the phosphate-binding region and the "activation loop" of the domain with varying degrees of associated resistance. Some mutations, such as at amino acids 351 and 355, do not affect response to dasatinib or nilotinib but confer low levels of resistance to imatinib.

Molecular studies of circulating tumor cells have detected resistance-mediating kinase mutations prior to initiation of therapy, particularly in patients with Ph+ acute lymphoblastic leukemia (ALL) or CML in blastic crisis. This finding strongly supports the hypothesis that drug-resistant cells arise through spontaneous mutation and expand under the selective pressure of drug exposure. Mutations may become detectable in the peripheral blood of patients receiving imatinib in the accelerated phase and in the late (>4 years from diagnosis) chronic phase of CML, heralding the onset of drug resistance.

Mechanisms other than BCR-ABL kinase mutation play a minor role in resistance to imatinib. Amplification of the wild-type kinase gene, leading to overexpression of the enzyme, has been identified in tumor samples from patients resistant to treatment. The multidrug resistant (MDR) gene, which codes for a drug efflux protein, confers resistance experimentally but has not been implicated in clinical resistance. Finally, Philadelphia chromosome-negative clones lacking the BCR-ABL translocation and displaying the karyotype of myelodysplastic cells may emerge in patients receiving imatinib for CML and may progress to myelodysplasia (MDS) and to acute myelocytic leukemia (AML). Their origin is unclear.

(Continued)

Targeted Anticancer Therapies — CHAPTER 46

d. **What other cancers and diseases are effectively treated with imatinib?**

Imatinib has efficacy in diseases in which the ABL, kit, or PDGFR protein kinases have dominant roles in driving the proliferation of the tumor, reflecting the presence of a mutation that results in constitutive activation of the kinase, either by fusion with another protein or via point mutations. Thus, imatinib shows remarkable therapeutic benefits in patients with chronic-phase CML (BCR-ABL), GIST (*kit* mutation-positive gastrointestinal stromal tumor), chronic myelomonocytic leukemia (EVT6-PDGFR translocation), hypereosinophilia syndrome (FIP1L1-PDGFR), and dermatofibrosarcoma protuberans (constitutive production of the ligand for PDGFR). It is the agent of choice for GIST patients with metastatic disease and as adjuvant therapy of *c-kit*-positive GIST. GIST biology is particularly instructive, as patients with an exon 11 mutation of *kit* have a significantly higher partial response rate (72%) than those with no detectable *kit* mutations (9%).

e. **What are the common and important side effects of therapy with imatinib, dasatinib, and nilotinib?**

Imatinib, dasatinib, and nilotinib cause GI distress (diarrhea, nausea, and vomiting), but these symptoms usually are easily controlled. All 3 drugs promote fluid retention, which may lead to dependent edema, and periorbital swelling. Dasatinib may cause pleural effusions. Nilotinib may prolong the QT interval, and should be used with caution in patients with underlying heart disease or arrhythmias, although ventricular arrhythmias have not been reported. Significant myelosuppression occurs infrequently but may require transfusion support, dose reduction, or discontinuation of the drug. All 3 drugs in this class can be associated with hepatotoxicity. Most nonhematological adverse reactions are self-limited and respond to dose adjustments. After the adverse reactions such as edema, myelosuppression, or GI symptoms have been resolved, the drug may be reinitiated and titrated back to effective doses.

CASE 46-2

In a number of epithelial cancers, the epidermal growth factor receptor (EGFR) is overexpressed or is activated by mutations.

a. **What role does the EGFR play in these epithelial cancers?**

The EGFR belongs to the ErbB family of transmembrane receptor tyrosine kinases. EGFR, also known as ErbB1 or HER1, is essential for the growth and differentiation of epithelial cells. Ligand binding to the extracellular domain of EGFR family members causes receptor dimerization and stimulates the protein tyrosine kinase activity of the intracellular domain, resulting in autophosphorylation of several Tyr residues in the C-terminal domain. Recognition of the phosphotyrosines by other proteins initiates protein-protein interactions that result in stimulation of a variety of signaling pathways, including MAPK, PI3K/Akt, and STAT pathways (see Figures 46-2 and 46-5). In epithelial cancers, overexpression (or mutational activations) of the EGFR is a common finding and, to some extent, creates a dependence on EGFR signaling in these tumors.

b. **What drugs are available to target the EGFR in epithelial cancers?**

Two separate classes of drugs that target the EGFR pathway have become important agents in the therapy of solid tumors. The EGFR tyrosine kinase inhibitors erlotinib and gefitinib bind to the kinase domain and block the enzymatic function of EGFR. The monoclonal antibodies cetuximab and panitumumab (see Table 46-1) bind specifically to the extracellular domain of EGFR. They inhibit EGFR-dependent signaling through inhibition of ligand-dependent activation and receptor dimerization, downregulation of EGFR expression, and induction of antibody-dependent cell-mediated cytotoxicity.

(Continued)

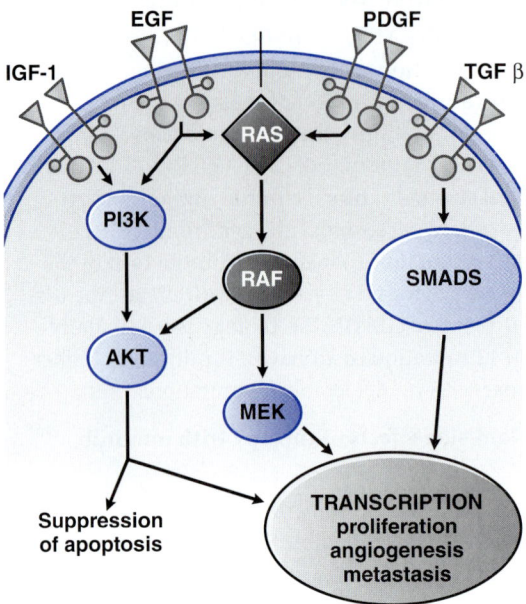

FIGURE 46-5 Growth factor signaling. Binding of agonist ligands to growth factor receptors causes receptor dimerization and activation of cytosolic protein kinase domains, leading to activation of multiple signaling pathways. Shown here are the RAS/MAPK/ ERK, PI3K, and SMAD pathways, each of which is activated by receptors or cross-talk from adjacent pathways. Their signals regulate proliferation, metabolism, survival, and the synthesis of other growth factors, such as the vascular endothelial growth factor (VEGF).

c. **What kinds of epithelial cancers are effectively treated with EGFR-targeted agents?**

Erlotinib is approved for first-line treatment of patients with locally advanced, unresectable, or metastatic pancreatic cancer in combination with gemcitabine, and is also approved for second-line treatment of patients with locally advanced or metastatic non–small cell lung cancer.

Gefitinib initially was approved for the third-line treatment of patients with non–small cell lung cancer based on promising results in 2 small clinical trials. However, a larger, randomized, placebo-controlled trial failed to show an effect on survival, leading the FDA to restrict its use to patients who have previously received clinical benefit from the drug. Gefitinib continues to be widely used outside the United States.

Retrospective analysis of multiple studies has revealed that patients who were nonsmokers, Asians, or women were most likely to respond to gefitinib. Tumors from these patients frequently have characteristic activating mutations in EGFR. These mutations mostly fall into 2 groups: (1) small in-frame deletions within exon 19 and (2) the L858R point mutation. Trials that randomized never- and light-smoking patients to first-line gefitinib or to chemotherapy demonstrated a 70% response rate to gefitinib in patients with an activating EGFR mutation, compared with responses in only 1% in patients without an EGFR mutation. In patients with EGFR-mutant tumors, the response rate to gefitinib was double the response to standard chemotherapy. Therefore, mounting evidence supports the use of gefitinib, and potentially erlotinib, as first-line therapy in patients selected for the presence of sensitizing EGFR mutations.

Cetuximab won FDA approval based on an improvement in overall survival when used in combination with radiation therapy for locally or regionally advanced squamous cell carcinoma of the head and neck (HNSCC). It received a second indication as monotherapy for patients with metastatic or recurrent HNSCC who had

(Continued)

failed platinum-based chemotherapy. It has become a useful agent in combination with cisplatin-based chemotherapy, where it has shown an improvement in survival compared to chemotherapy alone.

Panitumumab improves progression-free survival in patients with metastatic colorectal carcinoma, as demonstrated in patients with EGFR-expressing tumors who had 2 or more previous therapies.

d. What are the common and important toxicities of EGFR-targeted agents?

The most common adverse reactions in patients receiving erlotinib and gefitinib are diarrhea, an acneform rash, anorexia, and fatigue. Most adverse effects occur within the first month of therapy and are tolerable when managed with supportive medications and dose reductions. Cetuximab therapy is associated with infusion-related toxicity and skin rash in 75% of treated patients (see Table 46-2).

Serious or fatal interstitial lung disease, often associated with symptoms of cough and dyspnea, occurs with a frequency of 0.7 to 2.5%.

Hepatic function deserves close monitoring because serious or fatal hepatic failure due to erlotinib has been reported, particularly in patients with baseline hepatic dysfunction. Asymptomatic increases in liver transaminases with gefitinib may necessitate dose reduction or discontinuation of therapy.

Other rare but serious toxicities with erlotinib therapy include GI perforation, renal failure, arterial thrombosis, microangiopathic hemolytic anemia, hand-foot skin reaction, and corneal perforation or ulceration. Erlotinib therapy may cause rare cases of Stevens-Johnson syndrome/toxic epidermal necrolysis.

(Continued)

TABLE 46-2 Dose and Toxicity of Monoclonal Antibody-Based Drugs

DRUG	MECHANISM	DOSE AND SCHEDULE	MAJOR TOXICITY
Rituximab	ADCC; CDC; apoptosis	375-mg/m^2 IV infusion weekly for 4 weeks	Infusion-related toxicity with fever, rash, and dyspnea; B-cell depletion; late-onset neutropenia
Alemtuzumab	ADCC; CDC; apoptosis	Escalating doses of 3, 10, 30 mg/m^2 IV three times/week followed by 30 mg/m^2 three times/week for 4-12 weeks	Infusion-related toxicity, T-cell depletion with increased infection; hematopoietic suppression; pancytopenia
Trastuzumab	ADCC; apoptosis; inhibition of arrest HER2 signaling with G$_1$ arrest	Loading dose of 4-mg/kg infusion followed by 2 mg/kg weekly	Cardiomyopathy; infusion-related toxicity
Cetuximab	Inhibition of EGFR signaling; apoptosis; ADCC	Loading dose of 400-mg/kg infusion followed by 250 mg/kg weekly	Infusion-related toxicity; skin rash in 75%
Bevacizumab	Inhibition of angiogenesis/neovascularization	5 mg/kg IV every 14 days until disease progression	Hypertension; pulmonary hemorrhage; GI perforation; proteinuria; congestive heart failure
Denileukin diftitox	Targeted diphtheria toxin with inhibition of protein synthesis	9-18 µg/kg/day IV for the first 5 days every 3 weeks	Fever; arthralgia; asthenia; hypotension
Gemtuzumab ozogamicin	Double-strand DNA breaks and apoptosis	Two doses of 9 mg/m^2 IV separated by 14 days	Infusion-related toxicity; hematopoietic suppression; mucosal hepatic (VOD); skin toxicity
^{90}Y-ibritumomab tiuxetan	Targeted radiotherapy	0.4 mCi/kg IV	Hematological toxicity; myelodysplasia
^{131}I-tositumomab	Targeted radiotherapy	Patient-specific dosimetry	Hematological toxicity; myelodysplasia

ADCC, antibody-dependent cellular cytotoxicity; CDC, complement-dependent cytotoxicity; EGFR, epidermal growth factor receptor; intravenous; VOD, veno-occlusive disease.

e. **What are the mechanisms of resistance to EGFR-targeted agents?**

Patients with non–small cell lung cancer who initially respond to erlotinib or gefitinib have tumors that are dependent on the EGFR signaling pathway. Clinical response to these agents is strongly associated with the presence of sensitizing mutations in *EGFR* as described in the answer to part c above, but response is less strongly correlated with overexpression or amplification of EGFR.

Tumors containing mutations in *EGFR* initially respond to erlotinib and gefitinib but eventually progress. Resistance arises through several different mechanisms. A secondary mutation in the EGFR gatekeeper residue, T790M, prevents binding of drug to the kinase domain and confers resistance. Irreversible EGFR inhibitors currently are in clinical development to overcome this mechanism.

Amplification of the *MET* oncogene provides an alternative pathway to clinical resistance by activating cell growth signals downstream of EGFR. *MET*-amplified tumors respond in vitro to the simultaneous inhibition of EGFR and MET. Other potential mechanisms of resistance include activation of downstream mediators, efflux of drug, and altered receptor trafficking. The subset of non–small cell lung tumors harboring *k-ras* mutations and *EML4-ALK* translocations do not respond to EGFR inhibitors.

CASE 46-3

A 58-year-old woman is diagnosed with metastatic *Her2/neu*-positive (*Her2*⁺) breast cancer.

a. **What is *Her2/neu* and how does this patient's *Her2/neu*-positive status affect her prognosis and the available therapeutic options?**

Thirty percent of breast cancers overexpress the HER2/neu (ErbB2) receptor due to gene amplification on chromosome 17. Amplification of the receptor is associated with lower response rates to hormonal therapies and to most cytotoxic drugs, with the exception of anthracyclines. Patients with HER2/neu-amplified tumors have higher recurrence rates after standard adjuvant therapy and poorer overall survival, as compared to patients with HER2-nonamplified tumors. The internal domain of the HER2/neu glycoprotein encodes a tyrosine kinase that activates downstream signaling, enhances metastatic potential, and inhibits apoptosis.

Both antibodies (trastuzumab) and small molecules (lapatinib and others in clinical trial) have striking antitumor effects in patients with *Her2*-positive breast cancer, and have become essential therapeutic agents in combination with cytotoxic chemotherapy for this aggressive malignancy.

Currently, trastuzumab is approved for HER2/neu-overexpressing metastatic breast cancer, in combination with paclitaxel as initial treatment or as monotherapy following chemotherapy relapse. Trastuzumab synergizes with other cytotoxic agents in HER2/neu-overexpressing cancers. Lapatinib is FDA-approved for HER2-amplified, trastuzumab-refractory breast cancer, in combination with the fluoropyrimidine analog, capecitabine (see Chapter 45). As a small molecule, lapatinib crosses the blood-brain barrier more readily than inhibitor antibodies and has produced anecdotal responses in patients with brain metastases and decreased the incidence of brain metastases in its phase III trial.

b. **What are the mechanisms of action of the ErbB2-targeted agents?**

Trastuzumab exerts its antitumor effects through several putative mechanisms of action: inhibition of homo- or heterodimerization of receptor, thereby preventing receptor kinase activation and downstream signaling; initiation of Fcγ-receptor-mediated antibody-dependent cellular cytotoxicity; and blockade of the angiogenetic effects of HER2 signaling.

Small molecules can inhibit receptor tyrosine kinase activity of ErbB2 (HER2/neu) and have antitumor activity in patients who have developed progressive disease

(Continued)

Targeted Anticancer Therapies

CHAPTER 46

on trastuzumab. Lapatinib and other pan-HER inhibitors block both ErbB1 and ErbB2 and bind to an internal site on the receptor (usually the ATP-binding pocket), compared to the external binding site of trastuzumab. Lapatinib also inhibits a truncated form of the HER2 receptor that lacks a trastuzumab-binding domain. These differences may account for the activity of lapatinib in trastuzumab-resistant patients.

c. **What other types of cancers express HER2/neu?**

HER2/neu expression is also found in subsets of patients with gastric, esophageal, lung, and other solid tumors, but clinical studies of the effects of trastuzumab in these tumors have not yet been completed.

d. **What are the important toxicities of the HER2/neu-targeted agents?**

The infusional effects of trastuzumab are typical of other monoclonal antibodies and include fever, chills, nausea, dyspnea, and rashes. Premedication with diphenhydramine and acetaminophen is indicated.

The most serious toxicity of trastuzumab is cardiac failure (see Table 46-2); reasons for cardiotoxicity are poorly understood, although the HER2 antigen is highly expressed in the developing heart during embryogenesis, and HER2 knockout mice fail to survive because of cardiomyopathy. Cardiac failure is a potentially disabling or fatal side effect unless it is recognized early and the drug is discontinued. Before initializing therapy, baseline electrocardiogram and cardiac ejection fraction measurement should be obtained to rule out underlying heart disease, and patients deserve careful clinical follow-up thereafter for signs or symptoms of congestive heart failure, such as cough, weight gain, or edema. When trastuzumab is used as a single agent, less than 5% of patients will experience a decrease in left-ventricular ejection fraction, and 1% will have clinical signs of congestive failure. However, left-ventricular dysfunction occurs in up to 20% of patients who received the antibody in combination with doxorubicin and cyclophosphamide. The risk of cardiac toxicity is greatly reduced with taxane–trastuzumab combinations.

Lapatinib toxicities include mild diarrhea, cramping, and exacerbation of gastroesophageal reflux. When lapatinib is combined with capecitabine, diarrhea becomes a significant side effect in one-third of patients. Lapatinib's inhibition of ErbB1 (EGFR) causes an acneform rash in one-third of patients; the rash can be effectively controlled in most cases with topical or oral antibiotics and topical benzoyl peroxide gel.

Unlike trastuzumab, lapatinib has not produced a clear signal of cardiac toxicity. Nonetheless, because it targets ErbB2, lapatinib should be used with caution in combination with other cardiotoxic drugs and with careful surveillance in patients who have underlying heart disease.

CASE 46-4

Angiogenesis is an essential property of many solid tumors, and the target of a number of anticancer drugs. One clinically important angiogenic pathway involves vascular endothelial growth factor (VEGF) and its cognate receptors.

a. **What is VEGF and how is it important in tumor growth and survival?**

Cancer cells secrete angiogenic factors that induce the formation of new blood vessels and guarantee the flow of nutrients to the tumor cells. Angiogenic factors secreted by tumors include VEGF (vascular endothelial growth factor), FGF (fibroblast growth factor), TGF-β (transforming growth factor β), and PDGF (platelet-derived growth factor). Multiple tumor types overexpress these angiogenic factors.

The best studied of the angiogenic factors is VEGF. VEGF initiates endothelial cell proliferation when it binds to a member of the VEGF receptor (VEGFR) family, a group of highly homologous receptors with intracellular tyrosine kinase domains

(Continued)

that includes VEGFR1 (FLT1), VEGFR2 (KDR), and VEGFR3 (FLT4). The binding of VEGF to its receptor activates the intracellular VEGFR tyrosine kinase activity and initiates mitogenic and antiapoptotic signaling pathways within the endothelial cell.

b. What agents target the VEGF pathway and what are their mechanisms of action?

Antibodies targeting VEGF, such as bevacizumab, sterically hinder the interaction of VEGF with its receptor. As an alternative to VEGF antibody therapy, the investigational drug aflibercept (VEGF Trap), a recombinant molecule that utilizes the VEGFR1-binding domain to sequester VEGF, acts as a "soluble decoy receptor" for VEGF. Alternatively, the propagation of proangiogenic signals can be abrogated by the inhibition of the tyrosine kinase activity of VEGFR. Three small molecules (pazopanib, sorafenib, and sunitinib) that inhibit the kinase function of VEGFR-2 have been approved for clinical use.

c. What kinds of tumors are effectively treated with agents that target the VEGF pathway?

As a single agent, bevacizumab delays progression of renal-cell cancer, and, in combination with cytotoxic chemotherapy, effectively treats lung, colorectal, and breast cancers. Bevacizumab is also approved as a single agent following prior therapy for glioblastoma.

Sunitinib competitively inhibits the binding of ATP to the tyrosine kinase domain on the VEGFR-2, and also inhibits other protein tyrosine kinases (FLT3, PDGFR-α, PDGFR-β, RET, CSF-1R, and c-KIT). Sunitinib has activity in metastatic renal-cell cancer, producing a higher response rate (31%) and a longer progression-free survival than any other approved antiangiogenic drug. Sunitinib also is approved for treatment of advanced renal-cell carcinoma and GIST that have developed resistance to imatinib as a consequence of c-KIT mutations.

Sorafenib, like sunitinib, targets multiple protein tyrosine kinases (VEGFR1, VEGFR2, VEGFR3, PDGFR-β, c-KIT, FLT-3, and b-RAF). Sorafenib is the only drug currently approved for treatment of hepatocellular carcinoma. It is also generally the preferred first-line therapy in metastatic renal-cell cancer.

d. What are the important toxicities of the agents that target the VEGF pathway?

The main toxicities of bevacizumab (see Table 46-2) are shared by all antiangiogenic inhibitors, including sunitinib and sorafenib. Specifically, patients taking this class of antiangiogenic agents can experience bleeding, hypertension, proteinuria, and uncommonly, arterial thromboembolic events and intestinal perforation. However, because sunitinib is a multitargeted tyrosine kinase inhibitor, it has a broader side effect profile than bevacizumab.

A prominent concern with this class of agents is the potential for vessel injury and bleeding. Bevacizumab is contraindicated for patients who have a history of hemoptysis, brain metastasis, or a bleeding diathesis, but in appropriately selected patients, the rate of life-threatening pulmonary hemorrhage is less than 2%. The safety of operating on patients treated with bevacizumab continues to be a major concern because of the risk of bleeding and poor wound healing; elective surgery should be delayed for at least 4 weeks from the last dose of antibody, and treatment should not be resumed for at least 4 weeks after surgery.

Other toxicity characteristics of antiangiogenic drugs include hypertension and proteinuria. A majority of patients receiving bevacizumab require antihypertensive therapy, particularly those receiving higher doses and more prolonged treatment. The mechanism driving this hypertension is still unclear but may relate, in part, to decreased endothelial nitric oxide production. The blood pressure of all patients on bevacizumab should be carefully monitored and antihypertensives used when appropriate. Case reports describe patients with poorly controlled hypertension developing a reversible posterior leukoencephalopathy during bevacizumab

(Continued)

treatment. Bevacizumab also is rarely associated with congestive heart failure, probably secondary to hypertension. Proteinuria during bevacizumab treatment is usually an asymptomatic finding and rarely associated with nephrotic syndrome.

The most dreaded vascular toxicity of antiangiogenic agents is an arterial thromboembolic event (ie, stroke or myocardial infarction). To reduce the risk of arterial thromboembolic events, clinicians should carefully evaluate a patient's risk factors (age >65 years, clotting diathesis, a past history of arterial thromboembolic events) before starting the drug.

GI perforation, a potentially life-threatening complication of bevacizumab, has been observed with particular frequency (up to 11%) in patients with ovarian cancer, perhaps related to the presence of peritoneal carcinomatosis and to prior abdominal surgery. In colon cancer patients, colonic perforation occurs infrequently during bevacizumab treatment but increases in frequency in patients with intact primary colonic tumors, peritoneal carcinomatosis, peptic ulcer disease, chemotherapy-associated colitis, diverticulitis, or prior abdominal radiation treatment. The rate of colon perforation is less than 1% in breast and lung cancer patients receiving the antibody.

Fatigue, the most common side effect of sunitinib, affects 50 to 70% of patients and may be disabling.

Hypothyroidism occurs in 40 to 60% of patients. Bone marrow suppression and diarrhea also are common side effects; severe neutropenia (neutrophils <1000/mL) develop in 10% of patients. Less common side effects include congestive heart failure (usually in association with hypertension) and hand-foot syndrome. To monitor for these side effects, it is essential to check blood counts and thyroid function at regular intervals. Periodic echocardiograms also are recommended.

Common adverse effects of sorafenib include fatigue, nausea, diarrhea, anorexia, and rash; uncommonly, bone marrow suppression and GI perforation.

CASE 46-5

A 47-year-old patient diagnosed with renal cancer is being treated with temsirolimus, a congener of rapamycin (sirolimus).

a. What is the mechanism of action of rapamycin and its congeners?

The rapamycins inhibit an enzyme complex, mTORC1, which occupies a downstream position in the PI3 kinase pathway (see Figure 46-2). mTOR forms the mTORC1 complex with a member of the FK506-binding protein family, FKBP12. Among other actions, mTORC1 phosphorylates S6 kinase and also relieves the inhibitory effect of 4EBP on initiation factor elf-4E, thereby promoting protein synthesis and metabolism. The antitumor actions of the rapamycins result from their binding to FKBP12 and inhibition of mTORC1. Rapamycin and its congeners have immunosuppressant effects, inhibit cell-cycle progression and angiogenesis, and promote apoptosis.

b. What are the toxicities of the rapamycins?

The rapamycin analogs have very similar patterns of toxicity. The most prominent side effects are a mild maculopapular rash, mucositis, anemia, and fatigue, each occurring in 30 to 50% of patients. A minority of patients will develop leukopenia or thrombocytopenia with progressive cycles of treatment, and these effects are reversed if therapy is discontinued. Less common side effects include hyperglycemia, hypertriglyceridemia, and, rarely, pulmonary infiltrates and interstitial lung disease. Pulmonary infiltrates emerge in 8% of patients receiving everolimus and in a smaller percentage of those treated with temsirolimus. In patients showing minor radiological changes, but without symptoms, drug administration may be continued. If symptoms such as cough or shortness of breath develop or radiological changes progress, the drug should be discontinued. Prednisone may hasten the resolution of radiological changes and symptoms.

(Continued)

c. **What are the mechanisms of resistance to the effects of the rapamycins?**

Resistance to mTOR inhibitors is incompletely understood but may arise through the action of a second mTOR complex, mTORC2, which is unaffected by rapamycins and which regulates Akt kinase (see Figure 46-2). Experimental work suggests that inhibition of mTORC1 leads to mTORC2 activation of Akt kinase and the MAP kinase pathway, and these actions may be responsible for incomplete responses or resistance of rapamycins. Dual mTORC1 and mTORC2 inhibitors are in clinical development.

CASE 46-6

A 50-year-old woman has a small lump in one of her breasts removed. The pathology indicates it is an estrogen receptor-positive (ER⁺) breast cancer. Her oncologist starts her on a course of tamoxifen.

a. **What is the mechanism of action of tamoxifen in breast cancer and in noncancerous tissues?**

Tamoxifen is classified as a selective estrogen receptor modulator (SERM) (see Chapter 28). SERMs bind to the ER and exert either estrogenic or antiestrogenic effects, depending on the specific organ. Tamoxifen citrate is the most widely studied antiestrogenic treatment in breast cancer. The recent decline in breast cancer mortality in Western countries is believed to be partly due to the common use of tamoxifen, especially in the adjuvant setting. However, in addition to its estrogen antagonist effects in breast cancer, tamoxifen also exerts estrogenic agonist effects on nonbreast tissues, thus influencing the overall therapeutic index of the drug.

Tamoxifen is a competitive inhibitor of estradiol binding to the estrogen receptor (ER), of which there are 2 subtypes: ERα and ERβ. The 2 ER subtypes have different tissue distributions and can either homo- or heterodimerize. Binding of estradiol and SERMs to the estrogen-binding sites of the ERs initiates a change in conformation of the ER, dissociation of the ER from heat-shock proteins, and inhibition of ER dimerization. Dimerization facilitates the binding of the ER to specific DNA estrogen-response elements (EREs) in the vicinity of estrogen-regulated genes. Coregulator proteins interact with the receptor to act as corepressors or coactivators of gene expression. Differences in tissue distribution of ER subtypes, the function of coregulator proteins, and the various transcriptional activating factors likely explain the variability of response to tamoxifen in hormone receptor–positive (ER⁺) breast cancer and its agonist and antagonist activities in noncancerous tissues. Other organs displaying agonist effects of tamoxifen include the uterine endometrium (endometrial hypertrophy, vaginal bleeding, and endometrial cancer), the coagulation system (thromboembolism), bone metabolism (increase in bone mineral density [BMD]), and liver (alterations of blood lipid profile).

Metabolism of tamoxifen is complex (see Figure 46-3) and principally involves CYPs 3A4/5, and 2D6 in the formation of N-desmethyl tamoxifen, and CYP2D6 to form 4-hydroxytamoxifen, a more potent metabolite. Both metabolites can be further converted to 4-hydroxy-N-desmethyltamoxifen, which retains high affinity for the ER.

b. **What are the clinical uses of tamoxifen?**

Tamoxifen has become a standard agent as a result of its anticancer activity and good tolerability profile. Tamoxifen is prescribed for the prevention of breast cancer in high-risk patients, for the adjuvant therapy of early-stage breast cancer following primary tumor excision, and for the therapy of advanced (metastatic) breast cancer (see Table 46-3). It prevents the development of breast cancer in women at high risk based on a strong family history, prior nonmalignant breast pathology, or inheritance of the BRCA1 or BRCA2 genes.

(Continued)

Targeted Anticancer Therapies CHAPTER 46

TABLE 46-3 Clinical Uses for Anti-Estrogen Therapy in ER+ Breast Cancer

DRUG	DISEASE SETTING			
	ADJUVANT (premen)	ADJUVANT (postmen)	METASTATIC (premen)	METASTATIC (postmen)
Tamoxifen	Yes (5 yr)	Yes (before AI for 2-5 yr)	Yes	Yes
Fulvestrant	No	No	No	Yes (PD on TAM or AI)
Anastrozole	No	Yes (upfront or after TAM)	No	Yes
Letrozole	No	Yes (upfront or after TAM)	No	Yes
Exemestane	No	Yes (upfront or after TAM)	No	Yes
Toremifene	No	Yes	No	Yes

Premen, premenopausal; Postmen, postmenopausal; AI, aromatase inhibitor; PD, progressive disease; TAM, tamoxifen; ER, estrogen receptor.

c. **What are selective estrogen receptor downregulators (SERDs) and how do they differ from SERMs like tamoxifen?**

SERDs, also termed "pure anti-estrogens," include fulvestrant and a host of agents in experimental trials. SERDs, unlike SERMs, are devoid of any estrogen agonist activity. Fulvestrant is a steroidal antiestrogen that binds to the ER with an affinity more than 100 times that of tamoxifen. The drug inhibits the binding of estrogen but also alters the receptor structure such that the receptor is targeted for proteasomal degradation; fulvestrant also may inhibit receptor dimerization. Unlike tamoxifen, which stabilizes or even increases ER expression, fulvestrant reduces the number of ER molecules in cells, both in vitro and in vivo; as a consequence of this ER downregulation, the drug abolishes ER-mediated transcription of estrogen-dependent genes. Whereas tamoxifen is used in both premenopausal and postmenopausal women with breast cancer at early and late stages, fulvestrant is reserved for use in premenopausal women with metastatic breast cancer (see Table 46-3).

d. **What are the mechanisms by which tumors develop resistance to tamoxifen?**

Despite its benefits, initial or acquired resistance to tamoxifen frequently occurs. Polymorphisms in CYP2D6 that reduce its activity lead to lower plasma levels of 4-OH tamoxifen, a potent metabolite (see Figure 46-3), and are associated with higher risks of disease relapse and a lower incidence of hot flashes. CYP2D6 is also responsible for the activation of tamoxifen to its active metabolite endoxifen (see Figure 46-3).

Cross-talk between the ER and HER2/neu pathway also has been implicated in tamoxifen resistance. The paired box 2 gene product (PAX2) has been identified as a crucial mediator of ER repression of ErbB2 by tamoxifen. Interactions between PAX2 and the ER coactivator AIB-1/SRC-3 determine tamoxifen response in breast cancer cells.

e. **What are the toxicities and beneficial effects that this woman is likely to experience while on tamoxifen?**

The common adverse reactions to tamoxifen include vasomotor symptoms (hot flashes), atrophy of the lining of the vagina, hair loss, nausea, and vomiting. These may occur in less than or equal to 25% of patients and rarely are sufficiently severe to require discontinuation of therapy. Menstrual irregularities, vaginal bleeding and discharge, pruritus vulvae, and dermatitis occur with increasing severity in postmenopausal women.

Tamoxifen also increases the incidence of endometrial cancer by 2- to 3-fold, particularly in postmenopausal women who receive 20 mg/d for 2 years or more. In general, tamoxifen-associated endometrial cancers are reported as low-grade and

(Continued)

early-stage tumors. Standard practice guidelines from the National Comprehensive Cancer Network alert physicians to the evaluation of abnormal vaginal bleeding in women with an intact uterus.

Tamoxifen increases the risk of thromboembolic events, which increase with the age of a patient and also in the perioperative period. Hence, it often is recommended to discontinue tamoxifen prior to elective surgery. Because tamoxifen is associated with thromboembolism, some authorities suggest that the pretreatment evaluation of breast cancer patients should include screening for coagulation abnormalities (factor V Leiden, protein C, antithrombin defects) and for a history of thromboembolic disease. Presence of these risk factors should lead to exclusion of women from treatment.

Like estrogen, tamoxifen is a hepatic carcinogen in animals, although increases in primary hepatocellular carcinoma have not been reported in patients on the drug. Tamoxifen causes retinal deposits, decreased visual acuity, and cataracts in occasional patients, although the frequency of these changes is more common in patients on high doses of drug.

In addition to its ability to prevent recurrence or the development of primary breast cancer, tamoxifen has other end-organ benefits related to its partial estrogenic action. For example, it may slow the development of osteoporosis in postmenopausal women. Like certain estrogens, tamoxifen lowers total serum cholesterol, low-density-lipoprotein cholesterol, and lipoproteins, and raises apolipoprotein A-I levels, potentially decreasing the risk of myocardial infarction.

f. **After receiving tamoxifen therapy for 2 years, the patient is switched to anastrozole. What is the mechanism of action of this agent and what is the rationale for using it in this patient?**

Anastrozole is a potent and selective aromatase inhibitor. Aromatase inhibitors (AIs) block the function of the aromatase enzyme (CYP19) that converts androgens to estrogens. CYP19 is highly expressed in human placenta and in granulosa cells of ovarian follicles, where its expression depends on cyclical gonadotropin stimulation. Aromatase also is present, at lower levels, in several nonglandular tissues, including subcutaneous fat, liver, muscle, brain, and normal breast, and in breast-cancer tissue. The aromatase enzyme is responsible for the conversion of adrenal androgens and gonadal androstenedione and testosterone to the estrogens, estrone (E1) and estradiol (E2), respectively (see Figure 46-4). In postmenopausal women, this conversion is the primary source of circulating estrogens, while estrogen production in premenopausal women primarily is from the ovaries. In postmenopausal women, AIs can suppress most peripheral aromatase activity, leading to profound estrogen deprivation. This strategy of estrogen deprivation of ER+ breast cancer cells stands in contrast to the ER antagonist activity that SERMs and SERDs exert.

AIs now are considered the standard of care for adjuvant treatment of postmenopausal women with hormone receptor–positive breast cancer, either as initial therapy or sequenced after tamoxifen (see Table 46-3).

CASE 46-7

An 84-year-old gentleman has metastatic prostate cancer with symptoms that include bone pain. His oncologist recommends that he receive hormone therapy.

a. **What is hormone therapy?**

The growth of a number of cancers is hormone-dependent or regulated by hormones. Hormone analogs and antagonists are used for the treatment of both breast and prostate cancer, as well as several other cancers (see Table 46-4). These molecules interrupt the stimulatory axis created by systemic pools of androgens and estrogens, inhibit hormone production or binding to receptors, and ultimately

(Continued)

TABLE 46-4 Hormones and Antagonists

TYPE OF AGENT	NONPROPRIETARY NAMES	DISEASE
Adrenocortical suppressants	Mitotane (o,p'-DDD)	Adrenal cortex cancer
Adrenocortico-steroids	Prednisone (other equivalent preparations available)	Acute and chronic lymphocytic leukemia; non-Hodgkin's lymphoma; Hodgkin's disease; breast cancer, multiple myeloma
Progestins	Hydroxyprogesterone caproate, medroxyprogesterone acetate, megestrol acetate	Endometrial, breast cancer
Estrogens	Diethylstilbestrol, ethinyl estradiol (other preparations available)	Breast, prostate cancer
Anti-estrogens	Tamoxifen, toremifene	Breast cancer
Aromatase inhibitors	Anastrozole, letrozole, exemestane	Breast cancer
Androgens	Testosterone propionate, fluoxymesterone (other preparations available)	Breast cancer
Anti-androgen	Flutamide, casodex	Prostate cancer
GnRH analog	Leuprolide	Prostate cancer

block the complex expression of genes that promotes tumor growth and survival. These drugs have proven effective in extending survival and delaying or preventing tumor recurrence in breast cancer and prostate cancer.

b. What is the goal of hormone therapy in treating metastatic prostate cancer?

Localized prostate cancer frequently is curable with surgery or radiation therapy. However, when distant metastases are present, hormone therapy is the primary treatment. Standard approaches either reduce the concentration of endogenous androgens or inhibit their effects. Androgen deprivation therapy (ADT) is the standard first-line treatment. ADT is accomplished via surgical castration (bilateral orchiectomy) or medical castration (using gonadotropin-releasing hormone [GnRH] agonists or antagonists). Other hormone therapy approaches are used in second-line treatment and include antiandrogens, estrogens, and inhibitors of steroidogenesis (see Table 46-4).

ADT is considered palliative, not curative, treatment. ADT can alleviate cancer-related symptoms, produce objective responses, and normalize serum prostate specific antigen (PSA) in more than 90% of patients. ADT provides important quality-of-life benefits, including reduction of bone pain and reduction of rates of pathological fracture, spinal cord compression, and ureteral obstruction. It also prolongs survival.

c. This patient will receive androgen deprivation therapy (ADT) using a synthetic GnRH analog, leuprolide. What is the mechanism of action of GnRH agonists?

The biosynthesis of androgens, primarily in the testes and adrenals, is described in Chapter 28, and the regulation of Leydig cell synthetic activity by the hypothalamic–pituitary axis is considered there as well. In the United States, the most common form of ADT involves chemical suppression of the pituitary gland

(Continued)

with GnRH agonists. Synthetic GnRH analogs have greater receptor affinity and reduced susceptibility to enzymatic degradation than the naturally occurring GnRH molecule and are 100-fold more potent. GnRH (also termed luteinizing hormone–releasing hormone, LHRH) agonists bind to GnRH receptors on pituitary gonadotropin-producing cells, causing an initial release of both LH and FSH and a subsequent increase in testosterone production from testicular Leydig cells. After ~1 week of therapy, GnRH receptors are downregulated on the gonadotropin-producing cells, causing a decline in the pituitary response. The fall in serum LH leads to a decrease in testosterone production to castrate levels within 3 to 4 weeks of the first treatment. Subsequent treatments maintain testosterone at castrate levels.

d. **During the first few days of treatment with leuprolide, the patient complains that his bone pain has worsened. What is causing this worsening of his symptoms?**

   During the first few days of therapy with a GnRH agonist, there is transient rise in LH, and the resultant testosterone surge may induce an acute stimulation of prostate cancer growth and a "flare" of symptoms from metastatic deposits. Patients may experience an increase in bone pain or obstructive bladder symptoms lasting for 2 to 3 weeks. The flare phenomenon can be effectively counteracted with concurrent administration of 2 to 4 weeks of oral antiandrogen therapy (ie, combined androgen blockade), which may inhibit the action of the increased serum testosterone levels.

   Combined androgen blockade (CAB) requires administration of ADT with an antiandrogen. The theoretical advantage is that the GnRH agonist will deplete testicular androgens, while the antiandrogen component competes at the receptor with residual androgens made by the adrenal glands. CAB provides maximal relief of androgen stimulation. Numerous large trials have compared CAB with ADT monotherapy, with variable results. Several meta-analyses of these trials suggest a benefit for CAB in 5-year survival but not at earlier time points. Toxicity and costs associated with CAB are higher than with ADT alone.

   GnRH antagonists have been developed to suppress testosterone while avoiding the flare phenomenon of GnRH agonists. Other than avoidance of the initial flare, GnRH antagonist therapy offers no apparent advantage compared with GnRH agonists. The first available GnRH antagonist, abarelix, rapidly achieves medical castration. However, local reactions and anaphylaxis have discouraged its clinical acceptance and have led to its withdrawal from the market. A second GnRH antagonist, degarelix, is not associated with systemic allergic reactions and is approved for prostate cancer in the United States.

e. **After several months of treatment with leuprolide, the oncologist adds an additional agent, abiraterone to further reduce growth of the patient's tumor. What is the rationale for adding this agent?**

   In the castrate state, androgen receptor (AR) signaling, despite low steroid levels, supports continued prostate cancer growth. AR signaling may occur due to androgens produced from nongonadal sources, AR gene mutations, or AR gene amplification. Nongonadal sources of androgens include the adrenal glands and the prostate cancer cells themselves (see Figure 46-4). Androstenedione, produced by the adrenal glands, is converted to testosterone in peripheral tissues and tumors. Intratumoral de novo androgen synthesis also may provide sufficient androgen for AR-driven cell proliferation.

   Abiraterone is an irreversible inhibitor of both 17α-hydroxylase and C-17,20-lyase CYP17 activity (see Figure 46-4). The parent compound, abiraterone acetate, is orally bioavailable and has been well tolerated in castration-resistant prostate cancer patients as secondary hormone therapy in phase I and II studies. With continuous administration, abiraterone increases ACTH levels, resulting in mineralocorticoid excess. Glucocorticoids, such as prednisone, are administered to compensate for inhibition of adrenal steroidogenesis.

Targeted Anticancer Therapies

CHAPTER 46

KEY CONCEPTS

- Targeted anticancer therapies are designed to block the oncogenic pathways that cause specific cancers.
- The efficacy and specificity of targeted anticancer therapies depends on the expression of the molecular target in cancer cells.
- Resistance to targeted therapy can develop because of mutations in the molecular target, decreased expression of the target, alterations in target pathways, as well as changes in drug efflux and metabolism.
- Different agents (eg, antibodies and small molecule inhibitors) directed at the same molecular target can have very different spectra of antitumor activity.
- The growth and survival of many cancers, particularly breast and prostate cancer, are hormone-dependent or regulated by hormones; hormone therapy can extend survival and delay or prevent tumor recurrence in many patients.
- Targeted anticancer therapies are often used in combination with cytolytic anticancer agents to achieve higher response rates.

SUMMARY QUIZ

QUESTION 46-1 An important mechanism by which clinical resistance develops to imatinib in chronic myelogenous leukemia is

a. increased excretion in the urine.
b. increased hepatic metabolism.
c. decreased bioactivation in cancer cells.
d. spontaneous mutations in the BCR-ABL kinase.
e. increased efflux from tumor cells.

QUESTION 46-2 The molecular target of trastuzumab is

a. BCR-ABL.
b. VEGF.
c. ErbB1.
d. ErbB2.
e. CD20.

QUESTION 46-3 Rituximab is approved as a single agent for relapsed indolent lymphomas. Its molecular target is

a. the CD20 antigen on B cells.
b. the CD52 antigen on B cells.
c. the CD33 antigen on B cells and other hematopoietic cells.
d. BCR-ABL in lymphoblasts.
e. the IL-2 receptor on T cells.

QUESTION 46-4 Which of the following agents kills multiple myeloma (MM) cells by indirectly preventing the transcriptional activity of NF-κB?

a. Thalidomide
b. Lenalidomide
c. Bortezomib
d. Sorafenib
e. Sirolimus

SECTION VIII   Chemotherapy of Neoplastic Diseases

QUESTION 46-5 Aldesleukin is approved for use in metastatic renal-cell cancer and metastatic melanoma. Its mechanism of action in treating these cancers is to

a. antagonize IL-2 receptors on T cells.

b. antagonize IL-2 receptors on epithelial cells.

c. stimulate the proliferation of activated T cells.

d. stimulate the proliferation of activated B cells.

e. inhibit the secretion of cytokines by immune effector cells.

SUMMARY QUIZ ANSWER KEY

QUESTION 46-1 Answer is **d**. The most important mechanism of acquired resistance to imatinib and other tyrosine kinase inhibitors arises from point mutations in the kinase domain of BCR-ABL. Molecular studies of circulating tumor cells have detected resistance-mediating kinase mutations prior to initiation of therapy, particularly in patients with Ph+ acute lymphoblastic leukemia (ALL) or CML in blastic crisis. This finding strongly supports the hypothesis that drug-resistant cells arise through spontaneous mutation and expand under the selective pressure of drug exposure. Mutations may become detectable in the peripheral blood of patients receiving imatinib in the accelerated phase and in the late (>4 years from diagnosis) chronic phase of CML, heralding the onset of drug resistance.

Mechanisms other than BCR-ABL kinase mutation play a minor role in resistance to imatinib. Amplification of the wild-type kinase gene, leading to overexpression of the enzyme, has been identified in tumor samples from patients resistant to treatment. The multidrug resistant (MDR) gene, which codes for a drug efflux protein, confers resistance experimentally but has not been implicated in clinical resistance.

QUESTION 46-2 Answer is **d**. Trastuzumab is a humanized monoclonal antibody that binds to the external domain of HER2/neu (ErbB2).

QUESTION 46-3 Answer is **a**. Rituximab is a chimeric monoclonal antibody that targets the CD20 B-cell antigen (Tables 46-1 and 46-2). CD20 is found on cells from the pre–B cell stage through its terminal differentiation to plasma cells and is expressed on 90% of B-cell neoplasms. The biological functions of CD20 are uncertain, although incubation of B cells with anti-CD20 antibody has variable effects on cell-cycle progression, depending on the monoclonal antibody type. Monoclonal antibody binding to CD20 generates transmembrane signals that produce autophosphorylation and activation of serine/tyrosine protein kinases, induction of c-myc oncogene expression, and expression of major histocompatibility complex class II molecules. CD20 also may regulate transmembrane Ca^{2+} conductance through its function as a Ca^{2+} channel. It is unclear which of these actions relates to the pharmacological effect of rituximab.

QUESTION 46-4 Answer is **c**. Bortezomib, an inhibitor of proteasome-mediated protein degradation, has earned a central role in the treatment of MM. Bortezomib binds to the β5 subunit of the 20S core of the 26S proteasome and reversibly inhibits its chymotrypsin-like activity. This event disrupts multiple intracellular signaling cascades, leading to apoptosis.

A most important consequence of proteasome inhibition is its effect on NF-κB, a key transcription factor that promotes cell damage response and cell survival. Most NF-κB is found in the cytosol bound to IκB; in this form, NF-κB is restricted to the cytosol and cannot enter the nucleus to regulate transcription. In response to stress signals resulting from hypoxia, chemotherapy, and DNA damage, IκB becomes ubiquitinated and then degraded via the proteasome. Its degradation releases NF-κB, which enters the nucleus, where it transcriptionally activates a host of genes involved in cell survival (eg, cell adhesion proteins E-selectin, ICAM-1, and VCAM-1), as well as proliferative (eg, cyclin-D1) or antiapoptotic molecules (eg, cIAPs, BCL-2). NF-κB is highly expressed in many human tumors, including MM, and may be a key factor in tumor cell survival in a hypoxic environment and during chemotherapy. Bortezomib

(Continued)

Targeted Anticancer Therapies — CHAPTER 46

blocks proteasomal degradation of IκB, thereby preventing the transcriptional activity of NF-κB and downregulating survival responses.

QUESTION 46-5 Answer is **c**. Aldesleukin possesses the biological activities of human native IL-2. IL-2 stimulates the proliferation of activated T cells and the secretion of cytokines from NK cells and monocytes. IL-2 stimulation increases cytotoxic killing by T cells and NK cells. The mechanism of tumor cell killing has not been precisely defined but is presumed to be the result of enhanced killing by immune effector cells.

SUMMARY: TARGETED ANTICANCER DRUGS

CLASS AND SUBCLASSES	NAMES	CLINICAL USES	TOXICITIES COMMON	TOXICITIES UNIQUE; CLINICALLY IMPORTANT
Protein Tyrosine Kinase Inhibitors—ATP inhibitors	Imatinib mesylate Dasatinib Nilotinib Gefitinib Erlotinib Lapatinib Sunitinib Sorafenib	See Table 45-5. Imatinib, dasatinib, and nilotinib are efficacious in diseases in which the ABL, kit, or PDGFR have dominant roles in driving the proliferation of the tumor (eg, chronic myelogenous leukemia, GI stromal tumor [GIST]) reflecting the presence of a mutation that results in constitutive activation of the kinase, either by fusion with another protein or via point mutations. Gefitinib and erlotinib are used in patients with non-small lung cancer, especially cancers associated with activating mutations in EGFR. Erlotinib in combination with gemcitabine is first-line treatment of patients with locally advanced, unresectable, or metastatic pancreatic cancer. Lapatinib is used for HER2-amplified, trastuzumab-refractory breast cancer. Sunitinib is used for renal-cell cancer and GIST. Sorafenib is used for renal-cell cancer and is the only drug currently approved for treatment of hepatocellular carcinoma	Imatinib, dasatinib, and nilotinib cause GI distress (diarrhea, nausea, and vomiting), fluid retention, which may lead to dependent edema, and periorbital swelling. Dasatinib may cause pleural effusions. Nilotinib may prolong QT interval. Diarrhea and pustular/papular rash common in patients taking gefitinib and erlotinib; also GI effects, fatigue, dry skin, pruritus. Sunitinib and sorafenib are associated with vascular toxicities due to antiangiogenic effects (bleeding, hypertension, and arterial thromboembolic events, GI perforation), also fatigue, diarrhea, skin reactions. Sunitinib is associated with hypothyroidism (50%) and severe neutropenia (10%)	Imatinib, dasatinib, and nilotinib can be associated with hepatotoxicity; infrequently cause myelosuppression. Interstitial lung disease in <2% of patients taking gefitinib and erlotinib that may be fatal. Rare but serious toxicities with erlotinib include serious or fatal hepatic failure, GI perforation, renal failure, arterial thrombosis, microangiopathic hemolytic anemia, hand-foot skin reaction, corneal perforation or ulceration, Stevens-Johnson syndrome/toxic epidermal necrolysis
Monoclonal Antibodies—Growth Factor Receptors (EGFR, HER2/neu, VEGFRs, PDGFR) Antibodies	Cetuximab Panitumumab Trastuzumab	See Table 46-1. Cetuximab is used for squamous cell carcinoma of the head and neck (HNSCC), EGFR-positive metastatic colorectal cancer, and in combination with other agents for other metastatic colon cancers. Trastuzumab is used for HER2/neu-amplified breast cancer	See Table 46-2. Rash and dermatological toxicities are common with cetuximab and panitumumab; headache and diarrhea may also occur	See Table 46-2. Rare but serious adverse effects with cetuximab and panitumumab include interstitial lung disease, hypomagnesemia, cardiopulmonary arrest, and anaphylactoid reactions. The most serious toxicity of trastuzumab is cardiac failure; patients should be evaluated before therapy and afterward for changes in left ventricular function

(Continued)

SECTION VIII Chemotherapy of Neoplastic Diseases

CLASS AND SUBCLASSES	NAMES	CLINICAL USES	TOXICITIES	
			COMMON	UNIQUE; CLINICALLY IMPORTANT
Monoclonal Antibodies—Growth Factor (VEGF) Antibodies	Bevacizumab Ranibizumab	See Table 46-1 Bevacizumab is used in highly vascularized tumors, including renal-cell, lung, colorectal, and breast cancers, and glioblastoma Bevacizumab restores hearing in patients with progressive deafness due to neurofibromatosis type 2–related tumors Ranibizumab is used to treat wet macular degeneration (see Chapter 47)	See Table 46-2 Potential for vessel injury, bleeding, and poor wound healing following surgery Hypertension (a majority of patients require antihypertensive therapy) and proteinuria (usually asymptomatic)	See Table 46-2 Bevacizumab is associated with arterial thromboembolic events and GI perforation Bevacizumab is contraindicated in patients who have a history of hemoptysis, brain metastasis, or a bleeding diathesis; elective surgery should be delayed for at least 4 weeks from the last dose of antibody, and treatment should not be resumed for at least 4 weeks after surgery
Monoclonal Antibodies—CD20 Antibodies	Rituximab ^{131}I-Tositumomab ^{90}Y-Ibritumomab tiuxetan Ofatumumab	See Table 46-1 Rituximab is used as a single agent for relapsed indolent lymphomas and with chemotherapy for diffuse large B-cell lymphoma and other indolent B-cell non-Hodgkin lymphomas (NHLs) Rituximab is also used for autoimmune diseases, including rheumatologic disease, thrombotic thrombocytopenic purpura, autoimmune hemolytic anemias, cryoglobulin-induced renal disease and multiple sclerosis Ofatumumab is approved for treating patients with chronic lymphocytic leukemia (CLL)	See Table 46-2 The radioimmunoconjugates cause antibody-related hypersensitivity, bone marrow suppression, and secondary leukemias Ofatumumab's primary toxicities consist of immunosuppression and opportunistic infection, hypersensitivity reactions during antibody infusion, and myelosuppression	See Table 46-2 Rituximab infusion reactions can be life-threatening, but with pretreatment are usually mild and limited to fever, chills, throat itching, urticaria, and mild hypotension; severe mucocutaneous skin reactions, including Stevens-Johnson syndrome are rare May cause reactivation of hepatitis B virus or rarely, JC virus; should not be administered to patients with active infection Hypogammaglobulinemia and autoimmune syndromes may occur 1-5 months following treatment with rituximab
Monoclonal Antibodies—CD52 Antibodies	Alemtuzumab	See Table 46-1 Used to treat B- and T-cell low-grade lymphomas and CLL	See Table 46-2 Acute infusion reactions and serious myelosuppression, (all blood lineages) with significant risk of fungal, viral, and other opportunistic infections; patients should receive antibiotic and antiviral prophylaxis and be monitored for signs and symptoms of CMV and other infections	See Table 46-2 CD4$^+$ T-cell counts may remain profoundly depleted for 1 year Alemtuzumab does not combine well with chemotherapy in standard regimens because of significant infectious complications
Monoclonal Antibodies—CD33 Antibodies	Gemtuzumab ozogamicin	See Table 46-1 Currently is approved in patients >60 years with AML in first relapse	See Table 46-2 Myelosuppression in all patients, hepatocellular damage in 30-40% of patients	See Table 46-2 Causes a syndrome that resembles hepatic venoocclusive disease when patients subsequently undergo myeloablative therapy or when following, high-dose chemotherapy Prolonged myelosuppression, particularly delayed recovery of platelet counts

(Continued)

Targeted Anticancer Therapies — CHAPTER 46

CLASS AND SUBCLASSES	NAMES	CLINICAL USES	TOXICITIES COMMON	TOXICITIES UNIQUE; CLINICALLY IMPORTANT
Thalidomide and its Derivatives (Immunomodulatory analogs, IMiDs)	Thalidomide Lenalidomide	See Table 45-5 Used in newly diagnosed and heavily pretreated relapsed/refractory multiple myeloma (MM) patients Lenalidomide also used in 5q− myelodysplastic syndrome (MDS) and CLL	Sedation and constipation are common with thalidomide, but not with lenalidomide Lenalidomide causes significant leukopenia in 20% of patients Thromboembolic risk increases with both thalidomide and lenalidomide	Thalidomide-related peripheral sensory neuropathy (10-30% of patients); long-standing sensory loss may not reverse and caution is advised in patients with preexisting neuropathy Rarely, lenalidomide causes hepatotoxicity and renal dysfunction CLL patients taking lenalidomide should receive pretreatment hydration and allopurinol to avoid the consequences of tumor swelling and tumor lysis Thalidomide is teratogenic, but lenalidomide is not
Proteasome Inhibitors	Bortezomib	Initial therapy for MM and as therapy for MM after relapse from other drugs, relapsed or refractory mantle cell lymphoma, and myeloma	Thrombocytopenia (28%), fatigue, peripheral neuropathy (12%), GI distress, anemia and neutropenia, limb pain	Chronic peripheral neuropathy, especially in patients with history of neuropathy Cardiac toxicity and long QT are rare
mTOR Inhibitors	Rapamycin Temsirolimus Everolimus	See Table 45-5 [in previous chapter] Used for renal-cell cancer and may also be useful in mantle cell lymphomas and other cancers	Mild maculopapular rash, mucositis, anemia, and fatigue, each occurring in 30-50% of patients Leukopenia or thrombocytopenia with progressive cycles of treatment in some patients	Pulmonary infiltrates and interstitial lung disease; if symptoms such as cough or shortness of breath develop or radiological changes progress, the drug should be discontinued
Interleukin-2 (IL-2) Receptor Agonists	Aldesleukin Denileukin diftitox	See Table 45-5 Aldesleukin used for metastatic renal-cell cancer and metastatic melanoma Denileukin diftitox used for recurrent/refractory cutaneous T-cell lymphomas	Most patients develop a pruritic skin rash over most of the body See Table 46-2 for denileukin diftitox toxicities	Most significant toxicity with aldesleukin is capillary leak syndrome which can be life-threatening, but reversible with discontinuation of therapy; patients should have good hepatic and renal function before starting therapy Typical significant toxicities with denileukin diftitox include acute hypersensitivity reactions, vascular leak syndrome, and constitutional toxicities (see also Table 46-2)
Colony-Stimulating Factors	See Chapter 25	Used as supportive therapy to restore hematopoiesis following high-dose and combination therapies (see Chapter 25)	See Chapter 25	See Chapter 25

(Continued)

SECTION VIII: Chemotherapy of Neoplastic Diseases

CLASS AND SUBCLASSES	NAMES	CLINICAL USES	TOXICITIES	
			COMMON	UNIQUE; CLINICALLY IMPORTANT
Glucocorticoids	Prednisone Dexamethasone	See Table 46-4 Used as cytotoxic agents in the treatment of acute leukemia in children and malignant lymphoma in children and adults Used to control autoimmune hemolytic anemia and thrombocytopenia associated with CLL Used with radiotherapy to reduce edema related to tumors in critical areas such as the brain and spinal cord	See Chapter 29	See Chapter 29
Progestins	Medroxyprogesterone Megestrol acetate	See Table 46-4 Used as second-line hormonal therapy for metastatic hormone-dependent breast cancer and in endometrial carcinoma previously treated by surgery and radiotherapy	See Chapter 28	See Chapter 28
Estrogens and Androgens	See Chapter 28	See Table 46-4 Used in hormone-dependent neoplasms such as breast and prostate cancers	See Chapter 28	High-dose therapy has significant risk of thromboembolism (see Chapter 28)
Antiestrogens—Selective Estrogen-Receptor Modulators (SERMs)	Tamoxifen Toremifene Raloxifene	See Table 46-4 Used for prevention of breast cancer in high-risk patients, for the adjuvant therapy of early-stage breast cancer, and for the therapy of advanced breast cancer (estrogen receptor-positive [ER+] cancers are most responsive)	Vasomotor symptoms (hot flashes), atrophy of the lining of the vagina, hair loss, nausea, and vomiting Menstrual irregularities, vaginal bleeding and discharge, pruritus vulvae, and dermatitis are more severe in postmenopausal women	Increased risk of thromboembolic events Increased risk of endometrial cancer
Antiestrogens—Selective Estrogen-Receptor Downregulators (SERDs)	Fulvestrant	Used in postmenopausal women as antiestrogen therapy of hormone receptor-positive metastatic breast cancer after progression on first-line antiestrogen therapy such as tamoxifen	Nausea, asthenia, pain, vasodilation (hot flashes), and headache Risk of injection site reactions (7%) reduced by slow injection	
Antiestrogens—Aromatase (CYP19) Inhibitors	Anastrozole Letrozole Exemestane	See Table 46-4 Adjuvant hormonal therapy in postmenopausal women with early-stage breast cancer and as treatment for advanced breast cancer (ER+ and PR+)	Vaginal bleeding, vaginal discharge, hot flashes, but lower frequency of such side effects than tamoxifen	Lower risk of estrogen-related toxicities (including thromboembolism, endometrial cancer) than tamoxifen, but greater risk of musculoskeletal disorders and fractures

(Continued)

Targeted Anticancer Therapies CHAPTER 46

CLASS AND SUBCLASSES	NAMES	CLINICAL USES	TOXICITIES	
			COMMON	UNIQUE; CLINICALLY IMPORTANT
Gonadotropin-Releasing Hormone (GnRH) Agonists	GnRH Leuprolide Buserelin Nafarelin Histrelin Triptorelin Goserelin	See Table 46-4 Used for first-line androgen deprivation therapy (ADT) as palliative treatment to alleviate cancer-related symptoms (eg, bone pain), produce objective responses, and normalize serum prostate-specific antigen (PSA) in patients with metastatic prostate cancer	Vasomotor flashing, loss of libido, impotence, gynecomastia, fatigue, anemia, weight gain, decreased insulin sensitivity, altered lipid profiles, osteoporosis and fractures, and loss of muscle mass	Cause an initial release of LH and FSH resulting in a testosterone surge that may cause an acute stimulation of prostate cancer growth and a "flare" of symptoms from metastatic deposits; the flare phenomenon can be counteracted with concurrent administration of antiandrogen therapy (known as combined androgen blockade [CAB])
Gonadotropin-Releasing Hormone (GnRH) Antagonists	Cetrorelix Ganirelix Abarelix Degarelix	Used in a similar manner to GnRH agonists for ADT in patients with metastatic prostate cancer, but avoids the flare phenomenon of GnRH agonists	Same as GnRH agonists	
Antiandrogens—Steroidal	Cyproterone Megestrol	Most commonly used as secondary hormone therapy in prostate cancer or in CAB Cyproterone has inferior efficacy compared with other forms of ADT	Cause more gynecomastia, mastodynia, and hepatotoxicity but less vasomotor flashing, and loss of bone mineral density than GnRH agonists	Cyproterone is associated with liver toxicity
Antiandrogens—Nonsteroidal	Flutamide Bicalutamide Nilutamide	See Table 46-4 Used as secondary hormone therapy (in combination with other agents) or in CAB	Flutamide causes diarrhea, breast tenderness, and nipple tenderness; less commonly, nausea, vomiting, Nilutamide causes mild nausea, alcohol intolerance (5-20%), and diminished ocular adaptation to darkness (25-40%)	Flutamide is associated with risk of hepatotoxicity Nilutamide is associated rarely with interstitial pneumonitis
Estrogens	See Chapter 28	See Table 46-4 High-dose estrogen is used in patients with prostate cancer to reduce testosterone to castrate levels via negative feedback on the hypothalamic–pituitary axis Estrogen may also exert a cytotoxic effect on prostate cancer cells	Impotence, loss of libido, and lethargy	Increased risk of myocardial infarctions, strokes, and pulmonary emboli; increased mortality
Inhibitors of Steroidogenesis	Ketoconazole Abiraterone	Used to reduce nongonadal (eg, adrenal and tumor) androgen synthesis in castration-resistant prostate cancer	Ketoconazole causes significant diarrhea and hepatic enzyme elevations Abiraterone increases ACTH levels, resulting in mineralocorticoid excess	Glucocorticoids are administered to compensate for inhibition of adrenal steroidogenesis

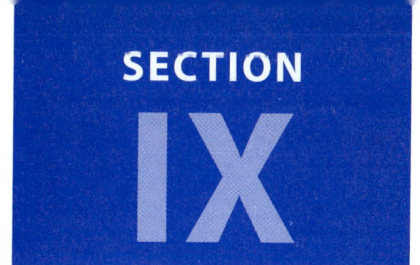

Special Systems Pharmacology

47. Ocular Pharmacology. 690

48. Dermatological Pharmacology 707

CHAPTER 47

Ocular Pharmacology

DRUGS INCLUDED IN THIS CHAPTER[a]

- Abobotulinumtoxin A (DYSPORT)
- Acetylcholine (MIOCHOL-E)
- Apraclonidine (IOPIDINE)
- Atropine (ATROPINE-CARE, ISOPTO ATROPINE)
- Azelastine (OPTIVAR)
- Bepotastine (BEPREVE)
- Betaxolol (BETOPTIC, others)
- Bevacizumab (AVASTIN)
- Bimatoprost (LUMIGAN, LATISSE)
- Brimonidine (ALPHAGAN, others)
- Brinzolamide (AZOPT)
- Bromfenac (XIBROM)
- Carbachol (MIOSTAT, ISOPTOCARBACHOL, others)
- Carteolol (OCCUPRES, others)
- Chondroitin sulfate (VISCOAT)
- Cromolyn sodium (CROLOM, others)
- Cyanoacrylate tissue adhesive (ISODENT, DERMABOND, HISTOACRYL)
- Cyclopentolate (CYCLOGYL, others)
- Cyclosporin A (RESTASIS)
- Dexamethasone (DEXASOL, others)
- Diclofenac (VOLTAREN, others)
- Difluprednate (DUREZOL)
- Dipivefrin (PROPINE, others)
- Dorzolamide (TRUSOPT, others)
- Echothiophate (PHOSPHOLINE IODIDE)
- Emedastine difumarate (EMADINE)
- Epinastine (ELESTAT)
- Fibrinogen glue (TISSEEL, EVICEL)
- Fluocinolone ophthalmic implant (RETISERT)
- Fluorescein sodium
- Fluorometholone (FML, others)
- Fluorouracil
- Flurbiprofen (OCUFEN, others)
- Homatropine (ISOPTO HOMATROPINE, others)
- Hyaluronate (HEALON, others)
- Hydroxyamphetamine + topicamide (PAREMYD)

(continues)

This chapter will be most useful after having a basic understanding of the material in Chapter 64, Ocular Pharmacology in *Goodman & Gilman's The Pharmacological Basis of Therapeutics*, 12th Edition. In addition to the material presented here, the 12th Edition contains:

- A detailed description of the anatomy of the eye and extraocular structures
- Table 64-1 Autonomic Pharmacology of the Eye and Related Structures
- Table 64-8 Vitreous Substitutes
- The mechanism of action of vitamin A in retinal physiology and vision
- Figure 64-7 Structural formula for β-carotene and structural formulas for the vitamin A family of retinoids
- Table 64-9 Ophthalmic Effects of Selected Vitamin Deficiencies and Zinc Deficiency
- Figure 64-8 Major steps in photoreceptor signaling

LEARNING OBJECTIVES

- ☑ Understand the principles of using drugs to treat ophthalmic disorders.
- ☑ Know the ocular toxicities of systemic drugs.
- ☑ Know the mechanisms of action, clinical uses, and toxicities of ophthalmic drugs.
- ☑ Describe how ophthalmic drugs administered topically can cause systemic side effects.
- ☑ Understand the pathophysiology of glaucoma and the role of pharmacotherapy in its management.

MECHANISMS OF ACTION OF DRUGS FOR OPHTHALMIC USE

DRUG CLASS	DRUG	MECHANISM OF ACTION
Autonomic Agents	Dipivefrin	Prodrug that is converted to epinephrine by esterases in the cornea (see Table 47-4, Figure 47-1, and Chapter 7)
	Apraclonidine Brimonidine	Selective α_2 adrenergic agonist (see Table 47-4 and Figure 47-1)
	Acetylcholine Carbachol Pilocarpine	Cholinergic agonist (see Table 47-4, Figure 47-1, and Chapter 6)
	Echothiophate	Organophosphate acetylcholinesterase inhibitor (see Table 47-4, Figure 47-1, and Chapter 6)
	Atropine Scopolamine Homatropine Cyclopentolate Tropicamide	Muscarinic antagonist (see Table 47-4, Figure 47-1, and Chapter 6)
	Phenylephrine Naphazoline Tetrahydrozoline	Sympathomimetic agent (see Table 47-4, Figure 47-1, and Chapter 7)

(Continued)

Ocular Pharmacology

CHAPTER 47

DRUG CLASS	DRUG	MECHANISM OF ACTION
	Betaxolol	β_1-Selective adrenergic receptor antagonist (see Table 47-4, Figure 47-1, and Chapter 7)
	Carteolol Levobunolol Metipranolol Timolol	Nonselective β adrenergic receptor antagonists (see Table 47-4, Figure 47-1, and Chapter 7)
Prostaglandin Analogs	Latanoprost Travoprost Bimatoprost	Prostaglandin analogs that lower intraocular pressure (IOP) by facilitating aqueous outflow through the accessory uveoscleral outflow pathway
Carbonic Anhydrase Inhibitors	Dorzolamide Brinzolamide	Inhibit carbonic anyhdrase found in the ciliary body epithelium; this reduces the formation of bicarbonate ions, which reduces fluid transport and, thus, IOP
Ophthalmic Glucocorticoids	Dexamethasone Prednisolone Fluorometolone Loteprednol Rimexolone Difluprednate Triamcinolone (intravitreal) Fluocinolone (implant)	Anti-inflammatory (see Chapters 22 and 29)
Nonsteroidal Anti-inflammatory Agents	Flurbiprofen Ketorolac Diclofenac Bromfenac Nepafenac	Anti-inflammatory (see Chapter 22)
Antihistamines and Mast Cell Stabilizers	Emedastine difumarate	H_1 receptor antagonist
	Cromolyn sodium Lodoxamide tromethamine Pemirolast	Mast cell stabilizer that prevents the release of histamine and other autocoids from mast cells
	Nedocromil	Mast cell stabilizer with some antihistamine properties
	Olopatadine Ketotifen fumarate Bepotastine Azelastine Epinastine	H_1 receptor antagonists with mast cell stabilizing activity
Immunosuppressive and Antimitotic Agents	Fluorouracil Mitomycin	Antineoplastic agents (see Chapter 45) that act by limiting the healing process and reduce the risk of scarring
	Cyclosporine A	Inhibits activation of T cells (see Chapter 23) and decreases inflammation in lacrimal gland
Agents Used in Ophthalmic Surgery	Povidone iodine	Antiseptic

(Continued)

DRUGS INCLUDED IN THIS CHAPTER (Cont.)

- Hydroxypropyl cellulose ophthalmic insert (LACRISERT)
- Hydroxypropylmethylcellulose
- Indocyanine green
- Ketorolac (ACULAR, others)
- Ketotifen fumarate (ZADITOR, ALAWAY)
- Latanoprost (XALATAN)
- Levobunolol (BETAGAN, others)
- Lodoxamide tromethamine (ALOMIDE)
- Loteprednol (ALREX, LOTEMAX)
- Metipranolol (OPTIPRANOLOL, others)
- Mitomycin (MUTAMYCIN)
- Naphazoline (AK-CON, ABALON, NAPHCON, others)
- Nedocromil (ALOCRIL)
- Nepafenac (NEVANAC)
- Olopatadine (PATANOL, PATADAY)
- Onabotulinumtoxin A (BOTOX)
- Pegaptanib (MACUGEN)
- Pemirolast (ALAMAST)
- Phenylephrine + cyclopentolate (CYCLOMYDRIL)
- Phenylephrine + scopolamine (MUROCOLL-2)
- Polydimethylsiloxanes (ADATOSIL 5000)
- Prednisolone (PRED FORTE, others)
- Povidone iodine (BETADINE OPHTHALMIC)
- Ranibizumab (LUCENTIS)
- Rimexolone (VEXOL)
- Scopolamine (ISOPTO HYOSCINE)
- Tetrahydrozoline (ALTAZINE, MURINE, VISINE, others)
- Timolol (TIMOPTIC, BETIMOL, others)
- Travoprost (TRAVATAN, TRAVATAN Z)
- Triamcinolone intravitreal formulations (TRIVARIS, TRIESENCE)
- Tropicamide (MYDRIACYL)
- Trypan Blue (VISIONBLUE, MEMBRANEBLUE)
- Tyloxapol (ENUCLENE)
- Verteporfin (VISUDYNE)

[a]Drugs included in this chapter have specific ophthalmic uses. Antimicrobial agents are listed in Tables 47-1 through 47-3. Their pharmacology is discussed in previous chapters.

SECTION IX

Special Systems Pharmacology

DRUG CLASS	DRUG	MECHANISM OF ACTION
	Hyaluronate Chondroitin sulfate Hydroxypropyl methylcellulose	Viscoelastic substances
	Cyanoacrylate Fibrinogen gel	Tissue adhesives
	Vitreous substitutes	See Table 64-8 Goodman and Gilman's The Pharmacological Basis of Therapeutics, 12th Edition
	Polydimethylsiloxanes	Tamponade of retina
Agents Used in the Treatment of Strabismus and Blepharospasm	Onabotulinumtoxin A Abobotulinumtoxin A	Prevent acetylcholine release at neuromuscular junction
Agents Used to Treat Macular Degeneration	Verteporfin	Activation by laser in the presence of oxygen generates free radicals, which cause vessel damage and occlusion of choroidal neovascularization
	Pegaptanib	Antagonist of VEGF (an inducer of angiogenesis)
	Bevacizumab Ranibizumab	Inhibitors of vascular proliferation and tumor growth by inhibiting VEGF-A (see Chapter 46)
Wetting Agents and Tear Substitutes	Tyloxapol Carboxymethylcellulose Hydroxyethyl cellulose Hydroxypropyl cellulose Hydroxypropyl methylcellulose Methylcellulose	Ophthalmic lubricants

TABLE 47-1 Topical Antibacterial Agents Commercially Available for Ophthalmic Use

GENERIC NAME (TRADE NAME)	FORMULATION[a]	TOXICITY	INDICATIONS FOR USE
Azithromycin (AZASITE)	1% solution	H	Conjunctivitis
Bacitracin	500 units/g ointment	H	Conjunctivitis, blepharitis, keratitis, keratoconjunctivitis, corneal ulcers, blepharoconjunctivitis, meibomianitis, dacryocystitis
Besifloxacin (BESIVANCE)	0.6% suspension		Conjunctivitis
Chloramphenicol	1% ointment	H, BD	Conjunctivitis, keratitis
Ciprofloxacin hydrochloride (CILOXAN, others)	0.3% solution; 0.3% ointment	H, D-RCD	Conjunctivitis, keratitis, keratoconjunctivitis, corneal ulcers, blepharitis, blepharoconjunctivitis, meibomianitis, dacryocystitis
Erythromycin (ILOTYCIN, others)	0.5% ointment	H	Superficial ocular infections involving the conjunctiva or cornea; prophylaxis of ophthalmia neonatorum

(Continued)

Ocular Pharmacology — CHAPTER 47

GENERIC NAME (TRADE NAME)	FORMULATION[a]	TOXICITY	INDICATIONS FOR USE
Gatifloxacin (ZYMAR)	0.3% solution	H	Conjunctivitis
Gentamicin sulfate (GARAMYCIN, GENOPTIC, GENT-AK, GENTACIDIN, OTHERS)	0.3% solution; 0.3% ointment	H	Conjunctivitis, blepharitis, keratitis, keratoconjunctivitis, corneal ulcers, blepharoconjunctivitis, meibomianitis, dacryocystitis
Levofloxacin (QUIXIN, IQUIX)	0.5% solution	H	Conjunctivitis
Levofloxacin (IQUIX)	1.5% solution	H	Corneal ulcers
Moxifloxacin (VIGAMOX)	0.5% solution	H	Conjunctivitis
Ofloxacin (OCUFLOX, OTHERS)	0.3% solution	H	Conjunctivitis, corneal ulcers
Sulfacetamide sodium (BLEPH-10, CETAMIDE, ISOPTO CETAMIDE, others)	1%, 10%, 15%, and 30% solution; 10% ointment	H, BD	Conjunctivitis, other superficial ocular infections
Polymyxin B combinations[b]	Various solutions and ointments		Conjunctivitis, blepharitis, keratitis
Tobramycin sulfate[c] (TOBREX, AKTOB, DEFY, others)	0.3% solution; 0.3% ointment	H	External infections of the eye and its adnexa

[a]For specific information on dosing, formulation, and trade names, refer to the *Physicians' Desk Reference for Ophthalmic Medicines*, which is published annually. [b]Polymyxin B is formulated for delivery to the eye in combination with bacitracin, neomycin, gramicidin, oxytetracycline, or trimethoprim. See Chapters 38-41 for further discussion of these antibacterial agents. [c]Tobramycin is formulated for delivery to the eye in combination with dexamethasone or loteprednol etabonate. H, hypersensitivity; BD, blood dyscrasia; D-RCD, drug-related corneal deposits.

TABLE 47-2 Antiviral Agents for Ophthalmic Use

GENERIC NAME (TRADE NAME)	ROUTE OF ADMINISTRATION	OCULAR TOXICITY	INDICATIONS FOR USE
Trifluridine (VIROPTIC, others)	Topical (1% solution)	PK, H	Herpes simplex keratitis and keratoconjunctivitis
Acyclovir (ZOVIRAX)	Oral, intravenous (200-mg capsules, 400- and 800-mg tablets)		Herpes zoster ophthalmicus[a] Herpes simplex iridocyclitis
Valacyclovir (VALTREX)	Oral (500- and 1000-mg tablets)		Herpes simplex keratitis[a] Herpes zoster ophthalmicus[a]
Famciclovir (FAMVIR)	Oral (125-, 250-, and 500-mg tablets)		Herpes simplex keratitis[a] Herpes zoster ophthalmicus[a]
Foscarnet (FOSCAVIR)	Intravenous Intravitreal[a]		Cytomegalovirus retinitis
Ganciclovir (CYTOVENE) (VITRASERT)	Intravenous, oral Intravitreal implant		Cytomegalovirus retinitis
Valganciclovir (VALCYTE)	Oral		Cytomegalovirus retinitis
Cidofovir (VISTIDE)	Intravenous		Cytomegalovirus retinitis

[a]Off-label use. For additional details, see Chapter 44. PK, punctate keratopathy; H, hypersensitivity.

SECTION IX

Special Systems Pharmacology

TABLE 47-3 Antifungal Agents for Ophthalmic Use

DRUG CLASS/AGENT	METHOD OF ADMINISTRATION	INDICATIONS FOR USE
Polyenes		
Amphotericin B[a]	0.1-0.5% (typically 0.15%) topical solution	Yeast and fungal keratitis and endophthalmitis
	0.8-1 mg subconjunctival	Yeast and fungal endophthalmitis
	5-µg intravitreal injection	Yeast and fungal endophthalmitis
	Intravenous	Yeast and fungal endophthalmitis
Natamycin	5% topical suspension	Yeast and fungal blepharitis, conjunctivitis, keratitis
Imidazoles		
Fluconazole[a]	Oral, intravenous	Yeast keratitis and endophthalmitis
Itraconazole[a]	Oral	Yeast and fungal keratitis and endophthalmitis
Ketoconazole[a]	Oral	Yeast keratitis and endophthalmitis
Miconazole[a]	1% topical solution	Yeast and fungal keratitis
	5-10 mg subconjunctival	Yeast and fungal endophthalmitis
	10-µg intravitreal injection	Yeast and fungal endophthalmitis

[a]Off-label use. Only natamycin (NATACYN) is commercially available and labeled for ophthalmic use. All other antifungal drugs are not labeled for ophthalmic use and must be formulated for the given method of administration. For further dosing information, refer to the *Physicians' Desk Reference for Ophthalmic Medicines*. For additional discussion of these antifungal agents, see Chapter 43.

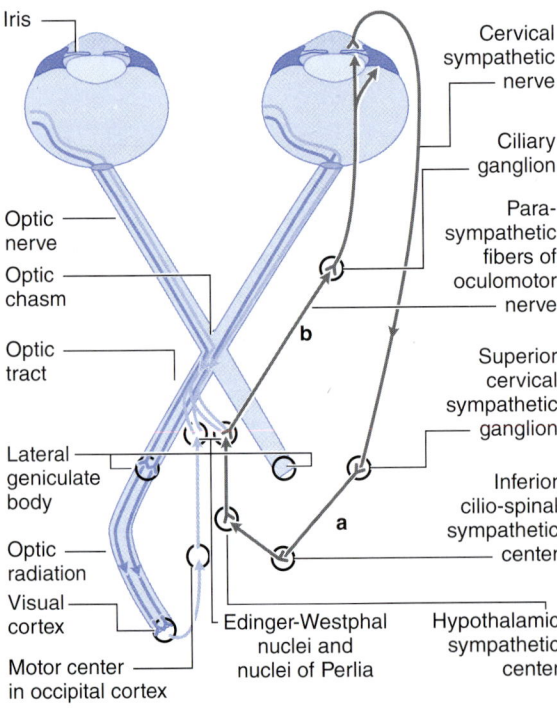

FIGURE 47-1 Autonomic innervation of the eye by the sympathetic (**a**) and parasympathetic (**b**) nervous systems. (*Adapted with permission from Wybar KC, Kerr-Muir M. Baillière Concise Medical Textbooks, Ophthalmology, 3rd ed. Baillière Tindall, New York, 1984. Copyright © Elsevier.*)

Ocular Pharmacology — CHAPTER 47

TABLE 47-4 Autonomic Drugs for Ophthalmic Use

DRUG CLASS (TRADE NAME)	FORMULATION	INDICATIONS FOR USE	OCULAR SIDE EFFECTS
Cholinergic agonists			
Acetylcholine (MIOCHOL-E)	1% solution	Miosis in surgery	Corneal edema
Carbachol (MIOSTAT, ISOPTO CARBACHOL, others)	0.01-3% solution	Miosis in surgery; Glaucoma[a]	Corneal edema, miosis, induced myopia, decreased vision, brow ache, retinal detachment
Pilocarpine (ISOPTO CARPINE, PILOCAR, PILAGAN, PILOPINE HS, PILOPTIC, PILOSTAT, others)	0.5%, 1%, 2%, 4%, and 6% solution; 4% gel	Glaucoma	Same as for carbachol
Anticholinesterase agents			
Echothiophate (PHOSPHOLINE IODIDE)	0.125% solution	Glaucoma; Accommodative esotropia	Retinal detachment, miosis, cataract, pupillary block glaucoma, iris cysts, brow ache, punctal stenosis of the nasolacrimal system
Muscarinic antagonists			
Atropine (ATROPINE-CARE, ISOPTO ATROPINE)	0.5%, 1%, and 2% solution; 1% ointment	Cycloplegia, mydriasis,[b] Cycloplegic retinoscopy,[a] Dilated funduscopic exam	Photosensitivity, blurred vision
Scopolamine (ISOPTO HYOSCINE)	0.25% solution	Cycloplegia, mydriasis[b]	Same as for atropine
Homatropine (ISOPTO HOMATROPINE, others)	2% and 5% solution		
Cyclopentolate (AK-PENTOLATE, CYCLOGYL)	0.5%, 1%, and 2% solution		
Tropicamide (MYDRIACYL, TROPICACYL)	0.5% and 1% solution		
Sympathomimetic agents			
Dipivefrin (AKPRO)	0.1% solution	Glaucoma	Photosensitivity, conjunctival hyperemia hypersensitivity
Phenylephrine (AK-DILATE, MYDFRIN, NEO-SYNEPHRINE, others)	0.12%, 2.5%, and 10% solution	Mydriasis, vasoconstriction, decongestion	Same as for dipivefrin
Apraclonidine (IOPIDINE)	0.5% and 1% solution	Ocular hypertension	
Brimonidine (ALPHAGAN-P, others)	0.1%, 0.15%, and 0.2% solution	Glaucoma, ocular hypertension	
Naphazoline (AK-CON, ALBALON, NAPHCON, others)	0.012%, 0.03%, and 0.1% solution	Decongestant	
Tetrahydrozoline (ALTAZINE, MURINE TEARS PLUS, VISINE, others)	0.05% solution	Decongestant	
α and β adrenergic antagonists			
Betaxolol (β₁-selective) (BETOPTIC, BETOPTIC-S, others)	0.25% and 0.5% suspension	Glaucoma, ocular hypertension	
Carteolol (β) (OCUPRESS, others)	1% solution		
Levobunolol (β) (BETAGAN, others)	0.25% and 0.5% solution		
Metipranolol (β) (OPTIPRANOLOL, others)	0.3% solution		
Timolol (β) (TIMOPTIC, TIMOPTIC XE, BETIMOL, others)	0.25% and 0.5% solution and gel		

[a]Off-label use. Refer to the *Physicians' Desk Reference for Ophthalmic Medicines* for specific indications and dosing information. [b]Mydriasis and cycloplegia, or paralysis of accommodation, of the human eye occurs after one drop of atropine 1%, scopolamine 0.5%, homatropine 1%, cyclopentolate 0.5% or 1%, and tropicamide 0.5% or 1%. Recovery of mydriasis is defined by return to baseline pupil size to within 1 mm. Recovery of cycloplegia is defined by return to within 2 diopters of baseline accommodative power. The maximal mydriatic effect of homatropine is achieved with a 5% solution, but cycloplegia may be incomplete. Maximal cycloplegia with tropicamide may be achieved with a 1% solution. Times to development of maximal mydriasis and to recovery, respectively, are: for atropine, 30-40 minutes and 7-10 days; for scopolamine, 20-130 minutes and 3-7 days; for homatropine, 40-60 minutes and 1-3 days; for cyclopentolate, 30-60 minutes and 1 day; for tropicamide, 20-40 minutes and 6 hours. Times to development of maximal cycloplegia and to recovery, respectively, are: for atropine, 60-180 minutes and 6-12 days; for scopolamine, 30-60 minutes and 3-7 days; for homatropine, 30-60 minutes and 1-3 days; for cyclopentolate, 25-75 minutes and 6 hours to 1 day; for tropicamide, 30 minutes and 6 hours.

SECTION IX

Special Systems Pharmacology

SYSTEMIC DRUGS WITH OCULAR SIDE EFFECTS

DRUG	SIDE EFFECT
Topiramate	Angle-closure glaucoma
Hydroxychloroquine	Central retinal toxicity
Tamoxifen	Crystalline maculopathy of the retina
Vigabatrin	Progressive and permanent bilateral concentric visual field constriction
Digoxin	A sign of elevated plasma concentrations is a yellow halo around objects
Phosphodiesterase (PDE5) inhibitors: sildenafil, vardenafil, and tadalafil	Seeing a bluish haze or experiencing light sensitivity
Ethambutol Chloramphenicol Rifampin	Toxic optic neuropathy with progressive bilateral scotomas and vision loss
Rifabutin	Iridocyclitis
Isotretinoin	Dry eye and meibomian gland dysfunction
Amiodarone Indomethacin Atovaquone, chloroquine, hydroxychloroquine	Corneal drug deposits
Chlorpromazine Thioridazine	Brown deposits in cornea
Gold	Gold deposition in cornea and conjunctiva (chrysiasis)
Tetracyclines	Yellow discoloration of light-exposed conjunctiva
Minocycline	Blue-gray scleral pigmentation

CASE 47-1

A 48-year-old man with a 10-year history of congestive heart failure following an acute myocardial infarction is treated with timolol eye drops for increased intraocular pressure (IOP). After using the eye drops for 1 week the patient notices increased fatigue and shortness of breath.

a. What kind of drug in timolol?

Timolol is a nonselective β adrenergic receptor antagonist (see Chapter 7). Its adverse systemic effects are bradycardia, negative cardiac inotropy, and decreased cardiac output. These effects would worsen this patient's congestive heart failure.

b. How is the timolol associated with a worsening of this patient's heart failure when the drug is being administered as drops to the eye?

All ophthalmic medications are potentially absorbed into the systemic circulation (see Figure 47-2; Table 47-5), so undesirable systemic side effects may occur. Topically administered drugs may undergo systemic distribution primarily by nasal mucosal absorption and possibly by local ocular distribution by transcorneal/transconjunctival absorption. Following transcorneal absorption, the aqueous humor accumulates the drug, which then is distributed to intraocular structures as well as potentially to the systemic circulation via the trabecular meshwork pathway (see Figures 47-2 and 47-3).

(Continued)

Ocular Pharmacology

CHAPTER 47

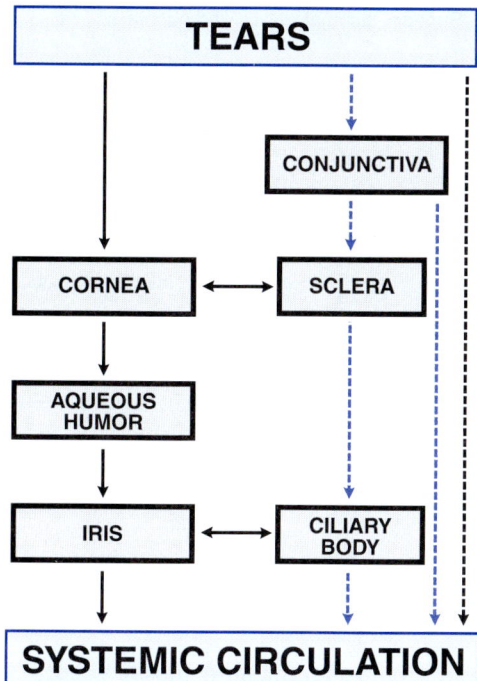

FIGURE 47-2 Possible absorption pathways of an ophthalmic drug following topical application to the eye. Solid black arrows represent the corneal route; dashed blue arrows represent the conjunctival/scleral route; the black dashed arrow represents the nasolacrimal absorption pathway. (*Adapted with permission from Chien DS et al. Curr Eye Res. 1990;9:1051–1059. Copyright © Taylor & Francis Group, http://www.informaworld.com.*)

Systemic absorption after ocular administration of β adrenergic receptor antagonists can induce all the side effects found with direct systemic administration. Absorption from the nasal mucosa avoids first-pass metabolism by the liver, and consequently, significant systemic side effects may be caused by topical medications, especially when used chronically. Possible absorption pathways of an ophthalmic drug following topical application to the eye are shown in Figures 47-2 and 47-3.

TABLE 47-5 Some Characteristics of Ocular Routes of Administration

ROUTE	ABSORPTION PATTERN	SPECIAL UTILITY	LIMITATIONS AND PRECAUTIONS
Topical	Prompt, depending on formulation	Convenient, economical, relatively safe	Compliance, corneal and conjunctival toxicity, nasal mucosal toxicity, systemic side effects from nasolacrimal absorption
Subconjunctival, sub-Tenon's, and retrobulbar injections	Prompt or sustained, depending on formulation	Anterior segment infections, posterior uveitis, cystoid macular edema	Local toxicity, tissue injury, globe perforation, optic nerve trauma, central retinal artery and/or vein occlusion, direct retinal drug toxicity with inadvertent globe perforation, ocular muscle trauma, prolonged drug effect
Intraocular (intracameral) injections	Prompt	Anterior segment surgery, infections	Corneal toxicity, intraocular toxicity, relatively short duration of action
Intravitreal injection or device	Absorption circumvented, immediate local effect, potential sustained effect	Endophthalmitis, retinitis, age-related macular degeneration	Retinal toxicity

SECTION IX Special Systems Pharmacology

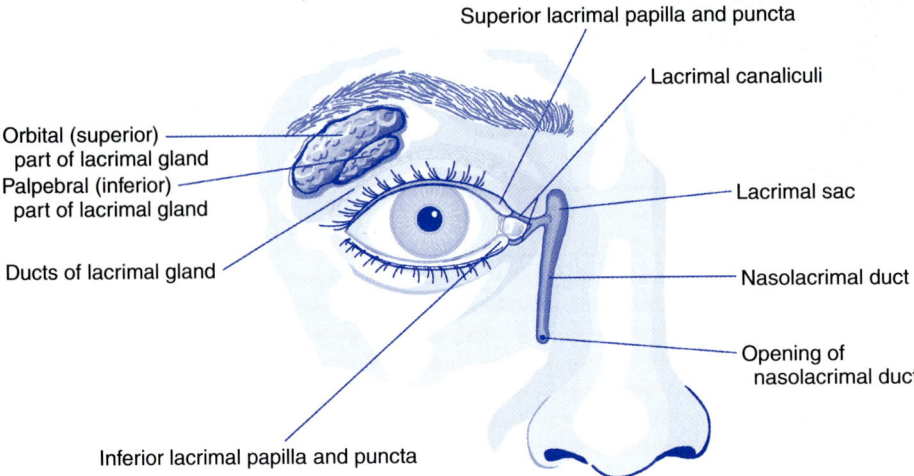

FIGURE 47-3 Anatomy of the lacrimal system.

CASE 47-2

A 17-year-old girl is brought to the emergency room after ingesting Jimson weed. Her main complaint is the bright lights that are an irritation to her eyes. Her pupils are dilated.

a. What is Jimson weed?

Jimson weed is commonly found in backyards and vacant lots. Its seeds contain belladonna alkaloids including atropine (see Chapters 3 and 6). The seeds are ingested to attain the CNS effects of atropine including mild hallucinations.

b. Why do antimuscarinic substances cause mydriasis?

The autonomic innervation of the eye by the sympathetic and parasympathetic nervous systems is shown in Figure 47-1. The effect of cholinergic agents on the pupil is constriction (miosis) (see Table 47-6). Thus, the effect of an anticholinergic agent such as atropine would be dilation (mydriasis). For further explanation see Chapter 6.

TABLE 47-6 Effects of Pharmacological Agents on the Pupil

CLINICAL SETTING	DRUG	PUPILLARY RESPONSE
Normal	Sympathomimetic drugs	Dilation (mydriasis)
Normal	Parasympathomimetic drugs	Constriction (miosis)
Horner's syndrome	Cocaine 4-10%	No dilation
Preganglionic Horner's	Hydroxyamphetamine 1%	Dilation
Postganglionic Horner's	Hydroxyamphetamine 1%	No dilation
Adie's pupil	Pilocarpine 0.05-0.1%[a]	Constriction
Normal	Opioids (oral or intravenous)	Pinpoint pupils

Topically applied ophthalmic drugs unless otherwise noted. [a]This percentage of pilocarpine is not commercially available and usually is prepared by the physician administering the test or by a pharmacist. This test also requires that no prior manipulation of the cornea (ie, tonometry for measuring intraocular pressure or testing corneal sensation) be done so that the normal integrity of the corneal barrier is intact. Normal pupils will not respond to this weak dilution of pilocarpine; however, an Adie's pupil manifests a denervation supersensitivity and is, therefore, pharmacodynamically responsive to this dilute cholinergic agonist.

Ocular Pharmacology

CHAPTER 47

CASE 47-3

A 53-year-old man has been told by his ophthalmologist that his intraocular pressure is increased and that he will need to be treated for glaucoma.

a. What is the pathophysiology of glaucoma?

The peripheral anterior chamber angle is an important anatomical structure for differentiating 2 forms of glaucoma: open-angle glaucoma, which is by far the most common form of glaucoma in the United States, and angle-closure glaucoma (see Figure 47-4). Current medical therapy of open-angle glaucoma is aimed at decreasing aqueous humor production and/or increasing aqueous outflow. The preferred management for angle-closure glaucoma is surgical iridectomy, by either laser or incision, but short-term medical management may be necessary to reduce the acute intraocular pressure (IOP) elevation and to clear the cornea prior to surgery. Long-term IOP reduction may be necessary, especially if the peripheral iris has permanently covered the trabecular meshwork.

(Continued)

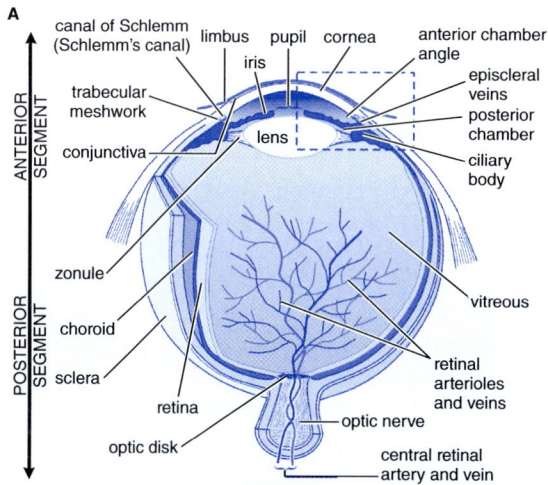

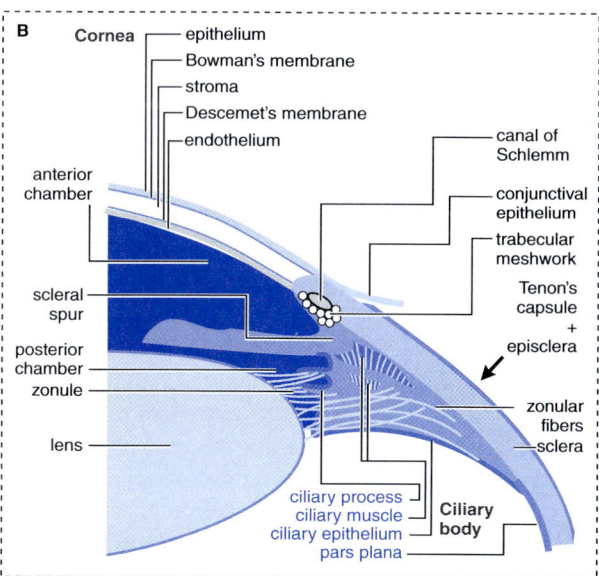

FIGURE 47-4 A. Anatomy of the eye. **B.** Enlargement of the anterior segment, revealing the cornea, angle structures, lens, and ciliary body. *(Adapted with permission from Riordan-Eva P. Anatomy and embryology of the eye. In, Vaughan & Asbury's General Ophthalmology, 17th ed. [Riordan-Eva P, Whitcher JP, eds.] McGraw-Hill, New York, 2008. Copyright © 2008 by The McGraw-Hill Companies, Inc. All rights reserved.)*

b. What are the options for therapy in this patient?

Table 47-4 lists the autonomic drugs for ophthalmic use. Current pharmacotherapies are targeted at decreasing the production of aqueous humor at the ciliary body and increasing outflow through the trabecular meshwork and uveoscleral pathways. The goal is to prevent progressive glaucomatous optic-nerve damage with minimum risk and side effects from either topical or systemic therapy. With these general principles in mind, a stepped medical approach may begin with a topical prostaglandin (PG) analog. Due to their once-daily dosing, low incidence of systemic side effects, and potent IOP-lowering effect, PG analogs have largely replaced β adrenergic receptor antagonists as first-line medical therapy for glaucoma. Modifications to the chemical structure of $PGF_{2\alpha}$ have produced analogs with a more acceptable side-effect profile.

The β adrenergic receptor antagonists now are the next most common topical medical treatment. There are 2 classes of topical β blockers. The nonselective ones bind to both $β_1$ and $β_2$ adrenergic receptors and include timolol maleate and hemihydrate (timolol hemihydrate is not available in the United States), levobunolol, metipranolol, and carteolol.

When there are medical contraindications to the use of PG analogs or β receptor antagonists, other agents, such as a $β_2$ adrenergic receptor agonist or topical carbonic anhydrase inhibitor (CAI), may be used as first-line therapy. Any of these drug classes can be used as additive second- or third-line therapy.

CASE 47-4

A 60-year-old man wakes up with a crusty discharge in both eyes. His ophthalmologist diagnoses blepharitis.

a. What is blepharitis?

Blepharitis is a common bilateral inflammatory process of the eyelids characterized by irritation and burning, usually associated with a *Staphylococcus* spp. infection. Local hygiene is the mainstay of therapy; topical antibiotics frequently are used, usually in gel, drop, or ointment form, particularly when the disease is accompanied by conjunctivitis and keratitis.

Conjunctivitis is an inflammatory process of the conjunctiva that varies in severity from mild hyperemia to severe purulent discharge. The more common causes of conjunctivitis include viruses, allergies, environmental irritants, contact lenses, and chemicals. The less common causes include other infectious pathogens, immune-mediated reactions, associated systemic diseases, and tumors of the conjunctiva or eyelid.

Keratitis, or corneal inflammation, can occur at any level of the cornea (eg, epithelium, subepithelium, stroma, and endothelium). It can be due to noninfectious or infectious causes. Numerous microbial agents have been identified as causes of infectious keratitis, including bacteria, viruses, fungi, spirochetes, cysts, and trophozoites. Severe infections with tissue loss (corneal ulcers) generally are treated more aggressively than infections without tissue loss (corneal infiltrates).

The mild, small, more peripheral infections usually are not cultured, and the eyes are treated with broad-spectrum topical antibiotics. In more severe, central, or larger infections, corneal scrapings for smears, cultures, and sensitivities are performed, and the patient is immediately started on intensive hourly, around-the-clock topical antibiotic therapy. The goal of treatment is to eradicate the infection and reduce the amount of corneal scarring and the chance of corneal perforation and severe decreased vision or blindness. The initial medication selection and dosage are adjusted according to the clinical response, and culture and sensitivity results.

b. What are the treatment options with this patient?

Table 47-1 shows the topical antibacterial agents available for ophthalmic use. See Chapters 38, 39, 40, and 41 for additional details about specific agents.

Ocular Pharmacology CHAPTER 47

CASE 47-5

A 33-year-old woman has developed a herpes simplex infection of her cornea (viral keratitis).

a. What is the pathophysiology of viral infections of the eye?

Viral keratitis, an infection of the cornea that may involve either the epithelium or stroma, is most commonly caused by herpes simplex type I and varicella zoster viruses. Less common viral etiologies include herpes simplex type II, Epstein-Barr virus, and cytomegalovirus (CMV). Topical antiviral agents are indicated for the treatment of epithelial disease due to herpes simplex infection. When treating viral keratitis topically, there is a very narrow margin between the therapeutic topical antiviral activity and the toxic effect on the cornea; hence, patients must be followed very closely.

b. What treatment options are available for this patient?

The various antiviral drugs currently used in ophthalmology are summarized in Table 47-2 (see Chapter 44 for additional details about specific agents).

The primary indications for the use of antiviral drugs in ophthalmology are viral keratitis, herpes zoster ophthalmicus, and retinitis. There currently are no antiviral agents for the treatment of viral conjunctivitis caused by adenoviruses, which usually has a self-limited course and typically is treated by symptomatic relief of irritation.

Topical glucocorticoids are contraindicated in herpetic epithelial keratitis due to active viral replication. In contrast, for herpetic disciform keratitis, which predominantly is presumed to involve a cell-mediated immune reaction, topical glucocorticoids accelerate recovery.

CASE 47-6

A 43-year-old woman who has been receiving chemotherapy for colon cancer is diagnosed with a fungal keratitis.

a. What treatment is available for this patient?

The only currently available topical ophthalmic antifungal preparation is a polyene, natamycin (NATACYN). Other antifungal agents may be extemporaneously compounded for topical, subconjunctival, or intravitreal routes of administration (see Table 47-3). The pharmacology and structures of specific antifungal agents are given in Chapter 43.

As with systemic fungal infections, the incidence of ophthalmic fungal infections has risen with the growing number of immunocompromised hosts. Ophthalmic indications for antifungal medications include fungal keratitis, scleritis, endophthalmitis, mucormycosis, and canaliculitis. Risk factors for fungal keratitis include trauma, chronic ocular surface disease, contact lens wear, and immunosuppression (including topical steroid use). In 2005 to 2006, there was a worldwide epidemic of *Fusarium* fungal keratitis related to a specific contact lens solution, which resolved when it was removed from the market. When fungal infection is suspected, samples of the affected tissues are obtained for smears, cultures, and sensitivities, and this information is used to guide drug selection.

KEY CONCEPTS

- The eye is relatively secluded from systemic access by blood-retinal, blood-aqueous, and blood-vitreous barriers; as a consequence, the eye exhibits some unusual pharmacodynamics and pharmacokinetic properties.
- Topically administered drugs may undergo systemic distribution primarily by nasal mucosal absorption and possibly by local ocular distribution by transcorneal/transconjunctival absorption.

(Continued)

- Drug absorption from the nasal mucosa avoids first-pass metabolism by the liver, and consequently, significant systemic side effects may be caused by topical medications.
- Individual variation may be an important consideration for ocular drug distribution due to drug-melanin binding to melanocytes in the iris.
- Classical pharmacokinetic theory based on studies of systemically administered drugs does not fully apply to all ophthalmic drugs administered topically or locally.
- After topical instillation of a drug, the rate and extent of absorption are determined by the time the drug remains in the cul-de-sac and precorneal tear film, elimination by nasolacrimal drainage, drug binding to tear proteins, drug metabolism by tear and tissue proteins, and diffusion across the cornea and conjunctiva.
- Several drug formulations prolong the time a drug remains on the surface of the eye and thus facilitate drug absorption.
- Appropriate selection of an antimicrobial and route of administration is dependent on the patient's symptoms, the clinical examination, and the culture/sensitivity results.

SUMMARY QUIZ

QUESTION 47-1 A 42-year-old man with a seizure disorder has developed glaucoma. It is possible that he has developed glaucoma from the use of

a. phenytoin.
b. topiramate.
c. carbamazepine.
d. lamotrigine.
e. valproic acid.

QUESTION 47-2 A 25-year-old woman with refractory seizures is started on vigabatrin. She should be counseled about

a. the development of glaucoma.
b. eye lid droop.
c. conjunctivitis.
d. permanent constriction of visual fields.
e. mydriasis.

QUESTION 47-3 A 53-year-old woman with type 2 diabetes has noticed that her blood sugar has been difficult to regulate after she started using glucocorticoid eye drops. It is likely that the glucocorticoid is being absorbed into the systemic circulation from the

a. nasal mucosa.
b. drops that spill from the eye and enter her oral cavity.
c. lens.
d. vitreous humor.
e. canal of Schlemm.

QUESTION 47-4 A 42-year-old man with glaucoma is treated with the α_2 adrenergic receptor agonist apraclonidine. Despite being a derivative of clonidine, apraclonidine does not cause systemic hypotension because it is

a. tightly bound to plasma proteins.
b. metabolized rapidly by the liver.
c. highly ionized at physiological pH.
d. not absorbed from the eye.
e. rapidly excreted by the kidney.

Ocular Pharmacology — CHAPTER 47

QUESTION 47-5 A 48-year-old man experiences a bluish haze and light sensitivity when he takes which of the following medications?

a. Tetracycline
b. Amoxicillin
c. Metoprolol
d. Ibuprofen
e. Tadalafil

QUESTION 47-6 A 65-year-old woman is being treated with verteporfin intravenously followed by laser light activation for age-related macular degeneration. She should be cautioned about which of the following side effects?

a. Photosensitization
b. Liver impairment
c. Kidney impairment
d. Chronic ophthalmic discharge
e. Yellowing of the sclera

QUESTION 47-7 Vitamin A plays an essential role in the function of the retina. Vitamin A deficiency interferes with

a. tear production.
b. vision in dim light.
c. color distinction.
d. peripheral vision.
e. vision in bright light.

SUMMARY QUIZ ANSWER KEY

QUESTION 47-1 Answer is **b**. The antiseizure drug topiramate frequently has been reported to cause choroidal effusions, thereby anteriorly rotating the ciliary body and causing angle-closure glaucoma.

QUESTION 47-2 Answer is **d**. The antiseizure drug vigabatrin causes progressive and permanent bilateral concentric visual field constriction in a high percentage of patients. The mechanism is not known, but vigabatrin is more effectively transported into the retina than into the brain, and consequently, elevations of retinal GABA concentrations may contribute to the vision loss.

QUESTION 47-3 Answer is **a**. Topically administered drugs may undergo systemic distribution primarily by nasal mucosal absorption and possibly by local ocular distribution by transcorneal/transconjunctival absorption (see Figures 47-2 and 47-3).

QUESTION 47-4 Answer is **c**. Apraclonidine is a relatively selective α_2 adrenergic agonist that is highly ionized at physiological pH and therefore does not cross the blood-brain barrier.

QUESTION 47-5 Answer is **e**. The 3 phosphodiesterase (PDE) inhibitors—sildenafil, vardenafil, and tadalafil—inhibit PDE5 in the corpus cavernosum to help achieve and maintain penile erection. The drugs also mildly inhibit PDE6, which controls the levels of cyclic GMP in the retina. Visually, this can result in seeing a bluish haze or experiencing light sensitivity.

QUESTION 47-6 Answer is **a**. Verteporfin is approved for photodynamic therapy of the exudative form of age-related macular degeneration (ARMD) with predominantly classic choroidal neovascular membranes. Verteporfin also is used in the treatment of predominantly classic choroidal neovascularization caused by conditions such as pathological myopia and presumed ocular histoplasmosis syndrome.

(Continued)

SECTION IX   Special Systems Pharmacology

Verteporfin is administered intravenously, and once it reaches the choroidal circulation, the drug is light-activated by a nonthermal laser source. Depending on the size of the neovascular membrane and concerns of occult membranes and recurrence, multiple photodynamic treatments may be necessary. Activation of the drug in the presence of oxygen generates free radicals, which cause vessel damage and subsequent platelet activation, thrombosis, and occlusion of choroidal neovascularization.

The potential side effects include headache, injection-site reactions, and visual disturbances. The drug causes temporary photosensitization, and patients must avoid exposure of the skin or eyes to direct sunlight or bright indoor lights for 5 days after receiving it.

QUESTION 47-7 Answer is **b**. Vitamin A deficiency interferes with vision in dim light, a condition known as night blindness (nyctalopia), as well as causing xerosis (dryness), and keratomalacia (corneal thinning), which may lead to corneal perforation. Nyctalopia may be reversed with vitamin A therapy; however, rapid, irreversible blindness ensues if the cornea perforates.

Following short-term deprivation of vitamin A, dark adaptation can be restored to normal by the addition of retinol to the diet. However, vision does not return to normal for several weeks after adequate amounts of retinol have been supplied. The reason for this delay is unknown.

SUMMARY: DRUGS USED FOR OPHTHALMIC DISORDERS

Class and Subclasses	Names	Clinical Uses	TOXICITIES Common	Unique; Clinically Important
Autonomic Agents	Dipivefrin	Second-line therapy for glaucoma	Localized irritation and hyperemia	Systemic effects of epinephrine (see Chapter 7)
	Apraclonidine	Treatment of glaucoma	Skin allergy	Systemic effects if absorbed (see Chapter 7) Does not cross the blood-brain barrier so systemic effects are less than with clonidine
	Brimonidine	Treatment of glaucoma	Skin allergy	Systemic effects if absorbed (see Chapter 7)
	Acetylcholine	Used to induce intraoperative miosis	Side effects and toxicity are generally related to systemic absorption (see Chapter 6)	
	Carbachol	Used to induce intraoperative miosis	Side effects and toxicity are generally related to systemic absorption (see Chapter 6)	
	Pilocarpine	Historically important glaucoma medication, but rarely used today	Side effects and toxicity are generally related to systemic absorption (see Chapter 6)	
	Echothiophate	Miotic agent that may be used to treat glaucoma	Quaternary ammonium compound that is poorly absorbed	
	Atropine Scopolamine Homatropine	Mydriasis, cycloplegia	Photosensitivity and blurred vision	Side effects and toxicity are generally related to systemic absorption (see Chapter 6)

(Continued)

Ocular Pharmacology — CHAPTER 47

Class and Subclasses	Names	Clinical Uses	TOXICITIES Common	Unique; Clinically Important
	Cyclopentolate Tropicamide	Mydriasis, cycloplegia Used to treat uveitis		
	Phenylephrine	Mydriasis, vasoconstriction, decongestant		Side effects and toxicity are generally related to systemic absorption (see Chapter 7)
	Naphazoline Tetrahydozoline	Decongestant		
	Betaxolol Carteolol Levobunolol Metipranolol Timolol	Used to treat glaucoma		Side effects and toxicity are generally related to systemic absorption (see Chapter 7)
Prostaglandin Analogs	Latanoprost Travoprost Brimatoprost	Used to treat glaucoma	Blurred vision, burning, stinging, conjunctival hyperemia, dry eyes	See Chapter 22
Carbonic Anhydrase Inhibitors	Dorzolamide Brinzolamide	Used to treat glaucoma		Side effects and toxicity are generally related to systemic absorption (see Chapter 15)
Ophthalmic Glucocorticoids	Dexamethasone Prednisolone Fluorometolone Loteprednol Rimexolone Difluprednate	Treatment of ocular inflammatory diseases	Side effects and toxicity are generally related to systemic absorption (see Chapter 29)	Development of cataracts, secondary infections, secondary open-angle glaucoma
	Triamcinolone (intravitreal)	Intravitreal formulation for ocular inflammatory conditions		
	Fluocinolone	Ophthalmic implant used for treatment of chronic noninfectious uveitis		
Nonsteroidal Anti-inflammatory Agents	Flurbiprofen Ketorolac Diclofenac Bromfenac Nepafenac	Used to treat ocular inflammation	Side effects and toxicity are generally related to systemic absorption (see Chapter 22)	Occasionally associated with corneal perforation
Antihistamines and Mast Cell Stabilizers	Emedastine difumarate Cromolyn sodium Lodoxamide tromethamine Pemirolast Nedocromil Olopatadine Ketotifen fumarate Bepotastine Azelastine Epinastine	Used to treat allergic conjunctivitis	Side effects and toxicity are generally related to systemic absorption (see Chapter 21)	
Immunosuppressive and Antimitotic Agents	Fluorouracil Mitomycin	Used in glaucoma surgery to limit the postoperative wound-healing process and prevent scarring		Can result in thin, ischemic, avascular tissue that is prone to breakdown
	Cyclosporine A	Treatment of chronic dye eye	Localized burning, tearing, discharge, itching Visual blurring	

(Continued)

SECTION IX — Special Systems Pharmacology

Class and Subclasses	Names	Clinical Uses	Common	Unique; Clinically Important
			TOXICITIES	
Agents Used in Ophthalmic Surgery	Povidone iodine	Ophthalmic solution used for preoperative preparation of periocular skin		Contraindicated in patients that are hypersensitive to iodine
	Hyaluronate Chondroitin sulfate Hydroxypropyl methylcellulose	Viscoelastic substances used to assist in ocular surgery		Transient elevation of IOP after surgery
	Cyanoacrylate Fibrinogen gel	Used as a tissue adhesive during ocular surgery Approved for cardiac, vascular, and general surgery, but not for the eye		
	Vitreous substitutes	Used for reattachment of the retina following vitrectomy and other retinal surgeries (see Table 64-8 *Goodman and Gilman's The Pharmacological Basis of Therapeutics,* 12th Edition)		
	Polydimethylsiloxanes	Used for long-term tamponade of the retina		Glaucoma, cataract formation, corneal edema, corneal band keratopathy, and retinal toxicity
	Trypan Blue	Used during ophthalmic surgery to visualize the lens and to guide the excision of tissue		
Agents Used in the Treatment of Strabismus and Blepharospasm	Onabotulinumtoxin A Abobotulinumtoxin A	Used in the treatment of strabismus and blepharospasm		Double vision, lid droop Potentially life-threatening distant spread of toxin (see Chapter 6)
Agents Used to Treat Macular Degeneration	Verteporfin	Approved for photodynamic therapy of the exudative form of age-related macular degeneration (ARMD)	Headache, injection site reactions, and visual disturbances	Temporary photosensitivity of the skin and eyes Patients must avoid direct sunlight or bright indoor lights for 5 days
	Pegaptanib	Treatment of neovascular (wet) ARMD	Side effects are related to the intravitreal injection	Monitor patients for increase IOP and endophthalmitis Rare cases of anaphylaxis
	Bevacizumab Ranibizumab	Used for the treatment of ARMD and off label to treat neovascularization caused by other diseases (see Chapter 46)	Risk of hemorrhage and infection from intravitreal injection	Associated with cerebrovascular accidents (see Chapter 46)
Wetting Agents and Tear Substitutes	Tyloxapol Carboxy-methylcellulose Hydroxylethyl cellulose Hydroxypropyl cellulose Hydroxypropyl methyl-cellulose Methylcellulose	Artificial tears and ophthalmic lubricants used for the management of dry eyes	Localized burning and irritation	

CHAPTER 48

Dermatological Pharmacology

This chapter will be most useful after having a basic understanding of the material in Chapter 65, Dermatological Pharmacology in *Goodman & Gilman's The Pharmacological Basis of Therapeutics*, 12th Edition. In addition to the material presented here, the 12th Edition contains:

- A detailed description of the structures of the skin and their pharmacological implications
- A discussion of antimicrobial therapy of skin disorders
- A discussion of the use of cytotoxic and immunosuppressive drugs in the treatment of skin disorders
- Tables 65-4 and 65-5 which are a listing of topical and systemic retinoids, respectively
- Chemical structures of drugs used to treat dermatological disorders

LEARNING OBJECTIVES

- ☑ Understand how drugs are absorbed through the skin.
- ☑ Know the mechanisms of action, therapeutic uses, and toxicities of topical and systemic drugs used to treat dermatological disorders.
- ☑ Know the principles of photochemotherapy of dermatological disorders.
- ☑ Know the science behind the use of sunscreen agents.

DRUGS INCLUDED IN THIS CHAPTER[a]

- Acitretin (SORIATANE)
- Adalimumab (HUMIRA)
- Adapalene (DIFFERIN)
- Alefacept (AMEVIVE)
- Alitretinoin (9-*cis*-retinoic acid) (PANRETIN)
- Aminolevulinic acid (ALA, LEVULAN KERASTICK)
- Azathioprine (IMURAN, others)
- Azelaic acid (AZELEX, FINACEA)
- Benzyl alcohol
- Bexarotene (TARGRETIN)
- Bleomycin (BLENOXANE)
- Calcipotriene (DOVONEX, others)
- Capsaicin (ZOSTRIX, CAPSIN)
- Carmustine (BICNU)
- Chloroquine (ARALEN, others)
- Crotamiton (EURAX)
- Cyclophosphamide
- Cyclosporine (NEORAL, GENGRAF, others)
- Dapsone (diaminodiphenylsulfone, DDS)
- Denileukin Diftitox (ONTAK)
- Doxorubicin (DOXIL, CAELYX)
- Efalizumab (RAPTIVA)
- Etanercept (ENBREL)
- Finasteride (PROPECIA, others)
- Fluorouracil (CARAC, others)
- Hydroquinone (TRI-LUMA)
- Hydroxychloroquine (PLAQUENIL, others)
- Imiquimod (ALDARA)
- Infliximab (REMICADE)
- Isotretinoin (13-*cis*-retinoic acid) (ACCUTANE)
- Ivermectin (STOMECTOL)
- Lindane
- Malathion (OVIDE)
- Mechlorethamine (MUSTARGEN)
- Mequinol (SOLAGE, in combination with tretinoin and vitamin C)

(continues)

MECHANISMS OF ACTION

DRUG CLASS	DRUG	MECHANISM OF ACTION
Glucocorticoids	Triamcinolone acetonide Triamcinolone hexacetonide Numerous other agents (Table 48-7)	See Chapter 29
Retinoids	Tretinoin Isotretinoin Acitretin Tazarotene Bexarotene Adapalene Alitretinoin	Exert their effect on gene expression by activating 2 families of receptors: retinoic acid receptors (RARs) and retinoid X receptors (RXRs) Bexarotene selectively binds RXRs
Vitamin Analogs	Calcipotriene	Vitamin D analog exerts its effects through the vitamin D receptor (VDR); upon binding the VDR, the drug receptor complex associates with RXR-α and binds to vitamin D response elements on DNA
Photochemotherapeutic Drugs (PUVA, Table 48-4)	Methoxsalen	Methoxsalen followed by ultraviolet radiation between 320-340 nm (UVA) results in 2 photoreactions: Type I reactions involve the oxygen-independent photoaddition of the psoralen to pyrimidine bases in DNA; Type II reactions are oxygen-dependent and involve the transfer of energy to molecular oxygen, creating reactive oxygen species (Table 48-4)

(continued)

707

SECTION IX

Special Systems Pharmacology

DRUGS INCLUDED IN THIS CHAPTER (Cont.)

- Methotrexate (RHEUMATRIX)
- Methoxsalen (OXSORALEN, others)—not marketed in the United States
- Methylaminolevulinate (MAL, VETVIXIA)
- Minoxidil (ROGAINE, others)
- Monobenzone (BENOQUIN)
- Mycophenolate mofetil (CELLCEPT)
- Permethrin (KLOUT shampoo)
- Pimecrolimus (ELIDEL)
- Podophyllin (podophyllum resin)
- Quinacrine (ATABRINE)
- Retapamulin (ALTABAX)
- Retinol (vitamin A)
- Tacrolimus (FK506, PROTOPIC)
- Tazarotene (TAZORAC, others)
- Thalidomide (TALOMID)
- Tretinoin (all *trans*-retinoic acid; vitamin A acid) (ATRALIN, others)
- Triamcinolone acetonide (KENALOG-10)
- Triamcinolone hexacetonide (ARISTOSPAN)
- Vinblastine (VELBAN)

[a]Drugs included in this chapter have specific dermatological uses. Antibiotics used to treat acne are listed in the Side Bar ANTIBIOTICS USED TO TREAT ACNE. Antimicrobials used to treat cutaneous infections are discussed in the cases; the pharmacology of specific drugs can be found in Chapters 35, 39, 40, 41, 43, and 44. Sunscreen agents are listed in the Table SUNSCREEN AGENTS.

DRUG CLASS	DRUG	MECHANISM OF ACTION
Photodynamic Therapy (Table 48-4)	Aminolevulinic acid Methylaminolevulinate	Prodrugs that are converted to protoporphyrin IX in living cells; in the presence of specific wavelengths of light (Table 48-4) and oxygen, protoporphyrin produces reactive oxygen species
Antimicrobial Agents	Various antibacterial, antifungal (Table 48-5), and antiviral agents	See Chapters 38, 39, 40, 41, 43, and 44
	Retapamulin	Selectively inhibits bacterial protein synthesis by interacting at a site on the 50S subunit of bacterial ribosomes
Agents Used to Treat Infestations	Permethrin	Interferes with insect sodium transport proteins causing neurotoxicity and paralysis
	Malathion	Cholinesterase inhibitor (see Chapter 6)
	Ivermectin	Anthelmintic (see Chapter 37)
	Lindane	A pesticide that interferes with GABA neurotransmitter function
	Crotamiton	Toxic to scabies mite by an unknown mechanism
	Benzyl alcohol	Inhibits lice from closing their respiratory spiracles causing asphyxiation
Antimalarial Agents	Chloroquine Hydroxychloroquine Quinacrine	Proposed mechanisms of action include stabilization of lysosomes, inhibition of antigen presentation, inhibition of prostaglandin synthesis, inhibition of inflammatory cytokine synthesis, photoprotection, inhibition of immune complex formation, and antithrombotic effects (see Chapter 35)
Antimetabolites	Methotrexate	Folic acid analog that competitively inhibits dihydrofolate reductase (see Chapter 45 and Table 48-8)
	Azathioprine	Impairs purine synthesis and cell proliferation (see Chapter 23 and Table 48-8)
	Fluorouracil	Interferes with DNA synthesis by blocking the methylation of deoxyuridylic acid to thymidylic acid (see Chapter 45 and Table 48-8)
Alkylating Agents	Cyclophosphamide Mechlorethamine Carmustine	See Chapter 45 and Table 48-8
Calcineurin Inhibitors	Cyclosporine Tacrolimus Pimecrolimus	See Chapter 23 and Table 48-8

(Continued)

Dermatological Pharmacology

CHAPTER 48

DRUG CLASS	DRUG	MECHANISM OF ACTION
Other Immunosuppressive and Anti-inflammatory Agents	Mycophenolate mofetil	Inhibits the enzyme inosine monoposphatase dehydrogenase (IMPDH) thereby depleting guanosine nucleotides essential for DNA and RNA synthesis (see Chapter 23 and Table 48-8)
	Imiquimod	Acts as a ligand at toll-like receptors in the innate immune system and induces the cytokines interferon-α (IFN-α), tumor necrosis factor-α (TNF-α) and IL-1, IL-6, IL-8, IL-10, and IL-12 (see Table 48-8)
	Vinblastine Bleomycin Doxorubicin	See Chapter 45 and Table 48-8
	Dapsone	See Chapter 42 and Table 48-8
	Thalidomide	See Chapter 23 and Table 48-8
Biological Agents (Table 48-3)	Alefacept	Binds to CD2 on the surface of T cells, thus blocking a necessary costimulation step in T-cell activation (see Figures 48-1 and Table 48-3)
	Efalizumab	Binds to CD11a on T cells and prevents binding of leukocyte function-associated antigen 1 (LFA-1) to intercellular adhesion molecule (ICAM)-1 on the surface of antigen-presenting cells, vascular endothelial cells, and cells in the dermis and epidermis, thereby interfering with T-cell activation (see Figures 48-1 and 48-2, and Table 48-3)
	Etanercept	Mouse-human chimera antibody that binds soluble and membrane-bound TNF and inhibits its action (see Chapter 23 and Table 48-3)
	Infliximab	Mouse-human chimera antibody that binds soluble and membrane-bound TNF-α and inhibits its action Induces complement-dependent and cell-mediated lysis (see Chapter 23 and Table 48-3)
	Adalimumab	Human antibody that binds soluble and membrane-bound TNF-α and inhibits its action Induces complement-dependent and cell-mediated lysis (see Chapter 23 and Table 48-3)
Agent Used for Treatment of Cutaneous T-Cell Lymphoma	Denileukin Diftitox	Fusion protein composed of diphtheria toxin fragments A and B and the receptor-binding portion of IL-2; once internalized by endocytosis the active fragment of diphtheria toxin is released into the cytosol, where it inhibits protein synthesis through ADP ribosylation (see Chapter 46)

(Continued)

SECTION IX

Special Systems Pharmacology

MECHANISMS OF PERCUTANEOUS ABSORPTION

The process of absorption of a topically applied drug consists of:

- Establishment of a concentration gradient
- Movement of drug into stratum corneum (partition coefficient)
- Diffusion of drug across layers of skin (diffusion coefficient)

The relationship of these factors is summarized in the following equation:

$$J \propto C_{veh} \cdot K_m \cdot D/X$$

where J is the rate of absorption; C_{veh} is the concentration of drug in the vehicle; K_m is the partition coefficient; D is the diffusion coefficient; and x is the thickness of the stratum corneum

DRUG CLASS	DRUG	MECHANISM OF ACTION
Sunscreens	Various chemicals (see Table SUNSCREEN AGENTS)	Absorb incident solar radiation in the ultraviolet B (UVB) or ultraviolet A (UVA) ranges and physical agents that contain particulate materials that can block or reflect incident energy and reduce its transmission to the skin
Drugs for Androgenic Alopecia	Minoxidil	Minoxidil is bioactivated to form minoxidil sulfate which relaxes arteriolar smooth muscle by activating ATP-modulated K$^+$ channels (K_{ATP} channels) (see Chapter 15)
	Finasteride	Inhibits the type II isozyme of 5α-reductase, the enzyme that converts testosterone to dihydrotestosterone (see Chapter 28)
Agents Used to Treat Hyperpigmentation	Hydroquinone Monobenzone Azelaic Mequinol	Decrease melanocyte pigment production by inhibiting the conversion of dopa to melanin through inhibition of the enzyme tyrosinase
Miscellaneous Agents	Capsaicin	Interacts with the transient receptor potential vanilloid (TRPV1) receptor on C-fiber sensory neurons TRPV1 is a ligand-gated nonselective cation channel Capsaicin first stimulates then desensitizes this channel to noxious stimuli

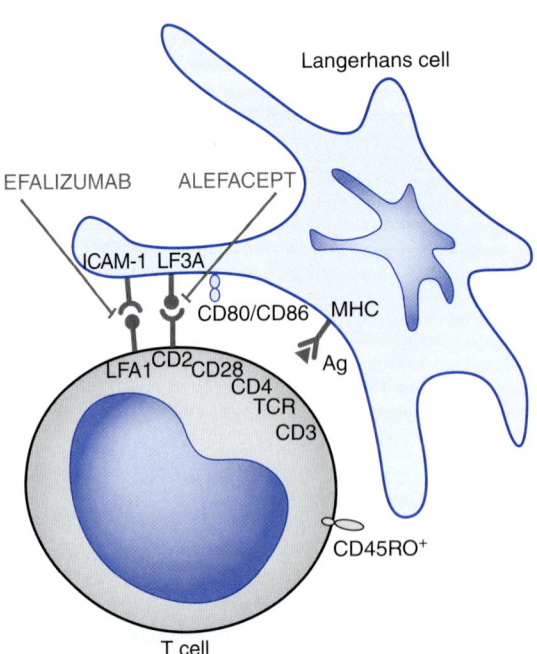

FIGURE 48-1 Mechanisms of action of selected biological agents in psoriasis. Newer biological agents can interfere with one or more steps in the pathogenesis of psoriasis, resulting in clinical improvement. See text in Chapter 65, Dermatological Pharmacology in *Goodman & Gilman's The Pharmacological Basis of Therapeutics*, 12th Edition for details. ICAM-1, intercellular adhesion molecule 1; LFA, lymphocyte function–associated antigen; MHC, major histocompatibility complex; TCR, T-cell receptor.

Dermatological Pharmacology

CHAPTER 48

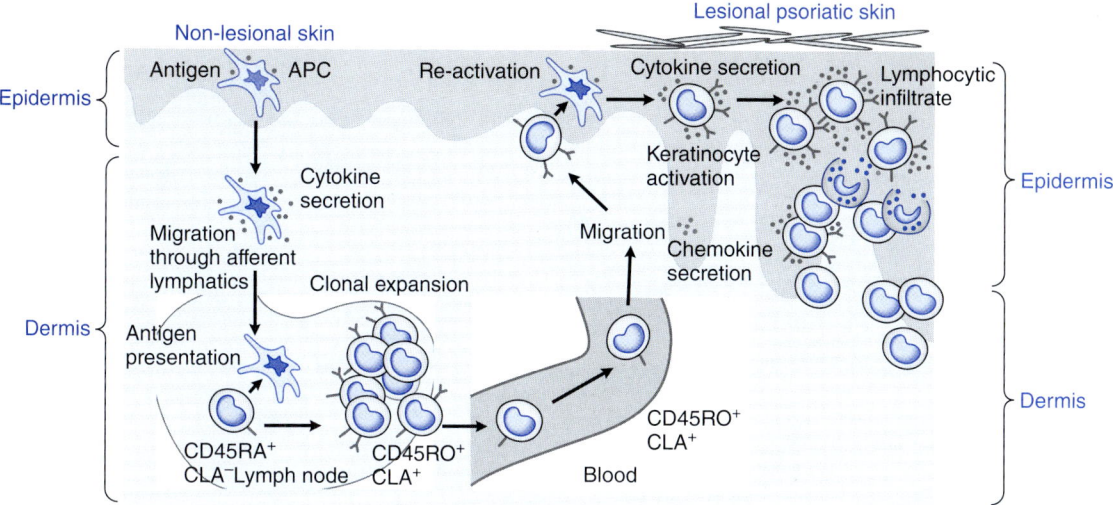

FIGURE 48-2 Immunopathogenesis of psoriasis. Psoriasis is a prototypical inflammatory skin disorder in which specific T-cell populations are stimulated by as-yet undefined antigen(s) presented by antigen-presenting cells. The T cells release proinflammatory cytokines, such as tumor necrosis factor-α (TNF-α) and interferon-γ (IFN-γ), that induce keratinocyte and endothelial cell proliferation. APC, antigen-presenting cell; CLA, cutaneous lymphocyte-associated antigen.

CASE 48-1

A 70-year-old woman has developed an infection from scratching an area on her leg. Despite her physician's recommendation for an oral antibiotic, she wishes to have a "cream" to put on it.

a. What is the process of absorption of the antibiotic through the skin?

Passage through the outermost layer is the rate-limiting step for percutaneous absorption. Figure 48-3 shows the structure and layers of the skin, and Figure 48-4 shows the compartments of skin as they relate to cutaneous drug delivery. The mechanisms of percutaneous absorption are shown in the Side Bar MECHANISMS OF PERCUTANEOUS ABSORPTION.

b. What are the important considerations when applying a drug to the skin?

The important considerations when applying a drug to the skin are shown in Table 48-1. In addition, the following considerations should be taken into account: *dosage*, under-application of a drug because of cost considerations often occurs when large amounts of skin are treated for a long time; *regional anatomical variation*, drug penetration is higher on the face, intertriginous areas, and perineum due to stratum corneum thickness (see Figures 48-3 and 48-4). Skin sites that are naturally occluded by apposing surfaces, such as the axillae, groin, and inframammary areas, are vulnerable to drug-related atrophy from potent topical glucocorticoids; *altered barrier function in disease*, in many dermatological diseases, the stratum corneum is abnormal and barrier function is compromised. In these

(Continued)

TABLE 48-1 Important Considerations When a Drug Is Applied to the Skin

What are the absorption pathways of intact and diseased skin?
How does the chemistry of the drug affect the penetration?
How does the vehicle affect the penetration?
How much of the drug penetrates the skin?
What are the intended pharmacological targets?
What host and genetic factors influence drug function in the skin?

SECTION IX
Special Systems Pharmacology

TABLE 48-2 Vehicles for Topically Applied Drugs

	CREAM	OINTMENT	GEL/FOAM	LOTION/SOLUTION/FOAM
Physical basis	Oil in water emulsion	Water in oil	Water-soluble emulsion	Solution-dissolved drug base Lotion-suspended drug Aerosol propellant with drug Foam drug with surfactant as foaming agent and propellant
Solubilizing medium	>31% water (up to 80%)	<25% water	Contains water-soluble polyethylene glycols	May be aqueous or alcoholic
Pharmacological advantage	Leaves concentrated drug at skin surface	Protective oil film on skin	Concentrates drug at surface after evaporation	
Advantages for patient	Spreads and removes easily No greasy feel	Spreads easily Slows water evaporation Gives a cooling effect	Nonstaining Greaseless Clear appearance	Low residue on scalp
Locations on body	Most locations	Avoid intertriginous areas	Foams well for scalp and other hairy locations	Solutions and foams are well accepted on scalp
Disadvantages	Needs preservatives	Greasy to very greasy Stains clothes	Needs preservatives High alcohol can be drying	
Occlusion	Low	Moderate to high Increases skin moisture		
Composition issues	Requires humectants (glycerine, propylene glycol, polyethylene glycols) to keep moist when applied Oil phase with long-chain alcohol for stability and smooth feel Has absorption bases—hydrophilic petrolatum	Needs surfactants to prevent phase separation Hydrocarbon (VASELINE)	Microspheres or microsponges can be formulated in gels	

settings, increased percutaneous absorption of potent topical steroids can cause systemic toxicity, such as hypothalamic–pituitary–adrenal (HPA) axis suppression; *vehicle*, drug vehicles are summarized in Table 48-2 and below in the answer to Case 1c; *age*, children have a greater ratio of surface area to mass than adults do, so the same amount of topical drug can result in a greater systemic exposure; *application frequency*, topical agents often are applied twice daily. For certain drugs, once-daily application of a larger dose may be equally effective as more frequent applications of smaller doses. For some drugs, the stratum corneum may act as a drug reservoir that allows gradual penetration into the viable skin layers over a prolonged period; *intralesional administration*, intralesional drug administration is used mainly for inflammatory lesions but also can be used for treatment of warts and selected neoplasms. Medications injected intralesionally have the advantages of direct contact with the underlying pathological process, no first-pass metabolism, and the opportunity for a slowly absorbed depot of drug.

c. **What vehicles are available for topically applied drugs?**

Vehicles for the topical administration of drugs are shown in Table 48-2. Newer vehicles include liposomes and microgel formulations. Liposomes are concentric

(Continued)

Dermatological Pharmacology

CHAPTER 48

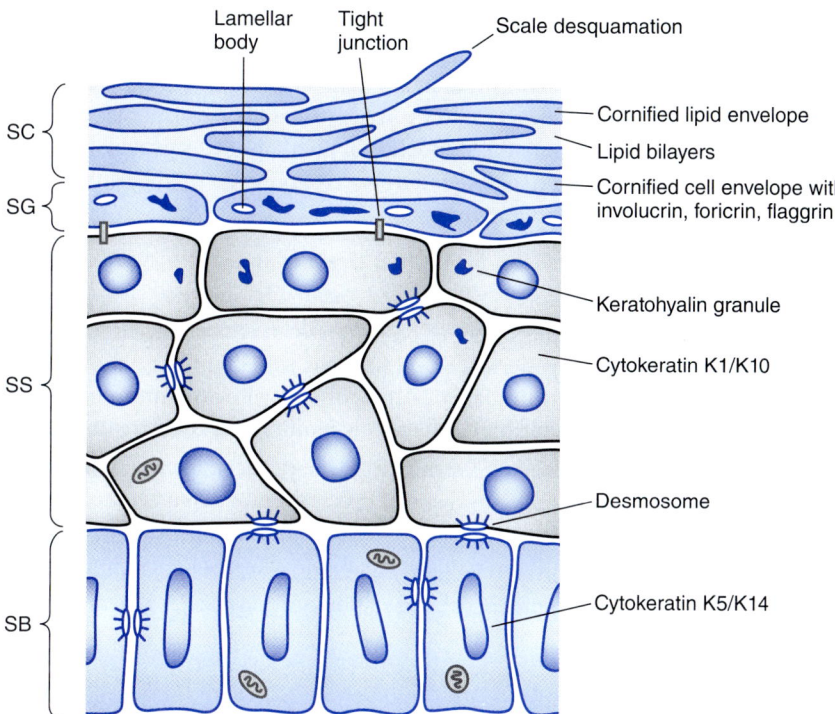

FIGURE 48-3 Structure of the epidermis. The epidermis matures progressively from the stratum basale (SB) to the stratum spinosum (SS), stratum granulosum (SG), and stratum corneum (SC). Important structural and metabolic proteins are produced at specific layers of the epidermis. *(Reproduced with permission from Wolff K et al (eds). Fitzpatrick's Dermatology in General Medicine, 7th ed. McGraw-Hill, Inc., 2008. Figure 45-2.)*

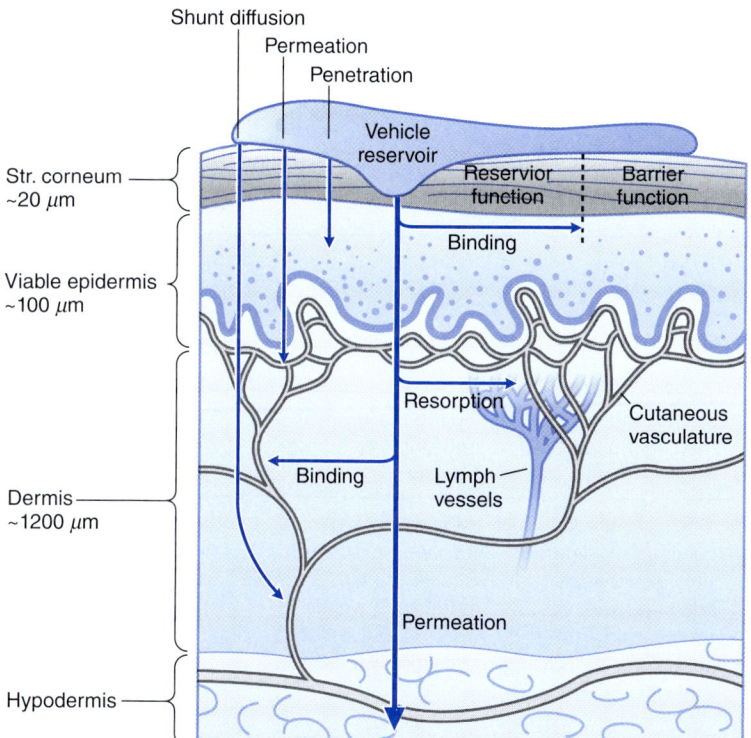

FIGURE 48-4 Cutaneous drug delivery. Diagrammatic representation of the 3 compartments of the skin as they relate to drug delivery: surface, stratum (Str.), and viable tissues. After application of drugs to the surface, evaporation, structural, and compositional alterations, which determine the bioavailability of drugs, occur in the applied formulation. The stratum corneum limits diffusion of compounds into the viable skin and body. After absorption, compounds either bind targets in viable tissues or diffuse within the viable tissue or into the cutaneous vasculature, where they may be carried to internal cells and organs. *(Reproduced with permission from Wolff K et al (eds). Fitzpatrick's Dermatology in General Medicine, 7th ed. McGraw-Hill, Inc., 2008. Figure 215-1.)*

spherical shells of phospholipids in an aqueous medium intended to enhance percutaneous absorption in normal and abnormal stratum corneum. Variations in size, charge, and lipid content can influence liposome function substantially. Transfersomes are a drug-delivery technology based on highly deformable, ultra-flexible lipid vesicles that penetrate the skin when applied nonocclusively. Microgels are polymers intended to enhance solubilization of certain drugs, thereby enhancing topical penetration and diminishing irritancy.

d. What concerns should the physician have when treating an infection of the skin with topical therapy?

Gram-positive organisms, including *Staphylococcus aureus* and *Streptococcus pyogenes*, are the most common cause of pyoderma. Skin infections with gram-negative bacilli are rare, although they can occur in diabetics and patients who are immunosuppressed; appropriate parenteral antibiotic therapy is required for their treatment.

Topical therapy frequently is adequate for impetigo, a superficial bacterial infection of the skin caused by *S. aureus* and *S. pyogenes*. Topical therapy often is employed for prophylaxis of superficial infections caused by wounds and injuries.

Deeper bacterial infections of the skin include folliculitis, erysipelas, cellulitis, and necrotizing fasciitis. Because streptococcal and staphylococcal species also are the

(Continued)

TABLE 48-3 Biological Agents Commonly Used in Dermatology

DRUG	ALEFACEPT	EFALIZUMAB	ADALIMUMAB	ETANERCEPT	INFLIXIMAB
Structural class	Receptor-antibody fusion protein	Humanized monoclonal antibody	Human monoclonal antibody	Receptor-antibody fusion protein	Chimeric monoclonal antibody
Components	LFA-3 and Fc IgG$_1$	Complementarity determining region of mouse monoclonal antibody on human IgG$_1$	IgG$_1$	p75 TNF receptor and Fc IgG$_1$	Variable region of mouse monoclonal antibody on human IgG$_1$
Binding site	CD2	CD11a subunit of LFA-1	TNF-α	TNF-α	TNF-α
Method of administration	IM	SC	SC	SC	IV
Dosing for psoriasis	15 mg weekly × 12 weeks, stop 12 weeks, then repeat	0.7 mg/kg first week, then 1 mg/kg weekly	80-mg loading dose, then 40 mg biweekly	50 mg twice weekly × 3, months then 50 mg weekly	5 mg/kg at weeks 0, 2, and 6, then every 6-8 weeks
FDA indications	Moderate-severe psoriasis	Moderate-severe psoriasis	Moderate-severe psoriasis; moderate-severe psoriatic arthritis; adult and juvenile rheumatoid arthritis; ankylosing spondylitis; Crohn's disease	Moderate-severe psoriasis; moderate-severe psoriatic arthritis; adult and juvenile rheumatoid arthritis; ankylosing spondylitis	Severe psoriasis; moderate-severe psoriatic arthritis; adult rheumatoid arthritis; ankylosing spondylitis; ulcerative colitis; Crohn's disease
Pregnancy category	B	C	B	B	B
Efficacy in psoriasis[a]	28-33%	27-39%	53%	47%	76-80%

[a]Probability (%) of Psoriasis Area and Severity Index (PASI) score of 75 after 12 weeks of therapy at the dosing described in the table. LFA, lymphocyte function—associated antigen; IgG, immunoglobulin G; TNF, tumor necrosis factor; IM, intramuscular; SC, subcutaneous; IV, intravenous.

Dermatological Pharmacology

CHAPTER 48

most common causes of deep cutaneous infections, penicillins (especially β-lactamase–resistant β-lactams) and cephalosporins are the systemic antibiotics used most frequently in their treatment (see Chapter 39). A growing concern is the increased incidence of skin and soft-tissue infections with hospital- and community-acquired methicillin-resistant *S. aureus* (MRSA) and drug-resistant pneumococci. Infection with community-acquired MRSA often is susceptible to trimethoprim–sulfamethoxazole. See previous chapters for the pharmacology of specific antibacterial agents.

CASE 48-2

A 35-year-old man has the diagnosis of psoriasis. He is being treated with methotrexate.

a. What is psoriasis?

Psoriasis is a disorder of Th1 cell-mediated immunity (see Figure 48-2), with the epidermal changes being secondary to the effect of released cytokines.

b. Why is methotrexate efficacious in the treatment of psoriasis?

The antimetabolite methotrexate is a folic acid analog that competitively inhibits dihydrofolate reductase (see Chapter 45). Methotrexate has been used for moderate to severe psoriasis since 1951. It suppresses immunocompetent cells in the skin, and it also decreases the expression of cutaneous lymphocyte-associated antigen (CLA)–positive T cells and endothelial cell E-selectin, which may account for its efficacy.

c. What adverse effects of methotrexate might limit its use?

Doses of methotrexate must be decreased for patients with impaired renal clearance. Methotrexate should never be co-administered with trimethoprim–sulfamethoxazole, probenecid, salicylates, or other drugs that can compete with it for protein binding and thereby raise plasma concentrations to levels that may result in bone marrow suppression. Fatalities have occurred because of concurrent treatment with methotrexate and nonsteroidal anti-inflammatory agents. Methotrexate exerts significant antiproliferative effects on the bone marrow; therefore, a complete blood count should be monitored serially. Physicians administering methotrexate should be familiar with the use of folinic acid (leucovorin) to rescue patients with hematological crises caused by methotrexate-induced bone marrow suppression. Careful monitoring of liver function tests is necessary but may not be adequate to identify early hepatic fibrosis in patients receiving chronic methotrexate therapy. Methotrexate-induced hepatic fibrosis may occur more commonly in patients with psoriasis than in those with rheumatoid arthritis. Consequently, liver biopsy is recommended when the cumulative dose reaches 1 to 1.5 g. A baseline liver biopsy also is recommended for patients with increased potential risk for hepatic fibrosis, such as a history of alcohol abuse or infection with hepatitis B or C. Patients with significantly abnormal liver function tests, symptomatic liver disease, or evidence of hepatic fibrosis should not use this drug. Many clinicians routinely administer folic acid along with methotrexate to ameliorate side effects; this does not reduce efficacy of the methotrexate. Pregnancy and lactation are absolute contraindications to methotrexate use.

d. What other therapeutic options are available for this patient?

Biological agents (see Chapter 23) are compounds derived from living organisms that target specific mediators of immunological reactions. Classes of biologicals include recombinant cytokines, interleukins, growth factors, antibodies, and fusion proteins. Currently, 5 biological agents are approved for the treatment of psoriasis (see Table 48-3). Biological therapies modify the immune response in psoriasis through (1) reduction of pathogenic T cells, (2) inhibition of T-cell activation, (3) immune deviation (from a Th1 to a Th2 immune response), and (4) blockade of the activity of inflammatory cytokines.

(Continued)

SECTION IX — Special Systems Pharmacology

TABLE 48-4 Photochemotherapy Methods

	PUVA	PHOTODYNAMIC THERAPY	PHOTOPHERESIS
Target	Broad cutaneous area	Focal cutaneous sites	Peripheral blood leukocytes
Photosensitizing agent	Methoxsalen (8-methoxypsoralen) Trioxsalen (4,5′,8-trimethylpsoralen) Bergapten (5-methoxypsoralen)	Protoporphyrin IX	Methoxsalen
Method of drug administration	Oral Topical lotion Bath water	Topical cream or solution of a prodrug (aminolevulinic acid or methylaminolevulinate)	To isolated plasma within photopheresis device
FDA-approved indications	Psoriasis Vitiligo	Actinic keratosis	Cutaneous T-cell lymphoma
Activating wavelength	UVA2 (320-340 nm)	417 nm and 630 nm	UVA2 (320-340 nm)
Adverse effects (acute)	Phototoxic reactions Pruritus Hypertrichosis GI disturbance CNS disturbance Bronchoconstriction Hepatic toxicity Herpes simplex recurrence Retinal damage	Phototoxic reactions Temporary dyspigmentation	Phototoxic reactions GI disturbance Hypotension Congestive heart failure
Adverse effects (chronic)	Photoaging Nonmelanoma skin cancer Melanoma[a] Cataracts[a]	Potential scarring	Loss of venous access after repeated venipuncture
Pregnancy category	C	C	FDA unrated

[a]Controversial. CNS, central nervous system; GI, gastrointestinal; UVA, ultraviolet A.

The appeal of biological agents in the treatment of psoriasis is that they specifically target the activities of T lymphocytes and cytokines that mediate inflammation versus traditional systemic therapies that are broadly immunosuppressive or cytotoxic. Thus, the use of these agents theoretically should result in fewer toxicities and side effects.

When evaluating the efficacy of biological agents, it is important to understand the standard measurement of efficacy in psoriasis treatment, the Psoriasis Area and Severity Index (PASI). The PASI quantifies the extent and severity of skin involvement in different body regions as a score from 0 (no lesions) to 72 (severe disease). To gain FDA approval for the treatment of psoriasis, a biological agent must decrease the PASI by 75%. Although such quantification is an essential element in controlled clinical trials, many patients in practice may gain clinically significant benefit from biological treatment without achieving this degree of PASI improvement.

CASE 48-3

Prior to his treatment with methotrexate, the patient in Case 48-2 was treated with photochemotherapy.

a. **What is photochemotherapy?**

Phototherapy and photochemotherapy are treatment methods in which UV or visible radiation is used to induce a therapeutic response either alone or in the presence of a photosensitizing drug. To be effective, the incident radiation must

(Continued)

be absorbed by a target or chromophore in the skin—which in phototherapy is endogenous and in photochemotherapy must be administered exogenously (see Table 48-4).

The action spectrum for oral psoralen (eg, methoxysalen) followed by ultraviolet light A (PUVA) is between 320 and 340 nm. Two distinct photoreactions take place. Type I reactions involve the oxygen-independent photoaddition of psoralens to pyrimidine bases in DNA. Type II reactions are oxygen-dependent and involve the transfer of energy to molecular oxygen, creating reactive oxygen species. Through incompletely understood mechanisms, these phototoxic reactions stimulate melanocytes and induce antiproliferative, immunosuppressive, and anti-inflammatory effects.

b. What are the potential toxicities of phototherapy and photochemotherapy and how should patients be monitored?

Patients treated with these modalities should be monitored for concomitant use of other potential photosensitizing medications before initiation of therapy. Such drugs include phenothiazines, thiazides, sulfonamides, nonsteroidal anti-inflammatory agents, sulfonylureas, tetracyclines, and benzodiazepines.

The major side effects of PUVA are listed in Table 48-4. Phototoxicity is characterized by erythema, edema, blistering, and pruritus. Ocular toxicity can be prevented by wearing UVA-blocking glasses the day of treatment. The risk of nonmelanoma skin cancer is dose-dependent, with the greatest risk in those receiving more than 250 treatments. A possible association of melanoma and extensive exposure to PUVA has been reported; however, several other studies have failed to confirm this association. As skin cancer may not develop for decades after exposure, annual skin examinations should be continued for years after completion of PUVA.

ANTIBIOTICS USED TO TREAT ACNE

TOPICAL	Clindamycin
	Erythromycin
	Benzoyl peroxide-antibiotic combination
	Sulfacetamide
	Sulfacetamide/sulfur combination
	Metronidazole
	Azelaic acid
SYSTEMIC	Tetracycline
	Doxycycline
	Minocycline
	Trimethoprim-sulfamethoxazole

CASE 48-4

A 17-year-old boy with noninflammatory acne is treated with a topical retinoid preparation.

a. What is acne?

Acne is believed to result from a combination of sebaceous gland hyperplasia, follicular hyperkeratosis, *Propionibacterium acnes* colonization, and inflammation. Though incompletely understood mechanisms, topical retinoids correct abnormal follicular keratinization, reduce *P. acnes* counts, and reduce inflammation, thereby making them the cornerstone of acne therapy. Topical retinoids are first-line agents for noninflammatory (comedonal) acne and often are combined with other agents in the management of inflammatory acne.

b. What is the mechanism of action of retinoids?

Retinoids exert their effects on gene expression by activating 2 families of receptors—retinoic acid receptors (RARs) and retinoid X receptors (RXRs)—that are members of the steroid receptor superfamily.

Unique therapeutic effects can be produced by targeting specific retinoid receptors. For example, retinoids that target RARs predominantly affect cellular differentiation and proliferation, whereas retinoids that target RXRs predominantly induce apoptosis. Hence, tretinoin, adapalene, and tazarotene, which target RARs, are used in acne, psoriasis, and photoaging (disorders of differentiation and proliferation), whereas bexarotene and alitretinoin, which target RXRs, are used in mycosis fungoides and Kaposi sarcoma (to induce apoptosis of malignant cells).

c. What retinoid preparations are available for this patient?

Topical and systemic retinoids are shown in Tables 65-4 and 65-5, respectively, in *Goodman and Gilman's The Pharmacological Basis of Therapeutics*, 12th Edition.

(Continued)

SECTION IX

Special Systems Pharmacology

TABLE 48-5 Recommended Cutaneous Antifungal Therapy

CONDITION	TOPICAL THERAPY	ORAL THERAPY
Tinea corporis, localized	Azoles, allylamines	—
Tinea corporis, widespread	—	Griseofulvin, terbinafine, itraconazole, fluconazole
Tinea pedis	Azoles, allylamines	Griseofulvin, terbinafine, itraconazole, fluconazole
Onychomycosis	—	Griseofulvin, terbinafine, itraconazole, fluconazole
Candidiasis, localized	Azoles	—
Candidiasis, widespread and mucocutaneous	—	Ketoconazole, itraconazole, fluconazole
Tinea versicolor, localized	Azoles, allylamines	
Tinea versicolor, widespread	—	Ketoconazole, itraconazole, fluconazole

d. **What adverse effects might this patient experience from retinoids?**

Acute retinoid toxicity is similar to vitamin A intoxication. Side effects of systemic retinoids include dry skin, nosebleeds from dry mucous membranes, conjunctivitis, reduced night vision, hair loss, alterations in serum lipids and transaminases, hypothyroidism, inflammatory bowel disease flare, musculoskeletal pain, pseudotumor cerebri, and mood alterations. RAR-selective retinoids are more associated with mucocutaneous and musculoskeletal symptoms, whereas RXR-selective retinoids induce more physiochemical changes. Suicide or suicide attempts have been associated with the use of isotretinoin. Thus, all patients treated with isotretinoin should be observed closely for symptoms of depression or suicidal thoughts.

Adverse effects of all topical retinoids include erythema, desquamation, burning, and stinging. These effects often decrease with time and are lessened by concomitant use of emollients. Patients also may experience photosensitivity reactions because of enhanced reactivity to UV radiation and have a significant risk for severe sunburn. See Summary Quiz Question 48-3 for a discussion of the avoidance of retinoids during pregnancy.

e. **What other drugs are available for the treatment of acne?**

Antibiotics are commonly used to treat acne. Commonly used antibiotics are shown in the Side Bar ANTIBIOTICS USED TO TREAT ACNE.

CASE 48-5

A 53-year-old woman has widespread tinea corporis infection in her skin that is causing irritation and itching. Her physician has prescribed oral fluconazole.

a. **What preparations are available for the treatment of cutaneous fungal infections?**

Table 48-5 shows the recommendations for cutaneous antifungal therapy.

(Continued)

b. What are the adverse effects of fluconazole?

The azoles interact with hepatic CYPs as substrates and inhibitors, providing myriad possibilities for the interaction of azoles with many other medications. See Chapter 43 for a complete discussion of the drug interactions with azole antifungal drugs.

Side effects in patients receiving more than 7 days of fluconazole, regardless of dose, include the following: nausea, headache, skin rash, vomiting, abdominal pain, and diarrhea. Use of high doses may be limited by nausea. Reversible alopecia may occur with prolonged therapy at 400 mg daily. Rare cases of deaths due to hepatic failure or Stevens-Johnson syndrome have been reported. Fluconazole is teratogenic in rodents and has been associated with skeletal and cardiac deformities in at least 3 infants born to 2 women taking high doses during pregnancy. Fluconazole is a Category C agent that should be avoided during pregnancy unless the potential benefit justifies the possible risk to the fetus.

SUNSCREEN AGENTS

ULTRAVIOLET A (UVA) SUNSCREEN AGENTS	ULTRAVIOLET B (UVB) SUNSCREEN AGENTS
Avobenzone (Parsol 1789)	*p*-Aminobenzoic acid (PABA) esters (padimate O)
Oxybenzone	Cinnamates (octinoxate)
Titanium dioxide	Octocrylene
Zinc oxide	Salicylates (octisalate)
Ecamsule (MEXORYL SX)	

CASE 48-6

A 23-year-old woman is planning a beach vacation. She asks you for advice on sunscreen agents.

a. What are sunscreens?

Photoprotection from the acute and chronic effects of sun exposure is readily available with sunscreens. The major active ingredients of available sunscreens include chemical agents that absorb incident solar radiation in the UVB and/or UVA ranges and physical agents that contain particulate materials that can block or reflect incident energy and reduce its transmission to the skin (see the Table SUNSCREEN AGENTS). Many of the sunscreens available are mixtures of organic chemical absorbers and particulate physical substances. Ideal sunscreens provide a broad spectrum of protection and are formulations that are photostable and remain intact for sustained periods on the skin. They also should be nonirritating, invisible, and nonstaining to clothing. No single sunscreen ingredient possesses all these desirable properties, but many are quite effective nonetheless.

The major measurement of sunscreen photoprotection is the sun protection factor (SPF), which defines a ratio of the minimal dose of incident sunlight that will produce erythema or redness (sunburn) on skin with the sunscreen in place (protected) and the dose that evokes the same reaction on skin without the sunscreen (unprotected). The SPF provides valuable information regarding UVB protection but is useless in documenting UVA efficacy. In 2007, the FDA proposed a consumer-friendly rating system for UVA products consisting of 1 to 4 stars representing low, medium, high, and highest UVA protection available in an OTC sunscreen product as an indicator of the product's ability to prevent tanning. The test proposed to determine UVA rating is analogous to the SPF test used to determine the effectiveness of UVB sunscreen products.

Except for total sun avoidance, sunscreens are the best single method of protection from UV-induced damage to the skin.

SECTION IX
Special Systems Pharmacology

TABLE 48-6 Agents Used for the Treatment of Pruritus

Pruritoceptive Pruritus: Itch originating in the skin due to inflammation or other cutaneous disease
- Emollients—Repair of barrier function
- Coolants (menthol, camphor, calamine)—Counter-irritants
- Capsaicin—Counter-irritant
- Antihistamines—Inhibit histamine-induced pruritus
- Topical steroids—Direct anti-pruritic and anti-inflammatory effects
- Topical immunomodulators—Anti-inflammatories
- Phototherapy—Reduced mast cell reactivity and anti-inflammatory effects
- Thalidomide—Anti-inflammatory through suppression of excessive tumor necrosis factor-α

Neuropathic Pruritus: Itch due to disease of afferent nerves
- Carbamazepine—Blockade of synaptic transmission and use-dependent sodium channels
- Gabapentin—Suppresses neuronal hyperexcitability by inhibiting voltage-dependent calcium channels
- Topical anesthetics (EMLA, benzocaine, pramoxine)—Inhibit nerve conduction via decreased nerve membrane permeability to sodium

Neurogenic Pruritus: Itch that arises from the nervous system without evidence of neural pathology
- Thalidomide—Central depressant
- Opioid-receptor antagonists (naloxone, naltrexone)—Decrease opioidergic tone
- Tricyclic antidepressants—Decrease pruritus signaling through alteration in neurotransmitter concentrations
- Selective serotonin reuptake inhibitors (SSRIs)—Decrease pruritus signaling through alteration in neurotransmitter concentrations

Psychogenic Pruritus: Itch due to psychological illness
- Anxiolytics (alprazolam, clonazepam, benzodiazepines)—Relieve stress-reactive pruritus
- Antipsychotic agents (chlorpromazine, thioridazine, thiothixene, olanzapine)—Relieve pruritus with impulsive qualities
- Tricyclic antidepressants—Relieve depression and insomnia related to pruritus
- SSRIs—Relieve pruritus with compulsive qualities

CASE 48-7

A 65-year-old woman has a complaint of itching on her arms and legs. Physical examination shows that she has broken skin on her legs from scratching.

a. What are the common causes of itching?

The term pruritus is derived from the Latin prurire, which means "to itch." Pruritus is a symptom unique to skin that occurs in a multitude of dermatological disorders, including dry skin or xerosis, atopic eczema, urticaria, and infestations. Itching also may be a sign of internal disorders, including malignant neoplasms, chronic renal failure, and hepatobiliary disease. In addition to treating the underlying disorder, a general approach to the treatment of pruritus can be made by classifying pruritus into one of four clinical categories (see Table 48-6).

b. What agents are available for itching when there is no obvious cause?

Agents useful in treating pruritus are listed in Table 48-6.

KEY CONCEPTS

➭ Drugs can be applied to the skin to directly treat disorders of the skin or to deliver drugs to other tissues.

➭ Effective and safe use of topical agents requires appreciation of the physical and physiological variables that influence the interactions of drugs and the skin, impacting absorption and transport.

(Continued)

Dermatological Pharmacology — CHAPTER 48

- There is a superficial capillary plexus between the epidermis and dermis that is the site of the majority of the systemic absorption of cutaneous drugs (see Figure 48-4).
- Passage through the outermost layer of skin (stratum corneum) is the rate-limiting step for percutaneous absorption.
- The unique therapeutic effects of retinoids can be produced by targeting specific retinoid receptors (RXR and RAR).
- Except for total sun avoidance, sunscreens are the best single method of protection from UV-induced damage to the skin.
- Cytotoxic and immunosuppressive drugs are used in dermatology for immunologically mediated diseases such as psoriasis, autoimmune blistering diseases, and leukocytoclastic vasculitis (see Table 48-8).
- Biological therapies modify the immune response in patients with psoriasis through (1) reduction of pathogenic T cells, (2) inhibition of T-cell activation, (3) immune deviation (from a Th1 to a Th2 immune response), and (4) blockade of the activity of inflammatory cytokines (see Table 48-3 and Figures 48-2 and 48-1).

SUMMARY QUIZ

QUESTION 48-1 The rate-limiting step in the absorption of drugs through the skin is passage through the

a. dermis.
b. epidermis.
c. stratum corneum.
d. hypodermis.
e. sweat glands.

QUESTION 48-2 A 35-year-old man has a fungal infection of his toenails. A systemic antifungal preparation, griseofulvin, is prescribed because

a. topical antifungal preparations are irritating.
b. topical antifungal agents are expensive.
c. systemic antifungal agents produce high drug concentrations in the nails.
d. systemic antifungal agents have no adverse effects.
e. topical antifungal preparation are easily washed off the nails.

QUESTION 48-3 A 23-year-old woman with recalcitrant acne is being treated with an oral dose of isotretinoin. She should be warned against

a. getting pregnant.
b. sun exposure.
c. close contact with her 1-year-old child.
d. flying in an airplane.
e. eating broccoli.

QUESTION 48-4 A 53-year-old woman with psoriasis is treated with methotrexate. Aside from monitoring her blood count for evidence of bone marrow suppression, she should also have careful monitoring of her

a. kidney function.
b. liver function.
c. sexual function.

(Continued)

SECTION IX Special Systems Pharmacology

d. cognitive function.

e. visual function.

QUESTION 48-5 A 76-year-old man has severe eczema on his legs for which a potent glucocorticoid ointment is prescribed. He should be warned not to use an occlusive dressing as it may result in

a. blistering.

b. decreased kidney function.

c. behavioral changes.

d. suppression of the hypothalamic-pituitary-adrenal axis.

e. breakdown of the glucocorticoid.

QUESTION 48-6 A 43-year-old woman with severe psoriasis is prescribed adalimumab. Adalimumab is an inhibitor of

a. T-cell activation.

b. IL-2.

c. CYP2D6.

d. β adrenergic receptors.

e. TNF-α.

SUMMARY QUIZ ANSWER KEY

QUESTION 48-1 Answer is **c**. Passage through the outermost layer (stratum corneum) is the rate-limiting step for percutaneous absorption. Permeability generally is inversely proportional to the thickness of the stratum corneum. Drug penetration is higher on the face, intertriginous areas, and perineum due to minimal stratum corneum thickness in these regions.

QUESTION 48-2 Answer is **c**. Systemic therapy is necessary for effective management of onychomycosis (see Chapter 43). Griseofulvin is deposited in keratin precursor cells; when these cells differentiate, the drug is tightly bound to, and persists in, keratin, providing prolonged resistance to fungal invasion. For this reason, the new growth of hair or nails is the first to become free of disease. As the fungus-containing keratin is shed, it is replaced by normal tissue.

QUESTION 48-3 Answer is **a**. Isotretinoin is approved for the treatment of recalcitrant and nodular acne vulgaris. Systemic retinoids are highly teratogenic. There is no safe dose during pregnancy. Common malformations include craniofacial, cardiovascular, thymic, and central nervous system (CNS) abnormalities. Although there appears to be minimal, if any, risk of retinoid embryopathy in fetuses conceived by males taking systemic retinoids, it is commonly recommended that men avoid retinoid therapy when actively trying to father children.

QUESTION 48-4 Answer is **b**. Careful monitoring of liver function tests is necessary but may not be adequate to identify early hepatic fibrosis in patients receiving chronic methotrexate therapy. Methotrexate-induced hepatic fibrosis may occur more commonly in patients with psoriasis than in those with rheumatoid arthritis. Consequently, liver biopsy is recommended when the cumulative dose reaches 1 to 1.5 g. A baseline liver biopsy also is recommended for patients with increased potential risk for hepatic fibrosis, such as a history of alcohol abuse or infection with hepatitis B or C. Patients with significantly abnormal liver function tests, symptomatic liver disease, or evidence of hepatic fibrosis should not use this drug.

(Continued)

Dermatological Pharmacology — CHAPTER 48

TABLE 48-7 Potency of Selected Topical Glucocorticoids

CLASS OF DRUG[a]	GENERIC NAME, FORMULATION	TRADE NAME
1	Betamethasone dipropionate cream, ointment 0.05% (in optimized vehicle) Clobetasol propionate cream, ointment 0.05% Diflorasone diacetate, ointment 0.05% Halobetasol propionate, ointment 0.05%	DIPROLENE TEMOVATE PSORCON ULTRAVATE
2	Amcinonide, ointment 0.1% Betamethasone dipropionate, ointment 0.05% Desoximetasone, cream, ointment 0.25%, gel 0.05% Diflorasone diacetate, ointment 0.05% Fluocinonide, cream, ointment, gel 0.05% Halcinonide, cream, ointment 0.1%	CYCLOCORT DIPROSONE, others TOPICORT FLORONE, MAXIFLOR LIDEX, LIDEX-E, FLUONEX HALOG, HALOG-E
3	Betamethasone dipropionate, cream 0.05% Betamethasone valerate, ointment 0.1% Diflorasone diacetate, cream 0.05% Triamcinolone acetonide, ointment 0.1%, cream 0.5%	DIPROSONE, others BETATREX, others FLORONE, MAXIFLOR ARISTOCORT A, others
4	Amcinonide, cream 0.1% Desoximetasone, cream 0.05% Fluocinolone acetonide, cream 0.2% Fluocinolone acetonide, ointment 0.025% Flurandrenolide, ointment 0.05%, tape 4 µg/cm^2 Hydrocortisone valerate, ointment 0.2% Triamcinolone acetonide, ointment 0.1% Mometasone furoate, cream, ointment 0.1%	CYCLOCORT TOPICORT LP SYNALAR-HP SYNALAR CORDRAN WESTCORT KENALOG, ARISTOCORT ELOCON
5	Betamethasone dipropionate, lotion 0.05% Betamethasone valerate, cream, lotion 0.1% Fluocinolone acetonide, cream 0.025% Flurandrenolide, cream 0.05% Hydrocortisone butyrate, cream 0.1% Hydrocortisone valerate, cream 0.2% Triamcinolone acetonide, cream, lotion 0.1% Triamcinolone acetonide, cream 0.025%	DIPROSONE, others BETATREX, others SYNALAR CORDRAN SP LOCOID WESTCORT KENALOG ARISTOCORT
6	Alclometasone dipropionate, cream, ointment 0.05% Desonide, cream 0.05% Fluocinolone acetonide, cream, solution 0.01%	ACLOVATE TRIDESILON, DESOWEN SYNALAR
7	Dexamethasone sodium phosphate, cream 0.1% Hydrocortisone, cream, ointment, lotion 0.5%, 1.0%, 2.5%	DECADRON HYTONE, NUTRICORT, PENECORT

[a]Class 1 is most potent; class 7 is least potent.

QUESTION 48-5 Answer is **d.** Chronic use of class 1 (see Table 48-7) topical glucocorticoids can cause skin atrophy, striae, telangiectasias, purpura, and acneiform eruptions. Occlusion increases the risk of HPA suppression (see Chapter 29).

QUESTION 48-6 Answer is **e.** Adalimumab is a human IgG$_1$ monoclonal antibody that binds soluble and membrane-bound TNF-α. Like infliximab, it can mediate complement-induced cytolysis on cells expressing TNF. Unlike infliximab, however, it is fully human, which reduces the risk for development of neutralizing antibodies.

SECTION IX
Special Systems Pharmacology

TABLE 48-8 Mechanism of Action for Selected Cytotoxic and Immunosuppressive Drugs

Methotrexate	Dihydrofolate reductase inhibitor
Azathioprine	Purine synthesis inhibitor
Fluorouracil	Blocks methylation in DNA synthesis
Cyclophosphamide	Alkylates and cross-links DNA
Mechlorethamine hydrochloride	Alkylating agent
Carmustine	Cross-links in DNA and RNA
Cyclosporine	Calcineurin inhibitor
Tacrolimus	Calcineurin inhibitor
Pimecrolimus	Calcineurin inhibitor
Mycophenolate mofetil	Inosine monophosphate dehydrogenase inhibitor
Imiquimod	Interferon-α induction
Vinblastine	Inhibits microtubule formation
Bleomycin	Induction of DNA strand breaks
Dapsone	Inhibits neutrophil migration, oxidative burst
Thalidomide	Cytokine modulation

SUMMARY: DRUGS USED TO TREAT DERMATOLOGIC DISORDERS

CLASS AND SUBCLASSES	NAMES	CLINICAL USES	TOXICITIES COMMON	TOXICITIES UNIQUE; CLINICALLY IMPORTANT
Glucocorticoids	Triamcinolone acetonide Triamcinolone hexacetonide Numerous other agents (see Table 48-7)	Anti-inflammatory and immunosuppression (see Table 48-7)	See Chapter 29	See Chapter 29
Retinoids	Tretinoin Isotretinoin Acitretin Tazarotene Bexarotene Adapalene Alitretinoin	Tretinoin, adapalene, and tazarotene, which target RARs, are used to treat acne, psoriasis, and photoaging Bexarotene and alitretinoin, which target RXRs are used to treat mycosis fungoides and Kapposi sarcoma Acitretin is used to treat the cutaneous manifestations of psoriasis Isotretinoin is approved for the treatment of recalcitrant and nodular acne vulgaris	Topical retinoids may cause erythema desquamation, burning, stinging, and photosensitivity Serum lipid elevation is a common laboratory abnormality of systemic retinoids	Systemic retinoids are highly teratogenic and their use is contraindicated in women who are pregnant, contemplating pregnancy, or breast feeding The use of topical retinoids should be avoided during pregnancy Systemic retinoids may also cause cheilitis, xerosis, cutaneous photosensitivity, photophobia, myalgia, nail fragility, and increased susceptibility to staphylococcal infections
Vitamin Analogs	Calcipotriene	Vitamin D analog used in the treatment of psoriasis	Perilesional irritation and mild photosensitivity	Hypercalcemia and hypercalcuria with high doses

(Continued)

Dermatological Pharmacology
CHAPTER 48

CLASS AND SUBCLASSES	NAMES	CLINICAL USES	TOXICITIES COMMON	UNIQUE; CLINICALLY IMPORTANT
Photochemotherapeutic Drugs	PUVA Methoxsalen	Approved for the treatment of vitiligo and psoriasis	Erythema, blistering, and pruritus (see Table 48-4)	See Table 48-4
	Photodynamic therapy Aminolevulinic acid Methyl-aminolevulinate	Approved for use to treat actinic keratosis Commonly used to treat thin nonmelanoma skin cancers, acne, and photo-damaged skin		
Antimicrobial Agents	Various antibacterial, antifungal, and antiviral agents	Treatment of cutaneous infections (see Chapters 38, 39, 40, 41, 43, and 44) (See Table 48-5 for antifungal agents	See Chapters 38, 39, 40, 41, 43, and 44	See Chapters 38, 39, 40, 41, 43, and 44
	Retapamulin	Approved for topical treatment of impetigo		
Agents Used to Treat Infestations	Permethrin	Treatment of scabies and lice infestations in infants ≥2 months of age	Irritation and burning	
	Malathion	Treatment of lice infestation in children ≥6 years of age	See Chapter 6	See Chapter 6
	Ivermectin	Oral anthelmintic approved for the treatment of onchocerciasis and stronglyoidiasis but used off-label for treatment of scabies and lice	See Chapter 37	See Chapter 37
	Lindane	Treatment of lice infestation		Neurotoxicity Contraindicated in premature infants and in patients with seizure disorders
	Crotamiton	Used to treat scabies and lice when lindane and permethrin are contraindicated		
	Benzyl alcohol	Approved for treatment of lice		
Antimalarial Agents	Chloroquine Hydroxychloroquine Quinacrine	Used in the treatment of cutaneous lupus erythematosus, cutaneous dermatomyositis, porphyria cutanea tarda, and sarcoidosis	See Chapter 35	See Chapter 35
Antimetabolites	Methotrexate	Used to treat psoriasis	See Chapter 45	See Chapter 45
	Azathioprine	Used off-label as a steroid-sparing agent for autoimmune and inflammatory dermatoses	See Chapter 23	See Chapter 23
	Fluorouracil	Used to treat actinic keratosis, actinic cheilitis, and superficial basal cell carcinomas	See Chapter 45	See Chapter 45

(Continued)

SECTION IX Special Systems Pharmacology

CLASS AND SUBCLASSES	NAMES	CLINICAL USES	TOXICITIES COMMON	UNIQUE; CLINICALLY IMPORTANT
Alkylating Agents	Cyclophosphamide Mechlorethamine Carmustine	Used for the treatment of cutaneous T-cell lymphoma	See Chapter 45	See Chapter 45
Calcineurin Inhibitors	Cyclosporine Tacrolimus Pimecrolimus	Cyclosporin is approved for the treatment of psoriasis Tacrolimus and pimecrolimus are approved for the treatment of atopic dermatitis in patients ≥2 years of age	See Chapter 23	See Chapter 23
Other Immunosuppressive and Anti-inflammatory Agents	Mycophenolate mofetil	Used to treat inflammatory and autoimmune diseases in dermatology	See Chapter 23	See Chapter 23
	Imiquimod	Approved for the treatment of genital warts and actinic keratoses	Irritant reactions including edema, vesicles, erosions, or ulcers	Minor flu-like symptoms
	Vinblastine Bleomycin Doxorubicin	Vinblastine and doxorubicin are used to treat Kaposi sarcoma Vinblastine is used to treat T-cell lymphoma Intralesional bleomycin is used for recalcitrant warts	See Chapter 45	See Chapter 45
	Dapsone	Approved for use in dermatitis herpetiformis and leprosy	See Chapter 42	See Chapter 42
	Thalidomide	Approved for treatment of erythema nodosum leprosum	See Chapter 23	See Chapter 23
Biological Agents and Tumor Necrosis Factor (TNF) Inhibitors	Alefacept Efalizumab Etanercept Infliximab Adalimumab	Treatment of psoriasis Infliximab is a mouse-human chimeric IgG$_1$ monoclonal antibody Etanercept is a fully human TNF receptor fusion protein Adalimumab is a human IgG$_1$ monoclonal antibody	See Table 48-3 and Chapter 23	See Table 48-3 and Chapter 23
Agent Used for Treatment of Cutaneous T-Cell Lymphoma	Denileukin difitox	Used to treat advanced cutaneous T-cell lymphoma	Pain, fever, chills, nausea, vomiting, and diarrhea (see Chapter 46)	Hypersensitivity reaction (hypotension, back pain, dyspnea, and chest pain) Capillary leak syndrome (edema, hypoalbuminemia, and hypotension) (see Chapter 46)
Sunscreens	Various chemicals (see Table SUNSCREEN AGENTS)	Used to provide protection against ultraviolet radiation	Local irritation and skin sensitivity	
Drugs for Androgenic Alopecia	Minoxidil	Used to treat hair loss	Allergic and contact dermatitis	See Chapter 15
	Finasteride	Used to treat hair loss	Decreased libido, erectile dysfunction, and ejaculation disorder See Chapter 28	Pregnant women should not be exposed to finasteride

(Continued)

Dermatological Pharmacology — CHAPTER 48

CLASS AND SUBCLASSES	NAMES	CLINICAL USES	TOXICITIES COMMON	UNIQUE; CLINICALLY IMPORTANT
Agents Used to Treat Hyperpigmentation	Hydroquinone Monobenzone Azelaic Mequinol	Used to treat hormonally or light-induced pigmentation within the epidermis	Dermatitis and ochronosis	Monobenzone may cause permanent hypopigmentation
Miscellaneous Agents	Capsaicin	Approved for the treatment of minor aches and pains associated with backpain, strains, and arthritis Used off-label for postherpetic neuralgia and painful diabetic neuralgia		
	Podophyllin	Treatment of anogenital warts	Irritation and ulcerative local reactions	Should not be used during pregnancy

INDEX

Page numbers followed by "f," "t," or "b" indicate figures, tables, or boxes respectively.

A

Abacavir, 601t, 603t, 607f, 608f, 621t
    adverse effects, 615
    mechanisms of action and resistance, 603t, 604f, 607f, 608f, 614–615
    structure, 607f
Abarelix, 665t, 687t
Abatacept, 368t, 381t, 387t
ABCB1 transporter, 23t, 24t, 25t, 38
ABCC1 transporter, 23t
ABCC2 transporter, 23t
ABCC3 transporter, 24t
ABCC4 transporter, 24t
ABCC5 transporter, 24t
ABCC6 transporter, 24t
ABCDE emergency care, 51, 52t
ABC emergency care, 63, 64
ABCG2 transporter, 24t
ABCG5 transporter, 25t
ABCG8 transporter, 25t
Abciximab, 323t, 324–325, 331–332, 332t
ABC transporters, 23t, 23t–25t
ABDE treatment, 52t
Abiraterone, 665t, 668f, 680, 687t
Abobotulinumtoxin A, ophthalmic, 692t, 706t
Absorption, 20b, 20f. *See also specific drugs and drug classes*
    children, 67b
    drug–drug interactions, 48t
    elderly, 73b, 73f, 73t–74t
    poisoning, 52
ABVD, 630f, 643t, 645–647
Acamprosate, 177t, 186–187, 186t, 193t, 257
Acarbose, 471t, 479t
Acceptors, 2b
Acebutolol, 126t, 128t, 146t
Acetaminophen, 28–29, 50–54, 50f
    actions, 371, 372
    drug–drug interactions, 48
    metabolism, 28–29, 50f, 207, 208
    oxycodone-acetaminophen, 207, 208
    pain target and site of action, 205t
Acetaminophen toxicity, 28–29, 50–54, 52t, 207, 208
    with alcohol, 366
    antidote, 42t
    diagnosis, 54
    metabolism and mechanisms, 50f, 53–54, 207, 208
    N-acetylcysteine therapy, 40t, 42t, 54, 65t
    symptoms, 366
    treatment, 54
Acetazolamide, 225t, 237t
Acetylcholine (ACh), 81f, 82f, 97f, 112t
    acetylcholinesterase hydrolysis, 104f
    Alzheimer's disease, 246, 250–252
    mechanisms of action, 95t
    neuromuscular junction, 105f
    on nicotinic receptors, 93, 94
    pharmacology, 83t–84t, 85, 92–94, 99t
    somatic neuromuscular junction, 82f, 93, 94
    synthesis enhancer, dexpanthenol, 498t, 507t
Acetylcholine receptor (AChR), 97f
Acetylcholine receptor (AChR) agonists, 106, 117t
Acetylcholinesterase (AChE), 97f, 104f
Acetylcholinesterase (AChE) inhibitors, 100t
Acetylcholinesterase (AChE) inhibitors, reversible, 114t–115t
Acetylcysteine, 40t, 42t, 54, 65t
Acetylsalicylic acid. *See* Aspirin
Acid urine, 20b, 21–22, 39
Acitretin, 707t, 724t
Acne, 717–718
    retinoids, 707t, 717–718, 717b
Acrivastine, 347t, 355t
Acromegaly, 423–424, 424f
Actinomycin D, 630f, 643t, 658t
Action potential, 90f
    cardiac, 312f, 313f
Activated complex (LR*), 6b
Activated protein C, 333t
    drotrecogin alfa, 323t, 333t
    mechanisms of action, 323t
Active ingredients, 3. *See also specific drugs*
Active transport, 19b, 19f
    drugs requiring, 20b
    membrane transporters, 23b
Acute coronary syndrome, 290t, 291f. *See also* Myocardial ischemia
    drugs, 296–297
    percutaneous coronary interventions, 297
Acute myocardial infarction, 290t. *See also* Myocardial ischemia
Acyclovir, 600t, 605–608, 619t
    adverse effects, 608
    antiherpes, 600t–601t, 604f–605f, 605–608, 605t, 617–618, 619t
    CMV retinitis, 617, 618
    mechanisms of action and resistance, 601t, 604f–606f, 606–607
Adalimumab
    Crohn's disease, 381
    dermatologic, 709t, 714t, 722, 723, 726t
    immunotherapy, 368t, 376t, 381, 383, 384, 386t
    inflammatory bowel disease, 499t, 509t
    mechanisms of action, 368t
    molecular target, 383, 384
    rheumatoid arthritis, 368t
Adapalene, 707t, 724t
Adaptive immunity, 376b
Addiction, drug, 254–265. *See also specific types*
    alcoholism, 256–257, 256t
    benzodiazepine, 257–258, 257t
    cannabis, 263
    cocaine, 262–263, 263t
    cocaine + ethanol (cocaethylene), 265, 266
    dependence, physical, 264, 266
    MDMA, 265, 266
    multiple simultaneous variables, 255, 255t
    negative reinforcement, 265, 266
    nicotine, 258–259, 259t
    opioids, 259–262, 260f, 261t
    oxycodone, 254–256, 255f, 264, 266
    tolerance, 255, 256t, 264, 265
Addison's disease, 461f, 465
Additive drug–drug interaction, 48b
Adefovir dipivoxil, 600t, 602t, 620t
Adenosine
    antiarrhythmic, 312t, 317t, 318, 322t
    electrophysiologic actions, 317t
    paroxysmal ventricular tachycardia, 314t, 318
Adenosine receptor agonists, antiarrhythmic, 312t, 322t
    adenosine, 312t, 317t, 318, 322t
Adie's pupil, 698t
Administration, repeated, 38b, 38f
Administration, routes, 20b, 21t. *See also specific drugs and routes*
    ocular, 697t
    skin, 710b, 711–715, 711t, 713f (*See also* Skin absorption)
Administrations, routes, 20b, 21t. *See also specific drugs and drug classes*
    inhaled, elderly, 74t
    intramuscular, 21t
        elderly, 74t
        neonates, infants, and children, 67b
    intranasal, elderly, 74t
    intravenous, 21t
    ocular, 697t
    oral, 21t
        elderly, 73t
        infant bioavailability, 72, 74
    rectal, elderly, 73t
    subcutaneous, 21t
        elderly, 74t
    sublingual, 22
        elderly, 73t
    topical (dermal), 710b, 711–715, 711t, 713f
        important considerations, 711–712, 711t
        on pharmacokinetics, 20b, 21t
        rate-limiting step, 721, 722
        systemic spread, 702, 703
        for topical infections, 714–715
        vehicles, 712–714, 712t
ADP receptor antagonists, 323t, 332t
    clopidogrel, 323t, 324, 325, 325t, 331–332, 332t
    mechanisms of action, 323t
    prasugrel, 323t, 324, 325, 325t, 332t
    ticlopidine, 323t, 332t
Adrenal cortex
    anatomy, 461f
    zona glomerulosa, 461f, 467, 468
Adrenal insufficiency, 461f, 465, 467, 468

728

Adrenergic neuron blocking agents,
   antihypertensives, 277t, 286t
   guanadrel, 277t, 287t
   reserpine, 277t, 286t
Adrenergic pharmacology, 139t
   acebutolol, 126t, 128t, 146t
   albuterol, 125t, 127, 135, 137, 143t
   alfuzosin, 119t, 140t
   α_1 adrenergic receptor antagonists, 119t, 121–124, 123f, 140t
   α_1-selective adrenergic receptor agonists, 119t, 122f, 123f, 139t
   α_2 adrenergic receptor antagonists, 120t, 123f, 141t
   α_2-selective adrenergic receptor agonists, 119t, 122f, 123f, 124–125, 139t–140t
   α adrenergic receptor agonists, 83t–84t, 93, 94, 123f, 136, 137
   α receptor antagonists, additional, 120t, 123f, 141t
   amphetamine, 120t, 135–136, 137, 141t
   apraclonidine, 119t, 140t
   arformoterol, 125t, 144t
   atenolol, 126t, 128t, 146t
   betaxolol, 126t, 128t, 145t
   β_1-selective adrenergic receptor antagonists, 123f, 128t, 145t–146t
   β_2-selective adrenergic receptor agonists, 123f, 127, 143t–144t
   β adrenergic receptor agonists, 123f, 142t
   β adrenergic receptor antagonists
      with additional cardiovascular effects, 123f, 128t, 146t
      for heart failure, 129–130, 286t, 302t, 304, 311t (See also Heart failure)
         mechanisms of action, 302t
         nonselective, 123f, 128t, 144t–145t
         third-generation, 123f, 129, 146t
         vasodilating, 126f
   bisoprolol, 126t, 128t, 145t
   bitolterol, 125t, 143t
   brimonidine, 119t, 140t
   bucindolol, 126t, 146t
   bunazosin, 120t, 141t
   carteolol, 125t, 128t, 144t
   carvedilol, 126t, 128t, 129, 146t
   catecholamine metabolism, 121f
   celiprolol, 126t, 128t, 146t
   classification, 123f
   clonidine, 119t, 124–125, 139t
   dexmedetomidine, 119t, 139t
   dexmethylphenidate, 120t, 141t
   dobutamine, 125t, 142t, 308t
   doxazosin, 119t, 140t
   epinephrine, 118t, 139t
   esmolol, 126t, 128t, 146t
   fenoterol, 125t, 143t
   formoterol, 125t, 144t
   guanabenz, 119t, 140t
   guanfacine, 119t, 140t
   indoramin, 120t, 141t
   isoetharine, 125t, 143t
   isoproterenol, 125t, 142t
   ketanserin, 120t, 133t, 141t
   labetalol, 126t, 128t, 146t
   levalbuterol, 125t, 143t
   levobetaxolol, 126t, 145t
   levobunolol, 125t, 144t
   lisdexamfetamine, 120t, 141t
   mechanisms of action, 119t–120t, 123f
   mephentermine, 119t, 139t
   metabolism, 123f
   metaproterenol, 125t, 143t
   metaraminol, 119t, 139t
   methamphetamine, 120t, 141t
   methyldopa, 119t, 140t
   methylphenidate, 120t, 141t
   metipranolol, 125t, 144t
   metoprolol, 126t, 127–129, 128t, 145t
   midodrine, 119t, 139t
   modafinil, 120t, 142t
   nadolol, 125t, 128t, 144t
   naphazoline, 120t, 142t
   nebivolol, 126t, 128t, 146t
   norepinephrine, 118t, 135, 137, 139t
   oxymetazoline, 120t, 136, 137, 142t
   pemoline, 120t, 141t
   penbutolol, 128t
   phenoxybenzamine, 120t, 136, 137, 141t
   phentolamine, 120t, 141t
   phenylephrine, 119t, 139t
   pindolol, 126t, 128t, 145t
   pirbuterol, 125t, 143t
   prazosin, 119t, 121–124, 123f, 140t
   procaterol, 125t, 143t
   propranolol, 125t, 128t, 136, 138, 144t
   propylhexedrine, 120t, 142t
   pseudoephedrine, 120t, 142t
   ritodrine, 125t, 144t
   salmeterol, 125t, 143t
   serotonin, norepinephrine, and dopamine reuptake inhibitors, 147t
   sibutramine, 147t
   silodosin, 119t, 140t
   sympathomimetic agonists, misc., 120t, 123f, 141t–142t
   synthesis, storage, and release, 122f
   tamsulosin, 119t, 140t
   terazosin, 119t, 140t
   terbutaline, 125t, 143t
   timolol, 126t, 128t, 145t
   transporters, catecholamine plasma membrane, 124t
   urapidil, 120t, 141t
   xylometazoline, 120t, 142t
   yohimbine, 120t, 141t
Adrenergic receptors, 122f
Adrenocortical steroid biosynthesis inhibitors
   aminoglutethimide, 459t, 469t
   etomidate, 459t, 469t
   ketoconazole, 459t, 469t
   mechanisms of action, 459t
   metyrapone, 459t, 466, 469t
Adrenocortical steroids, 468t. See also Corticosteroids; Glucocorticoids; specific agents
   adrenal insufficiency, 461f, 465, 467, 468
   conjunctivitis, bacterial, 466
   Crohn's disease, 465
   Cushing's syndrome, 465–466
   glucocorticoids, general principles, 464b
   hydrocortisone, 390t, 403t, 460t, 464, 464f
   mechanisms of action, 459t, 462f, 464
   names and preparations, 460t–461t
   physiologic functions and pharmacologic effects, 462t–463t
   potencies and equivalent doses, 463t
   rheumatoid arthritis, 463–465
   therapeutic uses, 463b
   toxicities, 464b
Adrenocortical suppressants, mitotane, 679t
   cancer, 644t, 659t
   pharmacology, 459t, 469t
Adrenocorticolytic agents, 459t
Adrenocorticotropic hormone (ACTH) analog, 459t, 461f, 468t
   cosyntropin, 459t, 461f, 468t
   mechanisms of action, 459t, 461f
Adriamycin. See Doxorubicin
Adverse drug events, 56–57, 57t
Adverse effects, 5b, 9–12. See also specific drugs and drug classes
   specificity, 9
Affinity (K_A), 6b, 8
   competitive antagonists, 7b, 16, 17
Aflatoxin B_1, 41t, 60–62, 61f
   hepatitis B from, 61
African-American heart failure therapy, 306, 306b, 309, 310
Agonism, quantification, 7f
Agonists, 3b, 8. See also specific types
   allosteric (allotropic), 4b, 5f, 8
   full, 4b, 4f, 7b, 9
   inverse, 4, 4b, 4f, 9
   partial, 4b, 4f, 7b, 9
   primary, 3b, 8
Akathisia, 172t
Albumin, 22b
Albuterol
   pharmacology, 125t, 127, 135, 137, 143t
   pulmonary, 389t, 402t
Alclometasone dipropionate, 460t. See also Corticosteroids
Alcohol. See Ethanol
Alcohol dehydrogenase (ALDH), 178f
   disulfiram on, 187
   genetic variants, 189, 190
Alcoholism
   detoxification, 257
   fetal effects, 182b, 187
   negative reinforcement, 265, 266
   neurochemical system impacts, 185t
   physiological system effects, 183, 183t–185t, 189, 190
   treatment, 186, 256–257, 256t
Alcoholism drugs, 177t, 186–187, 186t, 193t
   acamprosate, 177t, 186–187, 186t, 193t, 257
   disulfiram, 177t, 178f, 186–187, 186t, 193t, 257
   ethanol and methanol metabolism, 178f
   nalmefene, 177t, 193t
   naltrexone, 177t, 186–187, 186t, 203, 257
Alcohol withdrawal syndrome, 256, 256t

Aldesleukin
  anticancer, 663t, 682, 683, 685t
  immunostimulant, 381t, 388t
Aldicarb, 100t, 115t
Aldosterone antagonists. See K⁺-sparing diuretics, mineralocorticoid antagonists
Aldosterone receptor antagonists, 269t, 271t, 272f, 285t
  eplerenone, 269t, 280–281, 285t, 302t, 311t
  heart failure, 302t, 307, 311t
    eplerenone, 302t, 311t
    mechanisms of action, 302t
    spironolactone, 302t, 307, 311t
  spironolactone, 269t, 285t, 302t, 307, 311t
Alefacept, 376t, 386t
  dermatologic, 709t, 710f, 714t, 726t
  immunotherapy, 376t, 386t
  psoriasis, 709t, 710f
Alemtuzumab
  anticancer, 662t, 667t, 671t, 684t
  immunotherapy, 376t, 378, 386t
Alendronate, 481t, 488t
Alfentanil, 195t, 208t
Alfuzosin, 119t, 140t
Aliskiren, 273t, 282, 283, 286t
Alitretinoin, 707t, 724t
Alkaline urine, 20b, 21–22, 39
Alkaloids, natural, 99t
Alkylating agents, 626–635, 627t–628t, 651t–653t. See also specific types and agents
  activation, in vivo, 631, 631f
  alkylsulfonates, 627t, 651t
    busulfan, 627t, 632t, 651t
    mechanisms of action, 627t, 628b–629b, 630f
    mechanisms of resistance, 627t, 632–633, 632b
    toxicities, 632b–633b, 632t, 651t
  cell cycle specificity, 630f
  dermatologic, 708t, 724t, 726f
    carmustine, 708t, 724t, 726t
    cyclophosphamide, 708t, 724t, 726t
    mechlorethamine, 708t, 724t, 726t
  DNA repair mechanisms, 629b
  ethyleneimines and methylmelamines, 627t, 651t
    altretamine (hexamethylendiamine), 627t, 651t
    mechanisms of action, 627t, 628b–629b, 630f
    mechanisms of resistance, 627t, 632–633, 632b
    thiotepa, 627t, 632t, 651t
    toxicities, 632b–633b, 632t, 651t
  mechanisms of action, 626, 627t–628t, 628, 628b–629b, 630f
  mechanisms of resistance, 627t–628t, 632–633, 632b
  methylhydrazines, 629t, 652t
    mechanisms of action, 628b–629b, 628t, 630f
    mechanisms of resistance, 628t, 632–633, 632b

    procarbazine, 629t, 652t
    toxicities, 632b–633b, 652t
    uses, 629t
  nitrogen mustards, 627t, 651t
    activation, in vivo, 631, 631f
    bendamustine, 627t, 651t
    chlorambucil, 627t, 651t
    cyclophosphamide, 627t, 631f, 632t, 651t
    ifosfamide, 627t, 632t, 651t
    mechanisms of action, 626, 627t, 628, 628b, 630f
    mechanisms of resistance, 627t, 632–633, 632b
    mechlorethamine HCl, 627t, 651t
    melphalan, 627t, 632t, 651t
    toxicities, 632b–633b, 632t, 651t
    uses, 629t
  nitrosoureas, 652t
    carmustine, 632t, 652t
    lomustine, 652t
    mechanisms of action, 627t, 628b, 630f
    mechanisms of resistance, 627t, 632–633, 632b
    semustine, 652t
    streptozocin, 652t
    toxicities, 632b–633b, 652t
    uses, 629t
  platinum coordination complexes, 628t, 633–635, 653t
    carboplatin, 628t, 629t, 632t, 653t
    cell cycle specificity, 630f
    cisplatin, 628t, 629t, 632t, 653t
    mechanisms of action, 628b–629b, 628t, 630f, 633
    mechanisms of resistance, 628t, 632b, 634–635
    oxaliplatin, 628t, 629t, 653t
    toxicities, 632b–633b, 632t, 633–634, 653t
    uses, 629t, 653t
  toxicities, 631–632, 632b–633b
    dose-limiting, 631, 632t
  triazenes, 652t
    dacarbazine, 628t, 629t, 630f, 645–647, 652t
    mechanisms of action, 628b, 628t, 630f
    mechanisms of resistance, 628t, 632–633, 632b
    temozolomide, 652t
    toxicities, 632b–633b, 652t
  uses, 629t
Alkyl Sulfonates, 627t, 651t
  busulfan, 627t, 632t, 651t
  mechanisms of action, 627t, 628b–629b, 630f
  mechanisms of resistance, 627t, 632–633, 632b
  toxicities, 632b–633b, 632t, 651t
  uses, 629t
Allergic reactions, 46t. See also specific drugs and drug classes
  case study, 3–6
  urticaria, H₁ antihistamines for, 351, 352
Allopurinol, 369t, 370–372, 373t

Allosteric agonists, 4b, 5f, 8
Allosteric antagonists, 4b, 9
Allosteric site, 8
Allotropic agonists, 4b, 5f, 8
Allotropic antagonists, 4b, 9
Allotropic site, 8
All-trans retinoic acid (ATRA), 645t, 646t, 659t
Almotriptan, 130t, 147t
Alogliptin, 471t, 472f, 479t
Alopecia, androgenic, 710t, 726t
  finasteride, 710t, 726t
  minoxidil, 710t, 726t
Alosetron, 498t, 505, 506, 508t
  antidiarrheal, 505, 506
  pharmacology, 130t, 147t
1α-Hydroxycholecalciferol, 481t, 488t
1α-Hydroxylase, 482f, 486, 487
5α-Reductase inhibitors, 442t, 458t
  dutasteride, 442t, 458t
  finasteride, 442t, 456, 457, 458t
$α_1$-Acid glycoprotein, 22b
$α_1$ Adrenergic receptor antagonists, 119t, 121–124, 140t
  antihypertensives, 277t
    doxazosin, 277t, 286t
    prazosin, 277t, 286t
    terazosin, 277t, 286t
  classification, 123f
  mechanisms of action, 119t, 123f
  pharmacology, 140t
  prazosin, 121–124, 123f
$α_1$-Selective adrenergic receptor agonists, 119t, 124–125, 139t
  classification, 123f
  clonidine, 124–125
  mechanisms of action, 119t, 123f
  pharmacology, 122f, 139t
$α_2$ Adrenergic receptor agonists
  classification, 123f
  mechanisms of action, 119t
$α_2$ Adrenergic receptor antagonists, 120t, 123f, 141t
  antihypertensives, 277t, 286t
    clonidine, 277t, 286t
    guanabenz, 277t, 286t
    guanfacine, 277t, 286t
  classification, 123f
  pharmacology, 141t
$α_2$-Selective adrenergic receptor agonists, 119t, 124–125, 139t–140t
  classification, 123f
  mechanisms of action, 119t, 122f, 139
  pharmacology, 122f, 139t–140t
α Adrenergic receptor agonists, 123f, 136, 137
  airflow resistance, 136, 137
  classification, 123f
  pharmacology, 83t–84t, 93, 94
α Adrenergic receptor antagonists, 120t, 123f, 141t
  classification, 123f
  mechanisms of action, 120t
  pharmacology, 141t
α-Glucosidase inhibitors, 471t, 479t
  acarbose, 471t, 479t
  mechanisms of action, 471t

α-Glucosidase inhibitors (*Cont.*)
   miglitol, 471t, 479t
   voglibose, 471t, 479t
Alprazolam, 92, 176t, 180, 191t, 192t
   addiction, 257–258, 257t
   withdrawal syndrome, 257–258, 257t
Alteplase, 323t, 329–330, 329f, 333t
Altretamine, 627t, 651t
   mechanisms of action, 627t, 628b–629b, 630f
   mechanisms of resistance, 627t, 632–633, 632b
   toxicities, 632b–633b, 651t
Alvimopan, 498t, 507t
Alzheimer's disease, 245–246, 246f
   acetylcholine deficiency, 246, 250–252
Alzheimer's disease drugs, 239t, 245–248, 247t, 253t
   behavioral, 247–248
   cognitive, 246–247, 247t
   donepezil, 239t, 246, 247t, 250–252, 253t
   galantamine, 239t, 246, 247t, 253t
   memantine, 239t, 246–247, 251, 252, 253t
   rivastigmine, 239t, 246, 247t, 253t
   tacrine, 239t, 247t, 253t
Amanita muscaria, 97, 100
Amanita phalloides, 97
Amantadine
   anti-influenza, 601t, 602t, 604f, 612–613, 620t
     adverse effects, 613
     influenza A prophylaxis, 612
     mechanisms of action and resistance, 602t, 604f613
   Parkinson's disease, 239t, 242t, 245, 253t
Ambenonium chloride, 97f, 100t, 104–105, 105f, 106f, 114t
Ambrisentan, pulmonary, 391t, 398–400, 399f, 404t
Amcinonide, 460t. *See also* Corticosteroids
Amebic colitis, 532–533
   paromomycin, 531t, 532–533, 535t
Amethopterin. *See* Methotrexate
Amikacin, 559–566, 559b, 567t
Amiloride, 269t, 284t
Aminocyclitols, 569t, 576t
Aminoglutethimide, 459t, 469t
Aminoglycosides, 559–567
   amikacin, 565, 566, 567t
   + β-lactam antibiotics, 559, 560f
   dosing
     maintenance, 562
     schedule, 515, 560–561, 561f
   gentamicin, 566t
   kanamycin, 567t
   mechanisms of action, 559b
   monitoring, plasma concentrations, 561–562, 563, 564–565
   neomycin, 567t
   nephrotoxicity, 563–564
   netilmicin, 567t
   ototoxocity, 562–563
   penetration, intracellular, 564–566
   penicillin inactivation, 565, 566
   postantibiotic effect, 564, 565
   on protein synthesis, 559, 560f
   with renal dysfunction, 562
   resistance, 559–560, 559b
   streptomycin, 567t
   tobramycin, 566t
Aminolevulinic acid photodynamic therapy, 708t, 725t
Amiodarone, 312t, 321t
   electrophysiologic actions, 317t
   iodine-induced hypothyroidism, 435t, 438, 439
   ventricular fibrillation, 316
   ventricular tachycardia, 318
Amitriptyline, 150t, 152–154, 152f, 168, 169, 173t, 205t
Amlodipine
   antihypertensive, 277t, 282, 287t, 294
   myocardial ischemia, 290t, 294–295, 298, 299, 300t
Amobarbital, 177t, 181t, 192t
Amoxapine, 150t, 173t
Amoxicillin, 552t, 555t
   for duodenal ulcer, 492, 494t
Amphetamine, 120t, 135–136, 137, 141t. *See also specific types*
   alertness, 135–136, 137
   toxidrome, 53t
Amphotericin B, 530t, 534, 535t, 588t, 589–590
   adverse effects, 590
   formulations and pharmacokinetics, 589–590, 589t, 596t
   mechanisms of action, 588t, 589f, 590
   mechanisms of resistance, 588t
   pharmacokinetic properties, 589t
   uses, 596t
Amphotericin B (C-AMB), 588t, 589–590, 589f, 589t, 595, 596, 596t
Amphotericin B colloidal dispersion (C-ABCD), 588t, 589–590, 589f, 589t, 596t
Amphotericin B lipid complex (ABLC), 588t, 589–590, 589f, 589t, 596t
Amphotericin B liposomal (L-AMB), 588t, 589–590, 589f, 589t, 596t
Ampicillin, 552t, 555t
Amprenavir, 601t, 603t, 608f, 609f, 622t
Amylin agonists
   mechanisms of action, 471t
   pramlintide, 471t, 479t
Amyotrophic lateral sclerosis (ALS), 239t, 249, 253t
   baclofen, 239t, 249, 253t
   dantrolene, 239t, 249, 253t
   riluzole, 239t, 249, 251, 252, 253t
   tizanidine, 239t, 249, 253t
Anakinra
   immunotherapy, 376t, 386t
   rheumatoid arthritis, 368t
Analgesic anesthetic adjuncts, 211t, 217, 223t
Anandamide, 263
Anaphylaxis, 56
Anastrozole, 442t, 458t
   anticancer, 664t, 677t, 679t, 686t
   mechanisms of action, 442t, 664t, 678
Androgen deprivation therapy, 679–680
Androgenic alopecia, 710t, 726t
   finasteride, 710t, 726t
   minoxidil, 710t, 726t
Androgen receptor antagonists, 442t, 458t
   bicalutamide, 442t, 458t
   flutamide, 442t, 454, 456, 457, 458t, 679t
   nilutamide, 442t, 458t
Androgens, 442t, 452–454, 458t
   anticancer, 664t, 679t, 686t
   biosynthesis, 679
   drugs against (*See* Antiandrogens)
   structures, 453f
   testosterone, 442t, 458t
   testosterone buccal tablet, 442t, 458t
   testosterone cypionate, 442t, 458t
   testosterone enanthate, 442t, 458t
   testosterone gel, 442t, 458t
   testosterone patch, 442t, 458t
   testosterone undecanoate, 442t, 458t
Anemia
   megaloblastic, 417–418, 537–540
   pernicious, 417–418
Anesthesia, general, 211–214
   anesthetic state, components, 211b
   first time, 211–212
   general principles, 211–212, 212b
   inducing agents, 212f, 213–214, 213f, 213t (*See also* Anesthetic agents, parenteral)
   mechanisms, 211b, 212–213
   types, 212
Anesthesia, spinal, 217–219
Anesthetic adjuncts
   analgesics, 211t, 217, 223t
   benzodiazepines, 211t, 216–217, 223t
   dexmedetomidine, 211t, 223t
   neuromuscular blocking agents, 211t, 223t
Anesthetic agents, 210–224
   endotracheal intubation, 216–217
   mechanisms of action, 210t–211t
Anesthetic agents, inhalational, 222t–223t
   blood:gas partition coefficient, 215–216, 215f, 215t, 220, 221
   choices, 214
   CO_2 absorbent, 220, 221
   desflurane, 210t, 215t, 220, 221, 223t
   enflurane, 210t, 215t, 223t
   halothane, 210t, 215t, 222t
   isoflurane, 210t, 215t, 222t
   minimum alveolar concentration (MAC), 215, 215t
   nitrous oxide, 210t, 215t, 223t
   pharmacokinetics, 215, 215t
   potencies, 215, 215t
   sevoflurane, 210t, 215t, 223t
   speed of induction, 215–216, 215t, 216f
   uptake, 215t, 216, 216f
   xenon, 211t, 215t, 223t
Anesthetic agents, local, 224t
   administration
     routes, 217b, 219
     spinal, 217–219
   allergic reactions, 217, 220, 221

articaine, 224t
benzocaine, 224t
bupivacaine, 224t
Chloroprocaine, 224t
cocaine, 224t
dibucaine, 224t
dyclonine, 224t
epinephrine in, 217
    end artery tissues and gangrene, 220, 221–222
lidocaine, 224t
mechanisms of action, 217, 218f
mepivacaine, 224t
pramoxine, 224t
prilocaine, 224t
procaine, 224t
proparacaine, 224t
ropivacaine, 224t
sulfite (methylparaben) in, 220, 221
tetracaine, 224t
uses, 217b
on voltage-gated Na^+ channels, 217
Anesthetic agents, parenteral, 222t
  context-sensitive half-time, 214, 214f
  differences, 213t, 214
  etomidate, 210t, 213t, 214f, 222t
  fospropofol, 210t, 222t
  on $GABA_A$ receptor, 219–220, 221
  ketamine, 210t, 213t, 214f, 217, 222t
  methohexital, 210t, 213t, 222t
  pharmacokinetics, 212f, 213–214
  pharmacological properties, 213t
  propofol, 210t, 213t, 214f, 220, 221, 222t
  sodium thiopental, 210t, 213t, 214f, 222t
  termination and redistribution, 220, 221
  use, 213
Anesthetic state, 211b
Angina, 290t. *See also* Myocardial ischemia
Angina drugs
  myocardial ischemia (*See* Myocardial ischemia drugs)
  non-myocardial ischemia conditions, 293t–294t
Angioedema. *See also specific drugs*
  ACE inhibitors, 279
Angiogenesis, 673
Angiotensin-converting enzyme (ACE) inhibitors, 270t, 273t, 285t
  acute MI, 279
  adverse effects, 276
  angioedema, 279
  benzapril, 273t, 285t
  captopril, 273t, 279, 285t
  cautions, 274–276
  diabetics, 274
  enalapril, 273t, 274–276, 275f, 285t
  enalaprilat, 273t, 285t
  fosinopril, 273t, 285t
  heart failure, 272f, 276f, 279, 285t, 303–304, 310t
  mechanisms of action, 270t, 273t, 274–276, 275f, 301t
  lisinopril, 273t, 281, 282, 285t
  mechanisms of action, 273t, 274–276, 275f
  moexipril, 273t, 285t
  perindopril, 273t, 285t
  quinapril, 273t, 285t
  ramipril, 273t, 285t
  structure, 275f
  trandolapril, 273t, 285t
Angiotensin II (Ang II), effects, 274f
Angiotensin II (Ang II) receptor antagonists, 270t
Angiotensin (AT_1) receptor blockers (ARBs), 270t, 273t, 285t
  candesartan cilexetil, 273t, 285t
  diabetics, 274
  heart failure, 273t, 274, 279, 280, 285t, 301t, 310t
  ibuprofen on, 282, 283
  irbesartan, 273t, 285t
  losartan, 273t, 285t
  olmesartan medoxomil, 273t, 285t
  structure, 275f
  telmisartan, 273t, 285t
  valsartan, 273t, 280, 282, 283, 285t
Anidulafungin, 588t, 589f, 598t
Animal testing, 8
Antacids, 490t, 496t
Antagonism, 4b, 5f, 8–9. *See also specific receptors*
  allosteric (allotropic), 4b, 9
  chemical, 4b, 9, 48b
  dispositional, 48b
  drug–drug interaction, 48b
  mechanisms, 4b, 5f
  receptor, 48b
Antagonists, 4b, 5f, 8–9. *See also specific drugs*
  competitive, 4b, 5b, 5f, 7b, 16, 17
  functional, 4b
  noncompetitive, 4b, 5f
Anthelminthics, 536–541. *See also* Helminth infection drugs
Anthracenedione derivative immunostimulants, mitoxantrone, 382t, 388t
Anthracyclines and anthracenediones, 643t, 658t
  daunorubicin, 630f, 643t, 645b, 658t
  doxorubicin, 630f, 643t, 645–647, 645b, 658t
  epirubicin, 630f, 643t, 645b, 658t
  idarubicin, 630f, 643t, 645b, 658t
  mechanisms of action, 630f, 643t
  mechanisms of resistance, 643t, 645b
  mitoxantrone, 630f, 643t, 645b, 658t
  uses, 644t, 658t
  valrubicin, 630f, 643t, 645b, 658t
Antiandrogens, targeted anticancer
  nonsteroidal, 665t, 679t, 687t
    bicalutamide, 665t, 687t
    flutamide, 665t, 679t, 687t
    nilutamide, 665t, 687t
  steroidal, 665t, 687t
    cyproterone, 665t, 687t
    megestrol, 665t, 687t
Antiarrhythmic drugs, 312–322
  adenosine receptor agonists, 312t, 322t
  adenosine, 312t, 317t, 318, 322t
  angina, 293t
  atrial fibrillation, 315, 316
  cardiac action potential, 312f, 313f
  class IA (sodium channel blockers), 312t, 320t–321t
    disopyramide, 312t, 317t, 321t
    procainamide, 312t, 316, 317t, 320t
    quinidine, 312t, 317t, 320t
  class IB (sodium channel blockers), 312t, 321t
    lidocaine, 312t, 316, 317t, 319, 320, 321t
    mexiletine, 312t, 317t, 321t
  class IC (sodium channel blockers), 312t, 321t
    flecainide, 312t, 317t, 321t
    propafenone, 312t, 317t, 321t
  class II (β adrenergic receptor antagonists), 312t, 317t, 321t
    esmolol, 312t, 321t
    propranolol, 312t, 317t, 321t
    sotalol, 312t, 317t, 321t
  class III, 312t, 317t, 321t–322t
    amiodarone, 312t, 316, 317t, 318, 321t
    dofetilide, 312t, 317t, 322t
    dronedarone, 312t, 317t, 321t
    ibutilide, 312t, 317t, 322t
    sotalol, 312t, 321t
  class IV (Ca^{2+} channel blockers, nondihydropyridine), 312t, 322t
    diltiazem, 312t, 315, 317t, 322t
    verapamil, 312t, 317t, 322t
  drug–drug interactions, 319, 320
  electrophysiologic actions, 317t
  inhibitor concentration, 513–514, 514f
  long QT and torsade de pointes, 313–315, 314t, 315b
  magnesium sulfate, 317t, 322t
  mechanistic approach, 314t
  Na^+-K^+-ATPase inhibitors, 312t, 322t
    digoxin, 312t, 317t, 319, 320, 322t
  paroxysmal ventricular tachycardia (PSVT), 314t, 318
  premature ventricular beats, 314t
  post-MI, 314t, 319, 320
  tachyarrhythmia mechanisms, 313b
  ventricular fibrillation, 314t, 316
Antibiotics. *See* Antimicrobial agents
Antibiotics, anticancer, 630f, 643t, 658t
  actinomycins, dactinomycin, 630f, 643t, 658t
  anthracyclines and anthracenediones, 643t, 658t
    daunorubicin, 630f, 643t, 645b, 658t
    doxorubicin, 630f, 643t, 645–647, 645b, 658t
    epirubicin, 630f, 643t, 645b, 658t
    idarubicin, 630f, 643t, 645b, 658t
    mechanisms of action, 630f, 643t
    mechanisms of resistance, 643t, 645b
    mitoxantrone, 630f, 643t, 645b, 658t
    uses, 644t, 658t
    valrubicin, 630f, 643t, 645b, 658t
  bleomycin, 630f, 643t, 645b, 658t
  mechanisms of action, 643t
  mechanisms of resistance, 643t, 645b–646b

Antibiotics, anticancer (*Cont.*)
   mitomycin, 630f, 643t, 646b, 658t
   uses, 644t, 658t
Anticholinergic toxidrome, 53t
Anticholinesterase agents, 89
Anticholinesterase insecticides, 102, 102b, 103f, 103t, 104f. *See also specific types*
   antidotes, 40t, 65t, 102
      pralidoxime, 41t, 42t, 65t, 100t, 102
Anticoagulants. *See also specific drugs and drug classes*
   indications, 325t
   monitoring, 325, 325t, 330b
   toxicities, 325
Anticoagulants, oral
   direct factor Xa inhibitors, 323t, 333t
      apixaban, 323t, 328, 331, 333t
      mechanisms of action, 323t
      rivaroxaban, 323t, 328, 333t
   direct thrombin inhibitors, 333t
      dabigatran etexilate, 323t, 328, 333t
      mechanisms of action, 323t
   vitamin K antagonist, 333t
      mechanisms of action, 323t
      warfarin (*See* Warfarin)
Anticoagulants, parenteral
   activated protein C, 333t
      drotrecogin alfa, 323t, 333t
      mechanisms of action, 323t
   direct thrombin inhibitors, 323t, 333t
      argatroban, 323t, 330, 331, 333t
      bivalirudin, 323t, 333t
      desirudin, 333t
      mechanisms of action, 323t
   heparinoid, 323t, 325, 333t
      ardeparin, 323t, 325, 333t
      dalteparin, 323t, 325, 333t
      enoxaparin, 323t, 325, 333t
      fondaparinux, 323t, 325, 333t
      heparin, 323t, 325, 327f, 333t
      lovenox, 325–326, 326f
      low-molecular-weight heparins, 323t, 324–325, 325f, 333t
      mechanisms of action, 323t
      nadroparin, 323t, 325, 333t
      tinzaparin, 323t, 325, 333t
Anticonvulsants. *See also specific drugs and drug classes*
   pain target and site of action, 205t
Anticonvulsants, malaria, 151t, 175t
   carbamazepine, 151t, 164–165, 175t
   lamotrigine, 151t, 165, 175t
   valproic acid, 151t, 164–165, 169, 173, 175t
Antidepressants, 155t–156t
   actions and effects, 152–154, 152f
   adverse effects, 154
   disposition, 158t
   drug-related deaths, 51t
   elderly, 71, 72, 75
   initial treatment phase, 153
   long-term effects, 153
   maintenance phase, 154

   mood elevation, 152–153, 152f
   phases of treatment, 153–154
   sites of actions, 152f
   structures, dosing, and adverse effects, 155t–156t
   therapeutic lag, 153
Antidepressants, atypical, 150t, 156t, 174t
   atomoxetine, 150t, 174t
   bupropion, 150t, 174t
   mianserin, 150t, 174t
   mirtazapine, 150t, 174t
   nefazodone, 150t, 174t
   reboxetine, 150t, 174t
   structures, dosings, and adverse effects, 156t
   trazodone, 150t, 174t
Antidepressants, tricyclic (TCAs)
   adverse effects, 154
   elderly, 71, 72, 75
   pain target and site of action, 205t
   sites of actions, 152f
Antidiabetic agents, oral
   α-glucosidase inhibitors, 471t, 479t
      acarbose, 471t, 479t
      mechanisms of action, 471t
      miglitol, 471t, 479t
      voglibose, 471t, 479t
   amylin agonists
      mechanisms of action, 471t
      pramlintide, 471t, 479t
   biguanides, metformin, 470t, 479t
   bile acid sequestrants, 471t, 479t
      colesevelam, 471t, 479t
      mechanisms of action, 471t
   dipeptidyl peptidase-4 inhibitors, 471t, 472f, 476, 479t
      alogliptin, 471t, 472f, 479t
      mechanisms of action, 471t, 472f
      saxagliptin, 471t, 472f, 479t
      sitagliptin, 471t, 472f, 479t
      vildagliptin, 471t, 472f, 479t
   drug development, 6–9
   GLP-1 agonists, 471t, 472f, 476, 479t
      exenatide, 471t, 472f, 479t
      liraglutide, 471t, 472f, 479t
      mechanisms of action, 471t, 472f
   insulin secretagogues, nonsulfonylurea, 470t, 472f, 479t
      nateglinide, 470t, 472f, 479t
      repaglinide, 470t, 472f, 479t
   insulin secretagogues, sulfonylurea, 470t, 472f, 479t
      adverse effects, 475
      gliclazide, 470t, 472f, 479t
      glimepiride, 470t, 472f, 477, 478, 479t
      glipizide, 470t, 472f, 479t
      glyburide, 470t, 472f, 479t
      mechanisms of action, 470t, 477, 478
   mechanisms of action, 470t–471t
   thiazolidinediones, 470t, 475–476, 479t
      adverse effects, 476
      mechanisms of action, 470t
      pioglitazone, 470t, 475–476, 479t
      rosiglitazone, 470t, 475–476, 479t

Antidiarrheal agents, 498t, 508t
   alosetron, 498t, 505, 506, 508t
   bismuth, 498t, 508t
   carboxymethylcellulose, 498t, 508t
   cholestyramine, 498t, 508t
   clonidine, 498t, 508t
   difenoxin + atropine, 498t, 508t
   diphenoxylate + atropine, 498t, 500, 508t
   loperamide, 209t, 498t, 500–501, 508t
   mechanisms of action, 498t
   octreotide, 498t, 508t
Antidiarrheal agents, opioid, 209t
   difenoxin, 209t
   diphenoxylate (+ atropine), 209t, 498t, 500, 508t
   loperamide, 209t, 498t, 500–501, 508t
   mechanisms of action, 195t
Antidotes, 42t, 65t. *See also specific poisons*
Antiemetics. *See* Antinauseants and antiemetics
Antiestrogens, targeted anticancer
   aromatase inhibitors, 664t, 679t, 686t
      anastrozole, 664t, 677t, 679t, 686t
      exemestane, 664t, 677t, 679t, 686t
      letrozole, 664t, 677t, 679t, 686t
   selective estrogen-receptor downregulators, 664t
      fulvestrant, 664t, 677t, 686t
   selective estrogen-receptor modulators, 664t, 686t
      mechanisms of resistance, 664t
      raloxifene, 664t, 686t
      tamoxifen, 664t, 667f, 676–678, 677t, 679t, 686t
      toremifene, 664t, 677t, 679t, 686t
      uses, 677t, 686t
Antifolates. *See* Folic acid analogs (antifolates)
Antifungal agents, 588–599
   amphotericin B, 588t, 589–590, 589f, 596t
      adverse effects, 590
      amphotericin B (C-AMB), 595, 596, 596t
      amphotericin B colloidal dispersion (C-ABCD), 596t
      amphotericin B lipid complex (ABLC), 596t
      amphotericin B liposomal (L-AMB), 596t
      mechanisms of action, 588t, 589f, 590
      mechanisms of resistance, 588t
      pharmacokinetic properties, 589t
   butenafine, 599t
   ciclopirox olamine, 598t
   dermatologic, 708t, 721, 722, 725t
   echinocandins, 588t, 589f, 598t
      anidulafungin, 598t
      caspofungin, 588t, 589f, 593, 593f, 598t
      mechanisms of action, 588t, 593, 593f
      micafungin, 598t
   flucytosine, 588t, 589f, 595, 596, 596t
   griseofulvin, 588t, 593–596, 598t, 721, 722
   halprogin, 598t
   imidazoles and triazoles, 588t, 589f, 590, 597t
      CYP interactions, 590, 590t

drug interactions, 590t–592t
fluconazole, 588t, 590, 595, 596, 597t, 719
itraconazole, 597t
posaconazole, 597t
voriconazole, 588t, 589f, 590t–592t, 592–593, 595, 596, 597t
imidazoles and triazoles, topical, 588t, 597t–598t
butoconazole, 597t
clotrimazole, 597t
econazole, 597t
ketoconazole, 598t
miconazole, 594, 597t
oxiconazole, 598t
sertaconazole, 598t
sulconazole, 598t
terconazole, 597t
tioconazole, 597t
mechanisms and sites of action, 588t, 589f
naftifine, 589f, 599t
nystatin, 599t
ophthalmic, 694t, 701
terbinafine, 588t, 589f, 596, 598t
tolnaftate, 598t
undecylenic acid, 599t
Whitfield's ointment, 599t
Antiglucocorticoids
mechanisms of action, 459t
mifepristone, 459t, 469t
Antihepatitis agents, 600t–602t, 620t
adefovir dipivoxil, 600t, 602t, 620t
entecavir, 600t, 602t, 620t
hepatitis B, entecavir, 618, 619
hepatitis C, ribavirin-pegylated interferon, 613–614, 617, 618
interferons, 600t–602t, 606f, 620t
lamivudine, 600t, 602t, 607f, 620t
mechanisms of action and resistance, 602t
peginterferons, 601t
Antiherpes agents, 600t–602t, 605–608, 619t
acyclovir, 600t–601t, 604f–605f, 605–608, 605t, 617–618, 619t
cidofovir, 600t, 601t, 605, 619t
docosanol, 600t
fomivirsen, 600t, 602t, 609, 619t
foscarnet, 600t, 602t, 604f, 605, 609–612, 617, 618, 619t
ganciclovir, 600t, 602t, 604f, 605, 605f, 609, 617, 618, 619t
idoxuridine, 600t, 602t, 605–606, 619t
mechanisms of action and resistance, 601t–602t, 606–607, 606f
penciclovir, 600t, 602t, 604f, 605, 605f, 608, 619t
trifluridine, 601t, 602t, 606, 619t
valacyclovir, 601t, 605, 608
valganciclovir, 601t
Antihistamines. See Histamine receptor antagonists
Antihypertensive drugs, 269–270. See also specific drugs and drug classes
Ang II receptor antagonists, 270t

β adrenergic receptor antagonists, 277t, 286t (See also β adrenergic receptor antagonists)
Ca^{2+} channel blockers, L-type, 270t, 277t, 287t (See also Ca^{2+} channel blockers)
dihydropyridines, 277t, 282, 287t, 290t, 300t, 306 (See also Ca^{2+} channel blockers, L-type, dihydropyridine)
edema, 282
mechanisms of action, 277t
nondihydropyridines, 277t, 278, 287t (See also Ca^{2+} channel blockers, L-type, nondihydropyridine)
choice, 270, 270t
classification, 270t
diabetes with, 273–274
direct renin inhibitors/vasodilators, 270t
diuretics, 268t–270t, 269–272, 283t–285t (See also Diuretics)
ibuprofen on, 282, 283
mechanisms of action, 270t
nephrons, 270b
pregnancy, 277–278, 278f
renin-angiotensin system inhibitors, 270t, 273t, 274–276, 274f, 275f, 279, 281–282, 285t (See also Renin-angiotensin system (RAS) inhibitors)
treatment algorithm, 275f, 276f
vasodilators
arterial, 278t, 287t (See also Vasodilators, arterial)
arterial and venous, nitroprusside, Antifungal agents 278t, 287t
Antihypertensive drugs, sympatholytics, 270t, 277t
adrenergic neuron blocking agents, Antifungal agents 277t, 286t
guanadrel, 277t, 287t
reserpine, 277t, 286t
centrally acting adrenergic agents
methyldopa, 277t, 286t
$α_2$ adrenergic receptor antagonists, 277t, 286t
clonidine, 277t, 286t
guanabenz, 277t, 286t
guanfacine, 277t, 286t
mechanisms of action, 277t
$α_1$ adrenergic receptor antagonists, 277t
doxazosin, 277t, 286t
prazosin, 277t, 286t
terazosin, 277t, 286t
β adrenergic receptor antagonists, oxazosin, 277t
Anti-IgE monoclonal antibodies, omalizumab, 390t, 397, 404t
Anti-infectives. See Antimicrobial agents
Anti-inflammatories, dermatologic. See Immunosuppressants and anti-inflammatories, dermatologic
Anti-influenza agents, 601t, 602t, Antifungal agents 604f, 620t
amantadine, 601t, 602t, 604f, 612–613, 620t

mechanisms of action and resistance, 602t, 604f
oseltamivir, 601t, 602t, 604f, 620t
rimantadine, 601t, 602t, 604f, 620t
zanamivir, 601t, 602t, 604f, 620t
Antimalarials agents, dermatologic (See Malaria chemotherapy, dermatologic agents)
Antimetabolites, 635–642, 635t–636t, 653t–656t
dermatologic, 708t, 724t, 725t
5-fluorouracil, 708t, 724t, 725t
azathioprine, 708t, 724t, 725t
methotrexate, 708t, 715, 721–722, Antifungal agents 724t, 725t
folic acid analogs, 635t, 653t
high-dose methotrexate with leucovorin rescue, 635t, 638–640, 653t
lometrexol, 635t, 653t
mechanisms and sites of action, 635t
mechanisms of resistance, 635t, 638b, 640
methotrexate, 635t, 653t
pemetrexed, 635t, 653t
pharmacogenetics, 637f, 639
pralatrexate, 635t, 653t
raltitrexed, 635t, 653t
toxicities, 653t
trimetrexate, 635t, 653t
uses, 637t
mechanisms of action, 653t–656t
mechanisms of resistance, 638b–640b, 653t–656t
purine analogs, 636t, 641–642, 655t–656t
6-mercaptopurine, 630f, 636t, 641–642, 655t
6-thioguanine, 630f, 636t, 655t
cladribine, 630f, 636t, 655t
clofarabine, 636t, 655t
fludarabine phosphate, 630f, 636t, 655t
mechanisms of action, 630f, 636t, 641–642
mechanisms of resistance, 636t, 639b–640b
nelarabine, 636t, 655t
pentostatin, 636t, 656t
toxicities, 642, 655t–656t
uses, 637t, 655t–656t
pyrimidine analogs, 635t–636t, 640–641
5-fluorouracil (5-FU), 630f, 635t, 638b–639b, 638f, 640–641
azacytidine, 636t
capecitabine, 630f, 635t, 638f
cytarabine (Ara-C), 630f, 635t, 639b, 648, 649
decitabine, 636t
floxuridine (FUdR), 630f, 635t, 638b–639b, 638f
gemcitabine, 630f, 636t, 639b
mechanisms and sites of action, 630f, 635t–636t, 638f, 640
mechanisms of resistance, 635t–636t, 639b, 640–641
uses, 637t
uses, 637t

Antimicrobial, ocular, topical, 692t–693t
Antimicrobial agents. *See also specific drugs and drug classes*
  dermatologic, 708t, 725t
    antibacterials, 708t, 725t
    antifungals, 708t, 721, 722, 725t
    retapamulin, 708t, 725t
  mechanisms of action, 2b
Antimicrobial therapy principles, 512–519. *See also specific drugs and disorders*
  area under the curve, 514, 515f
  barrier penetration, 512–513, 513f
    blood-brain, 512 (*See also* Blood-brain barrier (BBB))
    blood-CSF, 24b, 28f, 94
  β-lactam antibiotic resistance, 516–517
  classification, 512b
  combination therapy, 517b, 518
  disease progression timeline, 516, 516f
  dosing schedule
    on concentration-time profile, 514, 515f
    resistance suppression, 515
  drug and dose regimen choice, microbial laboratory, 513–514, 514f
  drug penetration, 512–513, 512b
  efflux pumps, 515b, 517
  empiric therapy, 516f, 518–519
  endocarditis risk and prophylaxis, 515b, 516
  HIV combination therapy, 518, 519
  indices, most important, 514, 515f
  inhibitory sigmoid E_{max} curve, 513, 513f, 514, 514f
  peak plasma concentration, 514, 515, 515f, 519
  postantibiotic effect, 515
  pre-surgery prophylaxis, 515b, 516
  resistance, 515b, 517
  wound infection prophylaxis, 514b, 516
Antinauseants and antiemetics, 498t, 508t
  aprepitant, 498t, 502t, 508t
  choice, 501, 501f
  classification, 501, 502t
  dronabinol, 498t, 502, 502t, 508t
  mechanisms of action, 498t
  nabilone, 498t, 502, 508t
  ondansetron, 498t, 501, 502t, 505, 506, 508t
Antiplatelet agents
  GPIIb/IIIa, 323t, 324–325, 332t
    abciximab, 323t, 324–325, 331–332, 332t
    eptifibatide, 323t, 324–325, 332t
    mechanisms of action, 323t
    tirofiban, 323t, 324–325, 332t
  indications, 324t
  irreversible, ADP receptor antagonists, 323t, 332t
    clopidogrel, 323t, 324, 325, 325t, 331–332, 332t
    mechanisms of action, 323
    prasugrel, 323t, 324, 325, 325t, 332t
    ticlopidine, 323t, 332t
  irreversible, COX-1 inhibitors
    aspirin, 323t, 324–325, 332t, 371, 372
    mechanisms of action, 323t, 358f
    sites of action, 325f
Antiproliferative/antimetabolic agents, 375t, 385t. *See under* Biological immunosuppressants
  azathioprine, 368t, 375t, 380, 385t
  everolimus, 375t, 385t
  MPA, 375t, 385t
  mycophenolate mofetil, 375t, 383, 384, 385t
  sirolimus, 375t, 377f, 383, 384, 385t
Anti-protozoal drugs, 530–535. *See also* Protozoal drugs
Antipsychotics
  adverse effects, 172t
  elderly, 77b, 168, 169, 171
  nonpsychotic disorders, 163b
Antipsychotics, atypical, 151t, 160t–161t, 175t
  aripiprazole, 151t, 170t, 175t
  chemical structures, dosages, and maintenance, 160t–161t
  metabolism, 170t
  olanzapine, 151t, 165, 168, 170t, 171–172, 175t
  potencies, 162t
  quetiapine, 151t, 171t, 175t
  risperidone, 151t, 168, 169, 171t, 175t
Antipsychotics, typical, 151t, 160t, 175t
  asenapine, 151t, 170t, 175t
  chemical structures, dosages, and maintenance, 160t
  clozapine, 151t, 167–169, 170t, 172, 175t
  droperidol, 151t, 175t
  haloperidol, 151t, 159, 163f, 171t, 175t
  iloperidone, 151t, 170t, 175t
  loxapine, 151t, 175t
  metabolism, 170t
  molindone, 151t, 175t
  paliperidone, 151t, 170t, 175t
  potencies, 162t
  receptor occupancy and clinical response, 163f
  sertindole, 151t, 175t
  ziprasidone, 151t, 171t, 175t
Antipsychotics, typical, phenothiazines, 150t, 174t
  chlorpromazine, 150t, 171t, 174t
  fluphenazine, 150t, 174t
  perphenazine, 150t, 174t
  trifluoperazine, 150t, 174t
Antirigidity agents, cholinergic, 106t, 117t
Antiseizure drugs, 225–235
  acetazolamide, 225t, 237t
  adverse effects, 227b, 227t
  agents and principles, 227b, 228
  barbiturates, phenobarbital, 225t, 236t
  benzodiazepines, 225t, 237t
    clonazepam, 225t, 237t
    clorazepate, 225t, 237t
  choice, 227b
  dosage, 227b
  felbamate, 226t, 237t
  gabapentin, 225t, 237t
  general principles, 227b
  hepatic microsomal enzyme interactions, 227t
  iminostilbenes, 225t, 236t
    carbamazepine, 225t, 226f, 232–235, 236t
    oxcarbazepine, 225t, 236t
  lacosamide, 226t, 237t
  lamotrigine, 225t, 232, 237t
  Lennox-Gastaut syndrome, 232
  levetiracetam, 225t, 234–235, 237t
  mechanisms of action, 225t, 225t–226t, 226f–227f
    Ca^{2+} channel blockers, T-type, 225t, 225t–226t, 227f, 230–231
    $GABA_A$ receptor synaptic transmission, 225t, 225t–226t, 226f
    Na^+ channel inactivation, 225t, 225t–226t, 226f
  pregabalin, 225t, 237t
  rufinamide, 226t, 237t
  succinimides, 225t, 236t
    ethosuximide, 225t, 230–231, 234, 235, 236t
    methsuximide, 225t, 236t
  tiagabine, 226t, 237t
  topiramate, 226t, 235, 236, 237t, 702, 703
  valproic acid, 225t, 231–232, 234, 235, 236t
    with lamotrigine, 235
  zonisamide, 226t, 237t
Antispasmodics, bowel, 498t, 508t
  dicyclomine, 498t, 508t
  glycopyrrolate, 498t, 508t
  hyoscyamine, 498t, 508t
  mechanisms of action, 498t
  methscopolamine, 498t, 508t
Antispasticity agents, cholinergic, 106t, 117t
Antithymocyte globulin (ATG), 376t, 377f, 377t, 378, 385t
Antithyroid agents, 431t, 439t–440t. *See also* Thyroid and antithyroid drugs
  carbimazole, 431t, 440t
  compounds, 435t
  methimazole, 431t, 435–436, 438, 439, 440t
  propylthiouracil, 431t, 439t
Anti-thyroid hormone compounds, 435t
Anti-TNF reagents, 376t, 386t. *See also under* Biological immunosuppressants
  adalimumab, 368t, 376t, 381, 383, 384, 386t
  certolizumab pegol, 376t, 381, 386t
  etanercept, 376t, 380, 386t
  golimumab, 376t, 386t
  infliximab, 368t, 376t, 380, 381, 386t

Antitussives, 209t, 391t, 404t
   benzonatate, 209t, 210t, 391t, 404t
   mechanisms of action, 196t
   opioid
      codeine, 209t, 391t, 404t
      dextromethorphan, 391t, 404t
   OTC cough medicines, young children, 350
Antiviral agents, 600–624
   antihepatitis agents, 600t–602t, 620t
      adefovir dipivoxil, 600t, 602t, 620t
      entecavir, 600t, 602t, 620t
      interferons, 600t–602t, 606f, 620t
      lamivudine, 600t, 602t, 607f, 620t
      mechanisms of action and resistance, 602t
      peginterferons, 601t
   antiherpes, 600t–602t, 605–608, 619t
      acyclovir, 600t, 601t, 604f, 605–608, 605f, 605t, 617, 618, 619t
      cidofovir, 600t, 601t, 605, 619t
      docosanol, 600t
      fomivirsen, 600t, 602t, 609, 619t
      foscarnet, 600t, 602t, 604f, 605, 609–612, 617, 618, 619t
      ganciclovir, 600t, 602t, 604f, 605, 605f, 609, 617, 618, 619t
      idoxuridine, 600t, 602t, 605–606, 619t
      mechanisms of action and resistance, 601t–602t, 606–607, 606f
      penciclovir, 600t, 602t, 604f, 605, 605f, 608, 619t
      trifluridine, 601t, 602t, 606, 619t
      valacyclovir, 601t, 605, 608
      valganciclovir, 601t
   anti-influenza, 601t, 602t, 604f, 620t
      amantadine, 601t, 602t, 604f, 612–613, 620t
      mechanisms of action and resistance, 602t, 604f
      oseltamivir, 601t, 602t, 604f, 620t
      rimantadine, 601t, 602t, 604f, 620t
      zanamivir, 601t, 602t, 604f, 620t
   entry inhibitors, 601t, 603t, 608f, 611f, 616, 623t
      enfuvirtide, 601t, 603t, 608f, 611f, 616, 623t
      maraviroc, 601t, 603t, 608f, 611f, 623t
      mechanisms of action and resistance, 603t
   famciclovir, 605, 608
   integrase inhibitor
      mechanisms of action and resistance, 603t
      raltegravir, 601t, 603t, 611f, 623t
   mechanisms of action and resistance, 601t–603t
   non-nucleoside reverse transcriptase inhibitors (NNRTIs), 601t, 603t, 608f, 610f, 623t
      delavirdine, 601t, 603t, 608f, 610f, 623t
      efavirenz, 601t, 603t, 608f, 610f, 623t
      etravirine, 601t, 603t, 608f, 610f, 623t
      mechanisms of action and resistance, 603t, 608f, 610f

      nevirapine, 601t, 603t, 608f, 610f, 615, 622t
      structures, 610f
   nucleoside reverse transcriptase inhibitors (NRTIs), 601t, 603t, 607f, 608f, 621t
      abacavir, 601t, 603t, 607f, 608f, 621t
      adverse effects, 615
      didanosine, 601t, 603t, 607f, 608f, 621t
      emtricitabine, 601t, 603t, 607f, 608f, 621t
      HIV, 614–615
      lamivudine, 601t, 602t, 607f, 621t
      mechanisms of action and resistance, 602t–603t, 604f, 608f, 614–615
      stavudine, 601t, 603t, 607f, 608f, 621t
      structures, 607f
      tenofovir disoproxil, 601t–603t, 607f, 608f, 621t
      zalcitabine, 601t, 621t
      zidovudine, 601t, 602t, 607f, 608f, 621t
   ophthalmic, 693t, 701
   other
      imiquimod, 601t, 602t, 621t
      ribavirin, 601t, 602t, 620t
      telbivudine, 601t, 602t, 607f, 608f, 620t
      tenofovir disoproxil, 601t–603t, 607f, 608f
   protease inhibitors, 601t, 603t, 608f, 609f, 621t–622t
      amprenavir, 601t, 603t, 608f, 609f, 622t
      atazanavir, 601t, 603t, 608f, 609f, 622t
      darunavir, 601t, 603t, 608f, 609f, 622t
      indinavir, 601t, 603t, 608f, 609f, 621t
      lopinavir, 601t, 603t, 615, 622t
      mechanisms of action and resistance, 603t, 608f, 609f
      nelfinavir, 601t, 603t, 608f, 609f, 622t
      ritonavir, 601t, 603t, 608f, 609f, 615–619, 622t
      saquinavir, 601t, 603t, 608f, 609f, 621t
      tipranavir, 601t, 603t, 608f, 609f, 622t
   virus replication stages and targets, 612t
Anxiolytics
   benzodiazepine, 174t (See also Benzodiazepines)
   buspirone, 150t, 174t
Apixaban, 323t, 328, 331, 333t
APLs, universal, glatiramer acetate, 382t, 388t
Apomorphine, 130t, 148t
   Parkinson's disease, 239t, 242t, 253t
Apparent dissociation constant (K_{app}), 7b
Apraclonidine
   blood-brain barrier, 702, 703
   ophthalmic, 690t, 695t, 702, 703, 704t
   pharmacology, 119t, 140t
Aprepitant, 498t, 502t, 508t
Aprotinin, 347t
aPTT, 330b
Arachidonic acid metabolism, 358f
   cyclooxygenase pathway, 358f
   lipoxygenase pathways, 358f, 359f
Ardeparin, 323t, 325, 333t
Area under the curve (AUC), 514, 515f

Arformoterol
   pharmacology, 125t, 144t
   pulmonary, 390t, 402t
Argatroban, 323t, 330, 331, 333t
Arginine vasopressin, 423t, 424f, 429t
Aripiprazole, 130t, 148t, 151t, 170t, 175t
   adverse effects, 163
   mania prophylaxis, 165
   mechanisms of action, 162–163
Aromatase inhibitors, 664t, 679t, 686t
   anastrozole, 664t, 677t, 679t, 686t
   exemestane, 664t, 677t, 679t, 686t
   letrozole, 664t, 677t, 679t, 686t
Arrhythmia drugs. See Antiarrhythmic drugs
Arrhythmias, cardiac, angina drugs, 293t
Arsenic, 41t, 43t, 63, 64, 66t
Arsenic trioxide (ATO), 630f, 645t, 646t, 660t
Artemether, 520t, 529t
Artemether-lumefantrine, 520t, 521, 527, 529t
Artemisinin-based combination therapies (ACTs), 521
Artemisinin, 520t, 529t
   artemether, 520t, 529t
   artemether-lumefantrine, 520t, 521, 527, 529t
   artesunate, 520t, 529t
   dihydroartemisinin, 520t, 529t
Artesunate, 520t, 529t
Arthritis. See also Rheumatoid arthritis
   NSAIDs for, 366–368 (See also Nonsteroidal anti-inflammatory drugs (NSAIDs))
Articaine, 224t
ASA. See Aspirin
Asenapine, 151t, 170t, 175t
Aspergillus flavus, 60, 61
Aspirin, 357t, 358f, 360t, 365–366, 371, 372
   antiplatelet, 323t, 324–325, 332t
   COX-1 inhibitors or NSAIDs with, 365–366
   pain target and site of action, 205t
   pregnancy, 365
   prophylaxis, daily, 365
   toxidrome, 53t
Association rate ($k+1$), 6b
Asthma, 393–397, 396f
   mild, 393–394 (See also Pulmonary drugs)
   severe, 393–398
   symptoms and pathophysiology, 393
AT_1 receptor blockers. See Angiotensin (AT_1) receptor blockers (ARBs)
Atazanavir, 601t, 603t, 608f, 609f, 622t
   CP3A4 metabolism, 617
Atenolol
   myocardial ischemia, 300t
   pharmacology, 126t, 128t, 146t
Atomoxetine, 150t, 174t
Atorvastatin, 334t, 343t
Atovaquone, 520t, 529t
Atovaquone-proguanil, for malaria
   chemoprophylaxis, 521–522, 522t, 526
   chemotherapy, 520t, 527, 529t
ATP inhibitors. See Protein tyrosine kinase inhibitors

Atracurium, 106t, 107t, 116t
Atrial fibrillation, 315, 316. *See also* Antiarrhythmic drugs
  ablation, 314t, 316
  antiarrhythmics, 314t
  competitive amateur athlete, 316
  DC cardioversion, 314t, 316
  digoxin, 319, 320
  uncomplicated, drugs, 315
  warfarin, 327
Atrial flutter, antiarrhythmics, 314t
Atrial natriuretic peptide, 269t
  carperitide, 269t, 284t
  nesiritide, 269t, 280, 284t
Atrial tachycardia, antiarrhythmics, 314t
Atropine, 40t, 65t, 96t, 101–102, 101t, 112t
  adverse effects, 80–82, 112t
  effects, dose in, 101t
  mechanisms of action, 96t
  ophthalmic, 690t, 695t, 704t
  uses, 112t
Autonomic ganglia drugs, 106t
Autonomic ganglionic blockade, 107t
Autonomic nervous system, 80–85, 92
  anatomy, 81f
  effector organs, 83t–84t
  ganglionic blockade, 107t
  parasympathetic, 82f, 85, 92, 107t
  peripheral divisions, 80, 85b
  somatic motor and efferent nerves, 82f, 92
  sympathetic, 82f, 85, 92, 107t
AV nodal reentrant tachycardia (PSVT) anti-arrhythmics, 314t
Azacytidine (5-azacytidine), 636t, 654t
  mechanisms and sites of action, 630f, 636t, 638f, 640
  mechanisms of resistance, 636t
  toxicities, 637t, 654t
  uses, 637t, 654t
Azathioprine
  dermatologic, 708t, 724t, 725t
  idiosyncratic reaction, 504
  immunotherapy, 368t, 375t, 380, 385t
  inflammatory bowel disease, 498t, 502–503, 503f, 509t
  metabolism, 502–503, 503f
  rheumatoid arthritis, 368t, 375t, 380, 385t
  ulcerative colitis, 502–503, 506, 507
Azelaic, 710t, 727t
Azelastine, 347t, 355t
  ophthalmic, 691t, 705t
Azithromycin, 568t, 570f, 576t, 692t
Azlocillin, 552t
Aztreonam, 549t, 553, 558t

B

Bacillus Calmette-Guerin (BCG), 381t, 387t
Bacitracin, 569t, 573, 577t, 692t
Baclofen, 239t, 249, 253t
Bactrim allergy, 56–57
Balsalazide, 357t, 498t, 503f, 509t
Barbiturates, 177t, 180–182, 181t, 192t
  adverse effects, 182
  amobarbital, 177t, 181t, 192t
  butabarbital, 177t, 181t, 192t
  mechanisms of action, 180–181
  mephobarbital, 177t, 181t, 192t
  methohexital, 177t, 192t
  overdose treatment, 189, 190
  pentobarbital, 177t, 181t, 192t
  pharmacologic properties and uses, 181t
  phenobarbital, 177t, 181t, 189, 190, 192t, 225t, 236t
  secobarbital, 177t, 180, 192t
  structures, 181t
  thiopental, 177t, 181t, 192t, 214f
  tolerance and physical dependence, 181–182
  toxidrome, 53t
  trade names, 181t
Baroreceptor reflex, elderly, 77b
Barrier penetration, 512–513, 513f
  blood-brain, 512 (*See also* Blood-brain barrier (BBB))
  blood-CSF, 24b, 28f, 94
Basal ganglia
  Huntington's disease, 248, 248f
  Parkinson's disease, 240–241, 241f
Basiliximab, 376t, 386t
BCNU. *See* Carmustine (BCNU)
BCRP transporter, 24t
Beclomethasone dipropionate, 390t, 403t
Beers Criteria, 69–70, 78b
Belatacept, 381t, 387t
Belladonna atropa toxidrome, 53t
Belladonna, 101–102
Bendamustine, 627t, 651t
  activation, in vivo, 631, 631f
  mechanisms of action, 626, 627t, 628, 628b, 630f
  mechanisms of resistance, 627t, 632–633, 632b
  toxicities, 632b–633b, 651t
  uses, 629t
Bendroflumethiazide, 269t, 284t
Benzapril, 273t, 285t
Benznidazole, 530t–531t, 535t
Benzo[a]pyrene, 41t, 63–65
Benzocaine, 224t
Benzodiazepine
  addiction, 257–258, 257t
  withdrawal syndrome, 257–258, 257t
Benzodiazepine receptor agonists, 177t, 192t
  eszopiclone, 177t, 192t
  zaleplon, 177t, 192t
  zolpidem, 177t, 178–179, 192t
Benzodiazepine receptor antagonists, 192t
  flumazenil, 41t, 42t, 65t, 177t, 179–180, 192t
Benzodiazepines, 191t–192t
  alcohol withdrawal, 256–257
  alprazolam, 176t, 180, 191t, 192t, 257–258, 257t
  amyotrophic lateral sclerosis, 249
  anesthetic adjuncts, 211t, 216–217, 223t
  anticonvulsants, 190
  antidote, flumazenil, 42t, 65t, 177t, 179–180
  antiseizure, 225t, 237t
    clonazepam, 225t, 237t
    clorazepate, 225t, 237t
  anxiolytic, 174t
  categories, elimination-based, 178b
  chlordiazepoxide, 176t, 191t, 192t
  clonazepam, 176t, 191t, 192t
  clorazepate, 176t, 191t, 192t
  dependence and withdrawal, 180
  diazepam, 176t, 191t, 192t, 214f
  drug-related deaths, 51t
  elderly, 71, 77b
  estazolam, 176t, 191t, 192t
  flurazepam, 176t, 180, 191t, 192t
  with hepatic cirrhosis, 189, 190
  hypnotics choice, 189, 190, 191t
  lorazepam, 176t, 189, 190, 191t, 192t
  metabolic relationships among, 188f
  midazolam, 176t, 191t, 192t, 214f
  overdose treatment, flumazenil, 41t, 42t, 65t, 177t, 179–180, 192t
  oxazepam, 176t, 189, 190, 191t, 192t
  quazepam, 176t, 191t, 192t
  sedative-hypnotics, 176t, 178b, 180, 189–190, 191t–192t
  temazepam, 176t, 191t, 192t
  toxidrome, 53t
  triazolam, 176t, 191t, 192t
Benzonatate
  antitussive, 209t, 210t, 391t, 404t
  mechanisms of action, 391t
Benzoylecgonine, 262
Benztropine mesylate, 96t, 114t
Benzyl alcohol, dermatologic, 708t, 725t
Bepotastine, ophthalmic, 691t, 705t
Best Pharmaceuticals for Children Act of 2002 (BPCA), 71b
11β-Hydroxysteroid dehydrogenase, 464f, 467, 468
β Blockers. *See* β adrenergic receptor antagonists
Betamethasone preparations, 460t. *See also* Corticosteroids
Betaxolol, 126t, 128t, 145t
  ophthalmic, 691t, 695t, 704t
$β_1$-Selective adrenergic receptor antagonists, 128t, 145t–146t
  mechanisms of action, 123f, 126t
  pharmacology and pharmacokinetics, 123f, 128t, 145t–146t
$β_2$ Adrenergic receptor agonists, long-acting pulmonary, 390t, 402t
  adverse effects, 392b, 398
  arformoterol, 390t, 402t
  asthma, 393–394, 396–397, 402
    adverse effects, 392b
    bronchodilation, indirect actions, 391b
    mechanisms of action, 390t, 391f, 394
  COPD, 395
  formoterol, 390t, 402t
  indacaterol, 390t, 402t
  mechanisms of action, 390t, 391b, 391f, 394
  salmeterol, 390t, 402t

β_2 Adrenergic receptor agonists, short-acting, pulmonary, 389t, 401, 402t
  adverse effects, 392b
  albuterol, 389t, 402t
  asthma, 393–394
  levalbuterol, 389t, 402t
  mechanisms of actions, 389t, 391b, 391f, 394
  metaproterenol, 389t, 402t
  pirbuterol, 389t, 402t
  terbutaline, 389t, 402t
β_2-Selective adrenergic receptor agonists, 127, 143t–144t
  adverse effects, 127
  albuterol, 125t, 127, 135, 137, 143t
  mechanisms of action, 123f, 125t, 127
  pharmacology and pharmacokinetics, 123f, 128t, 143t–144t
β Adrenergic receptor agonists, 123f, 142t
  with additional cardiovascular effects, 123f, 128t, 146t
  adverse effects, 128–129
  antihypertensive, 286t
    doxazosin, 277t
  classification, 123f
  elderly, 77b
  heart failure, 311t
    dobutamine, 302t, 307–308, 308t, 311t
    dopamine, 302t, 307–308, 308t, 311t
    mechanisms of action, 302t, 307–308
  for heart failure, 129–130, 286t, 302t, 304, 311t
  intrinsic sympathomimetic activity, 15, 16
  mechanisms of action, 125t, 127–128, 128t
  metoprolol
    heart failure, 306, 309, 310
    myocardial ischemia, 300t
    pharmacology, 126t, 127–129, 128t, 145t
  myocardial ischemia, 289t, 291f, 292–294, 300t
    atenolol, 300t
    with nitrates, 294
    propranolol, 300t
    timolol, 300t
  nonselective, 123f, 128t, 144t–145t
    mechanisms of action, 125t–126t
    pharmacology and pharmacokinetics, 123f, 128t, 144t–145t
  ophthalmic, 690t–691t, 695t, 700
  pharmacokinetics, 128t
  pharmacology, 123f, 128t, 142t
  pheochromocytoma, 136, 137
  third-generation, 123f, 129t, 146t
    mechanisms of action, 126t
    pharmacology, 123f, 146t
    vasodilating, 129t
  vasodilating, 126f
β Adrenergic receptor antagonists
  antiarrhythmic, 312t, 317t, 321t
    esmolol, 312t, 321t
    propranolol, 312t, 317t, 321t
    sotalol, 312t, 317t, 321t
  heart failure, 286t, 304, 310t
    bisoprolol, 301t, 309, 310, 310t
    carvedilol, 301t, 309, 310, 310t
    mechanisms of action, 301t
    metoprolol, 301t, 303–304, 306, 310t
β Cell, pancreatic, 471f, 472f, 473
β-Lactam antibiotics, 549–558. *See also specific agents and drug classes*
  + aminoglycosides, 559, 560f
  amoxicillin-clavulanic acid, 555, 558t
  aztreonam, 549t, 553, 558t
  β-lactamase inhibitors, 549t, 553, 558t
  carbapenems, 549t, 553
  cephalosporins, 549t, 550b, 553–555, 556t–558t (*See also* Cephalosporins)
  clavulanic acid, 555, 558t
  doripenem, 558t
  efflux pumps, 551f
  enzyme classes, 550b
  ertapenem, 558t
  imipenem, 558t
  imipenem-cilastatin, 554–555
  mechanisms of action, 549t
  meropenem, 558t
  penicillins, 549t, 550–556, 555t–556t (*See also* Penicillins)
  resistance, 516–517, 549t, 550b
  on *Staphylococcus aureus*, 550f
β-Lactamase, 517, 519
β-Lactamase inhibitors, 549t, 553, 558t
  clavulanic acid, 558t
  resistance, 549t
  sulbactam, 558t
  tazobactam, 558t
β-Lactam enzyme classes, 550b
Bethanechol, 95t, 99t, 112t
  mechanisms of action, 95t
  pharmacology, 99t, 112t
Bevacizumab, 662t, 671t, 674–675, 684t
Bexarotene, 707t, 724t
Bezafibrate, 335t, 344t
Bicalutamide, 442t, 458t, 665t, 679t, 687t
BiDil, 306, 306b
Biguanides, 470t, 479t
Bile acid–binding resins (sequestrants), 334t, 339, 340, 343t
  cholestyramine, 334t, 342–343, 343t
  colesevelam, 334t, 340, 343t, 471t, 479t
  colestipol, 334t, 342–343, 343t
  diabetes mellitus, 471t, 479t
  mechanisms of action, 334t, 471t
Bimatoprost, ophthalmic, 691t, 705t
Binding, 20f
  in vitro studies, 8
  plasma protein, 22b
    children, 68b
    elderly, 74b, 75t
  tissue, 22b–23b
    elderly, 75t
Bioavailability, 20b, 33b. *See also specific drugs and drug classes*
  elderly, 73b, 73f, 73t–74t
  infant, oral drug, 72, 74
  volume of distribution, 30, 33b, 34b
Biological immunosuppressants, 385t–386t
  anti-TNF reagents, 376t, 386t
    adalimumab, 368t, 376t, 381, 383, 384, 386t
    certolizumab pegol, 376t, 381, 386t
    etanercept, 376t, 380, 386t
    golimumab, 376t, 386t
    infliximab, 368t, 376t, 380, 381, 386t
  dermatologic, 709t, 714t, 715–716, 726t
    adalimumab, 709t, 714t, 722, 723, 726t
    alefacept, 709t, 710f, 714t, 726t
    efalizumab, 709t, 710f, 714t, 726t
    etanercept, 709t, 714t, 726t
    infliximab, 709t, 714t, 726t
  disease-modifying anti-rheumatic drugs
    abatacept, 368t, 381t, 387t
    adalimumab, 368t
    anakinra, 368t
    certolizumab, 368t
    golimumab, 368t
    infliximab, 368t, 376t, 380, 386t
    rituximab, 368t
  IL-1 inhibitors, 376t, 386t
    anakinra, 376t, 386t
    canakinumab, 376t, 386t
    rilonacept, 376t, 386t
  LFA-1 & LFA-3 inhibitors
    alefacept, 376t, 386t
    efalizumab, 376t, 386t
  monoclonal antibody, anti-CD3, muromonab-CD3, 376t, 378, 385t
  monoclonal antibody, anti-CD25, 376t, 379, 386t
    basiliximab, 376t, 386t
    daclizumab, 376t, 386t
  monoclonal antibody, anti-CD52, alemtuzumab, 376t, 378, 386t
  polyclonal antibodies, immune globulin preparations, 376t, 377f, 377t–378t, 378, 385t
Biotransformation, 20b, 28b
Biotransforming enzymes, 29b, 29t
Bipolar disorder, 164–166
Bisacodyl, 498t, 508t
Bismuth, 490t, 496t, 498t, 508t
Bisoprolol
  heart failure, 301t, 309, 310, 310t
  pharmacology, 126t, 128t, 145t
Bisphosphonates, 481t, 488t
  adverse effects, 485, 487, 488t
  alendronate, 481t, 488t
  etidronate sodium, 481t, 488t
  for hypercalcemia, 481t, 485, 488t
    pamidronate, 481t, 488t
    zoledronate, 481t, 485, 488t
  ibandronate, 481t, 485, 488t
  jaw osteonecrosis from, 481t, 485, 488t
  mechanisms of action, 481t
  for Paget disease, 481t, 488t
  pamidronate, 481t, 488t
  risedronate, 481t, 488t
  tiludronate, 481t, 488t
  zoledronate, 481t, 485, 488t
Bitolterol, 125t, 143t
Bivalirudin, 323t, 333t
Bleomycin, 643t, 658t
  dermatologic, 709t, 724t, 726t
  mechanisms of action, 630f, 643t, 647
  mechanisms of resistance, 645b
Blepharitis, 700

Blepharospasm agents, 692t, 706t
  abobotulinumtoxin A, 692t, 706t
  onabotulinumtoxin A, 692t, 706t
Blood-brain barrier (BBB), 24b, 28f
  drug diffusion, 94
  elderly, 74b
  infants, 68b
  penetration, 512
  pH on diffusion, 19–20, 19b–20b, 19f, 20f, 35, 37–38, 90
Blood coagulation reactions, 325–326, 326f
Blood-CSF barrier, 24b, 28f, 94
Blood:gas partition coefficient, 215–216, 215f, 215t, 220, 221
BNP, human recombinant. *See* Nesiritide (BNP)
Bone remodeling cycle, 482f, 485
Bone turnover disorder drugs, 480–489
  bisphosphonates, 481t, 488t
    alendronate, 481t, 488t
    etidronate sodium, 481t, 488t
    ibandronate, 481t, 485, 488t
    mechanisms of action, 481t
    pamidronate, 481t, 488t
    risedronate, 481t, 488t
    tiludronate, 481t, 488t
    zoledronate, 481t, 485, 488t
  hormones
    calcitonin, 480t, 483–484, 483f, 486, 487
    teriparatide, 480t
  hypercalcemia, 483–484
  mechanisms of action, 480t–481t
  monoclonal antibody, denosumab, 481t, 488t
  phosphate binders, 481t, 484, 488t
    lanthanum carbonate, 481t, 484, 488t
    mechanisms of action, 481t, 488t
    renal osteodystrophy, 482f, 484
    sevelamer hydrochloride, 481t, 484, 488t
  renal osteodystrophy, 482f, 484
  vitamin D and analogs, 481t, 482f, 484, 488t
    1α-hydroxycholecalciferol, 481t, 488t
    22-oxacalcitrolparicalcitol, 481t, 488t
    calcipotriol, 481t, 488t
    calcitriol, 481t, 482f, 488t
    dihydrotachysterol, 481b
    doxercalciferol, 481b
    ergocalciferol, 481t, 488t
    intestinal bypass surgery, 486, 487
    paricalcitol, 481t, 488t
    therapeutic uses, 481b
Bortezomib, 663t, 681, 682–683, 685t
Bosentan, 391t, 398–400, 399f, 404t
Botulinum toxins, 106t, 117t
  abotulinum toxin A, 692t, 706t
  onabotulinum toxin A, 106t, 117t, 692t, 706t
  rimabotulinum toxin B, 106t, 117t
Bowel disorder drugs, 497–508
  acetylcholine synthesis enhancer, dexpanthenol, 498t, 507t
  antidiarrheal, 498t, 508t
    alosetron, 498t, 505, 506, 508t
    bismuth, 498t, 508t
    carboxymethylcellulose, 498t, 508t
    cholestyramine, 498t, 508t
    clonidine, 498t, 508t
    difenoxin + atropine, 498t, 508t
    diphenoxylate + atropine, 498t, 500, 508t
    loperamide, 209t, 498t, 500–501, 508t
    mechanisms of action, 498t
    octreotide, 498t, 508t
  antinauseants and antiemetics, 498t, 508t
    aprepitant, 498t, 502t, 508t
    choice, 501, 501f
    classification, 501, 502t
    dronabinol, 498t, 502, 502t, 508t
    mechanisms of action, 498t
    nabilone, 498t, 502, 508t
    ondansetron, 498t, 501, 502t, 505, 506, 508t
  antispasmodics, 498t, 508t
    dicyclomine, 498t, 508t
    glycopyrrolate, 498t, 508t
    hyoscyamine, 498t, 508t
    mechanisms of action, 498t
    methscopolamine, 498t, 508t
  inflammatory bowel disease, 498t–499t, 509t
    adalimumab, 499t, 509t
    azathioprine, 498t, 502–503, 503f, 509t
    balsalazide, 498t, 503f, 509t
    budesonide, 498t, 509t
    certolizumab pegol, 499t, 509t
    cyclosporine, 499t, 509t
    infliximab, 499t, 509t
    mechanisms of action, 498t–499t
    mesalamine, 498t, 503f, 509t
    methotrexate, 499t, 509t
    natalizumab, 499t, 509t
    olsalazine, 498t, 503f, 506, 507, 509t
    sulfasalazine, 381, 498t, 502, 503f, 505, 507, 509t
  laxatives, 498t, 507t–508t
    bisacodyl, 498t, 508t
    bowel effects, 500t
    classification, 500t
    docusate sodium, 498t, 508t
    lactulose, 497t, 505, 506–507, 507t
    magnesium citrate, 497t, 507t
    magnesium hydroxide, 497t, 507t
    magnesium sulfate, 497t, 507t
    mechanisms of action, 498b, 498t, 499
    polyethylene glycol, 497t, 507t
    saline, 497t, 507t
    sodium phosphate, 497t, 507t
  opioid antagonists
    alvimopan, 498t, 507t
    mechanisms of action, 498t
    methylnaltrexone, 498t, 499, 505, 506, 507t
  prokinetics, 497t, 507t
    cisapride, 497t, 504, 506, 507t
    domperidone, 497t, 507t
    erythromycin, 497t, 507t
    lubiprostone, 497t, 507t
    mechanisms of action, 497
    metoclopramide, 497t, 504, 506, 507t
    prucalopride, 497t, 507t

Bradykinin, 347t
Bradykinin antagonists
  kallikrein inhibitors, 347t
  kinin receptor antagonists, 347t, 355t
Brain. *See also specific agents and disorders*
  signal transduction, 88f
Brater's algorithm, 275f, 276f, 283
Breast cancer. *See also* Cancer chemotherapy and cytotoxics; *specific agents*
  ER+, 676–679
  Her2/neu-positive, 672
  tamoxifen, 442t, 451, 456, 457, 458t, 664t, 667f, 676–678, 677f
Breastfeeding, FDA drug rules, 72b
Brimonidine, ophthalmic, 690t, 695t, 704t
Brinzolamide, ophthalmic, 691t, 705t
Bromfenac, 357t, 373t
  ophthalmic, 691t, 705t
Brimonidine, 119t, 140t
Bromocriptine, 422t, 426, 428t
  Parkinson's disease, 242t
  pharmacology, 130t, 148t
Brompheniramine maleate, 346t, 354t
BSEP transporter, 23t, 24t, 25t, 38
Bucindolol, 126t, 146t
Budesonide, 381, 460t. *See also* Corticosteroids
  Crohn's disease, 465
  inflammatory bowel disease, 498t, 509t
  pulmonary, 390t, 402, 403t, 460t
Bumetanide, 269t, 282, 283, 284t
Bunazosin, 120t, 141t
Bupivacaine, 224t
Buprenorphine, 194t, 195t, 200t, 203, 209t
  for opioid addiction, 261–262
  for opioid dependence, 203
Buprenorphine/naloxone, 261–262
Bupropion, 150t, 174t
  for smoking, 259
Buserelin, 664t, 687t
Buspirone, 130t, 133t, 136, 138, 147t, 150t, 174t
Busulfan, 627t, 632t, 651t
  mechanisms of action, 627t, 628b–629b, 630f
  mechanisms of resistance, 627t, 632–633, 632b
  toxicities, 632b–633b, 632t, 651t
  uses, 629t
Butabarbital, 177t, 181t, 192t
Butenafine, 599t
Butoconazole, 588t, 597t
Butorphanol, 194t, 195t, 200t, 203, 209t

C

Ca^{2+} channel blockers
  adverse effects, 295
  contraindications, 295
  toxidrome, 53t
Ca^{2+} channel blockers, L-type, 270t, 277t, 287t
  chemical structures and cardiovascular effects, 295t–296t
  contraindications, 295
  edema, 282
  mechanisms of action, 277t
  myocardial ischemia, 290t, 294–295, 298–299, 300t
  with nitrates, 297

739

Ca^{2+} channel blockers, L-type, dihydropyridine
antihypertensive, 277t, 282, 287t, 290t, 300t
amlodipine, 277t, 282, 287t, 290t, 294–295, 298, 299, 300t
clevidipine, 277t, 287t, 290t, 300t
felodipine, 277t, 287t, 290t, 300t
isradipine, 277t, 287t, 290t, 300t
nicardipine, 277t, 287t
nifedipine, 277t, 287t, 290t, 300t
nisoldipine, 277t, 287t, 290t, 300t
heart failure, 290t, 300t, 306
nimodipine, 290t, 300t
Ca^{2+} channel blockers, L-type, nondihydropyridine
antiarrhythmic, 312t, 315, 317t, 322t
diltiazem, 312t, 315, 317t, 322t
verapamil, 312t, 317t, 322t
antihypertensive, 277t, 287t
diltiazem, 277t, 278, 287t, 290t, 300t
verapamil, 277t, 287t, 290t, 300t, 306
Ca^{2+} channels, 86, 87f, 89t
T-type, antiseizure drugs on, 225t, 225t–226t, 227f, 230–231
Cabergoline, 130t, 148t, 422t, 426, 428t
Cadmium, 41t, 43t, 65t
Calcimimetics. *See* Cinacalcet
Calcineurin, 383–384
Calcipotriene, 707t, 724t
Calcipotriol, 481t, 488t
Calcitonin, 480t, 483–484, 483f, 486, 487
hypercalcemia, 480t, 481t, 483–484, 483f, 488t
Paget disease, 481t, 488t
PTH in, 483f
regulation, 486, 487
Calcitriol, 481t, 482f, 488t
Calcium sensor mimetics. *See* Cinacalcet
Camptothecin analogs, 643t, 657t
irinotecan, 630f, 643t, 644b–645b, 649–651, 657t
mechanisms of action, 630f, 643t, 649–651
mechanisms of resistance, 643t, 644b–645b
topotecan, 630f, 643t, 644b–645b, 649–651, 657t
toxicities, 657t
uses, 644t, 657t
Canakinumab, 376t, 386t
Cancer chemotherapy and cytotoxics, 626–660. *See also specific drugs and drug classes*
alkylating agents, 626–635, 627t–628t, 651t–653t (*See also* Alkylating agents)
antimetabolites, 635–642, 635t–636t, 653t–656t
cell cycle specificity, 630f
cytotoxic natural products, 630f, 642t–644t, 645–647
cytotoxics with diverse mechanisms of action, 644t–646t, 659t–660t (*See also* Cytotoxics with diverse mechanisms of action)
targeted, 661–687 (*See also* Targeted anticancer therapies)

Candesartan cilexetil, 273t, 285t
Candidiasis
esophageal, 589f, 590t–592t, 594–596
oral, 467, 468
vaginal, 594
Cannabinoid receptors, 263, 358f
Cannabis, 263
Capecitabine, 635t, 654t
mechanisms of action, 630f, 635t, 638f
uses, 637t, 654t
Capreomycin, 579t, 587t
Capsaicin, 710t, 727t
Captopril, 273t, 279, 285t
Carbachol, 95t, 99t, 112t
mechanisms of action, 95t
ophthalmic, 690t, 695t, 704t
pharmacology, 99t, 112t
Carbamate insecticides, 100t, 102, 115t
atropine for, 42t, 65t (*See also* Atropine)
Carbamazepine
alcohol withdrawal, 257
anticonvulsants, 151t, 164–165, 175t
antiseizure, 225t, 226f, 232–235, 236t
for glossopharyngeal and trigeminal neuralgias, 233
Huntington's disease, 248
for lightning-type pain, 233
Carbapenems, 549t, 553
Carbaryl, 100t, 115t
Carbenicillin, 552t, 556t
Carbidopa, 238t, 244f
Carbidopa/levodopa, 238t, 242, 250, 251, 252t
Carbimazole, 431t, 440t
Carbinoxamine, 346t, 353t
Carbon dioxide gas, therapeutic, 211t, 223t
Carbonic anhydrase inhibitors
antihypertensive, 268t, 271t, 272f, 283t
acetazolamide, 268t, 283t
brinzolamide, 283t
dichlorphenamide, 268t
dorzolamide, 283t
methazolamide, 268t
ophthalmic, 691t, 705t
brinzolamide, 691t, 705t
dorzolamide, 691t, 705t
Carboplatin (CBDCA), 628t, 653t
mechanisms of action, 628b–629b, 628t, 630f, 633
mechanisms of resistance, 628t, 632b, 634–635
toxicities, 632b–633b, 632t, 633–634, 653t
uses, 629t, 653t
Carboxymethylcellulose, 498t, 508t
ophthalmic, 692t, 706t
Carcinogens, 43t, 60–62, 60f, 61f. *See also specific types*
aflatoxin B$_1$, 41t, 60–62, 61f
initiation and promotion, 60, 60f
Cardiac action potential, 312f, 313f
Cardiac arrhythmias, drugs. *See* Antiarrhythmic drugs
Cardiovascular disease risk
assessment, 335–336, 338
LDL-C treatment guidelines, 336, 336t
prevention guidelines, 335, 335b, 338

Carisoprodol, 177t, 193t
Carmustine (BCNU), 627t, 652t
degradation, 631f
dermatologic, 708t, 724t, 726t
mechanisms of action, 627t, 628b, 630f
mechanisms of resistance, 627t, 632–633, 632b
toxicities, 631f, 632t, 652t
uses, 629t
Carteolol, 125t, 128t, 144t
ophthalmic, 691t, 695t, 704t
Carvedilol
heart failure, 301t, 309, 310, 310t
MI patients, 279
pharmacology, 126t, 128t, 129, 146t
Caspofungin, 588t, 589f, 593, 593f, 598t
Catecholamines. *See also specific types and drugs*
endogenous, 118t, 139t
metabolism, 121f
transporters, plasma membrane, 124t
Catechol-*O*-methyltransferase (COMT), 240f, 243, 250, 251
levodopa metabolism, 243, 243f, 244f
Catechol-*O*-methyltransferase (COMT) inhibitors, 238t, 242t, 244, 244f
CBDCA. *See* Carboplatin (CBDCA)
CCNU. *See* Lomustine (CCNU)
Cefaclor, 556t
Cefadroxil, 556t
Cefdinir, 557t
Cefditoren pivoxil, 557t
Cefepime, 558t
Cefixime, 557t
Cefmetazole, 557t
Cefoperazone, 557t
Cefotaxime, 557t
Cefotetan, 556t
Cefoxitin, 556t
Cefpodoxime proxetil, 557t
Cefprozil, 556t
Ceftazidime, 553, 557t
Ceftibuten, 557t
Ceftizoxime, 557t
Ceftriaxone, 554, 555, 557t
Cefuroxime, 556t
Cefuroxime axetil, 556t
Celecoxib, 357t, 358f, 363t, 371, 372, 373t
cardiovascular risk, 357, 365b, 371, 372
Celiprolol, 126t, 128t, 146t
Centrally acting adrenergic agents, antihypertensive
α$_2$ adrenergic receptor antagonists, 277t, 286t
clonidine, 277t, 286t
guanabenz, 277t, 286t
guanfacine, 277t, 286t
methyldopa, 277t, 286t
Central nervous system (CNS), 92
distribution, 24b
drugs, 91–92 (*See also specific drugs*)
neurotransmitters, 86b, 91–92, 91t
Cefadroxil, 556t
Cephalexin, 556t

Cephalosporins, 553–555, 556t–558t
　mechanisms of action, 549t
　mechanisms of resistance, 549t, 550b
Cephalosporins, first-generation, 556t
　cefadroxil, 556t
　cephalexin, 556t
　cephazolin, 556t
Cephalosporins, fourth-generation, cefepime, 558t
Cephalosporins, second-generation, 556t–557t
　cefaclor, 556t
　cefmetazole, 557t
　cefotetan, 556t
　cefoxitin, 556t
　cefprozil, 556t
　cefuroxime, 556t
　cefuroxime axetil, 556t
　loracarbef, 557t
Cephalosporins, third-generation, 553, 554, 555, 557t
　cefdinir, 557t
　cefditoren pivoxil, 557t
　cefixime, 557t
　cefoperazone, 557t
　cefotaxime, 557t
　cefpodoxime proxetil, 557t
　ceftazidime, 553, 557t
　ceftibuten, 557t
　ceftizoxime, 557t
　ceftriaxone, 554, 555, 557t
Cephazolin, 556t
Certolizumab (pegol)
　Crohn's disease, 381
　immunotherapy, 376t, 381, 386t
　inflammatory bowel disease, 499t, 509t
　rheumatoid arthritis, 368t
Cetirizine, 347t, 348, 348b, 351–352, 355t
　children, 351, 352
　motion sickness, 352
　pregnancy and lactation, 348, 348b, 351–352
Cetrorelix, 423t, 429t, 665t, 686t
Cetuximab, 662t, 667t, 669–672, 683t
Cevimeline, 95t, 112t
Channels, ion, 3. See also specific types
Chelators, heavy metal, 66t. See also specific agents
Chemical antagonism, 4b, 9, 48b
Chemotherapy, cancer. See Cancer chemotherapy and cytotoxics; specific drugs and drug classes
Children. See also specific drugs and disorders
　gray baby syndrome, 68
　infant oral drug bioavailability, 72, 74
　kernicterus, 68
　medication safety and FDA, 71b–72b
　morphine
　　infant dosing, 72, 74
　　metabolism, 68
Children, pharmacokinetics
　absorption, 67b
　distribution, 68b
　excretion, 69b
　metabolism, 70b

Chlamydia, cycloserine, 579t, 587t
Chloral hydrate, 177t, 193t
Chlorambucil, 629t
Chloramphenicol, 568t, 569f, 571, 576t, 692t
Chlordiazepoxide, 176t, 191t, 192t
Chloride channels, 86
2-Chloro-2'-fluoro-arabinosyladenine. See Clofarabine (2-chloro-2'-fluoro-arabinosyladenine)
2-Chlorodeoxyadenosine (2-CdA. See Cladribine
Chlorophyllin, 62
Chloroprocaine, 224t
Chloroquine
　dermatologic, 708t, 725t
　malaria chemotherapy, 521t, 522t, 523–524, 526, 529t
　P. falciparum resistance, 523–524, 523f
　toxicities, 524
Chloroquine/hydroxychloroquine, 521t, 522t, 523–524, 526, 529t
Chloroquine phosphate, 522t
Chlorothiazide, 269t, 284t
Chlorpheniramine, 346t, 354t
Chlorpromazine, 150t, 171t, 174t
Chlorpyrifos, 100t, 103t, 115t
Chlorthalidone, 269t, 284t
Cholesterol absorption inhibitors
　ezetimibe, 335t, 344t, 350
　ezetimibe/simvastatin, 344t, 350
Cholesterol level classification, 337t
Cholestyramine
　antidiarrheal, 498t, 508t
　on drug absorption, 342–343
Choline acetyl transferase (ChAT), 97f
Choline esters, 99t
Cholinergic antagonists, pulmonary muscarinic, 390t, 401–402, 403t. *See also specific drugs and drug classes*
　adverse effects, 395
　asthma, severe, 397
　COPD, 394–395
　ipratropium bromide, 390t, 402, 403t
　mechanisms of action, 390t
　tiotropium bromide, 390t, 401–402, 403t
Cholinergic crisis, 105
Cholinergic pharmacology, 95–116. *See also specific drugs and drug classes*
　acetylcholine, 95t, 97f, 99t, 112t
　acetylcholine receptors, 97f
　acetylcholinesterase, 97f
　acetylcholinesterase inhibitors, 100t
　aldicarb, 100t, 115t
　alkaloids, natural, 99t
　Amanita muscaria, 97, 100
　Amanita phalloides, 97
　ambenonium chloride, 97f, 100t, 104–105, 105f, 106f, 114t
　atracurium, 106t, 107t, 116t
　atropine, 96t, 101–102, 101t, 112t
　autonomic ganglionic blockade, 107t
　belladonna, 101–102
　benztropine mesylate, 96t, 114t
　bethanechol, 95t, 99t, 112t

carbachol, 95t, 99t, 112t
carbamate insecticides, 100t, 102
carbaryl, 100t, 115t
cevimeline, 95t, 112t
chlorpyrifos, 100t, 103t, 115t
choline acetyl transferase, 97f
choline esters, 99t
cholinergic crisis, 105
cisatracurium, 106t, 107t, 117t
cyclopentolate hydrochloride, 96t, 114t
dantrolene, 106t, 117t
darifenacin, 96t, 101t, 113t
diazinon, 100t, 103t, 115t
dicyclomine hydrochloride, 96t, 113t
donepezil, 100t, 115t
doxacurium, 106t, 107t, 117t
edrophonium, 100t, 104–105, 104f, 114t
fesoterodine, 96t, 101t, 113t
flavoxate, 96t
galantamine, 100t, 115t
glycopyrrolate, 96t, 113t
homatropine hydrobromide, 96t, 114t
ipratropium, 96t
jimson weed, 101–102, 101t
mecamylamine, 106t, 117t
mechanisms of action
　muscarinic agonists, 95t
　muscarinic antagonists, 96t
methacholine, 99t, 112t
methscopolamine bromide, 96t, 114t
mivacurium, 106t, 107t, 117t
muscarinic acetylcholine receptors, 98t–99t
muscarinic receptor antagonists, 99t, 100, 101b, 101t
muscarinic receptors, 97f
mushrooms, 97, 100
neostigmine bromide, 100t, 114t
neostigmine methylsulfate, 100t, 114t
neuroeffector junction, 97f
neuromuscular blocking agents
　classification, 107t
　mechanisms, 106t
nicotine gum or lozenge, 106t, 108, 108b, 117t
nicotine nasal spray or vapor inhaler, 106t, 108, 108b, 117t
nicotine transdermal patch, 106t, 108, 108b, 117t
nicotinic acetylcholine receptors, 98t
onabotulinum toxin A, 106t, 117t
organophosphates, 100t, 102, 102b, 103t, 104f
oxybutynin, 96t, 99t, 100, 101b, 101t, 113t
Panaeolus, 97
pancuronium, 97f, 105f, 106f, 106t, 107t, 116t
physostigmine salicylate, 100t, 102, 114t
pilocarpine, 95t, 99t, 112t
pilocarpine hydrochloride, 95t, 99t, 112t
pipecuronium, 97f, 105f, 106f, 106t, 107t, 116t
pralidoxime, 41t, 42t, 65t, 100t, 102, 116t
propoxur, 100t, 115t
Psilocybe, 97
psilocybin, 97

pyridostigmine bromide, 100t, 114t
rimabotulinum toxin B, 106t, 117t
rivastigmine, 100t, 115t
rocuronium, 97f, 105f, 106f, 106t, 107t, 117t
sarin, 100t, 103t, 115t
scopolamine, 96t, 112t
solifenacin, 96t, 101t, 113t
soman, 100t, 103t, 116t
succinylcholine, 97f, 105f, 107t, 108, 116t
summary table, 112t–117t
tabun, 100t, 103t, 116t
tiotropium, 96t, 113t
tolterodine, 96t, 101t, 113t
trihexyphenidyl hydrochloride, 96t, 114t
trimethaphan, 106t, 117t
tropicamide, 96t, 114t
trospium chloride, 96t, 101t, 113t
varenicline, 106t, 117t
vecuronium, 97f, 105f, 106f, 106t, 107t, 108, 116t
Cholinergic toxidrome, 53t
Cholinesterase inhibitor, 89
Cholinesterase reactivators, 41t, 42t, 65t, 102, 104f, 116t
Chondroitin sulfate, ophthalmic, 692t, 706t
Choriogonadotropin alfa, 423t, 427, 428, 430t
Chromium, 41t, 43t, 66t
Chronic myelogenous leukemia, Ph+, 664–669
  first-line treatment, 665–666
  molecular mechanism, 665–666
Chronic obstructive pulmonary disease (COPD), 394–395
  pathophysiology, 394
  treatments, 394–395 (See also Pulmonary drugs)
Chronic renal failure, diuresis, 282, 283
Chylomicrons, metabolic pathways, 335f
Ciclesonide, 460t. See also Corticosteroids
  pulmonary, 390t, 403t
Ciclopirox olamine, 598t
Cidofovir, 600t, 601t, 605, 619t, 693t
Cigarette addiction. See Smoking
Cilastatin, 554–555
Cilostazol, 295b
Cimetidine
  gastric acid disease, 491, 494, 495
  structure, 492f
  tolerance, 491, 494, 495
Cinacalcet, 481t, 486, 487, 488t
  hyperparathyroidism, 481t, 488t
  hypocalcemia, 481t, 488t
Cinchonism, 524
Ciprofibrate, 335t, 344t
Ciprofloxacin, 544, 544f, 545, 548t, 692t
Cisapride, 133t
  bowel disorders, 497t, 504, 506, 507t
  nausea and vomiting, 504, 506
  postmarketing surveillance, 47–48
Cisatracurium, 106t, 107t, 117t
Cisplatin, 628t, 653t
  mechanisms of action, 628b–629b, 628t, 630f, 633

mechanisms of resistance, 628t, 632b, 634–635
toxicities, 632b–633b, 632t, 633–634
uses, 629t, 632t, 653t
Citalopram, 130t, 146t, 150t, 174t
Citrovorum factor, 406t, 416, 417–418, 420t
Cladribine (2-chlorodeoxyadenosine, 2-CdA), 630f, 636t, 655t
  mechanisms of action, 630f, 636t, 641–642
  mechanisms of resistance, 636t
Clarithromycin, 568t, 570f, 571, 576t
  duodenal ulcer, 492, 494t
  peptic ulcer disease, 571
  toxicities, 571
Claudication, 295b
Claudication treatment, 295b
Clavulanic acid, 549t, 553, 558t
Cl⁻ channels, 86
Clearance (CL), 33b, 35, 35b–36b, 36f, 39
  elderly, 75b, 76f, 76t–77t, 77f
  first-order kinetics, 36b
  infants and children, 69b
  plasma concentration-time curves, 36b, 37f
Clemastine fumarate, 346t, 353t
Clevidipine
  antihypertensive, 277t, 287t
  myocardial ischemia, 290t, 300t
Clindamycin, 568t, 574, 575, 576t
Clobetasol propionate, 460t. See also Corticosteroids
Clocortolone propionate, 460t. See also Corticosteroids
Clofarabine (2-chloro-2′-fluoro-arabinosyl-adenine), 630f, 636t, 655t
  mechanisms of action, 630f, 636t, 641–642
  mechanisms of resistance, 636t
  uses, 637t
Clofazimine, 579t, 583, 587t
Clofibrate, 335t, 344t
Clomethiazole, 177t, 193t
Clomiphene, 442t, 452, 455–457, 458t
Clomipramine, 150t, 173t
Clonazepam, 176t, 191t, 192t
  amyotrophic lateral sclerosis, 249
  antiseizure, 225t, 237t
Clonidine
  antidiarrheal, 498t, 508t
  antihypertensive, 277t, 286t
  for opioid addiction, 261
  pharmacology, 119t, 124–125, 139t
Clopidogrel, 323t, 324, 325, 325t, 331–332, 332t
  bioactivation, 22, 28, 325t
  dosing, 22, 28
    patient-to-patient variability, 331–332
  drug interactions, 28
  mechanisms of action, 323t, 330, 331
Clorazepate, 176t, 191t, 192t
  antiseizure, 225t, 237t
Clotrimazole, 588t, 597t
Clotting cascade, 325–326, 326f

Cloxacillin, 551, 552t, 554, 555, 555t
Clozapine, 130t, 147t, 151t, 167–169, 170t, 172, 175t
CO_2 absorbent, 220, 221
Cocaethylene, 265, 266
Cocaine
  addiction, 262–263
  drug-related deaths, 51t
  ethanol with, 265, 266
  local anesthetic, 224t
  toxidrome, 53t
  withdrawal, 263, 263t
Cockcroft-Gault equation, 76b
Codeine, 195t, 200t, 206, 208, 208t
  antitussive, 209t, 391t, 404t
Colchicine, 369t, 370, 373t
Cold medicines. See also specific drugs and ingredients
  alcohol with, 366
  OTC, young children, 350
Colesevelam, 471t, 479t
  on drug absorption, 343
Colestipol, on drug absorption, 342–343
Colitis, amebic, 532–533
  paromomycin, 531t, 532–533, 535t
Colitis, ulcerative
  azathioprine, 502–503, 503f, 506, 507
  sulfasalazine, 381, 502
  thiopurine methyltransferase, 502–503, 503f, 506, 507
Colony-stimulating factors, 663t, 685t. See also specific types
Combination therapy, antimicrobial, 517b, 518
Combined androgen blockade, 680
Competitive antagonists, 4b, 5b, 5f, 16, 17
  affinity, 7b
Competitive neuromuscular blocking agents, 97f, 105f, 106f, 106t, 107t, 116t–117t
Concentration–response (curve), 6b, 6f
  quantal, 11f, 12
Concentration–time curves, plasma, 36b, 37f
  dose administration schedule, 514, 515f
  elderly, 73f
Conduction abnormalities
  angina drugs, 293t
  arrhythmia drugs (See Antiarrhythmic drugs)
Congestive heart failure. See Heart failure
Conivaptan, 279t, 281, 288t
Conjugated equine estrogens, 441t, 445t
Conjugated estrogen + medroxyprogesterone acetate, 441t
Conjugation, phase 2, 28–29, 28b, 33f, 35, 39
  neonatal, 70b
Conjugation reactions, drug metabolism, 32t
Conjunctivitis, 700
  adrenocortical steroids in, 466
Constipation
  fluid volume, 499, 499f
  laxatives, 498b, 498t, 499, 499f, 507t–508t
  from morphine, 92

Context-sensitive half-time, anesthetic, 214, 214f
Contraceptives, oral, 448–450, 458t
 brand names and formulations, 443t–444t
 desogestrel, 443t
 drospirenone, 441t, 443t, 444t
 emergency, 452
 ethinyl estradiol formulations, 441t, 443t–444t, 457t
 levonorgestrel, 443t, 444t
 mechanisms of action, 441t, 441t–442t
 migraine history, 455, 456–457
 norethindrone, 441t, 443t, 444t
 norgestrel, 443t, 444t
 options, 448–450
 progesterone, 450
 progestin-only, 450, 458t
 risks and adverse effects, 450–451
 ulipristal, 442t, 444t, 452, 458t
Copper supplement, 406t, 419t
Corneal inflammation, 700
Coronary heart disease, risk factors, 335, 335b
Corticorelin, 459t, 461f, 468t
Corticosteroids, 468t. *See also specific agents*
 carbohydrate and protein metabolism, 467, 468
 Crohn's disease, 465
 dexamethasone suppression test, 465–466
 dose tapering, 465
 general principles, 464b
 mechanisms of action, 459t, 462f
 names and preparations, 460t–461t
 physiologic functions and pharmacologic effects, 462t–463t
 potencies and equivalent doses, 463t
 rheumatoid arthritis, 463–465
 therapeutic uses, 463b
 toxicities, 464b
Corticosteroids, inhaled pulmonary, 390t, 403t
 adverse effects, 393b, 397–398
 asthma, 393–397
 beclomethasone dipropionate, 390t, 403t
 bioavailability, 467, 468
 budesonide, 390t, 402, 403t, 460t
 candidiasis, oral, 467, 468
 ciclesonide, 390t, 403t, 460t
 COPD, 395
 flunisolide, 390t, 403t, 460t
 fluticasone, 390t, 403t
 mechanisms of action, 390t, 392f, 393f
 mometasone, 390t, 403t, 461t
 triamcinolone, 390t, 403t, 461t
Corticosteroids, systemic pulmonary, 390t, 403t
 hydrocortisone, 390t, 403t, 460t, 464, 464f
 mechanisms of action, 390t, 392f, 393f
 methylprednisolone, 390t, 403t, 460t–461t
 prednisolone, 390t, 403t, 461t
Corticotropin-releasing hormone (CRH), 459t, 461f, 468t
 corticorelin, 459t, 461f, 468t
 mechanisms of action, 459t, 461f
Cortisol, 11β-hydroxysteroid dehydrogenase on, 464f, 467, 468

Costimulatory blockade, 380b, 380f
Cosyntropin, 459t, 461f, 468t
Cough, 400
Cough medicines. *See* Antitussives
COX-1/2 inhibitors
 aspirin, 323t, 324–325, 332t
 COX-1 inhibitors or NSAIDs with, 365–366
 irreversible
  aspirin, 357t, 358f, 360t, 365–366, 371, 372
  mechanisms of action, 357t, 358f
COX-1 inhibitors
 mechanisms of action, 323t, 357t, 358f
 selective, 357t, 358f
 ulcers from, 492
COX-2 inhibitors
 mechanisms of action, 358f
 pain target and site of action, 205t
 selective
  cardiovascular hazard, 357, 365b, 371, 372
  celecoxib, 357t, 358f, 363t, 371, 372, 373t
  etoricoxib, 363t
  lumiracoxib, 363t
  menstrual cramping, 364
  parecoxib, 363t
  risks, 357
Creatine clearance, loading dose, 34
Crohn's disease agents, 381
 adalimumab, 381
 adrenocortical steroids, 465
 azathioprine, 503–504
 budesonide, 465
 certolizumab, 381
 infliximab, 381, 503
 prednisone, 465, 467, 468
 sulfasalazine, 381, 498t, 502, 503f, 505, 507, 509t
Cromolyn sodium, ophthalmic, 691t, 705t
Crotamiton, 708t, 725t
Cryptosporidia
 diarrhea, 532
 nitazoxanide, 530t, 532, 535t
Cupric sulfate, 406t, 419t
Cushing's syndrome, 466
Cutaneous T-cell lymphoma agents, 709t, 727t
Cyanoacrylate, ophthalmic, 692t, 706t
Cyanocobalamin, 406t, 414–415, 417–418, 420t
Cyclic nucleotide–gated nonspecific cation channel inhibitors, 269t
 carperitide, 269t, 284t
 nesiritide, 269t, 280, 284t
Cyclizine, 346t, 350, 352, 354t, 502t
Cyclooxygenase-1 (COX-1), 324, 324f, 325f, 358f
Cyclopentolate, ophthalmic, 690t, 695t, 705t
Cyclopentolate hydrochloride, 96t, 114t
Cyclophosphamide, 627t, 631f, 632t, 651t
 activation, in vivo, 631, 631f
 cancer chemotherapy, 626, 628–633
 metabolism, 631f

 toxicities, 631f, 632b–633b, 632t, 651t
 dermatologic, 708t, 724t, 726t
 mechanisms of action, 626, 627t, 628, 628b, 630f
 mechanisms of resistance, 627t, 632–633, 632b
 rheumatoid arthritis, 368t
 toxicities, 631–632, 631f, 632b–633b, 632t, 651t
 uses, 629t
Cycloserine
 Mycobacterium avium complex, 579t, 587t
 tuberculosis, 579t, 587t
Cyclosporine, 368t, 375t, 377f, 380, 382–383, 385t
 dermatologic, 708t, 724t, 726t
 inflammatory bowel disease, 499t, 509t
 mechanisms of action, 375t, 382–383
 ophthalmic, 691t, 705t
 rheumatoid arthritis, 368t, 376t, 385t
CYP (cytochrome P-450 superfamily), 29b, 29t, 30, 30b–31b, 33f
 antiseizure drug interactions, 227t
 drug–drug interactions, 30b
 genes, 30b
 genetic polymorphisms, 27t, 28, 31b
 imidazole and triazole interactions, 590, 590t
 induction, 31b
 reaction catalysis, 30b, 32t
 SSRIs on, 133
CYP2C9, 27t, 30b–31b, 595, 596
 azole antifungals on, 590, 590t
 polymorphisms, 10t, 12–14, 13f
CYP2C19, 27t, 30b–31b, 595, 596
 clopidogrel bioactivation, 22, 28, 325t, 331–332
 isoniazid on, 582, 585, 586
 isoniazid + phenytoin on, 585, 586
 prasugrel bioactivation, 325t
CYP2D6, 27t, 30b–31b
 fluoxetine, 157
 isoniazid on, 582, 585, 586
 paroxetine, 157
 SSRIs on, 133
CYP2E, isoniazid on, 582
CYP3A4, 27t, 30b–31b, 595, 596
 atazanavir metabolism by, 617
 azole antifungals on, 590, 590t
 isoniazid on, 582, 585, 586
 lopinavir metabolism, 618, 619
 macrolides, 572
 quinupristin/dalfopristin, 572, 575
 ritonavir on, 617–619
 St. John's wort on, 619
CYP3A5, 27t, 30b–31b
CYP3A7, 27t, 30b–31b
Cyproheptadine, 346t, 354t
Cyproterone, 665t, 687t
Cytarabine (cytosine arabinoside, Ara-C), 635t, 648, 649, 654t
 mechanisms of action, 630f, 635t
 mechanisms of resistance, 635t, 639b
 toxicities, 637t, 654t
 uses, 637t, 654t

Cytochrome P-450 superfamily. See CYP (cytochrome P-450 superfamily)
Cytokine–cell interactions, 408f
Cytokines, recombinant, 381t. See also *specific agents*
    aldesleukin, 381t
    interferon-α-2b, 381t
    interferon-β-1a, 381t, 382
    interferon-β-1b, 381t, 382
    interferon-γ-1b, 381t
Cytotoxic natural products, 630f, 642t–644t, 645–647
Cytotoxics
    cancer (See Cancer chemotherapy and cytotoxics; *specific drugs and drug classes*)
    natural products (See Natural products, cytotoxic)
Cytotoxics with diverse mechanisms of action, 644t–646t, 659t–660t
    adrenocortical suppressants, mitotane, 644t, 659t, 679t
    differentiating agents
        arsenic trioxide, 630f, 645t, 646t, 660t
        HDAC inhibitors, 645t, 660t
            romidepsin, 645t, 660t
            vorinostat, 645t, 646t, 660t
        retinoids, 645t, 646t, 659t
    substitutes urea, hydroxyurea, 630f, 645t, 646t, 659t

D
Dabigatran etexilate, 323t, 328, 333t
Dacarbazine (DTIC), 628t, 629t, 630f, 645–647, 652t
    mechanisms of action, 628b, 628t, 630f, 647
    mechanisms of resistance, 628t, 632–633, 632b
    toxicities, 632b–633b, 652t
    uses, 629t
Daclizumab, 376t, 386t
Dactinomycin, 630f, 643t, 658t
Dalteparin, 323t, 325, 333t
Dantrolene
    amyotrophic lateral sclerosis, 239t, 249, 253t
    pharmacology, 106t, 117t
Dapsone
    dermatologic, 709t, 724t, 726t
    leprosy, 579t, 581f, 583–586, 587t
Daptomycin, 569t, 570f, 573, 575, 577t
    dosing schedule, 515
    mechanisms of action, 569t, 573
Darbepoetin alfa, 405t, 406–409, 418t
Darifenacin, 96t, 101t, 113t
Darunavir, 601t, 603t, 608f, 609f, 622t
Dasatinib
    anticancer, 661t, 668, 683t
    mechanisms of resistance, 668
    pharmacodynamics, 15
Daunorubicin, 643t, 658t

    mechanisms of action, 630f, 643t, 645–647
    mechanisms of resistance, 645b
DDAVP, 279t, 288t
Deaths, drug-related, 51, 51t. See also *specific drugs*
Decitabine (2'-deoxy-5-azacytidine), 636t, 654t
    mechanisms and sites of action, 630f, 636t, 638f, 640
    mechanisms of resistance, 636t
    toxicities, 637t, 654t
    uses, 637t, 654t
Deferasirox, 41t, 65t
Deferoxamine, 40t, 42t, 55, 65t
Degarelix, 665t, 686t
Dihydroartemisinin, 520t, 529t
Delavirdine, 601t, 603t, 608f, 610f
    mechanisms of action and resistance, 603t, 608f, 610f
    structure, 610f
Delirium tremens, 256t
Δ-9-THC, 265, 266
Denileukin diftitox
    anticancer, 663t, 671t, 685t
    cutaneous T-cell lymphoma agents, 709t, 727t
Denosumab, 481t, 488t
2'-Deoxy-5-azacytidine. See Decitabine (2'-deoxy-5-azacytidine)
2'Deoxycoformycin, 636t, 637t, 641–642, 656t
Dependence, 264, 266. See also Addiction; Opioid addiction; *specific drugs*
    barbiturates, 181–182
    benzodiazepines, 180
    opioid, buprenorphine for, 203
Depolarizing neuromuscular blocking agents, 97f, 105f, 107t, 108, 116t
Depression
    drug-induced
        acute, 92
        hyperexcitability after, 89–90, 94
    drugs (See Antidepressants)
Depsipeptide, 645t, 660t
Dermal absorption. See Skin absorption
Dermal administration
    elderly, 74t
Dermatologic disorders
    eczema, 720, 722, 723
    impetigo, 714
    pruritus, 720, 720t
    psoriasis, 709t, 710f, 715–716
    pyoderma, 714
    tinea corporis, 719
    topical administration, 714–715
Dermatologic therapies, 707–727
    alkylating agents, 708t, 724t, 726f
        carmustine, 708t, 724t, 726t
        cyclophosphamide, 708t, 724t, 726t
        mechlorethamine, 708t, 724t, 726t
    androgenic alopecia, 710t, 726t
        finasteride, 710t, 726t
        minoxidil, 710t, 726t
    antimalarial agents, 708t, 725t
        chloroquine, 708t, 725t

        hydroxychloroquine, 708t, 725t
        quinacrine, 708t, 725t
    antimetabolites, 708t, 724t, 725t
        5-fluorouracil (FU), 708t, 724t, 725t
        azathioprine, 708t, 724t, 725t
        methotrexate, 708t, 715, 721–722, 724t, 725t
    antimicrobial agents, 708t, 725t
        antibacterials, 708t, 725t
        antifungals, 708t, 721, 722, 725t
        retapamulin, 708t, 725t
    biologic agents, 709t, 714t, 715–716, 726t
        adalimumab, 709t, 714t, 722, 723, 726t
        alefacept, 709t, 710f, 714t, 726t
        efalizumab, 709t, 710f, 714t, 726t
        etanercept, 709t, 714t, 726t
        infliximab, 709t, 714t, 726t
    calcineurin inhibitors, 708t, 724t, 726t
        cyclosporine, 708t, 724t, 726t
        pimecrolimus, 708t, 724t, 726t
        tacrolimus, 708t, 724t, 726t
    capsaicin, 710t, 727t
    cutaneous T-cell lymphoma agents, denileukin diftitox, 709t, 727t
    glucocorticoids, 707t, 722, 723, 724t
        adverse effects, 723, 724t
        potency, 723t
        triamcinolone acetonide, 707t, 723t, 724t
        triamcinolone hexacetonide, 707t, 723t, 724t
    H_1 blockers
        first-generation, 718t
        second-generation, 718t
    H_2 blockers, 718t
    hyperpigmentation, 710t, 727t
        azelaic, 710t, 727t
        hydroquinone, 710t, 727t
        mequinol, 710t, 727t
        monobenzone, 710t, 727t
    immunosuppressives and anti-inflammatories, other, 709t, 724t, 726t
        bleomycin, 709t, 724t, 726t
        dapsone, 709t, 724t, 726t
        doxorubicin, 709t, 726t
        imiquimod, 709t, 724t, 726t
        mycophenolate mofetil, 709t, 724t, 726t
        thalidomide, 709t, 724t, 726t
        vinblastine, 709t, 724t, 726t
    infestation agents, 708t, 725t
        benzyl alcohol, 708t, 725t
        crotamiton, 708t, 725t
        ivermectin, 708t, 725t
        lindane, 708t, 725t
        malathion, 708t, 725t
        permethrin, 708t, 725t
    percutaneous absorption, 710t, 711–715, 711t, 713f (See also Skin absorption)
    photochemotherapeutic, 707t, 716t, 725t
        methoxsalen, 707t, 716t, 725t
        photopheresis, 716t
        PUVA, 716–717, 716t, 725t
        trioxsalen, 716t
    photodynamic therapy, 708t, 716t, 725t

Dermatologic therapies (Cont.)
    aminolevulinic acid, 708t, 725t
    methyl aminolevulinate, 708t, 725t
  podophyllin, 727t
  rate-limiting step, 721, 722
  retinoids, 707t, 717–718, 717b, 724t
    acitretin, 707t, 724t
    adapalene, 707t, 724t
    alitretinoin, 707t, 724t
    bexarotene, 707t, 724t
    isotretinoin, 707t, 721, 722, 724t
    pregnancy warning, 721, 722, 724t
    tazarotene, 707t, 724t
    tretinoin, 707t, 724t
  sunscreens, 710t, 719b, 726t
  vitamin analogs, calcipotriene, 707t, 724t
Desflurane, 210t, 215t, 220, 221, 223t
Desiccated thyroid, 431t, 439t
Desipramine, 150t, 173t
Desirudin, 333t
Desloratadine, 347t, 355t
Deslorelin, 664t
Desmopressin (DDAVP), 279t, 288t
Desonide, 460t. *See also* Corticosteroids
Desvenlafaxine, 130t, 147t, 150t, 174t
Detoxification. *See* Addiction; *specific drugs*
Dexamethasone, 460t. *See also* Corticosteroids
  anticancer, 664t, 686t
  ophthalmic, 691t, 705t
Dexamethasone suppression test, 465–466
Dexlansoprazole, 490t, 496t
Dexmedetomidine
  anesthetic adjunct, 211t, 223t
  pharmacology, 119t, 139t
Dexmethylphenidate, 120t, 141t
Dexpanthenol, 498t, 507t
Dextromethorphan, 209t, 210t, 391t, 404t
Diabetes mellitus
  antihypertensives, 273–274
  diagnostic criteria, 473, 473t
  drugs promoting, 477t
  glucocorticoids, 467, 468
  hypertension with, 273–274
  type 1, 473–474 (*See also* Insulin)
  type 2, 473t, 474–476, 475f (*See also* Antidiabetic agents, oral)
Diabetes mellitus pharmacotheapy, 470–479
  antidiabetic drugs (*See* Antidiabetic agents, oral)
  comprehensive care, 473, 473f
  drug development, 6–9
  hemoglobin A_{1c}, 473, 474t, 475–476
  insulin, 470–474
  therapeutic goals, 473, 474t
Dialysis disequilibrium syndrome, 283t
Diarrhea
  causes, 499b
  drugs, 498t, 508t (*See also* Antidiarrheal agents)
  Giardia intestinalis, 500–501
Diazepam, 176t, 191t, 192t
  context-sensitive half-time, 214f
  elderly, 71
Diazinon, 100t, 103t, 115t

Diazoxide
  hypertension and edema, 278t, 287t
  hypoglycemia, 471t, 472f, 476, 479t
Dibucaine, 224t
Diclofenac, 357t, 362t, 371, 372, 373t
  ophthalmic, 691t, 705t
Dicloxacillin, 551t, 552t, 554, 555, 555t
Dicyclomine (hydrochloride)
  bowel antispasmodic, 498t, 508t
  pharmacology, 96t, 113t
Didanosine, 601t, 603t, 607f, 608f, 621t
  mechanisms of action and resistance, 603t, 607f, 608f
  structure, 607f
Difenoxin, 209t
Difenoxin + atropine, 498t, 508t
Differentiating agents
  arsenic trioxide, 630f, 645t, 646t, 660t
  HDAC inhibitors, 645t, 660t
    romidepsin, 645t, 660t
    vorinostat, 645t, 646t, 660t
  retinoids, 645t, 646t, 659t
Diffusion. *See also* Blood-brain barrier (BBB); Blood-CSF barrier
  facilitated, 19b, 19f
  ionized molecules, 19b, 19f
  lipid membrane, 19–20, 20f
  nonionized molecules, 19–20, 19b–20b, 19f, 20f, 35, 37–38
  passive, 19b, 19f
Diflorasone diacetate, 460t. *See also* Corticosteroids
Diflunisal, 357t, 360t, 373t
2′,2′-Difluorodeoxyuridine. *See* Gemcitabine
Difluprednate
  ophthalmic, 691t, 705t
Digoxin
  antiarrhythmic, 312t, 317t, 319, 320, 322t
  atrial fibrillation, 319, 320
  electrophysiologic actions, 317t
  heart failure, 301t, 306, 307, 308t, 311t
  maintenance dose, steady state, 30–31, 34
  pharmacokinetics, 30–34
  pharmacology, 308t
  therapeutic index, 31, 306
  toxicity, 306, 309, 310
  volume of distribution, 30
Dihydrotachysterol, 481b
Dihydrotestosterone, 449f
Diisopropyl fluorophosphate (DFP), 103t, 104f
Diltiazem
  antiarrhythmic, 312t, 315, 317t, 322t
  antihypertensive, 277t, 278, 287t
  electrophysiologic actions, 317t
  myocardial ischemia, 290t, 300t
Dimenhydrinate, 352
Dimercaprol, 41t, 42t, 66t
Dimercaptosuccinic acid (DMSA), 41t, 66t
Dimethoxymethamphetamine (DOM), 266
Dipeptidyl peptidase-4 (DPP-4) inhibitors, 471t, 472f, 476, 479t
  Alogliptin, 471t, 472f, 479t
  mechanisms of action, 471t, 472f
  saxagliptin, 471t, 472f, 479t

  sitagliptin, 471t, 472f, 479t
  vildagliptan, 471t, 472f, 479t
Dimenhydrinate, 346t, 353t
Diphenhydramine, 19–22, 40t, 42t, 65t
  adverse effects, 89–90, 347
  for allergic reaction, food, 349–350
  antidote use, 42t, 65t
  antihistamine, 3–6
  elderly, 69
  H_1 receptor antagonist, 3–6, 346t, 347–350
  lipid membrane diffusion, 19–20, 20f
  mechanisms of action, 346t, 347
  motion sickness, 350
  pharmacodynamics, 3–6
  pharmacokinetics, 19–22
  pregnancy, 352
  toxidrome, 53t
Diphenoxylate, 209t
Diphenoxylate + atropine, 498t, 500, 508t
Diphyllobothrium latum, 537–540
Dipivefrin, ophthalmic, 690t, 695t, 704t
Direct factor Xa inhibitors, 323t, 333t
  apixaban, 323t, 328, 331, 333t
  mechanisms of action, 323t
  rivaroxaban, 323t, 328, 333t
Direct renin inhibitors, 270t, 273t, 286t
  aliskiren, 273t, 282, 283, 286t
  mechanisms of action, 273t
  structure, 275f
Direct renin inhibitors/vasodilators, 270t
Direct thrombin inhibitors, 323t, 333t
  argatroban, 323t, 330, 331, 333t
  bivalirudin, 323t, 333t
  dabigatran etexilate, 323t, 328, 333t
  desirudin, 333t
  mechanisms of action, 323t
Disease models, 7
Disease-modifying anti-rheumatic drugs (DMARDs), 368b, 368t, 379–380
  biologicals
    abatacept, 368t
    adalimumab, 368t
    anakinra, 368t
    certolizumab, 368t
    golimumab, 368t
    infliximab, 368t, 376t, 380, 386t
    rituximab, 368t
  rheumatoid arthritis, 368b, 368t, 379–380
  small molecules
    azathioprine, 368t, 375t, 380, 385t
    cyclophosphamide, 368t
    cyclosporine, 368t, 376t, 380, 385t
    hydroxychloroquine, 368t
    leflunomide, 368t
    methotrexate, 368b, 368t, 380
    minocycline, 368t
    sulfasalazine, 368t
Disease progression timeline, antimicrobial therapy, 516, 516f
Disopyramide
  antiarrhythmic, 312t, 317t, 321t
  electrophysiologic actions, 317t
Dispositional antagonism, 48b
Dissociation rate (k_{-1}), 6b

Distribution, 20f, 21b. *See also specific drugs and drugs classes*
   children, 68b
   CNS, 24b
   definition, 21b
   elderly, 74b, 75t
   phases, 21b
   poisoning, 52
   rate, 20f, 36b–37b, 37f
   tissue, 21b
   transmembrane, weak electrolytes, 19–20, 19b–20b, 19f, 20f, 35, 37–38
Disulfiram, 177t, 178f, 186–187, 186t, 193t, 257
Diuretics, 268t–269t, 269–272, 270t, 283t–285t. *See also specific types*
   atrial natriuretic peptide, 269t
      carperitide, 269t, 284t
      nesiritide, 269t, 280, 284t
   carbonic anhydrase inhibitors, 268t, 271t, 272f, 283t
      acetazolamide, 268t, 283t
      brinzolamide, 283t
      dichlorphenamide, 268t
      dorzolamide, 283t
      methazolamide, 268t
   classification, 270t, 272f
   excretory and renal hemodynamic effects, 271t
   heart failure, 284t–285t, 301t, 304, 311t
   ibuprofen on, 282, 283
   K$^+$-sparing, mineralocorticoid antagonists, 269t, 271t, 272f, 285t
      eplerenone, 269t, 280–281, 285t
      spironolactone, 269t, 285t, 307
   K$^+$-sparing, Na+-channel inhibitors, 269t, 271t, 272f, 284t
      amiloride, 269t, 284t
      triamterene, 269t, 282, 283, 284t
   loop, 269t, 271t, 272f, 284t
      bumetanide, 269t, 282, 283, 284t
      ethacrynic acid, 269t, 284t
      furosemide, 269t, 280, 284t, 306
      torsemide, 269t, 284t
   mechanisms and sites of action, 268t–269t, 270b–271b, 270t, 271t, 272f
   nephrons, 270b
   NSAIDs and resistance, 274b
   osmotic, 268t, 271t, 283t
      glycerin, 268t, 283t
      isosorbide, 268t, 283t
      mannitol, 268t, 283t
      urea, 268t, 283t
   renin release pathways, 272f
   resistance, 274b
   therapy, 274b
   thiazide/thiazide-like, 269t, 271, 271t, 272f, 284t
      bendroflumethiazide, 269t, 284t
      chlorothiazide, 269t, 284t
      chlorthalidone, 269t, 284t
      hydrochlorothiazide, 269t, 271, 273–274, 282, 283, 284t
      hydroflumethiazide, 269t, 284t
      indapamide, 269t, 284t
      methyclothiazide, 269t, 284t
      metolazone, 269t, 284t
      polythiazide, 269t, 284t
      quinethazone, 269t, 284t
      trichlormethiazide, 269t, 284t
   treatment algorithm, 275f, 276f
DMSA, 41t, 66t
DNA
   drug binding, 2b
   repair mechanisms, 629b
DNase (dornase alfa), mucolytic, 390t, 404t
DNA virus replicative cycles, 604f
Dobutamine, 125t, 142t
   heart failure, 302t, 307–308, 308t, 311t
   mechanisms of action, 307–308
Docetaxel, 642t, 648–650, 656t
   mechanisms of action, 630f, 642t, 648–650
   mechanisms of resistance, 642t, 644b
   toxicities, 656t
   uses, 644t, 656t
Docosanol, 600t
Docusate sodium, 498t, 508t
Dofetilide
   antiarrhythmic, 312t, 317t, 322t
   electrophysiologic actions, 317t
Dolasetron, 130t, 147t
DOM, 266
Domperidone, 497t, 507t
Donepezil
   Alzheimer's disease, 239t, 246, 247t, 250–252, 253t
   pharmacology, 100t, 115t
Dopamine (DA), 118t, 139t
   derivatives, 118t, 139t
   heart failure, 302t, 307–308, 308t, 311t
   Parkinson's disease, 240–241, 241f
   postsynaptic effect, 136–137, 138–139, 138f
   storage and release, 122f
   synthesis, 122f, 239, 240f
Dopamine (DA) agonists, endocrine, 422t, 428t
   bromocriptine, 422t, 426, 428t
   cabergoline, 422t, 426, 428t
   prolactin-secreting pituitary adenoma, 426
   quinagolide, 422t, 426, 428t
Dopamine (DA) receptors, 122f
Dopaminergic pharmacology
   apomorphine, 130t, 148t
   aripiprazole, 130t, 148t, 162–163, 165
   bromocriptine, 130t, 148t
   cabergoline, 130t, 148t
   dopamine, 118t, 139t
   dopamine derivatives, 118t, 139t
   dopaminergic receptor agonists, 130t, 148t, 422t, 426, 428t
   dopaminergic receptor antagonists, 130t, 148t
   dopexamine, 118t, 139t
   fenoldopam, 118t, 139t
   mechanisms of action, 130t
   pergolide, 130t, 148t
   pramipexole, 130t, 148t
   ropinirole, 130t, 148t
   rotigotine, 130t, 148t
   serotonin, norepinephrine, and dopamine reuptake inhibitors, 147t
   serotonin synthesis and inactivation, 131f
   sibutramine, 147t
Dopaminergic (DA) receptor agonists, 130t, 148t
Dopaminergic (DA) receptor antagonists, 130t, 148t
Dopaminergic terminal, 138–139, 138f
Dopexamine, 118t, 139t
Doripenem, 558t
Dornase alfa, mucolytic, 390t, 404t
Dorzolamide, ophthalmic, 691t, 705t
Dose. *See also specific drugs and drug classes*
   effective *vs.* lethal, 44f
Dose-dependent reactions, 46t
Dose-response curves (relationship), 4f–7f, 6b, 6f, 8–9, 44f, 45
   graded *vs.* quantal, 45
   toxicity, 44f, 45
Dosing interval, 31, 38b–39b
Dosing rate, 31, 35b, 38, 38b, 38f, 39
Dosing schedule. *See also specific agents*
   on concentration-time profile, 514, 515f
   resistance suppression, 515
Doxacurium, 106t, 107t, 117t
Doxapram, 391t, 404t
Doxazosin
   antihypertensive, 277t, 286t
   pharmacology, 119t, 140t
Doxepin, 150t, 173t, 346t, 353t
Doxercalciferol, 481b
Doxorubicin, 643t, 645–647, 658t
   dermatologic, 709t, 726t
   mechanisms of action, 630f, 643t, 645–647
   mechanisms of resistance, 645b
Doxycycline, 568t, 569f, 571, 574, 575, 576t
   malaria chemoprophylaxis, 522t
   mechanisms of action, 568t, 571
   MRSA infections, 571
DPP-4. *See* Dipeptidyl peptidase-4 (DPP-4) inhibitors
Dronabinol
   for anorexia, 266
   antidiarrheal, 498t, 502, 502t, 508t
   for nausea and vomiting, 502, 502t
   chemotherapy-related, 265, 266
Dronedarone
   antiarrhythmic, 312t, 317t, 321t
   electrophysiologic actions, 317t
Droperidol, 151t, 175t
Drospirenone, 441t, 443t, 444t, 446t
Drotrecogin alfa, 323t, 333t
Drugability, 7
Drug addiction. *See* Addiction, drug; Opioid pharmacology; *specific drugs*
Drug approval process, FDA, 44f, 45t, 46–48, 46t
Drug development, 6–9
Drug–drug interactions, 48. *See also specific drugs and drug classes*
   on absorption, 48t
      acetaminophen, 48

Drug–drug interactions (*Cont.*)
  additive, 48b
  antiarrhythmics, 319, 320
  classification and description, 48b, 48t
  CYP, 30b
  on drug metabolism, 48, 48b, 48t
Drug interactions, 47f. *See also specific drugs and drug classes*
Drug overdose, 63, 64
Drug penetration, 512–513, 512b
Drug receptor, 2b, 3t. *See also* Receptor, drug; *specific drugs and receptors*
Drug-receptor complex (*LR*), 6b
Drug-receptor complex conformational change (*LR**), 6b
Drug–receptor interactions, 3b–5b, 4f, 6b
Drug-related deaths, agents, 51t
Drug target, 2b
Drug testing, new drug, 44f, 45, 45t
DTIC. *See* Dacarbazine (DTIC)
Duloxetine, 130t, 147t, 150t, 174t
Duodenal ulcers
  proton pump inhibitor + clarithromycin + metronidazole or amoxicillin, 492, 494t, 495, 571
  proton pump inhibitors, 492, 493, 494t, 495
Duration of action, 36f
Dutasteride, 442t, 458t
Dyclonine, 224t
Dyslipidemia
  classification, 337t
  high-risk, 335b, 337t
  LDL-C treatment guidelines, 336t
Dyslipidemia drugs, 334–344
  bile acid–binding resins, 334t, 339, 340, 343t
    cholestyramine, 334t, 342–343, 343t
    colesevelam, 334t, 340, 343t
    colestipol, 334t, 342–343, 343t
    mechanisms of action, 334t
  cholesterol absorption inhibitor
    ezetimibe, 335t, 344t, 350
    ezetimibe/simvastatin, 344t, 350
  fibric acid, 335t, 339, 344t
    bezafibrate, 335t, 344t
    ciprofibrate, 335t, 344t
    clofibrate, 335t, 344t
    fenofibrate, 335t, 341, 342, 344t
    gemfibrozil, 335t, 344t
  HMG-CoA reductase inhibitors, 334t, 343t
    adverse effects, 338
    atorvastatin, 334t, 343t
    choice, 342, 343
    fluvastatin sodium, 334t, 343t
    lovastatin, 334t, 341, 342, 343t
    mechanisms of action, 334t, 337
    other drugs with, 339
    pitavastatin calcium, 334t, 343t
    pravastatin calcium, 334t, 343t
    pregnancy risks, 340
    rosuvastatin calcium, 334t, 338, 343t
    simvastatin, 334t, 343t
  LDL-C treatment guidelines, 336t
  mechanisms of action, 334t–335t
  for metabolic syndrome, 339–340
  multiple-agent therapy, 339
  nicotinic acid, 335t, 343t
    mechanisms of action, 335t
    niacin, 335t, 340, 341, 342, 343t
  pregnancy risk, 340
  vytorin, 339, 340
Dystonia, acute, 172t

E
Ebastine, 347t, 355t
Echinocandins, 588t, 589f, 598t
  anidulafungin, 598t
  caspofungin, 588t, 589f, 593, 593f, 598t
  mechanisms of action, 588t, 593, 593f
  micafungin, 598t
Echothiophate, ophthalmic, 690t, 695t, 704t
Econazole, 588t, 597t
Eczema, 720, 722, 723
Edema drugs
  diuretics (*See* Diuretics)
  tolvaptan, 279t, 281, 288t
Edrophonium, 100t, 104–105, 104f, 114t
EDTA CaNa$_2$, 41t, 42t, 63, 64, 66t
Efalizumab
  dermatologic, 709t, 710f, 714t, 726t
  immunotherapy, 376t, 386t
  psoriasis, 709t, 710f
Efavirenz, 601t, 603t, 623t
  mechanisms of action and resistance, 603t, 608f, 610f
  structure, 610f
Effective concentration, half-maximal (EC$_{50}$), 6f, 7b, 9
Effective dose, 44f
  vs. lethal dose, 44f
  median (ED$_{50}$), 44f, 45
Effector organs, autonomic, 83t–84t
Effector tone
  parasympathetic, 107t
  sympathetic, 107t
Efferent nerves, autonomic nervous system, 82f
Efficacious, 7b
Efficacy
  full, 4b, 4f
  relative, 7b, 7f, 9
Efflux pumps, 515b, 517
  antimicrobial agent, 516b
  resistance, 515b, 517
Efflux transporters, 24b
  blood-brain and blood-CSF barriers, 24b, 28f
Eflornithine, 530t, 535t
EGFR (ErbB1), 667t
Elderly, 68–69, 72, 75
  benzodiazepines, 71, 77b
  diphenhydramine, 40t, 65t, 69
  drug response, 77b
  inappropriate medications, 69–70, 78b
  NSAIDs, 68–69, 72, 75
  optimizing drug regimens, 77b
  therapeutic window, 11f, 12, 12f
  tricyclic antidepressants, 72, 75
Elderly pharmacokinetics
  absorption and bioavailability, 73b, 73f, 73t–74t
  clearance, 75b, 76f, 76t–77t, 77f
  distribution and volume of distribution, 74b, 75t
  excretion, 76b, 78t
  first-pass clearance, 73t–74t
  half-life, 77f
  metabolism, 73t–74t, 75b
  plasma concentration–time curves, 73f, 73t
Electrolytes, weak
  plasma–gastric juice partitioning, 19b–20b, 20f, 21–22
  transmembrane distribution, 19–20, 19b–20b, 19f, 20f, 35, 37–38
Eletriptan, 130t, 147t
11β-hydroxysteroid dehydrogenase, 464f, 467, 468
Elimination, 35b. *See also* Clearance; *specific drugs*
  first-order kinetics, 36b
  poisoning, 52
Elimination $t_{1/2}$, 34b, 37f, 39b
  elderly, 77f
Eltrombopag, 406t, 419t
Emedastine difumarate
  ophthalmic, 691t, 705t
Emesis. *See* Antinauseants and antiemetics
Emetic stimuli, 501, 501f
Empiric therapy. *See also specific drugs and disorders*
  antimicrobial, 516f, 518–519
Emtricitabine, 601t, 603t, 621t
  mechanisms of action and resistance, 603t, 607f, 608f
  structure, 607f
Enalapril, 273t, 274–276, 275f, 285t
Enalaprilat, 273t, 285t
Endocannabinoids, 358f
Endocarditis risk and prophylaxis, 515b, 516
Endocrine pancreas and pharmacotherapy, insulin
  secretion regulation, 470t, 472f
  signaling pathways, 470t, 471f
Endothelin-1 receptor antagonists, pulmonary, 391t, 404t
  adverse effects, 400
  ambrisentan, 391t, 398–400, 399f, 404t
  bosentan, 391t, 398–400, 399f, 404t
  mechanisms of action, 391t
  pulmonary artery hypertension, 398–400, 399f
Endotracheal intubation, neuromuscular blocking drugs, 216. *See also* Neuromuscular blocking agents
Enflurane, 210t, 215t, 223t
Enfuvirtide, 601t, 603t, 608f, 611f, 616, 623t
  adverse effects, 616
  HIV, 617–618
  mechanisms of action and resistance, 603t, 608f, 611f, 616
Enolic acid derivatives
  meloxicam, 357t, 363t, 373t
  nabumetone, 357t, 363t, 373t
  piroxicam, 357t, 363t, 373t
Enoxaparin, 323t, 325, 333t
Entacapone
  antiviral, 600t, 602t, 620t
  Parkinson's disease, 238t, 242t, 244f, 251, 252t

747

Enteric nervous system, 82–83
Entecavir
    antihepatitis, 600t, 602t, 620t
    HIV + chronic HBV, 618, 619
Enterobius infection, 536, 539, 540
Entry inhibitors, 601t, 603t, 608f, 611f, 616, 623t
    enfuvirtide, 601t, 603t, 608f, 611f, 616, 623t
    maraviroc, 601t, 603t, 608f, 611f, 623t
    mechanisms of action and resistance, 603t
Environmental toxicity. *See* Toxicity, clinical and environmental
Enzymes. *See also specific types*
    biotransforming, 29b, 29t
    intracellular, 3t
    transmembrane, 3t
    xenobiotic metabolizing, 29b, 29t
Epidermal growth factor receptor (EGFR), in epithelial cancers, 669
Epidermal growth factor receptor (EGFR) targeting agents, 669–671
    adverse effects, 671
    cetuximab, 662t, 669–672, 683t
    classes, 669
    epithelial cancers treated, 670–671
    erlotinib, 661t, 670–672, 683t
    gefitinib, 661t, 670–672, 683t
    mechanisms of resistance, 672
Epidermis, 713f
Epilepsy
    drug choice, 227b
    early diagnosis and treatment, 228
    general principles, 227b
    pharmacotherapy (*See* Antiseizure drugs)
    seizure classification, 228, 229t
    treatment principles, 227b, 228
Epinastine, ophthalmic, 691t, 705t
Epinephrine (E)
    adverse effects, 217
    for allergic reactions, 349–350
    anaphylaxis, 56
    end artery tissues, gangrene, 220, 221–222
    in local anesthetics, 217
    metabolism, 121f
    pharmacology, 118t, 139t
    synthesis, storage, and release, 122f
Epinephrine (E) receptors, 122f
Epipodophyllotoxins, 643t, 657t
    etoposide, 630f, 643t, 645b, 657t
    mechanisms of action, 630f, 643t
    mechanisms of resistance, 643t, 645b
    teniposide, 630f, 643t, 645b, 657t
    toxicities, 657t
    uses, 644t, 657t
Epirubicin, 643t, 658t
    mechanisms of action, 630f, 643t, 645–647
    mechanisms of resistance, 645b
Epithelial cancers, EGFR overexpression/activation, 669–672
Eplerenone, 269t, 280–281, 285t, 302t, 311t
Epoetin alfa, 405t, 406–409, 418t

Epoprostenol
    adverse effects, 400
    pulmonary, 391t, 398–400, 399f, 404t
Epothilones, 643t, 644b, 650, 657t
Eptifibatide, 323t, 324–325, 332t
Equilibration, 20f, 36b–37b, 37f
Equilibrative transport, membrane transporters, 23b
Equilibrium association constant (K_A), 6b, 8
Equilibrium dissociation constant (K_D), 6b, 8, 16, 17
ErbB2-targeted agents, 672–673
ER⁺ breast cancer, 676–679
Ergocalciferol, 481t, 488t
Ergot alkaloids and derivatives, 120t, 141t, 147t
Erlotinib, 661t, 670–672, 683t
Ertapenem, 558t
Erythromycin, 568t, 570f, 576t
    bowel disorders, 497t, 507t
Erythropoietin (EPO), 407t, 408f
Escherichia coli, cycloserine, 579t, 587t
Escitalopram, 130t, 146t
Esmolol
    antiarrhythmic, 312t, 321t
    pharmacology, 126t, 128t, 146t
Esomeprazole, 490t, 495, 496t
Estazolam, 176t, 191t, 192t
Estradiol cypionate, 441t, 457t
Estradiol + drospirenone, 441t, 444t, 457t
Estradiol micronized, 441t, 457t
Estradiol nonmicronized, 441t, 457t
Estradiol + norethindrone, 441t, 443t, 444t, 446t, 457t
Estradiol, testosterone effects, 449f
Estradiol transdermal/topical gel, 441t, 445t, 457t
Estradiol vaginal ring/vaginal tablets, 441t, 445t, 457t
Estradiol valerate, 441t, 457t
Estramustine, 630f, 643t, 650, 657t
Estrogen antagonists, 442t, 458t
    clomiphene, 442t, 452, 455–457, 458t
    fulvestrant, 442t, 458t
    mechanisms of action, 442t
Estrogen esterified esters, 441t
Estrogen receptor, 448f
Estrogens, 441t, 457t
    anticancer, 664t, 665t, 679t, 686t, 687t
    biosynthetic pathways, 446f
    conjugated equine estrogens, 441t, 445t
    conjugated estrogen + medroxyprogesterone acetate, 441t
    drospirenone, 441t, 443t, 444t, 446t
    estradiol cypionate, 441t, 457t
    estradiol + drospirenone, 441t, 444t, 457t
    estradiol micronized, 441t, 457t
    estradiol nonmicronized, 441t, 457t
    estradiol + norethindrone, 441t, 443t, 444t, 446t, 457t
    estradiol transdermal/topical gel, 441t, 445t, 457t
    estradiol vaginal ring/vaginal tablets, 441t, 445t, 457t
    estradiol valerate, 441t, 457t
    estrogen esterified esters, 441t

    estropipate, 441t, 445t
    ethinyl estradiol, 441t, 457t
    gonadotropin secretion, 447f
    hormone replacement therapy, 441t–442t, 445t–446t, 446–448, 455–457, 458t
    levonorgestrel, 443t, 444t, 446t
    mechanisms of action, 441t–442t
    oral contraceptives, 441t–444t, 448–450 (*See also* Contraceptives, oral)
    selective estrogen receptor modulators, 442t, 458t
        raloxifene, 442t, 458t
        tamoxifen, 442t, 451, 456, 457, 458t, 667f
        toremifene, 442t, 458t
    synthetic conjugated estrogens, 441t
Estrogen synthesis inhibitors, 442t, 458t
    anastrozole, 442t, 458t, 664t, 678
    exemestane, 442t, 458t
    formestane, 442t, 458t
    letrozole, 442t, 458t
Estropipate, 441t, 445t
Eszopiclone, 177t, 192t
Etanercept
    dermatologic, 709t, 714t, 726t
    immunotherapy, 376t, 380, 386t
Ethacrynic acid, 269t, 284t
Ethambutol
    Mycobacterium avium complex, 578t, 583, 587t
    tuberculosis, 578t, 583, 587t
Ethanol. *See also* Alcoholism
    abstention, 183
    with acetaminophen, 366
    alcohol dehydrogenase 2*2, 178f, 189, 190
    antidote, 42t, 50, 65t
    cocaine with, 265, 266
    coronary heart disease protection, 182–183
    drug-related deaths, 51t
    fetal alcohol syndrome, 182b, 187
    metabolism, 49f, 178f
    metronidazole with, 533, 534
    neurochemical system impacts, 185t
    physiological system effects, 183, 183t–185t, 189, 190
    poisoning, 41t, 49f, 65t
    teratogenic effects, 182b, 187
    toxicity, 41t, 65t
Ethinyl estradiol, 441t, 457t
Ethionamide, 579t, 587t
Ethosuximide, 225t, 230–231, 234, 235, 236t
Ethylene glycol antidote
    ethanol, 65t
    fomepizole, 42t, 65t, 178f
Ethyleneimines and methylmelanines, 627t, 651t
    altretamine, 627t, 651t
    mechanisms of action, 627t, 628b–629b, 630f
    mechanisms of resistance, 627t, 632–633, 632b
    thiotepa, 627t, 632t, 651t
    toxicities, 632b–633b, 632t, 651t

Etidronate sodium, 481t, 488t
Etodolac, 357t, 361t, 373t
Etomidate, 459t, 469t
　anesthetic, 210t, 213t, 214f, 222t
　context-sensitive half-time, 214f
　parenteral anesthetic, 210t, 213t, 222t
　sedative-hypnotic, 177t, 193t
Etoposide (VP-16-213), 643t, 657t
　mechanisms of action, 630f, 643t
　mechanisms of resistance, 643t, 645b
　toxicities, 657t
　uses, 644t, 657t
Etoricoxib, 363t
Etravirine, 601t, 603t, 608f, 610f, 623t
　mechanisms of action and resistance, 603t, 608f, 610f
　structure, 610f
Everolimus
　anticancer, 663t, 685t
　immunotherapy, 375t, 385t
Excitatory postsynaptic potential (EPSP), autonomic, 106f
Excretion, 20f
　children, 69b
　elderly, 76b, 78t
　pH, 20b
　weak acid, 36, 39
Exemestane
　anticancer, 664t, 677t, 679t, 686t
　estrogen synthesis inhibitor, 442t, 458t
Exenatide, 471t, 472f, 479t
Exercise-induced angina, 290t, 291f
Exertional angina, 290t, 291f
Expectorants, 390t, 404t
Eye
　anatomy, 699f
　autonomic innervation, 694f
Eythropoiesis-stimulating agents (ESAs), 405t, 418t
　darbepoetin alfa, 405t, 406–409, 418t
　epoetin alfa, 405t, 406–409, 418t
　indications, 406–409
　iron deficiency from, 409
　mechanisms of action, 405t
　toxicities and hazards, 409

F

Facilitated diffusion, 19b, 19f
Facilitated transport, 23b
Factor Xa inhibitors, direct, 323t, 333t
　apixaban, 323t, 328, 331, 333t
　mechanisms of action, 323t
　rivaroxaban, 323t, 328, 333t
Famciclovir, 605, 608
Famotidine
　gastric acid disease, 490t, 496t
　structure, 492f
FDA
　children, 71b–72b
　drug approval process, 44f, 45t, 46–48, 46t
　pregnancy and breastfeeding, 72b
FDA Safety and Innovation Act of 2012, 72b
Febuxostat, 369t, 370, 374t
Felbamate, 226, 237t

Felodipine
　antihypertensive, 277t, 287t
　myocardial ischemia, 290t, 300t
Fenamates
　flufenamic acid, 362t, 373t
　meclofenamate, 357t, 362t, 373t
　mefenamic acid, 357t, 362t, 373t
Fenofibrate, 335t, 341, 342, 344t
Fenoldopam
　hypertension and edema, 278t, 287t
　pharmacology, 118t, 139t
Fenoterol, 125t, 143t
Fentanyl
　heroin with, 260
　pharmacology, 194t, 195t, 203, 205–207, 208t
Ferrous aspartate, 406t, 413–414, 419t
Ferrous fumarate, 406t, 413–414, 419t
Ferrous gluconate, 406t, 413–414, 419t
Ferrous salts, 406t, 413–414, 419t
Ferrous succinate, 406t, 413–414, 419t
Ferrous sulfate, 406t, 413–414, 419t
Fertility agents, 442t, 452, 455–457, 458t
Ferumoxytol, 406t, 419t
Fesoterodine, 96t, 101t, 113t
Fetal alcohol syndrome, 182b
Fexofenadine, 347t, 355t
Fibric acid (fibrates), 335t, 339, 344t
　bezafibrate, 335t, 344t
　ciprofibrate, 335t, 344t
　clofibrate, 335t, 344t
　fenofibrate, 335t, 341, 342, 344t
　gemfibrozil, 335t, 344t
Fibrin clot formation, 325–326, 326f
Fibrinolysis, 329, 329f
Fibrinolytics, tPA, 323t, 333t
　alteplase, 323t, 329–330, 329f, 333t
　mechanisms of action, 323t
　reteplase, 323t, 333t
　tenecteplase, 323t, 333t
Fibrogen gel, ophthalmic, 692t, 706t
Filgrastim. See G-CSF (filgrastim)
Finasteride, 442t, 456, 457, 458t
　androgenic alopecia, 710t, 726t
First-pass effect, 20b, 35, 36–37
　elderly, 73t–74t
　nitroglycerin and nitrates, 22, 291, 299
Fish tapeworm, 537–540
5-ASA, 498t, 503f, 509t
5-Fluorouracil (5-FU), 635t, 640–641, 654t. See also 5-Fluorouracil
5-LOX inhibitors, 390t, 403t
5α-reductase inhibitors, 442t, 458t
　dutasteride, 442t, 458t
　finasteride, 442t, 456, 457, 458t
FK506-binding protein-12 (FKBP-12), 383, 384
Flavoxate, 96t
Flecainide
　antiarrhythmic, 312t, 317t, 321t
　electrophysiologic actions, 317t
Floxuridine (FUdR, fluorodeoxyuridine), 635t, 640–641, 654t
　mechanisms and sites of action, 630f, 635t, 638f, 640

　mechanisms of resistance, 638b–639b, 640–641
　toxicities, 637t, 641, 654t
　uses, 637t, 654t
FLT-3 ligand (FL), 407t, 408f
Fluconazole, 588t, 589f, 590, 597t
　adverse effects, 719
　formulations and actions, 597t
　mechanisms of action and resistance, 588t, 590
　tinea corporis, 719
　warfarin interaction, 595, 596
Flucytosine, 588t, 589f, 595, 596, 596t
Fludarabine phosphate, 630f, 636t, 655t
　mechanisms of action, 630f, 636t, 641–642
　mechanisms of resistance, 636t, 638b–640b
　toxicities, 642
　uses, 637t
Fludrocortisone acetate, 460t
Flumazenil, 41t, 42t, 65t, 177t, 179–180, 192t
Flu medicines. See also specific agents and ingredients
　alcohol with, 366
Flunisolide, 460t. See also Corticosteroids
　pulmonary, 390t, 403t
Fluocinolone, ophthalmic, 691t, 705t
Fluocinolone acetonide, 460t
Fluocinonide, 460t
Fluorodeoxyuridine. See Floxuridine (FUdR, fluorodeoxyuridine)
Fluorometholone, 460t
Fluorometholone acetate, 460t
Fluorometolone, ophthalmic, 691t, 705t
5-Fluorouracil, 635t, 640–641, 654t
　activation pathways, 638f
　agents combined with, 648, 649
　dermatologic, 708t, 724t, 725t
　mechanisms and sites of action, 630f, 635t, 638f, 640
　mechanisms of resistance, 635t, 638b–639b, 640–641
　ophthalmic, 691t, 705t
　topical, precancerous skin lesions, 640–641
　toxicities, 637t, 641, 654t
　uses, 637t, 654t
Fluoxetine
　on CYP2D6, 157
　Huntington's disease, 248
　pharmacology, dopaminergic and serotonergic, 130t, 131–133, 131f, 133t, 146t
　psychopharmacology, 150t, 157, 174t
Fluphenazine, 150t, 174t
Flurandrenolide, 460t. See also Corticosteroids
Flurazepam, 176t, 180, 191t, 192t
Flurbiprofen, ophthalmic, 691t, 705t
Flutamide
　androgen receptor antagonist action, 442t, 454, 456, 457, 458t, 679t
　anticancer, targeted, 665t, 679t, 687t
　prostate cancer, 442t, 454, 456, 457, 679t
Fluticasone, 390t, 403t

749

Fluvastatin (sodium), 334t, 343t
Fluvoxamine, 130t, 146t, 150t, 174t
Folate deficiency, 412f, 413b, 414–415
    pregnancy, 416, 417
    trimethoprim-sulfamethoxazole, 543, 543f
Folate metabolism, 543f
Folic acid analogs (antifolates), 635t, 653t
Folic acid and derivatives, 406t, 412f, 415b, 420t
    absorption and distribution, 412f
    deficiency, 412f, 413b, 414–415
    folic acid, 406t, 412f, 414–417, 414b, 415b, 420t
    folinic acid, 406t, 416, 417–418, 420t
    general principles, 414b
    mechanisms of action, 406t
    vitamin B_{12} interactions, 410b, 412f
Folic acid deficiency, 412f, 413b, 414–415
    pregnancy, 416, 417
Folinic acid, 406t, 416, 417–418, 420t
Follicle-stimulating hormone (FSH), 423t, 429t
    follitropin α, 423t, 430t
    follitropin β, 423t, 430t
    menotropin, 423t, 429t
    urofollitropin, 423t, 429t
Follitropin α, 423t, 430t
Follitropin β, 423t, 430t
Fomepizole, 41t, 42t, 65t, 178f
Fomivirsen, 600t, 619t
    antiherpes, 600t, 602t, 609, 619t
    CMV retinitis, 609
    mechanisms of action and resistance, 602t
Fondaparinux, 323t, 325, 333t
Formestane, 442t, 458t
Formoterol
    pharmacology, 125t, 144t
    pulmonary, 390t, 402t
Forward rate (k_{+1}), 6b
Foscarnet, 600t, 609–612, 619t
    adverse effects, 612, 617, 618
    antiherpes, 600t, 602t, 604f, 605, 609–612, 617, 618, 619t
    CMV retinitis, 609–612
    herpes simplex virus, 605
    mechanisms of action and resistance, 602t, 604f, 610–612
Fosinopril, 273t, 285t
Fosphenytoin, 225t, 236t
Fospropofol, 210t, 222t
Fractional occupancy (f), 7b, 8
Frovatriptan, 130t, 147t
FUdR. See Floxuridine (FUdR, fluorodeoxyuridine)
Full agonists, 4b, 4f, 7b, 9
Full efficacy, 4b, 4f
Fulvestrant, 442t, 458t
    anticancer, 664t, 677t, 686t
    estrogen antagonist, 442t, 458t
Fumagillin, 530t, 535t
Functional antagonists, 4b
Functional iron deficiency, 409
Functionalization, phase 1, 28b, 33f, 35, 38

neonatal, 70b
Fungal infections. See also specific types
    agents (See Antifungal agents)
    aspergillosis, invasive, 595, 596
    candidiasis
        esophageal, 589f, 590t–592t, 594–596
        oral, 467, 468
        vaginal, 594
    coccidioidal meningitis, 590, 592t–593t, 595, 596
    cryptococcal meningitis, 595, 596
    eye, 701
    mucormycoses, 589–590
    onychomycosis, 595–596, 721, 722
    tinea, 593–594
Furosemide, 269t, 280, 284t, 304t

G

GABA
    on $GABA_A$ receptor, 226f
    metabolism, antiseizure drugs, 225t–226t, 226b, 226f
$GABA_A$ receptor
    anesthetics on, 219–221
    antiseizure drugs on, 225t, 225t–226t, 226f
    binding sites, 178f
    flumazenil, 179
    GABA on, 226f
    sedative-hypnotics on, 178f, 179
Gabapentin, 205t, 225t, 237t
Galantamine
    Alzheimer's disease, 239t, 246, 247t, 253t
    pharmacology, 100t, 115t
Ganciclovir, 600t, 619t
    antiherpes, 600t, 602t, 604f, 605, 605f, 609, 617, 618, 619t
    CMV retinitis, 609, 617, 618
    herpes simplex virus, 605
    mechanisms of action and resistance, 602t, 604f, 605f
Ganglionic blocking drugs, 106t, 117t
Ganglionic stimulating agents, nicotine, 106t, 108, 108b, 117t
Ganirelix, 423t, 429t, 665t, 687t
Gases, therapeutic, 211t, 223t–224t. See also specific agents
    carbon dioxide, 211t, 223t
    helium, 211t, 224t
    nitric oxide, 211t, 223t
    oxygen, 211t, 223t
Gastric acid disease drugs, 490–496
    antacids, 490t, 496t
    bismuth, 490t, 496t
    cytoprotective agents, sucralfate, 490t, 496t
    H_1 receptor antagonists, 490t, 491f, 496t
        cimetidine, 491, 492t, 494, 495
        famotidine, 490t, 492f, 496t
        mechanisms of action, 490t, 491f
        nizatidine, 490t, 492f, 496t
        ranitidine, 490t, 492f, 496t
        tolerance, 491, 494, 495

    prostaglandin analog, misoprostol, 490t, 493, 494, 495, 496t
    proton pump inhibitors, 490t, 491f, 492, 493f, 496t
        dexlansoprazole, 490t, 496t
        esomeprazole, 490t, 495, 496t
        gastroesophageal reflux disease, 492, 493f
        iron deficiency from, 495
        lansoprazole, 490t, 493f, 496t
        mechanisms of action, 490t, 491f, 495
        omeprazole, 490t, 493f, 496t
        pantoprazole, 490t, 493f, 496t
        rabeprazole, 490t, 493f, 496t
        structures, 493f
    for ulcers, 492, 493, 494t, 495
    vitamin B_{12} absorption, 492
Gastric emptying, neonates and infants, 67b
Gastric secretion, regulation, 491f
Gastroesophageal reflux disease (GERD), 400. See also Pulmonary drugs
    cimetidine, 491
    management guidelines, 493f
    pregnancy, 494, 495
    proton pump inhibitors, 492
    treatments, 400
G-CSF (filgrastim), 405t, 407t, 408f, 409–410, 416, 417, 418t
    indications, 409–410, 416, 417
    mechanisms of action, 405t, 407t
    sites of action, 408f
G-CSF, pegylated recombinant (pegfilgrastim), 405t, 407t, 408f, 409–410, 418t
Gefitinib, 661t, 670–672, 683t
Gemcitabine, 630f, 636t, 654t
    mechanisms and sites of action, 630f, 636t, 638f, 640
    mechanisms of resistance, 635t, 639b
    toxicities, 637t, 654t
    uses, 637t, 654t
Gemfibrozil, 335t, 344t
Gemtuzumab ozogamicin, 662t, 667t, 672t, 684t
Genetic polymorphisms
    CYP, 27t, 28, 31b
    drug response, 10t, 12–14, 13f
Genotoxic effects, 46t
Gentamicin, 559–566, 559b, 566t
Giardia intestinalis, 500–501
Giardiasis, 531–532
    diarrhea, 500–501
    metronidazole, 530t, 532–533, 535t
Glargine. See also Diabetes mellitus
    vs. lispro, 478
Glatiramer acetate, 382t
Glaucoma, 699–700, 699f
Gliclazide, 470t, 472f, 479t
Glimepiride, 470t, 472f, 477, 478, 479t
Glimepiride + metformin, 477, 478
Glipizide, 470t, 472f, 479t
GLP-1 agonists, 471t, 472f, 476, 479t
    exenatide, 471t, 472f, 479t
    liraglutide, 471t, 472f, 479t
    mechanisms of action, 471t, 472f
Glucocorticoid receptors, 462f

Glucocorticoids. *See also specific drugs and drug classes*
   anticancer, targeted, 664t, 679t, 686t
      dexamethasone, 664t, 686t
      prednisone, 664t, 679t, 686t
   carbohydrate and protein metabolism, 467, 468
   dependence, 505–506, 507
   dermatologic, 707t, 722, 723, 724t
      adverse effects, 723, 724t
         potency, 723t
         triamcinolone acetonide, 707t, 723t, 724t
         triamcinolone hexacetonide, 707t, 723t, 724t
   dexamethasone, 664t, 686t
   dose tapering, 465
   drug interactions and dosing, 464
   drugs against (*See* Antiglucocorticoids)
   general principles, 464b
   gout, 369t, 370
   immunotherapeutic, 375t, 384t
   ophthalmic, 691t, 705t
      dexamethasone, 691t, 705t
      difluprednate, 691t, 705t
      fluocinolone, 691t, 705t
      fluorometholone, 691t, 705t
      loteprednol, 691t, 705t
      prednisolone, 691t, 705t
      rimexolone, 691t, 705t
      triamcinolone, 691t, 705t
   osteoarthritis and diabetes type II, 467, 468
   prednisone, 664t, 679t, 686t
   rheumatoid arthritis, 463–465
   topical, 465
   toxicities, 464b
Glucose-6-phosphate (G6PD), 586
Glucose-6-phosphate (G6PD) deficiency
   dapsone with, 584, 585–586
   primaquine with, 527, 528
Glucuronidation, neonatal, 70b
Glucuronosyl transferase, infants, 68
Glyburide, 470t, 472f, 479t
Glycerin diuretic, 268t, 283t
Glycopeptides
   teicoplanin, 569t, 570f, 577t
   vancomycin, 569t, 570f, 572–575, 577t
Glycopyrrolate
   bowel antispasmodic, 498t, 508t
   pharmacology, 96t, 113t
GM, 405t, 407t, 408f, 409–410, 418t
GnRH. *See* Gonadotropin-releasing hormone (GnRH)
Goiter, 437, 438
Golimumab
   immunotherapy, 376t, 386t
   rheumatoid arthritis, 368t
Gonadotropin-releasing hormone (GnRH), 422t, 429t, 680
   anticancer, 664t, 680, 687t
Gonadotropin-releasing hormone (GnRH) agonists, 680
   anticancer, 664t, 679–680, 687t
      buserelin, 664t, 687t
      deslorelin, 664t
      GnRH, 664t, 680, 687t
      goserelin, 664t, 687t
      histrelin, 664t, 687t
      leuprolide, 664t, 679t, 680, 687t
      nafarelin, 664t, 687t
      triptorelin, 664t, 687t
   pharmacology and actions
      androgen secretion, 425
      GnRH, 422t, 429t, 680
      goserelin, 422t, 429t
      histrelin, 423t, 429t
      leuprolide, 423t, 425–426, 429t
      nafarelin, 422t, 427, 428, 429t
      triptorelin, 422t, 429t
Gonadotropin-releasing hormone (GnRH) antagonists, 423t, 429t
   anticancer, 665t, 687t
      abarelix, 665t, 687t
      cetrorelix, 665t, 687t
      degarelix, 665t, 687t
      ganirelix, 665t, 687t
   pharmacology and actions
      cetrorelix, 423t, 429t
      ganirelix, 423t, 429t
Gonadotropins
   for gynecomastia, 427, 428
   neuroendocrine control, 447f
   secretion, 447f
Goserelin
   anticancer, 664t, 687t
   pharmacology and actions, 422t, 429t
Gout, 369t, 370
Gout drugs, 368b, 369–370, 369t, 374
   glucocorticoids, 369t, 370
   microtubule disruptors, 369t
      colchicine, 369t, 370, 373t
   NSAIDs, 369t
   urate oxidase, recombinant, 369t
      rasburicase, 369t, 374t
   uricosuric agents, 369t, 370
      probenecid, 369t, 370, 374t
   xanthine oxidase inhibitors, 369t
      allopurinol, 369t, 370–372, 373t
      febuxostat, 369t, 370, 374t
GPIIb/IIIa antiplatelet agents, 323t, 324–325, 332t
   abciximab, 323t, 324–325, 331–332, 332t
   eptifibatide, 323t, 324–325, 332t
   mechanisms of action, 323t
   tirofiban, 323t, 324–325, 332t
G protein-coupled receptors (GPCRs), 3t, 4
Granisetron, 130t, 147t
Graves disease, 432t, 434t, 435–439
Gray baby syndrome, 68
Griseofulvin, 588t, 593–596, 598t, 721, 722
Growth factor signaling, 670f. *See also specific growth factors and agents*
Growth hormone (GH), 423, 424f
   antagonist drug, pegvisomant, 422t, 424, 425f, 428
   receptor antagonism, 423, 425f
   recombinant, 422t, 427, 428, 428t
   secretion and actions, 423, 424f
Guaifenesin, 390t, 404t

Guanabenz
   antihypertensive, 277t, 286t
   pharmacology, 119t, 140t
Guanadrel, 277t, 287t
Guanfacine
   antihypertensive, 277t, 286t
   pharmacology, 119t, 140t
Gynecomastia treatment
   gonadotropin, 427, 428
   testosterone, 456, 457

H

H_1 receptor antagonists
   adverse effects, 4–6, 347, 350
   gastric acid disease, 490t, 491f, 496t
      cimetidine, 491, 492f, 494, 495
      famotidine, 490t, 492f, 496t
      mechanisms of action, 490t, 491f
      nizatidine, 490t, 492f, 496t
      ranitidine, 490t, 492f, 496t
      tolerance, 491, 494, 495
   uses, 6
H_1 receptor antagonists, first generation, 19–22, 346t, 352–354t
   adverse effects, 89–90, 347
   brompheniramine maleate, 346t, 354t
   carbinoxamine, 346t, 353t
   chlorpheniramine, 346t, 354t
   clemastine fumarate, 346t, 353t
   cyclizine, 346t, 350, 352, 354t, 502t
   cyproheptadine, 346t, 354t
   dermatologic, 718t
   dimenhydrinate, 346t, 353t
   diphenhydramine, 3–6, 346t, 347–350
   doxepin, 346t, 353t
   drowsiness, 19–20
   elderly, 69
   hydroxyzine, 346t, 354t
   ionization and lipid membrane diffusion, 19–20, 20f
   mechanisms of action, 346t, 347
   meclizine, 346t, 350, 352, 354t
   motion sickness, 350, 352
   phenindamine, 346t, 354t
   pregnancy and lactation, 348
   promethazine, 346t, 350–352, 354t
   pyrilamine, 346t, 353t
   vs. second generation, 347b–348b
   tripelennamine, 346t, 353t
H_1 receptor antagonists, second generation, 347t, 355t
   acrivastine, 347t, 355t
   advantages, 348
   azelastine, 347t, 355t
   cetirizine, 347t, 348, 348b, 351–352, 355t
   dermatologic, 718t
   desloratadine, 347t, 355t
   ebastine, 347t, 355t
   fexofenadine, 347t, 355t
   vs. first generation, 347b–348b
   ketotifen fumarate, 347t, 355t
   levocabastine, 347t, 355t
   levocetirizine, 347t
   loratadine, 347t, 348, 348b, 351–352, 355t
   mechanisms of action, 347t

mizolastine, 347t, 355t
nonionization and brain concentrations, 20, 38
olopatadine, 347t, 355t
pregnancy and lactation, 348, 348b, 351–352
H_1 receptors, 4
H_2 receptor antagonists
  dermatologic, 718t
  elderly, 73b
  mechanisms of action, 347t, 491, 491f
  structure, 491, 492f
  tolerance, 491, 494, 495
H_2 receptors, 4
H_3 receptor antagonists, 347t
H_3 receptors, 4
H_4 receptor antagonists, 347t
H_4 receptors, 4
Haemophilus influenzae meningitis prophylaxis, rifamycins, 578t, 579f–580f, 581–586, 586t. *See also* Rifamycins
Halcinonide, 460t. *See also* Corticosteroids
Half-life ($t_{1/2}$), 34b, 37f, 39b
  elderly, 77f
Half-maximal effective concentration (EC_{50}), 6f, 7b, 9
Half-time, context-sensitive, anesthetic, 214, 214f
Haloperidol, 151t, 159, 163f, 171t, 175t
Halothane, 210t, 215t, 222t
Halprogin, 598t
HDAC inhibitors, 645t, 660t
  romidepsin, 645t, 660t
  vorinostat, 645t, 646t, 660t
HDL-C levels, 337t
HDL-C metabolism, 335f
Heart failure
  African-American, 306, 306b, 309, 310
  BiDil, 306, 306b
  Brater's algorithm, 270t, 273t, 276f, 285t
  characteristics and causes, 302b, 302f
  comorbidities, 302b
  hypertension and diabetes risk, 304–305
  ibuprofen risk, 304
  pulmonary congestion and peripheral edema, 305–306
  stages, 303, 303b, 305f
  symptoms, 302b
  verapamil on, 306
Heart failure drugs. *See also specific drugs and drug classes*
  aldosterone receptor antagonists, 311t
    eplerenone, 302t, 311t
    mechanisms of action, 302t
    spironolactone, 302t, 307, 311t
  for angina, 294t
  angiotensin-converting enzyme inhibitors, 272f, 276f, 279, 285t, 303–304, 310t (*See also* Angiotensin converting enzyme (ACE) inhibitors)
    mechanisms of action, 270t, 273t, 274–276, 275f, 301t
  angiotensin receptor blockers, 273t, 274, 279, 280, 285t, 301t, 310t (*See also* Angiotensin (AT_1) receptor blockers (ARBs))

β adrenergic receptor agonists, 311t
  dobutamine, 302t, 307–308, 308t, 311t
  dopamine, 302t, 307–308, 308t, 311t
  mechanisms of action, 302t
  mechanisms of action, heart, 307–308
β adrenergic receptor antagonists, 286t, 304, 310t (*See also* β adrenergic receptor antagonists)
  bisoprolol, 301t, 309, 310, 310t
  carvedilol, 301t, 309, 310, 310t
  mechanisms of action, 301t
  metoprolol, 301t, 303–304, 306, 310t
Brater's algorithm, 270t, 273t, 276f, 285t
diuretics, 284t–285t, 301t, 304, 311t (*See also* Diuretics)
eplerenone, 269t, 280–281, 285t
mechanisms of action, 301t–302t
Na^+-K^+-ATPase inhibitors, 303f, 311t
  digoxin, 301t, 306, 307, 311t
  mechanisms of action, 301t
natriuretic peptide receptor agonists
  mechanisms of action, 302t
  nesiritide, 302t, 311t
nesiritide, 269t, 280, 284t
phosphodiesterase 3 inhibitors, 307, 309, 310, 311t
  inamrinone, 302t, 308, 308t, 311t
  mechanisms of action, 302t, 308
  milrinone, 302t, 308, 308t, 311t
  pharmacology, 308t
rationale, 303b, 305f
sites of action, 302f, 303
tolvaptan, 279t, 281, 288t
vasodilators, 304t, 311t
  arterial, 278t, 287t (*See also* Vasodilators, arterial)
  mechanisms of action, 301t
Heavy metal chelators, 66t
Heavy metals, 41t, 43t, 65t–66t
Helicobacter pylori triple therapy, 492, 494t, 495
Helium gas, therapeutic, 211t, 224t
Helminth infection drugs, 536–541
  benzimidazoles, 540t
    albendazole, 536, 540t
    mebendazole, 536, 540t
  diethylcarbamazine, 538–540, 540t
  doxycycline, 540t
  ivermectin, 537–540, 540t
  metrifonate, trichlorfon, 541t
  niclosamide, 539, 540, 541t
  oxamniquine, 541t
  piperazine, 541t
  pork tapeworm, 539, 540
  praziquantel, 537, 539, 540, 540t
  pyrantel pamoate, 536, 539, 540, 541t
Helminth infections
  Brugia malayi, 538
  fish tapeworm, 537, 538–539
  incidence, 537f
  onchocerciasis, 537–540
  pinworm, 536, 539, 540
  schistosomiasis, 537, 539, 540, 540t
  Wuchereria bancrofti, 538

Hematopoietic agents, 405–420, 405t–406t, 419t
  copper supplement, 406t, 419t
  cupric sulfate, 406t, 419t
  cytokine–cell interactions, 408f
  erythropoiesis-stimulating agents, 405t, 418t
    darbepoetin alfa, 405t, 406–409, 418t
    epoetin alfa, 405t, 406–409, 418t
    indications, 406–409
    iron deficiency from, 409
    mechanisms of action, 405t
    toxicities and hazards, 409
  hematopoietic growth factors, 407t
    erythropoietin, 407t, 408f
    FLT-3 ligand, 407t, 408f
    interleukins, 407t, 408f
    mechanisms of action, 407t, 408f
    sites of action, 408f
    stem cell factor, 407t, 408f
  iron supplements, oral, 406t, 419t
    ferrous aspartate, 406t, 413–414, 419t
    ferrous fumarate, 406t, 413–414, 419t
    ferrous gluconate, 406t, 413–414, 419t
    ferrous salts, 406t, 413–414, 419t
    ferrous succinate, 406t, 413–414, 419t
    ferrous sulfate, 406t, 413–414, 419t
    infants and children, 413
    mechanisms of action, 405t
    optimizing effects, 413–414
    polysaccharide ferrihydrite complex, 406t, 413–414, 419t
    pregnancy, 413–414
  iron supplements, parenteral, 406t, 419t
    ferumoxytol, 406t, 419t
    iron dextran, 406t, 419t
    iron sucrose, 406t, 419t
    mechanisms of action, 406t
    sodium ferric gluconate, 406t, 419t
  myeloid growth factors, 405t, 407t, 418t
    G-CSF, 405t, 407t, 408f, 409–410, 416, 417, 418t
    G-CSF, pegylated recombinant, 405t, 407t, 408f, 409–410, 418t
    GM-CSF, 405t, 407t, 408f, 409–410, 418t
    indications and choice, 409–410
    mechanisms of action, 405t, 407t
    sites of action, 408f
  thrombopoietic growth factors, 405t, 406t, 407t, 419t
    eltrombopag, 406t, 419t
    IL-11 (oprelvekin), 406t, 410–411, 419t
    mechanisms of action, 405t, 407t, 408f
    romiplostim, 406t, 417, 418, 419t
  vitamins, B_{12}, 406t, 420t
    absorption and distribution, 412f
    cyanocobalamin, 406t, 420t
    deficiency, 411b, 412f, 413b, 414–415, 417–418
    folate interactions, 410b, 412f
    general principles, 411b–412b
    hydroxycobalamin, 406t, 420t
    mechanisms of action, 406t, 420t

Hematopoietic agents (Cont.)
vitamins, folic acid and derivatives, 406t, 412f, 415b, 420t
absorption and distribution, 412f
deficiency, 412f, 413b, 414–415
folic acid, 406t, 412f, 414–417, 414b, 415b, 420t
folinic acid, 406t, 416, 417–418, 420t
general principles, 414b
mechanisms of action, 406t
vitamin B_{12} interactions, 410b, 412f
vitamins, pyridoxine, 406t, 419t
mechanisms of action, 406t
pyridoxine, 406t, 419t
riboflavin, 406t, 419t
Hematopoietic growth factors, 407t. *See also* Hematopoietic agents; *specific types*
erythropoietin, 407t, 408f
FLT-3 ligand, 407t, 408f
interleukins, 407t, 408f
mechanisms of action, 407t, 408f
sites of action, 408f
stem cell factor, 407t, 408f
Heme biosynthesis, 58f
Hemoglobin A_{1c}, 473
for monitoring diabetes mellitus, 473, 474t, 475–476
Henderson-Hasselbalch equation, 19b
Heparin, 323t, 325, 327f, 333t
Heparin-induced thrombocytopenia (HIT), 325, 330, 331
Heparinoid anticoagulants, parenteral, 323t, 325, 333t
ardeparin, 323t, 325, 333t
dalteparin, 323t, 325, 333t
enoxaparin, 323t, 325, 333t
fondaparinux, 323t, 325, 333t
heparin, 323t, 325, 327f, 333t
lovenox, 325–326, 326f
low-molecular-weight heparins, 323t, 324–325, 325f, 333t
mechanisms of action, 323t
nadroparin, 323t, 325, 333t
tinzaparin, 323t, 325, 333t
Hepatic metabolism and clearance. *See also specific drugs and drug classes*
elderly, 75b, 76f, 76t–77t, 77f
Hepatic microsomal enzymes. *See also specific types*
antiseizure drug interactions, 227t
Hepatitis
agents (*See* Antihepatitis agents)
fulminant, 231
hepatitis B, 61
hepatitis C, chronic, 613–614
Her2/neu, 672–673
Heroin. *See also* Opioid pharmacology
fentanyl with, 260
vs. methadone responses, 260, 260f
overdose, 203–204
tolerance, 260
toxidrome, 53t
Heroin addiction, 259–262, 260f, 261t
addictability, 259–261
overdose, 260
tolerance, 260

treatment, 260–262
withdrawal, 260, 261t
Herpes simplex virus (HSV) infection agents (*See* Antiherpes agents)
eye, 701
Hexamethylendiamine, 627t, 651t
mechanisms of action, 627t, 628b–629b, 630f
mechanisms of resistance, 627t, 632–633, 632b
toxicities, 632b–633b, 651t
High-dose methotrexate with leucovorin rescue (HDM-L), 635t, 638–640, 653t
mechanisms and sites of action, 620f, 635t, 637f, 638
mechanisms of resistance, 638b, 640
pharmacogenetics, 635t, 637f, 638–640, 639
toxicities, 653t
uses, 637t
High (narrow) specificity, 5b, 9
Histamine
actions, 3
in allergic reactions, 349–350
CNS neurotransmitter, 4–5
structure, vs. H_2 receptor antagonists, 492f
triple response of Lewis, 347b, 348
Histamine receptor antagonists and mast cell stabilizers, 3. *See also* H_1 receptor antagonists; *specific types*
actions and adverse effects, 4–6
active ingredient, 3
allergy, 351–352
drug class, 3
ophthalmic, 691t, 705t
azelastine, 691t, 705t
bepotastine, 691t, 705t
cromolyn sodium, 691t, 705t
emedastine difumarate, 691t, 705t
epinastine, 691t, 705t
ketotifen fumarate, 691t, 705t
lodoxamide tromethamine, 691t, 705t
nedocromil, 691t, 705t
olopatadine, 691t, 705t
pemirolast, 691t, 705t
Histamine receptors, 3t, 4
Histrelin
anticancer, 664t, 687t
GnRH agonist pharmacology, 423t, 429t
HMG-CoA reductase, 337
HMG-CoA reductase inhibitors (statins), 334t, 343t
adverse effects, 338
atorvastatin, 334t, 343t
choice, 342, 343
fluvastatin sodium, 334t, 343t
lovastatin, 334t, 341, 342, 343t
mechanisms of action, 334t, 337
other drugs with, 339
pitavastatin calcium, 334t, 343t
pravastatin calcium, 334t, 343t
pregnancy risks, 340
rosuvastatin calcium, 334t, 338, 343t
simvastatin, 334t, 343t
Hodgkin's lymphoma, ABVD regimen, 630f, 643t, 645–647
Homatropine, ophthalmic, 690t, 695t, 704t

Homatropine hydrobromide, 96t, 114t
Hormesis, 6b
Hormone replacement therapy, 441t–442t, 445t–448t, 446–448, 455–457, 458t
brand names and formulations, 445t–446t
estrogen/progestin, 446t, 455, 457, 458t
ethinyl estradiol/progesterone formulations, 441t, 446t, 447, 457t
indications and effects, 456, 457
mechanisms of action, 441t–442t
risks, 447–448
Horner's syndrome, 698t
Human chorionic gonadotropin (hCG), 423t, 427, 428, 430t
choriogonadotropin alfa, 423t, 427, 428, 430t
Human immunodeficiency virus (HIV), 614–619. *See also* Antiviral agents; *specific drugs and drug classes*
atazanavir-ritonavir, 617–619
combination therapy, 518, 519, 617, 618
drug resistance, 614
enfuvirtide, 617–618
lopinavir, 618, 619
replicative cycle, 608f
treatment principles, 614
treatment recommendations, 614
zidovudine-lamivudine-abacavir, 604f, 608f, 614–615
Human solute carrier (SLC) superfamily transporters, 23b–24b, 25t–26t
Huntington's disease, 248–249, 248f
tetrabenazine for, 239t, 249, 253t
Hyaluronate, ophthalmic, 692t, 706t
Hydantoins, antiseizure, 225t, 236t
fosphenytoin, 225t, 236t
phenytoin, 225t, 231, 234, 235, 236t
Hydralazine, 278t, 287t
Hydrochlorothiazide, 269t, 271, 273–274, 282, 283, 284t
Hydrocodone, 195t, 200t, 208t
structure and activity of, 464f
tolerance, 264, 265
Hydrocortisone, 460t, 464, 464f. *See also* Corticosteroids
adrenal insufficiency, 461f, 465
drug interactions and dosing, 464
general principles, 464b
mechanisms of action, 460t
physiologic functions and pharmacologic effects, 462t–463t
pulmonary, 390t, 403t
toxicities, 464b
trade names and preparations, 460t
Hydroflumethiazide, 269t, 284t
Hydrolysis reactions, drug metabolism, 32t
Hydromorphone, 194t, 195t, 200t, 208t
Hydroquinone, for hyperpigmentation, 710t, 727t
Hydroxychloroquine
dermatologic, 708t, 725t
malaria chemotherapy, 521t, 522t, 523–524, 526, 529t
rheumatoid arthritis, 368t

753

Hydroxychloroquine sulfate, 522t
1α-Hydroxycholecalciferol, 481t, 488t
Hydroxycobalamin, 406t, 414–415, 417–418, 420t
Hydroxyethyl cellulose, ophthalmic, 692t, 706t
Hydroxyprogesterone caproate, 679t
Hydroxyprophyl methylcellulose, ophthalmic, 692t, 706t
Hydroxypropyl cellulose, ophthalmic, 692t, 706t
Hydroxypropyl methylcellulose, ophthalmic, 692t, 706t
11β-Hydroxysteroid dehydrogenase, 464f, 467, 468
Hydroxyurea (HU), 630f, 645t, 646t, 659t
Hydroxyzine, 346t, 354t
Hyoscyamine, 498t, 508t
Hypercalcemia, 483–484
    bisphosphonates, 483
        pamidronate, 481t, 488t
        zoledronate, 481t, 485, 488t
    calcitonin, 480t, 481t, 483–484, 483f, 488t
    lung cancer, 483–484, 486, 487
    vitamin D and analogs for, 481t, 488t
Hypercortisolism, 465–466
Hyperglycemia. See also Antidiabetic agents; Diabetes mellitus
    drugs promoting, 477t
Hyperparathyroidism agents, 481t, 488t
Hyperphosphatemia agents
    lanthanum, 481t, 488t
    sevelamer, 481t, 488t
Hyperpigmentation agents, 710t, 727t
    azelaic, 710t, 727t
    hydroquinone, 710t, 727t
    mequinol, 710t, 727t
    monobenzone, 710t, 727t
Hypersensitivity reactions. See also specific drugs
    immediate, 349–350
    penicillins, 550f, 552, 554, 555
Hypertension
    criteria, 270t
    diabetes with, 273–274
    drugs (See Antihypertensive drugs)
    licorice, 467, 468
    pregnancy, 277–278, 278f
    progression, 269–270, 270t
Hyperthyroidism, 432t, 434t, 435–439
Hypertrophic cardiomyopathy, angina drugs, 294t
Hyperuricemia, 370
Hypnotics and sedative-hypnotics, 176–193, 191t–193t. See also specific types
    adverse effects, 179
    barbiturates, 177t, 180–182, 181t, 192t (See also Barbiturates)
    benzodiazepine receptor agonists, novel, 177t, 192t

        eszopiclone, 177t, 192t
        zaleplon, 177t, 192t
        zolpidem, 177t, 178–179, 192t
    benzodiazepine receptor antagonists, flumazenil, 41t, 42t, 65t, 177t, 179–180, 192t
    benzodiazepines, 176t, 178b, 180, 189–190, 191t–192t (See also Benzodiazepines)
    carisoprodol, 177t, 193t
    chloral hydrate, 177t, 193t
    clomethiazole, 177t, 193t
    etomidate, 177t, 193t
    $GABA_A$ receptor, 178f, 179
    insomnia categories, 178b, 179
    long-term use, 179
    melatonin congeners, ramelteon, 177t, 189, 190, 192t
    meprobamate, 177t, 193t
    paraldehyde, 177t, 193t
    propofol, 177t, 193t
    toxidrome, 53t
Hypocalcemia, cinacalcet, 481t, 488t
Hypochlorhydria, age-related, 73b
Hypoglycemia
    drugs promoting, 477t
    recurring, 476
Hypoglycemia agents, 471t, 479t
    diazoxide, 471t, 472f, 476, 479t
    glucagon, 471t
    mechanisms of action, 471t
Hypogonadism, 456, 457
Hypothalamic-pituitary axis, 422–430, 461f. See also specific hormones and regulators
    organs, hormones, and targets, 426f
Hypothalamic-pituitary axis agents, 422–430
    dopamine agonists, 422t, 428t
        bromocriptine, 422t, 426, 428t
        cabergoline, 422t, 426, 428t
        prolactin-secreting pituitary adenoma, 426
        quinagolide, 422t, 426, 428t
    follicle-stimulating hormone, 423t, 429t
        follitropin α, 423t, 430t
        follitropin β, 423t, 430t
        menotropin, 423t, 429t
        urofollitropin, 423t, 429t
    gonadotropin-releasing hormone agonists on androgen secretion, 425
        GnRH, 422t, 429t, 680
        goserelin, 422t, 429t
        histrelin, 423t, 429t
        leuprolide, 423t, 425–426, 429t
        nafarelin, 422t, 427, 428, 429t
        triptorelin, 422t, 429t
    gonadotropin-releasing hormone antagonists, 423t, 429t
        cetrorelix, 423t, 429t
        ganirelix, 423t, 429t
    growth hormone antagonist, pegvisomant, 422t, 424, 425f, 428t
    growth hormone, recombinant, 422t, 427, 428t

    human chorionic gonadotropin, 423t, 427, 428, 430t
        choriogonadotropin alfa, 423t, 427, 428, 430t
    insulin-like growth factor-1, mecasermin, 422t, 428t
    luteinizing hormone, lutropin alfa, 423t, 430t
    organs, hormones, and targets, 426f
    posterior pituitary hormones, 423t, 429t
        arginine vasopressin, 423t, 424f, 429t (See also Vasopressin)
        oxytocin, 423t, 424f, 430t
    prolactin-secreting pituitary adenoma, 426
    somatostatin analogs, 422t, 428t
        lanreotide, 422t, 428t
        octreotide, 422t, 428t
Hypothyroidism, 431t, 432–434, 432t, 433f, 434t
    diagnosis, 432, 432t, 433f
    iodine-induced, 432, 434t, 435t, 438, 439
    levothyroxine for, 431t, 432–434, 433f, 434t, 437–439, 439t
    subclinical, 437–439

I

^{131}I, 431t, 435, 437–439, 440t
Ibandronate, 481t, 485, 488t
    for osteoporosis, 481t, 485, 488t (See also Bisphosphonates)
Ibuprofen
    on antihypertensive drugs, 282, 283
    heart failure risk, 304
    menstrual cramping, 364
    pain target and site of action, 205t
Ibutilide
    antiarrhythmic, 312t, 317t, 322t
    electrophysiologic actions, 317t
Icatibant, 347t, 355t
Idarubicin, 643t, 658t
    mechanisms of action, 630f, 643t, 645–647
    mechanisms of resistance, 645b
Idiosyncratic reactions, 46t
IDL-C metabolism, 335f
Idoxuridine, 600t, 602t, 605–606, 619t
Ifosfamide, 627t, 632t, 651t
    activation, in vivo, 631, 631f
    mechanisms of action, 626, 627t, 628, 628b, 630f
    mechanisms of resistance, 627t, 632–633, 632b
    toxicities, 631–632, 632b–633b, 632t, 651t
    uses, 629t
IgE antibodies, in anaphylaxis, 56
IL-1, 407t, 408f
IL-1 inhibitors, 376t, 386t. See also under Biological immunosuppressants
    anakinra, 376t, 386t
    canakinumab, 376t, 386t
    rilonacept, 376t, 386t
IL-2, 407t, 408f
IL-3, 407t, 408f
IL-4, 407t, 408f

IL-5, 407t
IL-6, 407t, 408f
IL-7, 407t
IL-8, 407t
IL-9, 407t
IL-10, 407t
IL-11
  mechanisms of action, 407t, 408f
  therapeutic, 406t, 410–411, 419t
IL-12, 407t
Iloperidone, 151t, 170t, 175t
Iloprost, 391t, 404t
Imatinib (mesylate), 661t, 666–669
  adverse effects, 669
  anticancer, targeted, 661t, 666–669, 681, 682, 683t
  cancers, 669
  chronic myelogenous leukemia, Ph+, 661t, 666–668
  mechanisms of resistance, 666–668, 681, 682
  pharmacodynamics, 14–15
Imidazoles and triazoles, 588t, 589f, 590, 597t
  CYP interactions, 590, 590t
  drug interactions, 590t–592t
  fluconazole, 588t, 590, 595, 596, 597t, 719
  itraconazole, 597t
  posaconazole, 597t
  voriconazole, 588t, 589f, 590t–592t, 592–593, 595, 596, 597t
Imidazoles and triazoles, topical, 588t, 597t–598t
  butoconazole, 597t
  clotrimazole, 597t
  econazole, 597t
  ketoconazole, 598t
  miconazole, 594, 597t
  oxiconazole, 598t
  sertaconazole, 598t
  sulconazole, 598t
  terconazole, 597t
  tioconazole, 597t
Iminostilbenes, antiseizure, 225t, 236t
  carbamazepine, 225t, 226f, 232–235, 236t
  oxcarbazepine, 225t, 236t
Imipenem, 558t
Imipenem-cilastatin, 554–555
Imipramine, 150t, 173t
Imiquimod
  antiviral, 601t, 602t, 621t
  dermatologic, 709t, 724t, 726t
Immediate hypersensitivity reactions, 349–350
Immune globulin preparations, 376t, 377f, 377t–378t, 378, 385t
  agents, synonyms, and origins, 377t–378t
  mechanisms of action, 376t
  toxicities, 385t
  uses, 377b, 385t
Immune response, 376b. *See also* Hypersensitivity reactions; *specific types*
Immune (idiopathic) thrombocytopenic purpura (ITP), 406t, 417, 418, 419t

Immunity
  adaptive, 376b
  innate, 376b
Immunization, passive, 377t–378t, 381t
Immunomodulators, 381t–382t. *See also specific drugs and drug classes*
Immunostimulants, 381t
  anthracenedione derivative, mitoxantrone, 382t
  Bacillus Calmette-Guerin, 381t
  monoclonal antibody, natalizumab, 382t
  passive immunization, 377t–378t, 381t
  recombinant cytokines, 381t
    aldesleukin, 381t
    interferon-α-2b, 381t
    interferon-β-1a, 381t, 382
    interferon-β-1b, 381t, 382
    interferon-γ-1b, 381t
  thalidomide and analogs
    lenalidomide, 381t
    thalidomide, 381t
  universal APLs, glatiramer acetate, 382t
Immunosuppressants and anti-inflammatories, dermatologic, 709t, 724t, 726t
  bleomycin, 709t, 724t, 726t
  dapsone, 709t, 724t, 726t
  doxorubicin, 709t, 726t
  imiquimod, 709t, 724t, 726t
  mycophenolate mofetil, 709t, 724t, 726t
  thalidomide, 709t, 724t, 726t
  vinblastine, 709t, 724t, 726t
Immunosuppressants, ocular, 691t, 705t
  5-fluorouracil (FU), 691t, 705t
  cyclosporine A, 691t, 705t
  mitomycin, 691t, 705t
Immunotherapeutic agents, 375–388
  antiproliferative/antimetabolic, 375t, 385t
    azathioprine, 368t, 375t, 380, 385t
    everolimus, 375t, 385t
    MPA, 375t, 385t
    mycophenolate mofetil, 375t, 383, 384, 385t
    sirolimus, 375t, 377f, 383, 384, 385t
  biological immunosuppressants
    adverse effects, 378b
    anti-TNF reagents, 376t, 386t
      adalimumab, 368t, 376t, 381, 383, 384, 386t
      certolizumab pegol, 376t, 381, 386t
      etanercept, 376t, 380, 386t
      golimumab, 376t, 386t
      infliximab, 368t, 376t, 380, 381, 386t
    IL-1 inhibitors, 376t, 386t
      anakinra, 376t, 386t
      canakinumab, 376t, 386t
      rilonacept, 376t, 386t
    LFA-1 & LFA-3 inhibitors
      alefacept, 376t, 386t
      efalizumab, 376t, 386t
    monoclonal antibody, anti-CD3, muromonab-CD3, 376t, 378, 385t
    monoclonal antibody, anti-CD25, 376t, 379, 386t
      basiliximab, 376t, 386t
      daclizumab, 376t, 386t

    monoclonal antibody, anti-CD52, alemtuzumab, 376t, 378, 386t
    polyclonal antibodies, immune globulin preparations, 376t, 377f, 377t–378t, 378, 385t
    risks, 379
  calcineurin inhibitors, 375t, 385t
    cyclosporine, 368t, 375t, 377f, 380, 382–383, 385t
    mechanisms of action, 375t, 377f
    tacrolimus, 375t, 377f, 383, 385t
  Crohn's disease, 381
  glucocorticoids, 375t, 384t
  immunological tolerance and costimulatory blockade, 380b, 380f
  immunosuppressants and anti-inflammatories, dermatologic, 709t, 724t, 726t (*See also* Immunosuppressants and anti-inflammatories, dermatologic)
  mechanisms of action, 375t–376t
  organ transplant, 378–379
  rheumatoid arthritis, severe, 380–381
Impetigo, 714
Implantable cardioverter-defibrillator (ICD)
  ventricular fibrillation, 316
  ventricular tachycardia, 318
Inactive conformation, 4, 5f
Inamrinone, 302t, 308, 308t, 311t
Indacaterol, 390t, 402t
Indapamide, 269t, 284t
Indinavir, 601t, 603t, 608f, 609f, 621t
Indomethacin, 357t, 361t, 373t
Indoramin, 120t, 141t
Inducing agents, anesthesia, 212f, 213–214, 213f, 213t. *See also* Anesthetic agents, parenteral
Induction speed, anesthesia, 215–216, 215t, 216f
Infants. *See* Children
Infestation agents, dermatologic, 708t, 725t
  benzyl alcohol, 708t, 725t
  crotamiton, 708t, 725t
  ivermectin, 708t, 725t
  lindane, 708t, 725t
  malathion, 708t, 725t
  permethrin, 708t, 725t
Inflammatory bowel disease agents, 498t–499t, 509t
  adalimumab, 499t, 509t
  azathioprine, 498t, 502–503, 503f, 509t
  balsalazide, 498t, 503f, 509t
  budesonide, 498t, 509t
  certolizumab pegol, 499t, 509t
  cyclosporine, 499t, 509t
  infliximab, 499t, 509t
  mechanisms of action, 498t–499t
  mesalamine, 498t, 503f, 509t
  methotrexate, 499t, 509t
  natalizumab, 499t, 509t
  olsalazine, 498t, 503f, 506, 507, 509t
  sulfasalazine, 381, 498t, 502, 503f, 505, 507, 509t

Inflammatory response, 357b
Infliximab
　Crohn's disease, 381, 503
　dermatologic, 709t, 714t, 726t
　immunotherapy, 368t, 376t, 380, 381, 386t
　inflammatory bowel disease, 499t, 509t
　rheumatoid arthritis, 368t, 376t, 380, 386t
Influenza agents. See Anti-influenza agents
Inhaled administration. See also specific drugs and drug classes
　elderly, 74t
Inhalers, combination, 395, 397, 398, 401–402
Inhibitory concentration (IC), 513–514, 514f
Inhibitory postsynaptic potential (IPSP), 86, 86f, 106f
Inhibitory sigmoid E_{max} curve, 513, 513f, 514, 514f
Innate immunity, 376b
Inotropic agents. See also Digoxin; Dobutamine; Dopamine (DA); Phosphodiesterase 5 (PDE5) inhibitors
　mechanisms of action, 307–308
　pharmacology, 30–34, 308t
INR, 328, 330b
Insecticides. See also specific types
　aldicarb, 100t, 115t
　anticholinesterase, 102, 102b, 103f, 103t, 104f
　　antidotes, 40t, 41t, 42t, 65t, 100t, 102
　carbamate, 100t, 102, 115t
　　treatment, 42t, 65t
　carbaryl, 100t, 115t
　diazinon, 100t, 103t, 115t
　malathion, 100t, 102, 115t
　organophosphate, 100t, 102, 102b, 103f, 103t, 104f, 115t
　propoxur, 100t, 115t
Insomnia
　categories, 178b, 179
　zolpidem, 177t, 178–179, 192t
Insulin
　glargine, 476
　　vs. lispro, 478
　hospitalized, 477, 478
　mechanisms of action, 470t, 471f, 472f, 473
　secretion regulation, 470t, 472f
　sensitivity, 477, 478
　signaling pathways, 471f
Insulin-like growth factor-1 (IGF-1), 422t, 428t
Insulin-like growth factor-1 (IGF-1) receptor signaling pathway, 666f
Insulin secretagogues
　nonsulfonylurea, 470t, 472f, 479t
　　nateglinide, 470t, 472f, 479t
　　repaglinide, 470t, 472f, 479t
　sulfonylurea, 470t, 472f, 479t
　　adverse effects, 475
　　gliclazide, 470t, 472f, 479t
　　glimepiride, 470t, 472f, 477, 478, 479t
　　glipizide, 470t, 472f, 479t

　　glyburide, 470t, 472f, 479t
　　mechanisms of action, 470t, 477, 478
Integrase inhibitor
　mechanisms of action and resistance, 603t
　raltegravir, 601t, 603t, 611f, 623t
Interactions. See Drug interactions; specific drugs
Interceptor molecules, 62
Interferons (IFNs), antihepatitis, 600t–602t, 606f, 620t
　adverse effects, 614
　hepatitis C, chronic, 613–614
　IFN differences, 613–614
　mechanisms of action and resistance, 602t, 606f, 613
Interferon-α-2b, 381t
Interferon-β-1a, 381t, 382
Interferon-β-1b, 381t, 382
Interferon-γ-1b, 381t
Interleukin-2 (IL-2) receptor agonists, anticancer, 663t, 685t
　aldesleukin, 663t, 682, 683, 685t
　denileukin diftitox, 663t, 671t, 685t
　mechanisms of resistance, 663t
Interleukins. See also IL entries
　hematopoietic growth factors, 407t, 408f
　mechanisms of action, growth factor, 407t
Intestinal bypass surgery, 486, 487
Intracellular enzymes, 3t
Intramuscular administration, 21t
　elderly, 74t
　neonates, infants, and children, 67b
Intranasal administration, elderly, 74t
Intravenous administration, 21t
Intrinsic cellular responses, 2b
Intrinsic sympathomimetic activity (ISA), 15, 16
Inverse agonists, 4, 4b, 4f, 9, 16, 17
In vitro binding studies, 8
Iodide, 431t, 440t
Iodine
　drugs with, 434t
　high levels, 437, 438
　hypothyroidism from, 435t, 438, 439
　radioactive, 438–439
　radioactive (131I), 431t, 435, 437–439, 440t
　supplementation, post-thyroidectomy, 437, 438
Iodine deficiency (goiter), 437, 438
Ion channels, 3, 3t, 86, 86f–88f, 89t. See also specific types and drug classes
　Ca^{2+}, 86, 87f, 89t
　Cl^-, 86
　K^+, 86, 87f
　ligand-gated receptor structure, 88f
　Na^+, 86, 87f
　voltage-dependent, 86, 87f
Ionic thyroid inhibitors, 431t, 440t
　iodide, 431t, 440t
　sodium iodide, 431t, 440t
Ionization
　kidney tubules, 21–22
　plasma–gastric juice partitioning, 19b–20b, 20f, 21–22
Ionized molecules, diffusion, 19b, 19f

Iontophoresis, 203
Ion trapping, 20b
Ipratropium (bromide)
　COPD, 390t, 402, 403t
　pharmacology, 96t
　pulmonary, 390t, 402, 403t
Irbesartan, 273t, 285t
Irinotecan (CPT-111), 643t, 649–651, 657t
　mechanisms of action, 630f, 643t, 649–651
　mechanisms of resistance, 630f, 643t, 644b–645b, 649–651
Iron
　recommended dietary allowances, nonvegetarians, 411t
　requirement, daily, 411t
Iron deficiency
　functional, 409
　from proton pump inhibitors, 495
Iron dextran, 406t, 419t
Iron poisoning, 54–55
　deferasirox, 41t, 65t
　deferoxamine, 42t, 55, 65t
Iron sucrose, 406t, 419t
Iron supplements, oral, 406t, 419t
　ferrous aspartate, 406t, 413–414, 419t
　ferrous fumarate, 406t, 413–414, 419t
　ferrous gluconate, 406t, 413–414, 419t
　ferrous salts, 406t, 413–414, 419t
　ferrous succinate, 406t, 413–414, 419t
　ferrous sulfate, 406t, 413–414, 419t
　infants and children, 413
　mechanisms of action, 405t
　optimizing effects, 413–414
　polysaccharide ferrihydrite complex, 406t, 413–414, 419t
　pregnancy, 413–414
Iron supplements, parenteral, 406t, 419t
　ferumoxytol, 406t, 419t
　iron dextran, 406t, 419t
　iron sucrose, 406t, 419t
　mechanisms of action, 406t
　sodium ferric gluconate, 406t, 419t
ISDN, 289t, 300t
ISMN, 289t, 298, 299, 300t
Isocarboxazid, 130t, 147t, 150t, 173t
Isoetharine, 125t, 143t
Isoflurophate, 103t, 104f
Isoflurane, 210t, 215t, 222t
Isoniazid
　adverse effects, 582, 585, 586
　drug interactions, 582, 583t
　mechanisms of action, 578t, 580f
　tuberculosis, 578t, 580f, 582, 583t, 587t
　vitamin B_6 with, 582
Isoniazid-resistant tuberculosis, 583
Isoprostanes, 358f
Isoproterenol, 125t, 142t
Isosorbide, 268t, 283t
Isosorbide-5-mononitrate (ISMN), 289t, 298, 299, 300t
Isosorbide dinitrate (ISDN), 289t, 300t
Isotretinoin, 707t, 721, 722, 724t
Isradipine
　antihypertensive, 277t, 287t
　myocardial ischemia, 290t, 300t

^{131}I-tositumomab, 662t, 671t, 684t
Itraconazole, 588t, 589f, 590, 597t
Ivermectin, 708t, 725t
Ixabepilone, 643t, 644b, 650, 657t

J
Jaw osteonecrosis, bisphosphonate, 481t, 485, 488t
Jimson weed, 101–102, 101t, 694f, 698, 698t

K
K_A, 6b, 8
Kallikrein inhibitors, 347t
Kanamycin, 559–566, 559b, 567t
K^+ channels, 86, 87f
K_D, 6b, 8
Keratitis, 700
    fungal, 701
    viral, 701
Kernicterus, 68
Ketamine,
    analgesics, 217
    anesthetic, 210t, 213t, 214f, 217, 222t
Ketanserin, 120t, 133t, 141t, 147t
Ketoconazole, 459t, 469t, 588t, 598t
    anticancer, 665t, 687t
    mechanisms of action, 668f
Ketorolac, 357t, 361t, 373t
    ophthalmic, 691t, 705t
Ketotifen fumarate, 347t, 355t
    ophthalmic, 691t, 705t
Kidney
    passive diffusion, excretion, and pH, 20b
    tubule ionization, 21–22
Kinin receptor antagonists, 347t, 355t
K^+-sparing diuretics, 269t, 271t, 272f, 285t
    mineralocorticoid antagonists
        eplerenone, 269t, 280–281, 285t
        spironolactone, 269t, 285t, 307
    Na^+-channel inhibitors, 269t, 271t, 272f, 284t
        amiloride, 269t, 284t
        triamterene, 269t, 282, 283, 284t

L
LABAs. See β_2 adrenergic receptor agonists, long-acting
Labetalol, 126t, 128t, 146t
Lacosamide, 226t, 237t
Lacrimal system, 698f
Lactation, FDA rules, 72b
Lactulose, 497t, 505, 506–507, 507t
Lambert-Eaton syndrome, 104
Lamivudine, 601t, 602t, 607f, 621t
    adverse effects, 615
    antihepatitis, 600t, 602t, 607f, 620t
    mechanisms of action and resistance, 602t, 604f, 607f, 608f, 614–615
    structure, 607f
Lamotrigine, 225t, 232, 237t
    anticonvulsants, 151t, 165, 175t
    valproic acid with, 235
Lanreotide, 422t, 428t
Lansoprazole, 490t, 493f, 496t
Lanthanum, 481t, 488t
Lanthanum carbonate, 481t, 484, 488t

Lapatinib, 661t, 673, 683t
L-asparaginase (L-ASP), 630f, 643t, 644t, 648–650, 659t
Latanoprost, ophthalmic, 691t, 705t
Laxatives, 497t, 498t, 507t, 507t–508t
    bisacodyl, 498t, 508t
    bowel effects, 500t
    classification, 500t
    docusate sodium, 498t, 508t
    lactulose, 497t, 505, 506–507, 507t
    magnesium citrate, 497t, 507t
    magnesium hydroxide, 497t, 507t
    magnesium sulfate, 497t, 507t
    mechanisms of action, 497t–498t, 498b, 498t, 499
    polyethylene glycol, 497t, 507t
    saline, 497t, 507t
    sodium phosphate, 497t, 507t
LDL-C levels
    classification, 337t
    treatment, 336t
LDL-C metabolism, 335f
Lead, 41t, 43t, 57–58, 57b, 58f, 63, 64, 65t
Lead poisoning, 43t, 63, 64, 65t
    dimercaprol, 41t, 42t, 66t
    dimercaptosuccinic acid, 41t, 42t, 66t
    EDTA CaNa2, 41t, 42t, 63, 64, 66t
    health effects, 57b
    heme biosynthesis, 58f
    mechanisms, 41t
Leflunomide, 368t
Left ventricular dysfunction, angina drugs, 293t
Leishmaniasis, visceral, 534
Lenalidomide, 381t
    anticancer, 663t, 666f, 685t
    immunostimulant, 381t
Lennox-Gastaut syndrome, 232
Leprosy drugs
    clofazimine, 579t, 583, 587t
    combination therapy, 583–584
    dapsone, 579t, 581f, 583–586, 587t
    therapeutic principles, 584b
    TMC-207, 579t, 587t
Lethal dose, 44f
    vs. effective dose, 44f
    median (LD50), 44f, 45
Letrozole
    anticancer, 664t, 677t, 679t, 686t
    pharmacology, 442t, 458t
Leucovorin. See High-dose methotrexate with leucovorin rescue (HDM-L)
Leukotriene antagonists, pulmonary, 390t, 403t–404t
    5-LOX inhibitors, zileuton, 390t, 403t
    asthma, severe, 396f, 397
    leukotriene antagonists, 390t, 404t
        montelukast, 390t, 404t
        zafirlukast, 390t, 404t
    mechanisms of action, 390t, 396f
Leukotrienes, 358f
Leucovorin calcium, 406t, 416, 417–418, 420t
Leuprolide
    anticancer, targeted, 664t, 679t, 680, 687t
    prostate cancer, 423t, 425–426, 429t
Levalbuterol
    pharmacology, 125t, 143t
    pulmonary, 389t, 402t

Levetiracetam, 225t, 234–235, 237t
Levobetaxolol, 126t, 145t
Levobunolol, 125t, 144t
    ophthalmic, 691t, 695t, 704t
Levocabastine, 347t, 355t
Levocetirizine, 347t
Levodopa, 238t, 242, 243–245, 243f, 244f, 252t
Levofloxacin, 544, 544f, 545, 548t
Levonorgestrel, 443t, 444t, 446t
Levorphanol, 194t, 195t, 200t, 209t
Levothyroxine, 431t, 432–434, 434t, 436–439, 439t
    adverse effects, 434
    factors in, 434t
    hypothyroidism
        pregnancy dosing, 437–439
        subclinical, 437, 438–439
        therapeutic goals, 432
    mechanisms of action, 431t
    thyroid cancer, 436
Licofelone, 358f
Licorice, 467, 468
Lidocaine, 224t
    antiarrhythmic, 312t, 316, 317t, 319, 320, 321t
    electrophysiologic actions, 317t
    ventricular fibrillation, 316
    ventricular tachycardia, 319, 320
Ligand-gated receptors, 88f
Lincosamides, 568t, 574, 575, 576t
Lindane, 708t, 725t
Linezolid, 569t, 576t
Liotrix, 431t, 439t
Lipid membrane diffusion, 19–20, 20f
Lipopeptides, 569t, 570f, 573, 575, 577t
Lipoxins, 358f
Lipoxygenase pathways, 358f, 359f
Liraglutide, 471t, 472f, 479t
Lisdexamfetamine, 120t, 141t
Lisinopril
    heart failure, 306, 309, 310
    pharmacology and actions, 273t, 281, 282, 285t
Lispro. See also Diabetes mellitus; Insulin
    vs. glargine, 478
Lithium, 151t, 164–166, 175t
    adverse effects, 164t
    elderly, 165–166
    ibuprofen, 165, 168, 169
    lithium carbonate, 151t, 175t
    lithium citrate, 151t, 175t
    overdose, 166–167
Lithium carbonate, 151t, 175t
Lithium citrate, 151t, 175t
Liver metabolism and clearance. See also specific drugs and drug classes
    elderly, 75b, 76f, 76t–77t, 77f
L-methyl folate. See Folic acid and derivatives
LMWH. See Low-molecular-weight heparins (LMWHs)
Loading dose, 39b
    creatine clearance, 34
Local anesthetics. See Anesthetic agents, local; specific agents

Lodoxamide tromethamine, ophthalmic, 691t, 705t
Lometrexol, 635t, 653t
  mechanisms of action, 635t
  mechanisms of resistance, 638b
Lomustine (CCNU), 627t, 630f, 652t
  mechanisms of action, 627t, 628b, 630f
  mechanisms of resistance, 627t, 632–633, 632b
  toxicities, 652t
  uses, 629t
Long QT syndrome, 313–315, 315b
Loop diuretics, 269t, 271t, 272f, 284t
  bumetanide, 269t, 282, 283, 284t
  ethacrynic acid, 269t, 284t
  furosemide, 269t, 280, 284t, 306
  torsemide, 269t, 284t
Loperamide
  antidiarrheal, 209t, 498t, 500–501, 508t
  mechanisms of action, 498t
Lopinavir, 601t, 603t, 615, 622t
  adverse effects, 615
  CYP3A4 metabolism, 618, 619
  drug interactions, 615
  HIV, 618, 619
  mechanisms of action and resistance, 603t, 615
Loracarbef, 557t
Loratadine, 89–90
  H_1 receptor antagonist, 347t, 348, 348b, 351–352, 355t
  pregnancy and lactation, 348, 348b, 351–352
Lorazepam, 176t, 189, 190, 191t, 192t
Losartan, 273t, 285t
Loteprednol, ophthalmic, 691t, 705t
Lou Gehrig's disease. See Amyotrophic lateral sclerosis (ALS)
Lovastatin, 334t, 341, 342, 343t
Lovenox, 325–326, 326f
Low-molecular-weight heparins (LMWHs), 323t, 324–325, 325f, 333t. See also specific agents
  indications, 325
  lovenox, 325–326, 326f
  mechanisms of action, 325
  monitoring, 325, 330b
Low (broad) specificity, 5b, 9
Loxapine, 151t, 175t
5-LOX inhibitors, 390t, 403t
Lubiprostone, 497t, 507t
Lumiracoxib, 363t
Lumbar puncture
  sequelae, 219
  spinal anesthesia, 217–219
Lung cancer, hypercalcemia in, 483–484, 486, 487
  calcitonin for, 480t, 483–484, 488t
Luteinizing hormone (LH) therapy, 423t, 429t
Lutropin alfa, 423t, 430t
Lymphocyte function-associated antigen (LFA-1 & LFA-3) inhibitors
  alefacept, 376t, 386t
  efalizumab, 376t, 386t

Lymphocyte immune (ALG), 376t, 377f, 378, 378t, 385t

M

Macrolides and ketolides, 568t, 570f, 576t
  azithromycin, 568t, 570f, 576t
  clarithromycin, 568t, 570f, 571, 576t
  drug interactions, macrolide, 572
  erythromycin, 568t, 570f, 576t
  telithromycin, 568t, 570f, 576t
  toxicities, 571
Macrophage colony stimulating factor (M-CSF), 407t, 408f
Macular degeneration agents, 692t, 706t
  bevacizumab, 692t, 706t
  pegaptanib, 692t, 706t
  ranibizumab, 692t, 706t
  verteporfin, 692t, 703, 706t
Magnesium citrate, 497t, 507t
Magnesium hydroxide, 497t, 507t
Magnesium sulfate
  antiarrhythmic, 317t, 322t
  electrophysiologic actions, 317t
  laxative, 497t, 507t
Malaria chemoprophylaxis, 521–522, 522t
  atovaquone-proguanil, 521–522, 522t, 526
  chloroquine phosphate, 522t
  doxycycline, 522t
  general advice, 526–527
  hydroxychloroquine sulfate, 522t
  mefloquine, 522t, 524
  primaquine, 522t, 525–526
Malaria chemotherapy, 520–529, 520t–521t, 529t
  artemisinin, 520t, 529t
    artemether, 520t, 529t
    artemether-lumefantrine, 520t, 521, 527, 529t
    artesunate, 520t, 529t
    dihydroartemisinin, 520t, 529t
  atovaquone, meprone, 520t, 529t
  atovaquone-proguanil, 520t, 527, 529t
  chemoprophylaxis, 521–522, 522t, 526
  chloroquine/hydroxychloroquine, 521t, 522t, 523–524, 526, 529t
  chloroquine-resistant *P. falciparum*, 523f, 524
  cinchonism, 524
  dermatologic agents, 708t, 725t
    chloroquine, 708t, 725t
    hydroxychloroquine, 708t, 725t
    quinacrine, 708t, 725t
  endemic countries, 523, 523f
  mechanisms of action, 520t–521t
  mefloquine, 521t, 522t, 524, 527, 529t
  pregnancy, 527
  primaquine, 521t, 522t, 525–526, 526t, 527, 529t
  proguanil, 520t, 529t
  pyrimethamine-sulfadoxine, 521t, 529t
  quinine/quinidine, 521t, 524, 527, 529t
  sulfadoxine, 521t, 529t, 543t, 548t
  treatments of choice, 526–527
Malaria parasite
  developmental stages, 525, 526
  life cycle, 525–526, 525f

Malathion, 89
  dermatologic, 708t, 725t
  pharmacology, 100t, 102t, 115t
Mannitol, 268t, 283t
MAO inhibitors
  5-HT concentration altering, 130t, 147t
  food contraindications, 135, 137
  with SSRIs, 133
Maprotiline, 150t, 173t
Maraviroc, 601t, 603t, 608f, 611f, 623t
Marijuana, 263
  medicinal effects, 265, 266
  withdrawal syndrome, 263, 263t
Mast cell stabilizers. See Histamine receptor antagonists and mast cell stabilizers
MDR1 transporter, 23t, 24t, 25t, 38
MDR3 *(ABCB4)* transporter, 25t
Mecamylamine, 106t, 117t
Mecasermin, 422t, 428t
Mechlorethamine, dermatologic, 708t, 724t, 726t
Mechlorethamine HCl, 627t, 651t
  mechanisms of action, 626, 627t, 628, 628b, 630f
  mechanisms of resistance, 627t, 632–633, 632b
  toxicities, 632b–633b, 651t
  uses, 629t
Meclizine, 346t, 350, 352, 354t
Median effective dose (ED50), 44f, 45
Median lethal dose (LD_{50}), 44f, 45
Medication errors, 56–57, 57t
Medroxyprogesterone, targeted anticancer therapy, 664t, 679t, 686t
Medroxyprogesterone acetate (MPA) conjugated estrogen +, 441t
  hormone replacement therapy, 442t, 458t
MedWatch, 47
Mefloquine, malaria
  chemoprophylaxis, 522t, 524
  chemotherapy, 521t, 522t, 524, 527, 529t
Megaloblastic anemia, 417–418. See also Vitamin B_{12} deficiency
  fish tapeworm, 537–540
Megestrol, anticancer, 665t, 687t
Megestrol acetate, 442t, 458t
  anticancer, 664t, 679t, 686t
Melarsoprol, 530t, 534, 535t
Melatonin congeners, 177t, 189, 190, 192t
Melphalan, 627t, 632t, 651t
  mechanisms of action, 626, 627t, 628, 628b, 630f
  mechanisms of resistance, 627t, 632–633, 632b
  toxicities, 632b–633b, 632t, 651t
  uses, 629t
Memantine, 239t, 246–247, 251, 252, 253t
Menotropin, 423t, 429t
Menstrual cramping, 364–365
Meperidine, 195t, 200t, 204, 208t
  MAO inhibitors contraindication, 204
  toxicity, 204, 206, 208
Mephentermine, 119t, 139t
Mephobarbital, 177t, 181t, 192t
Mepivacaine, 224t

Meprobamate, 177t, 193t
Meprone, 520t, 529t
Mequinol, 710t, 727t
6-Mercaptopurine (6-MP), 636t, 641–642, 655t
  mechanisms of action, 630f, 636t, 641–642
  mechanisms of resistance, 636t, 639b, 642
  toxicities, 642, 655t
  uses, 637t, 655t
Mercury, 41t, 43t, 59–60, 59f, 65t
Meropenem, 558t
Mesalamine, 357t, 373t
Mesalamine (5-ASA), 498t, 503f, 509t
Metabolic syndrome, 339–340. *See also* Dyslipidemia drugs
Metabolism, drug, 20b, 28b. *See also specific drugs and drug classes*
  acetaminophen, 28–29, 50–54, 50f, 52t, 207, 208
  children, 70b
  CYP superfamily, 30, 30b–31b, 32t, 33f
  drug–drug interactions on, 48, 48b, 48t
  elderly, 73t–74t, 75b
  nuclear receptors inducing, 33t, 34f
  phase 1, 28b, 33f, 35, 38
    neonatal, 70b
  phase 2, 28–29, 28b, 33f, 35, 39
  poisoning, 52
  reactions, 32t
Metals, heavy (toxic), 41t, 43t, 65t–66t. *See also specific types*
  chelators, 66t
Metaproterenol
  pharmacology, 125t, 143t
  pulmonary, 389t, 402t
Metaraminol, 119t, 139t
Metformin, 470t, 479t
  diabetes mellitus type 2 after, hemoglobin A$_{1c}$, 475–476
  + glimepiride, 477, 478
Methacholine, 99t, 112t
  mechanisms of action, 95t
  pharmacology, 99t, 112t
Methadone, 194t, 195t, 200t, 201–203, 202t, 208t
  cancer pain, 201–203, 202t
    routes of administration, 202–203
  conversion guidelines, oral morphine to methadone, 202t
  vs. heroin responses, 260, 260f
  for opioid addiction, 260–261
Methamphetamine, 120t, 141t
Methanol, 42t, 49–50, 49f
  metabolism and poisoning, 49–50, 49f, 178f
Methanol antidote
  ethanol, 42t, 50, 65t
  fomepizole, 41t, 42t, 65t, 178f
Methenamine, 548t
Methicillin, 551, 552t, 554, 555, 555t
Methicillin-resistant *Staphylococcus aureus* (MRSA), 551, 571
  doxycycline, 571
  minocycline, 571

skin, treatment, 714–715
  tetracyclines, 571
Methimazole, 431t, 435–436, 438, 439, 440t
Methohexital, 177t, 192t
  anesthetic, 210t, 213t, 222t
  mechanisms and sites of action, 635t
Methotrexate, 635t, 653t
  + 5-FU, 648, 649
  anticancer
    mechanisms and sites of action, 630f, 635t, 637f, 638–639
    mechanisms of resistance, 635t, 638b, 640
  dermatologic, 708t, 715, 721–722, 724t, 725t
    psoriasis, 715–716, 721–722
  folinic acid with, 416, 417–418
  inflammatory bowel disease, 499t, 509t
  mechanisms and sites of action, 635t
  mechanisms of resistance, 638b, 640
  pharmacogenetics, 637f, 639
  rheumatoid arthritis, 368b, 368t, 380
  toxicities, 653t
  uses, 637t
Methoxsalen photochemotherapy, 707t, 716t, 725t
6-Methoxy-arabinosyl-guanine. *See* Nelarabine
Methscopolamine, 498t, 508t
Methscopolamine bromide, 96t, 114t
Methsuximide, 225t, 236t
Methylaminolevulinate photodynamic therapy, 708t, 725t
Methyl-CCNU. *See* Semustine (methyl-CCNU)
Methylcellulose, ophthalmic, 692t, 706t
Methyclothiazide, 269t, 284t
Methyldopa
  antihypertensive, 277t, 286t
  pharmacology, 119t, 140t
Methylenedioxymethamphetamine (MDMA)
  5-HT$_2$ receptor affinity, 265, 266
L-Methyl folate. *See* Folic acid and derivatives
Methylhydrazines, 629t, 652t
  mechanisms of action, 628b, 628t, 630f
  mechanisms of resistance, 628t, 632–633, 632b
  procarbazine, 629t, 652t
  toxicities, 632b–633b, 652t
  uses, 629t
Methylmelamines, 627t, 651t. *See also* Ethyleneimines and methylmelamines
Methylnaltrexone
  bowel disorders, 498t, 499, 505, 506, 507t
  constipation, opioid, 199, 498t, 499, 505, 506, 507t
  mechanisms of action, 498t
  opioid receptor antagonism, 195t, 199, 209t
Methylparaben, 220, 221
Methylphenidate, 120t, 141t
Methylprednisolone, 460t. *See also* Corticosteroids
  pulmonary, 390t, 403t

Methylxanthines, pulmonary, 390t, 403t
  COPD, 395
  mechanisms of action, 390t
  theophylline, 390t, 392f, 397, 403t
Methysergide, 130t, 147t
Metipranolol, 125t, 144t
  ophthalmic, 691t, 695t, 704t
Metoclopramide
  antiemetic, 502t, 504, 506
  bowel disorders, 497t, 504, 506, 507t
Metolazone, 269t, 284t
Metoprolol
  heart failure, 301t, 303–304, 306, 309, 310, 310t
  myocardial ischemia, 300t
  pharmacology, 126t, 127–129, 128t, 145t
Metronidazole, 530t, 532–534, 535t
  alcohol reaction, 533, 534
  amebic colitis, 530t, 532–533, 535t
  duodenal ulcer, 492, 494t
  giardiasis, 530t, 532–533, 535t
Metyrapone, 459t, 466, 469t
Mexiletine
  antiarrhythmic, 312t, 317t, 321t
  electrophysiologic actions, 316
Mezlocillin, 552t, 556t
Mianserin, 150t, 174t
Micafungin, 588t, 589f, 598t
Michaelis-Menten equation, 35b
Miconazole, 588t, 594, 597t
Microtubule-damaging agents. *See also* Colchicine; Taxanes; Vinca alkaloids
  estramustine, 630f, 643t, 650, 657t
  ixabepilone, 643t, 644b, 650, 657t
Microtubule disruptors, 369t
  colchicine, 369t, 370, 373t
Midazolam, 176t, 191t, 192t, 214f
Midodrine, 119t, 139t
Mifepristone, 442t, 458t, 459t, 469t
Miglitol, 471t, 479t
Migraine
  5-HT in, 133–134, 133t
  oral contraceptives with, 455, 456–457
Milnacipran, 150t, 174t
Milrinone, 302t, 308, 308t, 311t
Miltefosine, 530t, 534, 535t
Milnacipran, 130t, 147t
Mineral ion homeostasis disorder drugs, 480–489
  calcimimetics, cinacalcet, 481t, 486, 487, 488t
  hormones
    calcitonin, 480t, 483–484, 483f
    teriparatide, 480t
  hypercalcemia, 483–484
  vitamin D and analogs, 481t, 488t
    1α-hydroxycholecalciferol, 481t, 488t
    22-oxacalcitrolparicalcitol, 481t, 488t
    calcipotriol, 481t, 488t
    calcitriol, 481t, 482f, 488t
    dihydrotachysterol, 481b
    doxercalciferol, 481b
    ergocalciferol, 481t, 488t
    paricalcitol, 481t, 488t
    therapeutic uses, 481b

759

Mineralocorticoid receptor antagonists (K+-sparing), 269t, 271t, 272f, 285t
    eplerenone, 269t, 280–281, 285t
    spironolactone, 269t, 285t, 307
Minimum alveolar concentration (MAC), 215, 215t
Minimum effective concentration (MEC), 36f
Minimum inhibitory concentration (MIC), 513
Minocycline
    MRSA, 571
    rheumatoid arthritis, 368t
Minoxidil
    androgenic alopecia, 710t, 726t
    hypertension and edema, 278t, 287t
Miosis, 698, 698t
Mirtazapine, 150t, 174t
Misoprostol, 490t, 493, 494, 495, 496t
    gastric acid disease, 490t, 493, 494, 495, 496t
    GERD in pregnancy, 494, 495
    with NSAID-induced duodenal ulcer, 493
Mitomycin, ophthalmic, 691t, 705t
Mitomycin (mitomycin-C), 630f, 643t, 646b, 658t
Mitotane, 679t
    anticancer, 644t, 659t
    pharmacology, 459t, 469t
Mitoxantrone
    anticancer, 630f, 643t, 645b, 658t
    immunostimulant, 382t
Mivacurium, 106t, 107t, 117t
Mizolastine, 347t, 355t
Modafinil, 120t, 142t
Moexipril, 273t, 285t
Molindone, 151t, 175t
Mometasone, 390t, 403t
Monoamine oxidase inhibitors (MAOIs), 150t, 157, 173t. *See also specific agents*
    isocarboxazid, 150t, 173t
    meperidine contraindication, 204
    phenelzine, 150t, 173t
    selegiline, 150t, 173t
    SSRI after, 157
    structures, dosing, and adverse effects, 156t
    tranylcypromine, 150t, 173t
Monobenzone, 710t, 727t
Monoclonal antibodies (mAbs)
    anti-CD3, muromonab-CD3, 376t, 378, 385t
    anti-CD25 (anti-IL-2 R), 376t, 379, 386t
    basiliximab, 376t, 386t
    daclizumab, 376t, 386t
    anti-CD52, alemtuzumab, 376t, 378, 386t
    CD20, anticancer, 662t, 667t, 684t
        ^{99}Y-ibritumomab, 662t, 671t, 684t
        ^{131}I-tositumomab, 662t, 671t, 684t
        dose and toxicities, 671t, 684t
        mechanisms of resistance, 662t
        ofatumumab, 662t, 684t
        rituximab, 662t, 671t, 681, 682, 684t
    CD33, anticancer, 662t, 684t
        gemtuzumab ozogamicin, 662t, 667t, 672t, 684t
        mechanisms of resistance, 662t
    CD52, anticancer, 662t, 667t, 671t, 684t
        alemtuzumab, 662t, 667t, 671t, 684t
        mechanisms of resistance, 662t
    denosumab, 481t, 488t
    growth factor antibodies (VEGF), anticancer, 662t, 673–675, 684t
        bevacizumab, 662t, 671t, 674–675, 684t
        dose, 671t
        ranibizumab, 662t, 684t
        toxicities, 671t, 674–675, 684t
    growth factor receptor, anticancer, 662t, 683t
        cetuximab, 662t, 669–672, 683t
        dose and toxicities, 671t
        EGFR targeting, 669–672
        HER2/neu, 667t, 682t
        panitumumab, 662t, 669–672, 683t
        trastuzumab, 662t, 671t, 672–673, 681, 682, 683t
    natalizumab, 382t
Monocyte/macrophage colony stimulating factor (M-CSF, CSF-1), 407t, 408f
Montelukast, 390t, 404t
Morphine, 194t, 195t, 200t, 206–208, 208t
    constipation from, 92
    conversion guidelines, oral morphine to methadone, 202t
    infant dosing, 72, 74
    metabolism
        children, 68
        first-pass, 206, 207
        morphine-6-glucuronide, 206, 207–208
Morphine-6-glucuronide, 206, 207–208
Mosquito bite, 347b, 348
Motion sickness, 350, 352
Moxifloxacin, 544, 544f, 545, 548t
MPA. *See* Medroxyprogesterone acetate (MPA)
MPA immunotherapy, 375t, 385t
MRP1 (*ABCC1*) transporter, 23t
MRP2 (*ABCC2*) transporter, 23t
MRP3 (*ABCC3*) transporter, 24t
MRP4 (*ABCC4*) transporter, 24t
MRP5 (*ABCC5*) transporter, 24t
MRP6 (*ABCC6*) transporter, 24t
MRSA. *See* Methicillin-resistant *Staphylococcus aureus* (MRSA)
MTA. *See* Pemetrexed (MTA)
mTOR, 384
mTOR inhibitors, 663t, 685t
    everolimus, 663t, 685t
    mechanisms of action, 663t, 675
    mechanisms of resistance, 663t, 676
    rapamycin, 663t, 675–676, 685t
    temsirolimus, 663t, 675–676, 685t
Mucolytics, 390t, 404t
    DNase (dornase alfa), 390t, 404t
    N-acetylcysteine, 390t, 404t
Multiple myeloma, bortezomib, 663t, 681, 682–683, 685t
Multiple sclerosis (MS)
    IFN-β-1a and IFN-β-1b, 381t
    pathophysiology, 382
Mupirocin, 569t, 573, 577t
Muromonab-CD3, 376t, 378, 385t
Muscarine
    mushrooms, 97
    pharmacology, 99t
Muscarinic acetylcholine receptors (mAChRs), 98t–99t
Muscarinic receptor agonists, 99t, 112t. *See also specific types*
    bethanechol, 95t, 99t, 112t
    mechanisms of action, 95t
Muscarinic receptor antagonists, 99t, 100, 101b, 101t, 112t–114t. *See also specific types*
    mechanisms of action, 96t
    overactive bladder, 100, 101t
Muscarinic receptors, 82f, 97f
    atropine, 80–82
    muscarine, 97, 99t
Mushrooms, catecholaminergic, 97, 100
Mussels, saxitoxin, 221, 222
MXR transporter, 24t
Myasthenia gravis, 104–105, 105f
Mycobacterium avium complex drugs
    cycloserine, 579t, 587t
    ethambutol, 578t, 583, 587t
    therapeutic principles, 584b
    TMC-207, 579t, 587t
Mycobacterium intracellulare, 579t, 583, 584, 584b, 587t
Mycobacterium kansaii
    ethambutol, 578t, 583, 587t
    TMC-207, 579t, 587t
Mycobacterium spp., TMC-207, 579t, 587t
Mycobacterium tuberculosis drugs. *See* Tuberculosis drugs
Mycophenolate mofetil (MMF)
    dermatologic, 709t, 724t, 726t
    immunotherapy, 375t, 383, 384, 385t
    mechanisms of action, 375t, 383, 384
Mydriasis, 694f, 698, 698t
Mydriasis agents, 694f, 698, 698t
Myeloid growth factors, 405t, 407t, 418t
    G-CSF, 405t, 407t, 408f, 409–410, 416, 417, 418t
    G-CSF, pegylated recombinant, 405t, 407t, 408f, 409–410, 418t
    GM-CSF, 405t, 407t, 408f, 409–410, 418t
    indications and choice, 409–410
    mechanisms of action, 405t, 407t
    sites of action, 408f
Myocardial infarction
    aspirin prophylaxis, daily, 365
    drugs, 324–325, 324f (*See also* Thromboembolic disorder drugs)
    platelet adhesion and aggregation, 324, 324f (*See also* Antiplatelet agents)
Myocardial ischemia
    classification, 290t
    percutaneous coronary interventions, 297
    stents, drug-eluting coronary, 297, 297b
    symptoms, 289b–290b

Myocardial ischemia drugs, 289–300. *See also specific drugs and drug classes*
  β adrenergic receptor antagonists, 289t, 291f, 292–294, 300t
  Ca^{2+} channel antagonists, 290t, 294–295, 295t–296t, 297–299, 300t
  claudication, 295b
  mechanisms of action, 289t–290t
  Na$^+$ channel blocker, ranolazine, 290t, 298, 299, 300t
  nitrate vasodilators, organic, 22, 289t, 291–292, 291b, 291f, 294, 297–299, 300t
  peripheral vascular disease, 295b
  phosphodiesterase 5 inhibitors, 291b, 292, 300t
  unstable angina, 296–297
  variant angina, 297
  vasospastic angina with sinus bradycardia, 297, 298

N

Na$^+$-2Cl$^-$ symporter inhibitors. *See* Thiazide/thiazide-like diuretics
Na$^+$ balance disorder agents, 279t, 280–281, 281f. *See also* Diuretics
Nabilone, 498t, 502, 508t
Nab-paclitaxel, 642t, 648–650, 656t
  mechanisms of action, 630f, 642t, 648–650
  mechanisms of resistance, 642t, 644b
  toxicities, 656t
  uses, 644t, 656t
N-acetylcysteine (NAC), 40t, 42t, 54, 65t
  mucolytic, 390t, 404t
Na$^+$ channel blockers
  antiarrhythmic, 312t, 320t–321t
    disopyramide, 312t, 317t, 321t
    flecainide, 312t, 317t, 321t
    lidocaine, 312t, 316, 317t, 319, 320, 321t
    mexiletine, 312t, 317t, 321t
    procainamide, 312t, 316, 317t, 320
    propafenone, 312t, 317t, 321t
    quinidine, 312t, 317t, 320
  myocardial ischemia, ranolazine, 290t, 298, 299, 300t
Na$^+$ channels, 86, 87f
  antiseizure drug-enhanced inactivation, 225t, 225t–226t, 226f, 232
  voltage-gated
    local anesthetics on, 217
    structure and function, 218f
Nadolol, 125t, 128t, 144t
Nadroparin, 323t, 325, 333t
Nafarelin, 422t, 427, 428, 429t, 664t, 686t
Nafcillin, 551, 552t, 554, 555, 555t
Naftifine, 589f, 599t
Na$^+$-K$^+$-2Cl$^-$ symporter inhibitors. *See* Loop diuretics
Na$^+$-K$^+$-ATPase inhibitors
  antiarrhythmic, 312t, 322t
    digoxin, 312t, 317t, 319, 320, 322t
  heart failure, 303f, 311t
    digoxin, 301t, 306, 307, 311t
    mechanisms of action, 301t

Na$^+$-K$^+$ exchange, sarcolemmal, 303f
Nalbuphine, 195t, 200t, 209t
Nalmefene, 177t, 193t
Naloxone, 16, 17, 41t, 42t, 65t, 195t, 203–204, 205, 207, 209t
  opioid overdose, 203–204, 205, 207
  precautions, 203
  route of administration, 205, 207
  toxicity use, 41t, 42t, 65t
Naltrexone
  alcoholism, 177t, 186–187, 186t, 203, 257
  for opioid addiction, 262
  opioid receptor antagonism, 193t, 195t, 209t
Naphazoline, 120t, 142t
  ophthalmic, 690t, 695t, 705t
NAPQI (*N*-acetyl-*p*-benzoquinone imine), 29, 48, 53
Naratriptan, 130t, 147t
Natalizumab, 382t
Nateglinide, 470t, 472f, 479t
Natriuresis, 270b
Natriuretic agents
  atrial natriuretic peptide, 269t, 280, 284t
  diuretics (*See* Diuretics)
Natriuretic peptide receptor agonists, heart failure
  mechanisms of action, 302t
  nesiritide, 302t, 311t
Natural products, cytotoxic, 642t–644t, 645–647
  antibiotics, anticancer, 630f, 643t, 658t
    bleomycin, 630f, 643t, 645b, 658t
    mechanisms of action, 643t
    mechanisms of resistance, 643t, 645b–646b
    mitomycin (mitomycin-C), 630f, 643t, 646b, 658t
    uses, 644t, 658t
  antibiotics, anticancer: actinomycins, dactinomycin, 630f, 643t, 658t
  antibiotics, anticancer: anthracyclines and anthracenediones, 643t, 658t
    daunorubicin, 630f, 643t, 645b, 658t
    doxorubicin, 630f, 643t, 645–647, 645b, 658t
    epirubicin, 630f, 643t, 645b, 658t
    idarubicin, 630f, 643t, 645b, 658t
    mechanisms of action, 630f, 643t
    mechanisms of resistance, 643t, 645b
    mitoxantrone, 630f, 643t, 645b, 658t
    uses, 644t, 658t
    valrubicin, 630f, 643t, 645b, 658t
  enzymes
    L-asparaginase (L-ASP), 630f, 643t, 644t, 648–650, 659t
    pegaspargase (PEG-L-asparaginase), 643t, 659t
    uses, 644t
  mechanisms of action, 630f, 642t–643t
  mechanisms of resistance, 644b–646b
  microtubule-damaging agents
    epothilones: ixabepilone, 643t, 644b, 650, 657t
    estramustine, 630f, 643t, 650, 657t

  microtubule-damaging agents: taxanes, 642t, 648–650, 656t
    docetaxel, 630f, 642t, 644b, 648–650, 656t
    mechanisms of action, 630f, 642t, 648–650
    mechanisms of resistance, 642t, 644b
    nab-paclitaxel, 630f, 642t, 644b, 648–650, 656t
    paclitaxel, 630f, 642t, 644b, 648–650, 656t
    toxicities, 656t
    uses, 644t, 656t
  microtubule-damaging agents: vinca alkaloids, 642t, 656t
    mechanisms of action, 630f, 642t
    mechanisms of resistance, 642t, 644b
    toxicities, 656t
    uses, 644t, 656t
    vinblastine sulfate, 630f, 642t, 644b, 644t, 656t
    vincristine sulfate, 630f, 642t, 644b, 644t, 656t
    vinorelbine, 630f, 642t, 644b, 644t, 656t
  topoisomerase inhibitors: camptothecin analogs, 643t, 657t
    irinotecan, 630f, 643t, 644b–645b, 649–651, 657t
    mechanisms of action, 630f, 643t, 649–651
    mechanisms of resistance, 643t, 644b–645b
    topotecan, 630f, 643t, 644b–645b, 649–651, 657t
    toxicities, 657t
    uses, 644t, 657t
  topoisomerase inhibitors: epipodophyllotoxins, 643t, 657t
    etoposide, 630f, 643t, 645b, 657t
    mechanisms of action, 630f, 643t
    mechanisms of resistance, 643t, 645b
    teniposide, 630f, 643t, 645b, 657t
    toxicities, 657t
    uses, 644t, 657t
  trabectedin, 643t, 659t
  uses, 644t
Nausea drugs. *See* Antinauseants and antiemetics
Nebivolol, 126t, 128t, 146t
Nedocromil, ophthalmic, 691t, 705t
Nefazodone, 150t, 174t
Negative reinforcement, 265, 266
Nelarabine, 636t, 655t
  mechanisms of action, 630f, 636t, 641–642
  uses, 637t
Nelfinavir, 601t, 603t, 608f, 609f, 622t
Neomycin, 559–566, 559b, 567t
Neosporin, 573
Neostigmine, 104f
Neostigmine bromide, 100t, 114t
Neostigmine methylsulfate, 100t, 114t
Nepafenac, 357t, 361t, 373t
  ophthalmic, 691t, 705t

761

Nephrons, 270b
Nerve gases
　organophosphate, 100t, 103t, 116t
　sarin, 100t, 103t, 115t
　soman, 100t, 103t, 116t
　tabun, 100t, 103t, 116t
Nerve impulse transmission, 85–86, 85b, 86f
Nerve injury pain, 197b, 197f
Nesiritide (BNP), 269t, 280, 284t, 302t, 311t
Netilmicin, 559–566, 559b, 567t
Neurodegenerative disease drugs, 238–253. *See also specific diseases and drugs*
　Alzheimer's disease, 239t, 245–248, 253t
　amyotrophic lateral sclerosis, 239t, 249, 253t
　Huntington's disease, 239t, 248–249, 248f, 253t
　Parkinson's disease, 238t–239t, 239–245, 239b, 242t, 250–251, 252t–253t
Neuroeffector junction, 97f
Neuroleptic malignant syndrome, 172t
Neuromuscular blocking agents
　anesthetic adjuncts, 211t, 223t
　classification, 107t
　competitive, 97f, 105f, 106f, 106t, 107t, 116t–117t
　depolarizing, 97f, 105f, 107t, 108, 116t
　mechanisms of actions, 106t
Neuromuscular junction
　acetylcholine, 105f
　drugs at, mechanisms of action, 106t
　sites of action, 105f
　somatic, neurotransmitters, 82f, 93, 94
　(*See also specific types*)
Neuropeptides, 91t
Neuropeptide Y (NPY), 122f
Neurotransmission, 80–94
　alprazolam, 92
　atropine, 80–82
　autonomic nervous system, 80, 81f, 82f, 85b
　blood-brain barrier, 94
　brain signal transduction, 85, 86b, 86f
　cholinergic antagonist, 81f, 82f, 83t–84t, 93, 94, 95t
　cholinesterase inhibitor, 89
　CNS drugs, 91–92
　diphenhydramine *vs.* loratadine, 89–90
　drug-induced sedation/depression, hyperexcitability after, 89–90, 94
　enteric nervous system, 82–83
　excitatory and inhibitory, 86, 86f
　ion channels, 86, 86f–88f, 89t
　morphine, constipation, 92
　muscarinic receptors, 82f
　nerve impulse, 85–86, 85b, 86f
　neuropeptides, 91t
　neurotransmitters, 85, 86b, 86f, 89, 90f, 91–92
　nicotinic receptors, 82f, 93, 94
　receptors, 89b
　somatic nerves, 82f, 85, 92
　sympathetic *vs.* parasympathetic nervous systems, 82f, 85, 92

Neurotransmitters, 85, 86b, 86f
　actions and termination, 89, 90f
　CNS, 86b, 91–92, 91t
　PNS, 83t–84t, 86b, 92
　receptors, 89b
Nevirapine, 601t, 603t, 615, 622t
　HIV, 615
　mechanisms of action and resistance, 603t, 608f, 610f, 615
　structure, 610f
New drug testing, 44f, 45, 45t
　phases, 45t
Niacin, 335t, 340, 341, 342, 343t
　adverse effects, 341, 342
Nicardipine, 277t, 287t
Nicotine
　addiction, 258–259
　negative reinforcement, 265, 266
　poisoning, acute, 106t, 108, 108b
　withdrawal syndrome, 258–259, 259t
Nicotine gum or lozenge, 106t, 108, 108b, 117t, 259
Nicotine nasal spray or vapor inhaler, 106t, 108, 108b, 117t, 259
Nicotine transdermal patch, 106t, 108, 108b, 117t, 259
Nicotinic ACh receptor agonists, 106, 117t
Nicotinic acid, 335t, 343t
　mechanisms of action, 335t
　niacin, 335t, 340, 341, 342, 343t
Nicotinic receptors, 82f, 93, 94
Nifedipine
　antihypertensive, 277t, 287t
　myocardial ischemia, 290t, 300t
Nifurtimox, 531t, 535t
Nilotinib
　mechanisms of resistance, 668
　pharmacodynamics, 15
Nilutamide, 442t, 458t, 665t, 679t, 687t
Nimodipine, 290t, 300t
Nisoldipine
　antihypertensive, 277t, 287t
　myocardial ischemia, 290t, 300t
Nitazoxanide, 530t, 532, 535t
Nitrates
　first-pass effect, 22, 291, 299
　PDE5 inhibitor interactions, 291b, 292, 298, 299
Nitrate vasodilators, myocardial ischemia, 289t, 291f, 300t
　with Ca^{2+} channel blockers, 297
　isosorbide-5-mononitrate, 289t, 298, 299, 300t
　isosorbide dinitrate, 289t, 300t
　nitroglycerin, 22, 289t, 291–292, 291b, 291f, 300t
　PDE5 inhibitor interactions, 291b, 292, 298, 299
Nitric oxide gas, therapeutic, 211t, 223t
Nitrofurantoin, 545, 546, 547, 548t
Nitrogen mustards, 627t, 651t
　activation, in vivo, 631, 631f
　bendamustine, 627t, 651t
　cyclophosphamide, 627t, 631f, 632t, 651t
　ifosfamide, 627t, 632t, 651t
　mechanisms of action, 626, 627t, 628, 628b, 630f

　mechanisms of resistance, 627t, 632–633, 632b
　mechlorethamine HCl, 627t, 651t
　melphalan, 627t, 632t, 651t
　toxicities, 632b–633b, 632t, 651t
　uses, 629t
Nitroglycerin
　administration, timing, 291–292
　adverse effects, 292
　angina prevention, 291
　first-pass effect, 22, 291, 299
　myocardial ischemia, 22, 289t, 291–292, 291b, 291f, 300t
　PDE5 inhibitor interactions, 291b, 292, 298, 299
　pharmacology, 22, 289t
Nitroprusside, 278t, 287t
Nitrosoureas, 652t
　carmustine, 632t, 652t
　lomustine, 652t
　mechanisms of action, 627t, 628b, 630f
　mechanisms of resistance, 627t, 632–633, 632b
　semustine, 652t
　streptozocin, 652t
　toxicities, 632b–633b, 652t
　uses, 629t
Nitrous oxide, 210t, 215t, 223t
Nizatidine
　gastric acid disease, 490t, 496t
　structure, 492f
Nocardia, 579t, 587t
Nociception. *See also* Opioid pharmacology; Pain
　acute, 197b, 197f
Noncompetitive antagonists, 4b, 5f
Nonionized molecules
　blood-brain barrier, 19–20, 19b–20b, 19f, 20f, 35, 37–38
　diffusion, 19–20, 19b–20b, 19f, 20f, 35, 37–38
Non-nucleoside reverse transcriptase inhibitors (NNRTIs), 601t, 603t, 608f, 610f, 623t
　delavirdine, 601t, 603t, 608f, 610f
　efavirenz, 601t, 603t, 608f, 610f, 623t
　etravirine, 601t, 603t, 608f, 610f, 623t
　mechanisms of action and resistance, 603t, 608f, 610f
　nevirapine, 601t, 603t, 608f, 610f, 615, 622t
　structures, 610f
Nonsteroidal anti-inflammatory drugs (NSAIDs), 356–373
　acetic acid derivatives
　　bromfenac, 357t, 373t
　　diclofenac, 357t, 362t, 371, 372, 373t
　　etodolac, 357t, 361t, 373t
　　indomethacin, 357t, 361t, 373t
　　ketorolac, 357t, 361t, 373t
　　nepafenac, 357t, 361t, 373t
　　sulindac, 357t, 361t, 373t
　　tolmetin, 357t, 361t, 373t
　adverse effects, 364t, 365b, 367–368
　arthritis, 366–368
　balsalazide, 357t
　choice and dosing, 366–367

Nonsteroidal anti-inflammatory drugs (Cont.)
  classification, 360f, 361t–363t
  diflunisal, 357t, 360t, 373t
  mesalamine, 357t, 373t
  olsalazine, 357t, 373t
  ophthalmic, 691t, 705t
    bromfenac, 691t, 705t
    diclofenac, 691t, 705t
    flurbiprofen, 691t, 705t
    ketorolac, 691t, 705t
    nepafenac, 691t, 705t
  rheumatoid arthritis, 380
  salicylate, 357t, 373t
  salsalate, 357t, 373t
  sulfasalazine, 357t, 368t, 373t, 381
  ulcers from, 492
Non-ST–segment-elevation myocardial infarction, 290t, 291f. *See also* Myocardial ischemia
  drugs, 296–297
  percutaneous coronary interventions, 297
Norepinephrine (NE), 85, 93, 118t, 135, 137, 139t
  on bronchial airflow, 135, 137
  metabolism, 121f
  synthesis, storage, and release, 122f
Norepinephrine (NE) receptors, 122f
Norfloxacin, 544, 544f, 545, 548t
Nortriptyline, 150t, 173t
Nuclear factor of activated T lymphocytes (NFAT), 383
Nuclear receptors, 3t. *See also specific types*
  drug metabolism, 33t, 34f
Nucleoside reverse transcriptase inhibitors (NRTIs), 601t, 603t, 607f, 608f, 621t
  abacavir, 601t, 603t, 607f, 608f, 621t
  adverse effects, 615
  didanosine, 601t, 603t, 607f, 608f, 621t
  emtricitabine, 601t, 603t, 607f, 608f, 621t
  HIV, 614–615
  lamivudine, 601t, 602t, 607f, 621t
  mechanisms of action and resistance, 602t–603t, 604f, 608f, 614–615
  stavudine, 601t, 603t, 607f, 608f, 621t
  structures, 607f
  tenofovir disoproxil, 601t–603t, 607f, 608f, 621t
  zalcitabine, 601t, 621t
  zidovudine, 601t, 602t, 607f, 608f, 621t
Nystatin, 599t

O
Octreotide, 422t, 428t
  antidiarrheal, 498t, 508t
Ocular administration, elderly, 74t
Ocular pharmacology, 690–706
  absorption pathways, 697f
  antibacterials, topical, 692t–693t
  antifungals, 694t, 701
  antihistamines and mast cell stabilizers, 691t, 705t
    azelastine, 691t, 705t
    bepotastine, 691t, 705t
    cromolyn sodium, 691t, 705t
    emedastine difumarate, 691t, 705t
    epinastine, 691t, 705t
    ketotifen fumarate, 691t, 705t
    lodoxamide tromethamine, 691t, 705t
    nedocromil, 691t, 705t
    olopatadine, 691t, 705t
    pemirolast, 691t, 705t
  antivirals, 693t, 701
  autonomic agents, 690t–691t, 695t, 700, 704t–705t
    acetylcholine, 690t, 695t, 704t
    apraclonidine, 690t, 695t, 702, 703, 704t
    atropine, 690t, 695t, 704t
    betaxolol, 691t, 695t, 704t
    brimonidine, 690t, 695t, 704t
    carbachol, 690t, 695t, 704t
    carteolol, 691t, 695t, 704t
    cyclopentolate, 690t, 695t, 705t
    dipivefrin, 690t, 695t, 704t
    echothiophate, 690t, 695t, 704t
    homatropine, 690t, 695t, 704t
    levobunolol, 691t, 695t, 704t
    metipranolol, 691t, 695t, 704t
    naphazoline, 690t, 695t, 705t
    phenylephrine, 690t, 695t, 705t
    pilocarpine, 690t, 695t, 704t
    scopolamine, 690t, 695t, 704t
    tetrahydrozoline, 690t, 695t, 705t
    timolol, 691t, 695t, 696–697, 697f, 704t
    tropicamide, 690t, 695t, 705t
  carbonic anhydrase inhibitors, 691t, 705t
    brinzolamide, 691t, 705t
    dorzolamide, 691t, 705t
  glucocorticoids, 691t, 705t
    dexamethasone, 691t, 705t
    difluprednate, 691t, 705t
    fluocinolone, 691t, 705t
    fluorometolone, 691t, 705t
    loteprednol, 691t, 705t
    prednisolone, 691t, 705t
    rimexolone, 691t, 705t
    triamcinolone, 691t, 705t
  immunosuppressives and antimitotics, 691t, 705t
    5-fluorouracil (FU), 691t, 705t
    cyclosporine A, 691t, 705t
    mitomycin, 691t, 705t
  Jimson weed, 694f, 698, 698t
  macular degeneration agents, 692t, 706t
    bevacizumab, 692t, 706t
    pegaptanib, 692t, 706t
    ranibizumab, 692t, 706t
    verteporfin, 692t, 703, 706t
  mydriasis, 694f, 698, 698t
  NSAIDs, 691t, 705t
    bromfenac, 691t, 705t
    diclofenac, 691t, 705t
    flurbiprofen, 691t, 705t
    ketorolac, 691t, 705t
    nepafenac, 691t, 705t
  prostaglandin analogs, 691t, 705t
    bimatoprost, 691t, 705t
    latanoprost, 691t, 705t
    travoprost, 691t, 705t
  route of administration, 697t
  strabismus and blepharospasm agents, 692t, 706t
    abobotulinumtoxin A, 692t, 706t
    onabotulinumtoxin A, 692t, 706t
  surgery agents, ophthalmic, 691t–692t, 706t
    chondroitin sulfate, 692t, 706t
    cyanoacrylate, 692t, 706t
    fibrogen gel, 692t, 706t
    hyaluronate, 692t, 706t
    hydroxypropyl methylcellulose, 692t, 706t
    polydimethylsiloxanes, 692t, 706t
    povidone iodine, 691t, 706t
    vitreous substitutes, 692t, 706t
  systemic drugs with ocular adverse effects, 696t
  wetting agents/tear substitutes, 692t, 706t
    carboxymethylcellulose, 692t, 706t
    hydroxyethyl cellulose, 692t, 706t
    hydroxypropyl cellulose, 692t, 706t
    hydroxypropyl methylcellulose, 692t, 706t
    methylcellulose, 692t, 706t
    tyloxapol, 692t, 706t
Ocular route of administration, 697t
Ofatumumab, 662t, 684t
Office of Pediatric Therapeutics (OPT), FDA, 72b
Off-target interactions, 5b
Ofloxacin, 544, 544f, 545, 548t
Olanzapine, 130t, 147t, 151t, 165, 168, 170t, 171–172, 175t
Olmesartan medoxomil, 273t, 285t
Olopatadine, 347t, 355t
  ophthalmic, 691t, 705t
Olsalazine, 357t, 373t
  inflammatory bowel disease, 498t, 503f, 506, 507, 509t
  NSAID properties, 357t, 373t
Omalizumab, 390t, 397, 404t
Omeprazole, 490t, 493f, 496t
Onabotulinum toxin A, 106t, 117t
Onabotulinumtoxin A, 692t, 706t
Onabotulinumtoxin, A ophthalmic, 692t, 706t
Onchocerciasis (*Onchocerca volvulus*), 537–540
Ondansetron
  antidiarrheal, 498t, 501, 502t, 505, 506, 508t
  chemotherapy prophylaxis, 505, 506
  mechanisms of action, 498t
  pharmacology, 130t, 133t, 147t
1α-Hydroxycholecalciferol, 481t, 488t
1α-Hydroxylase, 482f, 486, 487
Onychomycosis, 595–596, 721, 722
Ophthalmic, brinzolamide, 691t, 705t
Ophthalmic pharmacology. *See* Ocular pharmacology
Ophthalmic surgery agents, 691t–692t, 706t
  chondroitin sulfate, 692t, 706t
  cyanoacrylate, 692t, 706t
  fibrogen gel, 692t, 706t
  hyaluronate, 692t, 706t

hydroxypropyl methylcellulose, 692t, 706t
polydimethylsiloxanes, 692t, 706t
povidone iodine, 691t, 706t
vitreous substitutes, 692t, 706t
Opiates. See also Opioid pharmacology; specific types
   adverse effects
      constipation, 198–199
      mood, reward, and addiction, 197–198, 198f
      respiratory depression, 196b, 199
   elderly, 71, 77b
Opioid addiction, 259–262, 260f, 261t
   overdose, 260
   tolerance, 260
   withdrawal, 260, 261t
Opioid addiction treatment, 260–262
   buprenorphine and buprenorphine/naloxone, 261–262
   clonidine, 261
   detoxification, 260–261
   methadone, 260–261
   naltrexone, 262
Opioid antagonists, bowel disorders
   alvimopan, 498t, 507t
   mechanisms of action, 498t
   methylnaltrexone, 498t, 499, 505, 506, 507t
Opioid pharmacology. See also specific drugs and drug classes
   actions and receptor selectivities, 194t–195t
   adverse effects
      constipation, 198–199
      respiratory depression, 196b, 199, 201
   antidiarrheals, 195t, 209t
   antitussives, 196t, 209t, 210t
   dosing data, 200t
   drug-related deaths, 51t
   mechanisms of action, 195t–196t
      analgesia, 196–197, 196f, 197f
      mood, reward, and addiction, 197–198, 198f
   metabolism, first-pass, 206, 207
   pain
      guidelines, 201t
      target and site of action, 205t
   pain, cancer
      methadone, 201–203, 202t
      routes of administration, 202–203
   pain states, 197b, 197f
   tolerance, 206, 207
   toxidrome, 53t
   withdrawal, 260, 261t
Opioid receptor agonist/antagonists and partial agonists, 194t–195t, 209t
   actions and receptor selectivities, 194t–195t
   buprenorphine, 194t, 195t, 200t, 203, 209t
   butorphanol, 194t, 195t, 200t, 203, 209t
   dosing, 200t
   mechanisms of action, 195t
   nalbuphine, 195t, 200t, 209t
   pentazocine, 195t, 209t

Opioid receptor agonists, 194t–195t, 201–208, 202t, 208t–209t
   actions and receptor selectivities, 194t–195t
   adjuvant analgesic use, 205, 207
   alfentanil, 195t, 208t
   codeine, 195t, 200t, 206, 208, 208t
   dosing, 200t
   fentanyl, 194t, 195t, 203, 205–207, 208t
   hydrocodone, 195t, 200t, 208t
   hydromorphone, 194t, 195t, 200t, 208t
   levorphanol, 194t, 195t, 200t, 209t
   mechanisms of action, 195t
   meperidine, 195t, 200t, 204, 208t
   methadone, 194t, 195t, 200t, 201–203, 202t, 208t
   morphine, 194t, 195t, 200t, 206–208, 208t
   oxycodone, 195t, 200t, 208t
   oxymorphone, 195t, 200t, 208t
   propoxyphene, 195t, 200t, 208t
   remifentanil, 195t, 208t
   sufentanil, 194t, 195t, 205, 207, 208t
   tapentadol, 195t, 209t
   tramadol, 195t, 200t, 209t
Opioid receptor antagonists, 203–205, 209t
   actions and receptor selectivities, 195t
   mechanisms of action, 195t
   methylnaltrexone, 195t, 199, 209t
   naloxone, 195t, 203–204, 205, 207, 209t
   naltrexone, 193t, 195t, 209t
   therapeutic uses, 203–204
Oprelvekin, 406t, 410–411, 419t
Oral administration, 21t. See also specific agents
   bioavailability, infant, 72, 74
   elderly, 73t
Oral contraceptives, 441t–444t, 448–450, 458t. See also Contraceptives, oral; Estrogen antagonists; Estrogens; specific agents
Organic anion-transporting polypeptide (OATP), 24b, 38
Organophosphates, 53t, 63, 64, 102, 102b, 103f, 103t, 104f
   diphenhydramine, 40t, 42t, 65t
   insecticides, 100t, 102, 102b, 103t, 104f, 115t
   mechanisms, 100t
   nerve gases, 100t, 103t, 116t
   poisoning, 63, 64
   symptoms, 102, 102b
   toxidrome, 53t
Organ transplant therapy
   general principles, 378b
   immunosuppressant risks/adverse effects, 378–379, 378b, 379
   immunotherapeutic agents (See Immunotherapeutic agents; specific agents)
   pre-transplantation, 378
   rejection prophylaxis, 378–379
Orthostatic hypertension, 306, 306b
Orthosteric site, 3b
Oseltamivir, 601t, 602t, 604f, 620t
Osmotic diuretics, 268t, 271t, 283t
   glycerin, 268t, 283t
   isosorbide, 268t, 283t

   mannitol, 268t, 283t
   urea, 268t, 283t
Osteoclast formation, RANKL, 482f
Osteodystrophy, renal, 482f, 484
   vitamin D, 481t, 482f, 484, 488t
Osteomalacia, 484
Osteonecrosis of jaw, bisphosphonate, 481t, 485, 488t
Osteoporosis. See also Bisphosphonates
   denosumab, 488t
   ibandronate, 481t, 485, 488t
   teriparatide, 481t, 488t
   types and pathophysiology, 482f, 484–485
   zoledronate, 481t, 485, 488t
22-Oxacalcitrol, 481t, 488t
Oxacillin, 551, 552t, 554, 555, 555t
Oxaliplatin, 628t, 653t
   mechanisms of action, 628b–629b, 628t, 630f, 633
   mechanisms of resistance, 628t, 632b, 634–635
   toxicities, 632b–633b, 633–634
   uses, 629t, 653t
Oxazepam, 176t, 189, 190, 191t, 192t
   alcohol withdrawal, 256
Oxazolidinones, 569t, 576t
Oxcarbazepine, 225t, 236t
Oxiconazole, 588t, 598t
Oxidative reactions, metabolic, 32t
Oxybutynin, 96t, 99t, 100, 101b, 101t, 113t
Oxycodone, 195t, 200t, 208t
   concerns, 254
   dependence, physical, 264, 266
   dose doubling, 255, 255t
   dose-response curves, idealized, 255, 256f
   long-acting, 256
   tolerance, 255, 256t
   toxidrome, 53t
Oxycodone-acetaminophen toxicity, 28–29, 50–54, 50f, 52t, 207, 208
Oxygen gas, therapeutic, 211t, 223t
Oxymetazoline, 120t, 136, 137, 142t
Oxymorphone, 195t, 200t, 208t
Oxytocin, 424f

P

PA-824, 579t, 587t
Paclitaxel, 642t, 648–650, 656t
   mechanisms of action, 630f, 642t, 648–650
   mechanisms of resistance, 642t, 644b
   toxicities, 656t
   uses, 644t, 656t
Paget disease
   bisphosphonates, 481t, 488t (See also Bisphosphonates)
   calcitonin, 481t, 488t
Pain
   breakthrough, 202, 206, 207
   incident, 202
   mechanisms, 196–197, 196f, 197f
   targets and sites of action, 205t
Pain, cancer
   methadone, 201–203, 202t
   routes of administration, 202–203

Pain management. *See also specific agents*
　　anticonvulsants, 205t
　　COX-2 inhibitors, 205t
　　drug targets and sites of action, 205t
　　morphine and opiates, 192f, 196b, 197, 199, 205t (*See also* Opioid pharmacology)
　　NSAIDs, 205t
　　opioid (*See* Opioid pharmacology)
　　tricyclic antidepressants, 205t
Pain states, 197b, 197f. *See also* Opioid pharmacology
Paliperidone, 151t, 170t, 175t
Palonosetron, 130t, 147t
2-PAM, 41t, 42t, 65t
Pamidronate, 481t, 488t
Panaeolus, 97
Pancreatic β cell, 471f, 472f, 473
Pancuronium, 97f, 105f, 106f, 106t, 107t, 116t
Panitumumab, 662t, 669–672, 683t
Pantoprazole, 490t, 493f, 496t
Papillary thyroid cancer, 436
Para-aminophenol derivative. *See* Acetaminophen
Paracellular transport, 19b, 19f
Paraldehyde, 177t, 193t
Parasympathetic nervous system, 82f, 85, 92, 107t
Parathion, 101t
Parathyroid hormone (PTH), 483
Parecoxib, 363t
Paricalcitol, 481t, 488t
Parkinsonism, 172t
Parkinson's disease, 239–245, 250–251
　　basal ganglia, 240–241, 241f
　　cardinal features, 239b
　　dopamine neurotransmission, 240–241, 241f
　　dopamine synthesis, neuronal, 239, 240f
　　pathophysiology, 239
　　prognosis, 241
Parkinson's disease drugs, 239–245, 250–251, 252t–253t
　　amantadine, 239t, 242t, 245, 253t
　　apomorphine, 239t, 242t, 253t
　　bromocriptine, 242t
　　carbidopa, 238t, 244f
　　carbidopa/levodopa, 238t, 242, 250, 251, 252t
　　dosing, 242t
　　early treatment options, 242–243, 242t, 252t–253t
　　entacapone, 238t, 242t, 244f, 251, 252t
　　levodopa, 238t, 242–245, 243f, 244f, 252t
　　mechanisms of action, 238t–239t
　　pramipexole, 238t, 242t, 245, 250–252, 252t
　　rasagiline, 239t, 242t, 244f, 245, 253t
　　ropinirole, 238t, 242t, 245, 250, 251, 252t
　　selegiline, 238t, 242t, 244f, 245, 250, 251, 253t
　　tolcapone, 238t, 242t, 244f, 252t
　　trihexyphenidyl HCl, 242t
Paromomycin, 531t, 532–533, 535t
Paroxetine, 130t, 146t, 150t, 157, 174t

Paroxysmal ventricular tachycardia (PSVT), 314t, 318
Partial agonist, 4b, 4f, 7b, 9
Passive diffusion, 19b, 19f
　　kidney, 20b
Passive immunization, 377t–378t, 381t
Passive transport, 19b, 19f
Pathological toxicity, 46t
Patient-controlled analgesia (PCA), 202
Peak effect, 36f
Peak plasma concentration, 514, 515, 515f, 519
Pediatric Research Equity Act of 2003 (PREA), 71b
Pediatrics. *See* Children
Pegaspargase (PEG-L-asparaginase), 643t, 659t
Pegfilgrastim, 405t, 407t, 408f, 409–410, 418t
Peginterferon alpha, 613–614
Peginterferons, 601t
Pegvisomant, 422t, 424, 425f, 428t
Pegylated recombinant GCSF (pegfilgrastim), 405t, 407t, 408f, 409–410, 418t
Pemetrexed (MTA), 635t, 638b, 640, 653t
　　mechanisms and sites of action, 630f, 635t, 639
　　mechanisms of resistance, 635t, 638b, 640
　　uses, 637t
Pemirolast, ophthalmic, 691t, 705t
Pemoline, 120t, 141t
Penbutolol, 128t
Penciclovir, 600t, 602t, 604f, 605, 605f, 608, 619t
Penetration, drug. *See* Barrier penetration
Penicillamine, 42t, 66t
Penicillin G, 552, 555t
Penicillins, 549t, 555t–556t
　　allergy, 550f, 552, 554, 555
　　aminoglycoside inactivation, 565, 566
　　amoxicillin, 552t, 555t
　　ampicillin, 552t, 555t
　　azlocillin, 552t
　　carbenicillin, 552t, 556t
　　classification, 552t
　　mechanisms of action, 549t, 550–551, 550f
　　mezlocillin, 552t, 556t
　　penicillinase-resistant, 554, 555
　　　　cloxacillin, 551, 552t, 555t
　　　　dicloxacillin, 551, 552t, 555t
　　　　methicillin, 551, 552t
　　　　nafcillin, 551, 552t, 554, 555, 555t
　　　　oxacillin, 551, 552t, 555t
　　penicillin G and V, 552, 555t
　　piperacillin, 552t, 556t
　　resistance, 549t, 550b, 551f
　　structures, 550f
　　ticarcillin, 552t, 556t
　　toxicity/allergy, 55–56
Penicillin V, 552, 555t
Pentamidine, 531t, 535t
Pentazocine, 195t, 209t
Pentobarbital, 177t, 181t, 192t
Pentostatin, 636t, 656t

　　mechanisms of action, 630f, 636t, 641–642
　　uses, 637t
Pentoxifylline, 295b
Peptic ulcer disease, 571
Percutaneous absorption, 710b, 711–715, 711t, 713f
　　elderly, 74t
　　important considerations, 711–712, 711t
　　rate-limiting step, 721, 722
　　for topical infections, 714–715
　　vehicles, 712–714, 712t
Pergolide, 130t, 148t
Perindopril, 273t, 285t
Perioral tremor, 172t
Peripheral nervous system (PNS) neurotransmitters, 83t–84t, 86b, 92
Peripheral vascular disease, 295b
Permethrin, 708t, 725t
Pernicious anemia, 417–418. *See also* Vitamin B_{12} deficiency
Peroxisome proliferator-activated receptors (PPARs), 341, 342
Perphenazine, 150t, 174t
Pesticide poisoning, 89
PGE1 analog, 356t
pH
　　diffusion, 19–20, 19b–20b, 19f, 20f, 35, 37–38
　　tissue uptake, 21b
　　urine, excretion, 20b, 21–22
Pharmacodynamics, 2–17. *See also specific drugs and drug classes*
　　active ingredient, 3
　　adverse effects, 4–6, 5b, 9–12
　　affinity (K_A), 6b, 8
　　allergy drug case study, 3–6
　　antihistamine, 3
　　competitive antagonists, 4b, 5b, 5f, 7b, 16, 17
　　concentration–response curve, 6b, 6f, 11f, 12
　　definition, 2b
　　dose–response curves, 4f–7f, 8–9
　　drug development, 6–9
　　drug–receptor interactions, 3b–5b, 4f
　　efficacy, 4b, 4f, 7b, 7f, 9
　　equilibrium association constant (K_A), 6b, 8
　　equilibrium dissociation constant (K_D), 6b, 8, 16, 17
　　fractional occupancy (*f*), 7b, 8
　　genetic polymorphisms, 10t, 12–14, 13f
　　half-maximal effective concentration (EC_{50}), 6f, 7b, 9
　　imatinib, 14–15
　　interindividual variability, 12
　　inverse agonists, 4, 4b, 4f, 9, 16, 17
　　ionization, kidney tubules, 21–22
　　postmarketing surveillance, 9–11, 46–48
　　resistance, 15
　　specificity, 5b, 9
　　therapeutic index, 11, 11f, 39b, 62, 64
　　therapeutic window, 11, 12, 12f, 16, 17, 35b, 36f
　　warfarin sensitivity, 10t, 12–14, 13f, 329b–330b

765

Pharmacogenetics. *See also* CYP (cytochrome P-450 superfamily); *specific drugs*
  folic acid analogs, 637f, 639
  high-dose methotrexate with leucovorin rescue (HDM-L), 635t, 637f, 638–640, 639
  methotrexate, 637f, 639
  warfarin dosing, 10t, 12–14, 13f
Pharmacokinetics, 18–39. *See also specific drugs and drug classes*
  absorption, 20b, 20f
  acetaminophen, 28–29, 50–54, 50f, 52t, 207, 208
  administration (*See also* Administration)
    repeated, 38b, 38f
    route of, 20b, 21t
  bioavailability, 20b, 33b
  biotransforming enzymes, 29b, 29t
  blood-brain barrier, 19–20, 19b–20b, 19f, 20f, 28f, 35, 37–38
  clearance, 33b, 35, 35b–36b, 36f, 37f, 39
  clinical, 33b–34b
  clopidogrel dosing, 22, 28, 331–332
  definition, 2b
  digoxin, 30–34, 308t
  diphenhydramine, 19–20, 40t, 65t (*See also* Diphenhydramine)
  distribution, 20f, 21b
    CNS, 24b
  dosing, 30–31
  drug interactions, 28
  elimination t1/2, 34b, 37f, 39b
  excretion, 20f
    weak acids, 36, 39
  first-pass effect, 20b, 22, 35, 36–37
  genetic polymorphisms, 10t, 12–14, 13f
  interindividual variability, 12
    drug response and toxicity, 22, 24b, 28, 34b
  ionization, plasma–gastric juice partitioning, 19b–20b, 20f, 21–22
  ionization state, 19–20, 19b–20b, 20f
  long-term therapy, rational, 35, 39
  metabolism, 20b, 28–29, 28b, 32t
    phase 1, 28b, 33f, 35, 38
  movement and availability characteristics, 18b
  nitroglycerin, first-pass effect, 22, 291, 299
  passive *vs.* active transport, 19b, 19f
  pH and diffusion, 19–22, 19b–20b, 19f, 20f, 35, 37–38
  pK$_a$, 19b–20b, 20f
  plasma protein binding, 22b
  rate of distribution and equilibration, 20f, 36b–37b, 37f
  steady state, 19f, 30–31, 34, 38b
  St. John's wort, 29–30, 33f, 34f
  tissue binding, 22b–23b
  transporters
    ABC, 23t, 23t–25t
    membrane, 23b–24b, 23t–25t
    SLC superfamily, 23b–24b, 25t–26t

Pharmacokinetics, children
  absorption, 67b
  distribution, 68b
  excretion, 69b
  metabolism, 70b
  plasma protein binding, 68b
Pharmacokinetics, elderly
  absorption and bioavailability, 73b, 73t–74t
  clearance, 75b, 76f, 76t–77t, 77f
  distribution and volume of distribution, 74b, 75t
  excretion, 76b, 78t
  first-pass clearance, 73t–74t
  half-life, 77f
  metabolism, 73t–74t, 75b
  plasma concentration–time curves, 73f, 73t
  plasma protein binding, 74b, 75t
  tissue binding, 75t
Phase 1 functionalization, 28b, 33f, 35, 38
  neonatal, 70b
Phase 1 metabolism, 28b, 33f, 35, 38
  neonatal, 70b
Phase 2 conjugation, 28–29, 28b, 33f, 35, 39
  neonatal, 70b
Phenazopyridine, 548t
Phenelzine, 130t, 147t, 150t, 173t
Phenindamine, 346t, 354t
Phenobarbital, 177t, 181t, 189, 190, 192t
Phenoxybenzamine, 120t, 136, 137, 141t
Phentolamine, 120t, 141t
Phenylephrine, 119t, 139t
  ophthalmic, 690t, 695t, 705t
Phenytoin
  antiseizure, 225t, 231, 234, 235, 236t
  electrophysiologic actions, 316
Pheochromocytoma, 136, 137
Philadelphia chromosome-positive (Ph+) chronic myelogenous leukemia, 664–669
  first-line treatment, 665–666
  molecular mechanism, 665–666
Phosphate binders, 481t, 484, 488t
  lanthanum carbonate, 481t, 484, 488t
  mechanisms of action, 481t, 488t
  renal osteodystrophy, 482f, 484
  sevelamer hydrochloride, 481t, 484, 488t
Phosphodiesterase 3 (PDE3) inhibitors, heart failure, 307, 309, 310, 311t
  inamrinone, 302t, 308, 308t, 311t
  mechanisms of action, 302t, 308
  milrinone, 302t, 308, 308t, 311t
  pharmacology, 308t
Phosphodiesterase 5 (PDE5) inhibitors
  myocardial ischemia, 300t
    nitrate interactions, 291b, 292
    sildenafil, 300t
    tadalafil, 300t
    vardenafil, 300t
  ocular effects, 703
  pulmonary, 391t, 404t
    adverse effects, 398, 399f, 400
    mechanisms of action, 391t
    pulmonary artery hypertension, 398–400, 399f

    sildenafil, 391t, 398–402, 399f, 404t
    tadalafil, 391t, 398–402, 399f, 404t
Photochemotherapy, 707t, 716t, 725t
  methoxsalen, 707t, 716t, 725t
  photopheresis, 716t
  PUVA, 716–717, 716t, 725t
  trioxsalen, 716t
Photodynamic therapy, 708t, 716t, 725t
  aminolevulinic acid, 708t, 725t
  methyl aminolevulinate, 708t, 725t
Photopheresis, 716t
Physiological receptors, 2b, 3t
Physostigmine (salicylate), 41t, 100t, 102, 114t
  antidote, 42t, 65t, 102
  mechanisms of action, 100t
Pilocarpine, 95t, 99t, 112t
  mechanisms of action, 95t
  ophthalmic, 690t, 695t, 704t
  pharmacology, 99t
  uses and toxicities, 112t
Pilocarpine hydrochloride, 95t, 99t, 112t
Pimecrolimus, 708t, 724t, 726t
Pindolol, 126t, 128t, 145t
Pioglitazone, 470t, 475–476, 479t
Pipecuronium, 97f, 105f, 106f, 106t, 107t, 116t
Piperacillin, 552t, 556t
Piperazines, 352
Pirbuterol
  pharmacology, 125t, 143t
  pulmonary, 389t, 402t
Pitavastatin (calcium), 334t, 343t
Pituitary adenoma, prolactin-secreting, 426
Pituitary gland
  anterior, 424f
  posterior, 424f
Pituitary hormones, posterior, 423t, 429t
  arginine vasopressin, 423t, 424f, 429t (*See also* Vasopressin)
  oxytocin, 423t, 424f, 430t
pK$_a$, 19–20, 19b–20b, 20f, 35, 37–38
Plasma concentration–time curves, 36b, 37f
  elderly, 73f, 73t
Plasma–gastric juice partitioning, 19b–20b, 20f, 21–22
Plasma protein binding, 22b
  children, 68b
  elderly, 74b, 75t
Plasmodium falciparum treatment, 579t, 581f, 583–586, 587t
Platelet-activating factor (PAF), 359f
Platelet adhesion and aggregation, 324, 324f
Platelet drugs. *See* Antiplatelet agents
Platinum coordination complexes, 628t, 633–635, 653t
  carboplatin, 628t, 629t, 653t
  cell cycle specificity, 630f
  cisplatin, 628t, 629t, 632t, 653t
  mechanisms of action, 628t, 630f, 633
  mechanisms of resistance, 628t, 632b, 634–635
  oxaliplatin, 628t, 629t, 653t
  toxicities, 632b–633b, 632t, 633–634, 653t
  uses, 629t, 653t

Plicamycin, 481t, 488t
Podophyllin, 727t
Poisoning. *See also* Toxicity, clinical and environmental; *specific poisons*
   ABDE treatment, 52t
   initial treatment, 63, 64
   largest number fatalities, 52t
   management, 50–52
      initial, 63, 64
      principles, 50–52
   most common substances, 51t
   most frequent substances, 51, 51t
   pharmacokinetics, 52
   prevention, children, 62–64
Polyclonal antibodies, 376t, 377f, 377t–378t, 378, 385t
Polycystic ovary syndrome, 452
Polydimethylsiloxanes, ophthalmic, 692t, 706t
Polyethylene glycol, 497t, 507t
Polymixins, 573
   polymyxin B, 569t, 576t
   polymyxin E, 569t, 576t
Polymorphisms, genetic
   CYP, 27t, 28, 31b (*See also* CYP (cytochrome P-450 superfamily))
   drug response, 10t, 12–14, 13f, 27t
Polymyxin-bacitracin-neosporin, 569t, 573, 576t, 577t
Polysaccharide ferrihydrite complex, 406t, 419t
Polythiazide, 269t, 284t
Pork tapeworm, 539, 540
Posaconazole, 588t, 589f, 590, 597t
Postantibiotic effect (PAE), 515
   cephalosporins, 564, 565
Posterior pituitary hormones, 423t, 429t
   arginine vasopressin, 423t, 424f, 429t (*See also* Vasopressin)
   oxytocin, 423t, 424f, 430t
Postmarketing surveillance, 9–11, 46–48
Postsynaptic potentials, autonomic, 106f
Potency, 7b, 7f
Potency, relative, 7f
Potentiation
   drug–drug interaction, 48b
   mechanisms, 4b, 5f
Povidone iodine, ophthalmic, 691t, 706t
Pralatrexate, 635t, 639, 653t
Pralidoxime chloride (2-PAM), 41t, 42t, 65t, 100t, 102, 116t
   mechanisms of action, 100t, 104f
   uses and toxicities, 41t, 42t, 65t, 100t, 102, 116t
Pramipexole
   Parkinson's disease, 238t, 242t, 245, 250, 251, 252, 252t
   pharmacology, 130t, 148t
Pramlintide, 471t, 479t
Pramoxine, 224t
Prasugrel, 323t, 324, 325, 325t, 332t
   bioactivation, 325t
   mechanisms of action, 323t, 330, 331

Pravastatin (calcium), 334t, 343t
Prazosin
   antihypertensive, 277t, 286t
   pharmacology, 119t, 121–124, 123f, 140t
Precocious puberty, 422t, 427, 428, 429t
Prednisolone
   ophthalmic, 691t, 705t
   pulmonary, 390t, 403t
Prednisone. *See also* Corticosteroids
   adverse effects, 467, 468
   cancer
      chemotherapy, 664t, 679t, 686t
      target, 664t, 679t, 686t
   cessation, adverse effects, 465
   Crohn's disease, 465, 467, 468
   dose tapering, 465
   pulmonary, 390t, 403t
   rheumatoid arthritis, 463–465
Pregabalin, 225t, 237t
Pregnancy, 365
   FDA rules, 72b
   iron supplements, 406t, 413–414, 419t
Prehypertension, 269–270, 270t
Premature ventricular beats, 314t
   post-MI, 314t, 319, 320
Pre-surgery prophylaxis, 515b, 516
Prilocaine, 224t
Primaquine
   G6PD deficiency, 527, 528
   malaria
      chemoprophylaxis, 522t, 525–526
      chemotherapy, 521t, 522t, 525–526, 526t, 527, 529t
      mechanisms of action, 521t
      parasite development stage, 526t
      regimens, 522t
Primary agonists, 3b, 8
Primary site, 3b, 8
Prinzmetal angina, 290t, 291f, 297. *See also* Myocardial ischemia
Probenecid, 369t, 370, 374t
Procainamide, 312t, 317t
   antiarrhythmic, 312t, 316, 317t, 320t
   electrophysiologic actions, 317t
   ventricular fibrillation, 316
Procaine, 224t
Procarbazine, 628t, 652t
   mechanisms of action, 628b–629b, 628t, 630f
   mechanisms of resistance, 628t, 632–633, 632b
   toxicities, 632b–633b, 652t
   uses, 629t, 652t
Procaterol, 125t, 143t
Prodrugs, 28b
Progesterone micronized, 442t, 445t, 458t
Progesterone receptor antagonists, 442t, 458t
Progesterone receptor modulator, selective, ulipristal, 442t, 444t, 452, 458t
Progesterone slow-release intrauterine device, 442t, 458t
Progesterone vaginal gel, 442t, 458t
Progesterone vaginal insert, 442t, 458t
Progestins
   anticancer, 664t, 679t, 686t

      hydroxyprogesterone caproate, 679t
      medroxyprogesterone, 664t, 679t, 686t
      megestrol acetate, 664t, 679t, 686t
   hormone replacement therapy, 442t, 458t
   mechanisms of action, 442t, 458t
   medroxyprogesterone acetate (MPA), 442t, 458t
   megestrol acetate, 442t, 458t
   progesterone micronized, 442t, 445t, 458t
   progesterone slow-release intrauterine device, 442t, 458t
   progesterone vaginal gel, 442t, 458t
   progesterone vaginal insert, 442t, 458t
   structural features, 451f
Proguanil, 520t, 529t
Prokinetics, bowel disorders, 497t, 507t
   cisapride, 497t, 504, 506, 507t
   domperidone, 497t, 507t
   erythromycin, 497t, 507t
   lubiprostone, 497t, 507t
   mechanisms of action, 497
   metoclopramide, 497t, 504, 506, 507t
   prucalopride, 497t, 507t
Prolactin
   GH receptor antagonism, 423, 425f
   secretion and actions, 424f, 425f
Prolactin-secreting pituitary adenoma, 426
Promethazine, 350–352, 354t
   antiemetic, 351, 352, 502t
   cold medication, 346t, 350
   mechanisms of action, 346t
   motion sickness, 352
Propafenone
   antiarrhythmic, 312t, 317t, 321t
   electrophysiologic actions, 317t
Proparacaine, 224t
Propionic acid derivatives, 362t–363t, 373t
   fenoprofen, 362t, 373t
   flurbiprofen, 357t, 363t, 373t
   ibuprofen, 357t, 362t, 364–365, 373t
   ketoprofen, 357t, 363t, 373t
   naproxen, 357t, 362t, 373t
   oxaprozin, 357t, 363t, 373t
Propofol
   anesthetic, 210t, 213t, 214f, 220, 221, 222t
   context-sensitive half-time, 214f
   sedative-hypnotic, 177t, 193t
   use, common, 220, 221
Propoxur, 100t, 115t
Propoxyphene, 195t, 200t, 208t
Propranolol
   antiarrhythmic, 312t, 317t, 321t
   electrophysiologic actions, 317t
   myocardial ischemia, 300t
   pharmacology, 125t, 128t, 136, 138, 144t
Propylhexedrine, 120t, 142t
Propylthiouracil, 431t, 439t
Prostacyclin (PG_{I2}) and analogs, 391t, 404t
   adverse effects, 400
   epoprostenol, 391t, 398–400, 399f, 404t

iloprost, 391t, 404t
mechanisms of action, 391t
treprostinil, 391t, 404t
Prostaglandins and analogs
  mechanisms of action, 356t–357t
  ophthalmic, 691t, 705t
    bimatoprost, 691t, 705t
    latanoprost, 691t, 705t
    travoprost, 691t, 705t
  PGE_1, 356t, 372t
    alprostadil, 356t, 372t
  PGE_1 analog, 356t, 372t
    misoprostol, 356t, 372t
  PGE_2, 356t, 372t
    dinoprostone, 356t, 372t
  $PGE_2\alpha$ analog, 356t, 372t
    bimatoprost, 356t, 372t
    carboprost, 356t, 372t
    latanoprost, 356t, 372t
    travoprost, 356t, 372t
    tromethamine, 356t, 372t
  PGI_2, 357t, 372t
    prostacyclin, 357t, 372t
  PGI_2 analog, 357t, 372t
    iloprost, 357t, 372t
    treprostinil, 357t, 372t
Prostate cancer
  flutamide, 442t, 454, 456, 457, 679t
  leuprolide, 423t, 425–426, 429t
  metastatic, 678–680
Protease inhibitors, 601t, 603t, 621t–622t
  amprenavir, 601t, 603t, 608f, 609f, 622t
  atazanavir, 601t, 603t, 608f, 609f, 622t
  darunavir, 601t, 603t, 608f, 609f, 622t
  indinavir, 601t, 603t, 608f, 609f, 621t
  lopinavir, 601t, 603t, 615, 622t
  mechanisms of action and resistance, 603t, 608f, 609f
  nelfinavir, 601t, 603t, 608f, 609f, 622t
  ritonavir, 601t, 603t, 608f, 609f, 615–619, 622t
  saquinavir, 601t, 603t, 608f, 609f, 621t
  tipranavir, 601t, 603t, 608f, 609f, 622t
Proteasome inhibitors, 663t, 681, 682–683, 685t
Protein binding, drug–drug interactions on, 48t
Protein drug receptors, 2b
Protein synthesis inhibitors, 568–577
  aminocyclitols, spectinomycin, 569t, 576t
  bacitracin, 569t, 577t
  chloramphenicol, 568t, 569f, 571, 576t
  lincosamides, clindamycin, 568t, 574, 575, 576t
  macrolides and ketolides, 568t, 570f, 576t
    azithromycin, 568t, 570f, 576t
    clarithromycin, 568t, 570f, 571, 576t
    drug interactions, 572
    erythromycin, 568t, 570f, 576t
    telithromycin, 568t, 570f, 576t
    toxicities, 571
  mechanisms of action, 568t–569t, 569f, 570f
  MRSA, 571
neosporin, 573
Oxazolidinones, linezolid, 569t, 576t
streptogramins, quinupristin/dalfopristin, 568t, 572, 575, 576b
tetracyclines, 568t, 569f, 576t
  doxycycline, 568t, 569f, 571, 576t
  food contraindications, 574, 575
  MRSA infections, 571
  photosensitivity, 574, 575
  tetracycline, 568t, 569f, 576t
  tigecycline, 568t, 569f, 576t
Protein tyrosine kinase inhibitors, 661t, 683t
  dasatinib, 661t, 668, 683t
  erlotinib, 661t, 670–672, 683t
  gefitinib, 661t, 670–672, 683t
  imatinib mesylate, 661t, 666–669, 681, 682, 683t
  lapatinib, 661t, 673, 683t
  mechanisms of resistance, 661t
  nilotinib, 661t, 668, 683t
  sorafenib, 661t, 674, 683t
  sunitinib, 661t, 674, 683t
Prothrombin time (PT) assay, 328, 330b
Proton pump inhibitors, 490t, 491f, 492, 493f, 496t
  dexlansoprazole, 490t, 496t
  elderly, 73b
  esomeprazole, 490t, 495, 496t
  gastroesophageal reflux disease, 492, 493f
  iron deficiency from, 495
  lansoprazole, 490t, 493f, 496t
  mechanisms of action, 490t, 491f, 495
  omeprazole, 490t, 493f, 496t
  pantoprazole, 490t, 493f, 496t
  rabeprazole, 490t, 493f, 496t
  structures, 492, 492f, 493f
  for ulcers, 492, 493, 494t, 495
  vitamin B_{12} absorption, 492
Protozoal drugs, 530–535
  amebic colitis, 532–533
  amphotericin (B), 530t, 534, 535t
  benznidazole, 530t–531t, 535t
  cryptosporidia diarrhea, 532
  eflornithine, 530t, 535t
  fumagillin, 530t, 535t
  giardiasis, 531–532
  leishmaniasis, visceral, 534
  mechanisms of action, 530t–531t
  melarsoprol, 530t, 534, 535t
  metronidazole, 530t, 532–534, 535t
  miltefosine, 530t, 534, 535t
  nifurtimox, 531t, 535t
  nitazoxanide, 530t, 532, 535t
  paromomycin, 531t, 532–533, 535t
  pentamidine, 531t, 535t
  sodium stibogluconate, 531t, 534, 535t
  toxoplasmosis, 532b
  Trichomonas vaginalis, 533, 534
  Trypanosoma brucei rhodesiense, 534
  trypanosomiasis, 533, 534
Protriptyline, 150t, 173t
Prucalopride, 497t, 507t
Pruritus, 720, 720t
Pseudoephedrine, 120t, 142t
Psilocybe, 97
Psilocybin, 97
Psoriasis, 715–716
  adalimumab, 709t, 714t, 722, 723
  biologic agent mechanisms of action, 710f
  immunopathogenesis, 711f
  methotrexate, 715–716, 721–722
Psychopharmacology, 149–175. *See also specific drugs and drug classes*
  anticonvulsants, malaria, 151t, 175t
    carbamazepine, 151t, 164–165, 175t
    lamotrigine, 151t, 165, 175t
    valproic acid, 151t, 164–165, 169, 173, 175t
  antidepressants
    actions and effects, 152–154, 152f
    adverse effects, 154
    disposition, 158t
    phases of treatment, 153–154
    sites of actions, 152f
    structures, dosing, and adverse effects, 155t–156t
  antidepressants, atypical, 150t, 156t, 174t
    atomoxetine, 150t, 174t
    bupropion, 150t, 174t
    mianserin, 150t, 174t
    mirtazapine, 150t, 174t
    nefazodone, 150t, 174t
    reboxetine, 150t, 174t
    structures, dosings, and adverse effects, 156t
    trazodone, 150t, 174t
  antipsychotics
    adverse effects, 172t
    elderly, 77b, 168, 169, 171
    nonpsychotic disorders, 163b
  antipsychotics, atypical, 175t
    aripiprazole, 151t, 170t, 175t
    chemical structures, dosages, and maintenance, 160t–161t
    metabolism, 170t
    olanzapine, 151t, 165, 168, 170t, 171–172, 175t
    potencies, 162t
    quetiapine, 151t, 171t, 175t
    risperidone, 151t, 168, 169, 171t, 175t
  antipsychotics, typical, 151t, 175t
    asenapine, 151t, 170t, 175t
    chemical structures, dosages, and maintenance, 160t
    clozapine, 151t, 167–169, 170t, 172, 175t
    iloperidone, 151t, 170t, 175t
    metabolism, 170t
    paliperidone, 151t, 170t, 175t
    potencies, 162t
    sertindole, 151t, 175t
    ziprasidone, 151t, 171t, 175t
  antipsychotics, typical, other, 151t, 175t
    droperidol, 151t, 175t
    haloperidol, 151t, 159, 163f, 171t, 175t
    loxapine, 151t, 175t
    molindone, 151t, 175t

Psychopharmacology (Cont.)
  receptor occupancy and clinical response, 163f
  antipsychotics, typical, phenothiazines, 150t, 174t
    chlorpromazine, 150t, 171t, 174t
    fluphenazine, 150t, 174t
    perphenazine, 150t, 174t
    trifluoperazine, 150t, 174t
  anxiolytics, benzodiazepine, 174t
  anxiolytics, non-benzodiazepine, 150t, 174t
    buspirone, 150t, 174t
  bipolar disorder, 164–166
    elderly, 77b
  lithium, 151t, 164–166, 175t
    adverse effects, 164t
    elderly, 165–166
    ibuprofen, 165, 168, 169
    lithium carbonate, 151t, 175t
    lithium citrate, 151t, 175t
    overdose, 166–167
  monoamine oxidase inhibitors (MAOIs), 150t, 157, 173t
    isocarboxazid, 150t, 173t
    phenelzine, 150t, 173t
    selegiline, 150t, 173t
    SSRI after, 157
    structures, dosing, and adverse effects, 156t
    tranylcypromine, 150t, 173t
  psychosis, acute, 160t–161t
  schizophrenia
    chemical structures, dosages, and maintenance, 160t–161t
    with drug abuse history, 159, 162–163
  selective serotonin reuptake inhibitors (SSRIs) (See Selective serotonin reuptake inhibitors (SSRIs))
  serotonin/norepinephrine reuptake inhibitors (SNRIs), 150t, 154, 157, 174t
    delay of onset, 157
    desvenlafaxine, 150t, 174t
    disposition, 158t
    duloxetine, 150t, 174t
    milnacipran, 150t, 174t
    venlafaxine, 150t, 154, 157, 174t
  serotonin/norepinephrine reuptake inhibitors (SNRIs), secondary amine tricyclics, 150t, 173t
    amoxapine, 150t, 173t
    desipramine, 150t, 173t
    maprotiline, 150t, 173t
    nortriptyline, 150t, 173t
    protriptyline, 150t, 173t
    structures, dosing, and adverse effects, 155t
  serotonin/norepinephrine reuptake inhibitors (SNRIs), tertiary amine tricyclics, 150t, 173t
    amitriptyline, 150t, 152–154, 152f, 168, 169, 173t
    clomipramine, 150t, 173t
    disposition, 158t
    doxepin, 150t, 173t
    imipramine, 150t, 173t
    structures, dosing, and adverse effects, 155t
    trimipramine, 150t, 173t
Psychosis drugs. See Antipsychotics
Pteroylglutamic acid (PteGlu). See Folic acid and derivatives
PTH-related protein (PTHrP), 483f
Pulmonary artery hypertension (PAH), 398–400, 399f
Pulmonary drugs, 389–404
  anti-IgE monoclonal antibodies, omalizumab, 390t, 397, 404t
  antileukotrienes, 390t, 403t–404t
    5-LOX inhibitors, zileuton, 390t, 403t
    asthma, severe, 396f, 397
    leukotriene antagonists, 390t, 404t
      montelukast, 390t, 404t
      zafirlukast, 390t, 404t
    mechanisms of action, 390t, 396f
  antitussives, 209t, 391t, 404t
    benzonatate, 391t, 404t
    codeine, 209t, 391t, 404t
    dextromethorphan, 391t, 404t
    mechanisms of action, 391t
  asthma, 393–397, 396f
  β_2 adrenergic receptor agonists, long-acting, 390t, 402t
    adverse effects, 392b, 398
    arformoterol, 390t, 402t
    asthma, 393–394, 396–397, 402
    COPD, 395
    formoterol, 390t, 402t
    indacaterol, 390t, 402t
    mechanisms of action, 390t, 391b, 391f, 394
    salmeterol, 390t, 402t
  β_2 adrenergic receptor agonists, short-acting, 389t, 401, 402t
    adverse effects, 392b
    albuterol, 389t, 402t
    asthma, 393–394
    levalbuterol, 389t, 402t
    mechanisms of actions, 389t, 391b, 391f, 394
    metaproterenol, 389t, 402t
    pirbuterol, 389t, 402t
    terbutaline, 389t, 402t
  combination inhalers, 395, 397, 398, 401–402
  COPD, 394–395
  corticosteroids, inhaled, 390t, 403t
    adverse effects, 393b, 397–398
    asthma, 393–394, 395–397
    beclomethasone dipropionate, 390t, 403t
    bioavailability, 467, 468
    budesonide, 390t, 402, 403t, 460t
    candidiasis, oral, 467, 468
    ciclesonide, 390t, 403t
    COPD, 395
    flunisolide, 390t, 403t
    fluticasone, 390t, 403t
    mechanisms of action, 390t, 392f, 393f
    mometasone, 390t, 403t
    triamcinolone, 390t, 403t
  corticosteroids, systemic, 390t, 403t
    hydrocortisone, 390t, 403t
    mechanisms of action, 390t, 392f, 393f
    methylprednisolone, 390t, 403t
    prednisolone, 390t, 403t
    prednisone, 390t, 403t
  endothelin-1 receptor antagonists, 391t, 404t
    adverse effects, 400
    ambrisentan, 391t, 398–400, 399f, 404t
    bosentan, 391t, 398–400, 399f, 404t
    mechanisms of action, 391t
    pulmonary artery hypertension, 398–400, 399f
  expectorants, guaifenesin, 390t, 404t
  gastroesophageal reflux disease (GERD), 400
  methylxanthines, 390t, 403t
    COPD, 395
    mechanisms of action, 390t
    theophylline, 390t, 392f, 397, 403t
  mucolytics, 390t, 404t
    DNase (dornase alfa), 390t, 404t
    N-acetylcysteine, 390t, 404t
  muscarinic cholinergic antagonists, 390t, 401–402, 403t
    adverse effects, 395
    asthma, severe, 397
    COPD, 394–395
    ipratropium bromide, 390t, 402, 403t
    mechanisms of action, 390t
    tiotropium bromide, 390t, 401–402, 403t
  phosphodiesterase 5 inhibitors, 391t, 404t
    adverse effects, 398, 399f, 400
    mechanisms of action, 391t
    pulmonary artery hypertension, 398–400, 399f
    sildenafil, 391t, 398–402, 399f, 404t, 703
    tadalafil, 391t, 398–402, 399f, 404t
  prostacyclin (PGI_2) and analogs, 391t, 404t
    adverse effects, 400
    epoprostenol, 391t, 398–400, 399f, 404t
    iloprost, 391t, 404t
    mechanisms of action, 391t
    treprostinil, 391t, 404t
    pulmonary artery hypertension, 398–400, 399f
  ventilatory stimulants, doxapram, 391t, 404t
Pulmonary edema, 303. See also Edema drugs; Heart failure
Pupil effects, 698, 698t
Purine analogs, 636t, 641–642, 655t–656t
PUVA photochemotherapy, 716–717, 716t, 725t
Pyoderma, 714
Pyrazinamide, 578t, 580b, 586t
Pyridostigmine bromide, 100t, 114t
Pyridoxine, 406t, 419t
  mechanisms of action, 406t
  pyridoxine, 406t, 419t
  riboflavin, 406t, 419t
Pyrilamine, 346t, 353t

Pyrimethamine-sulfadoxine, 521t, 529t
Pyrimidine analogs, 635t–636t, 640–641, 654t
   5-fluorouracil (5-FU), 630f, 635t, 638b–639b, 638f, 640–641, 654t
   azacytidine, 636t, 654t
   capecitabine, 630f, 635t, 638f, 654t
   cytarabine (Ara-C), 630f, 635t, 639b, 648, 649, 654t
   decitabine, 636t, 654t
   Floxuridine (FUdR), 630f, 635t, 638b–639b, 638f, 654t
   gemcitabine, 630f, 636t, 639b, 654t
   mechanisms and sites of action, 630f, 635t–636t, 638f, 640
   mechanisms of resistance, 638b–639b, 640–641
   toxicities, 637t, 654t
   uses, 637t, 654t

Q
QT interval, long, 313–315, 315b
Quantal dose-response phenomenon, 44f, 45
Quazepam, 176t, 191t, 192t
Quetiapine, 130t, 147t, 151t, 171t, 175t
Quinacrine, 708t, 725t
Quinagolide, 422t, 426, 428t
Quinapril, 273t, 285t
Quinethazone, 269t, 284t
Quinidine, antiarrhythmic, 312t, 317t, 320t
Quinine/quinidine, malaria, 521t, 524, 527, 529t
Quinolones, 544, 544f, 545, 548t
   ciprofloxacin, 544, 544f, 545, 548t
   levofloxacin, 548t
   mechanisms of action, 544f, 545
   moxifloxacin, 548t
   norfloxacin, 548t
   ofloxacin, 548t
   resistance, 544
Quinupristin/dalfopristin, 568t, 572, 575, 576b

R
Rabbit syndrome, 172t
Rabeprazole, 490t, 493f, 496t
Radioactive iodine (^{131}I), 431t, 435, 437–439, 440t
Raloxifene
   anticancer, 664t, 686t
   SERM, 442t, 458t
Raltegravir, 601t, 603t, 611f, 623t
Raltitrexed, 635t, 653t
Ramelteon, 177t, 189, 190, 192t
Ramipril, 273t, 285t
Ranibizumab, 662t, 684t
Ranitidine
   gastric acid disease, 490t, 496t
   structure, 492f
Ranolazine, 290t, 298, 299, 300t
Rapamycins
   anticancer, 663t, 675–676, 685t
   congeners, temsirolimus, 663t, 675–676
   mechanisms of action, 662t, 675
   toxicities, 675–676

Rasagiline, 239t, 242t, 244f, 245, 250, 251, 253t
Rasburicase, 369t, 374t
Rate of distribution, 20f, 36b–37b, 37f
Reboxetine, 150t, 174t
Receptor, drug. *See also specific drugs and receptors*
   conformation-selective drugs, 4, 4f
   definition, 2b
   drug–drug interactions, on binding, 48t
   functions, 2b
   nervous system, 89b
   nuclear, 3t, 33t, 34f
   physiological, 2b
   primary (orthosteric) site, 3b, 8
Receptor antagonism, 48b
Receptor for activating NF-κB ligand (RANKL), 482f
Receptor occupancy theory, 6b
Rectal administration, elderly, 73t
Reinforcement, negative, 265, 266
Relative efficacy, 7b, 7f, 9
Relative potency, 7f
Remifentanil, 195t, 208t
Renal epithelial Na$^+$-channel inhibitors, 269t, 271t, 272f, 284t
   amiloride, 269t, 284t
   triamterene, 269t, 282, 283, 284t
Renal function
   elderly, 76b, 78t
   infants and children, 69b
Renal osteodystrophy, 482f, 484
   vitamin D, 481t, 484, 488t
Renin-angiotensin system (RAS) inhibitors, 270t
   ACE inhibitors, 270t, 273t, 285t
   acute MI, 279
   adverse effects, 276
   angioedema, 279
   benzapril, 273t, 285t
   captopril, 273t, 279, 285t
   cautions, 274–276
   diabetics, 274
   enalapril, 273t, 274–276, 275f, 285t
   enalaprilat, 273t, 285t
   fosinopril, 273t, 285t
   lisinopril, 273t, 281, 282, 285t, 306, 309, 310
   mechanisms of action, 270t, 273t, 274–276, 275f
   moexipril, 273t, 285t
   perindopril, 273t, 285t
   quinapril, 273t, 285t
   ramipril, 273t, 285t
   structure, 275f
   trandolapril, 273t, 285t
   angiotensin II effects, 274f
   angiotensin receptor blockers (ARBs), 270t, 273t, 285t
   candesartan cilexetil, 273t, 285t
   irbesartan, 273t, 285t
   losartan, 273t, 285t
   olmesartan medoxomil, 273t, 285t
   structure, 275f
   telmisartan, 273t, 285t
   valsartan, 273t, 280, 282, 283, 285t

angiotensin (AT$_1$) receptor blockers (ARBs), diabetics, 274
   classification, 270t
   direct renin inhibitors, 270t, 273t, 286t
   aliskiren, 273t, 282, 283, 286t
   mechanisms of action, 273t
   structure, 275f
   effects, 273t, 274f
   mechanisms of action, 270t, 273t, 278t
   physiologic factors, 272f, 275b
   structures, 275f
   vasodilators, 270t, 278t
Renin inhibitors, direct, 270t, 273t, 286t
   aliskiren, 273t, 282, 283, 286t
   mechanisms of action, 273t
   structure, 275f
Renin inhibitors/vasodilators, direct. *See* Direct renin inhibitors
Renin release pathways, 272f
Repaglinide, 470t, 472f, 479t
Repeated administration, 38b, 38f
Reserpine, 277t, 286t
Resistance, 15, 515b, 517
   antimicrobial, 515b
   β-lactam antibiotics, 516–517
   β-lactamase, 517, 519
   dosing schedule, 515
   efflux pumps, 515b, 517
   mutations, 517
   suppression, dosing schedule, 515
Respiratory depression, opiate, 196b, 199, 201
Retapamulin, 708t, 725t
Reteplase, 323t, 333t
Retinoic acid receptors (RARs), 717
Retinoids, 707t, 717–718, 717b, 724t
   acitretin, 707t, 724t
   adapalene, 707t, 724t
   alitretinoin, 707t, 724t
   bexarotene, 707t, 724t
   cytotoxic actions and pharmacology, 645t, 646t, 659t
   isotretinoin, 707t, 721, 722, 724t
   pregnancy warning, 721, 722, 724t
   tazarotene, 707t, 724t
   tretinoin, 707t, 724t
Rheumatoid arthritis, 380
Rheumatoid arthritis drugs, 357, 368b, 368t
   disease-modifying anti-rheumatic drugs, 368b, 368t, 379–380
   (*See also* Disease-modifying anti-rheumatic drugs (DMARDs))
   immunotherapeutic agents, 380–381
   NSAIDs, 366–368, 380 (*See also* Nonsteroidal anti-inflammatory drugs (NSAIDs))
   prednisone, 463–465
Ribavirin, 601t, 602t, 620t
   adverse effects, 614
   hepatitis C, chronic, 613–614
Riboflavin, 406t, 419t
Rifabutin, 578t, 579f, 580f, 586t
Rifampin, 581–586, 586t
   adverse effects, 582

Rifampin (Cont.)
	H. influenzae meningitis prophylaxis, 578t, 579f, 581–582, 586t
	mechanisms of action, 578t, 579f
	mechanisms of resistance, 578t, 580f
	tuberculosis, 578t, 579f, 581–586, 586t
Rifamycins, 578t, 581–586, 586t
	H. influenzae meningitis prophylaxis, 578t, 581–586, 586t
	tuberculosis, 578t, 586t
		mechanisms of action, 578t, 579f
		mechanisms of resistance, 578t, 580f
		rifabutin, 578t, 586t
		rifampin, 578t, 579f, 581–586, 586t
		rifapentine, 578t, 586t
Rifapentine, 578t, 579f, 580f, 586t
Rigidity agents, cholinergic, 106t, 117t
Rilonacept, 376t, 386t
Riluzole, 239t, 249, 251, 252, 253t
Rimabotulinum toxin B, 106t, 117t
Rimantadine, 601t, 602t, 604f, 620t
Rimexolone
	ophthalmic, 691t, 705t
Rimonanbant, 98t
Risedronate, 481t, 488t
Risperidone, 130t, 147t, 151t, 168, 169, 171t, 175t
Ritodrine, 125t, 144t
Ritonavir, 601t, 603t, 608f, 609f, 615–619, 622t
	adverse effects, 615
	on CP3A4, 617–619
	drug interactions, 616
	mechanisms of action and resistance, 603t, 608f, 609f, 615
Rituximab
	anticancer, 662t, 671t, 681, 682, 684t
	rheumatoid arthritis, 368t
	toxicities, 684t
	uses, 684t
Rivaroxaban, 323t, 328, 333t
Rivastigmine, 100t, 115t
	Alzheimer's disease, 239t, 246, 247t, 253t
Rizatriptan, 130t, 147t
RNA virus replicative cycles, 604f
Rocuronium, 97f, 105f, 106f, 106t, 107t, 117t
Romidepsin (depsipeptide), 645t, 660t
Romiplostim, 406t, 417, 418t, 419t
Ropinirole
	Parkinson's disease, 238t, 242t, 245, 250, 251, 252t
	pharmacology, 130t, 148t
Ropivacaine, 224t
Rosiglitazone, 470t, 475–476, 479t
Rosuvastatin (calcium), 334t, 338, 343t
Rotigotine, 130t, 148t
Route of administration. *See* Administration, routes
Rubidomycin, 643t, 658t
	mechanisms of action, 630f, 643t, 645–647
	mechanisms of resistance, 645b
Rufinamide, 226t, 237t

S
Safety
	FDA Safety and Innovation Act of 2012, 72b
	medication, children, 71b–72b
Salbutamol
	pharmacology, 125t, 127, 135, 137, 143t
	pulmonary, 389t, 402t
Salicylate, 357t, 373t
Salicylate toxidrome, 53t
Saline laxative, 497t, 507t
Salmeterol
	pharmacology, 125t, 143t
	pulmonary, 390t, 402t
Salsalate, 357t, 373t
Saquinavir, 601t, 603t, 608f, 609f, 621t
Sargramostim, 405t, 407t, 408f, 409–410, 418t
Sarin, 100t, 103t, 115t
Saxagliptin, 471t, 472f, 479t
Saxitoxin, mussels, 221, 222
Schizophrenia
	drug abuse history, 159, 162–163
	drug structures, dosages, and maintenance, 160t–161t
Scopolamine
	antiemetic, 502t
	motion sickness, 346t, 350, 352
	ophthalmic, 690t, 695t, 704t
	pharmacology, 96t, 112t
Seafood allergies, 349–350
Secobarbital, 177t, 180, 192t
Sedation, drug-induced. *See also specific drugs*
	hyperexcitability after, 89–90, 94
Sedative-hypnotics, 176–193, 177t, 191t–193t. *See also* Hypnotics and sedative-hypnotics; *specific drugs and drug classes*
	adverse effects, 179
	barbiturates, 177t, 180–182, 181t, 192t
	benzodiazepine receptor agonists, novel, 177t, 192t
	benzodiazepine receptor antagonists, flumazenil, 41t, 42t, 65t, 177t, 179–180, 192t
	benzodiazepines, 176t, 178b, 180, 189–190, 191t–192t (*See also* Benzodiazepines)
	$GABA_A$ receptor, 178f, 179
	insomnia categories, 178b, 179
	long-term use, 179
	melatonin congeners, ramelteon, 177t, 189, 190, 192t
	toxidrome, 53t
Seizure disorders
	agents and principles, 227b, 228
	classification, 228, 229t
	drug choice, 227b
	early diagnosis and treatment, 228
	general principles, 227b
	treatment (*See* Antiseizure drugs)
Selective estrogen-receptor downregulators (SERDs), 664t
	fulvestrant, 664t, 677t, 686t

Selective estrogen receptor modulators (SERMS), 442t, 458t
	raloxifene, 442t, 458t
	tamoxifen, 442t, 451, 456, 457, 458t, 667f
	toremifene, 442t, 458t
Selective estrogen receptor modulators (SERMs), targeted anticancer, 664t, 686t
	mechanisms of resistance, 664t
	raloxifene, 664t, 686t
	tamoxifen, 664t, 667f, 676–678, 677t, 679t, 686t
	toremifene, 664t, 677t, 679t, 686t
	uses, 677t, 686t
Selective progesterone receptor modulator (ulipristal), 442t, 444t, 452, 458t
Selective serotonin reuptake inhibitors (SSRIs), 130t, 131–133, 131f, 136, 138, 146t
	case question, 136, 138
	citalopram, 150t, 174t
	delay of onset, 157
	disposition, 158t
	drug interactions, 157
	fluoxetine, 150t, 157, 174t
	fluvoxamine, 150t, 174t
	MAO inhibitors with, 133
	after MAOIs, 157
	mechanisms of action, 136, 138
	paroxetine, 150t, 157, 174t
	sertraline, 150t, 174t
	sites of actions, 152f
	structures, dosing, and adverse effects, 155t–156t
Selective T-cell costimulation blockers, 387t
Selegiline
	Parkinson's disease, 238t, 242t, 244f, 245, 250, 251, 253t
	psychopharmacology, 150t, 173t
Semustine (methyl-CCNU), 627t, 652t
	mechanisms of action, 627t, 628b, 630f
	mechanisms of resistance, 627t, 632–633, 632b
	toxicities, 652t
	uses, 629t
Serotonergic (5-HT) 5-HT receptor agonists, 130t, 133–134, 133t, 134f, 147t
Serotonergic (5-HT) 5-HT receptor antagonists, 130t, 131–133, 133t, 147t
Serotonergic (5-HT) pharmacology
	actions and clinical indications, 131–133, 133t
	adverse effects, 133
	almotriptan, 130t, 147t
	alosetron, 130t, 147t
	buspirone, 130t, 133t, 136, 138, 147t
	citalopram, 130t, 146t
	clozapine, 130t, 147t, 170t
	desvenlafaxine, 130t, 147t
	dolasetron, 130t, 147t
	drug interactions, 133
	duloxetine, 130t, 147t

771

eletriptan, 130t, 147t
ergot alkaloids and derivatives, 120t, 141t, 147t
escitalopram, 130t, 146t
fluoxetine, 130t, 131–133, 131f, 133t, 146t, 157
fluvoxamine, 130t, 146t
frovatriptan, 130t, 147t
granisetron, 130t, 147t
isocarboxazid, 130t, 147t
ketanserin, 133t, 147t
MAO inhibitors
    altering 5-HT concentrations, 130t, 147t
    foods prohibited, 135, 137
mechanisms of action, 130t
methysergide, 130t, 147t
milnacipran, 130t, 147t
naratriptan, 130t, 147t
olanzapine, 130t, 147t
ondansetron, 130t, 133t, 147t
palonosetron, 130t, 147t
paroxetine, 130t, 146t, 157
phenelzine, 130t, 147t
quetiapine, 130t, 147t
receptor subtypes, 132t
risperidone, 130t, 147t
rizatriptan, 130t, 147t
sertraline, 130t, 133t, 136, 138, 146t
sibutramine, 130t, 147t
sumatriptan, 130t, 133–134, 133t, 134f, 147t
tranylcypromine, 130t, 135, 137, 147t
venlafaxine, 130t, 147t
zolmitriptan, 130t, 147t
Serotonin (5-HT)
    in migraine, 133–134, 133t
    synthesis and inactivation, 131f
Serotonin, norepinephrine, and dopamine reuptake inhibitors, 130t, 147t
Serotonin/norepinephrine reuptake inhibitors (SNRIs), 130t, 147t, 150t, 154, 157, 174t
    delay of onset, 157
    desvenlafaxine, 150t, 174t
    disposition, 158t
    duloxetine, 150t, 174t
    milnacipran, 150t, 174t
    secondary amine tricyclics, 150t, 173t
        amoxapine, 150t, 173t
        desipramine, 150t, 173t
        maprotiline, 150t, 173t
        nortriptyline, 150t, 173t
        protriptyline, 150t, 173t
        structures, dosing, and adverse effects, 155t
    sites of actions, 152f
    tertiary amine tricyclics, 150t, 173t
        amitriptyline, 150t, 152–154, 152f, 168, 169, 173t
        clomipramine, 150t, 173t
        disposition, 158t
        doxepin, 150t, 173t
        imipramine, 150t, 173t

structures, dosing, and adverse effects, 155t
    trimipramine, 150t, 173t
    venlafaxine, 150t, 154, 157, 174t
Serotonin (5-HT) receptor agonists, 130t, 133–134, 133t, 134f, 147t
Serotonin (5-HT) receptor antagonists, 130t, 131–133, 133t, 147t
Serotonin (5-HT) receptors
    autoreceptor classes, 134, 134f
    subtypes, 132f
Serotonin (5-HT$_2$) receptors, MDMA and DOM affinity, 265, 266
Sertaconazole, 588t, 598t
Sertindole, 151t, 175t
Sertraline, 130t, 133t, 136, 138, 146t, 150t, 174t
Sevelamer, 481t, 488t
Sevelamer hydrochloride, 481t, 484, 488t
Sevoflurane, 210t, 215t, 223t
Short-acting inhaled β$_2$ agonists (SABAs). See β$_2$-adrenergic receptor agonists, short-acting
Sibutramine, 130t, 147t
Sildenafil
    myocardial ischemia, 300t
    ocular effects, 703
    pulmonary, 391t, 398–402, 399f, 404t
    pulmonary artery hypertension, 398–402
Silodosin, 119t, 140t
Simvastatin, 334t, 343t
Sinus bradycardia, vasospastic angina with, 297, 298
Sirolimus (rapamycin)
    immunotherapy, 375t, 377f, 383, 384, 385t
    mechanisms of action, 375t, 383, 384
Sitagliptin, 471t, 472f, 479t
6-Mercaptopurine (6-MP), 636t, 641–642, 655t
    mechanisms of action, 630f, 636t, 641–642
    mechanisms of resistance, 636t, 639b, 642
    toxicities, 642, 655t
    uses, 637t, 655t
6-Thioguanine (6-TG), 630f, 636t, 655t
    mechanisms of action, 630f, 636t, 641–642
    mechanisms of resistance, 636t
Skin absorption, 710b, 711–715, 711t, 713f
    important considerations, 711–712, 711t
    neonates, infants, and children, 67b
    rate-limiting step, 721, 722
    for topical infections, 714–715
    vehicles, 712–714, 712t
Skin disorders. See Dermatologic disorders
Skin structure, 713f
SLC superfamily transporters, 23b–24b, 25t–26t
Sleep apnea, opiates and respiratory depression, 196b, 199, 201
Sleeping sickness, 534
Small molecules, rheumatoid arthritis, 368t
Smoking, 258–259
    addiction, 258–259
    benzo[a]pyrene, 41t, 63–65

bupropion for, 259
    negative reinforcement, 265, 266
    withdrawal syndrome, 258–259, 259t
Sodium 2,3-dimercaptopropane sulfonate (DMPS), 41t, 66t
Sodium channel blockers. See Na$^+$ channel blockers
Sodium channels. See Na$^+$ channels
Sodium ferric gluconate, 406t, 419t
Sodium iodide, 431t, 440t
Sodium iodine (^{131}I), 431t, 435, 437–439, 440t
Sodium phosphate, 497t, 507t
Sodium stibogluconate, 531t, 534, 535t
Sodium thiopental, 210t, 213t, 214f, 222t
Solifenacin, 96t, 101t, 113t
Soman, 100t, 103t, 116t
Somatic motor nerves, 82f
    neurotransmitters, 82f, 93, 94 (See also specific types)
Somatic nervous system, 82f, 85, 92
Somatostatin (SST), 424f, 433f
Somatostatin (SST) analogs, 422t, 428t
    lanreotide, 422t, 428t
    octreotide, 422t, 428t
Sorafenib, 661t, 674, 683t
Sotalol
    antiarrhythmic, 312t, 317t, 321t
    electrophysiologic actions, 317t
Spasticity agents, cholinergic, 106t, 117t
Special populations, 67–78. See also Children; Elderly
Specificity. See also specific agents
    adverse effects, 9
    definition, 5b
    high (narrow), 5b, 9
    low (broad), 5b, 9
Spectinomycin, 569t, 576t
Spinal anesthesia, 217–219
Spironolactone, 269t, 285t
    adverse effects, 307
    heart failure, 302t, 307, 311t
Stable angina, 290t, 291f. See also Myocardial ischemia
Staphylococcus aureus treatment, cycloserine, 579t, 587t
Statins. See HMG-CoA reductase inhibitors (statins)
Stavudine, 601t, 603t, 621t
    mechanisms of action and resistance, 603t, 607f, 608f
    structure, 607f
Steady state
    dosing, 19f, 30–31, 34, 38b
    repeated administration, 38b, 38f
Stem cell factor (SCF), 407t, 408f
Stents, drug-eluting coronary, 297, 297b
Steroidogenesis inhibitors, 665t, 687t
    abiraterone, 665t, 668f, 680, 687t
    ketoconazole, 665t, 687t
Steroid synthesis pathways, 668f
St. John's wort
    on CYP3A4, 619
    pharmacokinetics, 29–30, 33f, 34f
Strabismus agents, 692t, 706t
    abobotulinumtoxin A, 692t, 706t
    onabotulinumtoxin A, 692t, 706t

Streptogramins, quinupristin/dalfopristin, 568t, 572, 575, 576b
Streptomycin, 559–566, 559b, 567t
Streptozocin (streptozotocin), 627t, 652t
    mechanisms of action, 627t, 628b, 630f
    mechanisms of resistance, 627t, 632–633, 632b
    uses, 629t
Stroke, tPA for, 323t, 329–330, 329f, 333t
Subcutaneous administration, 21t
    elderly, 74t
Suberoylanilide hydroxamic acid (SAHA), 645t, 646t, 660t
Sublingual administration, 22
    elderly, 73t
Succimer, 41t, 42t, 66t
Succinimides, antiseizure, 225t, 236t
    ethosuximide, 225t, 230–231, 234, 235, 236t
    methsuximide, 225t, 236t
Succinylcholine, 97f, 105f, 107t, 108, 116t
Sucralfate, 490t, 496t
Sufentanil, 194t, 195t, 205, 207, 208t
Sulbactam, 549t, 553, 558t
Sulconazole, 588t, 598t
Sulfadiazine, 543f, 543t, 547t
Sulfadoxine, 521t, 529t, 543t, 548t
Sulfamethoxazole, 56–57
    allergy, 56–57
    urinary tract infections, 543f, 543t, 547t
Sulfapyridine, 502, 503f, 505–506, 507
Sulfasalazine, 357t, 368t, 373, 381
    adverse effects, 368t
    Crohn's disease and ulcerative colitis, 381, 498t, 502, 503f, 505, 507, 509t
    inflammatory bowel disease, 381, 498t, 502, 503f, 505, 507, 509t
    rheumatoid arthritis, 368t
    structure, 503f
    sulfapyridine in, 502, 503f, 505, 507
Sulfation, neonatal, 70b
Sulfisoxazole, infants, 68
Sulfite, local anesthetics, 220, 221
Sulfonamides
    absorption and excretion kinetics, 543t
    bacterial vs. mammalian sensitivity, 546, 547
    mafenide, 546, 547, 548t
    pregnancy, 546, 547
    silver sulfadiazine, 543t, 547t
    structures, 543f
    sulfacetamide, 543f, 543t, 547t
    sulfadiazine, 543f, 543t, 547t
    sulfadoxine, 543t, 548t
    sulfamethoxazole, 543f, 543t, 547t
    sulfasalazine, 543t, 547t
    sulfisoxazole, 543f, 543t, 547t
Sulindac, 357t, 361t, 373t
Sumatriptan, 130t, 133–134, 133t, 134f, 147t
Sunitinib, 661t, 674, 683t
Sunscreens, 710t, 719b, 726t
Sympathetic nervous system, 82f, 85, 92, 107t
Sympatholytics, antihypertensive, 270t, 277t
    adrenergic neuron blocking agents, 277t, 286t
        guanadrel, 277t, 287t
        reserpine, 277t, 286t
    α_1 adrenergic receptor antagonists, 277t
        doxazosin, 277t, 286t
        prazosin, 277t, 286t
        terazosin, 277t, 286t
    β adrenergic receptor antagonists, doxazosin, 277t
    centrally acting adrenergics
        α_2 adrenergic receptor antagonists, 277t, 286t
        clonidine, 277t, 286t
        guanabenz, 277t, 286t
        guanfacine, 277t, 286t
        methyldopa, 277t, 286t
    mechanisms of action, 277t
Sympathomimetics, 120t, 123f, 141t–142t. See also α-Adrenergic receptor agonists
Sympathomimetic toxidrome, 53t
Synergistic drug–drug interaction, 48b
Synthetic conjugated estrogens, 441t
Syntopic interaction, 4b, 5f, 8

T
Tabun, 100t, 103t, 116t
Tachyarrhythmia
    drugs (See Antiarrhythmic drugs)
    mechanisms, 313b
Tacrine
    Alzheimer's disease, 239t, 247t, 253t
    pharmacology, 100t, 115t
Tacrolimus, 375t, 377f, 383, 385t
    dermatologic, 708t, 724t, 726t
    mechanisms of action, 375t, 383, 384
Tadalafil
    myocardial ischemia, 300t
    ocular effects, 703
    pulmonary, 391t, 398–402, 399f, 404t
    pulmonary artery hypertension, 398–402
Taenia solium, 539, 540
Tamoxifen, 442t, 451, 456, 457, 458t, 676–678
    anticancer, 664t, 667f, 676–678, 677t, 679t, 686t
    beneficial effects, 677–678
    mechanisms of action, 442t, 664t, 676
    mechanisms of resistance, 664t, 677
    structure and metabolites, 667f
    toxicities, 677–678, 686t
    uses, 676, 677t, 686t
Tamsulosin, 119t, 140t
Tapentadol, 195t, 209t
Tape test, 536
Tapeworm
    fish, 537–540
    pork, 539, 540
Tardive dyskinesia, 172t
Target
    drug, 2b (See also Receptor, drug)
    drugability, 7
    validity, 7
Targeted anticancer therapies, 661–687
    androgens, 664t, 679t, 686t (See also Androgens; *specific types*)
    antiandrogens, nonsteroidal, 665t, 679t, 687t
        bicalutamide, 665t, 687t
        flutamide, 665t, 679t, 687t
        nilutamide, 665t, 687t
    antiandrogens, steroidal, 665t, 687t
        cyproterone, 665t, 687t
        megestrol, 665t, 687t
    antiestrogens, aromatase inhibitors, 664t, 679t, 686t
        anastrozole, 664t, 677t, 679t, 686t
        exemestane, 664t, 677t, 679t, 686t
        letrozole, 664t, 677t, 679t, 686t
    antiestrogens, selective estrogen receptor downregulators (SERDs), 664t
        fulvestrant, 664t, 677t, 686t
    antiestrogens, selective estrogen receptor modulators (SERMs), 664t, 686t
        mechanisms of resistance, 664t
        raloxifene, 664t, 686t
        tamoxifen, 664t, 667f, 676–678, 677t, 679t, 686t
        toremifene, 664t, 677t, 679t, 686t
        uses, 677t, 686t
    colony-stimulating factors, 663t, 685t
    dose and toxicities, 671t
    EGFR (ErbB1), 667t
    estrogens, 664t, 665t, 679t, 686t, 687t (See also Estrogens)
    glucocorticoids, 664t, 686t
        dexamethasone, 664t, 686t
        prednisone, 664t, 679t, 686t
    gonadotropin-releasing hormone agonists, 664t, 679–680, 687t
        buserelin, 664t, 687t
        deslorelin, 664t
        GnRH, 664t, 680, 687t
        goserelin, 664t, 687t
        histrelin, 664t, 687t
        leuprolide, 664t, 679t, 680, 687t
        nafarelin, 664t, 686t
        triptorelin, 664t, 686t
    gonadotropin-releasing hormone antagonists, 665t, 686t
        abarelix, 665t, 687t
        cetrorelix, 665t, 687t
        degarelix, 665t, 687t
        ganirelix, 665t, 687t
    interleukin-2 receptor agonists, 663t, 685t
        aldesleukin, 663t, 682, 683, 685t
        denileukin diftitox, 663t, 671t, 685t
        mechanisms of resistance, 663t
    monoclonal antibodies: CD20, 662t, 667t, 684t
        [99]Y-ibritumomab, 662t, 671t, 684t
        ^{131}I-tositumomab, 662t, 671t, 684t
        dose and toxicities, 671t, 684t
        mechanisms of resistance, 662t
        ofatumumab, 662t, 684t
        rituximab, 662t, 671t, 681, 682, 684t
    monoclonal antibodies: CD33, 662t, 684t
        gemtuzumab ozogamicin, 662t, 667t, 672t, 684t
        mechanisms of resistance, 662t

monoclonal antibodies: CD52, 662t, 667t, 671t, 684t
  alemtuzumab, 662t, 667t, 671t, 684t
  mechanisms of resistance, 662t
monoclonal antibodies: growth factor antibodies (VEGF), 662t, 673–675, 684t
  bevacizumab, 662t, 671t, 674–675, 684t
  dose, 671t
  ranibizumab, 662t, 684t
  toxicities, 671t, 674–675, 684t
monoclonal antibodies: growth factor receptors, 662t, 683t
  cetuximab, 662t, 669–672, 683t
  dose and toxicities, 671t
  EGFR targeting, 669–672
  HER2/neu, 667t, 682t
  panitumumab, 662t, 669–672, 683t
  trastuzumab, 662t, 671t, 672–673, 681, 682, 683t
mTOR inhibitors, 663t, 685t
  everolimus, 663t, 685t
  mechanisms of action, 663t, 675
  mechanisms of resistance, 663t, 676
  rapamycin, 663t, 675–676, 685t
  temsirolimus, 663t, 675–676, 685t
progestins, 664t, 679t, 686t
  hydroxyprogesterone caproate, 679t
  medroxyprogesterone, 664t, 679t, 686t
  megestrol acetate, 664t, 679t, 686t
proteasome inhibitors, bortezomib, 663t, 681, 682–683, 685t
protein tyrosine kinase inhibitors, 661t, 683t
  dasatinib, 661t, 668, 683t
  erlotinib, 661t, 670–672, 683t
  gefitinib, 661t, 670–672, 683t
  imatinib mesylate, 661t, 666–669, 681, 682, 683t
  lapatinib, 661t, 673, 683t
  mechanisms of resistance, 661t
  nilotinib, 661t, 668, 683t
  sorafenib, 661t, 674, 683t
  sunitinib, 661t, 674, 683t
steroidogenesis inhibitors, 665t, 687t
  abiraterone, 665t, 668f, 680, 687t
  ketoconazole, 665t, 687t
thalidomide and derivatives, 663t, 685t
  lenalidomide, 663t, 666f, 685t
  mechanisms of action, 666f
  thalidomide, 663t, 666f, 685t
Taxanes, 642t, 648–650, 656t
  docetaxel, 630f, 642t, 644b, 648–650, 656t
  mechanisms of action, 630f, 642t, 648–650
  mechanisms of resistance, 642t, 644b
  nab-paclitaxel, 630f, 642t, 644b, 648–650, 656t
  paclitaxel, 630f, 642t, 644b, 648–650, 656t
  toxicities, 656t
  uses, 644t, 656t
Tazarotene, 707t, 724t
Tazobactam, 549t, 553, 558t

T-cell costimulation blockers, selective, 387t
Tear substitutes. See Wetting agents/tear substitutes
Teicoplanin, 569t, 570f, 577t
Telbivudine, 601t, 602t, 607f, 608f, 620t
Telithromycin, 568t, 570f, 576t
Telmisartan, 273t, 285t
Temazepam, 176t, 191t, 192t
Temozolomide, 652t
  mechanisms of action, 628b, 628t, 630f
  mechanisms of resistance, 628t, 632–633, 632b
  toxicities, 632b–633b, 652t
  uses, 629t
Temsirolimus, 663t, 675–676, 685t
Tenecteplase, 323t, 333t
Teniposide (VM-26), 643t, 657t
  mechanisms of action, 630f, 643t
  mechanisms of resistance, 643t, 645b
  toxicities, 657t
  uses, 644t, 657t
Tenofovir disoproxil, 601t–603t, 621t
  mechanisms of action and resistance, 602t, 603t, 607f, 608f
  structure, 607f
Terazosin
  antihypertensive, 277t, 286t
  pharmacology, 119t, 140t
Terbinafine, 588t, 589f, 596, 598t
Terbutaline
  pharmacology, 125t, 143t
  pulmonary, 389t, 402t
Terconazole, 588t, 597t
Teriparatide, 480t
  osteoporosis, 481t, 488t
Terlipressin, 279t, 288t
Tertiary amine tricyclics. See Serotonin/norepinephrine reuptake inhibitors (SNRIs), tertiary amine tricyclics
Testosterone, 442t, 458t
  adverse effects, 454
  effects, direct and mediated, 449f
  gynecomastia, 456, 457
  hypogonadism, 456, 457
  metabolism, 449f
  secretion, hCG, 422t, 427, 428, 429t
  synthesis, 449f
Testosterone buccal tablet, 442t, 458t
Testosterone cypionate, 442t, 458t
Testosterone enanthate, 442t, 458t
Testosterone gel, 442t, 458t
Testosterone patch, 442t, 458t
Testosterone replacement, 442t, 452–454, 453f
Testosterone supplement
  adverse effects, 454
  detection, 454
Testosterone undecanoate, 442t, 458t
Tetrabenazine, 239t, 249, 253t
Tetracaine, 224t
Tetracycline, 568t, 569f, 574, 575, 576t
Tetracyclines, 568t, 569f, 576t
  doxycycline, 568t, 569f, 571, 576t
  food contraindications, 574, 575
  MRSA infections, 571
  photosensitivity, 574, 575
  tetracycline, 568t, 569f, 576t
  tigecycline, 568t, 569f, 576t

Tetraethyl lead, 57
Tetrahydrozoline, ophthalmic, 690t, 695t, 705t
Thalidomide, 381t
  anticancer, 663t, 666f, 685t
  dermatologic, 709t, 724t, 726t
  immunostimulant, 381t
Theophylline
  asthma, 397
  pulmonary, 390t, 392f, 397, 403t
Therapeutic drug, 44f, 46, 46t
  monitoring, 39b
  toxicity, 44f, 46, 46t
Therapeutic gases. See Gases, therapeutic; specific agents
Therapeutic index, 11, 11f, 62, 64
  determining, 44f, 45
  digoxin, 31
  narrow, 22b, 31, 39b
Therapeutic window, 11, 12, 12f, 16, 17
  clearance, 35b
  in vitro binding studies, 8
  temporal characteristics, 36f
Thiazide/thiazide-like diuretics, 269t, 271, 271t, 272f, 284t
  bendroflumethiazide, 269t, 284t
  chlorothiazide, 269t, 284t
  chlorthalidone, 269t, 284t
  hydrochlorothiazide, 269t, 271, 273–274, 282, 283, 284t
  hydroflumethiazide, 269t, 284t
  indapamide, 269t, 284t
  methyclothiazide, 269t, 284t
  metolazone, 269t, 284t
  polythiazide, 269t, 284t
  quinethazone, 269t, 284t
  trichlormethiazide, 269t, 284t
Thiazide/thiazide-like diuretics (Na$^+$-2Cl$^-$ symporter inhibitors), 269t, 271, 271t, 272f, 284t
Thiazolidinediones, 470t, 475–476, 479t
  adverse effects, 476
  mechanisms of action, 470t
  pioglitazone, 470t, 475–476, 479t
  rosiglitazone, 470t, 475–476, 479t
Thienopyridines, 325t. See also Clopidogrel; Prasugrel; Ticlopidine
  bioactivation, 325t
  mechanisms of action, 323t, 330, 331
6-Thioguanine (6-TG), 636t, 655t
  mechanisms of action, 630f, 636t, 641–642
  mechanisms of resistance, 636t
Thiopental, 177t, 181t, 192t
  context-sensitive half-time, 214f
Thiopurine methyltransferase (TPMT), 502–503, 503f, 506, 507
Thiotepa, 627t, 632t, 651t
  mechanisms of action, 627t, 628b–629b, 630f
  mechanisms of resistance, 627t, 632–633, 632b
  toxicities, 632b–633b, 632t, 651t
Thrombin inhibitors, direct, 323t, 333t
  argatroban, 323t, 330, 331, 333t
  bivalirudin, 323t, 333t

Thrombin inhibitors (Cont.)
　　dabigatran etexilate, 323t, 328, 333t
　　desirudin, 333t
　　mechanisms of action, 323t
Thromboembolic disorder drugs, 323–333
　　anticoagulants (See Anticoagulants)
　　antiplatelets (See Antiplatelet agents)
　　fibrinolytics, 323t, 329–330, 329f, 333t
　　　　(See also Fibrinolytics, tPA)
Thrombopoietic growth factors, 405t, 406t, 407t, 419t
　　eltrombopag, 406t, 419t
　　IL-11 (oprelvekin), 406t, 410–411, 419t
　　mechanisms of action, 405t, 407t, 408f
　　romiplostim, 406t, 417, 418, 419t
Thrombopoietin (TPO, Mpl ligand), 407t, 408f
Thromboxane A_2, 324, 324t, 324f, 325f
Thyroid and antithyroid drugs, 431–440
　　antithyroid compounds, 435t
　　antithyroid drugs, 431t, 439t–440t
　　　　carbimazole, 431t, 439t
　　　　methimazole, 431t, 435–436, 438, 439, 440t
　　　　propylthiouracil, 431t, 439t
　　hyperthyroidism, 432t, 434t, 435–439
　　hypothyroidism, 431t, 432–434, 432t, 433f, 434t
　　ionic thyroid inhibitors, 431t, 440t
　　　　iodide, 431t, 440t
　　　　sodium iodide, 431t, 440t
　　mechanisms of action, 431t
　　papillary thyroid cancer, 436
　　radioactive iodine (^{131}I), 431t, 440t
　　thyroid hormones, 431t, 439t
　　　　desiccated thyroid, 431t, 439t
　　　　levothyroxine, 431t, 432–434, 434t, 436–439, 439t
　　　　liotrix, 431t, 439t
　　　　triiodothyroxine, 431t, 439t
Thyroid cancer, papillary, 436
Thyroid, desiccated, 431t, 439t
Thyroid disease
　　hyperthyroidism, 432t, 434t, 435–439
　　hypothyroidism, 431t, 432–434, 432t, 433f, 434t, 439t
　　symptoms, 432t
Thyroidectomy, 437, 438
Thyroid functions tests, 431t
Thyroid hormone, 431t, 439t
　　anti-thyroid hormone compounds, 435t
　　biosynthesis and release pathways, 433f
　　desiccated thyroid, 431t, 439t
　　levothyroxine, 431t, 432–434, 434t, 436–439, 439t
　　liotrix, 431t, 439t
　　mechanisms of action, 431t
　　secretion regulation, 433f
　　triiodothyroxine, 431t, 439t
Thyroid inhibitors, ionic, 431t, 440t
　　iodide, 431t, 440t
　　sodium iodide, 431t, 440t
Thyroid-stimulating hormone (TSH)
　　function test, 431t, 432, 437, 438
　　pathway and actions, 432, 433f

Thyrotoxicosis, 435
Thyrotropin-releasing hormone (TRH), 425f, 426, 432, 433f
Thyroxine (T_4)
　　function test, 431t
　　hypothyroidism, 432
Tiagabine, 226t, 237t
Ticarcillin, 552t, 556t
Ticlopidine
　　antiplatelet, 323t, 332t
　　bioactivation, 325
　　mechanisms of action, 323t, 330, 331
Tigecycline, 568t, 569f, 574, 575, 576t
Tiludronate, 481t, 488t
Timolol
　　myocardial ischemia, 300t
　　ophthalmic, 691t, 695t, 696–697, 697f, 704t
　　pharmacology, 126t, 128t, 145t
Tinea corporis, 719
Tinzaparin, 323t, 325, 333t
Tioconazole, 588t, 597t
Tiotropium, 96t, 113t
Tiotropium bromide, 390t, 401–402, 403t
Tipranavir, 601t, 603t, 608f, 609f, 622t
Tirofiban, 323t, 324–325, 332t
Tissue binding, 22b–23b
　　elderly, 75t
Tissue distribution, 21b
Tissue injury, pain, 197b, 197f
Tissue perfusion, elderly, 74b
Tizanidine
　　amyotrophic lateral sclerosis, 239t, 249, 253t
　　pharmacology, 119t, 140t
TMC-207
　　leprosy, 579t, 587t
　　Mycobacterium avium complex, 579t, 587t
Tobacco. See Smoking
Tobramycin, 559–566, 559b, 566t
Tolcapone, 238t, 242t, 244f, 252t
Tolerance
　　barbiturates, 181–182
　　heroin, 260
　　opioid, 206, 207
　　oxycodone, 255, 256t
Tolerogens, 381t
Tolmetin, 357t, 361t, 373t
Tolnaftate, 598t
Tolterodine, 96t, 101t, 113t
Tolvaptan, 279t, 281, 288t
Topical administration, 710b, 711–715, 711t, 713f
　　important considerations, 711–712, 711t
　　rate-limiting step, 721, 722
　　systemic spread, 702, 703
　　for topical infections, 714–715
　　vehicles, 712–714, 712t
Topiramate
　　antiseizure, 226t, 235, 236, 237t, 702, 703
　　glaucoma from, 702, 703
Topoisomerase inhibitors, 643t, 657t
　　camptothecin analogs, 643t, 657t

　　　irinotecan, 630f, 643t, 644b–645b, 649–651, 657t
　　　mechanisms of action, 630f, 643t, 649–651
　　　mechanisms of resistance, 643t, 644b–645b
　　　topotecan, 630f, 643t, 644b–645b, 649–651, 657t
　　　toxicities, 657t
　　　uses, 644t, 657t
　　epipodophyllotoxins, 643t, 657t
　　　etoposide, 630f, 643t, 645b, 657t
　　　mechanisms of action, 630f, 643t
　　　mechanisms of resistance, 643t, 645b
　　　teniposide, 630f, 643t, 645b, 657t
　　　toxicities, 657t
　　　uses, 644t, 657t
Topotecan, 643t, 649–651, 657t
　　mechanisms of action, 630f, 643t, 649–651
　　mechanisms of resistance, 643t, 644b–645b
Toremifene, 442t, 458t
　　anticancer, 664t, 677t, 679t, 686t
　　toxicities, 686t
　　uses, 686t
Torsade de pointes, 313–315, 315b
　　antiarrhythmics for, 314t
Torsemide, 269t, 284t
Toxicity, clinical and environmental, 40–66. See also specific substances
　　ABCDE emergency care, 51, 52t
　　ABCDE treatment, 52t
　　acetaminophen, 28–29, 50–54, 50f, 52t, 207, 208
　　acetylcysteine, 40t, 42t, 54, 65t
　　adverse drug events, 56–57
　　aflatoxin B_1, 41t, 60–62, 61f
　　anaphylaxis, 56
　　antidotes, 42t, 65t
　　arsenic, 41t, 43t, 63, 64, 66t
　　atropine, 40t, 65t
　　benzo[a]pyrene, 41t, 63–65
　　cadmium, 41t, 43t, 65t
　　carcinogens, 43t, 60–62, 60f, 61f
　　chelators, heavy metal, 66t
　　chromium, 41t, 43t, 66t
　　deaths, drug-related, 51, 51t
　　deferasirox, 41t, 65t
　　deferoxamine, 40t, 42t, 55, 65t
　　dimercaprol, 41t, 42t, 66t
　　dimercaptosuccinic acid, 41t, 66t
　　diphenhydramine, 40t, 42t, 65t (See also Diphenhydramine)
　　dose-response relationships, 44f, 45
　　drug–drug interactions, 48, 48b, 48t
　　drug interactions, 47f
　　drug overdose, initial management, 63, 64
　　drug-related deaths, agents, 51t
　　EDTA CaNa^2, 41t, 42t, 63, 64, 66t
　　effective vs. lethal dose, 44f
　　ethanol, 41t, 49f, 65t
　　ethanol antidote, 42t, 50, 65t
　　FDA drug approval process, 44f, 45t, 46–48, 46t

flumazenil, 41t, 42t, 65t, 177t, 179–180, 192t
fomepizole, 41t, 42t, 65t, 178f
iron poisoning, 54–55
largest number fatalities, 52t
lead, 41t, 43t, 57–58, 57b, 58f, 63, 64, 65t
management, 50–52
management, initial, 63, 64
medication errors, 56–57, 57t
mercury, 41t, 43t, 59–60, 59f, 65t
metals, heavy, 41t, 43t, 65t–66t
methanol, 42t, 49–50, 49f
most common substances, 51t
most frequent substances, 51, 51t
naloxone, 41t, 42t, 65t (See also Naloxone)
new drug testing, 44f, 45, 45t
organophosphates, 53t, 63, 64, 100t
penicillamine, 42t, 66t
penicillin, 55–56
pharmacokinetics, 52
physostigmine, 41t, 42t, 65t, 102
postmarketing surveillance, 9–11, 46–48
pralidoxime chloride, 41t, 42t, 65t, 100t, 102
prevention, children, 62–63, 64
sodium 2,3-dimercaptopropane, 41t, 66t
spectrum of effects, pharmaceutical, 44f
succimer, 41t, 42t, 66t
sulfamethoxazole, 56–57
therapeutic drug, 44f, 46, 46t
therapeutic index, 62, 64
toxidromes, 51, 53t
types, therapeutic drugs, 46, 46t
urine testing, 51–52
Toxidromes, 51, 53t. See also specific agents and types
Toxoplasmosis, 532b
tPA, 323t, 333t. See also Fibrinolytics, tPA
alteplase, 323t, 329–330, 329f, 333t
mechanisms of action, 323t
reteplase, 323t, 333t
tenecteplase, 323t, 333t
TPMT, 502–503, 503f, 506, 507
Trabectedin, 643t, 659t
Tramadol, 195t, 200t, 209t
Trandolapril, 273t, 285t
Transendothelial flux, 28b, 28f
Transepithelial flux, 28b, 28f
Transmembrane enzymes, 3t
Transport
active, 19b, 19f, 20b
paracellular, 19b, 19f
passive vs. active, 19b, 19f
Transporters. See also specific types
ABC, 23t, 23t–25t
catecholamine plasma membrane, 124t
efflux, 24b
elderly, 75t
plasma membrane, catecholamine, 124t
SLC superfamily, 23b–24b, 25t–26t
uptake, 24b
Tranylcypromine, 130t, 135, 137, 147t, 150t, 173t
Trastuzumab, 662t, 671t, 672–673, 681, 682, 683t

Travoprost, ophthalmic, 691t, 705t
Trazodone, 150t, 174t
Treprostinil, 391t, 404t
Tretinoin
cytotoxic, 645t, 646t, 659t
dermatologic, 707t, 724t
Triamcinolone, 390t, 403t
ophthalmic, 691t, 705t
Triamcinolone acetonide, 707t, 722, 723, 723t, 724t
Triamcinolone hexacetonide, 707t, 722, 723, 723t, 724t
Triamterene, 269t, 282, 283, 284t
Triazenes, 628t, 652t
dacarbazine, 628t, 629t, 630f, 645–647, 652t
mechanisms of action, 628b, 628t, 630f
mechanisms of resistance, 628t, 632–633, 632b
temozolomide, 652t
toxicities, 632b–633b, 652t
uses, 629t
Triazolam, 176t, 191t, 192t
Triazoles, 588t, 589f, 590, 597t. See also Imidazoles and triazoles
Trichlormethiazide, 269t, 284t
Trichomonas vaginalis, 533, 534
Tricyclic antidepressants (TCAs). See also Antidepressants
adverse effects, 154
elderly, 71, 72, 75
pain target and site of action, 205t
sites of actions, 152f
Trifluoperazine, 150t, 174t
Trifluridine, 601t, 602t, 606, 619t
Triglyceride levels, 337t
Trihexyphenidyl hydrochloride
Parkinson's disease, 242t
pharmacology, 96t, 114t
Triiodothyronine (T_3)
function test, 431t
hypothyroidism, 432
Triiodothyroxine, 431t, 439t
Trimethaphan, 106t, 117t
Trimethoprim-sulfamethoxazole, 542–543, 548t
allergy, 56, 543
bacterial vs. mammalian sensitivity, 546, 547
folate deficiency, 543, 543f
resistance, 543
structure, 543f
urinary tract infections, 56, 542–543, 543f, 546, 547, 548t
Trimetrexate, 635t, 640, 653t
Trimipramine, 150t, 173t
Trioxsalen photochemotherapy, 716t
Tripelennamine, 346t, 353t
Triple response of Lewis, 347b, 348
Triptorelin, 422t, 429t
anticancer, 664t, 686t
Tropicamide, 96t, 114t
ophthalmic, 690t, 695t, 705t
Trospium chloride, 96t, 101t, 113t
Trypanosoma brucei rhodesiense, 534
Trypanosomiasis, 533, 534

Tuberculin skin test reaction, 582, 585, 586
Tuberculosis drugs, 578–587, 578t–579t, 586t–587t
capreomycin, 579t, 587t
combination therapy, 581
cycloserine, 579t, 587t
definitive therapy, 581b
ethambutol, 578t, 583, 587t
ethionamide, 579t, 587t
isoniazid, 578t, 580f, 582, 583t, 587t
isoniazid-resistance, 583
mechanisms of action, 578t–579t, 579f
mechanisms of resistance, 578t–579t, 580f
PA-824, 579t, 587t
penetration, 585, 586
prophylaxis criteria, 580b
pyrazinamide, 578t, 580b, 586t
resistant and multidrug-resistant TB, 584, 584b
rifamycins, 578t, 581–586, 586t
mechanisms of action, 578t, 579f
mechanisms of resistance, 578t, 580f
rifabutin, 578t, 586t
rifampin, 578t, 579f, 581–586, 586t
rifapentine, 578t, 586t
tuberculin skin test reaction, 582, 585, 586
22-oxacalcitrolparicalcitol, 481t, 488t
2-PAM. See Pralidoxime chloride (2-PAM)
Tyloxapol, ophthalmic, 692t, 706t
Typical angina, 290t, 291f. See also Myocardial ischemia
Tyrosine kinase (TK) growth factor receptor signaling pathway, 666f

U

Ulcerative colitis
azathioprine, 502–503, 503f, 506, 507
sulfasalazine, 381, 502, 543t, 547f
thiopurine methyltransferase, 502–503, 503f, 506, 507
Ulcers
NSAID-induced, 492
proton pump inhibitors, 492, 493, 494t, 495 (See also Proton pump inhibitors)
Ulipristal, 442t, 444t, 452, 458t
Undecylenic acid, 599t
Unstable angina, 290t, 291f, 296–297. See also Myocardial ischemia
drugs, 296–297
percutaneous coronary interventions, 297
Uptake transporters, 24b
Urapidil, 120t, 141t
Urate oxidase, recombinant, 369t, 374t
Urea, diuretics for, 268t, 283t
Urea substitutes, 630f, 645t, 646t, 659t
Uric acid, 370
Uricosuric agents, 369t, 370, 374t
Uridine diphosphate-glucuronosyltransferase (UGT), antiseizure drugs and, 227t
Urinary tract infection agents, 542–548
analgesics, phenazopyridine, 548t

Urinary tract infection agents (Cont.)
  antiseptics
    methenamine, 548t
    nitrofurantoin, 545, 546, 547, 548t
  quinolones, 544, 548t
    ciprofloxacin, 544, 544f, 545, 548t
    levofloxacin, 548t
    mechanisms of action, 544f, 545
    moxifloxacin, 548t
    norfloxacin, 548t
    ofloxacin, 548t
    resistance, 544
    structures, 543f
    sulfadiazine, 543f, 543t, 547t
    sulfamethoxazole, 543f, 543t, 547t
    trimethoprim-sulfamethoxazole, 56, 542–543, 543f, 546, 547, 548t
    uncomplicated UTI, 542–543
Urinary tract infections, 548t
Urine
  acidification and alkalization, 39
  pH, 20b, 21–22
  testing, 51–52
Urofollitropin (uFSH), 423t, 429t

V

Valacyclovir, 601t, 605, 608
Valganciclovir, 601t. *See also* Acyclovir
Valproic acid
  anticonvulsants, 151t, 164–165, 169, 173, 175t
  antiseizure, 225t, 231–232, 234, 235, 236t
  with lamotrigine, 235
Valrubicin, 643t, 658t
  mechanisms of action, 630f, 643t, 645–647
  mechanisms of resistance, 645b
  uses, 644t, 658t
Valsartan, 273t, 280, 282, 283, 285t
Valvular heart disease, angina drugs, 294t
Vancomycin, 569t, 570f, 572–575, 577t
  empirical treatment, 572
  IV, hazards, 573, 574, 575
  mechanisms of action, 569t, 572
  resistance, 569t, 573
Vardenafil
  myocardial ischemia, 300t
  ocular effects, 703
Varenicline, 106t, 117t
  nicotine addiction, 259
Variant angina, 290t, 291f, 297. *See also* Myocardial ischemia
Vascular endothelial growth factor (VEGF)
  cancer angiogenesis, 673–674
  monoclonal antibodies targeting, 662t, 671t, 673–675
Vasodilators, 270t, 278t, 301t
  arterial, 278t, 287t
    diazoxide, 278t, 287t
    fenoldopam, 278t, 287t
    hydralazine, 278t, 287t
    hypertension and edema, 278t, 287t
    minoxidil, 278t, 287t
  arterial and venous, 278t, 287t
    nitroprusside, 278t, 287t
  heart failure, 301t, 304t, 311t
Vasopressin, 279t, 288t
Vasopressin receptor agonists, 288t
  mechanisms of action, 279t, 280f
  V_1 receptor, 279t, 288t
    terlipressin, 279t, 288t
    vasopressin, 279t, 288t
  V_2 receptor, 279t, 288t
    desmopressin, 279t, 288t
Vasopressin receptor antagonists
  mechanisms of action, 279t, 280f
  $V_{1a}R/V_2R$, nonselective, conivaptan, 279t, 281, 288t
  V_2 receptor, selective, tolvaptan, 279t, 281, 288t
Vasospastic angina, sinus bradycardia with, 297, 298
Vecuronium, 97f, 105f, 106f, 106t, 107t, 108, 116t
Venlafaxine, 130t, 147t, 150t, 154, 157, 174t
Ventilatory stimulants, 391t, 404t
Ventricular fibrillation, 314t, 316
  antiarrhythmics, 314t, 316 (*See also* Antiarrhythmic drugs)
  implantable cardioverter-defibrillator, 316
Ventricular tachycardia
  antiarrhythmics, 314t
  implantable cardioverter-defibrillator, 318
  nonsustained, 318
Verapamil
  antiarrhythmic, 312t, 317t, 322t
  antihypertensive, 277t, 287t
  electrophysiologic actions, 317t
  heart failure, 306
  myocardial ischemia, 290t, 300t
  toxidrome, 53t
Vildagliptin, 471t, 472f, 479t
Vigabatrin
  antiseizure, 226t, 235, 236, 237t, 702, 703
  ocular effects, 702, 703
Vinblastine (sulfate), 642t, 656t
  dermatologic, 709t, 724t, 726t
  mechanisms of action, 630f, 642t, 647
  mechanisms of resistance, 642t, 644b
  toxicities, 656t
  uses, 644t, 656t
Vinblastine sulfate, 630f, 642t, 644b, 644t, 656t
Vinca alkaloids, 642t, 656t. *See also specific types*
  mechanisms of resistance, 642t, 644b
  toxicities, 656t
  uses, 644t, 656t
Vincristine sulfate, 630f, 642t, 644b, 644t, 656t
  mechanisms of action, 630f, 642t
  mechanisms of resistance, 642t, 644b
  uses, 644t, 656t
Vinorelbine, 630f, 642t, 644b, 644t, 656t
  mechanisms of action, 630f, 642t
  mechanisms of resistance, 642t, 644b
  uses, 644t, 656t

Viral infections
  cytomegalovirus retinitis, 609–612, 617, 618
  drugs (*See* antiviral agents)
  eye, 701
  hepatitis C, chronic, 613–614
  herpes simplex virus, 605–608
  HIV, 614–619 (*See also* Human immunodeficiency virus (HIV))
  HSV, eye, 701
  influenza A, immunocompromised, 612–613
  replicative cycles, 604f
  varicella zoster virus (shingles), 608
  virus replication stages and targets, 612t
Vitamin A deficiency, 703, 704
Vitamin B_{12}, 406t, 420t
  absorption, 412f
    proton pump inhibitors on, 492
  cyanocobalamin, 406t, 420t
  distribution, 412f
  folate interactions, 410b, 412f
  general principles, 411b–412b
  hydroxycobalamin, 406t, 420t
  mechanisms of action, 406t, 420t
Vitamin B_{12} deficiency, 412f, 413b, 414–415, 417–418
  causes, 411b, 412f
  fish tapeworm, 537–540
Vitamin D 1α-hydroxylase, 482f, 486, 487
Vitamin D and analogs, 481t, 482f, 484, 488t
  1α-hydroxycholecalciferol, 481t, 488t
  22-oxacalcitrolparicalcitol, 481t, 488t
  calcipotriol, 481t, 488t
  calcitriol, 481t, 482f, 488t
  dihydrotachysterol, 481b
  doxercalciferol, 481b
  ergocalciferol, 481t, 488t
  hypercalcemia, 481t, 488t
  intestinal bypass surgery, 486, 487
  paricalcitol, 481t, 488t
  renal osteodystrophy, 481t, 482f, 484, 488t
  therapeutic uses, 481b
Vitamin K_1, warfarin antidote, 14, 42t
Vitamin K antagonist, 333t
  mechanisms of action, 323t
  warfarin (*See* Warfarin)
Vitamin K cycle, 327–328, 327f
Vitreous substitutes
  ophthalmic, 692t, 706t
VKORC1, 13–14, 13f
VLDL-C metabolism, 335f
VM-26. *See* Teniposide (VM-26)
Voglibose, 471t, 479t
Voltage-dependent ion channels, 86, 87f
Voltage-gated Na+ channels
  local anesthetics on, 217
  structure and function, 218f
Volume of distribution *(V)*, 30, 33b, 34b
  definition and equation, 34b
  digoxin, 30
  elderly, 74b, 75t
  variations, 34b
Vomiting drugs. *See* Antinauseants and antiemetics

777

Voriconazole, 588t, 590, 592–593, 595–596, 597t
    adverse effects, 593, 595, 596
    drug interactions, 590t–592t, 593
    mechanisms of action, 588t, 589f, 592
Vorinostat (SAHA), 645t, 646t, 660t
VP-16-213. *See* Etoposide (VP-16-213)
Vytorin, 344t, 350

W

Warfarin, 323t, 325–328, 333t
    altered activity, 329b
    altered anticoagulant activity, 329b–330b
    atrial fibrillation, 327
    counseling, 328
    food–drug interactions, 328
    indications, 325t
    mechanisms of action, 327–328, 327f
    monitoring, 325, 325t, 328, 330b
    post-stenting, 325
    risks and toxicities, 328
    therapeutic index, 329b
Warfarin sensitivity, 10t, 12–14, 13f
    vitamin K (K_1), 14, 42t

Weak electrolytes, transmembrane distribution, 19–20, 19b–20b, 19f, 20f, 35, 37–38
Wetting agents/tear substitutes, 692t, 706t
    carboxymethylcellulose, 692t, 706t
    hydroxyethyl cellulose, 692t, 706t
    hydroxypropyl cellulose, 692t, 706t
    hydroxypropyl methylcellulose, 692t, 706t
    methylcellulose, 692t, 706t
    tyloxapol, 692t, 706t
Whitfield's ointment, 599t
Wolff-Parkinson-White syndrome arrhythmias, 314t
Wound infection prophylaxis, 514b, 516

X

Xanthine oxidase inhibitors, gout, 369t
    allopurinol, 369t, 370–372, 373t
    febuxostat, 369t, 370, 374t
Xenobiotic metabolizing enzymes, 29b, 29t
Xenon, 211t, 215t, 223t
Xylometazoline, 120t, 142t

Y

^{99}Y-ibritumomab, 662t, 671t, 684t
Yohimbine, 120t, 141t

Z

Zafirlukast, 390t, 404t
Zalcitabine, 601t, 621t
    mechanisms of action and resistance, 601t
    structure, 607f
Zaleplon, 177t, 192t
Zanamivir, 601t, 602t, 604f, 620t
Zidovudine, 601t, 602t, 621t
    adverse effects, 615
    mechanisms of action and resistance, 517, 602t, 604f, 607f, 608f, 614–615
    structure, 607f
Zileuton, 390t, 403t
Ziprasidone, 151t, 171t, 175t
Zoledronate, 481, 485, 488t
Zolmitriptan, 130t, 147t
Zolpidem, 177t, 178–179, 192t
Zona glomerulosa, 461f, 467, 468
Zonisamide, 226t, 237t